CLINICAL MASSAGE THERAPY

UNDERSTANDING, ASSESSING AND TREATING OVER 70 CONDITIONS

Fiona Rattray, RMT
Linda Ludwig, B.A., RMT

First Published, March, 2000
02   12 11 10 9 8 7 6

Published by Talus Incorporated
55 Four Oaks Gate
Toronto, Ontario M4J 2X3
Canada
Phone: (416) 422-5459
Fax: (416) 422-5053

Editor: Laura Lee

Designed by: Gail Beglin, Laguna Graphics

Illustrations by: Gail Beglin

Set in Omni Book

Printed on recycled paper with vegetable-based inks

Printed in Canada

Canadian Cataloguing in Publication Data

Rattray, Fiona S. (Fiona Scott), 1958-
    Clinical Massage Therapy: Understanding, Assessing and Treating Over 70 Conditions
Includes bibliographical references and index.
ISBN 0-9698177-1-1
    1. Massage Therapy. I. Ludwig, Linda M. (Linda Maria), 1959-
II. Beglin, Gail. III. Title.
RM721.R38 2000 615.8'22 C99-901142-1

*To the one-fifty
and our families*

Acknowledgements

We finished writing this book on the day of the last solar eclipse of 1999; after a terrific thunderstorm with power interruptions, the sun came out, roofs were steaming in the heat and the trees were green and replenished. Some kind of turning point...

Many people have helped us, directly and indirectly, in the creation of this book. We would like to thank:

Tom Scanlan of Is Five Communications, for patience, putting together the team to make it all possible, expertise and a guiding hand in the process. We look forward to future projects.

Our editor, Laura Lee, for her thoroughness, enthusiasm and attention to detail which have been invaluable over the years it has taken to put this project together. Her insight and awareness of alternative health care move us to award her an honorary massage therapist diploma.

Gail Beglin of Laguna Graphics, our designer and illustrator; she has worked with us through *many* chapter versions to create "the look"; thanks for your patience, suggestions and perfectionism.

Evelyn Daicos, for inputting, enthusiasm, common sense and advice in the preparation of this book.

Leslie McIntyre, for inputting, troubleshooting and refereeing through Appendix C: Special Orthopedic Testing.

Elspeth Williams for answering legal questions.

Martina Davison Feistner and others for visuals.

Janet D'Arcy, DC, for professional insight and, with husband John Castellano, for a wonderful diversion and inspiration in allowing us the honour of attending the birth of the most fabulous Isabella.

Alex Daicos and Elizabeth Daicos, typeface consultants and opinion givers.

Kate and Ernest Ludwig, Steve Daicos and the Daicos family, Kathy Ludwig and Keith Dana for endless patience, support, a positive atmosphere and sustenance through too many holidays and weekends. We look forward to visits without the laptop. Let the champagne corks fly!

The memory, spirit and sense of humour of Catherine and John Rattray, who put a strong foundation in place.

James Astley, for sanity breaks: Bonaire, Bahamas and Roatan; and the entire family for providing real food and a calm space through the critical months.

Marley, black standard poodle extraordinaire, who hindered and helped us in his own special way and reminded us to remain playful (sas zx). And vivacious younger brother, Rodel, for insisting on long walks, chases and puddle jumping.

Dog walking friends, Madeleine, with Tristan, Tango and the late, sweet Shasta, for peace, fun and frolic.

Tanis Day, for integrating heart and spirit energy, and introducing the one-fifty.

CONTENTS

CONTENTS

ILLUSTRATIONS

v

ILLUSTRATIONS

ILLUSTRATIONS

PREFACE

Clinical Massage Therapy is designed for both the massage therapy student and the professional therapist in practice. The book covers the requirements of a treatment-based curriculum for a professional massage therapy training program that is a minimum of 2,200 hours in length. It also includes conditions that are frequently seen in clinical practice.

The word "client" is used in this book instead of the word "patient" to describe the person who is being treated. A client is a person who is able to make choices about health care.

Symbols used in this book:

✋ The open hand graphic denotes what the therapist does to treat the client.

✍ The writing hand graphic denotes what the therapist records or performs in an assessment, or writes down for the client to do as self-care.

Using This Text

Clinical Massage Therapy is designed to make the information necessary for an individual massage therapy treatment as accessible as possible. Most of the treatments in this text are organized in sections that follow a standard format:

✦ There are five "Strategies" chapters which provide a foundation for the chapters within that section of the book. It is recommended that these "Strategies" chapters be read in conjunction with the specific treatment in a particular section.

✦ Background information about the condition or disease is given first, so the student or therapist can understand the anatomy, process or pathology and medical intervention as it relates to the treatment.

✦ The Symptom Picture summarizes the client's symptoms.

✦ The Assessment section includes health history questions, observations, palpation and testing to be performed, and the expected results where relevant. Differential testing results are also listed to help the therapist rule out other conditions that the client may have. The student may use this as a guide for an assessment protocol; the therapist may use this as a reference or refresher with conditions she or he does not often treat.

✦ Contraindications to treatment are also highlighted.

✦ The Treatment Goals, Treatment Plan and Self-care information are treatment guidelines for the student or therapist.

✦ For some conditions, a brief treatment plan and contraindications only are described, because these are modifications of other treatments. These chapters are indicated in the text by a < > logo on the chapter number.

✦ The Appendices are reference tools.

✦ Appendix C: Special Orthopedic Testing comprises information compiled from orthopedic assessment textbooks, presenting the most agreed-upon versions of tests and their clinical results.

Manual medicine and massage therapy are in a state of growth and change. Some information, ideas and approaches to treatment are in conflict — either real or apparent. New information about the body, treatment protocols, medical approaches and medications are constantly being reported. A variety of massage therapy approaches are possible for a given condition; we describe treatment plans as samples that are effective based on research results, academic principles and clinical practice.

At the time of writing, the information in this book is as up-to-date as possible. We are happy to hear your comments and suggestions for future publications.

We have profound respect and love for this profession and are aware of the amazing impact that massage therapy has had for so many people. All kinds of health care — alternative and allopathic — have in their essence an underlying goal: health of body, mind and spirit.

We hope *Clinical Massage Therapy* can create a standard for the massage therapy profession. We also hope it can demonstrate the profound effects of massage therapy, and perhaps even provide a basis for research projects on the effects of massage in this new millennium.

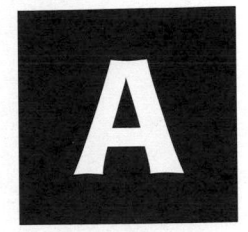

INTRODUCTION TO MASSAGE

A BRIEF HISTORY OF MASSAGE THERAPY

Fiona Rattray

The origin of the word "massage" is obscure. The word is derived from either the Arabic "mass", to touch, or the Greek "massein", to knead *(Basmajian, 1985)*. For thousands of years, literature from all over the world has mentioned kneading, pressing, anointing or rubbing as a healing practice. **The Yellow Emperor's Classics of Internal Medicine**, written in China in about 1000 BC and probably the oldest medical book in existence, mentions the treatment of paralysis and reduced circulation using massage. The information is attributed to Huang Ti, the Yellow Emperor who died in 2598 BC. During the T'ang dynasty (619-907 AD), there were professors of massage at the Imperial Medical Bureau. A three-year training program for doctors of massage included treatment of fractures, diseases, injuries and wounds. Massage was combined with breathing and postural exercises.

Hippocrates, circa 460-375 BC, discussed "gently rubbing" a dislocated shoulder following reduction to aid in healing *(Basmajian, 1985)*.

Massage, exercise and hydrotherapy were promoted by the Greek physician Asclepides. The ancient Greeks used massage on athletes before and after sport. It was thought to prepare the muscles before activity and remove extra fluid and metabolites after sport, a theory which is in use today. Galen of Rome (129-199 AD) wrote 16 books on frictions (the term for massage) and gymnastics (remedial exercise), describing the pressure, direction and frequency of treatment. Both rich and poor Romans used massage, which was often practised in the Roman baths. Massage was performed with the hands, and also with cloth of various textures, both rough and smooth. Instruments of bone or wood were also used to rub, polish or tap the skin, drawing circulation and warmth to the skin. Strigils were curved instruments, while ferrules were straight. A reference is also made to treating the edematous legs of pregnant women using massage with rose water *(DeLisa, Gans, 1993)*.

In India, a ninth century temple carving shows Bhudda being treated by a masseuse. The Hindi term *champna* (to press) means massage; it is likely the origin of the word shampooing. Used by English writers in nineteenth century India to describe massage, it now means to wash, rub or lather the hair *(Basmajian, 1985)*.

Massage terms in the Islands of Tonga include *fota* and *toogi-toogi*, while in Hawaii massage is called *lomi-lomi (Wood, Becker, 1981)*.

In Europe during the Dark and Middle Ages, massage and remedial exercise were barely mentioned in literature until the French surgeon Ambroise Pare (1510-1590) published a book on massage and its application for surgical patients *(DeLisa, Gans, 1993)*. He translated Galen's works on massage, and added information on treating those immobilized by their injuries; for example, the leg of a man whose femur had been fractured by a bullet was treated with light frictions and hydrotherapy to help resolve the congestion.

The pressure indicated for massage depends on the author cited *(Basmajian, 1985; Tappan, 1961; Wood, Becker, 1981)*. For example, vigorous and even painful techniques were advocated by Admiral Henry (1731-1823), while his contemporary, the physician Lorry, thought that techniques should be applied with gentleness. A balance between these extremes was suggested by William Beveridge of Edinburgh, who thought the therapist should adjust the pressure to the client's symptoms and tissue health.

The terminology currently used to describe the different techniques, such as petrissage, stroking and tapotement, gradually emerged during the eighteenth and nineteenth centuries in the writings of different authors. Per Ling, a fencer and physical education teacher in nineteenth-century Sweden, turned Stockholm into a centre for therapeutic exercise, which was called medical gymnastics, and massage therapy. The Royal Institute of Gymnastics was established in 1813 by the Crown to reward Ling's efforts. Medical gymnastics, including massage, were embraced by many physicians. Although Ling created a system for exercise and massage, he wrote little on the subject. However, one of his pupils, Augustus Georgii, published a book in French on Ling's system after his death in 1839. By the end of the nineteenth century, Swedish massage was internationally known thanks to his many enthusiastic followers *(Basmajian, 1985)*.

Johan Metzger, a physician in Amsterdam, successfully treated the Danish crown-prince for a chronic joint problem using massage. He helped move massage therapy into higher esteem among his European colleagues by combining physiology, pathology and anatomy with massage. His doctoral dissertation in 1868 was titled "The Treatment of Foot Sprain by Friction." Metzger moved to Germany in 1889 and interested many German physicians in what was now being called manual medicine.

In the United States, massage was being adopted due to the writings of the Boston physician Douglas Graham, and John Kellogg of Battle Creek, Michigan.

At the end of the nineteenth century, E. Kleen of Sweden wrote one of the earliest books that distinguishes massage from remedial exercise. Often, little distinction was made in earlier medical history between the two.

In the United Kingdom in the nineteenth century, massage became a specialized branch of nursing *(Boyling, Palastanga, 1994)*. This therapeutic practice quickly became popular. Unfortunately, it was plagued by a series of scandals involving poorly trained nurses who were lured into working in "houses of ill repute". In response, a group of nurses who recognized the therapeutic usefulness of massage therapy formed the Society of Trained Masseuses in 1895. This Society established training courses and examinations to standardize therapeutic massage practices. It is interesting that this group eventually became the Chartered Society of Physiotherapists.

The British physiotherapy profession initially relied solely on massage techniques and had incorporated remedial exercise and "medical electricity" by the end of the First World War. One example of a textbook for physiotherapists that combines remedial exercise and massage therapy is **Tidy's Massage and Remedial Exercises**. First published in 1932, it covers the treatment of pathologies and injuries.

Massage was advocated in the 1930s and 40s by Dr. James Mennell, an English physician specializing in the treatment of fractures. The connection between massage and physiotherapy remained strong in the U.K. As late as 1977, massage therapy was a core skill and was examinable material for British physiotherapists *(Boyling, Palastanga, 1994)*.

Massage therapy as a separate profession was formally introduced to the United States in 1917, when the Surgeon General set up a rehabilitation process for soldiers wounded in the First World War. Mary McMillan, an American trained in massage therapy in Britain, was appointed to set up this process, including the training of massage therapists to European standards *(Boyling, Palastanga, 1994)*.

Almost 50 years later, an American physiotherapist named Gertrude Beard wrote about massage therapy techniques for use by physical therapists, publishing the extensively researched **Beard's Massage.**

In many countries today, massage is a component of training for health care practitioners such as nurses, physiotherapists and athletic therapists. In some countries, massage therapy as a separate, legally recognized profession does not exist.

In other countries, massage therapy as a profession in its own right has existed for some time. For example in Ontario, Canada, massage therapy was first legislated and controlled under the *Drugless Practitioner's Act* (DPA) from 1924 to 1993. The DPA covered therapies that did not use medication in their scope of practice, but still required specific training and standards of practice. This changed on December 31, 1993, when the regulation of most professions covered under the DPA, including massage therapy, was transferred to another health care act. This new legislation, called the *Regulated Health Professions Act* (RHPA), brings massage therapy under the same legislation that governs nurses, doctors, dentists, pharmacists, chiropractors and physiotherapists. Later amendments to the act cover treatment plans and client consent, record keeping and standards for ongoing training for all professions under the RHPA *(Ontario, 1996, 1991a, 1991b)*. The inclusion of massage therapists with these other health care practitioners, all having recognized standards and obligations, further legitimizes massage therapy in Ontario as a respectable profession.

However, today's training standards, curriculums, accreditation and degree of acceptance by other health care practitioners are quite variable. In Britain, massage therapy training is at most a six-month program, and there is no single country-wide legislation standard for training. In America, massage practice laws vary from state to state; some states do not legislate massage while others do. In those with laws covering massage, entry level education requirements range from 300 to 750-plus hours of techniques, contraindications, supervised massage, anatomy, pathology, physiology, hygiene and ethics *(AMTA, 1999)*; some massage education programs considerably exceed these minimum requirements. In Canada also, some provinces and territories do not legislate massage therapy while others do. Entry level requirements in provinces legislating massage therapy also vary. Alberta has a 1,000-hour program that covers techniques, contraindications, supervised clinical time, anatomy, pathophysiology, hydrotherapy, hygiene and ethics; Ontario has a 2,200-hour (two year) program that covers the previously mentioned material plus massage treatments, assessment and remedial exercise; and British Columbia has a 3,000-hour (three-year) program. This treatment-oriented training is sometimes called medical massage therapy, to distinguish it from more relaxation-oriented massage. Modern massage therapy training seems to have caught up with the T'ang dynasty (619-907 AD).

Post-graduate training includes techniques from other disciplines such as osteopathy, athletic therapy and Eastern medicine, as therapists strive to make their work even more effective.

Why do we need these education standards and regulations for massage? What if a practitioner of massage wants to focus on relaxation only? The therapist has a responsibility to the public, to understand when massage is safe and appropriate and when to refer. Someone who wants "just relaxation" for their crampy, aching leg muscles may have tight muscles, fascia or trigger points causing the pain, in which case massage therapy is indicated. Or the pain source may be deep vein thrombosis in the legs, in which case massage is definitely not advisable as the client could be seriously harmed. In-depth training will allow the therapist to recognize contraindications and do no harm.

Another reason for standards and regulations is the public's increasing demand for complimentary therapies. Often the therapist is working with a client who has some type of soft-tissue pain and is seeking help to reduce the symptoms and return to normal function. Does the therapist not owe it to the client to be able to recognize what the problem likely is, as a result of his training, and be as effective as possible in treating the condition?

Higher standards of education, research on the effectiveness of the techniques, the existence of laws regulating the profession, as well as professional associations also signal to the public, other health care professionals and third-party payers that massage therapy is a respectable, effective profession.

2

THE EFFECTS OF MASSAGE THERAPY AND MASSAGE TECHNIQUES

Fiona Rattray, Linda Ludwig

"Many claims have been made for the use of massage. Some are based upon clinical experience, both objective reports and 'testimonials'. Some are rationalizations of hypotheses based on knowledge of anatomy and physiology. Some are based on controlled, carefully worked out laboratory studies, and some on what might be described as 'wishful thinking'" (Wood, Becker, 1981).

How Information Is Gathered

What are the effects of massage therapy and massage techniques? To answer that question requires an understanding of how research is done. Methods of gathering knowledge are usually described as being either empirical or scientific in origin.

The *empirical method* of research has been used for the majority of human history. This method is based on observation and experience recorded by the senses. Today this is called *qualitative research*: information is collected through open-ended interviews, direct observation and documentation. There is no difference between the observer and what is being observed; more than one reality is possible.

The *scientific method* began relatively recently, in the seventeenth century. In the current climate of increasing scientific knowledge and health research, it is now expected that every form of treatment should be provable using this methodology.

The scientific method is based on systematic observation, measurement and experiment. Today this is called *quantitative research*: a conclusion, or hypothesis, is made before all the facts are gathered; information is observed or measured; and the result is expressed in terms of numbers to test the hypothesis. Only one external reality exists. Certain rules must be followed to ensure the objectivity of the result: the result must be reproducible; it must not occur by chance or as a result of other explanations; and a certain action causes a specific result (cause and effect). The classical method is to use the double blind clinical trial, also called the *gold standard*, to prove or disprove a hypothesis *(Menard, 1994)*.

There is an abundance of literature supporting the effectiveness of numerous medical treatments. With the rise of scientific methods and medicine as a profession, multi-million dollar budgets and large facilities to perform research on medication and surgery have been available. However, in terms of scientific studies that demonstrate the effectiveness of specific techniques, many practitioners of manual medicine, such as massage therapists and physiotherapists, are in a similar situation: there is much less literature on the effectiveness of manual methods *(Stewart, 1996)*. In fact, much of the evidence for the effects and effectiveness of massage techniques has been empirical, based on centuries of observation and experience *(Basmajian, 1985)*.

This need not be viewed as a fault with massage therapy or other forms of manual medicine. One should keep in mind that "much of medicine practised today is based on principles of treatment that predates the [growth in scientific...research]. These therapeutic principles were the result of an accumulated body of empirical information based on the observations of clinical results by many different practitioners, and were — and still are — valid despite the fact that the underlying physiological processes involved were not studied and elucidated until relatively recently. This process of evolution from the empirical to the scientific has been the case with all of the widely accepted conventional forms of treatment" *(Yates, 1990)*. This likely holds true for massage therapy and other forms of manual medicine; we appear to be in a transition period in which the scientific model of research is on the increase.

Today's Massage Research

There seems to be a tendency today for some therapists to lament that there are no scientific studies to prove the effects of massage therapy, that the evidence is all empirical. Studies do exist, in English as well as other languages. For example, Yates's **A Physician's Guide to Therapeutic Massage** is based on over 200 articles in scientific, medical and health-sciences literature published from 1885 to 1987 on the effects of massage therapy *(Yates, 1990)*.

More recently, Dr. Tiffany Field of the Touch Research Institute at the Miami School of Medicine in Florida is researching the role of touch in health development and the treatment of disease *(Turnbull, 1994/5)*. She has published papers in leading pediatric and psychiatry journals, which she feels has contributed to the legitimacy of her research *(Knaster, 1994)*.

Examples of Field's current research include a study which examined the effect of 45 minutes of daily massage on premature babies. It reported that these babies had a 47 per cent weight gain compared to premature babies who received conventional treatment and who were not "unnecessarily handled" during hospital care. Another study, on the effects of massage on children with diabetes, revealed that 20 minutes of nightly massage for 30 days improved the subjects' blood glucose levels *(Field et al., 1997b)*.

Perhaps we, as massage therapists, have unrealistic expectations of massage and research in this field. For example, one issue that is questioned (often by the insurance industry) is the long-term effectiveness of massage; yet other common forms of treatment are not necessarily questioned, such as medication and the need for ongoing doses. Field notes that "we've been very concerned about convincing physicians sitting on committees [about this] and they don't care about long-term effects [of massage]. They want to know what happens immediately. [Physicians] know that if you want a drug to work, you have to keep taking it. They could be criticized if they said, 'How long...are the effects of [the drug]?' It's dose-dependent typically. Their reasoning is: would you expect if you stopped massaging someone that the positive effects of massage are going to go on any longer than if you stopped someone on a drug? They may have a point. It may be that you need to have a daily or weekly dose in order for the effects to persist. We do massage assessments on day one and then on day 30. If we look at baseline on day one versus baseline on day 30, the latter is better, suggesting an incremental effect of the month of therapy" *(Knaster, 1994)*.

The Future of Massage Research

At present in North America, there is an increasing focus on research into massage, to meet the standards of the medical model. In order to provide objective and scientific data on the effects of massage, the Ontario College of Massage Therapists, the Massage Therapy Associations of Ontario and British Columbia, the American Massage Therapy Association and the National Institute of Health in Maryland are currently providing funding for research.

Massage therapists, associations and schools are encouraged to employ research methods which encompass the science as well as the art of massage therapy and continue to evaluate its effectiveness.

Some concerns with studies that do exist on the effectiveness of massage therapy techniques are that they often neglect to mention which specific techniques are used and the pressure, rate, number of repetitions and areas of the body to which the techniques are applied. This makes the studies difficult to reproduce. The terminology used to describe techniques may vary. Studies also show a lack of consistency in approach so comparisons of techniques are difficult to make *(Zadai, 1992)*. To alleviate these problems, it is suggested that those who conduct massage therapy research be more specific in reporting techniques used and that they adopt a common language for techniques.

All this focus on research raises a concern for those therapists who feel that massage therapy is intuitive, that all its effects cannot be measured by scientific methods, nor should they be, and that massage is becoming too medicalized. Whether we like it or not, the public is seeing massage therapy not only as an alternative to traditional or allopathic medicine, but also as a respected therapeutic approach in its own right. As the public uses massage more frequently, and if we want to attract more people to using massage, the profession finds itself asked more frequently to "prove that massage works in medical terms".

Perhaps a compromise is to use both empirical and scientific methods, combining qualitative and quantitative research, because the positive effects of massage therapy are a combination of physiological and psychological factors.

Effects of Massage Therapy

The effects of massage are physiological and psychological in nature. The physiological effects are subdivided into mechanical effects — on adhesions and the vascular and lymphatic systems, for example — and its reflexive effects through the neurological systems — the central, perpheral and autonomic systems. It is often noted that all effects are interactive, even though they are divided into categories (DeLisa, Gans, 1993).

Massage therapy performed on a healthy person increases muscle flexibility and relaxation, and decreases stress levels. The psychological effects are the increased well being that usually occurs with positive touch. It is not clear from current studies exactly to what extent massage benefits a healthy person in addition to these factors, as physiological changes following massage are not always evident in tissue that is healthy (Yates, 1990).

The most profound changes from massage seem to occur in the body in areas that were experiencing pathology or trauma, such as tissue that was edematous, fibrosed, ischemic or painful. Psychological benefits are also most evident in those experiencing stress and depression.

Massage and Pain Control

Generally, massage is recognized as effective in reducing or managing pain. Pain from nerve receptors in the body is processed in the spinal cord and travels to the brain — the thalamus and cortex — where it is modulated. The person's perception of pain can be partially controlled by signals transmitted from the cerebellum down the spinal cord. These signals inhibit pain signal transmissions at the level where they enter the spinal cord, decreasing the person's level of pain sensitivity.

Massage affects pain in several different ways. Massage can address the source of the pain and stop the nociceptive (painful) nerve firing. Often there is a cycle of pain that begins with tissue ischemia. Tissue ischemia, or reduced local circulation, results from sustained muscle contraction (spasm) and fascial restriction. This reduces the blood flow and oxygen to the tissues in the constricted area, resulting in pain. The mechanism of ischemic pain is not clearly understood. It may be due to a reduction of available oxygen, a build-up of metabolites or a release of histamines or bradykinin from the constricted muscle cells.

Massage can break the pain cycle and eliminate the original source of the pain by increasing blood flow to the ischemic tissue (Kisner, Colby, 1996; Juhan, 1987). This increase in circulation to the affected tissue is created by the mechanical pressure of massage techniques on the veins and lymphatics. Cutaneous stimulation from the pressure may also cause reflex vasodilation of the blood vessels, further improving circulation. Pain from muscle spasm can also be reduced through techniques that can affect proprioceptors, such as movement of limbs, stretching and direct compression of the tissue (Yates, 1990). In one electromyographic muscle study, massage to the neck reduced muscle contraction and neck pain (Simons in Arat, 1973). Improving range of motion of affected joints and treating trigger points further break the pain cycle. A feeling of well being, which usually accompanies massage, reduces pain perception even more.

A study on the effects of massage on myofascial pain and muscle tension concluded that massage is beneficial. Massage was performed for 30 to 45 minutes on 26 patients, 10 times over a period of four weeks. Initially, in 21 of these patients, a significant increase was measured in concentrations of plasma myoglobin, an oxygen-binding protein. The myoglobin is thought to indicate a pathological process in the muscles; pain is a result of ischemia in the tissue, not due to myoglobin. Hypoxia, or a reduced amount of oxygen in the ischemic tissue, might damage the muscle cell membrane, allowing myoglobin to leak into the bloodstream. After several treatments, a gradual decline in plasma myoglobin concentration was noted along with a reduction of pain and muscle tension. At the end of the study there was a decline in pain and muscle tension in 21 of 26 patients. The remaining five did not have a reduction in their symptoms; they also did not have elevated myoglobin levels, suggesting that their symptoms were due to a different pathology (Danneskiold-Samsoe et al., 1986; Yates, 1990).

Massage can alter the processing of pain stimuli in the central nervous system. Opiate-like neurochemicals (endorphins and enkephalins) are produced in the brain. These substances are released in response to pain in order to control it. The Quebec Task Force on Spinal Disorders, 1987, recognized that the release of these neurochemicals through massage therapy could control or manage pain. Research does not present a clear picture. One study suggests that these chemicals are not released in healthy, pain-free clients during massage, but the researchers suggested further studies which would focus on the effects of massage on people in pain (Yates, 1990).

Massage can affect the processing of nociceptive firing by the peripheral nervous system. For example, cross-fibre frictions have been shown to create analgesic effects when used on tendon and ligament injuries (Boyling, Palastanga, 1994). A possible explanation is Melzack and Wall's gate control theory of pain. Simply put, the "gate" is a network of nerves in the region of the spine. When closed, the gate can block the transmission of the small-fibre, slower-moving pain impulses to the brain. This blocking occurs through stimulation of the proprioceptive and cutaneous nerve receptors which are supplied by larger, faster sensory nerve fibres. Therefore, pain intensity can temporarily be reduced over a period of minutes or hours through additional sensory input. This additional sensory input, or closing of the "gate", can be achieved through the instinctive massaging, rubbing or brushing of the skin that one does when injured (Porth, 1990), by deep, focal massage including frictions and with rhythmic movement of the body including the repetitive oscillations of joint play techniques (Hertling, Kessler, 1990; Wood, Becker, 1981; Yates, 1990).

In summary, massage reduces and manages pain that arises from a variety of sources, such as trauma, post-surgery, headache, fibromyalgia, arthritis and terminal illness.

Massage and Circulation

Massage has an effect on local blood flow as demonstrated in several studies, but the amount of increase in circulation is not agreed upon (Cafarelli, Flint, 1992).

The circulatory changes likely result from several factors: mechanical effects on the vasculature; local release of vasodilators; circulatory changes resulting from reflex responses of the autonomic nervous system; and changes in blood viscosity.

Mechanical centripetal pressure of techniques such as petrissage increases venous return (Basmajian, 1985). Massage can mechanically empty venous beds, lower venous pressure and increase capillary flow. Light massage causes a transient but immediate dilation of cutaneous capillaries; deeper pressure causes longer dilation of vessels (Wood, Becker, 1981). Deep stroking and kneading to the calf for 10 minutes demonstrated a doubling of blood flow, which lasted up to 40 minutes post-massage (Wood, Becker, 1981).

A more recent study showed that blood flow increased by 42 per cent following massage, as measured by the increase in washout of radioactive xenon *(Cafarelli, Flint, 1992)*. Further, it is often extrapolated that with massage there is a clearance of metabolic waste and by-products of tissue damage and inflammation, as well as the delivery of oxygen and nutrition to tissue cells through an increase in blood flow through the capillaries *(Yates, 1990)*.

The increase in blood flow, however, is transient; this is especially evident in healthy tissue where autoregulation and autonomic nervous system control of the arterioles ensure adequate blood supply to that tissue. This may be the case in one study which showed no change of blood flow in massage of a healthy resting limb *(Cafarelli, Flint, 1992)*. On the other hand, in tissue that has impaired circulation or venous stasis, massage seems to be more beneficial. For example, one study concluded that with deep stroking and kneading massage of limbs affected with flaccid paralysis, there was an increase in local circulation in the affected limb. No consistent changes were noted in the contralateral limb *(DeLisa, Gans, 1993)*. In the case of decreased blood flow and ischemia from secondary causes, such as muscle spasm or tight muscles and fascia, massage which addressed these specific causes was shown to improve local blood flow *(Yates, 1990)*.

Massage affects blood flow through the local release of vasodilators. The pressure of massage techniques stimulates the release of histamine and acetylcholine which then vasodilate the blood vessels. This is accompanied by a change in skin temperature *(Yates, 1990; Grodin, 1989)*. Rhythmical compression and decompression brought about improvement in colour and temperature in limbs paralysed by poliomyelitis *(Yates, 1990)*.

A variety of techniques was used to measure the effectiveness of massage on blood flow and the survival of ischemic flaps in laboratory animals over six days *(Winter, 1993/4)*. One hundred anesthetized rats had flaps incised through the skin on their backs to the first deep fascial layer; the flap was raised and then sutured back into position and blood flow was measured. Deep massage (using forceps to pinch the skin) was found more effective than acupressure (continuous deep pressure) or light stroking.

Deep massage was most effective three days post-surgery with a 72 per cent survival rate of the flaps. All techniques were found more effective after the procedure, perhaps indicating the beneficial effects of massage on injured tissue. Generally, it seems that superficial massage does not affect circulation to muscles but deeper massage creates an "effective increase" in blood flow to the muscles *(Wood, Becker, 1981)*.

Massage can result in circulatory changes due to reflex responses of the autonomic nervous system. Superficial or deep massage may cause changes in vascular tone through the sympathetic efferents. This may explain why areas, such as the hands and feet, experience increased blood flow and temperature after application of fascial techniques to other parts of the body. Fascial techniques also cause an increase in blood pressure, another indicator of the reflex effects of this type of massage *(Ebner, 1980)*.

The autonomic nervous is also involved as the client relaxes. There is a decrease in sympathetic nervous system firing that can lead to generalized vasodilation of peripheral vasculature and an increase in peripheral circulation.

Finally, blood and plasma viscosity and hematocrit (red blood cell) viscosity were decreased after a 20-minute massage treatment. This decrease in viscosity perhaps was due to an increased flow of interstitial fluid mechanically massaged from the tissues; or perhaps it was due to a vasodilator response to pressure *(Yates, 1990)*.

Massage and Blood Pressure

Several studies demonstrate that massage can reduce blood pressure.

Both systolic and diastolic blood pressure tended to decrease after a 20-minute back massage (technique depth, whether light or heavy, was not given) with a delayed effect of increase in systolic and a small additional decrease in diastolic. The net outcome was a decrease in blood pressure.

Another study demonstrated that a slow stroking back massage (60 strokes per minute, two inches on either side of spinous processes) lasting for six minutes (with a 10-minute rest before and after) decreased blood pressure and heart rate *(Yates, 1990)*.

In summary, massage has an effect on circulation, though the effect is transient. Local circulation is temporarily increased, with local hyperemia observed and an increase in temperature palpated. When dystrophy is apparent, massage improves tissue health. Blood viscosity decreases. Blood pressure can be affected, and therefore, massage, using appropriate techniques, is indicated for cardiac and hypertensive clients, as well as for stressed clients.

Massage and the Lymphatic System

Specialized massage techniques (Vodder's manual lymph drainage) are clearly proven to increase lymphatic flow in the superficial lymphatic capillaries. This increase may be as much as nine times the normal rate of flow *(Yates, 1990)*. Light Swedish techniques such as stroking and kneading, as well as elevation of a limb, are also shown to increase the flow of lymph *(Basmajian, 1985)*.

Massage techniques move lymph by mechanically pumping the lymphatic fluid through the lymphatic capillaries. Compression empties the capillaries, while decompression allows them to refill. Pressure within the capillaries is reduced, allowing the lymph to flow. Therefore, lymphatic drainage techniques reduce edema and pain in the area treated; also, these techniques reduce the build-up of excess fibrin which leads to scar tissue *(Wittlinger, Wittlinger, 1990)*. On people who had lymphedema, lymphatic drainage resulted in an increase in urine output — up to one litre of urine in one hour of massage. Urine concentrations of histamine, corticosteriods and noradrenaline increased. This suggests the techniques improve the clearance of these substances from edemetous tissues and, by extrapolation, other metabolic wastes *(Yates, 1990)*.

Experiments on animals reveal that there is little lymphatic flow in a muscle at rest, but drainage techniques were able to keep the lymph flowing continuously while applied. Proteins injected into joints and tracer isotopes in the skin were removed by massage *(DeLisa, Gans, 1993)*.

Interestingly, one study found that lymphatic massage techniques were more effective than passive range of motion at increasing lymphatic flow *(Wood, Becker, 1981)*. In addition, manual lymphatic drainage techniques have been found more effective in draining chronically edematous limbs than machines designed to reduce edema *(Swedborg, 1985; Casley-Smith, Casley-Smith, 1986)*.

In summary, massage improves lymphatic flow. It is used to reduce edema, ease pain secondary to edema, lower the chance of scar tissue formation and remove metabolic wastes secondary to edema and inflammation.

Massage and the Musculoskeletal System

The effects of massage have been studied on healthy, injured and denervated muscles. In healthy muscle, trunk and hip flexion was increased by the relaxation of back, gluteal and leg muscles following 30 minutes of Swedish techniques; and range of motion of hamstrings was increased after massage (DeLisa, Gans, 1993). Other research has found electromyographic evidence that slow stroking produced relaxation of back muscles (Yates, 1990).

Clinical applications of techniques that affect the gamma motor system, which controls muscle tone, are noted. Specifically, mechanical stimulation of Golgi tendon organs and muscle spindles decreases muscle spasm and increases the resting length of muscles (Gelb, 1985; DeLisa, Gans, 1993). Spasm is also reported to be reduced with joint play techniques (Kisner, Colby, 1990).

Massage is also effective at treating certain muscle dysfunctions. Trigger points were eradicated from muscles following 10 separate treatments of repetitive muscle stripping (Travell, Simons, 1992).

The amount of fibrosis and adhesion in muscle tissue that develops after injury, immobilization or denervation can be reduced (Boyling, Palastanga, 1994). Microscopic examination of animal muscles that had been subjected to crushing injury and then massaged revealed that the tissue appeared normal, with no hemorrhages, fibrous bands between muscle cells or fibrous thickening visible compared to a control group that received no massage. In a different study on denervated tissue, muscles were found to have less fibrosing and fewer adhesions following seven minutes of kneading, stroking and passive range of motion on a daily basis over a maximum period of six months (Wood, Becker, 1981).

Clinically, cross-fibre frictions are effective in reducing adhesions and fibrosis in subacute and chronic injuries (DeLisa, Gans, 1993).

In summary, massage can relax muscles, decrease spasms, improve resting length of muscles and reduce trigger points, fibrosis and adhesions.

Massage and Respiratory Function

Massage therapy, including tapotement, joint play, postural drainage and coughing techniques, has been shown to improve respiratory function and chest expansion and to clear mucus in respiratory pathologies. Massage therapy can also reduce the stress levels of those with asthma, in turn potentially reducing the frequency of attacks.

Tapotement techniques loosen mucus in the lungs (Kisner, Colby, 1996). When viewed with fibre optic bronchoscopy, percussion (tapotement) showed a "spattering of plugs" which blocked the bronchi (Barnes, 1988). Vibrations and shaking were noted as increasing peripheral secretion clearance in some studies, as well as increasing sputum production (Zadai, 1992). In another study, the forced expiratory volume of 11 children with mild to moderate asthma increased 10.3 per cent half an hour after tapotement (Rochester, Goldberg, 1980).

The combination of postural drainage, cough and tapotement was shown in another study to clear five times the mucus from the central and peripheral lung regions than was cleared on days when this therapy was not administered (Bateman et al., 1979).

Combinations of mobilizations and stretching the thorax have proven effective in increasing peak expiratory flow rates in patients with chronic obstructive pulmonary disease. Seven patients were treated for 30 minutes, twice a week for three weeks. Mobilization of the thoracic spine and costovertebral joints, as well as stretching of the intercostals, resulted in improved lung function after one treatment. The maximum oxygen uptake showed an increase of 20 per cent (Pryor, 1991). Chest expansion, vital capacity and respiratory rate were improved in another study on patients with bronchitis and emphysema. Rocking, mobilizing and passive movements were used in four 20-minute treatments (Yates, 1990).

A technique called productive coughing produced a greater amount of sputum than postural drainage or exercise alone in a study of eight patients with chronic bronchitis (Oldenberg et al., 1979).

Research on the effects of massage on younger children with asthma shows that pulmonary functions (including peak air flow) were improved during the study. In addition, the study group's levels of cortisol and anxiety decreased. The children were given 20 minutes of massage each night by their parents (trained in unspecified massage techniques) during the 30-day study (Field et al., 1997a).

Joint play, massage and fascial techniques also help to decrease asthma symptoms (Chapman, 1995; Ebner, 1980).

In summary, massage can improve respiratory function by loosening mucus and improving clearance of sputum, increasing chest expansion and vital capacity and decreasing stress levels.

Massage and the Immune System

Massage therapy appears to increase the activity of the immune system. One unpublished research paper from the Touch Research Institute shows that one month of daily massage increased the activity levels of white blood cells in people who were HIV positive, stimulating immunity. Although the volunteers' T-cell counts were unaffected, meaning that the progression of the HI virus was unchanged by massage, the study shows that massage may have helped fight some of the secondary infections associated with AIDS (Turnbull, 1994/5).

Stress is also shown to decrease the immune response, resulting in susceptibility to illness (Selye, 1974; Porth, 1990). Massage reduces stress levels and improves immune function.

In summary, massage can benefit the immune system.

Psychological Effects of Massage

Massage is able to reduce stress, anxiety and depression and give the client a feeling of well being. These effects are well documented.

A study on massage and job-related stress revealed that 15 minutes of on-the-job massage reduced saliva levels of cortisol, the stress hormone. The subjects of the study reported feeling more alert, which was borne out by an EEG study that showed brain waves consistent with increased alertness. Following the massage, the subjects were also able to solve computerized problems in half the time with 50 per cent fewer errors (Turnbull, 1994/5).

Ten 30-minute massage treatments were given to depressed adolescent mothers over a five-week period. Anxiety and salivary cortisol levels were lower in this group than in a control group who received relaxation therapy *(Field et al., 1995e).*

Massage has also been shown to have a positive effect on mood states in athletes. Tension, depression, fatigue, anger and confusion were significantly reduced *(Cafarelli, Flint, 1992).* In most cases, soothing touch creates a sense of well being for the client.

Finally, as massage changes stress levels, the person benefits, not only psychologically but physiologically as well. Field thinks that massage can be shown to have a positive effect on almost any condition. "I think that, bottom line, ultimately people are going to trace nearly all disease to stress, to disequilibrium in the physiology and biochemistry. I think that's why we invariably get reductions in cortisol levels and anxiety, because all of these conditions (asthma, depression, dermatitis, post-traumatic stress disorder) become more aggravated by knowing that you have a disease...It's almost as though the stress increases exponentially with the disease"*(Knaster, 1994).*

In summary, massage reduces emotional stress levels, giving people a sense of well being and relaxation.

What Massage Cannot Do

No evidence has been found to support claims that massage can increase muscle tone or directly increase muscle strength or bulk. Massage will also not directly decrease the amount of "cellulite" or adipose tissue. Further, with a permanent nerve lesion, massage will not prevent muscular atrophy in the denervated tissue *(Wood, Becker, 1981).*

B

TECHNIQUES AND APPLICATIONS

3

SWEDISH MASSAGE TECHNIQUES

Linda Ludwig, Fiona Rattray

Swedish massage techniques make up the classical manipulations used by a massage therapist. Through practise and conscious application, mastery of these soft tissue techniques "not only gives the therapist the tools to manipulate the soft tissue, it also facilitates the development and improvement of palpation skills so essential to the massage therapist" (Neumann, 1989). Swedish massage techniques are complimented by the use of non-Swedish techniques, remedial exercise and hydrotherapy to achieve physiological and psychological effects to treat the client's condition.

Technique Components

Swedish techniques can be categorized by the following components:

✦ **Direction** of movement:

- For relaxation or reduction of edema, the direction is centripetal (towards the heart) or in the direction of blood flow and, when possible, parallel with the muscle fibre direction.
- For treatment of fibrotic areas, the techniques are applied in a cross-fibre direction or in the direction of the restriction.

✦ **Pressure:**

- For relaxation, the pressure applied is usually light to moderate.
- Deeper pressure is used to reach deeper structures and for the treatment of adhesions.

✦ **Rhythm** of movement:

- An even rhythm should be used.

✦ **Rate** of movement:

- For relaxation, the rate of movement is slower and can be matched to the rate of respiration of the client.

- For a stimulating effect, techniques are applied more quickly.

✦ **Duration** of a technique:

- How long one applies a technique depends on the size of the area massaged, the pathological condition and the client's tolerance. For example, petrissage to an area of acute lumbar pain may only be tolerated for a short time before the tissue becomes irritated whereas, to reduce edema, a technique may be applied for 20 minutes or more.

✦ **Part** of the therapist's hand or arm that is used:

- Various parts of the hand or arm may be used to apply a technique. An elbow or thumb can achieve a more focused effect than the full surface of the palm, which applies more general pressure *(Wood, Becker, 1981; Boyling, Palastanga, 1994).*

Summary: To Achieve a Relaxing Effect

Generally, any technique applied in a slow, rhythmical and repetitive manner will evoke a relaxation response and decrease sympathetic nervous system firing. This is facilitated if the techniques are applied in a predictable pattern, at an even rate. Superficial techniques using light pressure tend to be relaxing but even techniques using deep pressure, if applied with a broad touch, such as the full palmar surface of the hand or the ulnar border of the forearm, can achieve this soothing effect.

Summary: To Achieve a Stimulating Effect

Techniques applied with briskness, in more erratic and less predictable patterns, will generally increase the sympathetic nervous system firing *(Basmajian, 1985).* Deeper pressure may also have this effect; this is especially true if the client experiences some discomfort with the work. When a smaller surface area is used to apply the techniques, such as thumbs, fingertips or olecranon, the sensation is concentrated and specific; the effect may be more stimulating for the client.

Terminology

The terminology used to describe massage techniques often varies from author to author *(Wood, Becker, 1981; Basmajian, 1985).* These inconsistencies of "terminology [have] unavoidably accompanied [massage therapists] throughout [their] history" *(Basmajian, 1985).*

The following technique definitions cover the terms used in this text for Swedish techniques. They are arranged in technique groups.

Stroking

Stroking is among the lightest techniques used for massage.

Uses of Stroking

Stroking is often used as an introductory or closing technique. This may pertain to working on a particular body part or on the whole body.

At the end of the massage, stroking from the head to the feet can create an awareness and sense of connection of the entire body.

Temperature differences can be palpated with stroking, but palpation of tone is not likely with the amount of pressure used for this technique.

How to Perform Stroking

- The palmar surface of the hand or the fingers is used; pressure is applied equally through the entire surface of the hand or fingers *(Basmajian, 1985)*.

- The technique is applied superficially. The tissue is not compressed and only the minimum amount of pressure is used to make contact with the tissue.

- The direction of stroking can be centripetal or centrifugal because the technique is so superficial.

- Stroking may be performed using long or short movements.

- It is not necessary to use a lubricant because there is little drag created with this technique.

- While stroking is generally applied on broad areas of the skin, it is also performed through the sheets.

Contraindications

- Stroking is not used over uncovered open or contagious skin lesions.

Effects of Stroking

- Generally, repetitive stroking is considered to be a soothing technique that decreases sympathetic nervous system firing and reduces pain perception *(Porth, 1990)*.

- It tends to have a reflexive effect on the circulatory system because of the lightness of the pressure.

Effleurage

Effleurage is from the French word "effleurer", to glide, stroke or touch lightly *(Basmajian, 1985)*.

Uses of Effleurage

Often effleurage is used early in a massage to spread the lubricant.

It can introduce the client to the therapist's touch.

Palpation of temperature, muscle tone and texture are incorporated with effleurage. Tenderness will not always be palpated unless the client's tissue is very tender or a very deep pressure has been used when applying the technique.

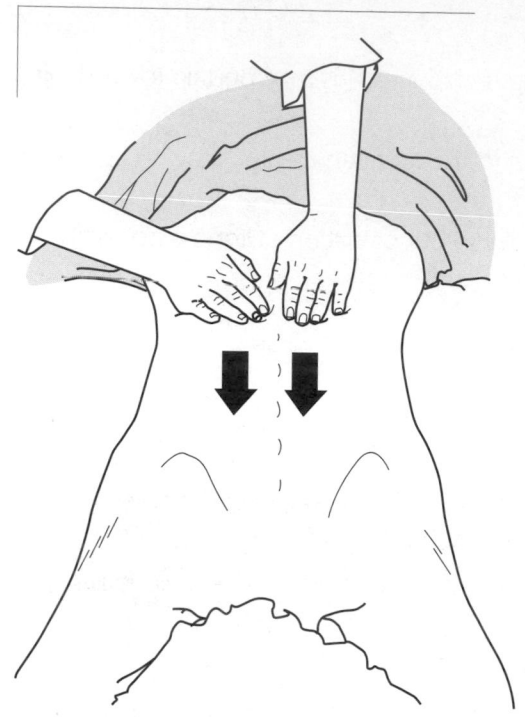

Figure 3.1
Effleurage.

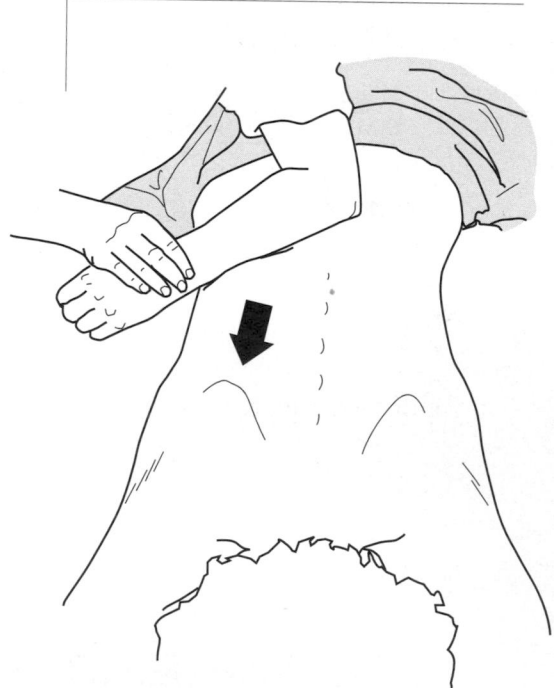

Figure 3.2
Effleurage using the middle of the ulnar border.

Effleurage prepares the tissue for deeper techniques.

It can be used as a transition stroke from one technique to another or when moving from one area of a limb or the trunk to another.

Because it is so general, this technique is often applied at the end of the massage of a particular body part, following the principles of massage described in the chapter on Sequence of Techniques.

How to Perform Effleurage

🖐 Most frequently, effleurage is applied using the hand, with fingers together *(Figure 3.1)*. The fingertips maybe used when applying effleurage to a small area such as the neck when the client is supine. The ulnar border of the forearm *(Figure 3.2)* may also be used, often when massaging over the larger muscle groups of the leg or over the back.

🖐 The surface of the hand, fingers or forearm should closely conform to the contours of the client's tissue or limb being touched.

🖐 The pressure is applied broadly and generally, through the entire surface of the structure used, whether it be the hand, fingers or forearm.

🖐 Effleurage is applied smoothly, using a light to moderate depth; the depth varies depending on the client's condition; lighter pressure is used if the client is more debilitated or tissue health is poor.

🖐 Effleurage is classically a long stroke, covering the length of the client's limb or thorax. The direction of effleurage is centripetal or towards the heart; therefore, while the therapist maintains contact on the return stroke, no pressure is used *(Wood, Becker, 1981)*.

Effects of Effleurage

✦ The effects vary depending on the depth, rate and rhythm of the technique; effleurage tends to have a more reflexive effect on circulation if less pressure is used and a more mechanical effect if deeper pressure is used. Repetitive and sweeping, effleurage is used to increase local venous and lymphatic return, to increase local circulation or to reduce edema.

Contraindications

♦ Effleurage is not used distal to an area of inflammation, distal to an injury in the acute and early subacute stage or distal to an area of infection.

♦ It is not used over uncovered or covered open or contagious skin lesions.

♦ This technique should not be performed repetitively on the limbs of clients with hypertension, heart disease, varicose veins or edema caused by a thrombus in a vein.

♦ Slow rhythmic effleurage has a sedative effect, decreasing sympathetic nervous system firing and, in turn, reducing pain and muscle hypertonicity.

♦ Quick and erratic effleurage is stimulating.

Petrissage

Petrissage is from the French "petrir" meaning to knead. These terms are often used interchangeably. In this text, kneading is considered a type of petrissage.

Uses of Petrissage

This group of techniques is used after the tissue is warmed up because of the increased pressure and focus of petrissage.

Petrissage makes up a key group of techniques used in treatment.

These techniques are applied to muscle groups, individual muscles or some part of a muscle.

How to Perform Petrissage

Types of petrissage include muscle squeezing, muscle stripping, wringing, picking up, skin rolling and, of course, a variety of kneading techniques. The part of the hand used varies, such as the palm, fingertip, thumb, forearm or knuckle. One or both hands may be used.

Generally, petrissage is any technique which rhythmically compresses and releases the tissue. This creates kneading and stretching of tissue layers relative to each other. Often petrissage is applied using short strokes of kneading, grasping, squeezing or pushing the tissue *(Wood, Becker, 1981; Basmajian, 1985)*. Contact is maintained with the client's tissue throughout the technique. The direction of the pressure of petrissage is variable. Some petrissage, such as all types of kneading, is performed centripetally. With other petrissage, the direction of pressure, whether more lateral or vertical once the initial lift is made, depends on the specific technique.

If pain is experienced, the pressure of the grasp is lessened or less of the underlying tissue is taken up.

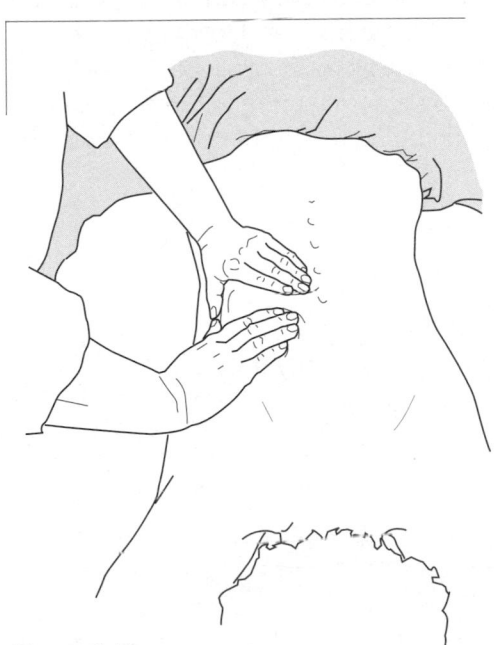

Figure 3.3
Petrissage: Muscle squeezing.

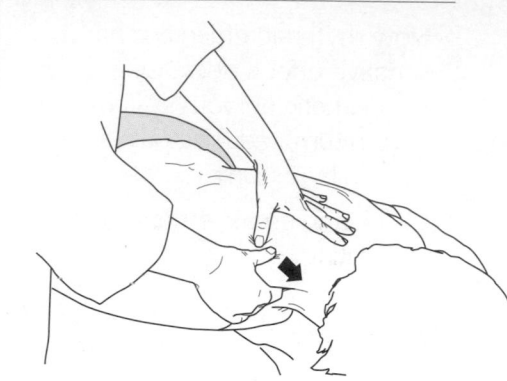

Figure 3.4
Petrissage: Muscle stripping using right thumb and fingers to upper trapezius.

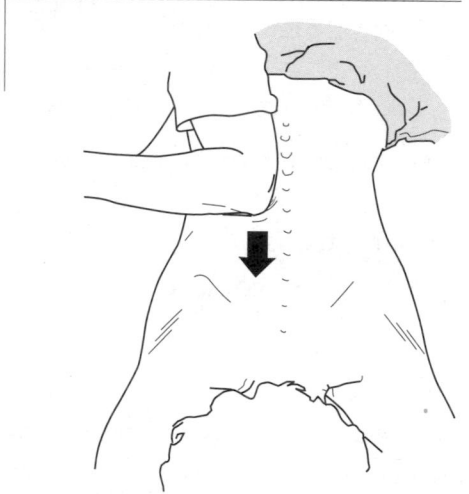

Figure 3.5
Petrissage: Muscle stripping using elbow to erector spinae.

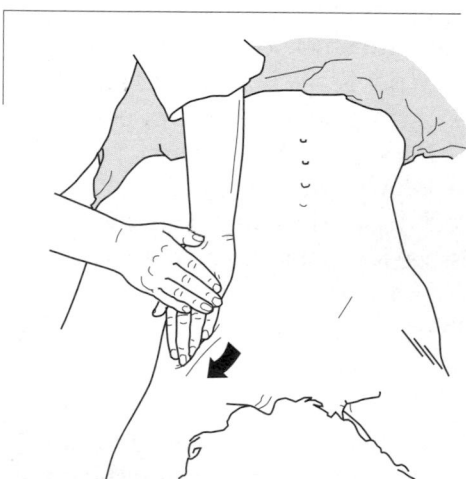

Figure 3.6
Petrissage: Muscle stripping using fingertips to infraspinatus

Types of Petrissage

- **Muscle squeezing:** The muscle is compressed between the palm and fingers or between both palms; the pressure is then directed slightly vertically *(Figure 3.3)*.

- **Muscle stripping:** The thumb *(Figure 3.4)*, elbow *(Figure 3.5)*, ulnar border of the hand or fingertips *(Figure 3.6)* are used. With moderate to deep pressure, the contours of muscles are followed, often from the distal to proximal muscle insertion. The pressure is applied along the fibre direction.

- **Wringing:** Both hands are used. They are placed on the area and allowed to conform to the tissue. Tension is created as each hand moves in an opposite direction and then back to the initial position *(Figure 3.7)*. The pressure changes during the technique, with more pressure used when the tissue is lifted and torqued, and less pressure at the beginning and end of the movement.

- **Picking up:** The fingers and thenar eminence or the palms of the hands squeeze the muscle, lifting it up from the underlying tissue using a vertical pressure *(Figure 3.8)*.

- **Skin rolling:** The skin is lifted between the thumb and fingers and gently rolled over the area being treated *(Figure 3.9)*. A slow speed is used so any superficially restricted areas are palpated. They can be addressed by slowly rolling the tissue back and forth over the adhesion in order to release it. It is possible to perform deeper skin rolling by grasping more tissue between the fingers and thumb and rolling the tissue.

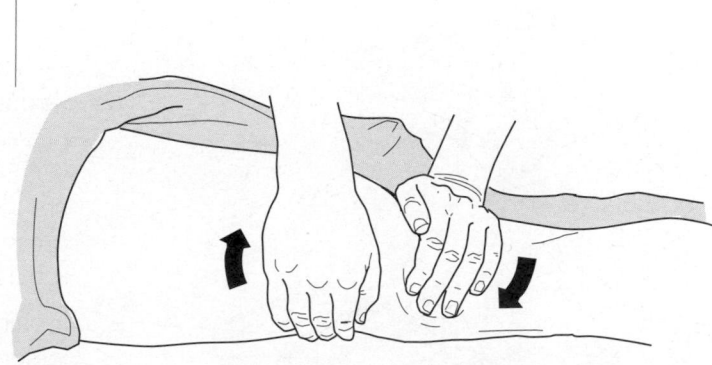

Figure 3.7
Petrissage: Wringing to hamstrings.

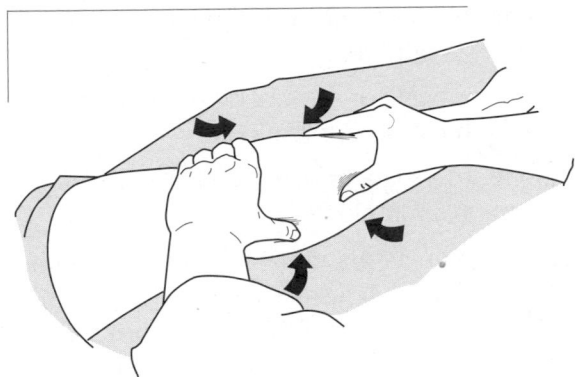

Figure 3.8
Petrissage: Picking up lifts muscle vertically from underlying tissue.

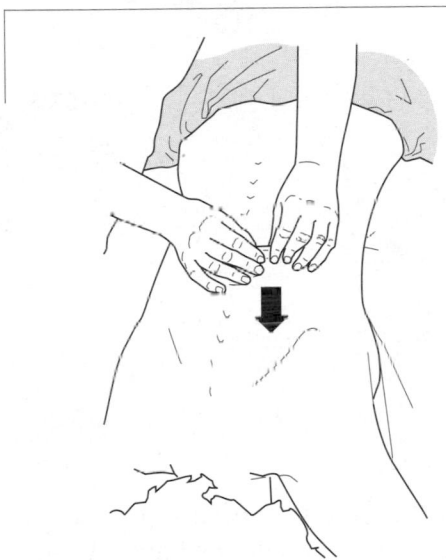

Figure 3.9
Petrissage: Skin rolling over erector spinae.

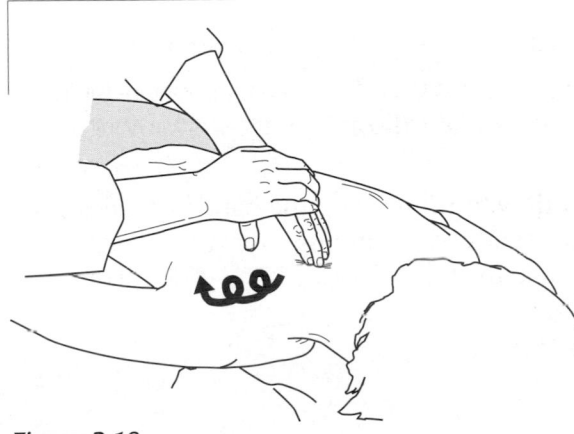

Figure 3.10
Petrissage: Fingertip kneading to supraspinatus.

Kneading: Using the thumb, fingertips *(Figure 3.10)*, palmar surface or ulnar border of the hand or forearm, the therapist performs short, rhythmical unidirectional or circular movements. The pressure peaks in the middle of the technique. Kneading can also be applied by alternating the circles. When deeper pressure is needed, the therapist can use one hand or thumb to perform the technique and the other hand for reinforcement and support *(Figure 3.11)*.

Effects of Petrissage

◆ All types of petrissage affect local circulation while they are being applied.

◆ Different techniques can achieve varying effects depending on the degree of pressure or compression and the amount of drag applied to the tissue.

◆ If increased drag is applied to the tissue, muscle fibre and connective tissue adhesions can be loosened *(DeLisa, Gans, 1993)*. If only the skin layer is engaged, only the superficial fascia is addressed.

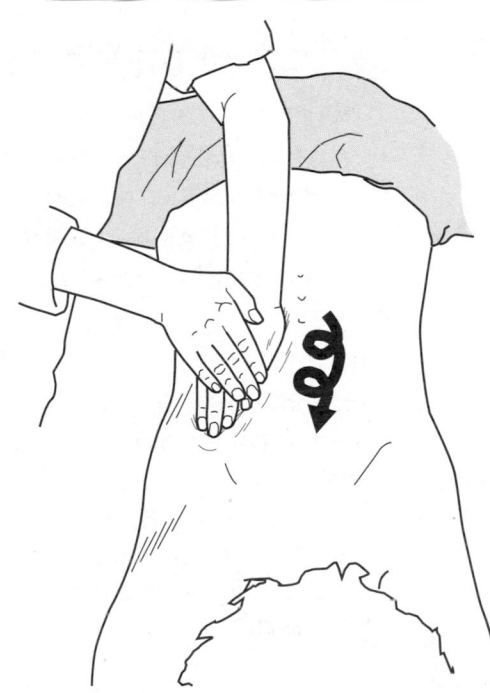

Figure 3.11
Petrissage: Reinforced palmar kneading to lower trapezius and latissimus dorsi.

Contraindications

✦ Petrissage is not used with most acute conditions and when local massage is contraindicated.

✦ With severely atrophied or atonic muscles, petrissage is not used because the drag of these techniques could damage tissue.

✦ Petrissage should not be used over moderate to severe varicosities.

✦ Muscle hypertonicity is reduced with the repetitive kneading movements of petrissage.

✦ Petrissage can be soothing or stimulating depending on the speed and rhythm of its application.

✦ Repetitive muscle stripping and skin rolling are used to treat trigger points in a muscle belly.

✦ Skin rolling is used as an assessment technique to check for superficial fascial restrictions *(Neumann, 1989; Ebner, 1980)* as well as for trigger points *(Travell, Simons, 1983)*. See the chapters on non-Swedish techniques and trigger points for more information.

Vibrations

Vibrations, or oscillations to the tissue, are probably one of the most difficult techniques to master; they require ongoing practise.

Uses of Vibrations

Vibrations are used at any time during the massage.

No lubricant is necessary when performing vibrations.

How to Perform Vibrations

🖐 This technique can be performed with one or both hands.

🖐 Once the hand is in contact with the tissue, the muscles of the forearm are alternately contracted and then relaxed to create a rhythmic movement through the hand. When the rhythmic movement is fast enough, a vibration is produced.

🖐 Vibrations may be easier to perform if the therapist keeps his upper arm and shoulder relaxed.

🖐 Once the vibration is initiated, it is directed into the area of the body to be treated.

🖐 Vibrations can be fine or course; **fine vibrations** are very short, fast, almost invisible oscillations of the arm and hand, whereas **coarse vibrations** are larger and more observable.

🖐 Vibrations can also be static or running. **Static vibrations** keep the hand in continuous contact with tissue without sliding over the client's skin. **Running vibrations** keep the hand in continuous contact with the tissue and then the vibrating hand glides over the client's skin.

Effects of Vibrations

✦ Vibrations can be used to create a different stimulation of the body because of their unusual feel; this is useful in painful areas and those which are hyposensitive or need sensory re-education — for example, after a cast has been removed.

✦ Fine vibrations are more soothing than coarse vibrations.

✦ Prolonged coarse or fine vibrations, when applied to the thorax, can assist in mechanically loosening the mucus present in respiratory conditions (*Wood, Becker, 1981*).

✦ Vibrations can be used to decrease muscle tone if they are applied to a muscle tendon for up to 30 seconds (*Fritz, Noltie, 1992*).

Tapotement

Tapotement is from the French "tapoter" meaning to rap, drum or pat.

Uses of Tapotement

Tapotement can be used at any time during the treatment, where it is appropriate.

If a heavier tapotement is required, it is applied in a sequence from light to heavier, then back to light, following the principles of massage described in the chapter on Sequence of Techniques.

No lubricant is needed with tapotement.

How to Perform Tapotement

There is a variety of ways to tapote the tissue. All types of tapotement are percussive and rhythmic, usually with the two hands alternately applying the pressure. It can be performed using fingertips, the ulnar borders of hands, the full palmar surfaces of the hands or the fists.

✦ **Light Tapotement**

The hands are light and springy, with the wrists relaxed; the technique is applied superficially with no force created beneath the skin.

Pincement: The tissue is gently plucked between the thumb and fingertips (*Figure 3.12*).

Tapping: The tissue is tapped with the fingertips (*Figure 3.13*).

✦ **Heavy Tapotement**

The hands are firm, with the wrists relaxed; a deeper force is used that carries below the skin surface.

Hacking: This is performed with the ulnar border of the hand. For less force the hand is relaxed; for

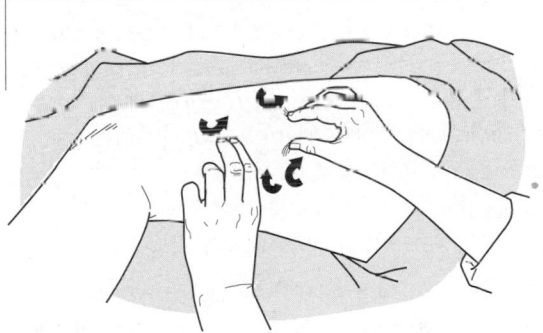

Figure 3.12
Tapotement: Pincement to lateral thigh.

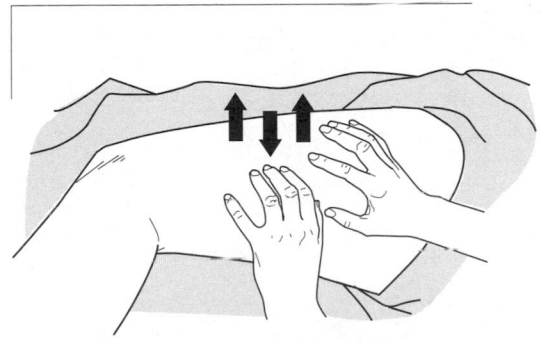

Figure 3.13
Tapotement: Tapping to lateral thigh.

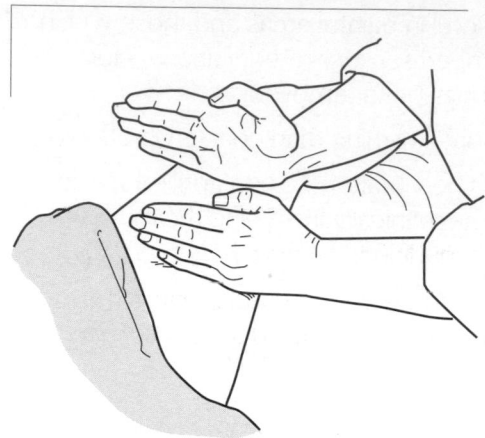

Figure 3.14
Heavy tapotement: Hacking to quadriceps.

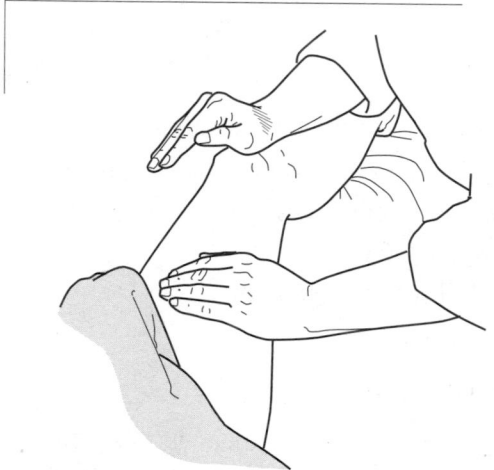

Figure 3.15
Heavy tapotement: Cupping to quadriceps.

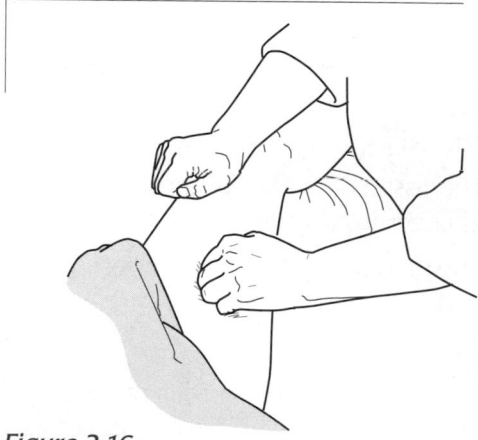

Figure 3.16
Heavy tapotement: Beating with extensor
surface of middle phalanges on quadriceps.

greater force the hand is stiff *(Figure 3.14)*.

🖐 **Clapping or Cupping:** The hand is held in a cupped position, with the fingers and thumb together; with the wrist pronated, the tissue is struck with alternating hands *(Figure 3.15)*. When done properly, there is an audible "clopping" noise.

🖐 **Beating:** The hand is held in a loose fist. Beating can be performed using the extensor surface of the phalanges of the digits (like rapping the knuckles *(Figure 3.16)* on a door) or the ulnar surface of the fist (as if pounding *(Figure 3.17)* on a table).

Effects of Tapotement

✦ The primary purpose of tapotement is to loosen mucus in clients with respiratory conditions.

✦ Heavy tapotement or prolonged light tapotement increases local circulation.

✦ Tapotement is generally stimulating and increases sympathetic nervous system firing; it can be used for clients with generalized fatigue.

✦ Heavy tapotement may elicit the stretch reflex of the muscles it is applied to, temporarily increasing their tone. Secondary to this, there is the reciprocal inhibition of the antagonist. For example, tapotement to the quadriceps may temporarily increase their tone but create a relaxation of the hamstrings, therefore facilitating stretching and lengthening of hamstrings *(Wood, Becker, 1981)*.

✦ Light tapotement is useful to stimulate hypotrophied muscles, though the pressure used is a reflection of the

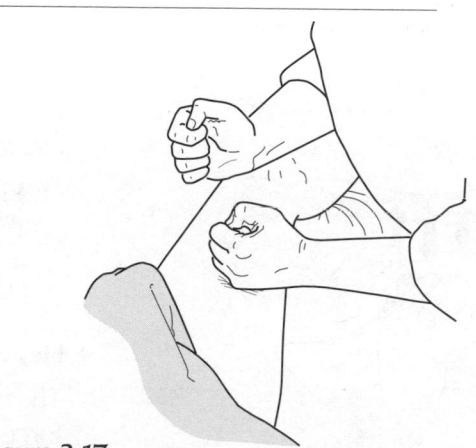

Figure 3.17
Heavy tapotement: Beating with ulnar surfaces
on quadriceps.

health of the muscles. It is also good for desensitizing areas such as amputation sites or tissue just after a cast is removed *(DeLisa, Gans, 1993)*.

Lubricants Used with Swedish Massage

The therapist uses some type of lubricant to reduce drag and to facilitate gliding over the skin. With a lubricant, different textures in the tissue may be more easily palpated, such as areas of denser or more fibrosed tissues. Lubricants themselves have different textures and viscosities, as well as rates of absorption into the skin.

The decision whether to use lotion, cream, gel or oil is based partly on the therapist's preference and partly on the client's needs. Of course, oils are not used with a client who has allergies or sensitivities to oil; instead a hypoallergenic lotion is chosen.

Oils

Oils are traditional massage lubricants. Their use dates back thousands of years; olive oil is commonly mentioned *(Basmajian, 1985)*. They are slow to be absorbed into the client's skin; a little goes a long way.

Vegetable or nut oils used in massage should be light in texture, as non-staining as possible, and have little odour of their own. An oil may be purchased unblended and in various-sized containers from food service or cosmetic industry suppliers. Sunflower and safflower oils are inexpensive; sweet almond and grape seed oils are more costly.

Commercially blended vegetable and nut oils may also be purchased; these usually contain an oil-dispersing agent (surfactant) which allows the oils to be laundered out of linens more easily. Blends may be unscented or have essential oils added for therapeutic effects.

Oils can stain a client's clothes unless wiped off after treatment. A client may not wish to get oil in her hair during a massage. Over time, oils without dispersants can accumulate on linens unless the linens are commercially laundered.

As oils can oxidize (become "off" or rancid) with exposure to air, heat and light, they should be stored away from sunlight.

If oils are purchased in smaller quantities, oxidization is reduced. An anti-oxidant such as vitamin E may be added by the therapist if oils are purchased in bulk; commercially blended oils may already contain anti-oxidants.

Jojoba oil may also be used as a lubricant. This is not an oil but a plant wax that is liquid at room temperature. As a wax, jojoba has the advantage of not oxidizing; it is light and odourless; however, it can be more costly than a vegetable oil.

Lotions, Creams and Gels

Lotions and cream- or gel-based lubricants are newer additions to massage therapy. They tend not to be staining and, for the most part, they do not oxidize. However, they may be rapidly absorbed into the skin, necessitating re-application while the therapist is working.

Lotions, creams and gels can be scent-free; they may have essential oils added for therapeutic effect. A hypoallergenic lotion should be available if the client needs one.

Other Additives and Topical Preparations

With the client's consent, other topical preparations may be used. Vitamin E oil may be added to an oil or cream to improve the client's tissue health and to decrease scar tissue formation *(Kirshmann, 1979)*.

Herbal extracts in a cream base may also be used for their therapeutic effects. For example, arnica montana helps to reduce pain and bruising.

Commercial gels or lotions that have either a topical cooling or heating effect may be applied to the client's skin after treatment; however, these do not have the same penetrating effect as a hydrotherapy application.

Essential oils can be added to the lubricant if the client agrees and has no allergies or sensitivities to them. These aromatic, highly concentrated plant extracts are derived from the petals, leaves, rinds and wood of various plants. The properties of essential oils have been widely researched and studied. Most essential oils are antiseptic, some are decongestants, others are calming. However, there are contraindications to the use of certain essential oils, and the therapist should have a reference text for choosing an appropriate oil *(Lawless, 1995; Watt, 1992; Valnet, 1990)*. Post-graduate training is also recommended.

In terms of massage, essential oils are not used straight out of the bottle due to their concentrated nature. They are diluted in a carrier oil, usually a nut oil such as sweet almond or grape seed oil. Specific dilutions of essential oils are noted in the text where appropriate. Petroleum-derived oils such as mineral oil should not be used as carrier oils because these seal the skin, preventing absorption of the essential oils.

4

NON-SWEDISH MASSAGE TECHNIQUES

Fiona Rattray, Linda Ludwig

Quick Reference for Non-Swedish Massage Techniques

The techniques described below are used in conjunction with Swedish massage; because they are not part of Per Ling's list of manipulations, this text refers to them as "non-Swedish". Many of these techniques have been developed in the last century, some of them within the last few decades, demonstrating the rapidly expanding nature of manual medicine.

The way in which originators of specific techniques created their manipulations appears to be a combination of necessity (no other technique existed), academic knowledge (anatomy and pathophysiology) and intuition (messages from the subconscious mind, the subliminal self *(Pirsig, 1974)*, the creative muse, the psyche, the divine spark, whatever one wants to call it).

For example, Elizabeth Dicke's connective tissue massage (Bindegewebsmassage) was created in the 1920s out of necessity. As a result of a neglected tooth abscess, Dicke developed general toxemia and a severe occlusion of the peripheral circulation in her right leg; she was advised to consider amputation of the limb. In addition to the pain in the leg, she suffered from backache. She found that by stroking with her fingertips over the painful areas in her back, the back pain diminished. Dicke continued to stroke over tight areas around her hip and noticed paresthesia in her affected limb, then warmth. The superficial circulation gradually reappeared in her thigh and leg; over three months of treatment the severe symptoms subsided. Dicke avoided amputation and was able to return to her occupation as a physiotherapist after one year *(Ebner, 1980)*. Many of today's direct fascial techniques are based on the system Dicke later researched and developed.

In contrast, Emil Vodder, another physiotherapist, visualized manual lymph drainage in a sudden instant of creativity. He had studied the immune system for a number of years in the 1920s at a time when it was first being recognized as the enormously important system that it is. "One day a client came to our physical therapy institute in Cannes for treatment of a nose and throat infection [and] migraine...As usual, I closed my eyes while I palpated the hard, swollen cervical lymph nodes. I suddenly imagined a nasal sinus covered with shimmering lymph vessels. In my mind I also saw...the lymph node chains that act as a natural draining system for the skin, mucosa and meninges, i.e., for all the organs and nodes in the head and neck. As far as I know, this complex had never previously been interpreted as a natural separate drainage apparatus for the entire head region." *(Wittlinger, Wittlinger, 1985)*. He went on to develop a highly effective system of lymphatic techniques for draining the whole body.

As complex systems of assessment and manual medicine evolved, some practitioners developed certain facets of these systems as therapies in their own right. For example, visceral manipulation, the muscle energy technique and craniosacral therapy originated from osteopathic concepts.

Manual therapists who trained under originators of specific techniques would often put their own stamp on the techniques after months or years of clinical experience. As the techniques were documented and taught in different locations, ideas cross-fertilized and new techniques were created, demonstrating the wonderful way that manual therapists have influenced each other over the centuries *(Basmajian, 1985)*.

The following chapter is by no means a comprehensive listing of non-Swedish techniques; it is meant to familiarize the reader with techniques that are described in the text. Therapists are encouraged to take professional post-graduate training in techniques in which they lack proficiency.

Diaphragmatic Breathing

Diaphragmatic breathing is a key part of every massage treatment. It is the easiest way for the client to achieve relaxation and to break the pain cycle; it also gives the client control over potentially uncomfortable techniques. Diaphragmatic breathing is regularly recommended as self-care.

The average person breathes 12 to 15 times per minute or 20,000 times per day *(Fried, 1990)*. Inefficient or inappropriate breathing patterns can lead to dysfunction, both structurally and physiologically.

Optimal Breathing

With relaxed inhalation, the respiratory diaphragm contracts and descends, compressing the abdominal viscera. The quadratus lumborum muscles stabilize the lower ribs and diaphragm. The external intercostal muscles contract and lift the ribs laterally, like the handle of a bucket. The scalene muscles along with the sternocleidomastoids contract to elevate the sternum and, primarily, the first two ribs. These actions increase space in the thoracic cavity and decrease air pressure within the lungs, which allows air to flow into the lungs.

Relaxed exhalation is a passive process and involves the relaxation of all the muscles of inspiration. Ideally, if the diaphragm is relaxed first, the largest volume of air can be expired easily. This is followed by relaxation of the intercostals, scalenes and sternocleidomastoids.

The diaphragm massages the viscera because it is located above the viscera. As it contracts, it descends and compresses the organs in the abdomen. The rhythmical action of the diaphragm creates a kind of vacuum in the thorax which facilitates the return of venous blood and lymphatic fluid from the legs and lower torso to the heart. Diaphragmatic breathing also allows the most efficient intake of oxygen and output of carbon dioxide.

Diaphragmatic breathing has many beneficial effects. It promotes relaxation by decreasing the effects of the sympathetic nervous system. Because muscles relax on exhalation and tighten when the breath is held, the therapist can use the client's conscious exhalation to relax muscles, increase the effectiveness of techniques and reduce the perception of pain. When using deeper techniques or working on painful areas, the therapist should encourage the client to "breathe into" the tissue and "breathe out" the pain.

Specific breathing exercises facilitate the post-isometric relaxation techniques used to stretch individual muscles. Refer to the chapter in this text on remedial exercise. See the stress reduction chapter for information on diaphragmatic breathing and stress reduction. Also see the chapters on respiratory conditions for breathing exercises.

Assessment

Diaphragmatic breathing is always encouraged. The therapist should not assume that a client can breathe diaphragmatically. It is important to assess for any dysfunctional breathing patterns. Breathing can be checked before and during the treatment.

- If the client is supine, the therapist places her hands on the client's abdomen, palpating and observing the motion as the client inhales and exhales. Next, the lateral motion of the ribs is palpated and observed, then the motion of the upper chest. This assessment may also be performed with the client sidelying or prone; in the prone position the therapist palpates the lower ribs and quadratus lumborum muscles instead of the abdomen.

Normal breathing patterns are as previously described: abdominal, lateral rib and upper chest movement.

Apical breathing is an inefficient breathing pattern, where the client mainly uses the upper chest, or apex of the lungs, to breathe; the lateral ribs move slightly; and the abdomen hardly moves at all. This pattern may be seen with respiratory dysfunctions such as asthma, with postural dysfunctions and when a client is in pain or under stress.

Paradoxical breathing occurs when the client's abdomen does not appear to rise as the client inhales. The abdominal muscles do not relax which holds the viscera somewhat immobile. The lateral rib motion and scalene muscles must compensate for the lack of visceral motion. Clients who must maintain a certain posture, such as dancers, figure skaters and gymnasts, are usually trained to breathe in this manner. Paradoxical respiration may also be indicative of a pathology — a pneumothorax or paralysis of the diaphragm (*Taber's Cyclopedic Medical Dictionary, 1981*).

The Diaphragmatic Breathing Technique

It is important to educate the client in proper breathing, preferably at the beginning of each treatment. The client is instructed to inhale through the nose, which warms and filters air before it enters the lungs, and exhale through the mouth.

Care is taken by the therapist when giving verbal instructions to the client, particularly avoiding suggestions. Instructions to the client such as "take a slow, deep breath, then another and another...good" are preferable to the implied finality of "take a breath, then another, then one last breath".

- There are three steps in showing the client diaphragmatic breathing. In the first step, while the client is supine, the therapist places her hands on the client's abdomen and asks the client to "lift up my hands with your breath". The client may respond better to a specific visualization, such as "imagine a balloon in your stomach that you are inflating with your inhalation". This should be done with as little upper chest movement as possible. Some clients have difficulty focusing on the diaphragm muscle. If the client seems anxious or frustrated, the therapist should move on to the next step in correct breathing.

- For the second step, the therapist places her hands on the lateral parts of the rib cage. The client is instructed to "move my hands out with your breathing". The therapist can apply some resistance against inhalation to increase the client's awareness of this aspect of correct breathing.

- In the third step, the therapist places the fingertips of one hand on the manubrium, just below the sternal notch. The client is asked to "breathe into this area and lift your sternum".

- For proper exhalation, the therapist can help by directing the client to relax the diaphragm first, followed by the intercostal muscles and then the neck muscles. This can be assisted by gently touching each area in the above order. As the client exhales,

34

✦ Contraindications to breathing exercises include long-term diabetes and kidney disease *(Fried, 1990)*.

full relaxation of the trapezius and scalene muscles should be encouraged by having the client think about bringing the shoulders "down". Diaphragmatic breathing should be slow, full and not forced. The client should not hyperventilate.

✦ Effects: Diaphragmatic breathing increases relaxation, lymphatic flow and efficiency of gas exchange, and facilitates stretching techniques; it also decreases pain and stress.

Manual Lymphatic Drainage (MLD)

Manual lymphatic drainage was researched and developed in the 1930s by Emil Vodder, a Danish physiotherapist. Numerous research studies have verified the efficacy of the technique since that time *(Foldi et al., 1985; Swedborg, 1985; Casley-Smith, Casley-Smith, 1986)*. Manual lymphatic drainage encourages lymph flow and reduces certain types of edema. The slow, repetitive, rhythmical nature of these techniques also decreases pain perception and the effects of the sympathetic nervous system.

With edema resulting from acute or subacute trauma, manual lymphatic drainage techniques are useful in reducing the formation of scar tissue. This is accomplished by the removal of fibrin from the initial lymphatics *(Casley Smith, Casley-Smith, 1986; Kurz, 1990)*.

Edema resulting from connective tissue restrictions such as post-surgical scarring can also be treated. Persons with lymphedema experienced an increase in urine output; urine concentrations of histamine, corticosteroids and noradrenaline also increased after lymphatic drainage, which suggests the techniques improve the clearance of these substances from edematous tissues and, by extrapolation, remove other metabolic wastes *(Yates, 1990)*.

The lymphatic system is largely a passive one. It relies primarily on surrounding skeletal muscles and the action of the diaphragm to move lymphatic fluid through its capillaries, nodes and ducts. The larger abdominal and thoracic ducts have contractile abilities and recent studies may indicate that the superficial lymphatic capillaries also have a minor capability to contract *(Immen, 1995)*.

The Manual Lymphatic Drainage Technique

Light, repetitive techniques are used to pump the lymphatic fluid through the superficial lymphatic capillaries. During the technique, the therapist's hands are soft and relaxed. No lubricant is needed, although talcum powder may be used to facilitate drag.

✋ Each manipulation must be repeated a minimum of five to seven times in order to pump the lymphatic fluid through the tissue. The strokes are unidirectional and overlapping. The pressure is applied centripetally, or towards the heart, in a rhythmic manner, starting at the proximal lymph nodes and working distally towards the edematous site. Thorough treatment of a single limb may take up to 20 minutes *(Wittlinger, Wittlinger, 1985)*.

A pressure of 20 to 40 mm Hg is used to avoid collapsing the superficial lymphatic capillaries. Pressure of more than 60 mm Hg will compress and temporarily collapse these vessels, which temporarily prevents the drainage of lymph. An average pressure of 30 mm

Contraindications

✦ Contraindications to lymphatic drainage techniques include chronic heart failure, acute conditions due to bacterial or viral infection, recent thrombosis, low-protein edemas due to kidney pathologies, malignancy and lymphatic obstruction by parasites *(Wittlinger, Wittlinger, 1990)*. See the chapter on edema for more details.

Hg has been found to have the greatest effect on moving the lymph *(Wittlinger, Wittlinger, 1990; Casley-Smith, Casley-Smith, 1986)*. In one study, the initial lymphatic vessels or capillaries took five seconds to refill after compression *(Casley-Smith, Bjorlin, 1985)*.

Complex decongestive physiotherapy, a combination of MLD, skin hygiene, bandaging and remedial exercises, is used effectively to treat lymphedema *(Foldi et al., 1985)*.

✦ Effects: Lymphatic drainage encourages lymph flow and reduces pain, edema, excess fibrin and metabolic products in the inflammatory process.

Other Lymphatic Drainage Techniques

Edema associated with an acute injury and chronic edema can also be treated with an adaption of some of the MLD techniques following the principles for pressure, repetition, direction and speed outlined above *(Wittlinger, Wittlinger, 1990)*.

The following techniques can be used to treat the entire body or just localized areas. To treat the local edema present at the acute or subacute stage of an injury, lymphatic drainage techniques are applied first. The therapist works from proximal to distal towards the localized edema. Deeper Swedish techniques are applied next, since these temporarily collapse the superficial lymphatic capillaries and inhibit the removal of edema. In treating chronic edema, the approach changes. Deeper Swedish and fascial techniques are applied proximal to the edematous site to release soft tissue restrictions that may inhibit lymphatic flow. In order for the lymphatic drainage to be most effective, a few minutes should elapse after the deeper Swedish techniques and before lymph drainage techniques are applied to allow the superficial lymphatic capillaries to refill.

In treating acute, subacute or chronic edema, **nodal pumping** or compression is applied to the lymphatic nodes of the most proximal part of the limb that has the edematous tissue. These nodes are also closest to the thoracic and right lymphatic ducts, which return lymph to the venous system. In the arm, these are the axillary lymph nodes *(Figure 4.1)*. In the leg, these are the inguinal lymph nodes. To massage the nodes, the palmar surface of the hand is used and pressure is applied in a wave-like motion, from just distal to the node in a proximal direction. This action compresses the capillaries

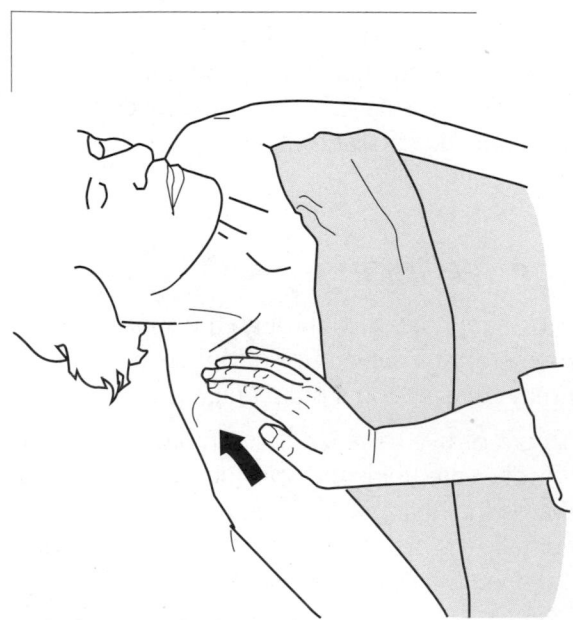

Figure 4.1
Lymphatic drainage techniques: Axillary nodal pumping.

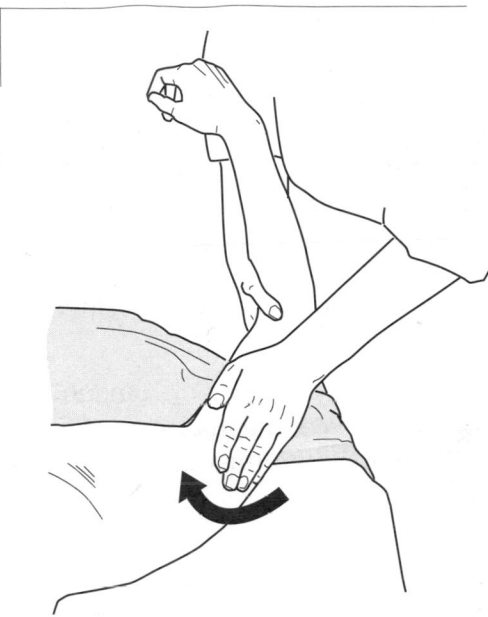

Figure 4.2
Lymphatic drainage techniques: Stationary circles.

distal to the node, moving the lymph proximally into the duct.

- 🖐 **Stationary circles** are used to treat larger areas of the limb between the edema and the proximal nodes. The palmar surface of one or both hands, including the fingers, rotate or spiral into and out of the tissue *(Figure 4.2)*.

- 🖐 Finally, the tissue immediately proximal to the edema is treated with the **local technique.** The ulnar borders of the hands, the web between the thumb and index finger *(Figure 4.3)* or the broad surface of the entire thumbs *(Figure 4.4)* are used to stroke the tissue in a proximal direction. Tissue distal to the lesion site is not treated with lymphatic drainage until the edema that is congesting the site itself is decreased.

Contraindications

✦ The contraindications to MLD also apply to these lymphatic drainage techniques.

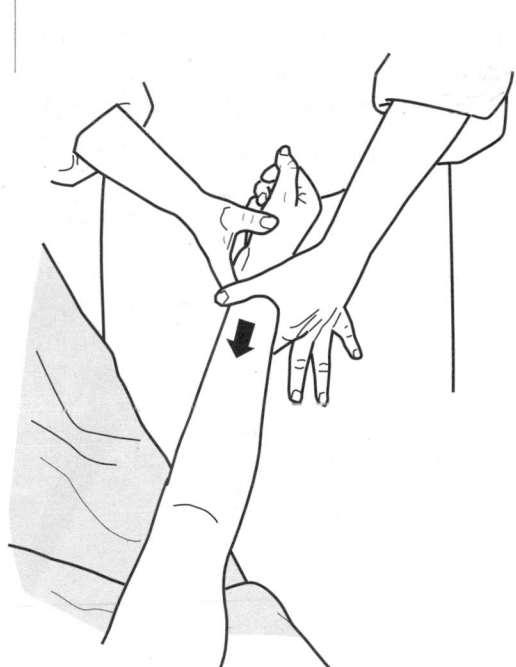

Figure 4.3
Lymphatic drainage: Local technique with web between thumb and index finger of left hand; working proximal to wrist edema.

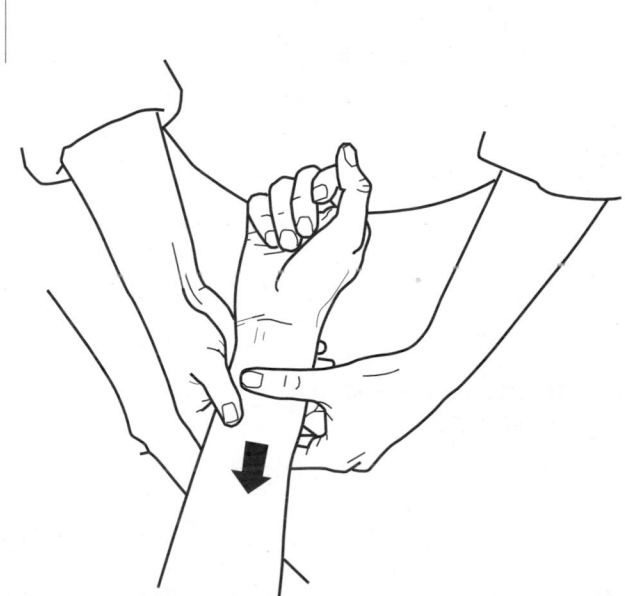

Figure 4.4
Lymphatic drainage: Local technique with broad surface of both thumbs.

Static Pressure Techniques

Golgi Tendon Organ (GTO) Release

A kinesiology technique, Golgi tendon organ release seems to have originated with physiotherapists *(Gelb, 1985)*. The Golgi tendon organs are proprioceptive nerve receptors or minute sensory organs located in the tendons near the junction with the muscle *(Guyton, 1984)*. Hundreds of these receptors detect the "load" placed on the tendons. The Golgi tendon organs are part of a muscle tension-monitoring system. They moderate the muscle contraction through a neuronal loop and, therefore, the effective strength of the muscular contraction.

Specifically, alpha motor neuron firing maintains muscle contraction. The Golgi tendon organ is able to slow this alpha neuronal firing, causing relaxation of the muscle *(Guyton, 1984; Chaitow, 1988)*. This inhibitory effect on muscle contraction is referred to as the lengthening reaction *(Chaitow, 1988)*.

Golgi tendon organs are also part of a protective reflex to prevent muscle injury or rupture through relaxation of the muscle; this reflex is activated when an excessive load or stretch is placed on a tendon.

Golgi tendon organ release can be used to reduce muscle spasm and tone, especially when on-site massage is too painful. The technique is most effective on muscles whose tendons are long and easily palpable, such as the Achilles tendon and hamstring tendon at the ischial tuberosity. It is also used on the suboccipital tendons between the occiput, C1 and C2.

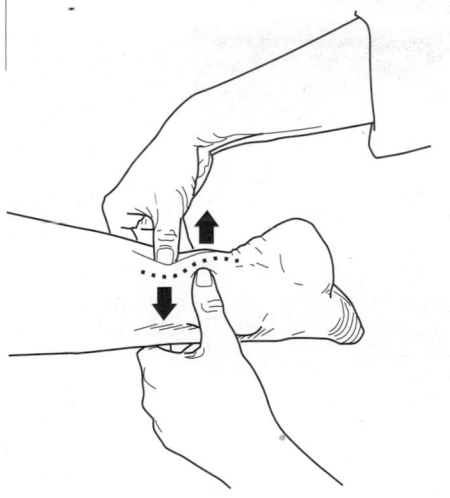

Figure 4.5
Golgi tendon organ release technique: S-bowing to Achilles tendon.

The Golgi Tendon Organ Release Technique

Direct compression placed on the tendon near the junction with the muscle will yield the best results. This is the area of greatest Golgi tendon organ concentration *(Mastalgia, Walton, 1982)*.

🖐 The therapist uses reinforced thumbs or fingers, holding for a minimum of 30 seconds or until the muscle relaxes. The tendon may also be bowed into an "s" or "c" shape *(Figure 4.5)*.

The rate is slow and the pressure is moderate to deep. One source states that muscle tension or spasm may be reduced by applying approximately two pounds of pressure on the Golgi tendon organs in the tendon in a direction away from the belly of the muscle *(Gelb, 1985)*.

✦ Effects: Golgi tendon organ release reduces muscle tone and spasm.

Contraindications

✦ Contraindications to GTO release are locally painful conditions, local acute conditions affecting the tendon to be treated, hypotonic or atonic muscles, tissue fragility, pathologies of connective tissue and skin lesions including healing incisions.

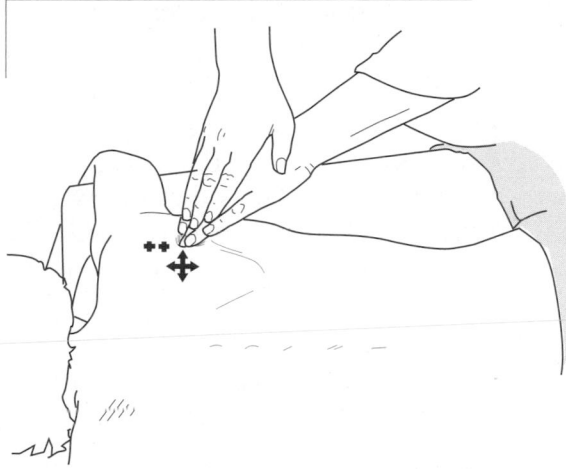

Figure 4.6
Origin and insertion technique to infraspinatus, medial attachment; small plus signs are made along the muscle attachment.

Contraindications

✦ Contraindications to the origin and insertion technique are the same as for Golgi tendon organ release.

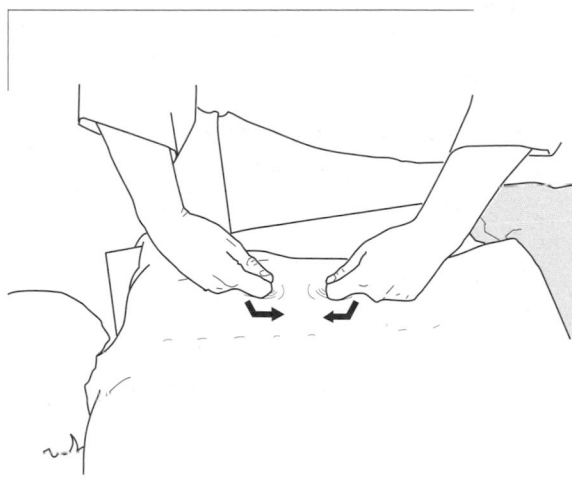

Figure 4.7
Muscle approximation to erector spinae; compressing the attachments of the muscles onto the bony structures below.

The Origin and Insertion Technique

The origin and insertion technique is a variation of Golgi tendon organ release, used when the tendon to be treated is short, such as the medial attachment of the infraspinatus muscle. It is also used to reduce spasm and tone in a muscle when direct work on the muscle belly is uncomfortable. As with the previous technique, stimulation of the Golgi tendon organs in the musculotendinous junction reduces muscle tone by inhibiting the alpha neuron firing which causes the muscle contraction in the first place *(Kisner, Colby, 1990).*

✍ The therapist thoroughly treats the origin (attachment) of the muscle using either reinforced finger or thumb kneading. Cross-fibre and then with-fibre strokes, like a little plus sign, are made on the same location *(Figure 4.6)*. The therapist then moves several centimetres along the origin to repeat the technique, continuing to make plus signs along the entire origin. The insertion (attachment) of the muscle is treated in the same manner. The rate is slow and the pressure is moderate to deep.

✦ Effects: The origin and insertion technique reduces muscle tone and spasm.

Muscle Approximation

Another kinesiology technique, muscle approximation, also seems to have originated with physiotherapists *(Gelb, 1985)*. The muscle spindles are proprioceptive nerve receptors or minute sensory organs located in the muscle belly. They monitor muscle length and help control muscle movements by detecting the amount of stretch placed on a muscle. Muscle spindles protect the muscle from being overstretched *(Guyton, 1984)*. They also set different levels of tone in a muscle in response to activity or stress, by increasing the gain or frequency of gamma efferent nerve firing *(Kisner, Colby, 1990)*.

It is speculated that each muscle has a resting length that is remembered by the amount of contraction of the spindle cells and the amount of relaxation of the Golgi tendon organs *(Gelb, 1985)*.

The technique of muscle approximation uses the reflex effect of muscle spindles to reduce tone or spasm in a muscle. Approximating, or bringing the ends of the muscle closer together, lessens the stretch on the

Contraindications

✦ Contraindications to muscle approximation are locally painful conditions, local acute conditions affecting the tendon to be treated, hypotonic or atonic muscles, tissue fragility, pathologies of connective tissue and skin lesions including healing incisions.

muscle spindles. This decreases gamma firing and reduces muscle tone and spasm.

🖐 The therapist can either compress the origin and insertion (attachments) onto the bony structures below, then approximate (*Figure 4.7*), or use a pincer grasp on the muscle attachments, and bring the ends towards each other. An average of two pounds of pressure is applied from each end towards the muscle belly (*Gelb, 1985*).

🖐 The rate is slow. The therapist takes care not to slide over the surface of the skin. Approximation is held until the muscle relaxes. The technique is primarily used on short muscles such as sections of the erector spinae group.

✦ Effects: Muscle approximation reduces muscle tone and spasm.

Myofascial Trigger Point (TrP) Techniques

Trigger points are treated by a variety of techniques, such as skin rolling, repetitive muscle stripping (described in Swedish Techniques), ischemic compression, intermittent cold distraction and stretch, percussion and stretch, and post-isometric relaxation.

🖐 An **ischemic compression** is a static compression applied by the therapist's thumbs, fingertips or olecranon to the trigger point. The pressure used is sufficient to temporarily cause local ischemia in the tissue that is compressed, while staying within the client's pain tolerance. The length of time the compression is held varies from seven seconds to one minute. The reactive hyperemia that follows the release of pressure may help to flush metabolites from the tissue (*Travell, Simons, 1983*).

🖐 **Intermittent cold distraction and stretch** is a brief application of cold to the skin over the muscle containing the trigger point. This is followed by a slow, careful stretch of the affected muscle to just before the onset of pain.

🖐 **Percussion and stretch** is a slow tapping of the trigger point using a reflex hammer, followed by a pain-free stretch (*Travell, Simons, 1992*).

Refer to the chapter on trigger points for definitions of trigger points, specific application of the techniques, the post-treatment hydrotherapy application of **heat** followed by **pain-free stretch** or full active free range of motion and the contraindications to the techniques.

The Pressure Point Technique

Compression then release of painful tissue creates a temporary local ischemia followed by reactive hyperemia. It is speculated that this helps to flush out the metabolites that cause nerve irritation and pain (*Travell, Simons, 1983*). Once the pain cycle is broken, hypertonicity and spasm also diminish. Compression over the frontal or maxillary sinuses is used to encourage drainage when treating sinusitis.

Eastern therapy systems such as acupressure, shiatsu and reflexology also use pressure point techniques. The pressure is applied to locations that are not based on the

Contraindications

✦ Contraindications for the pressure point technique are acute conditions, hypotonic or atonic muscles, painful conditions and tissue "lumps" such as lipomas, cysts and ganglions.

musculoskeletal system, but rather on the meridian system or lines of energy that flow through the body. The pressure is used to normalize the energy flow.

🖐 The pressure point technique is the gradual application of tolerable, static pressure to painful tissue. The fingers, reinforced thumbs, knuckles or elbow are used. This pressure is maintained until the symptoms decrease or the muscle relaxes. The rate is slow and the pressure variable. Lotions or oils need not be used.

✦ Effects: The pressure point technique helps to relax muscles and treat sinus congestion.

Cross-fibre Frictions

Cross-fibre frictions were first described by James Cyriax, MD. The technique is specifically intended to disrupt and break down existing and forming adhesions in muscles, tendons and ligaments using compression and motion. The therapist's fingers or thumb do not slide over the skin; instead, the superficial tissues are moved over the deeper ones. While most modern authors credit Cyriax with discovering the technique, Cyriax himself notes that it is a rediscovery of an old technique for tendinitis, described by Hooker in 1849 (*Cyriax, Coldham, 1984*).

In some sources there is confusion surrounding the term frictions. In historical writings from ancient Greece and Rome, the terms *rubbing* and *friction* were used to describe massage itself (*Basmajian, 1985*), while more contemporary sources describe the technique as a small circular motion where the hands slide over the surface of the skin (*Wood, Becker, 1981*). This is quite a different concept from cross-fibre frictions; this text uses the terms *frictions* and *cross-fibre frictions* interchangeably to mean Cyriax's technique.

Cross-fibre frictions can be used in the subacute and chronic stages of healing to break down adhesions which prevent normal motion. These adhesions may be within muscle fibres and between structures such as ligaments and tendons. Breaking down adhesions helps to form a smaller, more mobile scar. Over a series of treatments, the collagen fibres of the developing scar tissue are thought to be realigned by repeated frictions, in a manner similar to repeatedly rolling the fingertips over a pile of toothpicks lying in a random, haphazard manner. Eventually the toothpicks will orient perpendicular to the direction in which the hand moves (*Hertling, Kessler, 1990*). In the late subacute stage, the collagen fibres are weaker and break more easily, while in the chronic stage, deeper, more vigorous frictions are required to break down collagen fibres.

Although Cyriax advocated their use in acute injury to muscle, ligament or tendon, frictions may be too painful and therefore not tolerable for the client at this stage. Cyriax noted this fact and suggested 10 to 20 minutes of effleurage and gentle friction beforehand (*Cyriax, Coldham, 1984*). Moreover, because the technique, by definition, breaks down tissue, frictions may cause further injury in the acute stage. Later authors reserve its application for chronic injuries (*Hertling, Kessler, 1996*). In this text, cross-fibre frictions are used in the late subacute and chronic stages; lymphatic drainage is used in the acute and early subacute stages to remove excess fibrin that leads to adhesions (*Casley-Smith, Casley-Smith, 1986; Kurz, 1990*).

As well as breaking down adhesions, cross-fibre frictions have other effects. The depth of pressure used is sufficient to cause minor tissue damage and inflammation, with the resulting release of histamine and bradykinin. These chemicals have an effect on the local circulation and on nerve receptors for pain. The local vasodilation that occurs likely accelerates tissue repair. The nociceptive chemicals released by the frictions will cause pain. While it may seem contradictory to use a painful technique in an already painful area, it is thought that the painful stimuli close the "pain gate"; the injury itself is painful and the additional discomfort of the technique modulates and reduces the perception of peripheral pain. In addition, pain-blocking chemicals such as endorphins may be released *(Boyling, Palastanga, 1994)*. The result is a temporary local analgesia during application of the technique.

Assessment

Sources stress the importance of assessing for the specific structure involved and the site of the adhesion, rather than just treating a painful area. This is because the area perceived as painful may be pain referred from another area, not the adhesion itself *(DeFranca, Levine, 1996; Boyling, Palastanga, 1994)*.

Palpation and testing are used on tendons, muscles and ligaments. For example, with a muscle injury, active free and passive relaxed range of motion are used to assess for pain in the muscle's range. Active resisted testing is used to pinpoint the adhesion. As the client contracts the muscle, stress is placed on it, painfully pulling on the adhesion site where the frictions need to be applied. Palpation is used to confirm the location of the painful adhesion before treatment.

Adhesions within a tendon are located with active resisted testing and palpation, while joint capsule adhesions are located with passive stretching and palpation. Knowledge of anatomy is essential to orient the technique at right angles to the fibres of the structure being treated.

The Cross-Fibre Friction Technique

A specific consent to treat is required prior to using this technique, because initially it can be painful and deep. Communication about pain levels continues throughout the technique. Preparatory techniques such as lymphatic drainage, effleurage, petrissage and fascial or connective tissue techniques are used to prepare the tissue beforehand. The client must be in a comfortable, supported position. The tissue containing the adhesions is placed in an accessible position. For example, the supraspinatus tendon is made accessible by internally rotating, extending and adducting the humerus to bring the tendon out from beneath the acromion.

In addition, the tissue to be treated is put under appropriate tension. For a muscle or tendon without a synovial sheath, this means placing the structure in a relaxed, shortened position. This allows a maximum separation between the fibres so adhesions are broken down. For a tendon with a synovial sheath, the tendon is put in a maximum stretch, so the technique can develop a maximum force between the tendon and sheath. It is thought that frictions smooth out the roughened surface of the tendon *(Cyriax, Coldham, 1984)*. For a ligament, the appropriate tension is achieved using a shortened position so the ligament is as free as possible to move over the adjacent tissues *(Boyling, Palastanga, 1994)*.

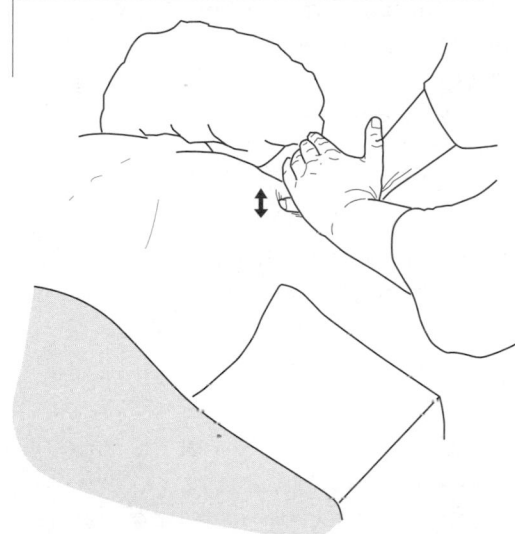

Figure 4.8
Cross-fibre frictions to the lateral tendon of infraspinatus; once the tendon is located using active resisted testing, the tendon is placed in a relaxed position; the adhesion is located; the treating thumb is reinforced by the therapist's other hand.

The therapist must be in a comfortable, biomechanically sound position, as the technique is applied over a number of minutes.

The technique is applied once the adhesion is located. This is often the most tender spot reported by the client. It is sometimes palpated as a different texture to the surrounding tissue.

- Reinforced fingers or thumbs are used to compress the superficial tissue over the adhesion. In illustrations of this method, the terminal phalanx of the index finger is applied to the skin, while the pad of the middle finger is placed on top of the index finger, reinforcing the treating finger from going into extension. In clinical practice, this is often not enough support; the heel of the therapist's other hand can also apply supportive pressure over the treating hand . Alternatively, if the thumb is used, the terminal phalanx is also reinforced by the heel of the therapist's other hand *(Figure 4.8)*.

Pressure and Direction

- The pressure used is sufficient to penetrate to the depth of the adhesion, while remaining within the client's pain tolerance. This will vary; for example, less pressure is required to reach adhesions in the more superficial common extensor tendon than in the deeper supraspinatus tendon. Cyriax states, "the least strength of friction which achieves [the] result is called for" *(Cyriax, Coldham, 1984)*. Less pressure is required for a relatively fragile subacute adhesion than for a tough chronic one.

- When the appropriate depth of tolerable pressure is achieved, the therapist moves her finger back and forth at right angles to the fibres of the tissue. The width of each movement, or sweep, is sufficient to produce movement between the superficial tissue and the adhesion, between the structure treated and the surrounding tissue, or across the width of the structure being treated, such as a ligament or tendon. The sweep is similar to taking a pencil eraser and rubbing out a single letter or number. The rate of movement is about two or three cycles per second *(Hertling, Kessler, 1996)*.

- While classic cross-fibre frictions are just that, cross fibre, minute circular movements may also be used, although these are not as effective *(Boyling, Palastanga, 1994)*.

- As mentioned previously, the therapist's fingers or thumb do not slide over the skin; instead, the superficial tissues are moved over the deeper ones. Any oil or lotion on the skin is removed to prevent sliding on the skin. If the finger does slide over the skin, a blister will form on the client's skin under the therapist's finger — not the effect that is wanted.

- Initially, the pressure is to the client's pain tolerance. After one or two minutes of treatment, the analgesic effect occurs and the client will report that the area is less tender. If the tenderness has not subsided, or if pain has increased, the technique is discontinued. Most commonly, the area is less tender and the therapist gradually increases the pressure to the client's new tolerance in order to "follow" the three-dimensional presentation of the adhesion. The frictions are continued at this deeper level, breaking down more adhesions while the analgesic effect is present.

Duration

✋ Depending on the client's tolerance, frictions may be applied initially with less pressure and for shorter periods of time over several sessions, gradually increasing the length of time the technique is used.

✋ In the literature, the recommended duration of the technique varies depending on the author: five, 10, 15 or up to 20 minutes *(Cyriax, Coldham, 1984; Hertling, Kessler, 1996; Boyling, Palastanga, 1994)*. Duration, like pressure, is also a factor of the stage of healing. A subacute injury may respond in one or two minutes, while a chronic one may take over two minutes or longer. However, longer applications cause bruising of the skin over the site and may be poorly tolerated by both the client and the therapist. In clinical experience, two to four minutes for a chronic adhesion is reasonable for each application.

Post-Technique Actions

After frictions, repetitive effleurage may be used to increase local circulation through the injury site and to decrease remaining pain perception.

✋ The injury site is reassessed after treatment. After the first session, there should be improvement; pain should be reduced in active resisted tests with muscle and tendon injuries, and in active and passive range of motion with ligament injuries *(Maigne, 1996)*.

✋ Next, the tissue that has been treated is mobilized or stretched through as much *pain-free range* as possible *(Cyriax in Basmajian, 1985)*. With muscles and tendons the stretch presumably normalizes the tissue length once the adhesions that reduce range are removed; with ligaments, mobilizing the ligaments over surrounding structures restores range and improves proprioception. With muscles or tendons, a pain-free passive stretch, or full passive relaxed or active free range of motion is used. With ligaments, pain-free full passive relaxed range, including distraction and overpressure (ligamentous stress), is used.

✋ Cyriax does not mention hydrotherapy applications in his original description. However, later sources mention an application of **ice** after frictions, presumably to control the inflammatory response *(Hecox et al., 1994; DeFranca, Levine, 1996)*. Because cold reduces tissue flexibility and pain perception, mobilizing is performed before the ice is applied.

After frictions are stopped, local hyperemia is present. Local tenderness may also arise the day after the first or second treatments. This is not uncommon after the technique and does not indicate a worsening of the client's symptoms unless other key symptoms related to the condition are also worse.

Contraindications

✦ Frictions are not used over peripheral nerves, with acute injury, rheumatoid arthritis, infective arthritis, structures that are too deep to be reached, client's use of anti-inflammatories, anticoagulants or high-dose long-term steroid medication, peripheral vascular disease, fragility of the skin or soft tissue to be treated and client discomfort with the technique.

Frequency

The number of sessions varies from six to 12 performed every other day *(Maigne, 1996)*. Another source indicates six to 10 sessions over two to three weeks *(Hertling, Kessler, 1996)*, with most overuse syndromes responding in two weeks to two months *(DeFranca, Levine, 1996)*. Injuries to ligaments likely heal in "as many weeks as... would otherwise have taken months" if the client had been using other rehabilitation methods than frictions *(Cyriax in Basmajian, 1985)*.

✦ Effects: Cross-fibre frictions break down adhesions found in late subacute and chronic injuries.

Fascial or Connective Tissue Techniques

Understanding Fascia

Connective tissue or fascia surrounds all muscles, muscle groups, bones and organs, holding them in place. Although it has various names depending on its anatomical location, fascia is, in fact, a continuous sheet of supportive tissue that envelops the entire body. It is strong yet mobile.

There are three categories of fascia: superficial, deeper and subserous. The superficial fascia lies just below the skin and is composed of loosely knit connective tissue combined with fat, vascular structures and nerve receptors. The superficial fascia is quite mobile and has potential for the accumulation of tissue fluids and metabolites. The deeper fascia is denser, tougher and tighter. It compartmentalizes the body and surrounds the muscles and viscera, contributing to the body's contours and function. The subserous fascia is a loose areolar tissue that covers the viscera. It supports the organs and provides lubrication so they may slide against each other *(Greenman, 1989; Ebner, 1980)*.

In general, fascia is oriented in a longitudinal direction, except for layers covering the lower opening of the pelvis (called the *pelvic diaphragm*), the thoracic diaphragm and at the junction of the thorax and cervical regions — termed either the *thoracic inlet* or *outlet*, depending on the source *(Greenman, 1989)*.

Fascial Assessment

Fascial shortening, adhesions or restrictions due to inflammation, trauma, surgery, pathology or postural imbalances create abnormal tension patterns. Symptoms that appear unrelated may actually be transmitted from one body part to another through fascial imbalances *(Upledger, Vredevoogd, 1983)*. Assessment is required to locate the restrictions prior to treatment.

Assessment methods include slow skin rolling, fascial glide and positional testing.

With **slow skin rolling,** any resistance in the superficial fascia is noted *(Ebner, 1980; Neumann, 1989)*. Areas of thickened, tender, hyperirritable skin, termed *panniculosis,* indicate fascial restrictions and sometimes the location of trigger points *(Travell, Simons, 1983).*

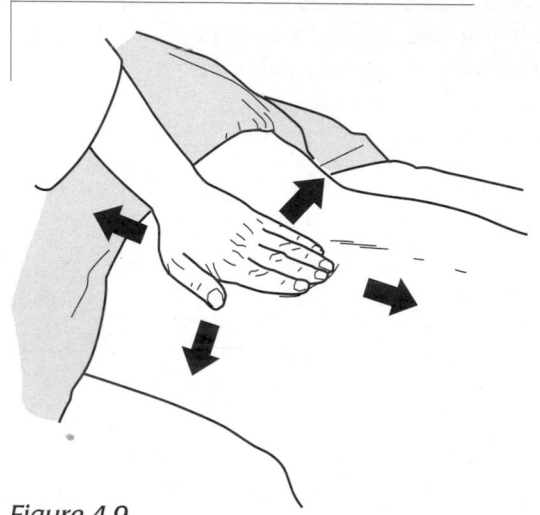

Figure 4.9
Fascial assessment: Fascial glide is performed on the cardinal planes to assess areas of restriction.

With **fascial glide,** the therapist's hands contact the skin and move or glide it over the deeper structures. The skin is moved on the cardinal planes, anteriorly, posteriorly, superiorly, inferiorly, laterally or medially *(Figure 4.9).* The pressure and direction of the glide vary depending on the fascia to be assessed; lighter pressure is used to assess more superficial fascia. The area and direction of greatest restriction to motion are noted.

With **positional testing,** the limb or body part is passively moved through its range until a barrier to motion is encountered. This barrier may be subtle or obvious. A fascial barrier occurs before a ligamentous or joint capsule barrier, which is called a capsular end feel. (For more information on end feel, see the Assessment chapter.) The fascia involved influences the quality and direction of the restriction of motion; knowledge of anatomy helps determine the location of the fascial restriction *(Greenman, 1989).*

There are numerous types of fascial or connective tissue techniques. They are divided into two main categories: direct techniques and indirect techniques.

Direct Fascial Techniques

Direct techniques take the fascia **towards** the restriction or adhesion. This engages the soft tissue barrier. The tissue is then carefully taken beyond the barrier, which breaks down the bonds between the connective tissue fibres *(Greenman, 1989; Lewit, 1993).* An example of intense, direct fascial techniques being inadvertently used is the painful burning feeling experienced with "rope burn" skin wringing — usually done on the forearm — perhaps familiar from childhood games.

This memory may remind the reader why it is important to obtain consent from the client before using direct fascial techniques and why it is important to work *within the client's pain tolerance* and to communicate about the discomfort levels during treatment.

Generally, direct techniques are based on the following concepts:

1) the appropriate level of fascia is reached by applying pressure to the tissue. The amount of pressure varies with the depth of the fascia;

2) a stretch is placed on the fascia to be treated, which takes the elastic slack out of the tissue;

3) the tissue is engaged by holding this stretch;

4) the stretch is held for a period of time sufficient to break some of the bonds

between the individual fibres of the connective tissue. A burning sensation is perceived by the client. Several minutes may be required to achieve successful tissue release;

5) successful release is indicated by hyperemia, a palpable release of heat, decrease of pain or other symptoms and a softening or lengthening of the tissue *(Greenman, 1989)*.

Little or no lubricant is used as these techniques rely on tissue drag for their effects. The pressure is moderate to deep and the speed is slow.

Skin rolling: The thumbs are placed on the skin next to each other while the fingers grasp the skin forming a line. The fingers are pulled towards the thumbs, raising the skin between them from the underlying layer. The thumbs are slowly pushed away from the therapist over the skin, engaging the tissue. At the same time, the fingertips are "walking" over the skin, gathering it up ahead of the thumbs and maintaining the raised roll of skin as the thumbs push forward. The rate is slow and the technique is performed in long sweeps. If oil is used, this is a petrissage technique.

Crossed-hands fascial stretch: The therapist's forearms are held parallel to each other with the elbows at 90 degrees of flexion. The palms of the hands contact the client's skin with the hands positioned so the fingers are pointing away from each other. The heels of the hands are a few inches apart. The appropriate depth is used to engage the fascia. Slack is taken out of the tissue by moving the hands away from each other; however, the palms should not slide over the skin. Once the tissue is engaged, the stretch is held until the tissue releases *(Figure 4.10)*.

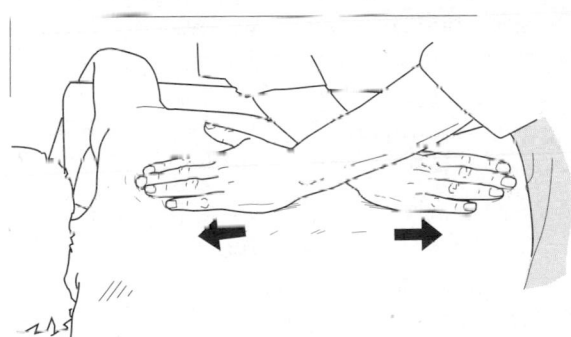

Figure 4.10
Direct fascial techniques: Crossed-hands fascial stretch.

Fascial spreading: The fingertips or thumbs of both hands may be used for this technique; it is important to hold the fingers of one hand together for support. The fingertips are placed on the skin at the required depth, then moved apart to take up the slack. The fingers continue to move apart, stretching the fascia between them. The stroke may be short or long, the hands moved away from each other or away from the therapist *(Figure 4.11)*.

Cutting technique: The therapist's fingers are held together for support, then placed on the skin at the required depth. The terminal phalanges are slightly flexed; the tissue is engaged by pulling towards the therapist. To treat, the fingertips, especially the middle fingertip, are pulled through the tissue towards the therapist in a cutting motion *(Ebner, 1980)*. Muscles may be outlined using progressively deeper strokes to the client's tolerance; then the fascia covering the muscles is loosened using oblique strokes *(Figure 4.12)*.

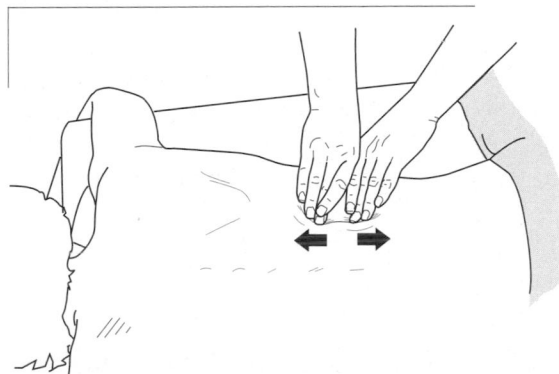

Figure 4.11
Direct fascial techniques: Fascial spreading using fingertips.

Fascial torquing: The tissue is raised between fingertips and thumbs of both hands to take up the slack, then pulled further off the underlying surface and twisted to engage it *(Figure 4.13)*.

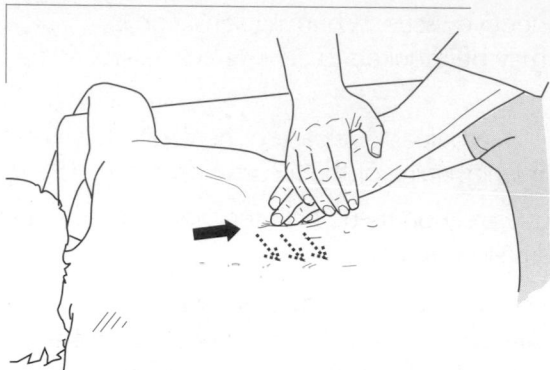

Figure 4.12
Direct fascial techniques: Cutting technique strokes outlining erector spinae; oblique strokes to loosen fascia shown as dotted arrows.

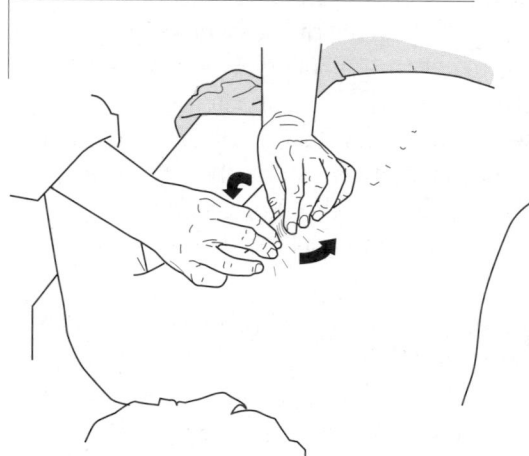

Figure 4.13
Direct fascial techniques: Fascial torquing.

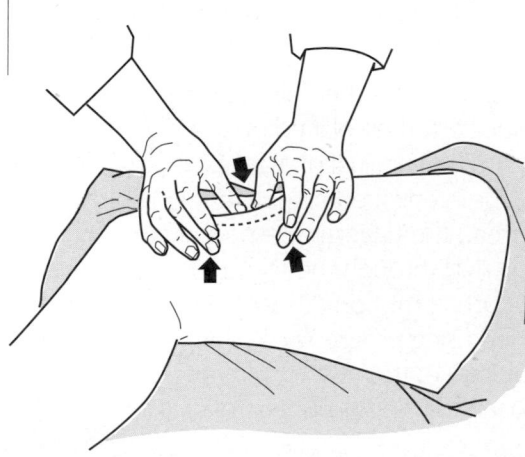

Figure 4.14
Direct fascial techniques: C-bowing to iliotibial band.

🖑 **S-bowing fascial technique:** The thumbs are placed on the skin parallel to, and pointing towards, each other, so when the thumbs are moved towards each other the fascia distorts in an S-shape. The usual concepts of engaging then holding the technique to release are followed. If the same thumb position is used on a tendon, it is called S-bowing Golgi tendon organ release.

🖑 **C-bowing fascial technique:** The thumbs are placed on the skin next to each other while the fingers grasp the skin forming a line. The fingers are pulled towards the therapist, with the little and ring fingers moving more than the index and middle fingers; at the same time the thumbs are pushed away from the therapist. This distorts the fascia into a C-shape, which is engaged and held to release *(Figure 4.14)*. If the same finger and thumb positions are used on a tendon, it is called C-bowing Golgi tendon organ release.

- An alternative position has one hand placed on the skin, thumb abducted so the hand is in a C-shape; the fingertips of the other hand engage the skin so they point into the web between thumb and index finger on the first hand. The tissue between the hands is distorted into a C-shape.

🖑 **J-stroke:** This is the deepest, most destructive direct fascial technique. It is used selectively after more superficial fascial techniques have been used, applied in an organized manner in lines or rows. The therapist makes a fist and places it on the tissue with the proximal phalanges contacting the tissue *(Figure 4.15)*. The appropriate depth is reached. The proximal interphalangeal joint of the index finger performs the technique, which is essentially drawing the knuckles towards the therapist to take up the slack, engaging the tissue, then making a small, J-shaped pull through the tissue. The proximal phalanges of the other fingers provide the distraction of pressure distributed over a wider area than just the knuckle of the index finger, making the technique more tolerable.

✦ Effects: Direct fascial techniques increase the excursion and flexibility of fascia by moving it towards, then beyond, the restriction.

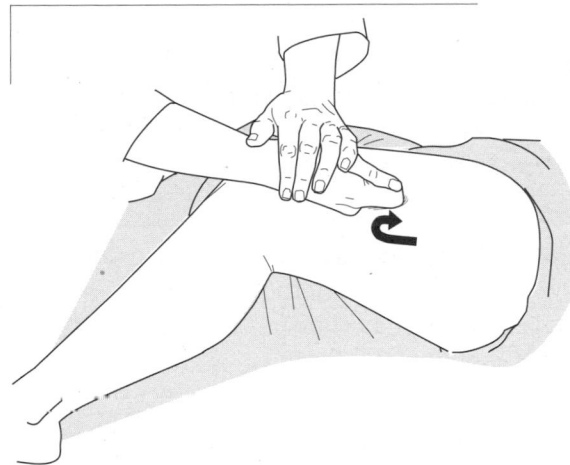

Figure 4.15
Direct fascial techniques: J-stroke to iliotibial band with left hand reinforcing the stroke.

Connective Tissue Massage

Elizabeth Dicke, a German physiotherapist, developed connective tissue massage (Bindegewebsmassage) in 1929 *(Ebner, 1980)*. Many similar principles and techniques have since been incorporated into other soft tissue manipulation systems, including the neuromuscular technique developed by Stanley Lief, a Latvian-born osteopath *(Chaitow, 1980 and 1988)*.

This type of direct fascial massage involves techniques such as **skin rolling** and **connective tissue cutting**. Restrictions in the fascia are assessed with one application of skin rolling, then treated with repeated skin rolling until the restriction is gone. Moderate to deep connective tissue cutting is also used to assess and treat restrictions. The therapist palpates for restrictions while outlining the various fascial compartments and muscles using the technique to stroke through the tissue. Repeated stroking along the restriction is performed until a tissue release is felt; the pressure is then increased to the client's pain tolerance.

Techniques are applied to the client's tolerance. Initially tenderness is noted; however, continued connective tissue cutting lessens muscular hypertonicity and pain, and increases local circulation. The autonomic nervous system appears to be affected; connective tissue changes on the surface of the body may correspond to internal organ pathologies *(Ebner, 1980)*.

Rate, pressure and direction all vary; no lubricant is used.

✦ Effects: Connective tissue techniques reduce pain and hypertonicity, and increase local circulation; the autonomic nervous system is also affected.

Neuromuscular Therapy (NMT)

Paul St. John, an American massage therapist, researched and developed the St. John Method of Neuromuscular Therapy and popularized it in 1978. He combined elements of Raymond Nimmo's "receptor tonus" system with Dicke's connective tissue techniques to create a system that treats regions of the body *(Calvert, 1992)*.

This should not be confused with neuromuscular therapy as defined by Schneider, Dvorak *et al.*, which is a form of manual medicine that improves mobility and stretches muscles using post-isometric relaxation, agonist and antagonist contraction, joint play and neuromuscular reflex mechanisms *(Schneider et al., 1988).*

Neuromuscular therapy is a system of evaluation and treatment for structural imbalances that cause pain. A thorough knowledge of functional anatomy is required. A complete postural assessment of the client is made before treatment begins to determine the specific muscles and fascia to be addressed. These are approached in a sequential and organized manner.

Contraindications

✦ Contraindications are the same as for other direct fascial techniques.

The system incorporates fascial techniques such as skin rolling and connective tissue cutting with passive range of motion, overpressure and stretching to lengthen tight or shortened tissues. Specific remedial exercises to stretch and strengthen the affected tissues are also included.

Rate, pressure and direction all vary. Minimal lubricant is used to facilitate tissue drag.

✦ Effects: Neuromuscular therapy reduces pain, hypertonicity and postural dysfunctions, and lengthens and strengthens tissues.

Indirect Fascial Techniques

Indirect techniques are thought to unhook the connective tissue. Similar to releasing two bungee cords hooked together, one must first push them together, exaggerating the elastic tension of the cords, before they can be disengaged.

The therapist applies pressure sufficient to contact the layer of fascia being treated; this pressure may be very light or moderately heavy. The therapist moves the tissue in the "direction of ease", or the direction the fascia will move most easily. This is usually opposite the direction of the restriction. The slack in the fascia is taken up. The fascia is then held in this position as the tissue attempts to return to its original position, which is palpated as a subtle sense of movement in the tissue.

As the tissue stops resisting the therapist's pressure, further slack will develop. This slack is taken up again, holding without pushing, until new slack develops. This is repeated through several cycles, until a tissue release is felt.

The direction of the perceived tissue motion may change but the therapist should not allow the tissue to return to the original position *(Upledger, Vredevoogd, 1983).*

The pressure is light to moderate and the rate is slow. No lubricant is used.

✦ Effects: Indirect fascial techniques increase the excursion and flexibility of fascia by moving it in the direction of ease, usually opposite to the restriction.

Contraindications

✦ Contraindications to indirect techniques include acute inflammation, undiagnosed lumps, recent head trauma and neurosurgery.

Visceral Manipulation

Visceral manipulation was developed by the French osteopaths Jean-Pierre Barral and Pierre Mercier. Their theory is that among the internal organs, or viscera, there is a relationship between the structure and function that is similar to the relationships of the components of the musculoskeletal system.

Visceral manipulation consists of assessment for visceral

motion, and direct and indirect fascial techniques to treat any dysfunctions found and restore normal visceral motion.

Healthy viscera should be able to slide over each other as the person breathes and moves. Restrictions between the fascia covering various internal organs can create dysfunctions, in the same manner that occurs in the musculoskeletal system. For example, scarring and adhesions following thoracic surgery create tensions and fascial restrictions that affect the movement of the thorax, lungs, and heart. Over time these visceral restrictions of motion can affect the fascia that runs from the thorax through the cervical spine, restricting neck movement. Eventually, if the body cannot adequately compensate for the restrictions, a structural problem such as scoliosis or head-forward posture may arise *(Barral, Mercier, 1988)*.

Healthy viscera have two types of motion. They move passively in response to the excursion of the diaphragm, termed *visceral mobility*; for example, the kidney moves three centimetres with each normal breath, which amounts to a cumulative motion of 600 metres per day *(Barral, Mercier, 1988)*. Each visceral component also has an inherent, characteristic motion around a particular axis, termed *motility*, which is independent of the motion imparted by outside sources such as the diaphragm. For example, the motility of the kidney in one subject was measured using intravenous pyelography, revealing an inherent kidney motion of three centimetres in a vertical and lateral direction. The subject held his breath during the measurement to remove diaphragmatic influences. In healthy viscera, the axes of mobility and motility are generally the same, while in dysfunctional viscera, the axes are often different.

Both mobility and motility are palpable as subtle motions. Assessment and techniques have met the scientific criteria of being reproducible on the same subject by several practitioners over several sessions. Also, the techniques produce the same results on different subjects. Barral and Mercier based visceral manipulation on extensive clinical experience and studies using ultrasound, radiology and dissection.

Contraindications

✦ Contraindications include acute inflammation, undiagnosed lumps and the general contraindications of direct fascial techniques.

A knowledge of anatomy and visceral symptoms, as well as subtle palpation skills are required. Techniques include recoil and release by positioning, described later in this chapter, as well as direct and indirect fascial techniques. Pressure varies with the tissue being treated. The rate of the manipulations depends on the speed of the connective tissue release. No lubricant is used.

✦ Effects: Visceral manipulation restores the motion and function of affected viscera.

Craniosacral Therapy

Craniosacral therapy is based on the research and clinical work of the American osteopath William Sutherland, who first noticed the subtle cranial rhythms in the 1940s. Later, work by John Upledger, DO, gave a plausible explanation for these motions and made this osteopathic technique a popular one.

The cranial bones have subtle, identifiable and patterned motions that are allowed by the cranial sutures. These motions have been thoroughly documented *(Pick, 1995; Basmajian, Nyberg, 1993; Upledger, Vredevoogd, 1983)*. This motion is a result of fluctuations in the production and flow of cerebrospinal fluid (CSF) which is contained within the meninges — cranial membranes — and bathes the brain and spinal cord. These membranes containing the brain, spinal cord and cerebrospinal fluid form a semi-closed hydraulic system. Since a fluid is not compressible the way a gas is, these CSF fluctuations have an effect on the meninges and, through them, the cranial bones. Attachments of the meninges covering the spinal cord to the sacrum influence motion of this bone. As fascia throughout the body is interconnected, the craniosacral rhythm is palpable in connective tissue throughout the body as well as through the cranial bones and sacrum *(Greenman, 1989).*

The rhythm consists of two movements, called cranial flexion and extension. In flexion (or expansion), which is active, there is a subtle, palpable increase in the width of the skull and body at the same time that the anteroposterior dimensions decrease. The limbs simultaneously move into a subtle external rotation.

In extension (or relaxation), which is passive, the opposite occurs. There is an equally subtle narrowing of the head and body, while the anteroposterior dimensions increase and the limbs move into subtle internal rotation.

This rhythm of flexion and extension occurs at a rate of six to 12 cycles per minute. The rhythm is used to assess for dysfunctions of the craniosacral system as well as to treat these dysfunctions *(Upledger, Vredevoogd, 1983).*

Dysfunctions can arise from fixations of any component of the craniosacral system as a result of trauma, either physical or emotional. Fixations are thought to increase the pressure within the semi-hydraulic craniosacral system. Dysfunction can, therefore, also occur to the tissues of the central nervous system contained within the meninges.

Contraindications

✦ Contraindications include brainstem tumour, recent aneurism or cranial fracture and concussion.

Subtle palpation skills and clear anatomical knowledge are required for addressing this system. Both indirect and direct fascial techniques are used. The pressure for many of the techniques is light (five grams) and the rate is slow. Tissue drag is required, so no lubricant is used.

✦ Effects: Craniosacral therapy is used to treat chronic pain, visceral dysfunctions, headache and temporomandibular joint dysfunction.

Myofascial Release

These techniques were developed by American osteopathic practitioners and from original work by Dr. A. J. Still, the founder of American osteopathy. A relatively recent addition to manual medicine, myofascial release combines soft tissue, craniosacral and muscle energy techniques, described later in this chapter. There are many technique combinations, and different practitioners have their own versions *(Greenman, 1989).* John Barnes, PT, has popularized one version.

These slow and subtle techniques can be used to release fascia and muscle throughout the body. The "tight-loose" concept is an integral part of myofascial release. Tightness creates shortness, compression and, therefore, asymmetry in the tissue. Looseness in another area permits this asymmetry. The tightness creates a tethering effect, which further restricts movement and allows for more tissue compression to occur *(Greenman, 1989; Basmajian, Nyberg, 1993).* Myofascial pain syndromes such as trigger points and tender points are also addressed. Tissue relaxation is achieved through the reflexive effects of the autonomic system and the application of appropriate techniques that stress the dysfunctional tissues.

An awareness of functional anatomy is important, as are palpation skills to assess tissue for looseness, tightness and inherent mobility. Both direct and indirect fascial techniques are combined for assessment and treatment of dysfunction.

Contraindications

✦ Contraindications are the same as for other direct and indirect fascial techniques.

Techniques include light to moderate traction, range of motion, appropriate tension and a twisting action to achieve biomechanical and reflex change *(Greenman, 1989)*.

✦ Effects: Myofascial release techniques reduce painful soft tissue dysfunctions.

Joint Mobilization Techniques

These techniques range from non-specific joint mobilizations such as rocking to very specific techniques to increase range of motion such as joint play. Because these techniques take a joint up to the limit of available motion and no further, they are sometimes called *mobilization without impulse.*

In contrast, chiropractic adjustments take the joint briefly past the limit of available motion. They are described as being high velocity, low amplitude thrust techniques, or *mobilization with impulse (Greenman, 1989)*. Mobilization with impulse is outside the scope of massage therapists.

Shaking

🖐 The therapist comfortably grasps either the muscle belly for **direct shaking,** or the distal limb for **indirect shaking,** and moves the tissue back and forth at an even rhythm.

Contraindications

✦ Contraindications include acute injuries to bones, joints, muscles or nerves.

Shaking is used with tight muscles. The increased sensory input from proprioceptive nerve afferents in muscles and joints during shaking reflexively reduces muscle tone, increasing the client's relaxation *(Hertling, Kessler, 1990)*.

The rate is variable, from gentle to vigorous.

✦ Effects: Shaking reflexively relaxes muscles. Indirect shaking creates successive action at the joint.

Rocking

🖐 The therapist moves the client's body part in a rhythmic manner and then allows it to return to its original position. The rocking motion is continued, allowing the adjacent joints to move. The rate is variable, from gentle to vigorous.

As with shaking, the increased sensory input from proprioceptors reflexively reduces muscle tone *(Hertling, Kessler, 1990)*. Rocking also helps mobilize the joint capsule. It increases the successive action present at a moving joint which helps to move synovial fluid necessary for joint nutrition.

Contraindications

✦ Contraindications include acute injuries to bones, joints, muscles or nerves.

Rocking can be used with hypertonic muscles or when treating chronic joint pathologies such as osteoarthritis.

✦ Effects: Rocking reflexively relaxes muscles, mobilizes the joint capsule and increases successive action.

Tractioning

🖐 The therapist grasps the client's occiput or distal limb without painfully squeezing the tissue. A slow pull along the axis of the body part (long-axis traction) is applied. The joint surfaces are distracted, or slightly pulled apart, by this action.

The ligamentous stability of the tractioned joint or the tone of muscles crossing it can be assessed with this technique, as can be the location of restrictions in the proximal tissue. For example, applying light traction to the ankle joint gives the therapist information on the tissue crossing that joint. Gradually and gently increasing the force of the traction takes the slack out of the ankle joint. Then the tibia and fibula are engaged, giving palpatory information about the knee. As the slack is taken out of this joint, the hip is engaged; eventually with gradually increasing force the technique can be taken up to the sacroiliac joint and lumbar spine.

To avoid jarring the tissue, it is important for the therapist not to let go of the occiput or limb suddenly. The length of time taken in applying the tractioning force should equal the length of time taken in releasing the tractioning.

Contraindications

✦ Contraindications to tractioning include acute injury, unhealed fractures, ruptured ligaments, rheumatoid arthritis, especially in the cervical spine at the C1 or C2 level, and with peripheral nerve lesions and hypermobile joints.

Successive action is increased in the joints tractioned. Proprioceptors in the joints are stimulated, decreasing tone of the surrounding muscles.

Tractioning or distracting a joint is the first step in joint play techniques, described later in this chapter.

✦ Effects: Tractioning increases successive action to the joint and decreases tone in muscles surrounding the joint.

Rhythmic Mobilizations

A system incorporating rhythmic mobilizations and remedial and breathing exercises to help reduce pain was developed by Milton Trager.

In rhythmic mobilizations, a series of passive rocking and shaking movements is used to mobilize joints. The client's own rhythm is used as a guide to the speed of the movements. To assess the required speed, the therapist initiates motion in the limb or torso and notes how long it takes to return to the starting position.

The amplitude of the movements is gradually increased by the therapist and is maintained for up to several minutes. The movements are then decreased just as gradually. During a series of rhythmic mobilizations for a particular area, such as the shoulder and neck, joints in the limbs and cervical spine are gradually moved through their range of motion.

Tractioning is also used during the movements.

Rhythmic mobilizations are used to assess possible restrictions of motion or holding patterns. They are also used to introduce a client to a massage treatment. If repeated for longer periods of time, they are used to reduce the hypertonicity of muscles, stretch the joint capsule, maintain range of motion and increase the succussive action of a joint.

During rhythmic mobilizations, while the joint capsule may be stretched either by positioning or by tractioning, the stretch is a general one; stretch is not applied to a specific part of the joint capsule as with joint play.

✦ Effects: Rhythmic mobilizations increase succussive action and maintain range of motion of the joint. They reduce hypertonicity of the muscles surrounding the joint.

Contraindications

✦ Contraindications include acute injury such as dislocations and fractures, recently healing peripheral nerve injuries, rheumatoid arthritis, osteoporosis, nausea, headaches and joints restricted by pins, screws, rods or surgical reduction of ligaments.

Recoil

Recoil techniques are a part of osteopathic techniques. They are used to reduce connective tissue adhesions and to mobilize joints and stretch fascia. Clear knowledge of anatomy, especially muscle attachments, and accurate palpation skills are required for these techniques.

🖐 After the therapist assesses for and locates the tissue to be mobilized, the tissue is positioned or stretched along the direction of the fibres that creates the greatest tension or barrier. Two hands are used. The position or stretch is held by the therapist while the client inhales fully and then exhales. On deep inhalation, the client's muscle tone increases and on exhalation it decreases. The increase in muscle tone may assist in mobilizing the joints that are correctly positioned at the restrictive barrier *(Neumann, 1989)*.

🖐 The therapist smoothly and quickly releases the stretch about one-quarter to one-third of the way through the client's subsequent inhalation. The tissue mobilizes itself as it rebounds to its original position.

The amount of pressure used varies from light to moderate, depending on the tissue type and number of restrictions to be reduced. The technique is usually repeated three to five times *(Barral, Mercier, 1988)*. For this technique to be effective, accuracy in aligning the fibres and speed in releasing the tension or stretch are essential.

🖐 Osteopaths use recoil techniques on adhered tissue anywhere in the body *(Barral, Mercier, 1988)* but the most familiar application of this technique by massage therapists is **rib springing** to mobilize the thorax. Rib springing can be used on the posterior, anterior or lateral part of the rib cage, depending on the location of restrictions. Some authors list rib springing as an assessment and joint play technique *(Magee, 1992)*, while others describe it as a mobilization technique *(Barral, Mercier, 1988; Pryor, 1991)*.

🖐 The therapist carefully compresses the client's rib cage with her hands during exhalation of a deep breath. The therapist then takes up the slack in the tissue, compressing it *to a soft-tissue end feel only.* This compression is maintained while the therapist instructs the client to inhale against the pressure of the compression. As the client's inhalation is about half completed, the therapist quickly and smoothly releases the compressive force. The client will often have an audible intake of breath, indicating a correct application of the technique.

Contraindications

✦ Contraindications to recoil techniques are hypermobile joints, joints restricted by pins, screws and wires, acute injury, rheumatoid arthritis, inflammation of costal cartilage and osteoporosis.

🖐 It is important that the client put effort into inhaling against the therapist's pressure as this will increase contraction of the intercostal muscles, increasing the effectiveness of these muscles in mobilizing the thorax. Rib springing can be repeated up to three times in one area. The therapist should allow the client enough time between deep breaths to avoid hyperventilation.

✦ Effects: Recoil techniques are used to increase tissue and joint mobility.

Joint Play

Robert Maigne, James Cyriax and John Mennell are the physicians who created the foundations of these techniques. Fred Kaltenborn, a Scandinavian physical therapist, has contributed greatly to this work. Peripheral joint mobilization techniques also evolved from osteopathic principles *(Hertling, Kessler, 1990; Kisner, Colby, 1990)*.

The small, accessory, intrinsic movements occurring at a joint were described by Mennell as *joint play*. These small movements must be possible in a joint for full, pain-free range of motion to occur *(Neumann, 1989)*.

Joint play techniques are passive joint mobilizations. The technique is used to both assess and treat a dysfunctional joint. A clear knowledge of anatomy, especially of the shape of joint surfaces, axes of motion and the range of motion of each joint, along with accurate palpation skills, are important for this technique to be applied safely. Once the area of dysfunction has been determined, an intermittent stretch is applied to the portion of the joint capsule to be mobilized.

Assessment

To assess the existing range of accessory movement, the therapist takes up the slack in the joint capsule and assesses for any dysfunctional physiological barriers to movement. The client must be fully relaxed.

🖐 The therapist uses one hand to stabilize proximal to the affected joint and the other hand to apply traction and movement.

🖐 The slack is taken out of the joint capsule by tractioning the joint, separating its articular surfaces. The term *long-axis traction* is used if traction is pulling on the long axis of the bone. The term *distraction* is used if the joint surfaces are pulled apart at right angles.

🖐 The therapist then makes small, specific gliding movements (called *glide*) to assess the motion present between the bones.

The direction of the movement is chosen according to the physiological motion allowed by the shape of the joint surfaces and the portion of the joint capsule to be stretched. A movement should never go into or through the point of pain.

Joint Play Techniques

Before joint play techniques are used for treatment, the soft tissue surrounding the joint is prepared with heat or massage. As with assessment, the client must be relaxed; the joint is stabilized proximally; slack is taken out of the joint and the joint surfaces are separated; small, specific gliding motions are made to stretch the joint capsule; and the movement should never go into or past the point of pain.

The techniques are applied rhythmically and slowly to allow the connective tissue time to respond. This affects joint proprioceptors, decreasing tone and spasm of muscles crossing the affected joint. Adhesions are reduced. In addition, joint health is promoted by the successive action of the techniques *(Hertling, Kessler 1996; Kisner, Colby, 1990)*.

If mobilizing the joint in the direction of restriction is too painful, the therapist should mobilize in a pain-free direction. This is progressed to mobilizing in the restricted direction as the pain decreases and the mobility improves.

To treat, two approaches are taken: graded oscillation and sustained translatory joint play.

🖐 Maitland's **graded oscillation technique** is used primarily for pain management and spasm in muscles that cross the joint being treated. Oscillations are applied smoothly at a rate of two or three per second for up to two minutes.

- In this system, Grade 1 or rhythmic, small-amplitude oscillations are used at the beginning of the soft tissue range, before tissue limitation. Grade 2 or rhythmic, large-amplitude oscillations are also performed before the end of soft tissue range is reached. Grade 3 or rhythmic, large-amplitude oscillations are used up to the limit of available motion and are then stressed into the tissue resistance. Grade 4 or rhythmic, small-amplitude oscillations are performed up to the limit of available motion and also stressed into the tissue resistance.

- The grade selected depends on the presentation of the dysfunction. With an acute injury, if joint play is appropriate, Grades 1 and 2 are used to reduce pain. With a chronic injury, Grades 3 and 4 are used to stretch the tissue. However, it is important to note that the addition of a high-velocity, small-amplitude thrust (a technique that is "with impulse") to joint play is outside the massage therapist's scope of practice.

🖐 Fred Kaltenborn's **sustained translatory joint play technique** is used primarily for regaining joint play movements and functional range of motion.

- To treat painful joints, intermittent distraction at right angles to the joint surfaces is applied for 10 seconds and then released, for several repetitions.

- To treat restricted joints, it is applied for six seconds and then partially released. This is repeated at three- to four-second intervals.

- In this system, Grade 1 small-amplitude distraction is applied to loosen the joint. No stress is placed on the capsule. Grade 2 distraction, then glide, is applied sufficiently to take up tissue slack and tighten the capsule. Grade 3 distraction, then glide, is applied sufficiently to place a stretch on the joint capsule. Grade 1 reduces pain, Grade 2 is used to assess the joint and Grade 3 is used to increase joint play *(Kisner, Colby, 1990)*. Kaltenborn suggests that when treatment is initiated the therapist goes up to a Grade 2 distraction only. The results are evaluated the next day. If pain or sensitivity has increased, Grade 1 distraction is used. However, if pain has decreased, the therapist progresses to Grade 3 distraction.

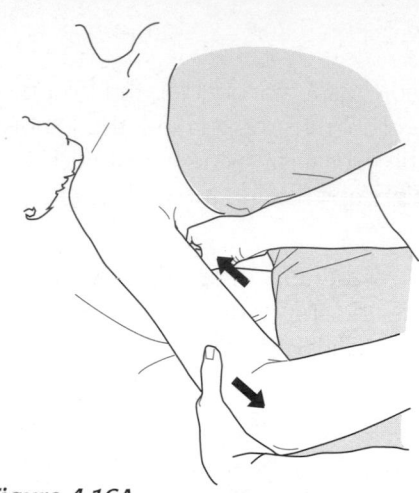

Figure 4.16A
Joint play: Inferior glenohumeral glide, using the fist to stabilize the scapula against the chest wall.

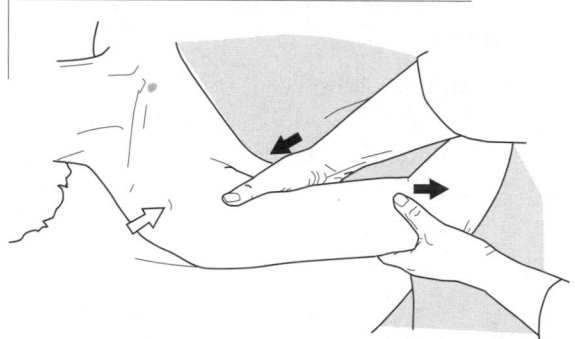

Figure 4.16B
Joint play: Inferior glenohumeral glide, using the back of the hand to stabilize the scapula; note dimple over dip at the humeral head (open arrow) as the humerus moves inferiorly.

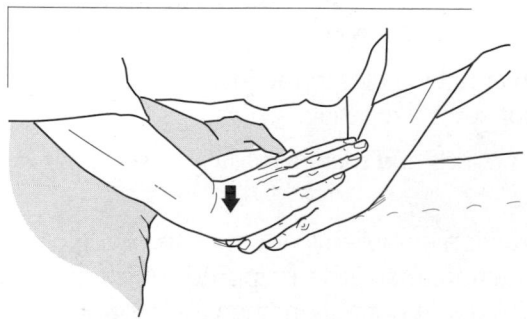

Figure 4.17
Joint play: Anterior spinous challenge, lumbar spine; the left hand isolates an individual spinous process while the right hand applies anterior pressure; this method is helpful when learning the technique; with practice, the heel of the palpating hand is sufficient.

Naming Joint Play Movements

Joint play movements are defined by the joint treated, the position of the joint and the direction of the glide. For example:

🖐 To apply **inferior glide** at the glenohumeral joint, the therapist stabilizes the scapula with one hand. The fist *(Figure 4.16A)* or the back of the hand *(Figure 4.16B)* can be used. The therapist's other hand distracts the joint and moves the humerus inferiorly

🖐 With the client prone, **anterior spinous challenge, or glide,** of the thoracic and lumbar spine begins by isolating one vertebral spinous process with the heel of the therapist's palpating hand *(Figure 4.17)*. This spinous process is then gently moved anteriorly. The therapist continues superiorly or inferiorly along the spine to assess or treat all vertebrae.

🖐 With the client supine, **anterior spinous challenge, or glide,** of the cervical spine is achieved by isolating one spinous process with the tips of both the therapist's middle fingers and gently moving the vertebrae anteriorly.

🖐 **Lateral spinous challenge, or glide,** is achieved by isolating one spinous process and gently gliding or challenging it laterally, to the left and to the right *(Figure 4.18)*. As before, the therapist continues superiorly or inferiorly along the spine to assess or treat all vertebrae.

🖐 **Spinous process oscillations** are performed by grasping the process and oscillating or wiggling it from side to side.

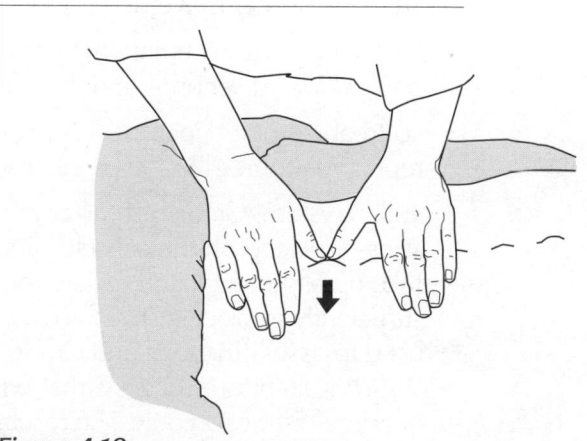

Figure 4.18
Joint play: Lateral spinous challenge to lumbar spine; thumbs isolate a spinous process and challenge it laterally.

✦ Effects: Joint play techniques assess joint dysfunctions, increase range of motion, stretch tight joint capsules, reduce adhesions, pain and spasm, and encourage the successive action of the joint.

Contraindications

✦ Contraindications to joint play are acute conditions, especially with joint effusion or infection, joints restricted by pins, screws, rods or surgical reduction of ligaments, joint hypermobility and with unhealed fractures. If inflammation is present, techniques that stretch the soft tissue are contraindicated, since they provoke pain and protective spasming.

✦ Extreme caution is used if performing these techniques on a client with osteoarthritis when osteophytes are present, and with other bone pathologies such as osteoporosis. Extreme caution is also used when weakened connective tissue is present. This may be the case with the use of certain medications such as corticosteroids, with systemic connective tissue disease such as inflammatory arthritides (during remission), after a period of disuse of the body part and with some elderly clients where there is weakened connective tissue and diminished circulation *(Kisner, Colby, 1990)*.

Muscle Energy

The muscle energy technique (MET) has been synthesized out of the work of osteopaths F. Mitchell Sr., Edward Stiles and others *(Chaitow, 1988)*. The technique is frequently used to normalize motion in the sacroiliac joints and the cervical, thoracic and lumbar spine, although it can be applied to any joint.

The technique is named after Mitchell's concept that instead of using the therapist's efforts to move the joint, the energy of the client's contracting muscles would be used to make the corrections. Muscle contractions can be isometric (no movement at the joint with contraction) or isotonic (joint movement occurs with contraction). Both are used with MET. Isometric techniques are the most widely applicable *(Basmajian, Nyberg, 1993)*. There is similarity between the light force isometric MET technique and post-isometric relaxation to lengthen muscles, discussed in the chapter on remedial exercise. Both involve submaximal contraction of a muscle for several seconds, followed by relaxation and then a comfortable stretch to lengthen the muscle.

A clear understanding of anatomy, muscle actions and joint motions and well developed palpation skills are necessary for these techniques.

Assessment

Accurate assessment of the dysfunctional joint through motion palpation is performed first. The therapist assesses for small, subtle and sensitive tissue motions using one hand to monitor, or "listen" to, the motions of the dysfunctional vertebral segment or tissue. With the other hand, the therapist moves the client's spine through flexion, extension, sidebending and rotation movements, introducing one movement at a time, until the motion barrier of the specific dysfunctional vertebral segment is found *(Basmajian, Nyberg, 1993; Chaitow, 1988)*.

Muscle Energy Techniques

Once the restriction is found, the client is positioned so the joint is at the barrier, or limit, of its dysfunctional range. This position is termed *localization*. The client is then instructed to resist the therapist's effort to move the client's body further into the barrier, so the antagonists are contracted, reciprocally inhibiting the shortened muscle. The contraction may be either isometric or isotonic, depending on the specific technique chosen by the therapist.

For example, to restore flexion and left sidebending and rotation at T7-8, the therapist stands at the left side behind the seated client. The therapist palpates between the spinous processes of T7-8 and then slightly flexes and left rotates the client's trunk until the barrier to motion is found to be localized at T7-8. The therapist instructs the client to hold that position, using minimum strength. Next, the therapist uses force equal to the client's resistance to attempt to rotate the trunk to the right. The client holds the isometric contraction for three to five seconds and then relaxes completely. The therapist localizes the new barrier for flexion and left sidebending and rotation. The technique is repeated a total of three times *(Boyling, Palastanga, 1994)*.

✦ Effects: Muscle energy technique restores joint motion in chronic conditions.

Contraindication

✦ A contraindication to muscle energy technique is acute injury, where edema and muscle strain may be present. This would be aggravated by isometric contraction.

Counterstrain

The American osteopath Lawrence Jones developed the counterstrain technique to relieve spinal or other joint pain *(Greenman, 1989; Jones, 1993)*. Dale Anderson has popularized it as the *hold and fold* method *(Anderson, 1992)*.

Jones discovered the technique by accident. He had unsuccessfully treated a patient with iliopsoas pain ("psoitis") using his regular manipulative techniques, for two months. In frustration, Jones tried to find a comfortable sleeping position for the patient. After passively moving the patient over a 20-minute period, a position of comfort was found. Jones left the patient in this position. Surprisingly, the patient was able to stand up comfortably after just this treatment. From this lucky accident, Jones experimented and developed counterstrain.

Passive indirect techniques such as counterstrain change the **interaction** of a dysfunctional vertebral segment with its neighbouring segments. These techniques are described as "release by positioning" *(Greenman, 1989)*. In contrast, a chiropractic adjustment changes the vertebral **position.**

Assessment

The therapist palpates for tender points in the muscle. Some of these points correspond to trigger points and acupressure points.

Contraindications

✦ Contraindications include hypermobile joints and acute joint inflammation.

The Counterstrain Technique

The therapist compresses the tender point while the client is placed in a position that moves the joint or limb *away* from the pain, shortens the muscle and almost completely reduces the pain *(Neumann, 1989)*. The compression and position are maintained for 90 seconds. After that the client *slowly* returns to a neutral posture and is reassessed.

✦ Effects: The counterstrain technique reduces pain, muscle spasm and hypertonicity of muscles surrounding a joint.

5

SEQUENCE OF TECHNIQUES:
The Principles of Massage

Linda Ludwig, Fiona Rattray

When performing a massage, the therapist utilizes a variety of Swedish and non-Swedish techniques in a manner that has one technique transitioning easily to another, as a particular part of the body is treated by any number of fluid movements.

Once the technical aspect of performing a technique is learned, the new therapist is faced with technique sequence: putting them together in a "routine" to address specific body parts and, eventually, to treat specific conditions. There are general sequencing principles that guide the application of massage techniques. These *principles of massage* describe the direction and progression of manipulations. They are:

General → specific → general

Superficial → deep → superficial

Proximal → distal → proximal

Peripheral → central → peripheral

The first two principles apply to every technique used by the massage therapist, be it a Swedish or non-Swedish technique.

+ **General to specific to general** and **superficial to deep to superficial** refer to how a group of techniques is applied to an area of the body. The first techniques are applied generally and superficially; these are followed by techniques that are more specific and deeper; the therapist then returns to more general and superficial techniques before moving to another area.

This sequencing has many effects: it accustoms the client to the therapist's touch; it allows the therapist to palpate through layers of tissue in a systematic manner; it prepares the tissue by increasing local circulation; it reduces sympathetic nervous system firing because it is performed in a predictable and systematic manner; and it prevents the subsequent techniques that require deeper pressure from being painful and feeling invasive. Without this approach, after deep work, the client may experience *kick-back* pain or post-treatment soreness for hours or days after the treatment.

- An example of the sequencing of techniques using the general–specific–general, peripheral–central–peripheral principles is as follows. An arm massage may begin with effleurage over the entire limb, then light petrissage, progressing to deep muscle stripping to specific hypertonic muscles, then finished with light petrissage, effleurage and stroking to the limb.

- In another example, tapotement is used on the thorax to remove mucus. The sequence of techniques begins with light tapotement, gentle tapping and pincement. This is followed by hacking — soft then hard. Cupping is used as the deepest and most specific technique. Reversing back through the techniques, hard then soft hacking is reapplied, followed by tapping or pincement, and finally some soothing effleurage.

A modification to these principles is used with direct fascial work. In order to prepare the tissue for these deeper and specific techniques, an application of heat is used to prepare the tissue in place of general and superficial massage techniques. For example, in treating postural conditions, the therapist applies heat and then treats the shortened connective tissue with direct fascial techniques. The drag necessary for effective fascial work is maximized, as a lubricant has not been applied. This work is followed by an application of lubricant and regular general and superficial Swedish massage techniques.

✦ **Proximal to distal to proximal** refers to how techniques are applied to the limbs in order to increase the local circulation of blood and lymph. When techniques are applied to the arms and legs, they are performed proximally or closer to the trunk. When a treatment is begun on structures closer to the trunk, hypertonicity and restrictions are reduced in these tissues, allowing for more efficient venous and lymphatic return from distal parts of the limb.

- For example, after the initial light effleurage to spread the lubricant over the entire posterior leg, various petrissage techniques are used on the muscles of the hip. These are started proximally at the iliac crest and progress over the gluteals to the attachments at the greater trochanter. Next, techniques are used on the posterior thigh muscles, working proximally from the ischial tuberosity and greater trochanter through the muscle bellies to their attachments at the knee. After this, the therapist moves distally to the lower leg then foot. Once this distal work is completed, deeper effleurage is used from the distal foot to the proximal hip, encouraging local venous return.

Both the pressure and the overall direction of techniques move towards the trunk and heart, or in a centripetal direction, promoting venous blood return *(Basmajian, 1985)*.

The pressure is lighter when the direction of manipulation is away from the heart, to prevent back pressure on the venous and lymph flow.

Some modifications to the principle of proximal–distal–proximal are made with the inflammatory process. With an injury in the acute or early subacute stage, the injury is considered the most distal point at which to perform techniques that affect the circulation and lymphatic flow. Therefore, massage is applied from the trunk to the injury site and back to the trunk. At this stage, massage over the injury site is generally not indicated. Massage distal to the injury site consists of stroking or gentle muscle squeezing. Techniques which increase venous and lymph return are avoided since painful congestion of the injury site is possible.

✦ The principle of **peripheral to central to peripheral** is used specifically when treating acute and subacute local injuries and scar tissue, and when approaching areas of apprehension or pain for the client.

By approaching healing tissue peripherally, the therapist can aid the removal of toxins and waste products that result from the inflammatory process. Scar tissue is generally more accessible and less adhered at the edges and, therefore, easier to break down. Only after the peripheral restrictions are released does the massage progress to the most adhered central area. Moving back to the periphery reduces the possibility of kick-back pain. Several treatments may be required before this central area can be addressed. This less direct approach to scar tissue is often more tolerable for the client.

The same peripheral to central approach is used to treat areas of apprehension and pain. Work directly to the most painful area is often very uncomfortable and invasive for the client, who may move away from the touch. The tissue will often respond reflexively by tightening and pushing the therapist's fingers out.

✦ **Treating the antagonist** of an affected muscle may be considered the fifth principle of massage. This principle relates to the reciprocal response between an agonist muscle and its antagonist. In treating only the agonist, potential sources of dysfunction in the antagonist may be overlooked. For example, with an anterior compartment syndrome, if the therapist focuses only on the painful, symptomatic tibialis anterior muscle, ignoring the potentially shortened gastrocnemius muscle, the source of the client's problem will not be addressed. A short, inflexible gastrocnemius muscle forces tibialis anterior to work harder to dorsiflex the ankle and thus reinforces the syndrome. A stretch or fascial work to the gastrocnemius will normalize the biomechanics of the ankle.

In another example, the antagonist may develop hypertonicity and trigger points secondary to the original lesion site. A shortened hip flexor such as psoas major will tip the pelvis anteriorly. In response, gluteus maximus develops increased tone, perhaps activating latent trigger points, as it attempts to stabilize the pelvis posteriorly. Working both agonist and antagonist treats all the symptoms.

6

HYDROTHERAPY APPLICATIONS

Fiona Rattray

> *Hydrotherapy uses water in its solid, liquid or gaseous form, for its therapeutic effects.*

The term hydrotherapy has been expanded to include thermal applications which are not pure water, such as wax baths, thermophores (moist electric heating pads), hydrocollators (gel-filled heat packs) and freezable gel packs. Besides Swedish and non-Swedish massage techniques, the therapist uses hydrotherapy and remedial exercise modalities during treatment.

The therapeutic use of water has a long history. Hot springs and healing baths have been used since ancient times *(Basmajian, 1985)*. The application of cold was mentioned by Hippocrates in the treatment of acute or overuse injuries *(Brukner, Khan, 1993)*.

More recently, Sebastian Kneipp of mid-nineteenth century Germany developed a therapy of water and herbal applications, exercise and diet called *water cures* to treat pathology and trauma *(Bruggeman, 1982; Boyle, Saine, 1988)*.

An old definition of hydrotherapy includes the idea that water may be applied internally as well as externally, such as in beverages (mineral or spring waters) and douches, the latter being outside the scope of massage therapy today *(Moor et al., 1964)*.

Hydrotherapy is a useful adjunct to any treatment. It can prepare the tissue before a treatment; for example, heat is used before applying fascial techniques to increase the flexibility of the fascia. It can be applied after certain techniques to modulate their effects; for example, cold is used after frictions to reduce the inflammatory response.

Hydrotherapy Principles

✦ Thermal effects occur with applications of water at temperatures above or below that

67

of the body. Generally, the greater the temperature difference, the more pronounced the effects.

✦ The effects of an application vary depending on the temperature and length of time it is applied *(Boyle, Saine, 1988)*.

 • For example, a brief application of cold (less than one minute) provokes the body to maintain thermal and circulatory equilibrium. Local vasoconstriction in the skin is followed by vasodilation, creating a perception of warmth, hyperemia, reflexively increased muscle tone and a feeling of general well being. Conversely, something of constant cold temperature left on the body for longer than one minute causes continued vasoconstriction and a perception of cold.

 • A short application of heat (less than five minutes) stimulates the circulation, with local cutaneous vasodilation followed by vasostasis. A prolonged application of heat longer than five minutes causes the metabolic rate to increase. This increases the circulatory rate, which places an extra stress on the circulatory system.

✦ Hydrotherapy may be used over the entire body or locally. A full-body application has a more profound effect than a small, local application *(Boyle, Saine, 1988)*.

 • For example, a hot full-immersion bath has an effect on the whole body, while a hot towel applied to one gastrocnemius muscle affects the local circulation.

✦ Generally, the client should rest following any full-body hydrotherapy treatment for at least the same length of time as the hydrotherapy was applied.

✦ The weight of an individual hydrotherapy application is considered before use. For example, a large, heavy ice pack may painfully compress an inflamed bursa whereas a thinner, lighter one may be more tolerable.

General Effects

The effects of hydrotherapy can be physiological or reflexive. Physiological effects occur as the body attempts to return to homeostasis, or the normal physiological state of balance, in response to the hydrotherapy application. For example, physiological effects of heat include an increase in blood flow and muscle relaxation, while physiological effects of cold include initial vasoconstriction and reduced pain.

Reflexive effects result from the influences of the nervous system in response to the application. These reflexive effects occur elsewhere in the body. For example, moist heat applied to the skin of the abdomen causes diminished intestinal activity, and heat applied to one limb causes an increase in the blood flow in the contralateral limb.

Heat

Effects of Heat

✦ Locally there is an increase in tissue temperature. Sources differ as to how deep this penetrates: 3.4 centimetres in one study, to the level of the superficial muscles *(Moor et al., 1964)*, yet not deeper than 3 to 5 millimetres below the surface of the skin in another source *(Buschbacher, 1994)*.

+ There is an increase in local vasodilation and blood flow to the skin and muscles below the heat source. This results in an increase in metabolism, oxygen and nutrient supply, capillary permeability, and an increase in sweat production. Applications of heat to the limbs cause a marked increase in blood flow: a twofold increase in flow was noted after a 30-minute application of heat to the forearm; this persisted approximately one hour after the application was removed (*Moor et al., 1964*). Distal to the heat source, there is also an increase in circulation to the skin.

+ Pain perception is decreased as a result of a decrease in nerve conduction velocity.

+ Muscle tone and spasm are also decreased, because heating muscle spindles causes them to decrease their sensitivity and rate of firing (*DeLisa, Gans, 1993*).

+ Heat between 42 and 45 degrees Celsius increases the extensibility of collagen tissue (*Buschbacher, 1994; Brukner, Khan, 1993*), making joints and muscles more flexible with stretching.

+ There is a reflex increase in blood flow in the contralateral limb.

+ Another reflex effect with heat applied to the abdomen is decreased gastrointestinal motility and gastric acid production.

+ Finally, a general sense of sedation and relaxation occurs with heat applications (*Buschbacher, 1994*).

Specific Heat Applications

The therapist should take care that the skin is not hyper- or hyposensitive to heat, that the application is not so hot as to burn the client, and also that the hydrotherapy is not applied for prolonged periods, again to prevent the possibility of burns. Between 36 and 38 degrees Celsius is considered warm, hot is over 39 degrees (*Bruggemann, 1982*). An application such as wax is tested on a small area first before being applied to a larger area.

• **Thermophore:** This electric moist-heat pad comes in different sizes, usually with a control for the client. A towel is placed between the thermophore and the client's skin; the client should never lie on the thermophore. Duration of application is up to 10 minutes.

• **Hydrocollator:** These gel-filled cloth packs are placed in a temperature-controlled water tank between uses. Tongs are used to lift the packs out of hot water. The therapist then wraps the hydrocollator pack in a towel before application. Duration of application is up to 10 minutes. The weight of the application is considered; a large, wet hydrocollator pack can be heavy. Packs should always be returned to the tank after use, otherwise they dry out and become hard. The water in the tank is kept clean according to the manufacturer's instructions.

• **Wax (paraffin) baths:** A commercial temperature-controlled paraffin bath contains melted paraffin wax. A small amount of mineral oil is added according to the manufacturer's instructions to keep the paraffin from crumbling once it is applied to the client's skin and dries. Before a wax application, the massage sheets should be protected from wax drops by placing plastic cling film over them. Paraffin can be applied to the client's skin in several methods. The client's clean hand or foot can be dipped in the wax six to 12 times, allowing the wax to cool between dippings. For applications of wax to other locations on the body, strips of cheesecloth or commercial cloth wipes are dipped into the wax, then applied in several layers over the skin.

Another method is to use a paint brush to apply the wax to the client's skin; however, this method is often messy and, as the brush cannot be left in the bath between treatments, it dries into a solid mass which must be warmed before use.

Once the wax is applied, the body part is covered first in plastic film, then in a towel to conserve heat. The wax is left on for up to 20 minutes, then removed before massage or fascial techniques are used.

- **Arm and foot baths:** This is a local immersion in water which covers either the forearms past the elbows or the feet past the ankles. The tub or container must be large enough to accommodate this. Temperatures over 39 degrees C are considered hot. Immersion times of up to 30 minutes are indicated. Afterwards the limbs are thoroughly dried.

- **Compresses:** Towels or cloths are immersed in hot water, wrung out and applied to the client's skin. The compress is covered with an insulating towel. The therapist must check that the compress has not become too cold and should replace it with another before this happens. The skin is dried after the application is finished.

- **Steam inhalation:** These can be pre-treatment or as self-care. A bowl is filled with water that has been boiled. The client sits in front of the bowl with a large towel covering the bowl and his head and shoulders. The client is instructed to close his eyes and inhale the steam. Care is taken not to come in contact with the hot water. Essential oils can be added to the water; see later in this chapter for details.

- **Full-body baths:** Often given as self-care, these may be up to 15 minutes in duration *(Bruggemann, 1982)*. Temperatures above 38 degrees C may be too stimulating, especially at night before bed time. A cool cloth for the forehead and drinking water are available for the client. Herbal extracts can be added to the bath water.

An epsom salts bath has up to 500 millilitres of epsom salts added to the water. The client soaks for up to 15 minutes. The bathtub plug is pulled and the water drains while he remains seated in the tub. The client then has a cool shower to rinse off the epsom salts.

- **Effects:** Heat is used with chronic conditions, to soften connective tissue and after treating trigger points. It increases vasodilation, local circulation, contralateral circulation, metabolism, collagen extensibility and overall relaxation; it decreases pain, spasm, hypertonicity and intestinal activity.

Contraindications

- Contraindications to heat applications are acute injury (heat will increase bleeding and swelling if used in the first 48 hours after injury), circulatory pathologies (especially with prolonged or full-body heat applications), sensory changes, acutely inflamed joints, acute infections, existing burns, hypersensitivity to heat and dependent limbs (a dangling position may cause edema in the limb). Heat applications can also cause burns if heat is left on the tissue for too long. For most people with multiple sclerosis, large applications are not well tolerated.

- For example, heat is contraindicated on the neck and shoulders of a client who has an acute ear infection. This could spread the infection and overload an already stressed lymphatic system. In another example, heat should not be placed on the shoulder or upper arm of a client who has decreased tissue health and chronic edema in the hand following third degree burns and skin grafts. The heat will add to congestion in the limb.

Cold

Cryotherapy is another term for the application of cold or ice.

Effects of Cold

✦ Cold applied locally reduces the temperature of the skin, muscle and joint it is applied to. Skin temperature decreases to a greater degree than muscle; however, depending on the length of time of the application, muscle tissue may stay cold for up to 45 minutes after the source is removed *(Brukner, Khan, 1993)*.

✦ Cold causes local vasoconstriction, decreasing blood flow; this allows cold to penetrate deeper into the tissue as there is little influx of fresh warm blood. A lower temperature increases blood viscosity, reducing bleeding. With injured tissue, this means decreased inflammation, swelling, edema and bleeding. Decreased cell metabolism and leukocyte migration are also noted with a prolonged application of cold, further decreasing inflammation *(Moor et al., 1964)*.

✦ Pain is decreased by cold either blocking pain transmission or acting as a counterirritant.

✦ Muscle spasm is decreased due to reduced muscle spindle firing *(DeLisa, Gans, 1993)*.

✦ Collagen extensibility is decreased with cold applications.

✦ Brief cold applications have a stimulating effect.

✦ Reflex effects of brief cold applications — less than 30 seconds — are a general peripheral vasoconstriction.

✦ If applied in less than two minutes after a deep burn, cold gives immediate pain relief, decreased tissue damage and hastened healing *(Buschbacher, 1994)*.

✦ In one study, cold applied to chronic inflammatory joint disease decreased pain and stiffness while increasing range of motion *(DeLisa, Gans, 1993)*.

Specific Cold Applications

At first, cold is often not as well tolerated as heat by the client; however, once accustomed to it, clients often get significant relief from pain and spasm.

An average duration of a gel-pack or ice application to reduce inflammation and pain is 25 to 30 minutes *(Buschbacher, 1994; Chatelaine, 1995)*. The therapist should take care that the application is not placed directly on the skin or left on so long as to cause frostbite. Between 13 and 18 degrees Celsius is considered cool; cold is between 0 and 12 degrees Celsius *(Bruggemann, 1982)*.

With a cold application, the client will experience the following stages over several minutes:

1) a sensation of cold;
2) tingling or itching;
3) aching or burning; then
4) numbness or analgesia *(Hooper, 1996)*.

It is important to inform a client who has not used cold hydrotherapy applications about these stages.

- **Ice packs:** These gel-filled plastic packs are kept in a refrigerator freezer until needed. The pack is wrapped in a towel before application to the affected area. Another towel is used to insulate the ice pack for the 25 to 30 minutes it is applied. Cold can be used following frictions and as self-care before or after exercise to decrease inflammation.

- **Ice massage:** Water is frozen in a paper or styrofoam cup; the edge of the cup is peeled back, giving the therapist an easier way to handle the ice than if it were just an ice cube. The ice is rubbed over the skin surface in a circular manner. The duration of the application varies according to different sources — either five to 10 minutes *(Brukner, Khan, 1993)* or 15 to 30 minutes *(Buschbacher, 1994)*. A brief application of ice is also used to treat trigger points as a distraction before stretch. See the chapter on trigger points for details *(Travell, Simons, 1983)*.

- **Arm and foot baths:** This local immersion in cool or cold water covers either the forearms past the elbows, or the feet past the ankles. Immersion times of up to a minute are indicated. Afterwards the limbs are thoroughly dried.

- **Compresses:** Towels or cloths are immersed in cold water, wrung out and applied to the client's skin. The compress is covered with an insulating towel. The therapist must check that the compress has not become too warm and replace it with another before this happens. The skin is dried after the application is finished.

Two less well-known cold hydrotherapy applications:

- A **cool wash** uses a cloth that has been folded into four and run under cold water. The therapist first washes over the tissue with one square of the cloth and then changes to a new square as the previously used one heats up.

- A **heating compress** will draw circulation to the area using the body's reflexes to warm a cold area. A cold cloth is placed over the area, then covered by a dry cloth. This remains in place until the body has heated the cold cloth to body temperature.

- Effects: Cold is used with acute conditions, after cross-fibre friction techniques or as a brief distraction when treating trigger points. It increases vasoconstriction and decreases local circulation, pain, inflammation, edema, spasm, metabolism and collagen extensibility; brief applications are stimulating.

Contraindications

- Contraindications to cold hydrotherapy are Raynaud's disease or other circulatory insufficiency, sensory changes (decreased skin sensitivity to temperature), cold sensitivity ("cold allergy"), debility and the client feeling chilled.

- For example, a cold foot bath is not used if the client feels cold, especially in winter. The cold will further decrease the client's body temperature.

Contrast

Effects of Contrast

Contrast hydrotherapy is a warm or hot application followed by a cool or cold application. This causes alternating vasodilation and vasoconstriction of the arterioles and capillaries. A marked increase in local circulation and venous return occurs; in one study a 30-minute contrast bath increased circulation in the lower body by 95 per cent *(Moor et al., 1964)*. This helps move metabolites, decrease edema and increase tissue healing.

A common ratio of time for each application of heat and cold is 3:1 — three minutes of hot, one minute of cold. However, local vasoconstriction occurs in 20 seconds, so the application of cold may be as brief as 30 seconds in duration *(Moor et al., 1964)*. Applications of heat and cold may be repeated several times for a stronger effect on local circulation. The greater the difference in temperature between the heat and cold, the greater the effect on local circulation. Contrast applications should always end with a cold application, encouraging vasoconstriction instead of congestion. Contrast applications may be used as self-care.

Contraindications

+ Contraindications to contrast hydrotherapy are acute conditions, decreased skin sensitivity to temperature, vascular pathologies and the client feeling chilled.

+ For example, a contrast arm bath of extreme temperature differences is contraindicated for a client with congestive heart failure. The increase in local circulation will place an excessive stress on the heart.

Specific Contrast Applications

For water applications, two containers are needed: one filled with hot water, the other with cold.

• Applications include **arm and foot baths** and **compresses.**

+ Effects: Contrast hydrotherapy is usually used for treating subacute conditions; it increases local circulation.

Hydrotherapy Additives

• **Essential oils** can be applied in various hydrotherapy modalities, such as in baths, compresses or steam inhalations. Essential oils are absorbed through the nasal epithelium and olfactory bulb to the brain and through the lungs and pores of the skin into the circulatory system, where they affect the body *(Lawless, 1995; Valnet, 1990)*. Specific hydrotherapy and essential oil applications are noted in the treatment chapters.

REMEDIAL EXERCISE

Fiona Rattray

Remedial exercise uses a combination of active and passive exercise to restore and improve the client's musculoskeletal health.

Remedial exercises fall into three main categories: range of motion, stretching and resistance exercise. Remedial exercise is used by the therapist *during* treatment and by the client *after* treatment as self-care.

✦ **Passive relaxed** and **active assisted ranges of motion** and **passive joint mobilization** all require that the therapist or another person help the client. They are usually included in a massage therapy treatment to stretch muscles and connective tissue, and to maintain joint health.

✦ **Stretching** can be performed during the treatment by the therapist and it may also be given as self-care.

✦ **Active free range of motion** and **active resisted exercise** are performed by the client, usually as self-care. This maximizes the therapist's hands-on treatment time.

Range of motion (active free and passive relaxed), passive joint mobilization and active resisted movement are used as both remedial exercises and assessment tools *(Kisner, Colby, 1990)*. See the chapter on assessment for more information.

Some remedial exercises that are specific to each condition are noted in the appropriate chapter. The therapist will need to refer to the sources listed in the bibliography for additional exercises.

Range of Motion (ROM)

The **range of motion of a joint** is the motion allowed by the shape of the joint and the soft tissue surrounding it. ROM occurs in planes of flexion, extension, abduction, adduction and internal and external rotation.

Body parts are moved either by the client actively contracting the muscles, by the therapist moving the body parts or by the force of gravity acting on the body part.

Each joint is capable of a specific range of motion and has an amount of movement available in that range. For example, in flexion, the knee joint normally moves through 0 to 135 degrees *(Clarkson, Gilewich, 1989)*.

Proprioceptive nerve receptors called Ruffini's end organs determine the degree of angulation of a joint by detecting the stretch placed on tissues and joint capsules; this information is transmitted to the brain, informing the person of the actual position of a joint or limb *(Guyton, 1984)*. Adhesions, especially within a joint capsule, leading to restricted range of motion alter this sense of proprioception, giving incorrect information about the position of the joint. Part of the remedial rehabilitation process involves restoring this sense correctly by restoring full range of motion where possible.

The **range of a muscle** is the distance that a muscle can shorten from the point of maximum lengthening to the point of maximum contraction *(Kisner, Colby, 1996)*. This is also called functional excursion.

When a muscle contracts, it moves the joint or joints that it crosses. The **inner range** of a muscle and the joint that it crosses is described as a position from where the muscle is completely shortened to where the muscle is half way through its full range *(Figure 7.1)*. The **outer range** of a muscle and the joint that it crosses is a position from half way through the full range to where the muscle is fully stretched. **Mid-range** is the segment from the midpoint of the inner range to the midpoint of the outer range *(Clarkson, Gilewich, 1989)*. It is necessary for the body part to be moved through all three available ranges in order to maintain the normal range of motion and full muscle strength *(Kisner, Colby, 1990)*.

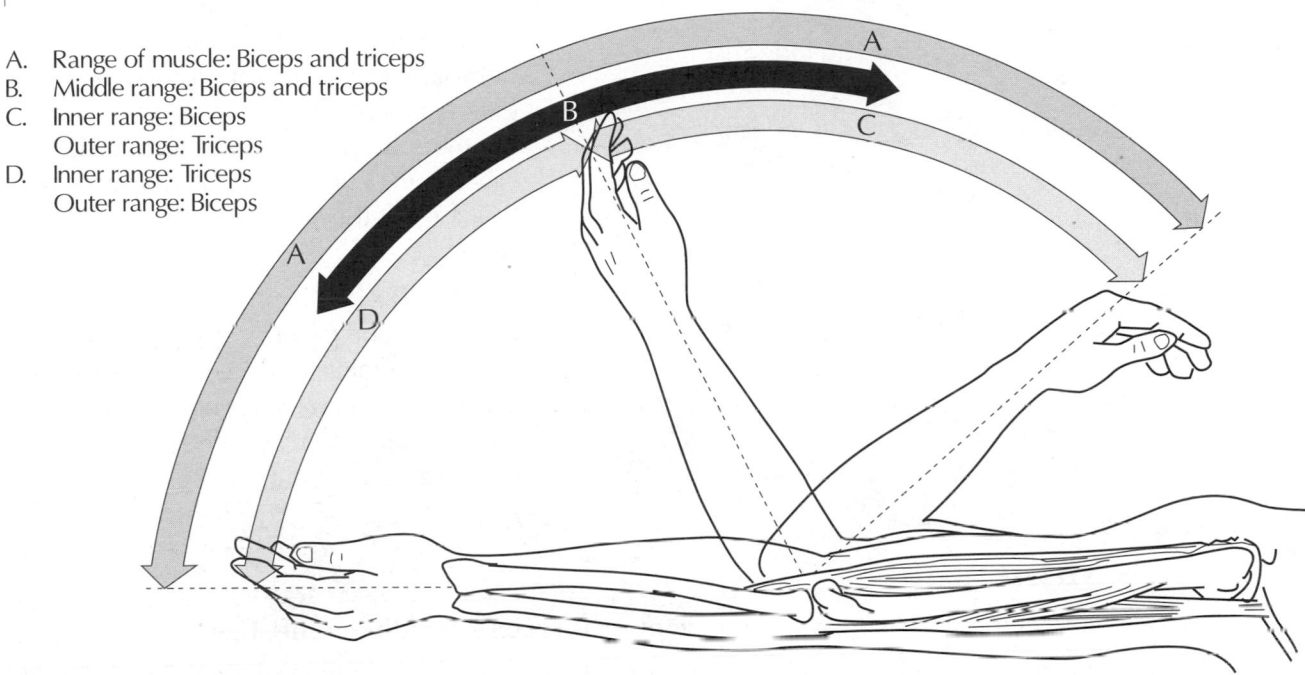

A. Range of muscle: Biceps and triceps
B. Middle range: Biceps and triceps
C. Inner range: Biceps
   Outer range: Triceps
D. Inner range: Triceps
   Outer range: Biceps

Figure 7.1
Muscle ranges.

Contraindications

✦ Contraindications to AF ROM are pain in the acute stage. Movement at a speed and range that do not cause pain is desired. Historically, any motion that may have been disruptive to the healing process was absolutely contraindicated. However, recent studies have shown the value of movement in the acute stage in preventing adhesions and decreasing the recovery time **as long as the movement is pain free** *(Kisner, Colby, 1990).*

Contraindications

✦ The contraindications for AA ROM are the same as for AF ROM.

Active Free (AF) ROM

🖑 **Active free range of motion** is performed when the client actively contracts the muscles crossing a joint, moving the joint through the unrestricted range.

✦ Effects: AF ROM maintains joint range of motion, proprioception, circulation and lymphatic flow, successive action of the joint and some muscle strength.

Active Assisted (AA) ROM

🖑 **Active assisted range of motion** is active free range of motion performed when assistance is required by the client to complete the active motion. It is used when a client has decreased muscle strength. The therapist can provide the assistance in completing the motion; or the client can use a pool, where water reduces the effects of gravity on the limb.

✦ Effects: AA ROM has the same effects as AF ROM.

Contraindications

✦ Contraindications to PR ROM include those for AF ROM, plus the following. Whenever motion may disrupt the acute stage of the healing process, motion is done in a **pain-free range**. During the subacute stage, the therapist should **stay within the client's pain tolerance, using reduced speed and the inner to mid-range** of joint movement. Increased pain or signs of inflammation following PR ROM indicate an overuse of this range. In chronic stages, the range is limited by the client's pain tolerance.

Passive Relaxed (PR) ROM

✋ Passive relaxed range of motion is movement within the unrestricted range of motion of a joint that is produced by an external force: the therapist, gravity or another part of the client's body. The client is **not** contracting the muscles. PR ROM is not the same as passive stretching.

✦ Effects: PR ROM maintains the joint range of motion and proprioception, assists in lymphatic drainage of a limb, increases the successive action of a joint and reduces the formation of adhesions and contractures.

Stretching

Stretching, performed by the client or therapist, lengthens soft tissue.

In order to properly stretch soft tissue, the therapist should understand the composition of soft tissue. Muscles, tendons, ligaments, fascia, joint capsules and skin are all soft tissue. Muscle fibres are contractile tissue and have the ability to contract and relax. Tendons, ligaments, fascia, joint capsules and skin are made up of **noncontractile tissue** (or connective tissue), which can neither contract nor relax. Noncontractile tissue is also interwoven throughout the contractile tissues of the muscle and is the *main source of resistance* to a passive stretch.

Noncontractile tissue is composed of collagen and elastin fibres as well as ground substance. Collagen fibres are the structural portion of the tissue, providing strength and stiffness. These wavy fibres are able to elongate when small loads are placed on them, but they stiffen and resist with increasing loads. Elastin fibres provide extensibility and are also able to elongate when small stress loads are placed on them. However, they will rupture with larger loads. Ground substance is a gel that transports nutrients and metabolites as well as reduces friction between the connective-tissue fibres. It is also likely that it prevents excess cross-linking between the individual collagen fibres *(Kisner, Colby, 1996)*.

The organizational pattern of collagen fibres dictates the relative strength of the noncontractile tissue and its ability to resist stress. Tendons have the greatest resistance to stress with their parallel arrangement of collagen fibres. Ligaments, fascia and joint capsules have moderate resistance to stress with a combination of both parallel and randomly arranged fibres. Skin has the least resistance to stress due to its random arrangement of collagen fibres.

Initially, when noncontractile tissue is stressed or stretched, the wavy collagen fibres straighten out. This is termed the *elastic range* of the tissue and is thought to be the slack that is taken out of the tissue during a stretch. If the stretch is released at this point, the collagen fibres will return to their original length. If the stretch is increased past the elastic range, the cross-links and bonds between the collagen fibres break and there is a release of heat (hysteresis); this is termed the *plastic range* of the tissue. If the stretch is released at this point, the tissue is permanently stretched (*Basmajian, Nyberg, 1993*).

Overstretching in the plastic range takes the tissue beyond the normal range of motion of a joint and its associated soft tissues. This results in hypermobility of the joint. If the stretch on the noncontractile tissue is continued past the plastic range, the tissue "fails" or ruptures.

Shortened muscles and connective tissue result in tight muscles. A tight muscle is a muscle that has undergone a mild adaptive shortening. This tightness is usually due to muscular inactivity and results in a decreased range of motion. A tight, shortened muscle becomes weaker as it is no longer able to develop peak tension. The muscle can be moderately lengthened, by activities of daily living, but not to its full range of extensibility without the client performing some type of stretching exercise.

Performing Any Stretch

✍ There are three categories of stretches: **active inhibition techniques, passive stretching** and **self-stretching.**

✍ Before any stretch, AF ROM or hot hydrotherapy should be used to help make the tissue as flexible as possible. Whether the stretch is performed by the therapist or by the client, it is done in a **slow, gentle and sustained manner.** The force is sufficient to stretch the tissues **without causing pain.** Rapid stretching and ballistic stretching ("bouncing" a stretch) engage the stretch reflex, causing a reflex contraction of the muscle; this should be avoided. An active inhibition technique (described below) is held for up to 10 seconds, while a passive stretch and self-stretch are held for at least 15 to 30 seconds. The tension in the muscle should gradually decrease during this time. Once this occurs, the muscle is taken a little farther into the stretch, again, without causing pain. Upon completion, a stretch is released **gradually.** The cycle can be repeated several times, with rests between each stretch.

✍ It may take several weeks to regain full flexibility. The therapist or client should not attempt to regain full range of motion in only one or two sessions (*Kisner, Colby 1990*).

✦ Effects: Stretching is used to lengthen soft tissue.

Contraindications

✦ Contraindications to all stretches — active inhibition techniques, passive stretch and self-stretch — are the acute stage of healing, especially with hematoma or recent fracture; acute joint inflammation due to trauma, infection or inflammatory arthritides; acute pain present with joint motion or stretching; joint motion restricted by bony end feel; joint hypermobility syndromes; and fascial or muscle contractures that provide joint stability in the absence of muscle strength or joint stability.

Active Inhibition Techniques

In active inhibition techniques, the client reflexively inhibits (relaxes) the muscle to be lengthened. A muscle that is inhibited has minimal resistance to being lengthened.

The client relaxes the contractile tissue in the muscle and then it is lengthened by either the client or the therapist. The noncontractile tissue is not as significantly affected unless the stretch is held for a prolonged time.

The muscle to be stretched must be normally innervated and under the client's control for active inhibition techniques to work. For example, a client with muscle flaccidity due to a severed peripheral nerve cannot contract the muscle. A client with spasticity cannot consciously relax the muscle.

Hold-relax, contract-relax, post-isometric relaxation and agonist contraction are examples of active inhibition techniques.

Hold-relax

The hold-relax technique uses maximal muscle contraction to facilitate muscle relaxation before stretching. The therapist comfortably and in a pain-free manner lengthens the tight muscle to the barrier. The client then **isometrically** (without moving the joint) and **maximally** (using full strength) contracts the muscle against the therapist's resistance for five to 10 seconds *(Kisner, Colby, 1990)*. When the muscle begins to fatigue, the client should fully relax the muscle. The therapist passively stretches the muscle by moving the limb through the range that has been gained to the new barrier. The procedure is then repeated until the desired length is achieved.

✦ Effects: Hold-relax lengthens soft tissue when **pain** and restricted ranges are present *(Basmajian, Nyberg, 1993)*.

Contract-relax

Contract-relax technique also uses maximal contraction and relaxation to facilitate a stretch. The therapist comfortably and in a pain-free manner lengthens the tight muscle. The client **concentrically** (contracting the muscle while it is shortening) and **maximally** contracts the tight muscle against the therapist's resistance for five to 10 seconds *(Kisner, Colby, 1990; McAtee, 1993)*. It should be noted that the client has the **intent** to move, although the therapist allows only **minimal** motion to occur *(Basmajian, Nyberg, 1993)*. As with the hold-relax technique, the fatigued muscle is relaxed by the client, then the therapist moves the limb through its new range. The technique is repeated. The stretch portion of this technique seems to cause the Golgi tendon organs to fire, relaxing (autogenically inhibiting) the muscle *(Kisner, Colby, 1996)*.

✦ Effects: Contract-relax is used to lengthen soft tissue when there is **no pain** present.

Post-isometric Relaxation (PIR)

Post-isometric relaxation was developed by Karel Lewit in the 1980s *(Lewit, Simons, 1984)*. It uses resisted minimal isometric contraction followed by relaxation and gentle stretch. Although the terms are often used interchangeably, PIR differs from hold-relax and contract-relax techniques in the force of the client's contraction, as well as in the use of breathing and specific eye movements which increase the stretch.

For PIR, the therapist slowly, passively stretches the muscle to the barrier, or onset of resistance only. The stretch is within a pain-free range. The client is then instructed to **gently, isometrically** and **submaximally** (using less than full strength) contract the muscle against the therapist's minimal resistance for up to 10 seconds, while **inhaling** slowly and deeply (*Lewit, 1993; Travell, Simons, 1992*). In a submaximal contraction, only a partial contraction is used, usually 10 to 25 per cent. An example of client instructions for maintaining a submaximal contraction are "contract this muscle with just a portion of your strength".

✋ The client then **completely relaxes** the muscle. This relaxation is helped by taking a full breath and then slowly **exhaling** through pursed lips, completely emptying the lungs. The therapist instructs the client to concentrate on total relaxation of the muscle during exhalation. Once full relaxation of the muscle has occurred, the therapist then gently stretches the muscle, stopping at the point of resistance, or barrier, and before pain. The stretch is not forced. The procedure is repeated three to five times and the therapist may not feel the muscle give way until the second or third repetition of the cycle (*Lewit, Simons, 1984; Chaitow, 1988*).

✋ The client can be instructed to add specific **eye movements** (or direct her gaze) to increase the range of PIR. In general, gazing in one direction facilitates movement in this direction and inhibits movement in the opposite direction. (The reader can experience this by looking to the left as the head is turned to the left. This is compared to the difficulty experienced when looking to the right as the head is turned to the left.) Flexion, extension and rotation of the head and trunk are facilitated by eye movements. For example, to increase the stretch to the right upper trapezius, the client is instructed to look to the left while exhaling (*Lewit, 1993*). Sidebending is not affected by the addition of eye movements.

✦ Effects: PIR lengthens soft tissue, helps to decrease muscle tone and symptoms of trigger points, and is highly specific in aligning the direction of force and individual muscle fibres.

Agonist Contraction

An active inhibition technique, agonist contraction relies on reciprocal inhibition — or the reflex relaxation of the muscle opposing the contracting muscle — and stretch.

The terminology of this technique may be confusing at first. In order for one muscle to contract, the opposing muscle must relax. The usual reference point is the tight or shortened muscle, which is called the *agonist*. The muscle that opposes it is usually called the *antagonist*. In this technique, however, the terminology is **reversed**, since the reference point is the muscle that **opposes** the tight or spasmed muscle. This opposing muscle, used as the reference point, is referred to in this technique as the *agonist*.

✋ Agonist contraction can be performed by the client, or by the therapist working with the client. In the first method, the **client** is instructed to **maximally** contract the muscle opposing the tight muscle (the former described in this case as the agonist). This contraction is held for five to 10 seconds. The tight muscle (described as the antagonist) is reciprocally inhibited, allowing it to relax and lengthen. This is especially useful when reducing muscle spasms. For example, a spasming gastrocnemius is reciprocally inhibited when the client is instructed to contract tibialis anterior by bringing her toes up towards her knee.

✋ In the second method, the **therapist** slowly, smoothly and **passively lengthens** the tight muscle (the antagonist) to a comfortable position that is pain free. The client **submaximally** and **concentrically** contracts the muscle opposing the tight muscle (the agonist) against the therapist's resistance. The contraction is held for five to 10 seconds while the limb moves in its range. Once again, the tight muscle is reciprocally inhibited, allowing it to lengthen *(Kisner, Colby, 1990)*.

✦ Effects: Agonist contraction is used to lengthen soft tissue when tightness, pain and spasm are present.

A Last Word about Active Inhibition Techniques

There is confusion surrounding terminology and the names of the many active inhibition techniques that exist. Active inhibition techniques started out as part of a larger system called Proprioceptive Neuromuscular Facilitation (PNF), which was developed in the 1940s by Herman Kabat, MD, and Margaret Knott, PT, to treat people with poliomyelitis. This system first assesses the patient for dysfunctional patterns of muscle strength, posture and movement. It helps to decrease pain as well as to regain stability, coordination and range of motion of the trunk and limbs. This is achieved through complex passive and active movement patterns of the whole body, isotonic and isometric resistance exercises to help regain mobility and strength, and hydrotherapy applications to reduce pain *(Basmajian, Nyberg, 1993)*. Physiotherapists and sports therapists have focused on the stretching aspect of this system *(Kisner, Colby, 1996; McAtee, 1993; Brukner, Khan, 1993)*.

Part of the confusion surrounding active inhibition techniques is in the type and force of the contraction used. The contraction may be isometric or isotonic, while the force can be submaximal or maximum, depending on the specific technique *(Basmajian, Nyberg, 1993; Chaitow, 1988; McAtee, 1993; Travell, Simons, 1983)*. Another area of confusion is definitions of certain terms. For example, the standard kinesiological definition of isotonic contraction differs from Kabat's PNF definition. Kinesiology defines isotonic contraction as a constant contraction **with** movement, whereas Kabat defines it as a constant contraction in which the patient has the "**intention**...to create movement" *(Basmajian, Nyberg, 1993)*. Finally, some techniques have undergone name changes over several years *(Kisner, Colby, 1996, 1990)*.

Passive Stretching

In a passive stretch, both contractile and noncontractile tissues are lengthened. Before passive stretching is performed, some form of active free movement, active inhibition technique or an application of heat is used to prepare the tissues. Passive stretching is performed while the client has relaxed the muscle to be stretched. The therapist can then stretch the muscle and the shortened connective tissues that are restricting the range of motion.

🖐 The therapist controls the direction and duration of the stretch, as well as the force and speed used. The stretch is applied slowly and held for between 15 and 30 seconds to ensure that the connective tissues are fully stretched beyond their resting length. This increases available range. The stretch is then repeated several times *(Kisner, Colby, 1990)*.

It is important to note that passive stretch is not the same as passive relaxed range of motion. A passive stretch is applied into the **restricted** range of motion, increasing the range, while passive relaxed range of motion is applied within the **unrestricted** available range.

✦ Effects: Passive stretching lengthens contractile and noncontractile soft tissue.

Passive Joint Mobilization

Passive joint mobilization (also called joint play techniques) is used to stretch the soft tissue crossing the joint and the joint capsule itself, increasing the joint range. Pain and spasm are also reduced in muscles crossing the treated joint.

🖐 The technique is performed by the therapist who gradually applies distraction and a controlled pressure at the end of the available passive joint range. See joint play in the non-Swedish massage techniques chapter for more details including contraindications.

✦ Effects: Passive joint mobilization (joint play techniques) stretch joint capsules, increase range and decrease pain and spasm.

Self-stretching

Self-stretch is usually a part of self-care. The client stretches her own soft tissue using her body weight as the stretch force. The client may also actively inhibit a muscle to increase its length using the principles of agonist contraction outlined above. The direction, duration, force and speed of the stretch are the same as passive stretching, but are controlled by the client. A stretch is held from 15 to 30 seconds without bouncing the muscle *(Kisner, Colby, 1990)*.

✦ Effects: In self-stretching, the soft tissue is lengthened by the client.

Resistance Exercise

A resistance exercise is any form of active exercise in which the client's muscular contraction is resisted by an outside force. The contraction may be static (isometric or without moving the joint) or dynamic (isotonic or with joint movement).

The resistance may be provided by the therapist, referred to as *manual resistance*. It may be provided by weights (either free weights or machines) or by other equipment (rubber tubing or Therabands).

Contraindications

✦ Contraindications to resistance exercises include the acute stage of healing, paralysis and severe pain on exercising.

Over time, resistance applied to a contracting muscle will increase its strength, endurance and overall physical function. Resistance exercises are used when pathology, immobilization or disuse result in muscle weakness.

✦ Effects: Resistance exercise increases the strength, function and endurance of a muscle.

Active Resisted (AR) Isometric Exercise

In AR isometric exercise, the muscle contracts statically or **isometrically**, without any visible joint motion or muscle shortening.

✐ Strength will increase if an isometric contraction is maintained against resistance for more than six seconds *(Kisner, Colby, 1990)*. The client can begin these exercises with submaximal contractions, using a portion of the muscle's strength only. However, strength will develop only at the position of the muscle in which the exercise is performed. If possible, the joint should be moved through its range, with the resistance applied at several points.

✦ Effects: Isometric exercises are used to maintain muscle strength and circulation when a joint is unstable or immobilized and in the early stages of healing when tissue is fragile.

Active Resisted (AR) Isotonic Exercise

In AR isotonic exercise, the muscle contracts dynamically or **isotonically**. A concentric contraction exercise occurs as the muscle shortens, while an eccentric contraction exercise occurs as the muscle lengthens. As the muscle lengthens or shortens through its available range of motion, the client resists against a constant or variable load.

✦ Effects: Isotonic exercises are used to increase muscle strength once full range of motion has been regained.

Suggested Progression of Remedial Exercise with Injury

The client's condition and the desired effects of the exercises should be considered by the therapist before incorporating remedial exercises into treatment or recommending a self-care program.

Consider two joint conditions: frozen shoulder, a condition of reduced motion, and dislocation, an overstretch injury. The range of motion of a frozen shoulder should be increased before the rotator cuff muscles are strengthened, since a muscle that cannot fully lengthen cannot regain full strength. In contrast, with a subacute shoulder dislocation, the strength of the muscles crossing the joint must be regained for joint stability before the range of motion is increased.

The term *progression of remedial exercise* includes the order in which remedial exercises are performed and the change in the range of motion and strength. Progression of remedial exercise is different depending on the injured tissue and the severity of the injury. Remedial exercise goals for an acute or severe injury are to maintain available range of motion and muscular strength. In the case of a chronic or mild injury, the focus is generally on increasing the range of motion and muscular strength.

With Muscle Injury

Early Stages of Muscle Healing

✦ **Passive relaxed** ROM in pain-free inner to mid-ranges is used to maintain joint range. Stretching is contraindicated to prevent further damage.

✦ **Active assisted** ROM is used if necessary, maintaining joint movement and some muscle strength.

✦ **Active free** ROM in a pain-free range is used to maintain joint range and some muscle strength.

◆ **Active resisted isometric** strengthening using a submaximal contraction is used to maintain or increase strength. Because the muscle is not changing length, this exercise will not stress the healing tissue *(Kisner, Colby, 1990)*.

Later Stages of Muscle Healing

◆ **Passive relaxed** ROM in pain-free middle to outer ranges is used to maintain joint range. This can progress to passive joint mobilization.

◆ **Passive joint mobilization** is used to stretch the joint capsule and ligaments if necessary.

◆ **Active free** ROM in a pain-free range, progressing to the onset of pain, is used to maintain joint mobility and some muscle strength.

◆ **Passive and active stretching** are used to lengthen the soft tissue.

◆ **Active resisted isometric** strengthening using a maximal contraction may be used to increase strength. This should progress to active resisted isotonic exercises.

◆ **Active resisted isotonic** strengthening is used to increase strength once joint range has been regained *(Kisner, Colby, 1990)*.

With Joint Injury

Early Stages of Joint Healing

◆ **Active resisted isometric** pain-free strengthening is used to maintain and increase the strength of muscles crossing the joint, increasing joint stability.

◆ **Passive relaxed** ROM is used to treat only the proximal and distal joints. The injured joint is **not** moved passively in the acute stage.

◆ **Active free** ROM is performed in a pain-free range.

Later Stages of Joint Healing

◆ **Passive relaxed** ROM is introduced only after the joint is stabilized by the muscles crossing it, usually in the late subacute stage. At first it is kept within mid-range of the joint, limited by pain, avoiding extremes of range. The affected range is introduced last. This is progressed as healing occurs.

◆ **Passive joint mobilization**, pain-free, is used to stress the ligament after frictions, to reduce any intra-articular adhesions and to restore joint biomechanics and proprioception.

◆ **Active assisted** ROM is introduced if necessary, maintaining joint range and some muscle strength.

◆ **Active free** ROM, to the onset of pain only, is used to maintain joint range and some muscle strength.

◆ **Active resisted isotonic** strengthening is used to increase strength once joint range has been regained, usually in the chronic stage. There should be no signs of inflammation *(Kisner, Colby, 1990)*.

Remedial Exercise as Self-care

✍ The client who is motivated to perform a self-care program becomes an active participant in her own health and recovery. The therapist designs an appropriate remedial exercise program after a thorough assessment of the client, checking for decreased range of motion in joints and for muscle weakness. The program should meet the client's current state of fitness and long-term goals. With the client's permission, the therapist should consult any other health care professionals, such as the physician, physiotherapist or chiropractor, who may have prescribed exercises or a specific exercise program. This will ensure a complementary and non-contradictory remedial exercise plan.

✍ The desired range of motion, numbers of repetitions and amount of resistance given for each exercise will depend on the client's degree of injury or postural dysfunction (mild, moderate or severe) and the presentation of pathology or injury (acute, subacute or chronic). For example, someone with a severe, acute injury is advised to move a limb in a pain-free active free range; in this early stage of rehabilitation, this may be only a small movement. A person with a mild, chronic injury will be advised to regain full range and strength. Before sending the client home with an exercise, the therapist should ensure that the client can perform it safely and correctly.

✍ Range of motion and strengthening exercises should progress from those requiring minimal tissue length and strength to those requiring maximum flexibility and strength. This decreases the chances of reinjury and overuse, while gradually increasing range of motion and strength. If pain or swelling is experienced the day after exercise, the exercise is too vigorous. The client is advised that, if this occurs, she should stop the program and apply ice to the area. The therapist then reassesses the exercise program; perhaps fewer repetitions, less force of contraction or less resistance are required.

✍ The program may also need to be adjusted to the client's progress and motivation. It is usually best to give a client two daily exercises, adding one or two more exercises on subsequent visits as the client's health improves. Only an unusually motivated client will comply with a complex exercise program.

✍ The therapist should use a positive and motivating approach to follow-up on the exercise and self-care program, particularly if reassessment shows that the client has not been doing the exercises. Guilt should not be used as a motivator. Phrases such as "Have you done your self-care exercises?" can embarrass the client. Instead, the therapist can remind the client of the usefulness of the exercises, by saying, for example, "I'd just like to remind you that you will improve faster if you are able to do your stretches".

ESTABLISHING THE GUIDELINES FOR TREATMENT

THERAPIST AND CLIENT BOUNDARIES

Linda Ludwig, Fiona Rattray

Boundaries in the context of therapeutic massage refer to the limits established by the therapist in relation to the client, before, during and after the treatment. They can be very concrete such as timing guidelines or more abstract such as the intention of touch. They can be very clear such as the decision not to treat a parent but murky around issues such as the effects of bartering massage for car repairs or a teacher assessing an injured student.

Boundaries are, in part, defined by the concept of the therapeutic relationship: the client arrives for treatment expecting a professional therapeutic process. The therapist has the responsibility to ensure that this trust is not broken. It is also the therapist's responsibility to make any adjustments necessary during the course of a treatment to safeguard proper client-therapist boundaries and professionalism, including referring the client to another therapist for treatment (Pavia, 1995). Boundaries are also governed by legislation for the profession about appropriate behaviour.

Establishing boundaries requires that a person be conscious of her thoughts and actions and the motivation behind the actions, and be able to analyze situations for possible harmful effects on the client or herself. This keeps the therapist from projecting her own beliefs or prejudices on the client. Preconceptions about race, gender, age, sexual orientation, body size, disease processes or people who get diseases can interfere not only with the therapeutic relationship but with the success of the treatment.

Good boundaries prevent the therapist from being triggered by clients, or over-identifying with them. For some therapists this can be especially difficult when treating clients who are terminally ill or elderly.

The client's sense of the healing process must be respected. For example, suggestions for self-care may not be carried out and the client's dysfunction is maintained. The therapist should try to be supportive, but also to explain the limitations in improvement that can be expected.

Some other boundary issues relate to the therapist's confidence in her skills and knowledge versus the client's requests. As a health care professional, the therapist should carry out treatments with confidence in the skill of techniques used, the effects of pressure and knowledge about tissue. For example, the therapist works with the tissue as it presents, using appropriate techniques and pressure, but the client wants ever-increasing pressure (the "no pain, no gain" mentality). If the pressure requested seems too deep or unsafe, the therapist must have the confidence to explain her sense of the tissue's limits and continue to massage at an appropriate depth. The client is then free to return for further treatment or choose another therapist.

Sometimes the client requests massage to an area that seems unsafe to the therapist. For example, massage to the calf is requested to address painful calf cramping. The therapist performs an assessment which might indicate a potentially dangerous condition such as deep vein thrombosis. The client should be informed why calf massage is inappropriate without alarming him. Appropriate treatment plan modifications are made. A referral to a physician is also recommended.

Occasionally, the client's request for increased pressure is from a distorted sense of the meaning of touch. For example, someone with an abuse history may request deeper pressure, causing pain, since the experience of touch is equated with pain. For the therapist to continue to use uncomfortable amounts of pressure just reinforces the abusive nature of touch for this person. If the therapist respects her own sense of appropriate depth, this scenario could be avoided.

The most effective work is done by the therapist who works neutrally — that is, without her own emotions, personal agenda or ego becoming engaged in the treatment. The therapist may think of it as leaving any personal agenda and her ego outside the treatment room. The client is, after all, coming to the therapist for treatment, not the other way around. In addition, the therapist's words and actions should reflect respect for the client and an awareness of the power differential inherent in the therapeutic relationship, both during and outside the treatment.

There is another important boundary concept which is sometimes overlooked. Massage therapists are thoroughly trained to create a respectful and safe environment for the client. The reciprocal side of this concept — in other words, the importance for the therapist to feel safe and to be treated in a respectful manner by the client — should not be forgotten. A student or therapist who feels unsafe during a treatment has the right to terminate the therapeutic relationship.

Timing

One area that is often overlooked in establishing boundaries is the time allotted to do a treatment, also referred to as *timing*. The therapist and the client agree upon a treatment duration — for example, one hour. A portion of that hour, perhaps 15 minutes, may be spent on assessing the client's condition, with the remaining 45 minutes spent on the massage itself. The entire treatment, including the assessment and massage, is, therefore, performed within the agreed-upon treatment duration. The therapist also needs a few minutes at the end of the treatment, before the next client arrives, to keep the first client's ongoing health history form up to date. It is the therapist's responsibility to create a treatment plan for each visit that stays within the agreed-upon time frame. This involves budgeting the time spent on any one area of the client's body so the entire treatment can be completed.

Of course, it is possible for the therapist and client to renegotiate the treatment duration if appropriate. If the half-hour treatment to relieve the effects of a fibrositic headache has not been sufficient, the therapist and client may choose to renegotiate an additional 15 minutes. However, the therapist must take into consideration her schedule for the rest of the day's massage appointments and the client's own schedule for that day.

It is important for the therapist not to go over time on a treatment because this can distort boundaries between the therapist and the client. If the client books a half-hour appointment and the therapist goes over time and performs a 40-minute treatment, the client may now have the expectation that the treatment duration is flexible. He may begin to expect an extra 10 minutes for the cost of a 30-minute treatment. In effect, the therapist is giving her time away at a reduced rate. The client may not necessarily appreciate the lack of boundaries and precision in the treatment duration, especially if he has a daily schedule to follow. If the client goes to a new therapist, he may have a distorted idea of treatment-duration boundaries and may bring these expectations to the new therapeutic relationship.

Emotions and Massage

Massage engages the entire person, physically and emotionally. When a client arrives for an appointment, he is often seeking relief from a physical complaint or stress. He may not even be aware of his emotional state or how the massage might affect this. Emotional releases may occur during a treatment. Several factors contribute to this. The therapist is providing a private space and creating a safe, respectful environment. The power of touch cannot be denied. There is also a phenomenon known as *tissue memory (Upledger, Vredevoogd, 1983; Barral, Mercier, 1988)* which can trigger an emotional response in the client.

Tissue memory is thought to be the remembrance of physical or emotional trauma that is stored in the tissues of the body, especially connective tissue. The fascia may somehow store the kinetic energy of the original injuring force. As the therapist works closer to the lesion site, the client may recall the pain and thoughts that were experienced when the injury first occurred; a release of emotions may result. It is not unusual for the rate of respiration to increase as the person goes into a sympathetic nervous system response.

Some clients seek the sanctuary of the treatment room to release tears and emotional stress they feel building up. For example, a client is aware of holding tension in his neck and shoulders after his house was damaged by fire. He seeks massage to reduce both his muscular and emotional tension. Others may not specifically seek massage for this, but during the treatment feel safe enough to let their emotions out. For example, a person has just experienced a death in the family; he is coping well but being away from everyone in the quiet space of the treatment room, he is able to relax and talk about the death, then begins to cry.

In all cases, it is essential that the therapist be supportive and make the experience safe for the client. The client should not be left alone. The therapist should stop the treatment and stand near the client. It is important that the therapist's own emotions do not become engaged or triggered. A therapist who does not consciously understand her own reactions to emotions is likely unable to put these emotions aside in the therapeutic setting. If, for example, the therapist habitually becomes withdrawn and uncomfortable when somebody cries, she may respond this way when a client cries during treatment. The client may perceive this as not only unsupportive but judgemental *(Haldane, 1984)*. The client should be reassured that his emotions are accepted and that emotional release during massage is not uncommon. If it seems appropriate, the therapist can maintain some gentle physical contact. For example, the therapist can gently place her hands on the client's shoulders. When the client is calm, the therapist should determine whether or not the client would like to continue the treatment.

If the therapist feels it necessary, she may inquire if the client has a support system or people he can talk to about personal issues. If not, a referral to a counsellor may be offered. It is beyond the scope of practice of massage therapists to counsel clients.

Confidentiality must be maintained by the therapist; this applies to anything said by the client during the course of the treatment. Being reminded of this fact can sometimes reassure a client who has revealed personal information during the treatment.

Dual Relationships

A dual relationship is one in which the therapist's professional relationship with the client is merged or blended with another form of relationship *(Pavia, 1995)*. It is essential that the therapist maintains the therapeutic relationship and preserves the integrity of the profession by not entering into a dual relationship with a client.

Such relationships create situations where it becomes increasingly difficult to maintain clear boundaries and the therapeutic process becomes distorted. There is a risk of harm for both parties.

While some dual relationships are clearly defined in legislation, in many cases there are no specific guidelines for dealing with them. The therapist must carefully weigh the benefits against the risks to herself and the client, if a particular relationship is entered into.

One difficult situation is the therapist who lives in a small town; treating acquaintances is unavoidable if a massage practice is to be maintained. The therapist in these circumstances must be ever vigilant of maintaining clear boundaries and setting clear expectations for treatments with clients.

Categorizing Dual Relationships

✦ Dual relationships can be categorized as low, moderate or high risk situations. An example of a **low risk** dual relationship is socializing with a client. Either the client or the therapist may develop minor expectations of the other when the person is seen outside the therapeutic relationship.

✦ **Moderate risk** situations include the therapist who treats a close friend or an immediate family member. The blurring of the therapeutic boundary may, for example, lead to the therapist feeling guilty if the client's health does not rapidly improve, or the client and therapist may emotionally trigger each other.

• Another example of a moderate risk situation is when a massage therapy instructor treats a student enrolled in her course. This example does not include a student volunteering to be the client in a classroom demonstration of techniques, but rather when the student books a series of appointments in the instructor's clinic. In some cases, it may be appropriate for a student to experience a single treatment from an instructor, so the student may directly learn from the instructor's methods. However, an ongoing therapeutic relationship crosses and distorts numerous boundaries including confidentiality, objectivity in grading (whether actual or perceived by other students), expectations for classroom interactions and financial issues.

✦ An example of a **high risk** situation is a sexual relationship between the therapist and the client, regardless of who initiates it. This situation is covered in detail in the following section on massage and sexuality. Sexualizing the therapeutic process or having a sexual relationship is prohibited due to the potential harm to the client. There are severe penalties for the therapist including the revocation of the licence to practise.

Massage and Sexuality

The therapist and client each have their own ideas about the meaning of touch and its relationship to sexuality. These ideas are influenced by cultural concepts about the body and by personal experiences. For many North Americans, the intimacy of touching is often seen primarily as sexual, a concept which is reinforced through the media. In response to this concept, the standards on this continent for secure draping and designation of appropriate areas to massage are well established. People from other cultures, such as many Europeans, are surprised when receiving massage in North America, because the draping covers so much of the body and breast massage is avoided.

While massage therapy itself is not, nor should it be, sexual, the environment may occasionally be challenging, because anywhere from 30 minutes to 90 minutes are spent in direct contact with the client. While both the client and the therapist are capable of creating sexual energy, it is the *therapist* who is responsible for maintaining appropriate professional boundaries and leaving sexual energy outside the treatment room.

During a therapeutic massage, the therapist and client are together often in a private environment. To avoid any obvious misconceptions, the treatment environment should be professional (this does not preclude an interesting decor), the lighting should be adequate (for example, candles can send a mixed message and are not appropriate), the therapist should dress professionally and interactions with the client are friendly but not overly familiar.

Therapist Feels Attracted to the Client

During the treatment, if the therapist feels sexual attraction to the client, as soon as the therapist is conscious of it, the therapist must shift this energy because that intent will be present in how she touches the client.

Control falls to the therapist regarding the intention behind the touch. The expectation of the massage is that the therapist's touch is not focused on sexual arousal, but on treatment of the client's presenting symptoms. It is an enormous breach of trust and a violation of the client on many levels for the therapist to introduce sexual energy or contact into a treatment.

To redirect the energy, the therapist breaks direct contact with the client and takes a few breaths. She focuses on something else. For example, she reviews the treatment plan agreed upon with the client. This refocusing is called *bracketing a thought*. The therapist then performs a new massage technique, so she refocuses her attention. Now refocused, the therapist completes the treatment.

Under no circumstances should a sexual intention be acted upon. It is not only unethical and poses a great risk for potential harm to the client but it is also illegal. For example, in Ontario, sexualization of the therapeutic relationship by the therapist is defined as sexual abuse and prohibited under the *Regulated Health Professions Act*. Sexual abuse of a client includes behaviour, remarks and touching of a sexual nature as well as physical sexual relations. It is *always* the therapist's responsibility to ensure that this abuse does not happen *(Ontario, 1991a; College of Massage Therapists of Ontario, 1996)*.

When the massage is finished the therapist must do some serious thinking about what occurred and why. Counselling should be sought if necessary. If the client rebooks, the therapist must determine for herself if she can maintain appropriate boundaries and intent. If this is not possible, the client should be referred to another therapist with a brief explanation of why. If the attraction is mutual, the therapeutic relationship must be terminated and the client should seek massage from another therapist.

Client Sexualizes Massage

A client can unconsciously or consciously sexualize a massage. Sexual arousal is a function of the parasympathetic nervous system response. Therefore, there is the potential for massage to create feelings of sexual arousal in the client any time sympathetic nervous system firing is decreased. Sexual arousal, however, is not purely physical: it also depends on tactile and psychological responses or intent *(Vander et al., 1994)*. There is a variety of ways to deal with the situation, depending on the therapist's sense of whether it is unintentional or intentional.

Unintentional

As the client relaxes, perhaps drifting in and out of sleep, the therapist perceives that sexual energy is present for the client as a product of relaxation. The therapist may choose to *redirect* the energy. The therapist should stop whatever technique is being performed and break contact with the client. A different technique is then used. It may be one that affects the sympathetic nervous system, such as brisk tapotement, or one that uses more focused pressure to a particular area, such as treating a trigger point. A stretch may be performed to create a different stimulus.

The *client's* focus is redirected to the treatment plan as the therapist begins to talk about the purpose of the techniques used and their effect on the tissue, or asks for feedback about the tenderness or tension in the area being worked on. Providing that the energy has shifted, the treatment is continued following the treatment plan.

Intentional

A client arriving for massage with the conscious intent to be aroused is not always obvious about it. Once treatment is underway, this intent may be indicated in a number of ways, such as rubbing the genitalia into the table. A male client may have an erection, genitalia may be exposed, a female client may move the draping to expose her breasts, inappropriate sexual comments may be made or stories may be related.

This is also a breach of the therapeutic relationship and a potentially harmful situation for the therapist, making her feel victimized or ashamed. In this situation the therapist must do more than shift the energy. There are different strategies for dealing with this.

The therapist can clearly state what she feels is happening in what is called an "I statement"; for example, "I feel that you are generating sexual energy". The therapist should let the client know that sexual energy is not appropriate in the context of therapeutic massage. Potentially, this allows the client to respond and clarify what is happening.

For some therapists it is difficult to state, "I feel you are generating sexual energy" or some similar statement. It may be more comfortable to say, "I think that the type of massage I do is not the kind of massage that you're looking for." This also allows the client to respond. If the client denies this is the case, the therapist needs to make a decision as to whether she feels safe about continuing the treatment. If the treatment continues, the strategies for redirecting energy are used. If the therapist does not feel safe, the treatment should be terminated. As with all treatments, the incident is objectively documented on the client's file.

Such situations are very difficult for the therapist, especially students and new therapists. Too often there is so much emphasis on the client's needs, that a therapist is reluctant to terminate both the massage and the client-therapist relationship, even when the therapeutic relationship is breached and the therapist's own boundaries are crossed. Termination of treatment should not be treated lightly but must be considered an option.

9

COMMUNICATION BETWEEN THERAPIST AND CLIENT

Linda Ludwig, Fiona Rattray

Background to Clear Communication

One of the strengths of massage therapy lies in the fact that massage therapists spend more time with the client than do most other health care practitioners. This abundance of clinical time allows the massage therapist to gather information from the client that is necessary to create an appropriate treatment. The therapist can explain to the client about her condition, what will happen during the massage treatment and what the client can do after the treatment to encourage the healing process. It is not uncommon for a therapist to hear a client say, "Oh, now I understand why I should put cold on an acute injury. No one has ever explained it to me before."

Gathering information and educating the client require clear communication. Communication involves both the information the therapist exchanges with the client and the manner in which this information is conveyed. Some components of clear communication include using an appropriate tone of voice, being non-judgemental, using accessible vocabulary and having good listening skills.

During all communications with the client a neutral voice is used. While communication can never be entirely objective and clear, using a neutral voice means asking a question or phrasing a statement in words that are as neutral as possible in tone, content and meaning. Care is taken not to lead the client or make assumptions about her symptoms. Generally, open-ended questions are used; these are questions that require more than a yes or no answer. The therapist should not be overbearing, especially if the client is uncertain about having some aspect of the massage performed. Likewise, an overly solicitous manner may seem condescending or diminishing to the client. A calm, confident tone of voice is especially important when working with a first-time client, who likely has no idea of what therapeutic massage entails and has questions about what will happen during the treatment.

The concept of initial neutrality is also important when responding to a client's health

97

history information. For example, a client reports that she is pregnant and the therapist replies, "That's great! Congratulations!" However, for whatever reasons, this may not be great for the client. The therapist's statement, no matter how sincere, is not initially neutral and the client may think that the therapist is not really going to listen to her concerns. The client is more likely to say what is true for her if the therapist responds instead with the neutral, "How do you feel about that?"

It is important for the therapist to choose language that does not convey negative stereotypes or have double meanings. For example, describing a limb as "uninjured" or "injured" avoids the judgemental terms "good side" and "bad side". When describing areas of the client's body that will be uncovered by the top sheet during the treatment, "uncover your leg" has less potential for misunderstanding than "expose your leg".

Avoiding language with negative stereotypes is also important with people who have physical or other disabilities. Labels such as "an epileptic" or "a hemiplegic" focus on the condition or disability, not on the person as a whole. The intention is to describe the person first rather than the disability. Examples of this type of respectful wording are "the person with epilepsy" and "the person with hemiplegia". Similarly, the phrase "uses a wheelchair" replaces "wheelchair-bound" and the phrase "person who experienced" replaces "victim of". The therapist can also listen to the language the client uses to describe herself and ask how the client prefers to be described. For more information see the communication skills chapter under conditions of the central nervous system.

Therapists are taught to understand and use anatomical and medical terminology. They are also expected to communicate with other therapists and health care professionals using proper vocabulary. The client, however, may not be familiar with this terminology. Instructions such as "extend your knee", "turn supine" or "I'd like to treat your pectorals" may not be clearly understood. One method of communicating clearly is to use lay terms or common words to describe things. The examples above then become "straighten your knee", "turn onto your back" and "I'd like to treat the muscles of your upper chest". Another method is to combine both the lay and medical terms, which may help to educate a client in medical wording. The last example above then becomes "I'd like to treat the muscles of your upper chest, or the pectoral muscles". The therapist may wish to point to these muscles on himself. An advantage of this method is that it does not assume the client is unfamiliar with medical vocabulary. It also allows for education in terminology if the client is unfamiliar with these words. Flip charts, diagrams and anatomical models can also be used to help the client visualize a particular structure.

Gathering information from the client about her health history before the treatment involves some additional skills. Some clients do not say much because they do not understand the relevance of their past health history to massage therapy or are impatient to start the massage. Other clients are very forthcoming about their health histories, sometimes giving an overabundance of details related (or unrelated) to their condition. The therapist may either have to coax information from the client, or redirect the client's flow of information. The therapist should acknowledge the client's needs: "You seem in a hurry to get the massage started" or "That's a great story. How about we finish this assessment and you can tell me the rest once you're on the table". This is followed by a brief explanation of why a complete assessment is necessary: "So that I can develop a safe and effective treatment plan for you".

Especially with a first-time client, the therapist should explain that all information given is confidential, unless the client gives specific written permission to share it with another health care practitioner or third party. Confidentiality is intended to prevent a client from feeling vulnerable about disclosing her health history. This confidentiality of the client's written records and verbal information is protected by law. Treating the client's health history information confidentially and respectfully also means refiling the paperwork after a treatment, instead of leaving the health history document lying about.

During the treatment, communication also involves information from the client to the therapist about sensation, such as pain, that the client may be experiencing. Some people are able to describe what they are feeling easily, especially if they have had massage before. Others may need to be offered examples and a possible vocabulary. In this case, the therapist might say, "When I'm working on these muscles in your neck, you may feel sensations in another part of your body; for example, discomfort or tingling into your arm." However, it takes a certain amount of skill to offer possibilities without leading the client to conclusions that are not what the client is really feeling.

It is important for the client and therapist to communicate during the treatment. The amount of talking should be directed by the client; some clients say very little during a massage, while others are more comfortable talking. However, continuous conversation can move the therapist's focus from the treatment, making the work less effective. It may also distract the client from feeling the massage. For people who like to talk, it is often comfortable to chat during part of the massage; and then the therapist directs the client to focus on her breathing or a specific area being treated. A comfortable balance for both the client and the therapist between complete silence and too much conversation is ideal for the effectiveness of the massage.

Consent to the Treatment Plan

Why Use a Treatment Plan?

A verbal treatment plan is simply an outline of what the therapist proposes to do in the treatment session, including the pre-treatment assessment, cost and the duration of the treatment, described in language that the client can understand. Consent to the treatment plan, often called *consent to treat* or *informed consent*, means that the client understands and agrees to what the therapist is suggesting.

For those therapists who are regulated under a health care act, consent to treat is required by law. Informed consent applies to other health care professions as well as massage therapy. Whether required by law or not, the purpose of the treatment description is to demystify health care procedures and to create informed health care consumers who, perhaps for the first time, are able to make choices on their method of treatment.

The importance of this concept can be illustrated if the reader remembers a personal situation where a health care provider either did not describe a particular procedure ahead of time or did not describe what the reader would experience during or after a procedure. While some people may not wish to know all the details, having enough information about the potential risks and benefits of a procedure gives the person a sense of control and choice in the situation.

Presenting the Treatment Plan

The process of creating and presenting a treatment plan begins when a prospective client phones to book an appointment; it is important to inform the client of the cost of the treatment and to request that she arrive a few minutes early to fill out a health history form. Cost and duration of treatment are part of the information the client needs to make a choice about the massage.

However, just because a client books an appointment does not mean she has automatically consented to massage; she may be gathering information about massage and may decide it is not for her.

After the client has arrived for the treatment and completed the paperwork, client and therapist proceed to the treatment room. The therapist refrains from asking personal health questions until in the privacy of the treatment room.

The therapist informs the client that all information is confidential and explains that gathering this information is necessary to create an effective and safe treatment. After taking a few moments to read over the client's health information, the therapist reviews the form with the client to be sure all the information is complete. For example, if a client has left the part on the health form that has to do with medication use blank, it may indicate several things. The client may indeed not be taking any medication; or she may be taking over-the-counter medication such as Aspirin and not interpret this as medication use; or she may be taking a herbal preparation and also not consider this medication use. Both the Aspirin and the herbal remedy could have an impact on certain techniques the therapist chooses, contraindicating their use. These are important pieces of information for the therapist to have in the creation of a safe, effective treatment plan.

At this time, the therapist may ask more questions to clarify and complete the information on the health history form and he may review why the client is there for treatment. See the chapter on assessment for details on health history forms.

Consent to Assess

Usually some form of assessment is required before the treatment plan can be determined. An assessment gives the therapist an idea of which soft tissue condition the client is most likely to be experiencing and which specific structures are involved. Even if the client's focus is relaxation with no specific condition to be treated, the therapist should at least assess the client's breathing patterns. Assessment includes the verbal health history information already obtained, as well as observations, palpation and testing done by the therapist; these involve looking closely at the client and touching or moving the client. In order to perform the rest of the assessment, the therapist needs to obtain consent to assess.

Consent to assess is a subcategory of consent to treat; it is used to inform the client of the assessment process and what the client may experience.

For example, if the therapist thinks that a postural assessment is necessary, the client is told that she will need to stand upright while the therapist observes how the client's body is aligned. It is often easier if the client wears shorts and a T-shirt for this, so she will need to know this also.

If palpation of a specific structure is needed — for example, to assess whether heat, tenderness or swelling is present — the therapist discusses why palpation is necessary and asks the client to let him know if the structure is tender. If testing is required, the therapist briefly describes the test position and movements, explains that testing may temporarily exacerbate the client's symptoms and asks the client to report any symptoms experienced.

The therapist asks the client if she has any questions (and answers them). He then gets the client's agreement to assess. See the chapters on assessment and preparation for treatment for more details on how to perform an assessment.

Consent to Assess Includes

+ Confidentiality of information
+ Why assessment is necessary
+ A brief description of what will happen
+ What the client will wear if different from street clothes
+ The areas to be observed, touched or moved
+ That assessment may temporarily exacerbate symptoms
+ That the client should describe any symptoms experienced during assessment
+ Does the client have any questions?
+ Does the client agree to the assessment?

Example of Consent to Assess Statement

"From your confidential health history information, I see that you have been experiencing low back pain. In order for me to figure out what structures are involved, and what I should treat, I'd like to perform some assessment. You can take your shoes off and sit on the table. I'll be asking you to move into certain positions, then placing you into certain positions. During the tests, your symptoms may temporarily return; please tell me if they do, at which point we'll stop the tests. Do you have any questions? Do you agree to the assessment?"

Consent to Treat

Now that the therapist has an idea of the client's health history, which structures need to be treated and what techniques are appropriate, the actual treatment plan is formulated. There are several components of the plan; these can be assembled in an order that suits the therapist.

The therapist lets the client know the goals of that day's treatment, such as reducing pain or increasing the range of motion of a particular joint.

Before the treatment begins, the client needs to know what position she will be in: prone, supine, sidelying or seated. If a face cradle is used, the client is instructed on how to position her head. If pillows are used, their position is described so the client knows where they go.

The therapist lists the areas of the client's body that will be treated in the proposed plan. A rationale may be needed to explain why certain areas are treated. For example, a client may not understand why the therapist wants to work on the client's abdomen to treat the back pain she is experiencing unless the therapist mentions that iliopsoas, a muscle palpated deep in the abdomen, can refer pain into the back.

If a client is uncomfortable having a particular area worked on, the description of areas to be treated allows her to ask that this area be omitted from today's treatment. For example, a person may have numbness and tingling around an old scar and be initially uncomfortable with it being touched. While lists can be made up of areas that some clients may find sensitive, such as the throat, abdomen and adductors, it is impossible to know what area a client will feel uncomfortable having treated, if in fact she feels this way at all. It is non-judgemental to just list the areas in the proposed plan and let the client choose. The only exceptions to this are nipples and genitalia which are never appropriate for massage therapy treatment and are outside the scope of practice for massage therapists.

Many first-time clients are worried about how much clothing to take off and whether they will be totally uncovered while they are on the table. The next part of the treatment plan addresses this concern. Depending on the areas that the therapist will be treating, the client is asked to take off as much clothing as is comfortable once the therapist has left the room. She is instructed to get between the sheets and cover herself with the top sheet (this prevents the therapist from returning to the treatment room and discovering that the client is lying on top of both the sheets). She is told that she will be covered, or draped, by the sheets during the treatment and that only the areas of the client's body that are being treated will be uncovered while the therapist is working on them.

Clients may worry that massage may be painful or uncomfortable. The client is informed that, during the treatment, the pressure can be adjusted so the client is comfortable. For some treatments, temporarily uncomfortable techniques, such as frictions, are useful to reduce symptoms, but ultimately techniques are used within the client's pain tolerance and may be stopped any time the client wishes. It is also possible that after the treatment the client may experience discomfort; the client is advised as to the self-care she can use to alleviate this possibility. Pain during or after treatment is an example of a risk of treatment.

What about the benefits or positive effects of massage? The client is informed of these, as, for example, when treatment may decrease pain and swelling around an injured joint.

If the therapist wants to use heat, cold or remedial exercise such as a stretch in the treatment, the client is informed of this also.

Once the client has a picture of the treatment, she is asked if she needs any assistance in getting on the table.

The therapist lets her know that this plan can be changed or stopped at any time, even during the treatment. She is given a chance to ask any other questions she may have before she agrees to the proposed treatment plan.

If the client hesitates over a particular aspect of a treatment plan, the therapist should not pressure the client to agree against her will, even if he perceives it as a key element to the success of the overall treatment. For example, the assessment reveals that the client's back pain is related to her flat feet and the therapist includes foot massage in the treatment plan. If the client says, "I'm a little uncomfortable having my feet massaged because they're ticklish", the therapist respects this limitation. He simply reviews the rationale for the approach and has the client consider it for next time, or offers some self-care that may also help with the foot concern.

Occasionally the health history information or the results of the testing will indicate contraindications or modifications to the treatment plan; or even that the client should be referred to another health care provider instead of having massage. In such a case, it is important to explain either the contraindications or modifications to the plan, or that massage is not appropriate that day, and refer the client appropriately.

Consent to Treat Includes

✦ Goal of treatment

✦ Position of client

✦ That the client will be covered (or draped) except for area worked on

✦ That the client will be between sheets

✦ Pillow position

✦ Areas of body treated and rationale for this

✦ That the client will remove clothes according to client comfort once therapist leaves the room

✦ That the amount of pressure used can be adjusted

✦ Risks of treatment

✦ Potential benefits of treatment

✦ Alternatives to plan (if needed)

✦ Hydrotherapy, stretching

✦ Contraindications (if present)

✦ Cost and duration

✦ Does the client need assistance getting on the table?

✦ Does the client have any questions?

✦ Does client consent to the plan?

Successfully Communicating the Treatment Plan

If unfamiliar with the concept of a treatment plan, the reader by now may be wondering how all this can be said in less than three minutes, let alone remembered by the client. The goal of the treatment plan is to inform the client so she feels more relaxed and has a sense of what will happen. It takes a bit of practice for the therapist to choose wording that makes the consent statement informative and concise, while using terms that are clear to the non-medically oriented client.

The information does not have to be in a particular order; indeed, some of the treatment plan components are said before the client is in the therapist's office; and consent to assess happens before the treatment plan.

Once the therapist practises a few times, the wording will be familiar and the tone more casual. The therapist can also keep in mind how he felt the first time he had a massage and the questions he had about what would happen during the treatment; this should help in how to convey the information.

Example of Consent to Treat Statement

The example below is one way to state a treatment plan once the client has been assessed. *The therapist should check local regulations, if any, concerning the specific contents of a treatment plan.*

"The results of the tests show that the muscles in the front of your hip and thigh are tight, which could be causing your low back pain by tipping your pelvis forward. Lengthening these muscles may help to reduce the back pain that you are experiencing.

"I'd like to start the treatment with you lying between the sheets face up on the massage table. This pillow goes under your knees. You will be covered at all times by a sheet, except for the part of your body I'm working on.

"In this half-hour treatment, I'd like to first work on the front of your thighs and then on a muscle called iliopsoas, which is deep in your abdomen and runs across the front of your pelvis. It can refer pain into your low back. (The therapist can point to the area on himself or on a muscle chart).

"Once these muscles are relaxed and stretched, I'd like you to turn over so that I can work on your low back and the muscles around your hip, which also seem to be tight.

"Let me know if the pressure I'm using is too light or too heavy and I'll adjust my pressure according to your tolerance. Also, if I press on an area and it gives you the same pain or sensation that you've been experiencing, or if it refers elsewhere in your body, please let me know. This tight point in the muscle, called a trigger point, may be contributing to your pain.

"You might feel a little bit sore tomorrow in areas that I've been working on; to help reduce this, you can take a hot bath at home and I'll show you some stretches after the treatment.

"If at any time you feel uncomfortable during the treatment and want me to stop or adjust it in any way, please let me know and I will do so. Is there anything you would like me to leave out? Do you have any questions? Do you agree to this treatment plan?" The therapist waits for the client's responses.

At present, the client's verbal consent to a treatment plan is sufficient. After the treatment, the therapist may wish to have the client initial the health history form beside that day's treatment notes, indicating that consent to the plan was given.

Changing the Plan

In massage therapy, the treatment plan is something that is developed by the therapist with some input from the client so her needs are met.

+ The *client* can modify or change the plan either before or during the treatment. The therapist may then suggest alternatives to the treatment plan, which are accepted or rejected by the client. For example, after hearing the proposed plan which includes a head, neck and shoulder massage, the client says, "Please don't massage my head, I'm going out after this and don't want my hair messed up". The therapist then adjusts the plan appropriately to avoid the head. In another example, the client does not agree to direct work on shortened adductor muscles. The therapist can propose alternatives, such as working through the sheets, a post-isometric stretching technique or self-care hydrotherapy and stretching to effect the changes needed; the client then consents to the plan that is comfortable for her.

✦ The *therapist* can also propose to change a treatment plan part way through a massage. For example, the client has consented to a one-hour full-body relaxation massage. During the treatment of the client's back, the increased tone in these muscles makes the therapist think that the focus needs to be on the upper body, not the legs. The client must consent to the proposed change to the plan, otherwise the original plan is followed.

During and After the Treatment

There are a few elements that are added either during testing, during the massage or at the end of the treatment, otherwise the treatment plan becomes too long and complicated and the client will likely forget what she is being asked to agree with.

These elements are specific information about extremes of pressure, remedial exercises, instructions about getting off the table and specific after-treatment self-care information. These are described just before the therapist is about to use the specific technique or just before the client is asked to perform a certain action.

✦ Extremes of pressure may be either deep or light. To establish a client's tolerance of deep pressure and pain prior to using a particular technique, a "one-to-10 pain scale" can be useful.

  • On this scale, one equals no pain, seven equals the client's pain tolerance and 10 equals extreme pain. The scale allows for differences in people's pain perception. One person's pain tolerance may be quite different from another's; a person's pain tolerance may vary from one day to the next; but a seven, whatever the acutal amount of pressure used, is always the client's maximum *tolerance*.

  • The therapist should not use pressures above a six for general treatment. The client is instructed to tell the therapist if the pain begins to approach a seven; at no point should the pressure cause pain to exceed this number. If the client indicates this level of pain has been reached, the therapist decreases the pressure until the client reports that it is comfortable. The pain scale is useful when treating trigger points or doing deeper fascial work.

  • A client may need information on techniques that use lighter pressure, as some people have a mistaken perception that only deep work is effective. For example, the therapist can explain that lymphatic drainage techniques to reduce swelling must be light to be effective; too much pressure will actually collapse the vessels that move the fluid, making drainage techniques ineffective.

✦ Specific instructions for remedial exercise during the treatment are given as the therapist is ready to use them; care is taken to use clear, accessible language.

✦ At the end of the treatment, the client may feel momentarily dizzy if she sits up quickly. The therapist instructs the client to take her time getting up when the therapist has left the room, to prevent this dizziness.

✦ If needed, specific post-treatment exercises may be demonstrated once the client is up off the table and dressed. The client lets the therapist know she is up and dressed, and the therapist returns to the room. At this point the client is able to watch the therapist demonstrate the exercise, then try the exercise herself while the therapist makes sure she is doing it correctly.

Consent with Repeat Clients

With repeat clients, a treatment plan can educate about massage to a different part of the body than she is used to, or about a new technique.

When treating a repeat client, the therapist reviews the client's health history with her to make sure there have been no changes in the client's health status or personal information since the last appointment.

✦ In terms of the treatment plan statement, the therapist may summarize the initial plan. He simply asks the client's response to the previous treatment and if the previous treatment approach is still acceptable; then he adds the details of any changes necessary for that day's treatment plan.

10

ASSESSMENT

Fiona Rattray, Linda Ludwig

An assessment is an educated evaluation of a client's condition and physical basis for his symptoms in order to determine a course of treatment.

Assessment is in the scope of practice of massage therapists in many places *(College of Massage Therapists of Ontario, 1996)* and is a component of post-graduate courses sanctioned by professional associations *(Lowe, 1995; American Massage Therapy Association, 1998)*. Assessment is in the orthopedic assessment texts written by doctors geared towards practitioners of manual medicine, such as physiotherapists and massage therapists, which clearly show how to perform and interpret the tests *(Brukner, Khan, 1993; Magee, 1992)*.

Massage therapists use the word *assessment* when evaluating the nature of a condition. It is essential to note that an assessment performed by a massage therapist is **not** a diagnosis. The term *diagnosis* is used by the medical profession. Making an assessment versus a diagnosis is the difference between investigating the nature of the condition versus naming that a specific condition is in fact present. Physicians use assessment and interpretation of both X-rays and other laboratory tests to make a diagnosis *(Taber's Cyclopedic Medical Dictionary, 1981)*. A massage therapist is not specifically trained to perform or interpret results of these last two diagnostic tools.

Why Do an Assessment?

An assessment is an essential tool of the massage therapist. The assessment process is about gathering information from the client. However, it involves more than just asking questions about the client's health. It can be a little like detective work: the therapist also looks at the client for clues to further define the client's problem, as well as making specific observations about posture, palpating the client's tissue and performing specific tests. In fact, the assessment for any treatment is divided into four components: health history questions, observations, palpation and orthopedic testing.

Through an assessment, the knowledge available to the therapist enables her to go beyond just treating where the pain is, but rather to treating causes and compensating structures. Without an assessment, of course, the client will feel better for being touched, but the results will be short-lived, because the origin of the client's pain or symptoms has not been determined and addressed. Too often a massage "treatment" involves a general massage of all structures, the therapist not worrying whether it is a muscle or joint or fascia that is the key, or if the pain is referred from somewhere else, or whether it is compensating for a problem elsewhere in the body.

The assessment provides the foundation for designing and performing a safe, knowledgeable and effective treatment. This type of approach — that is, addressing the cause — need not take away from a massage using respectful, intuitive touching with the focus on relaxing the client. Intuition is defined as the action of mentally examining, and looking into; immediate apprehension by the mind or senses without intervention or reasoning. Intuition comes from having accumulated knowledge and experience which then flows out of the person with little conscious effort *(Pirsig, 1974)*. Although many people naturally have caring hands and a nice touch, nothing replaces good training and the ability to perform a thorough assessment to address a client's health issues.

As an example, a therapist is dealing with someone with a history of shoulder dislocation. This therapist is afraid of, or does not see the necessity in, doing an assessment and in turn does not find out if the shoulder joint is stable. It is possible that she could take the arm through a range of motion that might reinjure the shoulder. She will likely not discover the muscles that are weak, in order to give self-care to strengthen them and support the joint. She might avoid movement of the shoulder joint and thus not promote successive action which contributes to good joint health.

On the other hand, another therapist who is very technically oriented performs a total assessment. While this is important, the therapist may be so focused on the results that she forgets to move the limb slowly and cautiously. She may lose sight of the fact that the injured shoulder is attached to a live human being; the client may be caused unnecessary discomfort or distress because the therapist does not observe the person's face or notice the tensing muscles when doing the testing. An effective therapist will balance the natural, caring approach and the technical investigative approach when performing the client assessment.

What if the Client Has Been Previously Diagnosed?

The massage therapist should always perform an assessment, even if the client has been previously diagnosed by another health care professional or has been assessed by another massage therapist. The therapist needs to achieve her own understanding of the client's condition as it relates to a safe, effective massage therapy treatment.

It is also possible that the previous diagnosis or assessment is incomplete or inaccurate. For example, from the authors' clinical experience, a prescription for treatment of a hamstring strain was made when the client actually had an injury to the quadriceps. Another clinical example is a client diagnosed with a common extensor tendinitis and a recommendation for frictions to the tendon; the client turned out after massage therapy assessment to have an extensor muscle strain. Frictioning the healthy tendon instead of treating the injured muscle belly would not have improved the client's condition.

✦ Assessment results give the following information:

- the history of the client's health
- the client's present symptoms and chief complaint
- overall tissue health
- functional ability such as walking or sitting and ability to move joints freely and comfortably
- specific structures involved such as muscles, tendons or joints
- an educated idea of the suspected condition
- contraindications: these could be absolute or require treatment modifications
- the need for referrals to other health care practitioners if symptoms suggest the condition is out of the scope of practice for massage therapy
- the need for referrals to complimentary therapy because the client needs more than just massage — for example, chiropractic treatments along with massage treatment.

The information gathered from the assessment enables the therapist to develop a treatment plan that is effective and safe.

After assessment, clear treatment goals are established, in consideration of any contraindications.

✦ The treatment plan includes decisions about:

- duration of the treatment
- positioning of the client
- treatment of symptoms and structures to be addressed
- specific techniques, both Swedish and non-Swedish
- hydrotherapy and remedial exercise to be used during the massage.

Standardizing Client Records: SOAP Notes

One challenge in gathering data about a person's state of health is how this information can best be organized, interpreted and used by health care professionals. If subjective information, test results, treatment plans and the person's responses to treatment are not clearly organized, the health care that the person needs may not be provided.

In the mid 1950s, Lawrence Weed, MD, began working with this organizational issue. By 1964, he had developed a system he called the Problem-Oriented Medical Record (POMR) for use by nurses and physicians (Weed, 1976). One portion of this system that is widely used today is the documentation method called SOAP notes.

SOAP is an acronym for **S**ubjective, **O**bjective, **A**ssessment, **P**lan. In Weed's original system, **subjective** data is the patient's perception of the current symptoms and his health history; **objective** data is the practitioner's observations, testing, and physical findings; **assessment** is the physician's assessment or diagnosis of the condition, including the severity and prognosis; and **plan** is what the practitioner does to treat the patient, including the overall treatment goals and patient education *(Weed, 1976; 1991)*. (Subjective and objective information are sometimes given the additional acronym "HOPS": History, Observations, Palpation and Special testing.)

As different health care practitioners — physiotherapists, massage therapists, osteopaths and occupational therapists — have used the SOAP note format, different interpretations have emerged for the various letters in the SOAP acronym. In one source, O stands for observations (what is looked for) while A stands for assessment of range of motion and orthopedic testing *(Magee, 1992)*. Osteopaths may include what they palpate, smell and hear in the O of observation *(Kuchera, Kuchera, 1993)*.

Another source defines the A of assessment as the changes in the person's condition, while the P of plan is the suggested future treatment *(Thompson, 1993)*. Some physiotherapists divide the A of assessment into several sub-categories which include a list of the person's problems, long- and short-term goal notes, progress notes and discharge notes *(Kettenbach, 1990)*.

✦ This text is organized to somewhat follow Weed's original definitions for SOAP notes. In the chapters on treatments, there is a **Subjective** information section detailing what the client says, including health history, the effects of previous treatment and self-care techniques and the results of visits to other health care professionals. There is an **Objective** information section that focuses on observations, palpation findings and orthopedic test results. In Weed's original format, an **Assessment** statement is the suspected condition or what the therapist *thinks it is* after combining the subjective and objective information. In this book, definitions of conditions are found at the beginning of each chapter. However, an assessment is also understood by many to *be* the subjective and objective information combined. This common understanding may be a cause for confusion with Weed's acronym. Finally, there is the treatment **Plan**, which in this book is the description of the treatment and the self-care program, including contraindications and referral to other practitioners, if necessary. The intent of this organization is to create categories of information that the therapist can easily insert into the SOAP note format.

Whatever method of collecting information the therapist uses, the health history form and ongoing treatment notes must be kept up to date. Therapists should check for local legal requirements pertaining to record keeping.

✦ Assessment information needs to be recorded in an organized fashion because:
  • the therapist wants a baseline to track the client's progress;
  • it increases the client's awareness and knowledge of his conditions and helps him to be a participant in the process;
  • it allows the therapist to communicate with other therapists in the same clinic who may be treating the client;
  • with the client's written permission, it can form a part of a medico-legal report to other health care professionals and to third-party payers, such as medicare plans or insurance companies;
  • it can provide the therapist with accurate information if the therapist is called to court as a witness.

Based on the fact that a massage therapist does not diagnose, the practitioner is faced with the dilemma of how to record the assessment results and treatment plan. Some statements might be "Assessment results indicate a *possible tendinitis* of the extensor tendons of the right arm" or a *"suspected tendinitis"*. Since the statement is not definitive it is not a diagnosis.

Interpreting the Assessment

An interpretation of the results takes practice and clinical experience; yet, even then, occasionally the test results and, therefore, the treatment plan are unclear. What should the therapist do if she does not have a definitive answer? She reviews the individual pieces of information that she does have. For example, the negative test results show the therapist what the condition is *not*. Individual positive results give data about some structures and perhaps what to do with them. For example, testing shows a client to have short hamstrings; however, the therapist cannot reproduce the source of the client's low back pain. In a case where the source is not obvious and the therapist is unable to suggest a possible cause, rather than getting frustrated and doing just a general low back massage, the therapist treats the short hamstrings to see how this affects the low back. The therapist may do some research between treatments and reassess the client with new questions and tests in subsequent sessions, to slowly build a clearer picture of the problem. It may also be appropriate to refer the client to another care health professional, if no improvement is made.

It is very important that the therapist assess the client with an open mind, avoiding the temptation to draw conclusions until the entire assessment is completed. Preconceptions about the structures affected and even the specific condition the client has can lead to missed information or misinterpreted data. This can result in an ineffective or unsafe treatment.

The new therapist needs to be patient with herself and the process of assessment. It takes practice to feel comfortable asking questions in an organized manner, observing a client's posture, moving a person's body parts around, figuring out what tests to do and the order to do them in and recording the information so it is not forgotten. Just like learning any other skill, it takes practice to perform a thorough assessment in a timely manner. The ultimate benefit of this process is that it provides the therapist with a road map so she has a clear sense of how to proceed with the treatment.

Reassessment

To judge the effectiveness of the therapist's treatment approach and massage, as well as to monitor the client's progress, the therapist should reassess the client **after** each treatment and at the **beginning** of the next one, recording this information on the health history form *(Coulter, 1994)*. The end-of-treatment reassessment does not have to include all of the tests that were initially performed, just the tests pertinent to the day's treatment. A total reassessment can be performed in a month to six weeks. For example, in reassessing a client with hyperlordosis due to short hip flexors, the therapist retests the length of the hip flexors and the pelvic tilt angle at the end of the day's treatment, while a full postural reassessment is performed in six weeks' time.

Health History Questions

Throughout the assessment, the client is encouraged to ask questions, so he can feel informed during this process.

Health history questions are asked by the therapist to gain *subjective information* from the client. These questions are asked before the client is positioned on the massage table and while the client is still clothed. There are several approaches to gaining this information. A portion of the information is obtained in a written health history form that the client fills out before treatment begins *(Figure 10.1)*. This form contains practical information such as the date, the client's name, address, phone number, age, occupation and source of referral as well as the name and phone number of the primary physician. The remainder of the form relates to specific health history information including surgery, allergies, medication use and other health care practitioners seen, past history of illness or injury and today's main symptoms (called the primary or *chief complaint*).

Some clients cannot see the necessity of revealing all their medical information if they "just want a massage"; the therapist should explain that the health history form is required by law, where massage therapy is regulated, and, most important, the information gathered will allow for the development of a treatment plan that will safely meet the needs of the client. The therapist gathers further information by asking the client a series of questions. These questions give the therapist more details which are added to the form.

A suggested method is to begin with questions that review the information on the health history form. With the client informed of this necessity, the therapist then confirms that the client has filled out the form completely. For example, upon noticing that the client has not filled in the section regarding previous injuries, the therapist might say, "I would just like to confirm that you have had no previous injuries".

Questions can be phrased as open-ended or closed-ended or a combination of both.

✦ An **open-ended** approach to questions does not restrict the client's responses as the therapist guides the discussion of the health history. An example of an open-ended question is, "What brings you in for a massage today?" This allows the client to relate the information he feels is important. The greatest challenge with this type of questioning is structuring the discussion carefully to obtain the information needed and to avoid long answers off topic *(Hertling, Kessler, 1990)*.

✦ Another approach is referred to as **closed-ended.** These are questions phrased so they require "yes" or "no" answers, such as, "Do you have a headache now?" While this method of asking health history questions is efficient, the therapist must ask the appropriate questions to elicit all the relevant information. For example, the person may have what he considers a headache but, in fact, it is a migraine. The client may attempt to cooperate by providing the information that is specific to the questions asked rather than elaborating on other information about his symptoms.

A combination of both these methods is often the most effective. Moving from open-ended to closed-ended questions is called the *funnel technique*. In addition to the types of questions, the therapist can also use paraphrasing to confirm data and further gather information *(Goodman, Snyder, 1990)*. Here the therapist repeats the information presented by the client. For example, the therapist may say, "You've told me that the symptoms are relieved by stretching. Are there any other activities or things that you do

Health History Form

This information is to help the therapist to create a safe and effective treatment plan.

Name: _____   Today's Date: _____

Address: _____   Date of Birth: _____

City: _____ Postal Code/ZIP_____   Occupation: _____

Phone: (_____)_____   Work Phone: (_____)_____

How did you hear about us? _____   Physician: _____

What is your chief complaint? _____   Phone: _____

Please check ☑ conditions you are experiencing and ⟨circle⟩ conditions you have experienced in the past.

SKIN
- ❑ rashes/bruise easily
- ❑ infectious skin conditions:
  _____
- ❑ Other: _____

MUSCLES/JOINTS
Indicate Left (L) or Right (R) where appropriate.
- ❑ neck
- ❑ upper back
- ❑ mid back
- ❑ lower back
- ❑ shoulder
- ❑ elbows
- ❑ arm
- ❑ wrist
- ❑ hand
- ❑ hip
- ❑ leg
- ❑ knee
- ❑ ankle
- ❑ foot
- ❑ weakness or loss of strength
- ❑ clumsiness
- ❑ osteoarthritis
- ❑ rheumatoid arthritis
- ❑ other arthritis:
  _____
- ❑ osteoporosis
- ❑ tendinitis:
  location_____ date_____
- ❑ strain:
  location_____ date_____
- ❑ joint sprain/dislocation
  location_____ date_____
- ❑ other injury:
  location_____ date_____

RESPIRATORY
- ❑ asthma
- ❑ bronchitis
- ❑ chronic cough
- ❑ difficult breathing
- ❑ emphysema
- ❑ shortness of breath
- ❑ smoking
- ❑ other: _____

CARDIOVASCULAR
- ❑ bleeding disorder
- ❑ high blood pressure:
  _____
- ❑ low blood pressure:
  _____
- ❑ heart attack
- ❑ heart disease
- ❑ angina
- ❑ stroke/cerebrovascular accident
- ❑ pacemaker
- ❑ varicose veins
- ❑ phlebitis
- ❑ poor circulation
- ❑ other:
  _____

HEAD/NECK
- ❑ visual impairment:
  _____
- ❑ hearing impairment:
  _____
- ❑ speech impairment:
  _____
- ❑ headache/migraine
- ❑ jaw pain (temporomandibular joint [TMJ] pain)
- ❑ sinus problems

GI CONDITIONS
- ❑ constipation
- ❑ diarrhea
- ❑ irritable bowel:
  _____
- ❑ hiatus hernia
- ❑ ulcers

OTHER CONDITIONS
- ❑ allergies
- ❑ cancer
- ❑ diabetes
- ❑ fainting
- ❑ fever
- ❑ insomnia
- ❑ numbness/tingling:
  _____
- ❑ seizures
- ❑ stress

INFECTIOUS CONDITIONS
- ❑ hepatitis: _____
- ❑ HIV
- ❑ TB

FRACTURE: No ❑   Yes ❑
  location_____ date_____

SURGERY: No ❑   Yes ❑
  for what?_____ date_____

MOTOR VEHICLE ACCIDENT:
  No ❑   Yes ❑
  symptoms_____
  _____ date_____

MEDICATIONS currently taken:
(This includes prescription drugs, over-the-counter and supplements)

OTHER HEALTH CARE received:
  _____
  _____

Figure 10.1 The health history form.

which relieve the symptoms?" This method also ensures the information given by the client is clearly understood by the therapist.

As already mentioned, the therapist must remember that clients do not always understand the relevance to massage therapy of their health history or medication use. The fact that a person fractured a leg as a child may not seem to have any bearing on today's low back pain until the therapist explains how a difference in leg lengths can throw off the balance in the client's pelvis, creating compensatory back pain. The client may neglect to mention on the health history form about taking over-the-counter remedies, herbal remedies and medications unless the therapist specifically asks about medication usage of any kind.

The client is encouraged to keep the therapist informed of any changes to his health. Regardless, health history questions should be reviewed before each treatment. This is a brief process whereby the therapist gives a short summary of the relevant facts for confirmation by the client, followed by asking if any changes have occurred since the last treatment. This includes effects of the last massage treatment and a review of current symptoms. For example, a client may be pregnant and have a different symptom picture as the condition progresses; likewise, a client with an injury such as whiplash will have changing symptoms as the tissue heals or if self-care is performed.

Additional Questionnaires

There are several standard questionnaires available to the therapist for documenting how the client feels or is capable of functioning. The Revised Oswestry Questionnaire deals with low back pain and its impact on the client's activities of daily living. The Roland-Morris form also deals with low back pain, while the Vernon-Minor Index assesses neck pain. All three questionnaires use descriptions of the client's daily activities and a pain scale *(Chapman-Smith, 1994)*. The McGill pain questionnaire asks the client to describe the pain experienced using sensory, affective and evaluative terms *(Goodman, Snyder, 1990)*. Salzmann's chart uses standardized pictographs and written descriptions to locate pain and tissue dysfunctions *(Coulter, 1994)*.

General Questions

The following are suggested general health history questions. Additional questions that are specific for certain conditions are located in the appropriate section of each chapter.

+ Does the client have any hearing or vision loss that may affect communication? If so, what can be done to help the situation? For example, if there is a hearing loss, the client may suggest talking more loudly or slowly and making eye contact when speaking.

+ How is the client's health in general?

+ Does the client have any pathological conditions, such as diabetes mellitus, hypertension or cancer? What treatment is the client receiving for this? Is the client on any medication for this condition?

+ Has the client had any major illnesses, injuries or surgery? The nature and time frame of each should be recorded.

+ Is there a family history of the presenting complaint?

+ What are the client's occupation, activities and hobbies? The client can describe or show his posture for each of these, such as sitting at a computer terminal.

✦ What is the client's sleeping posture, if known? Does the client sleep on his side, front or back?

✦ Are there any dietary contributions to the client's condition?

✦ What is the client's present level of stress? How long has this degree of stress been present?

Specific Questions

✦ Is there something in particular for which the client is coming for treatment? This is known as the *chief* or primary complaint.

✦ When did the trauma occur or the symptoms begin?

✦ Where is the affected area? The client is encouraged to point to the area or, if there is a body outline on the case form, to draw on it.

✦ Has this ever happened before?

✦ Can the client describe the mechanism of injury? Was the onset trauma-induced or gradual?

✦ If the injury was trauma-related, what was done at the time of injury? For example, was first aid applied or was an ice pack used?

✦ If onset was gradual, when were the symptoms first noticed?

✦ Have there been a physician's consultation and diagnosis?

✦ Was there medical treatment or other therapy given such as a cervical collar, cast, physiotherapy or chiropractic treatment?

✦ Is the client taking medication specific to the presenting complaint such as Aspirin or anti-inflammatories, including over-the-counter or herbal preparations?

✦ Are there any known complications to the present condition, such as fracture, vascular or nerve damage, thrombus formation or paralysis?

Pain Questions

Pain itself is poorly defined and understood, although it warns of injury or disease. Perhaps the best definition of pain is McCaffery's: "whatever the experiencing person says it is, existing whenever he says it does" *(Porth, 1990)*. The therapist needs to ask a thorough range of questions about pain being experienced by the client.

✦ Does the client have pain now?

✦ Where exactly is the pain?

✦ Does it move or refer to other areas? For example, does the pain start in one place such as the back of the head and then move to another place, such as the forehead?

✦ Can the client describe the pain? Or, more specifically, what is the nature of the pain? For example, is it sharp or diffuse? What is the type of pain? For example, is it hot, achy or bright?

✦ How painful is it, mild, moderate or severe? A pain scale may be useful. On a scale from one to 10, with one meaning mild pain and 10 meaning unbearable pain, what number would be given to this pain?

✦ How long does it last?

✦ How often does it occur?

✦ What relieves the pain?

✦ What aggravates the pain? What activities of daily living are limited, if any?

✦ Are there any other symptoms associated with this condition? For example, is there numbness, tingling, headache, nausea or autonomic phenomena?

Some Common Types of Pain

✦ **Radicular pain** is associated with nerve root compression. Sharp, shooting pain may be accompanied by other neurological signs such as paresthesia corresponding to a dermatome, or muscle weakness *(Brukner, Khan, 1993)*.

✦ **Cutaneous pain** is from superficial tissue damage. It is described as being sharp, bright, burning and well-localized.

✦ **Deep somatic pain** is from muscles, tendons, joints and periosteum. More diffuse than cutaneous pain, deep somatic pain can refer to other areas of the body. These referral patterns are based on the embryological development of the musculoskeletal system *(Hertling, Kessler, 1990)*.

✦ **Visceral pain** arises from visceral distension or ischemia or strong, abnormal gastrointestinal contractions. Visceral pain is often diffuse.

✦ **Referred pain** may come from cutaneous, deeper somatic and visceral tissue. It occurs in tissue that is remote from the original lesion or injury. Referred pain is well localized.

✦ **Functional or psychogenic pain** is believed to arise from the emotions or psyche, but is experienced as though it originates from an organic disorder.

The client's experience of pain can be influenced by his emotional state, culture, past experiences, learned behaviours and motivation *(Porth, 1990)*. Chronic pain in particular can be accompanied by depression and anxiety.

The client's pain experience may also be different from the therapist's experience. For example, as a child the client may have been socialized to freely express his feelings about pain, while the therapist may have grown up with the concept of just "grin and bear it". It is important not to disbelieve or belittle the client's perception of pain during assessment or treatment, for example, by saying, "I hardly moved your knee at all during that test, how could it be that painful?", or "Wow, doesn't that hurt, it looks like it should" or by thinking, "I didn't press *that* hard for him to jump like that". The therapist should instead non-judgementally note and record the client's pain perceptions, and adjust the movement, technique or pressure accordingly.

Any other questions specific to the particular condition are listed in the individual treatment chapters.

Blood Pressure

It is suggested that when a therapist sees a client for the first time, she take the client's blood pressure. How to take blood pressure is described in the chapter on hypertension. Current blood pressure is especially important when treating clients who are pregnant or who have cardiovascular concerns, as treatment modifications may be indicated due to hypertension.

Observations

Observations are the visual clues the therapist looks for in order to gain objective information about the client's condition.

Observations are recorded on the client's health history chart.

Observation begins as soon as the therapist meets the client; functional abilities such as ease of movement, changing positions or removing a coat are noted. Obvious aids are noted such as walking supports or a hearing aid. The facial expression of the client is observed; it may be relaxed, pained or medicated. It is difficult to observe emotions, unless the client states his feelings. If the massage therapist feels it is necessary to record perceived emotions, the wording must remain non-judgemental and should contain objective observations such as, "The client moved and talked slowly. He responded to questions in a monotone voice, with one- or two-word answers."

Postural and Gait Assessment

A more organized and detailed observation is achieved with a postural assessment. A postural assessment analyzes any imbalances in the client's posture that may contribute to the client's condition. A gait assessment analyzes any imbalances in how the client walks. Both of these assessments will require that the client wear either a gown or shorts and a T-shirt, and that the client consent to the assessment before it is performed. Obtaining **consent to perform a postural assessment** involves giving a brief description of why the assessment is necessary, what the procedure is and what the client will wear. See Appendix B for how to perform postural and gait assessments.

✍ When performing a postural or gait assessment, a general overview should be taken first, to look for gross, observable differences. Stepping back from the client, the therapist can bilaterally compare various structures, such as the levels of the shoulders, any rotation in the trunk or the shape of the negative spaces between the arms and the trunk and between the legs.

✍ The therapist also observes for antalgic posture. This is a posture that the client assumes in order to relieve pain. It may give clues as to which structures the client is using to compensate for the existing condition. If the painful condition is a temporary one, such as an ankle sprain, a postural assessment should be performed again once there is no longer any pain to see if the client has developed any compensatory postural changes. If the painful condition is a chronic one, such as osteoarthritis, the client should be periodically reassessed to keep track of any postural changes due to the pathology.

✍ The overview is followed by a detailed and specific postural assessment, described in Appendix B in this text.

117

ℹ Even if a full postural assessment is not performed, a general overview, noting any obvious asymmetries, is the least that should be done.

ℹ The client's gait can be observed. Lack of smooth movement is observed, limping or favouring of a body part is noted. Information is asked about the regular use of observed supports used such as a cane, a walker or a wheelchair.

Other Observations

ℹ Changes in soft tissue are detected as swelling, increased muscle bulk, nodules, tissue wasting or atrophy. Altered contours may be present, such as gaps in a muscle seen with more severe strains or the tunnelling between the phalanges that results with an ulnar nerve lesion.

ℹ Skin details are noted, such as colour (redness from inflammation or pallor from a lack of circulation) and texture (dry and scaly or oily).

ℹ Nail bed changes to look for include splitting, dry, discoloured or clubbed nails.

ℹ Any scars are noted. They may be surgical or traumatic.

ℹ Open wounds may indicate the need for a medical referral; the cause may be a trauma or something more insidious such as a decubitus ulcer or secondary to diabetes.

ℹ Any other observations specific to the particular treatment are listed in the appropriate chapter.

Palpation

Palpation is the placement of the therapist's hands on the client's tissues to assess their condition.

Palpation is a primary tool for the massage therapist. Palpation skills are refined and improved in every treatment the therapist performs. The greater the number of clients a therapist works on, the greater the variations in tissue quality the therapist will experience. This skill is cumulative and, like any skill, must be practised with conscious awareness, constantly.

✚ The three most common errors made while palpating to assess tissue are **lack of concentration** on what is being touched, **too much movement** of the palpating fingers and using **excessive pressure** *(Neumann, 1989)*.

An experienced therapist is able to feel very subtle differences in temperature, tone and texture of the client's muscles and skin. One study measured the accuracy of experienced physiotherapists in detecting temperature differences. When a small metal testing device that could be heated or cooled in a controlled manner was used, the therapists were able to detect absolute temperature differences of plus or minus 0.2 degrees C. In terms of the temperature gradients palpable in a large area of a person's skin, the therapists palpated the entire low backs of patients with low back pain. They were able to detect pathologically significant skin temperature differences of 1 degree C with 100 per cent accuracy *(Boyling, Palastanga, 1994)*.

Any palpation done before the treatment requires **consent from the client**. The process to obtain consent includes the description of the area to be palpated and instructions to the client to let the therapist know if a particular structure is tender or refers pain.

It is the therapist's refined palpation skills and knowledge of anatomy that facilitate the assessment of, among other things, fascial restrictions, adhesions, trigger points, muscle hypertonicity and inflammation. Palpation continues in the massage treatment as the therapist assesses the amount of resistance in the tissues and how they are responding to the treatment. As an example, the therapist considers the effort required to muscle strip the erector spinae muscles; any areas of increased or decreased tightness or fibrosity are noted; there should be awareness of any changes in the tissue, in response to treatment.

The therapist should notice if the client reacts to the pressure of palpation. Some clients will report pain, but others will need to be asked directly, "Is this tender or painful?" The therapist should be vigilant for any response that may indicate client discomfort, such as flinching away from the touch, increased rate of breathing, sweating or flushing.

How to Palpate Effectively

As with other parts of the assessment, palpation of structures, joint alignment and tissue health should be performed in a systematic way. Palpation is always performed **bilaterally**, starting on the unaffected side. Unaffected tissue is compared to the affected tissue. It is easiest if the therapist starts palpation by orienting herself with accessible bony prominences. Palpation is initiated using the palmar surface of the hand and light pressure *(Alexander, 1995);* this allows the bony landmark to be easily located by a broad, light touch. The therapist then palpates towards the specific soft tissue structure, using the fingertips and increasing the pressure.

An awareness of the anatomy and fibre direction of contractile and noncontractile tissue further helps to differentiate specific tissue. A more superficial ligament can be palpated by locating its attachments, then passively stressing it, causing it to become taut under the palpating fingers. A specific muscle can be palpated by locating its attachments, knowing its actions and then having the client submaximally contract the muscle against resistance, causing it to tighten under the palpating fingers. Active resisted isometric contraction is also used to differentiate a muscle from a ligament, because only the muscle is capable of contracting.

The Four "T's" of Palpation

The information gathered from palpation is often organized and recorded into four categories: **temperature, texture, tenderness** and **tone.** These are also referred to as the four "T's" of palpation.

✎ Temperature: Tissue may be hot, indicating inflammation, or cool, indicating ischemia.

✎ Texture: Swelling or edema is present. In an acute condition, this edema may be hard whereas in a chronic condition there is a boggy, congested edema. Healthy tissue has an even texture throughout. Trophic changes indicating muscle wasting may feel soft with little resilience in the tissue. Adhesions feel as if the tissue is stuck together and is less mobile. Crepitus is a palpable roughness in the joint or tendon that is noted with movement and sometimes accompanied by an audible "crunching".

✎ Tenderness: Pain can be indicated if the client winces or pulls away with tissue compression. Some structures may be too painful to be palpated. The therapist notes when the area experiencing pain, tenderness or usual sensation is reported by the client as being different from the area being compressed.

✍ Tone: Tissue may be hypertonic — that is, experiencing an increase in tone relative to nearby muscles — or hypotonic, which is a decrease in tone relative to nearby muscles. The tone should be compared throughout a muscle group.

Any other palpation information specific to the particular treatment is listed in the appropriate chapter.

Testing

Testing is the assessment of the client's current levels of function, using active free and passive relaxed ranges of motion, end feel, muscle length and strength, and a variety of specific orthopedic tests. Testing means looking at the person in a dynamic manner, compared to the static nature of questions and observation.

Tests may be **positive** or **negative** in outcome. A positive test provokes the client's symptoms or reproduces the pain, limitation or weakness the client is experiencing. A negative test does not provoke the symptoms.

When to Test

Testing is performed before the treatment begins, to assess the client's levels of function, to help differentiate the structures that are causing the client's symptoms and to determine whether massage therapy is appropriate for the client's symptoms or whether the client should be referred to another health care practitioner. Testing is also performed at the end of the treatment to assess the effectiveness of the work.

As the therapist becomes more experienced with performing the tests and having the client perform them, she will become more proficient at interpreting results and at determining whether they fall within normal limits for the test.

The client's consent to testing is required before it is performed. Obtaining **consent to test** involves giving a brief description of why the testing is necessary, what the client will wear (appropriately draped or wearing either a gown or shorts and a T-shirt), a brief explanation of the procedure itself, the instructions that the client should stop the test or that the therapist will stop the test if it is painful and that the procedure may temporarily aggravate the client's symptoms. Candour on the part of the therapist helps prepare the client for this potential consequence and subsequently builds the client's trust in the therapist's judgement. See the chapter on communication between therapist and client for specific consent to test phrasing.

Accuracy of Testing

Testing must be performed accurately. This process is assisted by clear instructions to the client before each test is performed. The therapist should take care that the structure to be assessed is accurately isolated; knowledge of anatomy and correct positioning of the therapist's hands are important.

It is also important for the therapist not to hurt herself through awkward or inefficient positioning while performing orthopedic testing. The therapist takes a comfortable and stable position before each test begins. For example, when assessing the ankle of a client seated on the end of the massage table, instead of squatting or bending over, the therapist sits on a chair or stool.

A textbook on anatomy or orthopedic assessment should be consulted for average statistics on active free and passive relaxed ranges of specific joints. In terms of range of motion test results, one source notes that if the testing is performed by the same therapist, an increase in the range of three or four degrees indicates improvement. If the testing is performed by two or more therapists, an increase of five or six degrees indicates improvement *(Clarkson, Gilewich, 1989)*. With overpressure assessment, one study found that the accuracy of experienced physiotherapists in assessing vertebral movement is sufficiently precise for recording purposes *(Boyling, Palastanga, 1994)*.

A test should not be repeated too many times in one assessment or inaccuracies will occur. A muscle length test that is repeated three or four times will begin to stretch the muscle, not just assess it. An active resisted strength test that is repeated more than three times will fatigue the muscle, giving the appearance of decreased strength.

There are several client positions possible for testing specific muscle lengths and end feels. For example, with gastrocnemius length tests the client may be either supine or prone. Whichever position for testing is chosen, it is important that the therapist use a consistent position from one client to the next, so the therapist develops a baseline for evaluation *(Fox, Del Pizzo, 1993)*.

Making Tests Safe

While symptoms may be temporarily exacerbated, testing in itself should not injure the client. For example, assessment of an acute severe muscle strain should not begin with maximal, active resisted strength testing. Overpressure may only be applied if active free movement is full and pain free *(Magee, 1992)*. Any contraindications to testing for a particular condition are listed in the appropriate chapter.

If the therapist uses abrupt passive movements to assess the integrity of a ligament, protective muscle spasm can occur in response to pain. To prevent this, the therapist gradually places the appropriate stress on the ligament and oscillates, or repeats this, several times. This stress and range of motion are increased up to, but not beyond, the point of pain *(Magee, 1992)*.

Measuring Range of Motion

When a joint does not have full range of motion, a goniometer or other measuring device can be used to more accurately record the range. There are two kinds of goniometers, a universal goniometer and an OB goniometer.

A universal goniometer is a 360-degree protractor with two arms that are joined by an axis or pivot point. One arm is stationary and one arm is movable *(Figure 10.2)*. The axis is placed on the joint to be measured and each arm is aligned with the long axis of the bones that comprise the joint. The client moves the joint through the range while the therapist holds the goniometer in place, the movable arm kept in alignment with the moving bone or bony prominence. At the end of the range of motion, the degrees of motion are then read off the protractor. The universal goniometer is relatively inexpensive. However, it has some

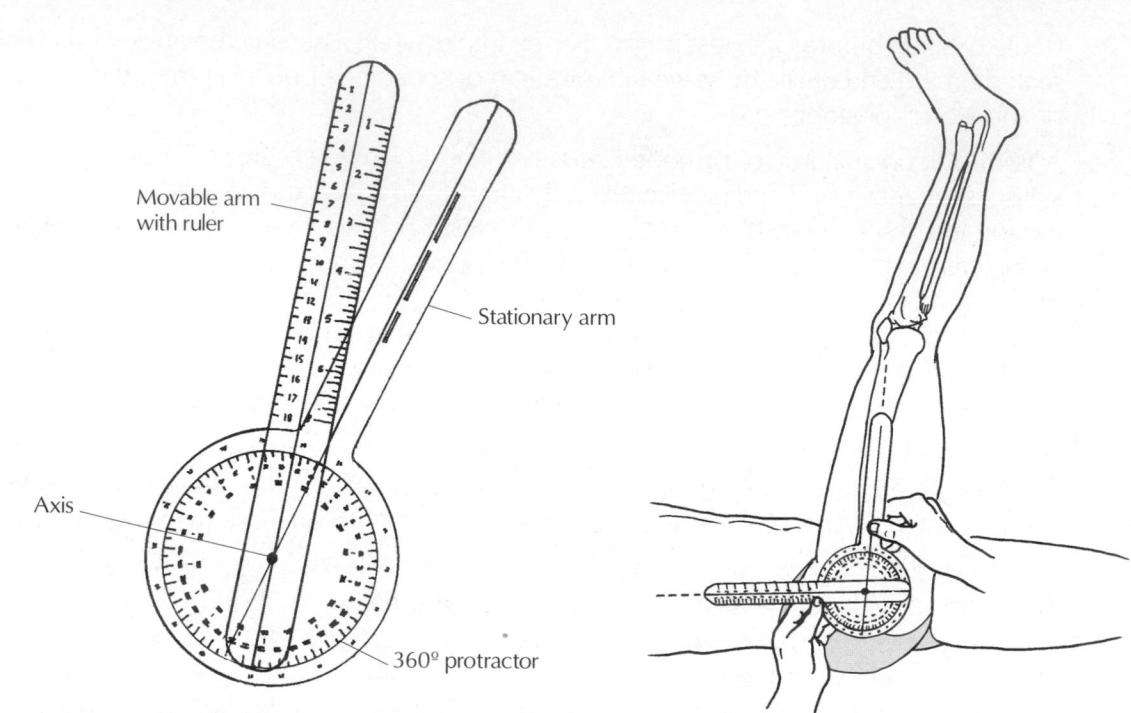

Movable arm
with ruler

Stationary arm

Axis

360º protractor

Figure 10.2
Universal goniometer measuring range of motion at the hip. The axis or pivot is placed over the greater trochanter.

drawbacks: it is not accurate for measuring range of motion of the spine; some errors may occur if the goniometer is not positioned carefully throughout the test; and the therapist initially needs to practise using the device to hold it in proper alignment (*Clarkson, Gilewich, 1989*).

An OB goniometer is a fluid-filled device with a 360-degree dial that can strap onto the body part to be assessed. The pointer on the dial responds to gravity and to magnetic north, so the OB goniometer can measure vertical as well as horizontal motion. While this goniometer is easier to use, it is more expensive and cannot be used to measure the small joints of the hand and foot.

A measuring tape may also be used to record ranges of motion of the spine *(Figure 10.3)* and to determine girth measurements of a limb when edema is present and to measure thoracic cage expansion.

✍ When range is recorded with a goniometer, it is important to avoid unclear or ambiguous notations. For example, a fully extended knee is at 0 degrees, not 180 degrees; a hyperextended knee is recorded as 15 degrees of hyperextension instead of -15 degrees (*Walker, Helewa, 1996*).

✍ The therapist may estimate the range of a joint by recording "less than quarter range", "quarter range", "less than half range", "half range", "less than three-quarters range", "three-quarters range", "less than full range" and "full range". However, this is not as accurate as measuring with a goniometer.

It is worth noting that joints usually become stiffer with age. Therefore, a reduced range may be appropriate with an elderly client. Younger children have more flexibility, which

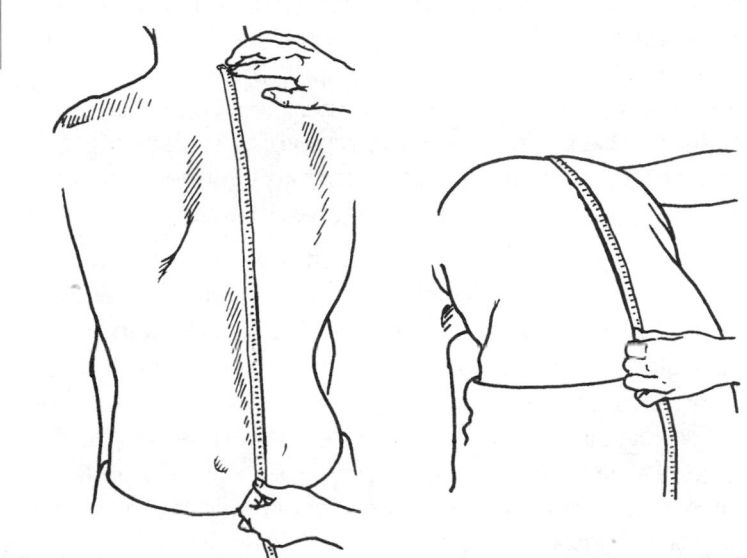

Figure 10.3
Using a tape measure to record flexion of the thoracolumbar spine.

decreases in adult life. Regardless of age, females are generally more flexible than males *(Beighton et al., 1989).*

Recording Test Results

✍ Test results are recorded on the health history form. Both positive and negative test results are recorded, as well as results that are within normal limits. A negative test result is just as important in determining the tissues that are affected as a positive result because a negative result can be used to rule out conditions. Moreover, should the therapist have to report to a third-party payer or find herself a witness in court, a complete set of test results including normal ranges and negative tests displays competency.

✍ The therapist should not have expectations for what a test result should be, but should record the results as they actually exist.

✍ The therapist's interpretation of the results leads to the modalities and techniques that are used in the treatment plan. Frequently, the interpretation of results and the techniques to use is straightforward. For example, a shortened rectus femoris should be lengthened. However, sometimes the results do not have clear interpretations or the source of the client's symptoms is not revealed in the initial testing. The therapist may have to repeat tests or perform new ones over a series of treatments to obtain a clearer picture of the structures that are involved.

How to Organize Testing

At first, a student therapist may be overwhelmed at the possibilities for arranging a testing protocol. Experienced therapists have had years to decide in what order to perform tests, and often develop protocols or sequences of tests for a particular area of the body, such as the neck or low back, that they have frequently worked with. As stated before, practice makes it easier to choose the order of tests and the selection of additional tests to confirm test results.

✍ There are some guidelines for safely sequencing tests. Active free range of motion, or what the client is able to do pain-free, is usually performed before other tests. This allows the therapist to note what the client cannot do and carefully approach these ranges when performing other tests. Passive relaxed range of motion and overpressure give information about the joints; these are usually performed next. Muscle strength and length tests and other specialized tests are then performed.

✍ In another method of sequencing tests, they may be chosen according to the client's symptoms; tests may suggest themselves to the therapist after observation and palpation have been completed. For example, the client reports pain, numbness and tingling in the thumb and index finger; the therapist notices some swelling in the hand. These suggest carpal tunnel syndrome. However, if the therapist jumps to this conclusion and performs tests only for carpal tunnel syndrome, she misses the possibility that other conditions may be the source of the symptoms, such as trigger points. The client may also have more than one condition, such as tight neck muscles or nerve compression at the neck, which add to the overall presentation.

✍ Another method of sequencing is *rule-out testing.* This concept was developed in order to catch any proximal dysfunction that may be causing symptoms in the limbs, perhaps unrelated to what the therapist suspects the condition to be. For example, with arm or hand pain, the therapist starts with tests for the head, then neck, then shoulder, then elbow and finally the hand itself. Since extremity symptoms may originate in the peripheral nervous system, neurological rule-out tests are often performed first to eliminate this tissue as a source of dysfunction. For example, upper limb tension tests and the cervical compression test, described in Appendix C, could be performed first, followed by other neck and shoulder tests.

✍ In some cases it is important to perform vascular or neurological tests immediately after active free range of motion to screen out potential vascular or neurological pathologies. For example, with a client who has unassessed neck pain in flexion and rotation, the vertebral artery test, then Kernig's or Brudzinski's neurological tests are performed before passive relaxed tests.

✍ Tests that differentiate between conditions that cause similar symptoms are listed under the heading "Differentiating Sources of...Pain" at the end of the testing section in the relevant chapters.

✍ Yet another method of organizing tests has the therapist arrange the testing for the client's comfort, with the most painful movements performed last. The therapist can perform all tests that have the client in one position, such as standing tests, then reposition the client for tests performed in another position, such as seated tests.

✍ Some combination of these methods is acceptable: active free range of motion followed by rule-outs and tests performed in one position.

✍ Regardless of the method of organizing tests, all testing is performed **bilaterally**, first on the unaffected side and then on the affected side, so the therapist will have a reference point from which to compare any compromised function.

✍ Range of motion (active free and passive relaxed), overpressure and active resisted strength testing can be used as both assessment and remedial exercise tools *(Kisner, Colby, 1990).* However, the progression of these actions differs, depending on the purpose to be achieved — either assessing an injured limb or rehabilitating it. The therapist may refer to the section on remedial exercise for more information.

Types of Tests

Active Free Range of Motion (AF ROM)

Active free range of motion is performed when the client moves the joint through the cardinal planes of motion that are normal for that joint. Any pain or crepitus present during the range is reported. The test assesses what the client is willing or able to do.

+ Effects: AF ROM gives only functional information about the client's willingness to move the body part. AF ROM is **limited by pain.**

Passive Relaxed Range of Motion (PR ROM)

Passive relaxed range of motion is performed when the therapist moves the joint passively through the cardinal planes of motion that are normal for the joint. The test assesses whether there is limitation (hypomobility) or excess (hypermobility) of range. Passive movement is done carefully and gently, to allow the client to fully relax the muscles while the tests are performed. Restriction or hypermobility in the range is noted. The client reports the point at which pain, if present, occurs. The therapist stops the motion at the point of pain.

+ Effects: PR ROM gives information about the joint capsule and ligaments. Normally, passive relaxed range of motion will be slightly greater than active free range. PR ROM also assesses the ligaments for joint hypomobility or hypermobility. PR ROM is **limited by pain.**

For further interpretation of limitation of motion, overpressure is applied.

Overpressure and End Feel

Overpressure is the term used when the therapist gradually applies more pressure when the end of the available passive range of joint motion is reached. The sensation transmitted to the therapist's hands by the tissue resistance at the end of the available range is the *end feel* of a joint *(Cyriax, 1991)*. The stretch on the soft tissues such as muscles, tendons, fascia and ligaments, as well as the arrangement of the joint surfaces, determine the range of motion of the joint and, therefore, the joint's normal end feel.

An end feel may be normal or abnormal. Normal end feel exists when the joint has full range of motion and the range is stopped by the anatomy of the joint. Abnormal end feel exists when the range of the joint is less or greater than normal, is painful, or when a structure other than the normal anatomy of the joint stops the motion. Information on the possible causes of the restriction or the hypermobility can be gained by assessing the quality of the end feel that is noted at the end range of painful, restricted or increased motion *(Cyriax, 1991; Hertling, Kessler, 1990)*.

+ Effects: End feel assesses the specific structure that is limiting movement or that is likely injured; muscle length is also assessed at the end of the range.

Types of End Feel

Sources vary as to the terms used for, and the descriptions of, end feels, both normal and abnormal *(Cyriax, 1991; Hertling, Kessler, 1990; Magee, 1992; Clarkson, Gilewich, 1989)*.

+ Normal end feels:

• **Soft tissue approximation** end feel occurs when the full range of the joint is restricted by the normal muscle bulk (especially so if muscular hypertrophy is present). For the therapist, normal soft tissue approximation has a feeling of soft compression. For the client, it is painless, as when elbow flexion is stopped by biceps muscle.

- **Muscular** or **tissue stretch** end feel, occurs at the extremes of muscle stretch, such as in the hamstrings during a straight leg raise or extension of the metacarpophalangeal joints. For the therapist, normal tissue stretch has a feeling of increasing tension, springiness or elasticity. The client may feel a stretching sensation, as in the hamstrings when the hip is flexed while the knee is in extension. Muscle length is also assessed when the muscle is fully lengthened; sometimes length tests are listed as special tests.

- **Capsular stretch** or **leathery** end feel occurs when the joint capsule is stretched at the end of its normal range, such as with external rotation of the glenohumeral joint. For the therapist, normal capsular stretch feels like stretching a piece of leather. For the client, it is painless.

- **Bony** end feel occurs when bone contacts bone at the end of normal range, as in extension of the elbow. Normal bony end feel is abrupt and hard.

✦ Abnormal end feels:

- **Empty** end feel occurs when there is no physical restriction to movement except the pain perceived by the client. This indicates acute bursitis or joint inflammation.

- **Muscle spasm** end feel occurs when passive movement stops abruptly with some springy rebound and pain. This is a result of reflexive muscle spasm, which is designed to prevent further injury. It also indicates synovial inflammation when felt with a capsular pattern of restriction (see capsular pattern below).

- **Boggy** or **soft** end feel occurs with joint effusion or edema. It has a mushy and soft quality to it, indicating acute inflammation. In the case of ligamentous injury, such as in a moderate to severe sprain, a softer end feel is encountered by the therapist, until the slack is taken up by other structures.

- **Springy block** or **internal derangement** end feel is a springy or rebounding sensation in a non-capsular pattern (see non-capsular pattern below). This indicates loose cartilage or meniscal tissue within the joint.

- **Capsular stretch** or **leathery** end feel occurring before normal range indicates capsular fibrosis if a capsular pattern of restriction is present with no inflammation (see capsular pattern below).

- **Bony** end feel occurring before normal range indicates bony changes, such as osteophytes present with degenerative joint disease or malunion of a joint following a fracture.

✦ A **capsular pattern** is the pattern of limitation of movement at an injured or affected joint. With injury to the joint capsule or the synovial lining, a pattern of proportional limitation will be noted as the therapist takes the joint through its passive range. The limitation is due either to fibrosing (thickening) of the joint capsule, to inflammation or to joint effusion (swelling). Each joint has its characteristic pattern of limitation due to the arrangement of the ligaments and joint surfaces. The glenohumeral joint has a different pattern of restriction, for example, than the knee joint. However, the capsular pattern of all glenohumeral joints is similar in that external rotation and abduction are most restricted. Only joints that are controlled by muscular movement have capsular patterns. The sacroiliac joint, for example, does not have a capsular pattern.

✦ A **non-capsular pattern** is limitation of movement of a joint but not in a capsular pattern. This restriction may be due to an intra-articular mechanical blockage from torn pieces of cartilage, menisci or intra-articular adhesions. It may be due to extra-capsular lesions, such as muscle contracture, myositis ossificans or acute bursitis.

Active Resisted (AR) Testing

Active resisted testing assesses the strength of the muscles. Muscle strength is influenced by the client's age, gender, body type and occupation *(Pedretti, Zoltan, 1990)*. The resistance to the client's muscles may be supplied by gravity or by the therapist.

The client's movements against gravity are performed on the vertical plane, directed away from the floor towards the ceiling. If the therapist adds extra resistance to the force of gravity, the client's movement is also on the vertical plane. Muscles of the neck, trunk and limbs are usually assessed in this manner. Tests for weaker muscles are performed on the horizontal plane, where the effects of gravity are decreased *(Kendall, McCreary, 1983)*. For specific muscle strength tests and the grading of muscle strengths see Appendix C.

✦ A **painful** contraction indicates an injury to the muscle or tendon, such as a muscle strain.

✦ A **weak** contraction can indicate a lack of muscular strength, a partial rupture of the muscle or tendon, or a peripheral nervous system injury when found in conjunction with positive neurological testing results.

✎ With **isometric resistance**, the muscle contracts but the joints that it crosses do not move. To isometrically test muscle strength, the therapist positions the client in such a way as to isolate the muscle and tendon to be assessed. The muscle is placed at a length that will allow the maximum contraction available. This is usually at mid-range (the middle point of the range) because a muscle that is fully lengthened or fully shortened does not have sufficient power to fully contract. Stabilization is required to prevent joint movement and to keep the client from recruiting other muscles to perform the contraction *(Kendall, McCreary, 1983)*.

✎ With **isotonic resistance**, the muscle contracts and moves the joints that it crosses through their ranges of motion. This allows the therapist to further assess the strength of the isolated muscle by resisting its action throughout the available range, rather than at only mid-point. Isotonic testing takes practice to perform correctly and safely. The therapist slowly applies resistance while the client meets this force, then the joint is moved. Care must be taken not to overpower the client in the inner and outer ranges, or to move into pain.

Alternatively, if the muscle is a weight bearing one — for example, the quadriceps group — the client can perform the resistance exercise, in this case by doing deep knee bends or squats. The client's body weight becomes the added resistance to motion. Any weakness and asymmetry in strength are noted by the therapist. The test may have to be repeated several times to fatigue the muscle sufficiently to observe any weakness present.

✦ Effects: Active resisted testing assesses contractile tissue for pain or weakness with muscle, tendon or peripheral nerve injury.

Special Orthopedic Tests

Special tests include muscle length tests, combinations of active, passive and resisted tests and neurological tests. These assessments isolate a specific structure or provoke a symptom that the client is experiencing. They may be named after the person who first described the test (such as Ober's and Apley's) or according to the action performed during the test (such as Wright's hyperabduction test of the glenohumeral joint).

Adson's test, for example, is a combination of passive relaxed extension and external rotation of the humerus, active free rotation of the neck and the client actively inhaling and holding the breath. All these actions place maximum compression on the neurovascular bundle supplying the arm and are designed to provoke the symptoms of thoracic outlet syndrome.

✦ Effects: Special orthopedic tests are used to isolate a specific condition.

In each chapter, orthopedic testing and the expected results that are specific to the condition are given. Appendix C gives a description of these tests, which are standard orthopedic tests, easily recognized by other health care professionals. There may be variations on a particular test to further differentiate among various dysfunctional structures. The therapist may refer to texts on orthopedic testing for more details.

11

PREPARATION FOR TREATMENT, POST-TREATMENT AND SELF-CARE

Fiona Rattray

Where Do Treatments Take Place?

Massage therapy may be performed in a separate treatment room in a clinical setting, such as an office building, a separate treatment room in a resort or spa setting, or in a therapist's residence. In an educational setting, supervised treatments occur in individual treatment rooms or private, curtained cubicles. In a clinical, resort or educational setting, there is usually a reception area where client health history forms are stored securely. Massage therapy may also be performed in a hospital setting or at an athletic event. No matter what the setting, there must be access to clean toilet facilities, disinfectant soap and water for hand washing.

The therapist's licences and credentials are clearly displayed somewhere in the treatment space.

The Treatment Room

A treatment room, whether in a clinical, residential or educational setting, should provide privacy for the client to get undressed. It should also be comfortable, clean and tidy. Good air circulation is important and the room is kept dust- and mold-free to avoid triggering clients with allergies and asthma. The floor, whether carpet or tile, is also kept clean.

The room should be warm and lighting should be adequate, not excessive. A dimmer switch or other adjustable light source is appropriate. Candles are not considered appropriate lighting (see Therapist and Client Boundaries chapter).

There are some safety concerns for clients. The treatment room should not be cluttered, so someone with mobility aids, such as a cane or wheelchair, can have clear access to the table. If the floor is tile, any oil, lotion or hydrotherapy spills must be cleaned up promptly to prevent slipping; a throw rug is not a good idea if it can slip and become a hazard.

Ideally, a treatment room is a quiet, relaxing environment. A music system can also provide calming background music.

Massage tables come in a variety of configurations, prices and materials: wooden or metal legs, portable or non-portable, different widths and lengths, adjustable split tables, adjustable hydraulic tables, ones with face cradles or arm rests. For in-chair massage, there is a variety of chairs that support the torso, arms and head. A new therapist on a budget might want to start off with a simple, sturdy table. Once he finds out what kind of clientele he will develop and what their needs are, an informed choice can be made about table styles and features.

An adjustable-height chair, with wheels, for the therapist is important. A sturdy, non-mobile chair is provided for the client to sit on while her health history is reviewed in the assessment process. A place for the client to put her clothes is also necessary.

Other items in the treatment room are a clean clinical gown (shorts and a t-shirt may be supplied by the client instead) for the client to wear during the assessment, and a plumb-line, goniometer and measuring tape, again for assessment purposes. A blood pressure cuff and stethoscope are also suggested; their use for monitoring blood pressure is described in the chapter on hypertension and congestive heart failure.

Hydrotherapy applications should be ready to use: the thermophore cover and wax bath clean; clean tubs for foot or arm baths; and a clean bowl for facial steams. A kettle for preparing facial steams and a refrigerator for ice packs are also useful.

The containers for lotions, oils or other lubricants are kept wiped down. The decision whether to use lotion or oil is partly the therapist's preference, partly the client's needs. Of course, a client with allergies or sensitivities to oil should have access to a hypoallergenic lotion. In terms of oil, a water-dispersable oil will help prevent oil stains.

A supply of vinyl gloves and facial tissues is necessary, along with a disinfectant for cleaning the table between clients.

Linens and Pillows

An adequate supply of clean sheets, towels, face cradle covers, pillowcases and blankets is necessary. Sheets should be large enough to completely cover the client. While therapists may frequently use smaller sheets because they provide adequate coverage at a reasonable cost, it is advisable that at least a few sets of large sheets are available for use with clients who are larger or with clients who are pregnant.

A supply of different-sized pillows, bolsters or a specially designed foam support system is necessary to support client positioning. For sanitary reasons, pillows need to be covered, either with clean pillowcases or towels, with each client.

Concepts for Table Set Up and Getting the Client on the Table

+ Two sheets and a top blanket are placed on the table; a face cradle cover is also used. The top sheet is neatly turned down over the blanket so no part of the blanket is in direct contact with the client.

+ When and where to place pillows depends on two factors: the assessment to be performed and the treatment plan that is chosen.

+ When a client is brought into the treatment room by the therapist, often she is asked to be seated on the chair while the therapist reviews the health history form with her. If necessary, the client's blood pressure is taken and recorded. Some type of an assessment is then performed and pillow placement becomes a factor. The therapist may select tests that require the client to lie on the table in a prone, supine, seated or sidelying position, and pillows already in place under the sheets may need to be moved to perform the tests. This is not a concern for an experienced therapist; he just moves the pillows around or removes them. Clinical experience has shown that a student in a supervised massage may be less inclined to move the pillows if they are already in place, feeling perhaps a subtle or not so subtle pressure to get the client on the table as soon as possible in the position already chosen by the pillowing layout. By not having pillows in place, just the two sheets and top blanket, the student has more incentive to choose tests and positioning according to a treatment plan and then, after the assessment, place the pillows accordingly.

+ The treatment plan that is chosen may begin with the client in either a supine, sidelying, prone or seated position. Whatever plan is chosen and consented to by the client, the therapist instructs the client on how to get on the table and the position she will be in.

+ The therapist tells her that once he leaves the room, she is to get undressed, removing as much clothing as she is comfortable with, and lie between the sheets, covering herself with the top sheet and blanket. The therapist also inquires if the client needs assistance in getting on the table or in getting undressed. Assistance may be required if the client has a central nervous system lesion; the client may be more comfortable leaving some or all of her clothing on if the therapist remains in the room to assist.

+ The therapist then leaves the room to give the client privacy to get undressed and on the table, unless specifically requested to assist the client in some way. Permission is requested to re-enter the room once the client is settled.

Pillowing and Positioning

Pillows can be positioned before the client gets on the table or afterwards; pillows can be added to further support the client at any point in the treatment. Positioning is adjusted for the client's comfort.

+ Prone
  • Pillows are placed between the table and the bottom sheet so they will be under the client's abdomen to reduce the lordotic curve and under the ankles to reduce plantarflexion.
  • If a face cradle is used, the client may need to be told how to place her head into it and the face cradle height may need to be adjusted for comfort. If no face cradle is used, the client turns her head to one side or the other. This position should be changed regularly to prevent neck discomfort while the client is prone. If the client has a respiratory condition that requires postural drainage, a wedge of several pillows is built up under the client's pelvis to raise the pelvis and lower the head (see the chapter on chronic bronchitis for details).
  • Three-quarters prone positioning requires pillows under one shoulder and the knee on the same side of the body.
+ Sidelying
  • The client gets between the sheets and lies with the side to be treated uppermost.

131

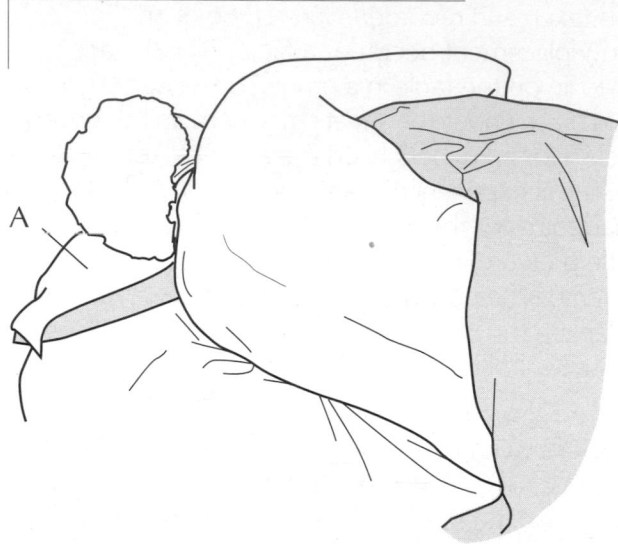

Figure 11.1
Sidelying pillowing: A pillow is placed under the client's head (A), supporting it in line with the rest of the spine.

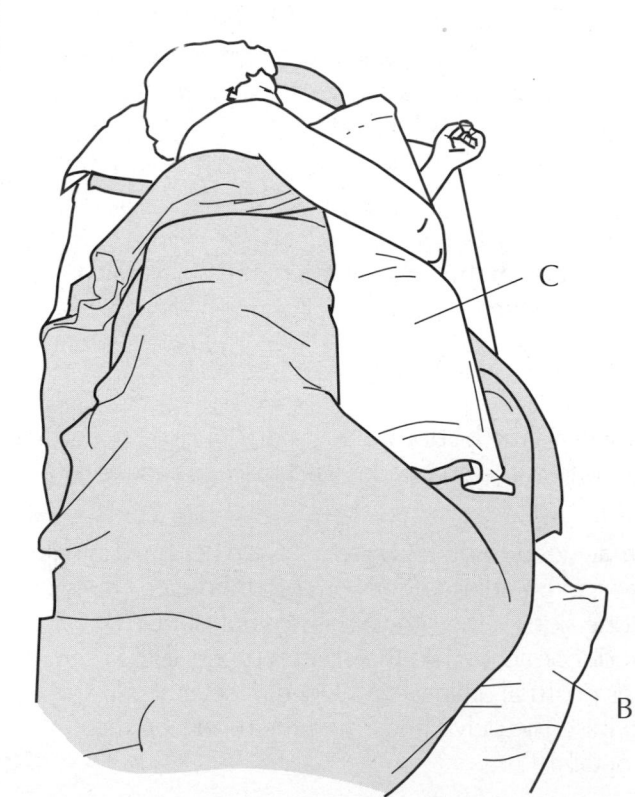

Figure 11.2
Sidelying pillowing: A pillow is placed between the client's knees (B), while the anterior chest and arm are supported with another pillow which the client hugs (C).

- When the therapist returns to the room, a pillow is placed under the client's head, supporting it in line with the rest of the spine *(Figure 11.1)*. Another pillow is placed between the client's knees. A third may be used to support the client's anterior chest and arm — the client hugs the pillow *(Figure 11.2)* — or to support under the abdomen of a pregnant client.

✦ Supine

- One or more pillows are placed between the table and the bottom sheet so they will be under the client's knees. More than one pillow is used if the therapist wants to neutralize the client's lumbar curve; the therapist can ask what is most comfortable for the client.

- If a client has a condition such as a hiatus hernia or hypertension, she may require extra pillows to support the trunk and head in a semi-seated position. These are placed between the table and the bottom sheet; the therapist can inquire as to the client's sleeping position for comfort guidelines.

✦ Seated

- The client is seated on a stool in front of the table, wearing a clinic gown or wrapped in a sheet.

- When the therapist returns to the room, pillows are placed on the table in front of the client to support her torso and head; she then leans forwards into them.

Additional Pillows for Drainage or Support

Multiple pillows can be used to elevate an edematous limb for drainage or to support an injured limb in a position that does not further stress injured tissue. These modifications are discussed in individual treatment chapters.

Draping

Draping the client, or covering the client with sheets or towels, is designed to make the client feel comfortable, secure and warm during the treatment.

+ Only the part of the client that is being worked on is uncovered.

+ The client may request that the draping be rearranged. If the draping then covers more of the client, the therapist may need to adjust the treatment plan to work through the sheets if the area to be addressed is no longer directly accessible. If the draping is more revealing, it is up to the therapist to decide if he is comfortable with it.

+ Under no circumstances are the client's genitalia and gluteal cleft exposed or touched.

+ When treating a female client, the therapist should ensure that the client's breasts are covered with a towel. If it is indicated to perform breast massage, and the client consents to this, the breast tissue is uncovered only when it is being directly worked on; the nipple and areola are not touched. Breast massage is indicated with general breast drainage problems, post-surgery to promote mobile scarring and for symptomatic relief of pain, such as pre- or post-menstrual, or discomforts of pregnancy or lactation.

+ Male clients may also feel more comfortable and secure having their chests draped. A towel is used for draping the chest when treating the abdomen. Regardless of whether a towel is used or not, the nipples are not touched.

+ The therapist's fingers or hands should not go below the draping; the line that the draping forms is a boundary for the client's security.

+ The draping should be neat and secure, especially if the limb is to be moved through a range of motion during the treatment.

+ The sheet is tucked securely yet non-invasively around the client's limb or trunk; if the client is wearing underwear, the draping is tucked neatly into it, so no underwear is visible.

+ The therapist must resecure the draping should it work loose during the treatment.

Draping Boundary Lines

Boundary lines created by draping allow the maximum amount of tissue to be uncovered while still securely covering the client.

+ Prone:
  • undrape the back to the PSIS levels;
  • undrape the leg to the greater trochanter so the gluteal muscles are accessible. Undraping to the lateral iliac crest may be indicated so gluteal attachments are accessible.

+ Sidelying:
  • undrape the back to the iliac crest;
  • undrape the leg to the greater trochanter, ensuring that the genital area and gluteal cleft are covered *(Figure 11.3)*. Undraping to the lateral iliac crest may be indicated so gluteal and tensor fascia lata attachments are accessible.

+ Supine:
  • undrape the pectoral muscles; with a female client, undrape to the rise of the breasts.

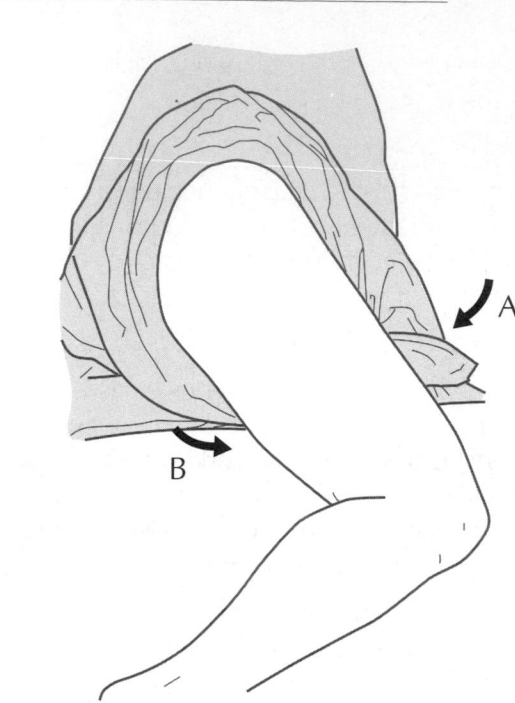

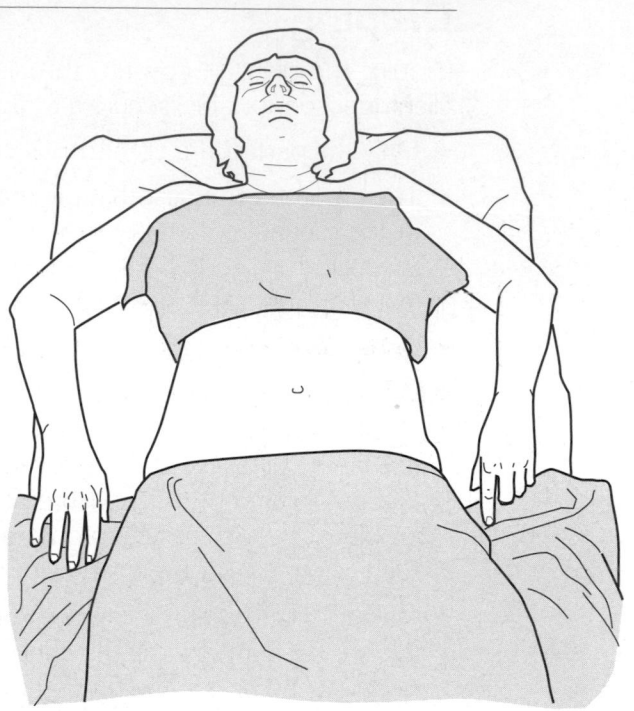

Figure 11.3
Sidelying draping for the leg: The client's leg is undraped to the knee; a pillow is placed between the knees; the corner of the sheet in front of the knee is brought under and behind the leg from (A); the corner of the sheet behind the knee is brought under and in front of the leg from (B); the draping is slid up the leg to above the greater trochanter and secured.

Figure 11.4
Supine draping for the abdomen: While the top sheet is still covering the client's torso, the towel may be placed on the sheet over the breasts. The client is asked to hold the upper edge of the towel in place while the therapist pulls the sheet downwards from underneath the towel; the therapist's hands are at the level of the abdomen; the draping is secured around the pelvis at ASIS levels.

This will differ with each client; ideally the therapist should be able to get one hand between the clavicle and line of the drape; however, the client must be comfortable with the draping line;

- undrape the abdomen to the ASIS levels; with a female client, the lines are the ASIS levels and the xiphoid process; a towel is used to cover the breasts *(Figure 11.4)*;

- undrape the legs to the greater trochanter, within a few inches of the adductor attachments.

Some Draping Examples

For the new therapist, it can take practice to feel comfortable moving the draping to uncover the part being massaged, moving the client's limbs around and tucking the draping in place. During the treatment the therapist should move the client's limbs carefully, securely and without sudden motions. This allows the client to relax fully and not hold or guard against unexpected movements. The therapist should also not be afraid to give the client instructions to assist with the draping — for example, to pull the sheet tight around the adductors, holding the draping in place while the leg is moved through a range of motion; or to hold the upper edge of the towel lying over the top sheet and blanket in place while the therapist lowers the sheets to the ASIS levels for an abdominal massage, thus keeping the breasts covered.

There are many ways to drape a client securely. Different educational institutions may show different draping styles; these styles can vary from teacher to teacher, or from one circumstance to another.

For example, during an athletic event, a client may be wearing shorts and a shirt; she leaves these on during a leg massage and the therapist uses a towel tucked into the leg of the shorts to keep the massage lotion from coming in contact with the clothing; no other draping is used as the client is securely covered by her clothing.

In another example, a client's symptoms indicate a short iliopsoas muscle. The usual treatment plan would be to undrape the abdomen for massage; however, in this case, the client, for cultural and personal reasons, is not comfortable with this plan. The therapist then suggests working through the sheets so the abdomen is not uncovered; if this is not acceptable, the therapist can do a stretch for the muscle or show the client a self-stretch.

After graduation, the therapist may develop his own style of draping or take post-graduate courses that show alternative draping procedures.

The main point of draping is that it is *secure during the treatment and covers the parts of the client not being worked on.* Instead of listing specific draping procedures, the following are some suggestions.

An Approach to Posterior Leg Draping

When working on the posterior of a client's right thigh and leg, the therapist first uncovers that leg only, dropping the edge of the sheet that was over the leg between the client's knees and ankles. The sheet is then tucked in at the client's hip, under the anterior superior iliac spine. Next the therapist flexes the client's right knee and extends the hip, holding the leg with one hand and arm. With the other hand, the therapist brings the right edge of the top sheet at the client's knee **under** the right thigh *(Figure 11.5).* The therapist then places the client's right leg on top of the top sheet. If necessary, the sheet can be tucked into the client's underwear (if she is wearing any) and adjusted superiorly to uncover the gluteal muscles. A towel placed over the gluteals and tucked into the underwear will help hold the draping in place *(Figure 11.6).*

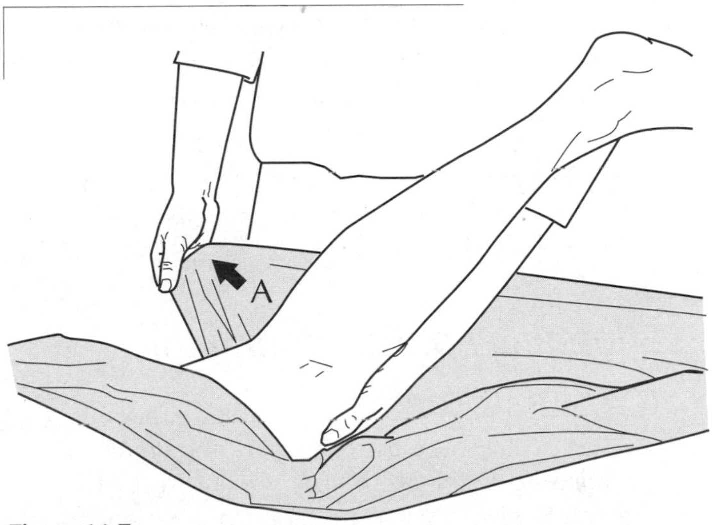

Figure11.5
Posterior leg draping: After uncovering the right leg to the knee, the therapist extends the client's right leg while bringing the top sheet laterally under the knee and thigh.

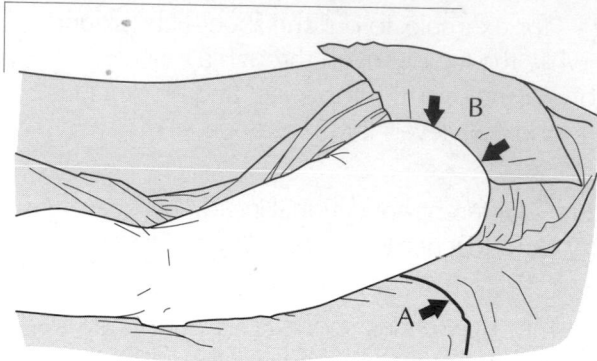

Figure 11.6
Posterior leg draping: The edge of the top sheet at (A) may be pulled higher to tighten adductor draping after the towel at (B) is tucked into the gluteal draping to hold it in place.

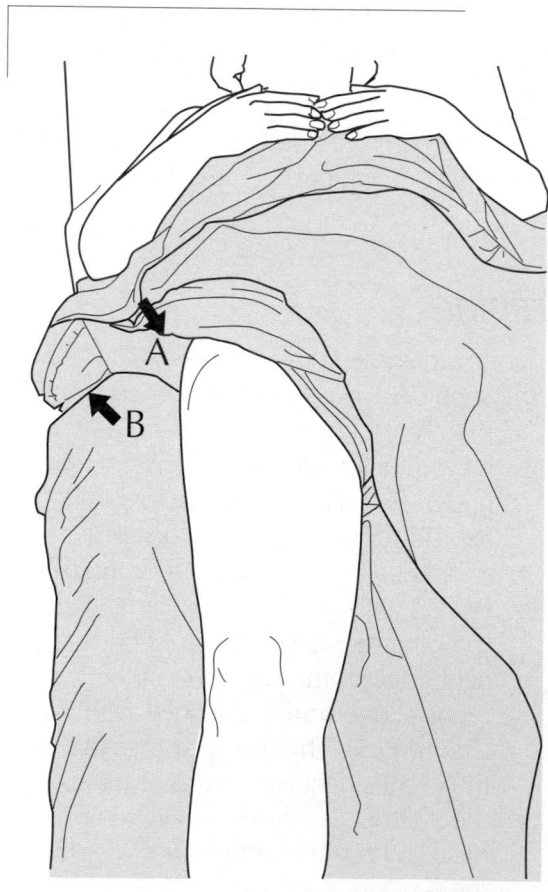

Figure 11.7
Anterior leg draping: The leg is covered to mid-thigh and the sheet is tucked under the client's hip at (A). The sheet is brought under the slightly flexed knee and leg to hang over the edge of the table at (B).

An Approach to Anterior Leg Draping

- The leg to be treated is uncovered by dropping the edge of the sheet that was over the leg between the client's knees and ankles as in the prone approach. The sheet is tucked in at the client's hip. The therapist flexes the client's knee and hip, holding the leg with one hand and arm. With the other hand, the top sheet is brought **under** the leg to hang over the edge of the table. The client's leg is then placed on top of the sheet *(Figure 11.7)*. If the therapist needs to move the hip through range of motion, the client is asked to hold onto the edge of the sheet that goes under the thigh, pulling it up and keeping the draping from gapping around the adductors.

An Approach to Seated Draping

- For a treatment in a seated position, the client leans forward onto the table, with three or four pillows piled up to support the trunk and head. The client may be given a clinical gown to put on while the therapist is out of the room, with the opening at the back. Alternatively, while the client is on the table between two sheets, the top sheet is wrapped around the client's body securely. The corners can be tied together at the client's shoulder, toga-fashion. Once the client is seated and leaning forward into the supporting pillows, the gown is untied at the back, or the sheet corners are unknotted at the shoulder, uncovering the client's back and neck for treatment. For more details, see the chapter on dislocations.

- Other specific draping variations are listed in appropriate chapters.

Changing Position during the Treatment

- After treatment of the body part, the draping is readjusted so the client's body is covered. The therapist gives clear instructions to the client about each positional change. For example, "Whenever you are ready, I'd like you to lift up in the middle so I can remove the pillow under your abdomen, then

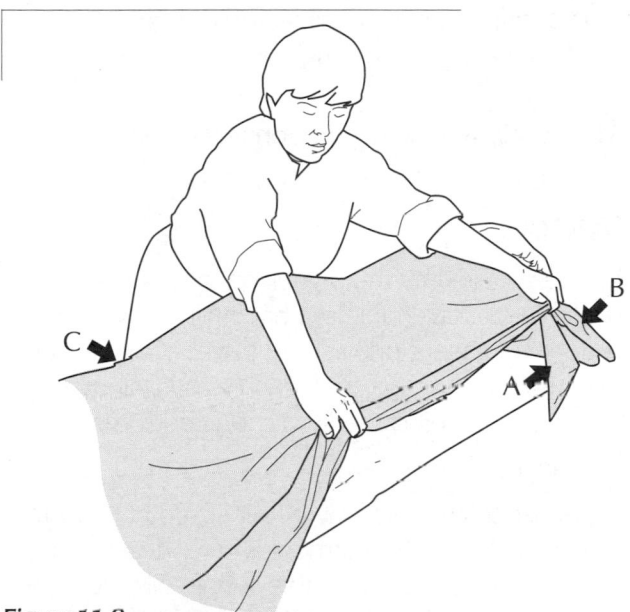

Figure11.8
Securing the sheets so the client may turn over: The
bottom sheet (A) and top sheet and blanket (B) are
held together by the therapist on the opposite side
of the table, while the sheets are held in place on
the therapist's side by leaning against the table (C).

I'll hold the sheets so you are covered. Take
your time turning onto your back." The
therapist then removes any pillows that may
restrict easy movement.

The sheets are secured so the client is not
uncovered as she changes position: the
therapist holds the edges of the top and
bottom sheets together on the side of the
table opposite him; the top and bottom
sheets and blanket on his side of the table are
secured by the therapist's legs leaning against
the table *(Figure 11.8)*. If the client keeps both
arms under the top sheet while turning, there
is less of a chance that the upper chest area
will be exposed; this is especially important
with female clients.

Although it may sound obvious, the therapist
should take care that the client does not fall
off the table when changing positions. Once
the client has changed position, pillows are
placed appropriately and the next stage of
the treatment begins.

In-chair Massage in Work Place Setting

The chair is set up in a quiet location, often in a separate room in an office or work place.
Client's health records must be stored confidentially. A portable container, for assessment
tools such as a goniometer and hydrotherapy applications such as a thermaphore, is useful.

The client remains clothed, although restrictive clothing is loosened and shoes are
removed. Sheets and pillows are not necessary. However, face cradle covers and
disinfectant cleaners should be used for sanitary reasons. Usually direct pressure techniques
are used, so no oils or lotions are required. The therapist often works in a standing position;
however, a portable stool can be useful for working on the client's legs and feet.

Massage in a Hospital Setting

Treatment occurs with the consent of the client and the treating physician. The client may
be in a private room or may share a room. It is important for the client to have as much
privacy as possible during the treatment; the curtains are drawn around the client's bed.
Since the client is in a hospital bed, linens and pillows are already available. Disinfectant
hand soap for the therapist and extra towels and pillows, oils or lotions for the treatment
can be carried in a bag. Health history forms must be stored in a secure place.

Care must be taken not to interfere with any medical equipment, intravenous tubes or
other lines connected to the client during the massage.

The use of essential oils must be cleared with the hospital staff; if more than one person is
in the room, the other patients must also be comfortable with the oils used.

It is also important for the therapist to be as comfortable as possible and not get into postures that strain or stress his own body. This may mean moving about or changing positions frequently.

For information on treating a client in a wheelchair, see the chapter on ambulation aids.

Massage at a Sporting Event

Tables, linens and heat and cold packs may be supplied by the organizers of the event; more commonly, the therapist brings a portable massage table or chair and his own supplies. These can include an adequate supply of sheets, pillows and towels. Case forms, lotions, disinfectant hand soap, table disinfectant, assessment tools such as a goniometer and tape measure, and hydrotherapy applications can be carried in a sports equipment bag.

Health history forms must be stored in a secure place.

Depending on the location of the sporting event, treatments may occur in separate rooms or in an area set aside for health care needs and first aid. If treatment is in a private room, the therapist proceeds as described in the previous sections for table set up, pillowing and draping. If the treatment occurs in an area set aside for health care needs, curtained private tables may or may not be available. In a case where the therapist is working in an open area, the client remains dressed during treatment. Often the client is wearing shorts and a sleeveless tank top, so lotions or oils can be used on uncovered skin. Otherwise, direct pressure is used through clothing. The table is covered by a single sheet and wiped down thoroughly with disinfectant cleanser between clients.

The therapist should be alert for athletic injuries and for hematoma, sudden swelling, spasm and other signs of inflammation. These concerns are covered in the musculoskeletal injuries section of this book.

End of Treatment

Once the treatment is concluded, the client is redraped. She is instructed to take a few moments to relax on the table. The therapist tells her that after he leaves the room, she can get up and get dressed, unless she needs assistance.

The client is also instructed to sit up slowly to prevent dizziness from occurring. This dizziness, if it occurs, may be due to positional hypotension; blood temporarily leaves the brain as the client sits up suddenly.

Self-care

✍ In general, a client recovers more rapidly and completely from a condition or injury when she participates actively in the healing process through a self-care plan. Self-care includes remedial exercise, hydrotherapy, self-massage, diaphragmatic breathing and referrals to other practitioners, self-help groups or exercise programs.

✍ Self-care suggestions should fit in with the client's abilities and lifestyle for the greatest likelihood of compliance. For example, one or two specific exercises that can be done first thing in the morning, perhaps in the shower, will more likely be done than a complex series of exercises.

✍ To help a client remember the self-care program, written take-home instructions for any hydrotherapy application or diagrams for remedial exercises are helpful. Commercially prepared stretching exercises printed on tear-off sheets are available for the therapist to purchase *(Anderson, 1980)* or the therapist may print up his own instructions.

✍ It is important that the client perform the exercises correctly and safely. The therapist should demonstrate the remedial exercise to the client after the treatment. The client then performs the exercise so the therapist can see if she is doing it safely and correctly.

Self-care for the Therapist

✍ Self-care during the treatment for the therapist includes keeping the body as relaxed as possible while working, without straining or torquing to reach over the client's body. It is important to use biomechanically sound positions during massage. The therapist uses his body weight for leverage, rather than just arm strength, and remembers to breathe while working.

✍ After the treatment, self-care for the therapist includes stretching, hydrotherapy and massage. For example, stretches for flexors and extensors of the wrist, pectoralis major and minor, and the scalene muscles are important. Hydrotherapy, such as regular contrast arm baths or wax baths, is helpful.

✍ The therapist is recommended to receive massage treatments focusing on the forearms, pectoral muscles and rotator cuff muscles using muscle stripping, trigger point techniques and fascial techniques including skin rolling, and joint play — just like the treatments recommended for the client. Classes that teach stretching, yoga, Tai Chi, correct postural movement or other exercise are also suggested.

✍ If the therapist develops overuse syndromes or has a postural dysfunction, the appropriate chapter for treatment applies to the therapist as well as the client. A therapist should have his own therapist for tissue maintenance and well being.

12

WORKING WITH THE CLIENT'S TISSUE

Fiona Rattray, Linda Ludwig

In order to perform an effective massage, the therapist must approach the treatment with a clear, focused mind. With a solid foundation in anatomy, physiology and pathology, as well as some clinical experience, the therapist can approach the massage intelligently while striving to apply the techniques in an artful manner. This blend will result in the therapist "making decisions as he goes along. For that reason, he'll be absorbed and attentive to what he's doing even though he doesn't deliberately contrive this. His motions...are in a kind of harmony" *(Pirsig, 1974)*.

A knowledge base of anatomy includes muscle actions, joint ranges, where muscles and fascia attach, fibre direction and the relation of muscles to one another and other tissues such as fascia, ligaments, tendons and bones. A knowledge of physiology is necessary to understand the relationship between structure and function. The therapist needs to understand the difference between healthy and dysfunctional tissue and the mechanisms of pathology that cause disease. This understanding of healthy and dysfunctional or pathological tissue is gained by touching a lot of tissue. After palpating 500 middle scalene muscles, the therapist gets a broad experience of what *middle scalene* is: for example, the differences in tone and texture, thickness, length, movement or lack of it, the difference in the muscle's orientation from one client to the next and how the muscles respond to the various techniques used on them.

Good communication skills are important when working with the client's tissue. The therapist shares what she is palpating, perceiving and doing; the client shares with the therapist what he is feeling while the work is being done; together the client and therapist communicate to maximize the effectiveness of the techniques. It is an unfortunate therapist who thinks she can, or should, feel everything and not use the rich resource of the client's experience.

Using Appropriate Pressure and Speed

Good palpation skills and the ability to choose techniques that are appropriate for the type of tissue, its state of health and the treatment plan are important. The therapist should remain alert as to whether the client is comfortable with the techniques and pressure being used during the treatment. The therapist should ask the client directly if the pressure is uncomfortable should the client breathe more rapidly or flinch from the touch. The judgement necessary to calculate the correct pressure and rate in applying techniques arises from experience.

✦ Ideally, the therapist uses the *minimum pressure and rate required to achieve the desired change in the tissue (Basmajian, 1985)*. While too little pressure may make a technique safe, it may be ineffective. However, the rapid application of too much pressure may be painful or unsafe. A successful treatment includes techniques that are both effective and safe.

Finely tuned palpation skills will reveal the appropriate pressure, whether light or heavy, that will affect a specific tissue layer. Pressure the therapist uses will vary from light to heavy to light again within the course of one treatment. It will likely even vary with the same client from treatment to treatment. The appropriate amount of pressure is a function of the client's perceived pain levels and the resistance of the tissue to palpation. An exercise in improving layer palpation skills is included at the end of this chapter.

✦ For the student massage therapist, the Granter-King grading system is one method of determining the appropriate pressure *(Brukner, Khan, 1993)*.

✦ The **client's** perception of pain is graded: 1 is no pain, 2 is onset of tolerable discomfort or pain, 3 is moderate pain and 4 is severe pain (used infrequently).

✦ The **therapist's** perception of tissue resistance is graded: "A" is no perceived tissue resistance, "B" is onset of tissue resistance and "C" is moderate tissue resistance.

• For an **acute** injury, the therapist uses a 1A depth (no pain and no tissue resistance) to avoid further tissue damage and to assess the client's response to the treatment.

• For an **early subacute** injury, the therapist uses a 1B depth (no pain and onset of tissue resistance).

• For a **late subacute** injury a 2B depth is appropriate (onset of tolerable discomfort or pain and onset of tissue resistance).

• For a **chronic** injury, 2C and 3C depths are used.

In terms of speed of a technique, all soft tissue has a rate at which it deforms (or can be manipulated) and a rate at which it reacts (by lengthening or by contracting). This rate varies from one tissue type to another and from client to client *(Greenman, 1989)*. Forcing the tissue faster than this rate can be painful for the client and can cause the surrounding tissue to become hypertonic, or tighter, a protective mechanism. If in pain, the client will sometimes unconsciously, sometimes consciously, tighten the muscles to "push" the therapist out.

Finally, the rate at which a tissue deforms is related to its health; adhesions are more bound down than healthy, flexible tissue.

Being *Deep* Without Being Forcible

Techniques may be *deep* without being forcible or invasive if the therapist works with the client's breathing. If a broad pressure is used initially to reach the psoas muscle with, for example, the therapist's palmar surface, the client can relax his abdominal muscles under the therapist's touch. As the muscles relax, the therapist then focuses the pressure into a narrower application with, for example, the fingertips. As the client exhales, the therapist compresses into the abdomen until resistance is felt in the tissue. This resistance may be pain-free or perhaps tolerably tender. The pressure is maintained as the client inhales. With each cycle of breathing, the therapist moves deeper into the tissue until the psoas is palpated. As the therapist gains palpation skills, the length of time it takes to reach the psoas decreases.

The therapist's hands should be relaxed yet moulded to the client's tissues. The concepts of *hard* and *soft* touch will enable the therapist to work deeper into the tissue without being invasive. If the therapist uses a hard touch, keeping the hands pokey, rigid and tense, the client is uncomfortable and tenses up. In contrast, if the therapist uses a soft touch, letting the hands be flexible and relaxed while maintaining the necessary pressure, the client is more comfortable and relaxed. Using a soft touch also allows the therapist to feel changes in the tissue more easily. To demonstrate this, the therapist tenses the hand while palpating any muscle, noting how little sensory information the palpating hand can receive while it is tense. The therapist repeats the exercise with a relaxed hand and notes the increase in sensory information. This relaxed approach is facilitated if the therapist is relaxed; diaphragmatic breathing is not only for the client's use.

Finally, the therapist's intent also influences any technique. If the therapist views the tissue as being mobile and fluid, working with its rate of release, she is more likely to reach the targeted structures efficiently and comfortably.

The Systematic Approach

It is important to develop a systematic approach to palpating and treating each muscle in a group of muscles that make up a body part. The therapist mentally reviews the anatomy of the region to be worked on, visualizing the structures under the hands in a three dimensional image. Each muscle in the group is first assessed in terms of tone, texture, temperature and tenderness. Any dystrophic or painful areas are noted. This assessment is **ongoing** while the therapist is treating the tissue.

Each muscle is treated from one tendinous attachment to the other, so nothing is missed. For example, when working the muscles of the upper back and shoulder, the therapist may start with an effleurage that covers the whole back, palpating for general differences in temperature, texture, tenderness and tone. Petrissage in the form of scooping is then applied to the upper fibres of the trapezius, working from the scapula to the cervical attachments. The rhomboids are treated with palmar kneading; deeper, more specific fingertip kneading and muscle stripping are focused on the erector spinae group and semispinalis. The deeper muscles attaching superior to the scapula, such as levator scapulae and supraspinatus, are muscle stripped from one attachment to the other. A similar pattern is followed with infraspinatus, teres major and teres minor. The deltoid is treated with picking up and kneading. The therapist then returns to an effleurage that covers the latissimus dorsi and the muscles surrounding the scapula that were just treated. Any areas that need more attention may now be treated more thoroughly. For example, the therapist may have noted crepitus at the levator scapula insertion at the scapula or fibrosing and trigger points within teres major. This systematic method ensures that no muscle is overlooked and that the client experiences a feeling of flow and continuity in techniques.

Overtreated Tissue

The therapist should be careful not to overtreat the tissue in any one session. Tissue that has been overtreated or overworked with massage techniques becomes tender, hyperemic and hot. It may remain this way for hours or even a day or two. The client may report post-treatment tenderness in the overworked muscles. To avoid this, the therapist should not become overly focused on one area of the body or lose track of how long she has spent on a given structure. It is important to remember that rarely is just one area the cause of the client's complaint.

If heat and hyperemia develop in tissue that has been treated for too long, repetitive effleurage and an application of cool or cold hydrotherapy may help to prevent post-treatment tenderness. The client may also be instructed to apply ice as self-care if the tissue remains warm or feels tender. The prolonged heat and hyperemia of overtreated tissue should not be confused with the temporary hyperemia and heat release associated with successful fascial techniques or with the desired inflammatory response to friction techniques (and that is controlled by an ice application). Nor should it be confused with the desired temporary hyperemia and warmth of tissue that follows techniques used to increase local circulation or the application of hot hydrotherapy.

Palpation Exercise

A simple exercise can be used to increase the therapist's palpation skills and awareness of tissue layers. Skin, subcutaneous tissue, vasculature, nerves, fascia, muscle, tendon, ligaments, bursa, joint space, bone, anatomical barriers to movement and end feel are all encountered in this exercise *(Neumann, 1989)*.

The exercise can be done by one therapist and another person or by two therapists simultaneously. The therapist and the person being palpated are both comfortably seated, facing each other across a table. If only one therapist is performing the exercise, the person is asked to supinate one forearm on the table so the flexor surface is uppermost. If two therapists are working together, both supinate the same side forearms on the table — for example, the right forearms — which become the surfaces to be palpated. The hands on the other side are the examining tools — for example, the left hands.

◆ The relaxed palm and fingers of the therapist's left hand make slow, gentle contact with the person's skin over the flexor surface. The therapist thinks "skin" and evaluates how warm, cool, thick, soft or rough the skin is.

◆ The therapist uses a bit more pressure to assess the subcutaneous tissues. By moving the tissue superiorly and inferiorly, medially and laterally, the therapist checks how loose or tight the subcutaneous tissue is. How thick is the layer? Can it be moved in one direction more easily than another? Arteries, veins and nerves can all be palpated in the subcutaneous tissue layer. Many tissue changes resulting from a somatic dysfunction can be palpated at this tissue level *(Neumann, 1989)*.

✦ The therapist increases the pressure to reach the deep layer of fascia over the muscles, while thinking "fascia". This layer can be described using terms such as firmness, softness, areas of thickening and continuity.

✦ The person being palpated is asked to open and close the left hand, while the therapist palpates the muscle layer under the fascia. Can the individual muscles and the septa covering them be noted? Are any muscle fibres palpable?

✦ The person is now asked to isometrically contract the flexors by making a fist, while the tone of the flexor muscles is noted. This approximates the tone present in a hypertonic muscle.

✦ While the person is making a fist, the therapist also tenses her own hand and notes what ability she has to evaluate the texture of the muscle, then the subcutaneous tissue and finally the skin when tension is held in the therapist's own hand.

✦ After relaxing her hand again, the therapist now follows the person's flexor muscles distally towards the wrist. At what point does the muscle become the musculotendinous junction? This area is often prone to injury. At what point does the width of the muscle become the round hardness of the flexor tendons?

✦ By following the tendons distally to the carpal bones and staying at the same depth of pressure, the therapist may palpate the transverse carpal ligament. This structure runs medially to laterally. How thick or firm is it? In what direction do the fibres run?

✦ The therapist now moves the right hand proximally to the person's elbow, while the person is asked to pronate the forearm and slightly flex the elbow. The therapist's index finger is placed on the olecranon and the thumb is placed on the head of the radius. Using more pressure, the therapist thinks "bone" and evaluates how hard the bone is and how it reacts to pressure. The person is asked to slowly supinate and pronate the forearm, while the therapist feels the difference between the moving head of the radius and the stationary olecranon. Under normal circumstances, the olecranon bursa cannot be palpated unless a bursitis is present.

✦ The therapist now moves the index finger to grasp the head of the radius, so the index finger moves into the joint space. The joint capsule is located here. Under normal circumstances it cannot be palpated unless a joint pathology is present.

✦ The person is asked to supinate and pronate the forearm again while the therapist feels for the anatomical barrier to the end range of active movement. Then the therapist passively supinates and pronates the person's forearm, noting the end feel of the joint. Is it leathery or springy?

✦ Finally, the therapist returns to the pressure originally used when first palpating the skin. Placing the hand over the flexor surface skin once more and moving the skin slightly distally, the therapist assesses the minimum amount of pressure needed for the person to report that the skin over the cubital fossa is being tugged on. How does this tissue resistance feel?

✦ Engaging the subcutaneous layer, the therapist feels the minimum amount of distal pressure needed for the person to feel drag in the skin over the biceps or over the deltoid. This proprioceptive sense of tissue drag and resistance can be used to palpate changes in the tissue while assessing and while treating.

✦ The exercise can also be performed by the therapist on her own arm.

13

CONTRAINDICATIONS AND MODIFICATIONS FOR SPECIFIC CONDITIONS AND MEDICATIONS

Fiona Rattray

A **contraindication** (CI) is a symptom or circumstance that makes a particular treatment inadvisable. In terms of massage therapy, a contraindication may be absolute; in other words, massage is an inappropriate method of treating a particular condition that affects either the whole body or a part of the body. For example, massage is an inappropriate treatment during an acute asthma attack, but is beneficial between attacks. It is also inappropriate and unsafe to massage locally over an open wound or over a local contagious skin condition; however, massage to other parts of the client's body is safe.

A treatment **modification** is a change to the initial treatment plan when massage is appropriate for the client, to allow for safe, effective treatment. Modifications may be made in technique choice, pressure and direction of technique, position of the client, hydrotherapy duration, location and temperature, area treated and duration of treatment. For example, with a peripheral nerve lesion, deep work and direct fascial techniques are not used on the flaccid muscles. However, light stroking over them is appropriate and safe. A person with multiple sclerosis may only tolerate a short local application of heat, such as following treatment of a trigger point. However, she could not tolerate a full-body application such as a bath.

The concepts of absolute contraindication and modifications of treatment are often combined in clinical usage into one catch-all phrase: *contraindications to treatment*. Contraindications to treatment noted in an assessment are discussed with the client before treatment begins so the necessary modifications can be made, or occasionally the client can be referred to another health care practitioner.

There are many reasons for massage therapy to be contraindicated. For example, a thrombus may be dislodged from a femoral vein by deep, vigorous local petrissage. Full-strength active resisted maximal isometric testing may further injure a moderate gastrocnemius strain. Deep moist heat applied to an area of acute inflammation will painfully congest the injury site, slowing the healing process. Joint play may damage a joint capsule weakened by long-term rheumatoid arthritis. The reasons for specific contraindications to massage therapy are listed in each chapter.

A therapist can stay current with the conditions that contraindicate massage through a local regulating body.

The following list contains absolute contraindications and treatment modifications that are a combination of recommendations from the College of Massage Therapists of Ontario, research and clinical practice (*College of Massage Therapists of Ontario, 1991*).

Absolute Contraindications to General Conditions

Massage therapy is not appropriate for a client with the following conditions.

✦ **Acute conditions requiring first aid or medical attention:** anaphylaxis, appendicitis, cerebrovascular accident, diabetic coma or insulin shock, myocardial infarction, pneumothorax, atelectasis, severe asthmatic attack, status asthmaticus, acute seizure or syncope (fainting)

✦ Acute pneumonia

✦ Advanced kidney failure, advanced respiratory failure or liver failure (a very modified treatment may be possible with medical consent)

✦ Diabetes with complications such as gangrene, advanced heart or kidney disease or very unstable or high blood pressure

✦ Eclampsia

✦ Hemophilia

✦ Hemorrhage

✦ Post-cerebrovascular accident or post-myocardial infarction where the condition has not stabilized

✦ Severe atherosclerosis

✦ Severe, undiagnosed headaches in those over 50 years of age

✦ Severe, unstable hypertension

✦ Shock

✦ Significant fever (38.5º C, 101.5º F)

✦ Some highly metastatic cancers not judged terminal

✦ Systemic contagious or infectious condition

Absolute Contraindications to Local Conditions

Massage therapy is not appropriate locally for any of the following conditions.

✦ Acute flare-up of inflammatory arthritides, such as rheumatoid arthritis, systemic lupus erythematosus or ankylosing spondylitis (the contraindication may be general depending on the presentation)

✦ Acute neuritis

✦ Acute trigeminal neuralgia

✦ Aneurisms deemed life-threatening — for example of the abdominal aorta (the contraindication may be general depending on the location)

+ Deep vein thrombosis, thrombophlebitis or arteritis (may be a general contraindication if located in a major circulatory vessel)

+ Ectopic pregnancy

+ Esophageal varicosities

+ Frostbite

+ Local contagious condition

+ Local irritable skin condition

+ Malignancy, especially if judged unstable

+ Open wound, sore, decubitus ulcer

+ Pain syndromes, such as causalgia or reflex sympathetic dystrophy

+ Radiation therapy site both during and up to several weeks post-radiation therapy (physician's consent is important)

+ Recent burn

+ Sepsis

+ Undiagnosed lump

+ Varicosities (up to 24 hours post-treatment with saline injection)

General Conditions Requiring Treatment Modifications

The following conditions require an awareness of possible adverse effects of massage therapy without appropriate and substantial treatment modifications. Consultation with the client's physician may be required with the client's written permission.

+ Any condition of spasticity (for example, cerebral palsy, hemiplegia, multiple sclerosis, spinal cord injury) or rigidity (Parkinsons)

+ Asthma

+ Cancer, ensuring that massage therapy is not in conflict with any other treatment being given

+ Congestive heart failure

+ Chronic kidney disease

+ Client who is immunosuppressed

+ Coma (may be an absolute contraindication depending on the cause)

+ Debilitation

+ Diagnosed atherosclerosis

+ Drug withdrawal

+ Emphysema

+ Fibromyalgia

+ Hypertension

+ Hypotension

+ Inflammatory arthritides
+ Major surgery or abdominal surgery
+ Medication use by client: anti-inflammatories, muscle relaxants, stimulants, anticoagulants, analgesics or any other medications that alter sensation, muscle tone, standard reflex reactions, cardiovascular function, kidney or liver function or emotions
+ Moderate diabetes mellitus (regarding tissue health and potential for hypoglycemic attack)
+ Osteoporosis or osteomalacia
+ Pregnancy and labour
+ Post-cerebrovascular accident or myocardial infarction
+ Recent head injury
+ Seizure disorders

Local Conditions Requiring Treatment Modifications

+ Acute disc herniation
+ Aneurysm (may be a general contraindication depending on the location)
+ Acute inflammatory conditions and injuries
+ Any anti-inflammatory injection site (target tissue and the immediate vicinity) for up to 21 days post-injection (Persad, 1995a)
+ Any chronic or long-standing thrombosis
+ Bell's palsy (possibility of eye infection)
+ Buerger's disease (may be a general contraindication if unstable)
+ Bursitis
+ Chronic arthritic conditions
+ Chronic abdominal or digestive disease
+ Chronic inflammation (such as sinusitis, chronic bronchitis)
+ Contusion
+ Diarrhea
+ Endometriosis
+ Flaccid paralysis or paresis
+ Flare-up of irritable bowel syndrome
+ Fracture while casted and post cast removal until muscle tone has returned and tissue fragility has decreased
+ Frozen shoulder
+ Hematoma
+ Hernia
+ Indwelling medication catheter (thorax)
+ Infection, including parasites (proximal drainage and circulation techniques are avoided)
+ Inflammatory bowel disease

- ✦ Joint instability or hypermobility
- ✦ Joint hypomobility due to pins, screws, wires, plates or surgical shortening of ligaments
- ✦ Lymphedema
- ✦ Kidney infection or kidney stones
- ✦ Mastitis
- ✦ Migraine
- ✦ Minor surgery
- ✦ Ostomy site
- ✦ Pelvic inflammatory disease
- ✦ Pitting edema
- ✦ Portal hypertension
- ✦ Prolonged constipation
- ✦ Raynaud's disease and phenomenon
- ✦ Recent abortion
- ✦ Recent vaginal birth
- ✦ Spasmodic torticollis
- ✦ Stress fracture site
- ✦ Temporomandibular joint dysfunction
- ✦ Tracheotomy site
- ✦ Trigeminal neuralgia between attacks
- ✦ Varicosities

Massage Therapy Contraindications to Specific Medication Use

Medication that the client is taking may necessitate modifications to the treatment plan. The client may not view the daily use of Aspirin or other over-the-counter medication as having an effect on the body that may contraindicate massage therapy, or she may not reveal certain medication use on a written health history form, such as antidepressants. Furthermore, the client's physician may be unaware that the client is receiving massage therapy or that there are some specific massage contraindications to medication use. An example is when a physician refers a client for frictions to treat a tendinitis while the client is also taking anti-inflammatory medication.

It is, therefore, important for the therapist to *ask the client* if she is taking any medication, including over-the-counter and herbal remedies. The length of time that a medication has its effect on the body varies, depending on the dosage and the client's tissue health and metabolism. Medication in capsule and tablet form generally enters the bloodstream within 30 minutes, with liquid oral dosages requiring slightly less time. Injections and inhalations are almost instantaneous in their action.

Muscle relaxant levels peak in the blood one to three hours after ingestion and may last for six to 12 hours *(Persad, 1995b)*. On the other hand, Aspirin reaches peak blood levels in two to four hours and may be present in reduced quantities 24 hours later *(Persad, 1995a)*. Some medications have multiple uses, such as Diazepam, which is both a muscle relaxant and an antidepressant, and Aspirin, which is an analgesic and anticoagulant *(Canadian Pharmaceutical Association, 1996)*. The client may also be on several medications for different conditions, which may complicate the massage contraindications.

Analgesics

Due to the nature of analgesic medication, the client is unable to give accurate information about the perception of pain. Deep pressure and extreme ranges of motion are contraindicated.

✦ Aspirin, Tylenol, Anaprox and Motrin are examples of non-narcotic analgesics.

Anti-asthmatic Medication

Anti-asthmatic drugs can cause an increase in sympathetic nervous system response, such as increased heart and respiration rates and an increase in blood pressure. If an increase in blood pressure is present, techniques that are vigorous, deep or painful and hydrotherapy applications of heat are contraindicated.

✦ Ventolin is an example of this medication type.

Anticoagulants

Anticoagulant medications slow the clotting process. It is possible that deep techniques such as deep, repetitive muscle stripping and frictions could lead to bruising.

✦ Aspirin, coumadin and heparin are anticoagulants.

Antidepressants

Antidepressants can alter the normal responses of the vasculature to temperature changes. Hydrotherapy applications should be at moderate temperatures and local in nature, and the client should be monitored both visually and by palpation for any adverse reactions. Full-body hydrotherapy applications are contraindicated.

✦ Diazepam (Valium), Prozac and Paxil are antidepressants.

Anti-inflammatories

The suppression of the inflammatory process can make an assessment inaccurate. Moreover, techniques such as frictions that rely on this response — which has been suppressed —are contraindicated.

✦ Aspirin, Tylenol and Clinoril are examples of this medication type.

Corticosteroids

Specialized anti-inflammatories such as corticosteroids appear in various forms including injections, tablets and creams. Injection sites are avoided for 14 to 21 days post-injection

(Persad, 1995a). Prolonged use of corticosteroids may lead to the following concerns. In general, tissue healing may be delayed and there may be decreased bone formation, leading to osteoporosis. With repeated injections, the injection site is tender and the connective tissue and muscle break down. A palpable gap in the muscle may be noticed in areas that have had repeated injections.

Prolonged use of skin creams containing corticosteroids may lead to atrophy of the skin and subcutaneous tissue. On palpation, the skin and muscle may feel inelastic. Techniques that stress the tissue, such as fascial techniques, frictions and joint play, are contraindicated.

✦ Topicort, Cortisol, Corticream and Aclovate are examples of this type of medication.

Muscle Relaxants

Muscle relaxant medications act on the neuromuscular junction, altering the stretch response of the muscles. The muscle may feel stretchy or loose on palpation. Deep techniques, extreme stretches and full-body hydrotherapy applications are contraindicated. Hydrotherapy should be moderate in temperature and local in application. The client should be instructed to get up off the table slowly, since postural hypotension and dizziness may be present with medication use.

✦ Flexeril, Diazepam (Valium) and Norflex are examples of muscle relaxants *(Canadian Pharmaceutical Association, 1996; Persad, 1995b).*

Other Important Considerations

Blood Pressure Precautions

It is suggested that when a therapist sees a client for the first time, he take the client's blood pressure. How to take blood pressure is described in the chapter on hypertension. It is also important to know current blood pressure especially when treating clients who are pregnant or who have cardiovascular concerns, since treatment modifications may be indicated due to hypertension. A client with hypotension should be instructed to get up from the table slowly to prevent post-treatment dizziness.

It is important to keep the stethoscope and blood pressure cuff wiped down with an alcohol wipe to prevent possible bacterial infection *(Globe and Mail, 1995).*

Possible Allergic Reactions

Health history questions should establish any known allergies the client may have.

Clients may be allergic to certain nut oils, such as peanut oil, to creams, or disinfectants used on the tables, or soaps and fabric softeners used on the sheets. The therapist must ask health history questions to determine this and avoid using such products with these clients.

Allergies or allergic reactions to dusts, molds and pollens mean a treatment room should be kept clean and free of such allergens.

The client may also have reactions to scents or perfumes. The therapist is advised to remain as scent-neutral as possible by not wearing perfumes or after-shave lotions while working.

In terms of essential oils, most allergic scent reactions are to any synthetic chemical components of a perfume rather than to natural, unadulterated essential oils used in massage therapy. However, allergic reactions to essential oils can occur. For example, pine, clove and cinnamon essential oils may provoke local skin irritation in some clients *(Watt, 1992)*. The therapist is advised to have the client smell an essential oil before it is used either in a treatment or in self-care. This helps the client determine if the essential oil is offensive to the client before it is applied to the skin.

Bergamot and lemon essential oils increase the photosensitivity of the client's skin to ultraviolet rays and may allow the skin to burn more readily when it is exposed to sunlight or other sources of ultraviolet light *(Watt, 1992)*. The therapist should advise the client to avoid skin exposure to sunlight or ultraviolet tanning beds for a few hours following the use of either of these essential oils. Alternatively, after the treatment the client may wash off the oils to avoid possible burns.

Preventing Possible Infection

Skin conditions or cuts on the therapist's hands or on the client's body require the therapist to wear single-use disposable gloves. Vinyl is recommended over latex for glove composition, because some people have serious allergies to latex. If the therapist wants to use latex gloves, health history questions to determine possible latex allergies should be asked before use.

For the therapist treating temporomandibular joint dysfunction, where intra-oral work is required, use of single-use, disposable vinyl gloves is also indicated to prevent transmission of bacterial or viral infection between the therapist and client.

Body fluid spills on sheets or tables — for example, blood or exudate from lesions — should be cleaned with the usual precautions to prevent viral or bacterial infection (universal precautions). A 9:1 solution of water and bleach (a 10 per cent bleach solution) is used for cleaning; the therapist wears vinyl gloves to clean up and disposes of the gloves and cleaning cloth afterwards.

Linens are bagged separately from other soiled linens in a plastic bag marked "contaminated with body fluids". If the therapist cleans her own linens, they are washed in hot soapy water separately from other soiled linens and dried on a hot setting. For more information on updated universal precautions, the therapist may contact the local board of health.

Consultations and Referrals

Massage therapists should know when to consult with physicians and other health care professionals, and how to do so. With the client's permission, the therapist may send a letter of introduction and a summary of the massage treatment plan to the other health care provider or providers. This professional courtesy contributes to building professional relationships with other health care providers. Local regulating bodies or health care professional associations can be resources for referrals to other practitioners.

Referrals may also be required with clients who have emotional or psychiatric conditions. This topic is beyond the scope of this text; however, therapists may refer to resources such as **Emotional First Aid** *(Haldane, 1984)* for more information.

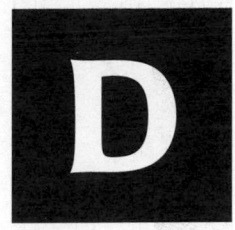

TREATMENT
FOUNDATIONS

14

STRESS REDUCTION AND RELAXATION:
The Essential Treatment

Linda Ludwig

> **Stress is defined as the body's non-specific response to any demand made upon it (Selye, 1974). Stress is not a disease but can contribute to ill health.**

The definition of stress was developed by Hans Selye, a world-renowned Canadian endocrinologist and a leading authority on stress and its effects. It may seem a fairly dry and innocuous definition for a condition that adversely affects most people at some point over the course of their lives. For the massage therapist, however, the components of a stress reduction massage are the basis of all treatments. This is because the emotional and physical effects of the body's stress response are pervasive and manifest to varying degrees whenever pain and worry are present. A detailed exploration of what happens to a person when stress is experienced ensures a clear understanding of the focus on reducing stress in every treatment.

Selye's definition refers to the fact that the internal environment of the body must be in balance, a state known as "homeostasis". Non-specific responses are required within the body to enable adaptation to the constantly changing demands placed on it. If the body is cold, a person shivers and blood vessels vasoconstrict to conserve heat; if the body is hot, a person sweats, the evaporation of sweat having a cooling effect. While these are specific reactions, the term "non-specific response" refers to the fact that the body must make some kind of adaptation to a problem no matter what the problem is. Even when a person is completely relaxed and comfortable, stress is experienced in the body with, for example, the digestion of food, the beating of the heart or the contraction of muscles that hold a person upright. Complete freedom from stress would mean death.

Selye differentiates between stress and distress. Stress includes the usual physiological activity required to maintain homeostasis and the healthy emotional stress that makes life interesting and exciting — the "spice of life". Distress is the term used to denote harmful aspects of physical and emotional stress. Unfortunately, this distinction has been lost. Through common usage, stress has come to signify the negative aspects of this state, physically or emotionally, such as physical injury, illness, pain, fear, challenge, grief or change.

Causes of stress vary for each individual but include:

➤ **emotions** such as anxiety, depression and fear;

➤ **threats to self-esteem**;

➤ **pain** from injury or disease;

➤ **excessive intake of a stimulant** such as caffeine or chocolate, or as a side effect of medication such as overuse of an inhaler for respiratory difficulties;

➤ **pathology** such as hypothyroidism or a tumour affecting the pituitary or thyroid glands;

➤ **environmental exposure** to toxins or to excessive heat or cold.

Stress is considered a combination of **stressors** and a person's **stress reactivity.** Stressors are defined as potential triggers to the stress response, also known as the "fight or flight response". Stressors can be environmental agents or events, within or outside the body. They include mental and physical effort, heat, cold, hunger, fatigue and everyday life experiences. Stress reactivity is very individual, relating to the body's physiological response to a trigger. In fact, stressors can cause uncontrolled and excessive responses in many systems of the body, many of which are not appropriate or necessary to the triggering situation.

Stress reactivity is usually affected by the **degree** and **duration** of the stressor. In the case of emotional stressors, the degree or intensity of the emotional state is the significant factor, not whether the emotion is negative or positive, pleasant or unpleasant. Emotions are connected to the limbic system, which is one system in the brain that can trigger the stress reponse. Therefore, emotional stresses cause the same biochemical and physical changes within the body as physiological stresses. If someone is told a loved one has died, he experiences intense grief. If that loved one is then found to be alive, intense joy is experienced. While the emotions are different, the readjustment to the new situation is the same.

✦ Duration of the stressor influences the person's reactivity to it:

  • *a brief acute event* that does not recur, such as the immediate act of jumping out of the way of an oncoming car: the body's response is rapid and efficient;

  • *a series of stressful secondary events that occurs as a result of an initiating event,* such as divorce or job loss: yields various regularly occurring stressful situations, which, over time, can increase the person's physiological responses to potential stressors;

  • *chronic intermittent stress,* such as school exams or work deadlines: requires frequent responses to a regularly occurring stressor;

  • *chronic and sustained stress;* for example, not having time for breakfast, then getting stuck in traffic, followed by being unprepared for a meeting, being put on hold on the telephone, having lunch served slightly cool, and so on, all in one day, compounded by underlying stresses such as financial, health or relationship issues: the most incapacitating. This continual exposure to stressors fatigues the stress response and impairs its effectiveness.

So, even though an acute situation elicits an intense response, the response is short lived and ultimately less debilitating than an unrelenting, low-intensity response to less aggravating stressors.

Selye put forth the concept of the **General Adaptation Syndrome** (GAS) which explains the effects of long-term stress on the body and helps to explain why stress can cause illness. GAS refers to the stages the body goes through according to the duration of the stressor.

✦ *Alarm* denotes the first exposure of the body to a particular stress. The body's cortisol (a stress hormone) levels are high and no one organ system is predominantly active *(Porth, 1990)*. A sufficiently severe stress, such as a third degree burn on a large portion of the body, can be fatal.

✦ *Resistance/Adaptation* occurs if exposure to the stress continues. The body tries to resist the stress and adapt to it; the initial alarm response diminishes and cortisol levels decrease. The body's resistance response rises to above its normal reaction level. The duration of this period depends on the body's innate ability to adapt and the intensity of the stressor.

  • The body has a limited amount of energy to adapt to stress. A person risks his health by ignoring the body's limitations and exposing it to too much stress. Working long hours, not sleeping enough, eating poorly and drinking to excess can lead to illness. Ways of conserving the body's adaptive energy include a good night's sleep. After a stressful time, a holiday can restore resistance and adaptive ability.

  • In a physiological sense, the body will use the most efficient and effective response to a stressor. Short-term responses will be used first, such as a temporarily increased heart rate to increase oxygen to tissues in need. If the situation becomes chronic, a long-term adaptation occurs, such as hypertrophy of the heart's left ventricle in response to systemic hypertension.

✦ *Exhaustion* results after long exposure to the same stressor. The body has adapted but eventually the adaptive energy is exhausted. Signs of acute stress response, as in the alarm stage, reappear.

  • At this point, the reaction spreads through other systems in the body. Originally, adaptation occurs in the most appropriate systems but, over time, wear and tear result and other areas are affected *(Porth, 1990)*.

While people generally have the same stress response when it is triggered and similar adaptation patterns in chronic situations, in fact, we do not all respond to the same stressors or have the same stress reactivity. Stressors have the *potential* to trigger a fight or flight response and are very individual.

One person may be happy and not feel stressed about a job promotion whereas another may be very fearful of the change. Likewise, one person looks forward to retirement and another is worried about it.

The varying degrees of stress reactivity are partly due to different conditioning factors. Currently, it is thought that exposure to severe stressors at an early age could cause a person to become increasingly sensitive to stressors later — similar to the process in which one develops an increased sensitivity to particular allergens with each exposure. Similarly, genetics, gender, age, medication side effects and diet, such as the amount of stimulant intake, can affect how reactive a person is to a stressor.

The Anatomy of the Fight or Flight Response

The stress response is caused by the body's instinct to defend itself. The instinct known as the fight or flight response is a programmed reaction to perceived danger. It could be a response to an internal physical stressor such as a virus or hypertension or an external stressor such as being in the path of a speeding car or being faced with a dangerous person or animal. This primitive, instinctive response could save a person's life and served the early hunter-gatherers well as they fled from a dangerous animal.

Physiologically, the body gains alertness, strength and speed, allowing for immediate life-saving action. Many systems in the body are involved in initiating and maintaining this complex response. The response relies on communication, in the central nervous system, among various brain structures such as the cerebral cortex, the limbic system, the thalamus and the hypothalamus. Also involved are the reticular formation and the reticular activating system (RAS), and their influence on the autonomic nervous system and the endocrine, immune and musculoskeletal systems. The hypothalamus is a key player in the stress response through modulation of the autonomic nervous system and the endocrine system.

The Autonomic Nervous System

The **autonomic nervous system** regulates the internal functions of the body, in order to maintain a consistent internal environment (homeostasis). Smooth muscle such as the muscles of the visceral organs, arteries, arterioles and veins, the heart and the glands, among others, are controlled by this system.

The autonomic system is divided into two parts: the parasympathetic nervous system and the sympathetic nervous system. Normally, there is a low rate of continual firing through all the fibres of both the sympathetic and parasympathetic nervous systems. This allows for at least some degree of tone in affected structures such as blood vessel walls or organ walls. With an increase in firing there is an increase in the tone and, conversely, if there is a decrease in firing there is a decrease in tone. This allows for more precise control over specific functions. For example, as there is already some vasoconstriction or tone in a blood vessel wall, increased sympathetic nervous system firing will cause further vasoconstriction. Decreased firing could result in vasodilation.

There are three main differences between the two autonomic systems: the origin and distribution of the nerves; the type of neurotransmitter used post-ganglion; and the effects exerted on innervated structures (often these are opposing effects).

The Parasympathetic Nervous System

The **parasympathetic nervous system** conserves energy and serves to restore resources and maintain organ function during times of minimal activity. This system conserves the body's energy by slowing the heart rate and promoting the digestion of food — the "rest and digest" functions.

The fibres of this system originate in the brain stem, in several cranial nerves, primarily the vagus nerve (CN X) which supplies parasympathetic fibres to the heart, lungs and most of the organs in the abdomen including the stomach, small intestine and colon. The third, seventh and ninth cranial nerves supply the head, including the lacrimal, nasal and submaxillary glands. There are also fibres from the middle three segments of the sacral cord (S2 to S4) which supply the bladder, lower colon and rectum.

✦ The parasympathetic nervous system is responsible for:

- reduction of the heart rate;
- constriction of the pupils;
- secretion from most of the glands such as the salivary glands in the mouth and the gastric glands in the stomach;
- facilitation of food transit through the gastrointestinal tract with promotion of peristalsis and a decrease in the tone of the gastrointestinal sphincters;
- emptying of the urinary tract by increasing pressure in the bladder walls while relaxing the urethral sphincter.

✦ The parasympathetic nerve endings exert their effect on the body through the secretion of acetylcholine.

The Sympathetic Nervous System

The **sympathetic nervous system** expends the body's energy. Increased firing of this system is commonly referred to as the fight or flight response. It is stimulated by the hypothalamus, the limbic system and the reticular activating system in response to stress. The sympathetic nerve fibres exit from the spinal cord, beginning at the thoracic segments and continuing down to the second or third lumbar segments. These nerves exit the sympathetic chains that run along either side of the spinal cord and travel to supply various structures. The head is supplied by thoracic fibres which join cervical nerves before distributing to the neck and head arteries. Sympathetic nerves also supply the visceral organs such as the colon as well as travelling throughout the body with spinal nerves to innervate blood vessels, sweat glands and the erector pili muscles. In the case of the hunter-gatherer fighting a dangerous animal, the effectiveness of this response is clear.

✦ The sympathetic nervous system causes:

- mental alertness;
- increases in cellular metabolism;
- release of glucose and fats from the liver for quick energy and fuel for the cells involved in this intense activity;
- increased heart rate, as much as three times the norm, and an increased force of heart contractions;
- controlled blood flow, causing vasodilation (or a reduction of constriction) in skeletal-muscle blood vessels to better support the muscles that will be engaged in fleeing to safety or fighting. Skin and abdominal blood vessels may be vasoconstricted to limit bleeding in the case of an injury;
- an elevation in blood pressure from the increased peripheral resistance in the circulatory system, due to increased vasoconstriction;
- dilation of the bronchioles and rapid, apical breathing to allow increased oxygen intake;
- dilation of the pupils to allow more light to enter and to increase visual acuity;

- changes in the digestive process, such as a dry mouth and slower transit of food through the gastrointestinal tract due to the inhibition of peristalsis and increased tone of the sphincters;

- a decrease in urine output because of constriction of the urinary sphincters (digestion, defecation and urination are not essential activities if a person's life is in danger);

- increased sweating to cool the body that is engaged in activity.

✦ Sympathetic nerve endings mainly secrete norepinephrine to achieve their effects on the body.

The **endocrine system** consists of glands that secrete hormones and some cells that are diffusely located throughout organs and tissues. Hormones modulate body and cellular responses *(Porth, 1990)*. The hypothalamus acts as a command post for this system using two main signalling hormones — those which inhibit functions and those which stimulate actions. The hypothalamus-pituitary-adrenal axis refers to a system of communication among these structures. The hypothalamus secretes a cortisol-releasing factor, which stimulates the nearby pituitary gland to release ACTH (adrenocorticotrophic hormone). This hormone communicates to the distant adrenal glands, located above the kidneys. The adrenal glands release cortisol and epinephrine (also known as adrenaline).

The body undergoes many changes in response to these chemicals. Cortisol is involved in maintaining glucose levels, facilitating fat metabolism and influencing vascular flow and breathing. Epinephrine circulates in the bloodstream, reaching many cells that have no direct sympathetic innervation. This dilates some blood vessels and increases cellular metabolism and heart activity.

The **limbic system** is the emotional centre of the brain. Almost any intense emotion — anger, excitement, agitation or fear — can trigger reactions throughout the body. It is interesting that smell can influence emotions because of the close proximity of the olfactory sensory receptors to the limbic system. Emotions excite the limbic system and, in turn, the hypothalamus and endocrine systems, which increase the activity of the reticular activating system. The RAS then promotes sympathetic nervous system activity.

The **reticular activating system**, found within the reticular formation of the brain, influences not only the autonomic nervous system but also mental alertness and the musculoskeletal system. The RAS is stimulated through a variety of sensory input — somatic, visual and auditory — as well as through signals from the cerebral cortex, the hypothalamus and the limbic system. When excited, the RAS moves the entire brain to activity or wakefulness, promotes sympathetic nervous system function and influences stimulation of the **musculoskeletal system**. Muscle tone is increased when signals from the RAS are sent down the spinal cord to influence the gamma efferent fibres and muscle spindles within the nerves that control muscle tone. Muscular hypertonicity and the subsequent development of trigger points in these muscles commonly lead to neck stiffness, low back pain and headaches.

While the stress response is appropriate in an emergency, it becomes obvious that it is not a useful reaction to life's daily challenges and changes *(College of Family Physicians of Canada, 1995b)*. The body will respond to symbolic stressors as if they are life threatening but the fight or flight response before a major exam is not appropriate. Strength and speed are not necessary nor are increases in blood pressure, muscular tension and stress chemicals *(Greenberg, 1996)*. It seems that the brain has not evolved sufficiently to respond more appropriately to the symbolic stressors of the modern world.

Positive feedback loops contribute to problems in dealing with symbolic stressors, as well as in the case of pain perception. If the limbic system is stimulated, there is a resultant excitation of the autonomic nervous system and autonomic nervous system stimulation causes limbic system stimulation. This type of loop is considered unstable because it can create vicious cycles in which the initiating stimulus produces more of the same response *(Porth, 1990)*. In the case of the stress response, stimulation of the reticular activating system will stimulate connected systems — increased blood pressure and heart rate, increased respiratory rate and muscle tone. These increases will promote further excitation of the RAS. Interestingly, these can also work in reverse. If one system can be calmed, it can have an inhibiting effect on other related systems. A relaxation massage attempts to break the positive feedback of excitation of the involved systems by focusing on reducing muscular tension and pain, promoting slow, full breathing and calming the person emotionally.

Stress Can Make Us Sick

Stress can cause health problems or make them worse. As the adaptation stage goes on, physical symptoms occur. The body expends a lot of energy during this stage but has no chance to refuel and rebuild. Insomnia is frequently experienced. This contributes to feelings of fatigue, anxiety, fear and tension.

Today, there is an increased interest in the role that stress plays in the development of disease. The area of the body affected by stressors — heart, kidney, gastrointestinal tract or brain — will depend on which area of the body is the weakest link. An increase in serum cholesterol during stressful periods may contribute to *hypertension* and *heart disease (Greenberg, 1996)*. And the stress response itself, acting through the sympathetic nervous system, increases blood pressure and heart rate.

The exact mechanism by which stress affects *the immune response* is unknown. It is likely dependent on genetic and environmental factors. It is known that the stress response induces hormonal activity that can suppress some aspects of the immune response. Selye noted the presence of increased corticosteroid levels and atrophy of the thymus with the stress response, both of which would result in suppression of the immune response *(Selye, 1974)*. There is a clear relation between the increase in herpes simplex 1 and periods of inadequate rest and emotional upset. Usually the herpes virus is kept in check by body defences — mostly T-lymphocytes — until a stressful event suppresses the immune response. In addition, elevated cortisol levels present in those who are stressed interfere with the immune response and are linked to an increased susceptibility to colds and flu *(Porth, 1990)*. This diminished immune response is implicated in the development of *rheumatoid arthritis* with those who are genetically predisposed, as well as in the development of *cancer*. With those who have *asthma*, emotional stress can trigger the hyper-responsive smooth muscle of the bronchioles causing spasms and an asthma attack *(Vander et al., 1994)*.

Therefore, stress may contribute directly to the development of disease. It can also cause behaviours that contribute to the development of disease. Many people respond to stressful events by overeating, eating an unhealthy diet, smoking and increasing alcohol consumption or drug use, all of which place further stresses on the body.

Anxiety Disorder and Panic Attacks

✦ *Anxiety disorder* is experienced as a chronic generalized sense of uneasiness and fear. Usually there is a lack of clear, specific cause for these emotions. People with anxiety disorder startle easily and experience chronic fatigue and headaches. There is a tendency for anxiety disorder to run in families. It may also be related to minor cardiac problems such as a mitral valve prolapse *(Balch, Balch, 1997)*.

In some cases, the person's fear is specific though not particularly rational. Some people fear being in public or being alone, others may be fearful of heights, of flying or of an animal, insect or reptile. When exposed to these particular situations or creatures, the person's anxiety levels increase and anxiety disorder is triggered.

✦ *Panic attacks* are much more abrupt and intense compared to an anxiety disorder. Severe anxiety, including a sense of impending disaster or death, is experienced, along with a multitude of symptoms including:

- heart palpitations and tachycardia, throbbing or stabbing chest pain, tightness in the chest;
- shortness of breath with a tendency to hyperventilate; dry mouth, excessive yawning;
- hot flashes, chills, sweating;
- gastrointestinal disturbances such as nausea, epigastric pain and the constant urge to urinate or defecate;
- muscular tension leading to headaches, low back pain and muscle spasms, numbness and tingling in the extremities; general weakness and fatigue;
- insomnia, waking at night and nightmares;
- a sense of apprehension and unreality;
- for women, possible changes in the menstrual cycle or premenstrual symptoms;
- feelings of experiencing a heart attack or stroke.

The attack may last for a few seconds to half an hour. Frequency is variable, from every day to every few weeks and can happen any time, day or night. These types of attacks are much more common than once thought. Fifteen per cent of the population in the United States will experience a panic attack in their lifetimes; three per cent have experienced an attack in the previous month *(Murray, 1995)*.

The causes of these attacks are similar to those of general stress, such as conscious or unconscious emotional stress and excessive stimulant intake. However, they result in a much stronger physical response.

There appears to be a chemical imbalance involving lactic acid associated with the response. Those who suffer panic attacks are more sensitive to lactic acid imbalances than those who do not experience attacks. To correct the imbalance, at a given lactic acid level, hyperventilation may be triggered to facilitate the release of carbon dioxide in the blood to reduce carbon dioxide's acid-forming potential *(Fried, 1990)*. The hyperventilation will, in turn, stimulate a panic attack. Furthermore, as part of this imbalance, there may be hyperactivity of various areas of the brain which causes the release of norepinephrine and, in turn, increased heart rate, blood pressure and respiratory rate *(Balch, Balch, 1997)*. Food allergies, hypoglycemia and nutritional deficiencies, such as low calcium, magnesium and B vitamins, can bring on attacks and are commonly found in those with the disorder.

Medically, people are frequently treated with tranquillizers or antidepressants. This condition responds well to the stress reduction self-care recommendations listed at the end of the chapter.

Post-traumatic Stress Disorder (PTSD)

Post-traumatic stress disorder is considered an anxiety disorder. It can occur after one feels physical vulnerability and then experiences a traumatic event that produces an intense emotional response. This condition differs from other anxiety disorders because the person has, in fact, been exposed to a recognizable stressor of severity sufficient to evoke an extreme response in almost anyone (*Settle, 1996*). The psychological trauma may or may not include physical injury and even a relatively minor injury can still result in post-traumatic stress disorder. Much has been learned about this disorder through the study of the impact of war on soldiers, described as "brain weariness" in the American Civil War and "shell shock" in the First World War.

With post-traumatic stress disorder, the person repeatedly experiences flashbacks to the traumatizing event. There are attempts to avoid anything that reminds him of the trauma. Emotional numbing or decreased involvement with the outside world occurs, the person is no longer interested in activities previously enjoyed and is unable to feel emotions, especially intimacy. Other symptoms may include increased sympathetic nervous system firing which contributes to headaches, gastrointestinal problems, decreased appetite, sweating, palpitations, muscle spasms, fatigue, insomnia, being easily startled, anxiety or depression. There may also be impotence, blackouts, impaired memory, unpredictable outbursts of aggressive behaviour, difficulty completing tasks and problems concentrating. The symptoms can lead to substance abuse, difficulty with interpersonal relationships and even suicide.

Anxiety and other symptoms may recur or intensify when particular situations trigger memories of the original event. Sometimes the anniversary of the trauma will have the same result.

Duration of the disorder is variable. It is considered acute if it lasts less than six months and chronic if it is experienced for longer than six months. It is found that the condition lasts longer if the trauma is related to a human cause as opposed to a natural disaster such as a flood (*Achauer, 1987*).

For those who feel they require help, early recognition and treatment can facilitate recovery. Treatment includes relaxation strategies, especially breathing and visualization techniques, massage, counselling, including family therapy, and medication such as antidepressants.

Coping with Stress

The body can respond to physical or emotional stress by actively engaging in the stress response or by passively accepting the situation. Sometimes it is better for the person to ignore a situation or to consciously anticipate a problem, therefore suppressing the fight or flight instinct. Since a certain amount of stress is inevitable and unavoidable, it makes sense to develop efficient coping strategies. Many books and articles have been written on increasing one's ability to cope with stress specifically by improving the ability to relax. To this end, lifestyle changes include decreasing stimulant intake, getting adequate rest, having a healthy diet and exercising regularly. Anticipating a potentially stressful event or recognizing the development of a stressful situation is useful since a person can then attempt to control the response.

Stress and Breathing

Breathing is one of the few physical processes of the stress response over which a person can exercise some conscious control. Under stress, breathing becomes more shallow and apical as the body attempts to increase oxygen intake. The person can break this cycle by performing full resting breathing. During **relaxed inhalation** — also known as resting inhalation — the diaphragm contracts and flattens. The external intercostal muscles contract, which lifts the ribs and increases the anteroposterior and transverse dimensions of the thorax. The scalene muscles become active towards the end of resting inspiration, elevating the first and second ribs *(Basmajian, 1985)*. **Relaxed exhalation** is a passive process. As the diaphragm relaxes it moves upward into a domed shape. The external intercostals and scalenes also relax, allowing the ribs to drop. This type of breathing combined with meditation — a quietening of the mind — has proven successful in reducing blood pressure in those with hypertension. Dr. Herbert Benson, author of ***The Relaxation Response***, considers the relaxation response to be the opposite to the stress response. When the body is in this relaxed state, the increased heart and respiratory rates of the stress response diminish. Ten to 20 minutes of meditation daily can evoke this relaxation response. One study group reduced their systolic pressure an average of 10 points to 137 mm Hg and their diastolic pressure an average of five points to 88.9 mm Hg. These reductions were only maintained if the breathing sessions were continued daily *(Benson, Klipper, 1975)*.

Stress and Massage

Massage therapy has a positive impact in reducing the effects of stress on the body. Massage studies have been carried out by the Touch Institute at the University of Miami using increased cortisol levels as indicators of increased sympathetic nervous system firing and stress. Massage was found to reduce the levels of cortisol in the body and to decrease the person's perceived stress and anxiety levels *(Field et al., 1995d)*. It increases the person's awareness of tense areas in the body which enables the person to develop more relaxed posture and better breathing.

Creating an Appropriate Physical Space

The therapist must consider the massage space and create a safe physical environment that promotes relaxation. The consent to treatment gives the client control over the treatment, contributing to reduced stress levels. The therapist's voice is kept soft and conversation is brought to a minimum once the treatment begins, conveying a sense of calm and confidence throughout the session.

Warmth, moderate lighting, gentle music — approved by the client — and cleanliness all contribute to a positive space. Pure essential oils, used with client approval, can enhance relaxation. Lavender or marjoram, among others, may be placed in a diffuser or used to enrich an oil or lotion *(Lawless, 1995)*. A diffuser allows the essential oil to be dispersed into the air to be inhaled by the client whereas its addition to a massage lubricant allows for absorption through the skin and by inhalation. A 2.5 per cent dilution is made by adding 25 drops of essential oil to 50 ml. of carrier oil.

Symptom Picture

+ A person who is experiencing stress for whatever reason will exhibit certain common symptoms as a result of predictable muscle tension patterns, breathing problems and a suppressed immune response. In addition, a variety of conditions and diseases are linked to stress.

+ Hypertonicity in the muscles of the neck leads to headaches. Tension in the muscles of the lumbar area causes back pain.

+ Temporomandibular joint syndrome (TMJ syndrome) commonly results from teeth grinding and jaw clenching secondary to feelings of stress *(Greenberg, 1996)*.

+ Apical breathing contributes to hypertonicity of the respiratory muscles of the neck, the scalenes and the sternocleidomastoid muscles. Shortness of breath may result; an asthma attack can occur in people predisposed to asthma.

+ Feelings of anxiety, depression and irritability are experienced.

+ The gastrointestinal tract is affected. Constipation, diarrhea or irritable bowel syndrome, upset stomach and nausea may result. Though peptic ulcers are caused by Helicobacter pylori bacteria (H. pylori) rather than distress, stress can exacerbate this condition.

+ Weight gain or loss may be noticed.

+ Skin eruptions such as eczema, acne and herpes simplex may be caused or exacerbated.

+ Insomnia is common.

+ A decreased immune response leads to increased susceptibility to illness generally and specifically to colds and flu.

+ Chronic stress has been linked to rheumatoid arthritis, allergies, asthma, cancer, diabetes, gastrointestinal disorders, hormonal imbalances, atherosclerosis, hypertension and heart attack.

+ Increased stress levels aggravate spasticity and other symptoms associated with central nervous system lesions such as hemiplegia, multiple sclerosis and spinal cord injuries.

+ Anxiety disorder or panic attacks may occur.

Subjective Information

HEALTH HISTORY QUESTIONS

◆ What is the client's general health? Conditions such as hypothyroidism can cause an increased stress response. Asthma attacks may be exacerbated by stress.

◆ Does the client have any painful conditions, either acute or chronic?

◆ Does the client feel he is under some stress? This may be either a new stress, a temporary stress or a chronic, ongoing stress. Is the stress a controllable one?

◆ Is the client doing anything to reduce the effects of stress such as exercise, meditation, reducing stimulant intake or taking medication?

◆ Does the client take any medication that may provoke a stress response or insomnia such as overuse of an inhaler with asthma?

◆ Does the client have poor sleeping patterns? Does he wake up in the morning feeling refreshed or exhausted?

◆ Does the client experience anxiety attacks with increased heart rate and shallow breathing? How frequently does this occur?

◆ Has the client seen a physician?

Objective Information

Observations

✍ Apical breathing patterns are often observed. A client under stress breathes shallowly from the upper chest rather than deeply using the diaphragm.
✍ The shoulders may be raised, the jaw clenched or the hands held in fists.
✍ The posture appears rigid.
✍ The client may have a look of exhaustion due to lack of sleep.

Palpation

✍ Hypertonicity, trigger points and tenderness due to ischemia may be palpated in a variety of muscles. The muscles of mastication are affected by jaw clenching. Apical breathing further contributes to hypertonicity and trigger points in the neck and shoulder muscles. Low back muscles may be tight from holding the body rigidly.

Testing

✍ **AF ROM** is performed on any area experiencing discomfort or stiffness. This may reveal reduced range of motion of, for example, the cervical spine, the temporomandibular joint or the lumbar spine.

✍ **PR ROM** is performed on any area experiencing discomfort or stiffness. This may reveal reduced range of motion of the affected area with long-term stress.

✍ **AR testing** is performed on any area experiencing discomfort or stiffness. Muscle weakness and pain are present with active trigger points.

Special Tests

✍ **Breathing assessment**: Observation and palpation of the client's natural breathing patterns will likely reveal areas of restriction. Apical breathing is often noted, though a lack of lateral or upper chest movement may also occur. Paradoxical breathing is also a possibility. See the Non-Swedish Techniques chapter for details.

✍ **Motion palpation of the spine, anterior and lateral spinous challenge** and **rib motion** and **rib palpation testing** are performed. Restrictions may be noted.

Contraindications

✦ Aggressive or stimulating techniques such as tapotement and fascial techniques are used sparingly in the treatment. Treating a trigger point will perhaps be uncomfortable at the time of treatment, but will relieve referred pain and decrease muscular tension. These aid relaxation.

✦ Pressure on the abdomen should not be applied to the abdominal aorta, usually palpated just medial and inferior to the xiphoid process. If the pulse of the abdominal aorta or of any artery is noticeable, the therapist simply moves off this point.

Treatment Goals

The stress reduction massage is the basis of every massage treatment performed, regardless of the condition being treated.

Reduce pain and muscular hypertonicity and facilitate immune system function, healing and a calmer emotional state.

Treatment Plan

🖐 A full-body stress reduction treatment is usually described as lasting one hour. Once the time taken to obtain consent, assess the client and get him on the table is factored in, the massage itself may last from 50 to 55 minutes. When stress reduction is combined with another treatment, elements of stress reduction are incorporated into the other treatment. For example, when treating asthma and stress, the specific techniques and areas of the body treated with asthma are addressed in the overall predictable, soothing manner of the stress reduction treatment. As well, the therapist intersperses specific uncomfortable work with soothing techniques. For example, fascial techniques can be interspersed with stroking, or a treatment of a painful area can be finished with soothing work to the client's head, neck and shoulders. Stress reduction elements are also introduced into treatments that are half-hour and three-quarter-hour lengths.

🖐 Through induced relaxation, the client becomes more aware of his body and of areas where tension is held. A full-body relaxation massage addresses each area of the body. All techniques are applied in a slow rhythmical manner. Techniques should be organized so the same order is followed on each limb or side of the back. This

Treatment Goals   Treatment Plan

predictability aids relaxation. The therapist may treat active trigger points. Over the long term, the client's pain and muscular hypertonicity will decrease, contributing to increased relaxation. The therapist is cautioned to avoid treating too many trigger points in one session. Otherwise, not enough time is spent on soothing techniques.

🖑 **Positioning:** The client is usually treated in the prone position first, then turned supine. In the prone position, one pillow is placed under the abdomen to support the low back and another pillow is placed under the ankles. In the supine position, a pillow is placed under the knees. Nothing needs to be placed under the person's neck. But if a head-forward posture is observed and the client is uncomfortable in the supine position, a small towel roll is positioned to support — not increase — the cervical lordotic curve of the neck. Pillows used to support the cervical spine have a tendency to increase the head-forward posture, allowing trigger points in the sternocleidomastoid and anterior scalene muscles to be activated.

🖑 **Hydrotherapy** usually consists of applications of heat. If possible, before the massage, a full-body application such as a whirlpool or steam cabinet is excellent in facilitating relaxation. Before the treatment, a thermophore can be placed on the massage table where the client's trunk will be positioned, so it is warm when he lies down. Local heat applications such as a thermophore or hydrocollator are placed over a particularly tight area such as the low back or neck. Heat on the feet or abdomen may also feel pleasant for some clients.

General Treatment

🖑 With the client in the prone position, the massage begins with rhythmic techniques and rocking of the body or full-body muscle squeezing.

🖑 The treatment usually begins on the back since this is not usually an invasive area for the client and facilitates relaxation. Generally, each area of the back — lumbar, thoracic and shoulder — is addressed thoroughly. In the lumbar region, Swedish massage techniques are applied to the erector spinae and quadratus lumborum. The erector spinae are treated using fingertip and palmar kneading in both cross-fibre and with-fibre directions. The entire length of these muscles is massaged from the sacrum to the cervical region.

🖑 The quadratus lumborum is massaged inferior to the twelfth rib, along the iliac crest. Trigger points are palpated for while the thumbs move in a cross-fibre direction along the muscle, under the erector spinae.

🖑 The soft tissue over the sacrum is treated using techniques such as fingertip kneading, vibrations and tapping. Gentle sacral pumping can

Decrease sympathetic nervous system firing. Decrease muscle hypertonicity and pain of the back and posterior legs.

170

Treatment Goals   Treatment Plan

be performed with the therapist positioned at the head of the client. Both arms of the therapist are extended, with relaxed hands cupped over the sacrum. A rhythmic compression is applied to the sacrum at an oblique angle towards the feet. This creates a gentle traction to the spine.

- Muscle stripping is used along the intercostal muscles that are involved in full breathing. Latissimus dorsi, serratus anterior, rhomboids, trapezius, serratus superior posterior and the accessible rotator cuff muscles are massaged in turn, using petrissage techniques. Mobilization of the ribs and spinous processes is also indicated.

- The gluteal muscles and posterior legs are massaged using a variety of Swedish techniques. If excessive tension is held in the gluteal area, reference to the chapter on piriformis syndrome is recommended.

Decrease sympathetic nervous system firing. Decrease muscle hypertonicity and pain of the head, neck and shoulders.

- After the client is turned to a supine position, a few approaches are possible. The therapist may begin at the legs and feet, followed by the abdomen, arms, head, neck and shoulders. The massage may also begin at the head, neck and shoulders. Starting with the upper body allows for easy but unobtrusive observation of the client's breathing. This is useful since the person often changes his breathing pattern when he knows it is being watched.

- The massage to the head and neck addresses the scalenes because of their role in inhalation. Posterior neck muscles and sternocleidomastoid muscles are frequently hypertonic. A few trigger points might be treated. Commonly affected by trigger points are the upper trapezius, levator scapula, supraspinatus, splenius capitis and cervicis as well as the suboccipital muscles.

- The therapist may wish to begin with the anterior chest, lateral neck, posterior neck and suboccipital areas.

Decrease hypertonicity in the muscles of the face.

- This can be followed by a scalp massage from the back of the head to the forehead and a face massage. The therapist must take care when performing a massage in the head area because the tissue is thin over the bones.

- Fingertip kneading or gentle pressure points are systematically applied to the forehead and gentle squeezing is used along the eyebrows. Using one finger from each hand, the therapist strokes the muscles around the eyes in a circular movement starting at the medial supraorbital ridge. Just inferior to the zygomatic arch, gentle kneading and static pressure are applied. The muscles affecting the temporomandibular joint, such as masseter and temporalis, are similarly massaged. This is followed by the application of a gentle distraction pressure to the joint, in an inferior then forward direction. Stroking downward from the temporomandibular joint, the therapist then kneads or squeezes along the jaw line. With one hand on each

171

Treatment Goals   Treatment Plan

side of the neck, the therapist applies a stroke down the lateral neck and scalenes, then distal to and along the clavicle, around the deltoids to the posterior shoulder, up the posterior neck to the occiput.

Stretch shortened neck muscles.

🖐 Smooth passive range of motion is performed on the cervical spine. **Passive stretching** is also applied to shortened muscles. For example, to stretch the posterior neck muscles, the head is drawn into flexion with the chin brought towards the chest. Levator scapula is stretched by rotating the head slightly to the opposite side and directing the chin towards the axilla. Lateral flexion of the neck while the shoulder is held in a neutral position places a stretch on the upper trapezius and middle scalene. PIR may also be used.

🖐 An arm and hand massage is very relaxing, especially if there is a tendency for the client to hold the hands in fists.

Specific Treatment

Decrease hypertonicity of the abdominal muscles and diaphragm.

🖐 The abdominal area and diaphragm are key areas to massage because of their effect on a person's ability to breathe fully. No tension is held in the therapist's hands while massaging the abdomen. Warm, relaxed hands are placed on the abdomen as the client exhales. Overhand palmar kneading is performed slowly and rhythmically in a clockwise direction.

🖐 A modified effleurage may be used. It is composed of four strokes performed in one fluid movement. The effleurage stroke is applied by moving both hands in a superior direction, from the lower abdomen to the xiphoid process. At this point, the hands rotate and separate so the pressure is now applied through each thumb. The thumbs glide firmly along each side of the costal borders and move towards the back. Care is taken to release the pressure as the thumb moves towards the floating ribs so the hands simply glide around the waist to the back. The hands are repositioned with the fingertips at the base of the spine. Each hand now draws along the superior edge of the iliac crest towards the anterior hips.

🖐 Fingertip kneading is applied in a circular manner over the entire abdomen, in a clockwise direction. With client consent, the therapist may apply slow gentle skin rolling to release any facial restrictions, over the costal borders and the anterolateral intercostal areas in particular.

🖐 Specific treatment to the diaphragm is performed with the therapist working across the body, using kneading and static pressure points along the costal border. The techniques are applied near the xiphoid process, working in a lateral direction. Pressure is applied in a superior direction in order to reach the diaphragm attachments on the underside of the ribs. The pressure is held constant as the client

Treatment Goals   Treatment Plan

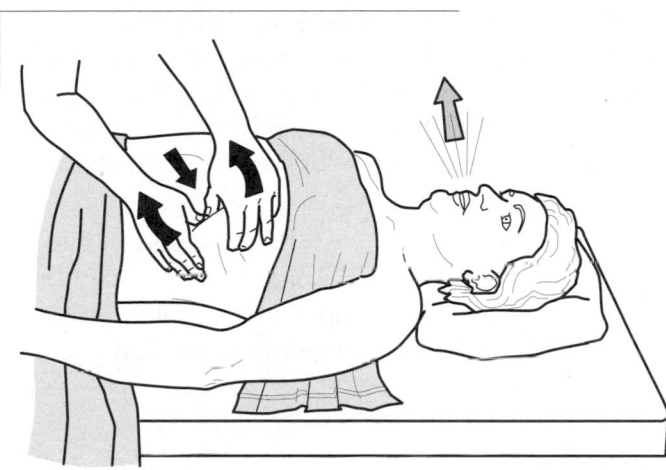

Figure 14.1
The lateral ribs are pulled medially as the client exhales to create slack. The therapist's thumbs move slowly under the costal margin to the diaphragm.

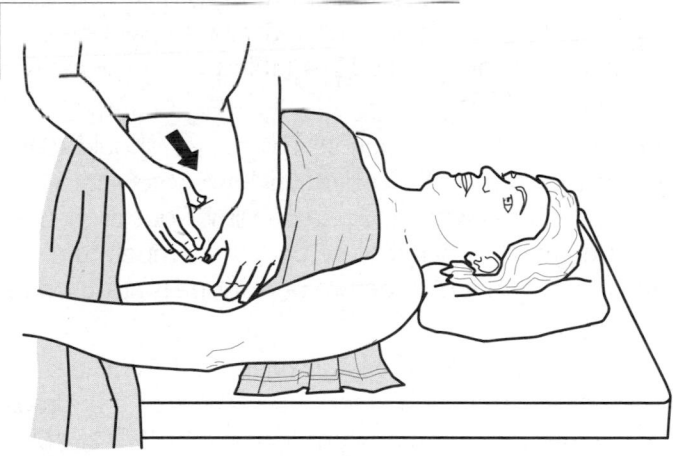

Figure 14.2
The left hand cups the lateral ribs while the right thumb reaches under the costal border to the diaphragm.

Educate about full breathing.
Encourage full breathing.

inhales, then increased when the client exhales, taking up the slack in the tissue. This is repeated up to three times in one area.

🖐 Care is taken if a pulse is palpated — usually to the left of the xiphoid process, indicating the abdominal aorta. In this case, the pressure is released and applied at a more lateral point. Tenderness on the right side could result with liver or gall bladder compression. Left side tenderness could result with clients who have a hiatus hernia or gastric ulcer.

🖐 The above principles are applied when working on the diaphragm, though the specific techniques may be different. The therapist can use the thumb of both hands under the costal border, while the fingers cup around the ribs *(Figure 14.1)*. The hands slowly pull up on the ribs from lateral to medial, creating slack at the medial costal border and space for the thumbs to massage the diaphragm. Another method has the therapist cupping the ribs in one hand and the thumb of the other hand reaching the diaphragm under the costal border *(Figure 14.2)*. The one hand draws the ribs lateral to medial, while the thumb applies pressure to the muscle.

🖐 Long strokes can be applied along the costal border in the same manner as the pressure points.

🖐 Continuing to work across the body, the therapist applies picking up and scooping strokes along the lateral trunk from the iliac crest to the lower ribs. Stripping of the accessible intercostal muscles and abdominal obliques is indicated.

🖐 The massage to the abdomen is completed using overhanded palmar kneading and vibrations.

🖐 After redraping the abdomen, the client is taught to breathe fully. The client inhales through the nose; the diaphragm is filled first; next, the ribs move laterally; and finally the sternum elevates slightly. Exhalation

173

Treatment Goals Treatment Plan

is through the mouth, releasing the air in the lower lungs first. Breathing is performed slowly and the therapist can direct the client by gently touching each area, in the above order. If it is difficult for the client to perform this type of breathing the exercise is stopped before it becomes stressful. It is then given as a self-care recommendation.

The treatment is finished by massaging the anterior legs and feet using a variety of Swedish techniques. After this, as therapist gently holds the feet, the client is asked to take a few full breaths. To connect the whole body, a continuous stroke may be applied bilaterally, starting at the shoulders, then along the arms and lateral legs to the feet.

Self-care Goals Self-care Plan

Educate the client.

✍ The client is educated to notice early signs of stress such as a stiff neck, raised shoulders, a clenched jaw or holding the hands in fists.

✍ **Hydrotherapy of both cold and hot applications is recommended.** Whirlpools or a steam cabinet, if available, allow for a hot, full-body treatment. Hot baths or foot baths, with additives, are suggested. Two cups of Epsom salt can be used; four to eight drops of lavender or juniper essential oil diluted in a tablespoon of vegetable oil are beneficial (*Lawless, 1995*).

✍ A hot bath before bed promotes relaxation. The person should soak for up to 20 minutes then remain in the bath until the water drains; this helps to prevent dizziness when the person climbs out of the tub. If the client is not used to a hot bath before bed, the temperature should be modified. A very hot bath before bed, if one is not used to it, can stress the body.

✍ Cool hydrotherapy can ultimately have a relaxing effect. A heating compress is applied to the abdomen before bed. Three or four drops of pure essential oil of lavender or marjoram (*Lawless, 1995*) can be added to the cold compress water. This cloth is covered by a dry towel and allowed to heat up naturally. This can aid sleep when a person has insomnia.

✍ Self-massage of the abdomen in a clockwise direction, followed by deep breathing, can also be used for insomnia. Lavender, marjoram, rose or ylang ylang pure essential oils at a one per cent dilution or 10 drops of the essential oil in 50 ml. of the carrier oil are indicated (*Lawless, 1995*). Two or three oils can be used in one mixture. For a one per cent dilution, the total number of drops in the blend should not exceed 10.

✍ Herbal teas such as chamomile, catnip, skullcap, passionflower or valerian can promote relaxation and sleep (*Balch, Balch, 1997*). An

174

Self-care Goals

Self-care Plan

herbalist or naturopath can also be consulted on appropriate herbs.

Educate the client in full diaphragmatic breathing.

✍ Full diaphragmatic breathing is encouraged. To practise, the client can be sitting or lying down. Any restricting clothing is loosened. One hand is placed on the stomach and the other is placed on the chest. The client inhales slowly through the nose, trying to bring the breath deep into the body, feeling the hand on the abdomen rise up. The upper chest should move very slightly. The breath is held for a second and then the air from the abdomen is exhaled slowly through the mouth.

Encourage stress reducing activities.

✍ Yoga or Tai Chi can be helpful.

✍ Meditation or visualization has proven beneficial. Meditation usually involves a quiet mind, where as visualization is a form of guided thought. Both are combined with deep breathing to allow for restoration of body and mind. Specifically designed tapes can be used or a person can simply sit in a quiet space. The clothes are loose, to allow for deep, unrestricted breathing. The exercise involves concentrating on the breathing process, inhaling deeply and slowly to the count of four, a pause for one second, and exhaling to the count of four. If a stray thought comes into the mind, the person gently nudges it away or stores it to be dealt with later. The person may wish to visualize a safe and special space — be it a beach, mountain, forest or wherever. Environmental music (of the ocean or other nature sounds) can contribute to relaxation.

✍ The above exercises are highly recommended for those suffering from anxiety disorder and panic attacks. Fear of an attack can be enough to trigger one. Slow, deep breathing used at the first sign of an attack can sometimes prevent it.

Encourage exercise, stretching and the progressive contract-relax technique.

✍ Exercise releases tension and works off accumulated stress hormones in the body.

• *Stretching* the entire body can relieve tension. The client should move the body part to be stretched until a gentle tension — not pain — is experienced. This is held for 20 to 30 seconds. The muscle can then be stretched a little further, without bouncing. An inhalation followed by an exhalation before trying for an additional stretch of the same muscle can be useful. See the Remedial Exercise chapter for more information about stretching.

• *Progressive contraction followed by relaxation* of each muscle in the body increases body awareness and facilitates stress reduction. The process usually begins at the feet. Without straining, the foot muscles are contracted for a few seconds, then, with exhalation, the muscles are relaxed. The person takes a moment to feel the difference between contraction and relaxation before moving on or repeating the contraction if there is still a sense of tension. Next,

175

Self-care Goals

Self-care Plan

the calf muscles are contracted and relaxed followed by the upper leg muscles, the buttocks and abdominals. The shoulders are raised then lowered. The hands are balled into fists then opened. The face muscles are contracted then relaxed.

Encourage the development of coping skills.

✍ Positive self-talk is very helpful. The person creates a series of positive statements which are repeated throughout the day, such as, "I am intelligent and creative", "I perform my job with excellence", "I am calm and serene". This positive reinforcement encourages the view that change and new situations are a challenge that can be handled, not a threat.

✍ The person is encouraged to determine what things would create a sense of control in typically stressful situations. For example, with a student, adequate preparation time before a presentation or an exam would help. For a mother, getting a babysitter for a few hours to allow time to oneself is positive. Along with realistic goals, the person needs to develop an awareness of things that cannot be controlled.

Refer the client.

✍ Finding a support network of people to talk to — there are specialized groups for those experiencing panic attacks — and getting help from friends or family are important. A referral to a counsellor may be useful.

✍ Stimulants should be avoided late in the day if they contribute to insomnia. Consultation with a naturopath or nutritionist can provide specific recommendations for supplements or dietary changes. These suggestions will help to support the body under stress and to limit dietary triggers that promote feelings of stress.

Treatment Frequency and Expected Outcome

One-hour treatments are optimal to allow the client sufficient time to unwind and relax into the massage.

If the stress is short term, the client is encouraged to come for massage during this time, once a week for one hour.

See also spasm, trigger points, hypertension, asthma, diabetes, constipation, irritable bowel syndrome, tension headache, migraine, fibromyalgia, temporomandibular joint dysfunction and inflammatory arthritides.

If the stress is chronic, regular appointments are appropriate. The client comes as often as he is able, every two or three weeks, for one hour.

If the stress is short term, massage facilitates the client's ability to cope more effectively.

If the stress is chronic, the client's ability to cope will depend on following the self-care recommendations and possibly making lifestyle changes and developing better coping mechanisms. Massage gives the body and mind rebuilding time and often helps the client to sleep better and experience less pain and stiffness, temporarily.

PREGNANCY

Linda Ludwig

Pregnancy is a state of wellness associated with many interrelated changes that occur throughout the woman's body as the fetus develops.

Changes that occur during pregnancy are physiological, affecting the musculoskeletal system and virtually every organ system. They are also emotional, with the woman adjusting to her changing body and lifestyle. These changes begin in the first weeks of gestation and continue throughout the pregnancy and often some months after delivery.

The main stages of the pregnancy are termed the first, second and third trimesters — that is, the first three months, the following four to six months and the last seven to nine months of pregnancy. Some changes may continue for six months and up to a year after the birth (especially with breast-feeding); this period after childbirth is referred to as "postpartum".

The massage therapist must be aware of the normal and potentially abnormal changes during pregnancy, with a view to preventative treatment, referrals to other health practitioners when necessary and maintenance of the client's wellness.

Pregnancy can be detected by a urine test. The test checks for high levels of the hormone chorionic gonadotropin that are present 35 days or earlier after conception *(Bourne, 1995)*.

First Trimester Symptoms

✦ **Nausea**, or the sensation of feeling sick, and **vomiting** are commonly referred to as morning sickness. These symptoms are not unusual in the early stages of pregnancy. They tend to be most severe in the early morning, but can occur in the evening and may last all day and night for a few unfortunate women. Both symptoms usually decrease by 10 weeks of pregnancy and are generally gone by the end of 14 weeks. Only rarely does this last through the entire pregnancy.

✦ **Frequent urination**, as often as every two hours during the day, is an early sign of pregnancy. It is initially due to the presence of the hormone progesterone which causes relaxation of the smooth muscle of the bladder. This tendency will decrease by the second trimester and increase again in the last stage of pregnancy, in part due to pressure of the enlarged uterus and notably when the baby's head is engaged in the pelvis.

✦ **Constipation** is common. This is primarily because the hormone progesterone causes relaxation in smooth muscle. The decreased tone of the smooth muscle of the intestine results in a slower transit time of the fecal matter through the system, as well as increased water absorption from the colon. Constipation may continue throughout the pregnancy. Mechanical pressure of the enlarging uterus contributes to the problem (*Knuppel, Drukker, 1993*).

✦ **Blood pressure** often falls in early pregnancy, specifically the diastolic pressure. This is also due to the presence of progesterone, which relaxes the muscular wall of the blood vessels. Vasodilation, combined with the placenta acting as an arteriovenous shunt, decreases peripheral resistance and slows the flow of the blood (*Chard, Lilford, 1998*). The woman may feel light-headed or faint, especially with prolonged standing. This is often combined with feelings of extreme fatigue or lack of energy. Blood pressure usually returns to normal during the 14th week of pregnancy.

✦ **Breast changes** begin during this stage. There is a sense of increased fullness as well as some tenderness and heightened sensitivity. This is experienced especially in the area at the front of the axilla and may continue, to varying degrees, throughout the pregnancy.

✦ **Musculoskeletal changes** result under the influence of estrogen, progesterone and relaxin. It is thought that estrogen prepares the sites for the action of relaxin. Relaxin is produced as early as two weeks into the pregnancy and is at its highest levels in the first trimester, then falls 20 per cent and remains at that level until labour. It affects the composition of collagen in the joint capsules, ligaments and fascia to allow greater elasticity. This enables more movement in the joints and creates more yield in the abdomen. While all joints are affected, those that are most vulnerable are those of the pelvis, such as the symphysis pubis and sacroiliac joint, and those which bear weight, such as the ankle and joints of the foot. The latter can lead to aching feet and pes planus (*Brayshaw, Wright, 1994*).

✦ **Taste and smell** are altered in the early stages of the pregnancy. Certain smells and food become disagreeable to the woman.

✦ **Mood swings** are most common in the first trimester but may continue throughout the pregnancy. Extreme fatigue during this time increases feelings of irritability or depression. Anxiety about the pregnancy, labour and delivery are natural, in both the woman and her partner, especially with a first pregnancy.

Second Trimester Symptoms

Months four through six are known as the quiet months. The risk of miscarriage is greatly reduced when the pregnancy reaches this stage. The woman experiences the reality of the fetus — hearing the fetal heartbeat, viewing the fetus through ultrasound (sonagram) and quickening, which is actually feeling the movement of the fetus in the womb. The woman begins to feel fetal movement, generally considered pleasant, between 18 and 21 weeks of pregnancy. It is also during this stage that women will receive test results indicating potential problems with the fetus. At the end of this trimester, by 23 weeks, the fetus can survive a premature birth *(Colman, Colman, 1991)*.

✦ **Edema** is common at any time during the pregnancy due to the retention of fluid. As the pregnancy advances, edema of the legs occurs in up to 40 per cent of women *(Chard, Lilford, 1998)*. The mechanical obstruction created by the uterus and its contents causes an increase in venous pressure distally, which then results in edema *(Knuppel, Drukker, 1993)*. While edema may be due to excessive weight gain, it may also be a symptom of pre-eclampsia. In the latter case, the midwife or physician should be informed.

✦ **Hypertension** can be chronic — existing before the pregnancy — or pregnancy-induced (PIH). PIH may also be referred to as pre-eclampsia, eclampsia or toxemia.

✦ Hypertension in pregnancy and its complications are a serious concern, being the second most common cause of maternal death. They can also contribute to fetal and neonatal morbidity (such as cerebral palsy and other mental and physical disabilities) and mortality. The baby is at risk when the blood flow through the vessels supplying the placenta is cut by half or more depending on the severity of the pre-eclampsia *(The American College of Obstetricians and Gynecologists, 1996)*.

• Pre-eclampsia is first detected by a sudden increase in blood pressure (the degree of elevation in blood pressure is considered more significant than the absolute values of the blood pressure). The diagnosis of pre-eclampsia is made when the increased blood pressure is in combination with proteinuria and generalized edema. Proteinuria is the presence of high concentrations of protein in the urine. The urine test will be regularly conducted by the midwife or a physician during the pregnancy.

• Edema in the face and hands is a better indicator of pre-eclampsia than the dependent edema found in the lower limbs. Of the 85 per cent of woman who develop generalized edema, only about 15 per cent develop pre-eclampsia *(Knuppel, Drukker, 1993)*. Pre-eclampsia affects seven out of 100 pregnant women *(The American College of Obstetricians and Gynecologists, 1996)*.

• Eclampsia includes all of the symptoms of pre-eclampsia with the addition of convulsions *(Knuppel, Drukker, 1993)*.

The cause of pre-eclampsia is unknown, but women who are predisposed are those with:

➤ a first pregnancy;

➤ a multiple pregnancy;

➤ chronic hypertension or long-term hypertension, pre-existing the pregnancy;

➤ hydatidiform mole, a degenerative process affecting the villi that connect to the part of the endometrium which gives rise to the placenta; it causes multiple cysts and hemorrhaging *(Taber's Cyclopedic Medical Dictionary, 1981)*;

➤ chronic renal disease;

➤ malnutrition;

➤ diabetes;

➤ a history of PIH in the family or in a previous pregnancy;

➤ younger than 20 years of age and older than 30;

➤ developing hydramnios, an excess of amniotic fluid.

✦ Taking accurate blood pressure during pregnancy requires greater care than usual because even slight changes in position can alter readings. Blood pressure readings are highest when the woman is standing or seated. They are somewhat lower in the supine position and lowest while the woman is sidelying. There can be a difference of 10 mm Hg between the inferior and superior arm while sidelying, with a lower reading achieved in the superior arm. Therefore, when blood pressure is taken, consistent positioning is important *(Knuppel, Drukker, 1993)*.

✦ **Supine hypotension** can occur as early as the fourth month and will continue until the end of the pregnancy. As the fetus grows, it compresses the aorta and inferior vena cava against the lumbar spine. This may cause the woman to feel faint when she is lying on her back.

✦ **Shortness of breath** may be experienced at any time during the pregnancy. This is due to a combination of both mechanical and physiological changes. Dyspnea becomes more likely as the uterus enlarges, pushing up on the abdominal contents which then push up on the diaphragm *(Fig. 15.1)*. The diaphragm is raised up to four centimetres and laterally expanded up to two centimetres. *(Chard, Lilford, 1998)*. The sub-sternal angle increases from approximately 70 degrees in the first trimester to 105 degrees at term, with the thoracic circumference increasing five to seven centimetres. *(Knuppel, Drukker, 1993)*. The resultant rib-flaring can cause pain along the anterior costal margin with associated thoracic back pain. Shortness of breath may be experienced when the woman exerts herself or lies flat.

✦ In the third trimester, after the baby's head has dropped into the pelvis, the woman may feel that breathing is easier. Physiologically, there is a 20 per cent increase in the required oxygen because of the increased basal metabolic rate of the pregnant woman. Breathlessness is experienced as the body adjusts to these changing requirements. An increase in inhaled oxygen results in an increase in carbon dioxide. The respiratory centre in the medulla oblongata responds to the concentrations of carbon dioxide when regulating breathing rate. In an attempt to reduce carbon dioxide levels,

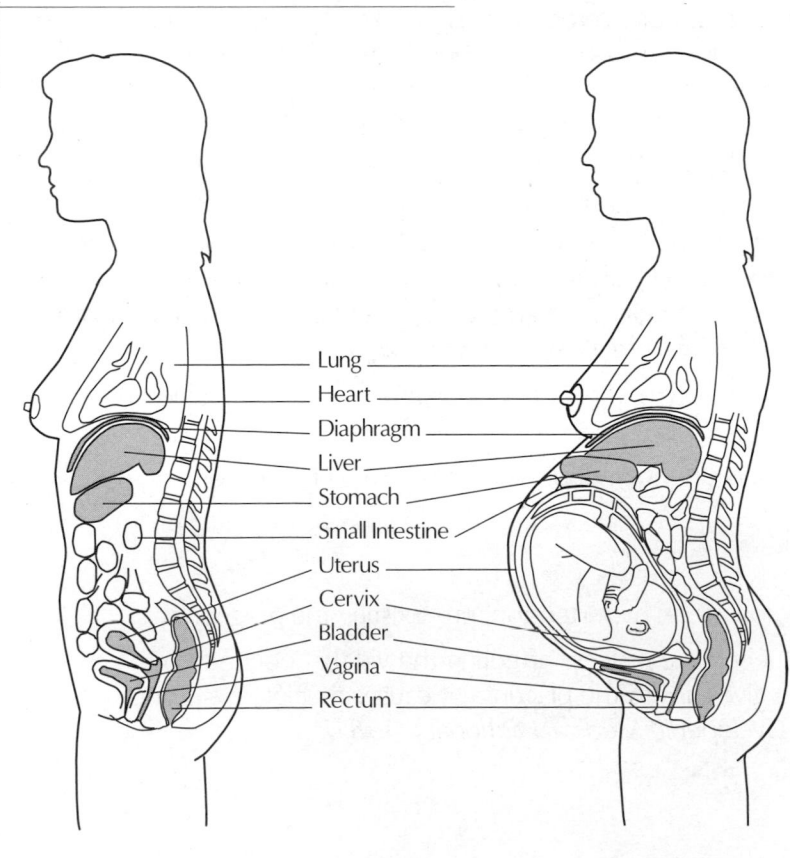

Lung
Heart
Diaphragm
Liver
Stomach
Small Intestine
Uterus
Cervix
Bladder
Vagina
Rectum

Early Pregnancy   Late Pregnancy

Figure 15.1
As the uterus grows during pregnancy, it compresses the digestive organs and pushes up on the diaphragm.

the rate of respiration is increased, especially with activity. This can occur at any time during the pregnancy *(Brayshaw, Wright, 1994)*.

✦ **Backache** is a common symptom. The softened and stretched ligaments and tendons supporting the pelvis and lumbar spine are particularly stressed with pregnancy. The excessive mobility in these areas can cause surrounding muscles to spasm in order to provide support. The woman's posture is altered as the increasing weight of the baby moves the centre of gravity anteriorly. These factors combine to result in poor posture such as **hyperlordosis** and **hyperkyphosis**, both of which can lead to and exacerbate back pain. Up to 88 per cent of women experience back pain at some time during their pregnancy. Other factors contributing to hyperlordosis are a lack of lumbar support by the stretched abdominal muscles, excessive weight gain during pregnancy, repeated changing from high heels to low heels and previous injury to the back and pelvis. Hyperkyphosis in the thoracic area is affected by the softening and stretching of local tendons and ligaments and aggravated by the increased weight and size of the breasts. Another contributing factor is lazy posture while standing and sitting, often accompanied by head-forward posture *(Kisner, Colby, 1996)*. These postural changes can begin as early as the fourth month and continue on through to the ninth month. They may persist for several months postpartum *(Brayshaw, Wright, 1994)*.

✦ **Abdominal pain** can be caused by all the same things that cause abdominal pain pre-pregnancy. The greatest concern is for previously unexperienced pain of sudden onset. Medical advice should be sought for this type of pain. The round ligament may be a source of discomfort. This ligament supports the uterus and is located along the side of the uterus passing from its upper regions down to the groin. Likewise, the linea alba and rectus abdominus muscles experience intense stretching as the pregnancy advances. Despite their increased suppleness through the actions of hormones, they may separate. This results in a condition called **diastasis recti**. Pain from this condition is most commonly experienced starting in the second trimester or at the start of the third trimester. It frequently stops by the 33rd week. This achy, nagging, occasionally sharp pain is more intense on the right side than the left.

✦ **Diastasis symphysis pubis** causes pain, of varying severity, over the pubic area and down the inner thigh. It is a separation of the pubic symphysis.

✦ **Varicose veins** may develop at any time during the pregnancy but are more likely as the pregnancy advances. The enlarging uterus compresses the veins in the pelvis. This obstructs venous return to the heart and increases pressure in the veins of the legs. Weight gain will also contribute to their development. Mild varicosities in the first pregnancy may improve or resolve through the first six months postpartum as the uterus shrinks, the woman loses weight and progesterone levels drop. More severe varicosities that develop during pregnancy may only partially regress postpartum. Unfortunately, varicose veins often return with increasing severity with each subsequent pregnancy.

✦ **Hemorrhoids** are varicose veins in and around the rectum, often secondary to straining and constipation. Just as with the veins in the leg, which experience increased pressure with the enlarged uterus, these rectal veins may enlarge for the same reason.

✦ **Pigmentation** changes may occur in the skin. Freckles may enlarge while birthmarks and moles may darken. In the latter half of gestation, the butterfly mask of pregnancy, also called "chloasma", may develop. This pigmentation spreads over the nose and cheeks like the wings of a butterfly. In many women, the line from the top to the bottom of the abdomen darkens, called the "linea nigra". Changes in pigmentation are of no medical concern and usually the affected areas return to their normal colour after delivery.

✦ **Stretch marks** may develop in tissue over the areas that rapidly enlarge such as the breasts and anterior abdomen. In cases of excessive weight gain, stretch marks may occur over the legs, buttocks and upper arms.

✦ **Other changes** include nosebleeds, gum bleeding and nasal congestion. Headaches at the front of the head as well as above the eyes are common. Migraine frequency can change, either increasing or slightly improving during pregnancy.

✦ **Emotionally**, the woman must deal with the many body changes that are occurring quite rapidly; the breasts enlarge, the waistline disappears and the abdomen grows larger. Most women have mixed feelings about these changes, excited about the life they are carrying, but also concerned about ever returning to their former body shape. Pregnancy can remind one of her own childhood; good memories may bring the woman closer to her parents but memories of conflicts may create stress in this relationship (*The American College of Obstetricians and Gynecologists, 1996*). The massage therapist needs to be respectful and non-judgemental of the woman's emotional state.

Third Trimester Symptoms

Many of the second trimester symptoms continue into the third trimester. As the pregnancy advances towards birth, physical discomfort increases, especially in the eighth month. The baby has almost reached its birth weight but has not yet positioned itself down into the pelvis. In the ninth month the woman may actually feel less physical discomfort and more energy after the baby's head drops into the pelvis, in preparation for birth.

✦ **Gestational diabetes** is a type of diabetes mellitus that develops during pregnancy. There are no known risk factors though frequently, late in the pregnancy, there are increased amounts of insulin in the blood because of an insulin resistance in the body (*Knuppel, Drukker, 1993*).

✦ Diabetes mellitus may have adverse effects on the pregnancy such as:

  • increased possibility of pre-eclampsia or eclampsia;

  • increased risk and severity of infection;

  • possibility of hydramnios (too much amniotic fluid) which can make it difficult for the mother to breathe and may also result in premature labour and delivery;

  • a difficult delivery or possible cesarean section due to increased size of the infant, known as "macrosomia" (babies may weigh 10 pounds or more);

  • a predisposition to postpartum hemorrhage (*Knuppel, Drukker, 1993*).

✦ **Ketoacidosis** is another danger secondary to diabetes. It is due to the increased stress experienced in the second and third trimesters and is more likely when the woman does not eat for long periods. Ketoacidosis has been associated with a maternal mortality rate of five to 15 per cent (*Knuppel, Drukker, 1993*). Therefore, diagnosis of gestational diabetes and education regarding its control are essential. Treatment is through diet and exercise or diet, exercise and insulin. While an abnormal glucose level may appear in pregnancy, glucose levels will usually return to normal after delivery. Unfortunately, gestational diabetes increases the woman's risk of developing diabetes later in life, particularly if the woman is over 30 and if she has a family history of diabetes. See the diabetes mellitus chapter for more information on this condition.

✦ **Edema** can occur in the legs, hands and especially fingers and face. In the morning, the hands may feel stiff and have the sensation of pins and needles. Compression syndromes may develop secondary to the edema. When hand and face edema occur, the woman may have pre-eclampsia and should see her midwife or physician.

✦ **Compression syndromes** such as thoracic outlet and carpal tunnel syndromes may occur secondary to arm and hand edema. Sciatic nerve compression may cause pain along the path of the nerve, down the leg to the ankle. Piriformis syndrome may occur as the legs rotate externally to accommodate the increasing girth of the abdomen. This condition may cause trigger points which refer into the buttock and down the posterior leg to the knee. Increased tone in the muscle may compress the sciatic nerve.

✦ **Backache** may increase because the centre of gravity shifts as the baby gets bigger and heavier, combined with the effects of the hormones progesterone and relaxin.

✦ **Sacroiliac sprain** can cause intense pain over the sacrum. It is often worse with rotational movements such as turning sideways in bed and may make walking difficult.

✦ **Leg cramps**, especially in the calf, become more frequent in the last trimester. They often occur at night. The pain is usually intense and can wake up the woman. Leg cramps can also be a sign of deep vein thrombosis during, and especially after, a cesarean section. The therapist should be aware of these risks and make appropriate referrals if this is suspected. See the chapters on spasms and circulatory pathologies.

✦ **Pelvic discomfort** is present in the last trimester. With a first pregnancy it often begins in the 30th to 32nd week. This is due to the softening of the ligaments of the pelvic girdle and the accompanying extra mobility of the joints. In the 36th week, after the baby's head is engaged, there is often a sensation of achiness and fullness in the abdomen. If the head compresses nerves, pain may be experienced on the anterior or inner thigh radiating down to the knee. The symphysis pubis, where the anterior pelvic bones are joined, may be tender and painful after exercise or when shifting weight from one leg to the other. This is not usually a serious condition, with rest often bringing relief. Pelvic discomfort may also occur if the baby kicks organs or pushes against the abdominal wall.

✦ **Costal margin pain** occurs as the pregnancy advances and the uterus compresses lower ribs. Usually experienced more on the right side, it begins in the 30th to 34th week. Relief may occur when the woman moves out of a sitting position and when the baby's head engages.

✦ **Frequent urination and incontinence** may occur with the increased pressure of the uterus on the bladder, with weight gain and with the influence of hormones on the urethra and pelvic floor muscles.

✦ **Fatigue** increases again in the third trimester as the woman becomes heavier.

✦ **Insomnia and restlessness** are common complaints. The woman may find it difficult to get in a comfortable position. Heartburn, fetal movement and the need to urinate frequently contribute to sleeping difficulties.

✦ **Emotionally**, by the third trimester, most women have resolved any ambivalent attitudes to the pregnancy. Some studies indicate that up to 50 percent of women in the first trimester admitted not wanting the baby but rarely expressed this feeling by the last trimester *(Colman, Colman, 1991).*

"Fourth Trimester" or Postpartum Period

✦ **Physical changes** in the woman's body linger after birthing, as time is needed to regain the balance of the body to its pre-pregnancy state. Immediately postpartum, the ligaments are at their longest and the joints at their most unstable *(Brayshaw, Wright, 1994)*; therefore, severe back pain may persist after delivery *(Buschbacher, 1994)*. Neck and shoulder pain continue due to poor posture while breast-feeding, lifting the baby up from a crib and carrying the baby for prolonged periods.

✦ **Post-surgical recovery** may arise from an episiotomy or a cesarean section. An episiotomy involves an incision in the perineum before the birth in order to prevent tearing in the area. Exercises can be performed by the woman during pregnancy to stretch this tissue in order to avoid having this surgery.

  • If a cesarean section was performed, the woman will be recovering from major abdominal surgery. If no complications are experienced, full recovery takes between four to six weeks, allowing the mother to resume her usual activities.

✦ **Breasts** may be sore with cracking around the nipples from breast-feeding.

✦ **Emotionally**, a woman may experience extreme joy but also sadness, fear, anger or anxiety. In a mild form, these latter feelings are called **postpartum blues**. Commonly felt by seven out of 10 mothers, they may last from a few hours to a few weeks. A more serious condition is **postpartum depression** which involves strong feelings of sadness, anxiety or hopelessness. Generally, counselling and treatment are required.

✦ Signs and symptoms of postpartum depression include:

  • postpartum blues that last more than two weeks or strong feelings of depression or anger a few months after childbirth;

  • increasingly intense feelings of anger, hopelessness and sadness that interfere with the mother's activities of daily life;

  • inability to sleep, even when tired, or sleeping most of the time even when the baby is awake;

  • extreme changes in appetite;

  • worrying about the baby excessively or taking little interest in the baby and family;

  • panic attacks;

  • fears of harming the baby or herself.

  (The American College of Obstetricians and Gynecologists, 1996)

✦ If a client appears to have postpartum depression the therapist should strongly recommend she see her physician for treatment.

Contraindications

✦ As a precaution, emmenagogic essential oils (those that induce uterine contraction) should not be used in the first three to four months of pregnancy. These include basil, bay, clary sage, cypress, fennel, frankincense, hyssop, jasmine, juniper, marjoram, myrrh, peppermint, rose, rosemary and thyme *(Tiran, 1996; Davis, 1998)*. Exceptions are chamomile, lavender and tangerine which may be used at a one per cent dilution — that is 10 drops of pure essential oil in 50 ml. of vegetable oil. This exception holds unless the woman has a risk of miscarriage due to her own history, a family history of miscarriage or because she is experiencing abnormal bleeding *(Davis, 1998)*.

✦ Abdominal and sacral massage is comprised of only light strokes or should be avoided, if the risk of miscarriage is present during the first trimester, as a precaution — even though there is no conclusive proof that this is a concern.

✦ Deep massage and fascial techniques are contraindicated over the low back during the first trimester.

✦ Care is taken when massaging over the abdomen during the entire pregnancy. After four months, a general but gentle abdominal massage is usually very enjoyable for both the mother and the growing baby.

✦ Fascia should be assessed for any stabilizing role in the client's posture before using techniques to stretch it.

✦ Aggressive joint play and mobilization techniques are avoided for the entire body, because of the increased joint laxity, during the whole pregnancy and up to six months after delivery.

✦ Avoid deep massage over varicose veins.

✦ Massage is contraindicated if a change in blood pressure is noted and if it is combined with other symptoms of pre-eclampsia. The client is recommended to see her midwife or physician immediately.

✦ If the client has diabetes, a snack or juice should be eaten just prior to the treatment to maintain blood sugar levels. The woman may wish to eat a snack shortly after the treatment as well. The client and therapist must remain vigilant for any signs or symptoms of ketoacidosis. See the diabetes mellitus chapter.

✦ In the second and third trimesters, the client must be carefully positioned on her back to avoid compression of the aorta and inferior vena cava. If nausea or discomfort is experienced, despite appropriate modifications, the position is changed to sidelying or seated, or the treatment is discontinued.

✦ When complicating postural concerns or compression syndromes are treated, the massage must be modified according to the previously listed contraindications.

✦ For women experiencing heartburn, two hours should elapse after a meal before having the massage *(Tiran, Mack, 1995)*. This prevents regurgitation of stomach acid, which can happen because of the stomach's upward displacement by the enlarged uterus *(Knuppel, Drukker, 1993)*.

Treatment Considerations

HEALTH HISTORY QUESTIONS

✦ How is the woman's general health? Is there a history of maternal cardiac, renal, thyroid, pulmonary, gastrointestinal or hepatic diseases or diabetes, placing the fetus or mother at some risk for complications ranging from low or high birth weight to potential early labour?

✦ At what stage is the pregnancy?

✦ Is there a history of previous pregnancies? Were there any complications?

✦ If known, what is the family history of pregnancies? Were there any complications in pregnancy or labour?

✦ What symptoms is the client experiencing at present?

✦ The therapist should take the client's blood pressure throughout the pregnancy. If signs of pre-eclampsia or eclampsia are present the woman is immediately referred to her midwife or physician.

WARNING SYMPTOMS — CONSIDERED SERIOUS AND WARRANTING IMMEDIATE REPORTING TO MIDWIFE OR PHYSICIAN:

✦ Vaginal bleeding especially in the first 24 weeks of pregnancy, but even after this time, could suggest a pregnancy at risk. Bedrest is recommended, with immediate notification of the physician.

✦ Severe continuous abdominal pain may be associated with premature placenta separation or other acute abdominal emergency.

✦ Breaking of water or rupture of membranes that precedes the onset of labour is the first symptom in 40 per cent of premature labours. Medical attention should be sought. After 34 weeks of pregnancy, this occurrance is of less concern for fetal health, but contact with the physician or midwife is important in order to arrange for delivery or hospital admission.

✦ Pre-eclampsia warning signs:

  • In the second trimester, mistiness, blurring or change in vision may signal pre-eclampsia or elevated blood pressure. Bedrest and notification of the physician are necessary.

  • Continuous severe headache usually over the front or the back of the head accompanied by visual disturbances may be a symptom of severe pre-eclampsia or hypertension. This is a headache that is not relieved by the usual remedies.

✦ Swelling of hands, especially the fingers, and face, should be reported to the physician or midwife.

✦ Pain on the upper right side of the abdomen should also be reported.

(Bourne, 1995)

THESE SYMPTOMS WARRANT EARLY REPORTING TO THE MIDWIFE OR PHYSICIAN (WITHIN 24 HOURS):

✦ Temperature of 38.5 degrees Celsius or more, even if the cause is known, should be checked.

✦ Frequency of urination and pain with urination can indicate a urinary tract infection.

✦ Absence of fetal movement is not unusual for periods of time, even up to 24 hours. During the 22nd to 24th weeks, it is possible that fetal movement may even stop for several days. Generally, as a precaution, if no movement is felt for longer than 24 hours the physician is notified.

✦ Excessive vomiting is not uncommon in the first trimester and occasionally in the last trimester. If it is of such severity and frequency that no food or fluids can be retained, medical attention is sought.

✦ Excessive itching, not the common generalized itching, may occasionally suggest a liver dysfunction (cholestasis) which requires notification of the physician.

Massage

🖑 The primary treatment goal is to promote a healthy pregnancy by including relaxation techniques and providing a supportive environment as part of every massage.

🖑 Hydrotherapy for any trimester:

- A warm foot bath with three to five drops of lemon essential oil may ease the aching of varicosities.

- Heat is used to decrease pain, to increase local circulation to hypertonic muscles and to relax the client. It will likely be used on the back, gluteals and neck.

- Contrast or cold baths or wraps to the feet and legs will help reduce edema.

- Cold figure-eight wraps around the breasts will decrease congestion and pain.

- Essential oils indicated for pregnant women after the first four months or for nursing women are lavender, which has a calmative effect, neroli, which helps decrease gastrointestinal smooth muscle spasm, and tangerine, which has an uplifting effect. These are used at a one per cent dilution only, which is 10 drops of pure essential oil per 50 ml. of carrier oil (Lawless, 1995).

- Essential oils indicated for labour are geranium, lavender and marjoram used before, during and after labour to relax muscles. These are also blended at a one per cent dilution. Arnica is also safe for muscle pain relief (Tiran, 1996).

First Trimester

🖑 **Positioning** can be prone, supine or sidelying. Some women may feel uncomfortable in the prone position by the end of the trimester, especially if their abdomen is noticeably enlarged.

🖑 General relaxation massage is appropriate, with an additional focus on areas requested by the client. Often these are not directly related to the pregnancy. The abdomen, low back and sacral areas are treated using only gentle stroking and petrissage; or they are not massaged at all.

Second and Third Trimesters

✋ The treatment addresses the individual woman's symptoms with the goal to decrease pain and postural discomforts while maintaining optimal wellness in preparation for labour. The massage focus is: to reduce trigger points, spasm and hypertonicity of muscles in the low back and gluteals; to treat the muscles involved in hyperlordosis and hyperkyphosis; to treat any compression syndromes; to relieve breast congestion and to reduce edema, if present. Specific treatments of postural dysfunction and compression syndromes are according to the usual protocol, with modifications made as necessary for the pregnancy (see contraindication section).

✋ **Positioning** in sidelying, supine and seated are appropriate. Supine hypotension may occur and can be relieved for a short time by placing a folded towel under the client's right hip. This repositions the weight of the fetus off the vascular structures. Positioning the woman on her left side will also effectively remove the pressure *(Brayshaw, Wright, 1994)*. Near the end of the second trimester until delivery, the client should also be pillowed in a semi-seated position while supine. Time spent in the supine position at this latter stage should not be longer than 10 to 15 minutes. The client is encouraged to let the therapist know if nausea or discomfort is felt in any way. If so, her position should be changed or the treatment discontinued. In the final month of pregnancy, positional changes may need to be made every 15 minutes or so to maintain client comfort. The treatment duration may also be shortened if the woman has difficulty changing positions or a seated position may be used for the entire treatment.

✋ The massage is performed in the context of a relaxation treatment.

✋ The treatment focus is on enhancing musculoskeletal health to assist with the added postural stress of an altered centre of gravity due to the growing fetus.

✋ Hyperlordosis is inevitable for the majority of women. A modified treatment is given while care is taken to avoid releasing supporting fascia. With the client in the sidelying position, the back is treated with a focus on the lumbar area, including quadratus lumborum and the lumbar erector spinae.

✋ Fingertip kneading along the iliac crest will help relax the abdominal oblique muscles.

✋ Stripping or spreading techniques are applied systematically along the intercostal muscles and serratus anterior muscles. Scooping may be applied along the lateral border of the latissimus dorsi muscle.

✋ The upper back and anterior chest are efficiently addressed in the sidelying position. A hyperkyphosis treatment is often necessary. Fascial techniques are gradually and gently applied to the anterior chest and lateral neck, if appropriate. Muscle stripping along the subclavius and pectoralis major and minor muscles is indicated. Care is taken around potentially tender breast tissue.

✋ A similar approach is taken to massage of the lateral neck, including upper trapezius and middle scalenes. PIR may be performed to upper trapezius muscle in the sidelying position with the therapist taking care to stabilize at the suboccipital insertion of the muscle.

✋ The periscapular muscles are treated systematically including subscapularis, infraspinatus, teres major and minor, supraspinatus, levator scapulae, rhomboids, middle trapezius and serratus posterior superior. A variety of petrissage techniques is used. If hyperkyphosis is present, the therapist must take care not to stretch the already fatigued and overstretched rhomboids and middle trapezius muscles.

🖐 Massage to the gluteal region is indicated with a focus on the piriformis muscle, using cross-fibre stripping and elbow compression. Specifically, techniques are applied along the sacroiliac joint and the greater trochanter to decrease hypertonicity in the gluteal muscles. In preparation for labour and delivery, fascial work and gentle PIR techniques may be indicated to lengthen the adductors and gluteals. Long circulatory strokes and lymphatic drainage techniques are applied on the legs to improve venous and lymphatic return. If varicosities are present the pressure is reduced. A pes planus treatment may be necessary. Foot massage is usually very relaxing and soothing for the client.

🖐 In a supine position, the head, neck and shoulders are massaged. Stretches are performed to the neck muscles and pectoralis major and minor. A face massage is usually very soothing for the client.

🖐 Compression syndromes of the shoulders and arms are treated, with appropriate modifications, by relieving the compression from its muscular or edematous origin.

🖐 Breast tenderness is treated by reducing congestion through cold hydrotherapy and lymphatic drainage techniques. Specific massage to pectoralis major and minor will also help to relieve breast congestion. The therapist must be aware that the anterior chest and axilla are likely to be very tender due to increased lymphatic activity. Specific consent from the client and a clear rationale from the therapist are required before treating breast tissue.

🖐 Abdominal massage is useful in treating constipation, to facilitate relaxation, to give the woman a sense of her entire body including the baby and to sooth and relax the growing baby. Techniques are applied in a clockwise direction over the abdomen. Broad hand contact is used to embrace the enlarged abdomen *(Figure 15.2)*. Gently applied but more specific stripping or pressure points may be used along the costal border and iliac crest to reduce some abdominal tension.

🖐 Passive joint range of motion is appropriate throughout the body to maintain joint health and movement. Aggressive joint play techniques are avoided, but carefully applied mobilization techniques to affected joints are possible, namely to the glenohumeral joint, the sacroiliac joints and the spine.

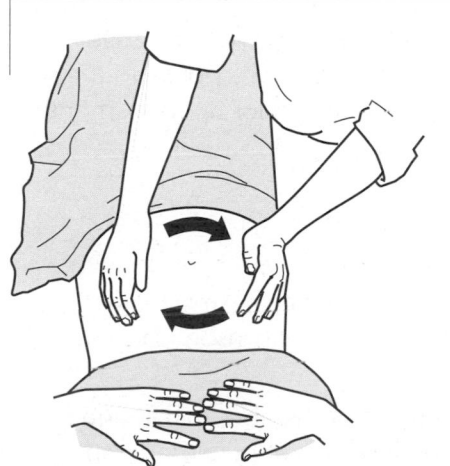

Figure 15.2
Massage to the pregnant woman's abdomen is performed clockwise.

Labour

🖐 The term "doula" seems to be becoming popular to describe a person, often experienced in childbirth, who gives support during labour. Massage therapists are increasingly providing this support. Actual experience is not necessary so much as knowledge of the process and an ability to remain calm and to stay focused in order to listen to the client's needs.

🖐 **Positioning** is however the woman wishes and usually changes frequently during the course of labour.

🖐 Some women prefer not to be touched during labour. For those who would like massage, it often provides a decrease in pain and anxiety, as well as a subsequent feeling of increased control during this time. Just a supportive touch will often help women feel calmer and better able to cope *(Stillerman, 1994)*. In some cases, the therapist may wish to guide the woman's partner in providing touch in order to include the partner in this process.

✋ In the early stages of labour, enriched oils may be used to facilitate contractions and to promote calmness in the woman. Massage over the sacrum with a blend of lavender and tangerine is useful when labour is not yet established *(Tiran, 1996)*. A compress of clary sage at the pubic bone and on the lower back can ease the aches of early labour.

✋ During active labour, a one per cent dilution of the essential oils of bergamot, chamomile, rose or ylang ylang may be helpful to the client. Lavender can enhance contractions and decrease the pain of established labour *(Tiran, Mack, 1995)*.

✋ Massage is directed by the woman and may be applied to the abdomen, back and other areas of tension such as the legs and forehead, to facilitate relaxation and diminish discomfort. Back labour, which is caused by the occipitoposterior position of the baby, is often relieved with massage. Firm circular strokes are applied with the heel of the hand over the sacral area. Gentle mobilization techniques at hypomobile spinous processes and pressure points, applied with the thumb along the spine, are also useful.

✋ During the transitional stage of labour, the pain intensifies. The therapist is again directed by the woman's needs, offering reassurance and support. During the birth itself, physical support may be given; application of compresses to the face and stroking between contractions are possible *(Snow, 1996/7)*.

✋ Immediately postpartum, an abdominal massage every four hours can assist in the involution of the uterus — that is, reduction of the size of the uterus after delivery *(Stillerman, 1994)*. Relaxation massage is appropriate in the weeks after the birth. Reducing feelings of stress will aid in milk production. Breast massage can also relieve feelings of local congestion.

✋ The long-term treatment goals after delivery focus on helping the woman to regain proper posture and biomechanics. Difficult deliveries (back labour) may contribute to long-lasting lower-back pain. Although the exact mechanism of injury or pain is unclear, the possibility of lumbo-sacral sprain or sacroiliac sprain is high *(Kisner, Colby, 1996)*. Difficult deliveries may cause injury to the pelvic joints or lumbar spine. In this case, specific assessment (sacroiliac joint motion palpation, hip passive relaxed range of motion, lumbar spine range of motion and muscle imbalance testing) is required before treatment.

✋ If cesarean surgery was performed, once the area has sufficiently healed, massage addresses the hyperlordotic postural compensation which occurs in response to the scar tissue. The therapist must keep in mind that joint laxity is a concern for up to six months after delivery.

Self-care during Pregnancy

✍ During pregnancy, relaxation exercises, deep diaphragmatic breathing, relaxation tapes and visualization will help the client feel more relaxed and help with insomnia. Mild herbal teas such as chamomile will assist sleep.

✍ Self-massage to the costal border, suprapubic attachments of the abdominals and perineum is recommended. A one per cent dilution or 10 drops of pure marjoram essential oil (only after the fourth month of pregnancy) or pure chamomile essential oil in 50 ml. of vegetable oil can be used.

✍ Stretching and lubricating the perineal area should begin in the last six weeks of the third trimester in preparation for birth. These exercises are given by the midwife or physician.

✍ Self-care for leg cramps includes circulatory exercises of the foot before bedtime, such as various active range of motion movements of the ankle, toes and knee. Once a cramp has occurred, active inhibition stretching techniques are used. The gastrocnemius is stretched by contracting the tibialis anterior through drawing the toes and foot upward into dorsiflexion; if necessary the client can assist the stretch with her hands or a towel around her foot. Massage of these muscles is also encouraged. This will relieve the cramp in a few minutes, but tenderness may remain for several hours to a few days.

✍ Self-care for varicose veins includes: avoidance of excessive weight gain; avoidance of standing still or crossing the legs for a prolonged period of time; avoidance of clothing that is tight around the upper leg or waist; wearing support hose if the varicose veins have already developed; elevation of the feet and legs when sitting; and performance of gentle passive relaxed range of motion exercises of the ankle and knees.

✍ A mild to moderate exercise program is encouraged throughout the pregnancy, when there is no evidence of an adverse effect on the fetus or pregnant woman (Buschbacher, 1994). Generally, activities enjoyed before pregnancy can be continued. However, strenuous exercise or exercise that includes jumping or risk of injury to the abdomen should be avoided. Increased joint laxity puts joints at risk for injury; therefore, caution must be exercised with flexibility training also. It is imperative that any exercise which causes faintness, nausea or pain, especially in the back or pubic area, should be stopped. Walking and swimming are good forms of exercise.

✍ During pregnancy, postural imbalances develop due to the enlarging fetus. After the birth, the woman is carrying an ever-growing baby — a kind of "progressive weight-lifting". To prepare for this, the woman is encouraged to stretch the scalenes, scapular protractors, shoulder internal rotators and levator scapulae, hip adductors, knee flexors and ankle plantar flexors. It is essential not to stretch these muscles beyond their normal range to prevent joint instability. Strengthening is performed for the upper neck flexors, shoulder extensors and external rotators, scapular retractors and depressors, hip extensors, knee extensors and ankle dorsiflexors (Kisner, Colby, 1996). The focus of the program is preventative and should be started early in the pregnancy.

✍ The client should be referred to a physiotherapist for specific exercises for diastasis symphysis pubis and diastasis recti. Generally, the client should be cautious with certain movements. Specifically, she should never do leg raises or sit-ups from a supine position.

✍ Self-care for frequent urination and incontinence includes regular exercise to strengthen the pelvic floor muscles. This involves resisting the passage of urine so it is released in small bursts, three to five seconds long. Or, while in a supine position, the client imagines doing this action up to a maximum of 10 repetitions. Eventually, the latter is performed in sitting or standing (Kisner, Colby, 1996).

Self-care after Delivery

✍ A specific remedial exercise program is recommended to restore postural alignment of the individual, based on a thorough assessment.

✍ Hydrotherapy, as appropriate, is encouraged. For example, heat may be applied to sore aching muscles and cold may be applied to inflamed muscles.

✍ Relaxation strategies such as breathing exercises, a support network and arranging "time out" are important for emotional well-being.

Baby Massage

🖐 Just as an adult can benefit from positive touch and massage, so too can infants. Over the years many studies have been performed examining babies' responses to touch or lack of touch. This has been especially demonstrated through the massage of preterm babies. One study examined the effects of 15 minutes of daily massage and passive movement on premature babies. First, the baby's neck, back or chest (depending on the position), legs, arms and head were gently rubbed for five minutes followed by five minutes of flexion and extension movements of the right arm, left arm, right leg, left leg and both legs together, then five more minutes of massage. It was reported that in a 10-day period the control group experienced an average weight loss of 48 grams, while infants that received massage and movement gained an average of 25 grams (Field et al., 1986). Food intake was increased with a resultant improvement in gastrointestinal functioning such as promotion of peristalsis and bowel movements. This, in turn, decreases gastric retention and abdominal distention. Sucking also seems to improve with better gastrointestinal function in preterm babies.

🖐 In another study, premature infants were given three sessions a day of 20 minutes of gentle massaging. Techniques were applied, using the palm and fingertips, to the head, shoulders, back, arms, legs and feet. Those babies that were massaged showed greater responsiveness to both tactile and visual stimuli than those preterm babies that were not given the added stimulation of touch and interaction; in fact, the performance of the massaged preterm babies in these areas was no different from full-term babies (Brown, 1984). Therefore, massage and tactile stimulation of the preterm baby improves growth which leads to an earlier discharge from the hospital.

🖐 Babies with special needs such as cocaine or HIV exposure or those born to depressed mothers also benefited from massage. This was indicated by improved weight gain, fewer stress behaviours (lower levels of stress hormones are found in the body after massage) and higher ratings in emotional, social and soothability scores as well as better alert responsiveness and attention scores (Wheeden et al., 1995; Scafidi, Field, 1995). Of course, healthy infants also respond well to massages showing improved temperament and physiological health, such as reduced colic and less fussiness. The parent can use a lotion or an enriched oil, such as 10 drops of pure lavender essential oil in 50 ml. of vegetable oil, for massaging. Babies seem to find abdominal stroking (in a downward or clockwise direction) and back stroking and kneading especially soothing

See also spasm, edema, stress reduction, hyperlordosis, hyperkyphosis, pes planus, constipation, carpal tunnel syndrome, thoracic outlet syndrome, piriformis syndrome, diabetes mellitus, hypertension, tension headaches, migraines and other circulatory concerns.

(Brown, 1984). The arms are kneaded in turn. This can be followed by the buttocks and each leg. The massage can be performed with the baby first in a supine position and then prone. The back and buttocks can also be massaged while the caregiver is holding the baby against her chest. Gentle and rhythmical movements may be included for the arms and legs, moving each joint in turn. An optimal time may be after changing diapers, after a bath or before a nap or bedtime. Massage of infants by the parents, in all cases, can provide an opportunity for positive interaction with the baby on all levels. It allows for emotional bonding between the infant and parent as well as affecting the infant's development for the better (Field, 1995).

16

SPASM

Fiona Rattray

> *A spasm is an involuntary, sustained contraction of a muscle.*
> *A cramp is a common or lay term for a painful, prolonged muscle*
> *spasm.*

There is a lack of a standardized terminology to describe the clinical presentation of soft tissue when it is dysfunctional. This confusion extends to the terms "spasm" and "tone", both in the literature and in common usage *(Janda, 1991; Travell, Simons, 1983)*. Perhaps this is due to the lack of focus that the medical model has regarding palpation of soft tissue. A quick glance through the indexes of many textbooks on neuromusculoskeletal injuries and conditions reveals few entries under "muscle spasm" or "muscle tone". The terms "tension" or "hypertonicity" are even rarer. Because massage therapists use these terms frequently, common definitions are important.

A **spasm** has been described as an involuntary muscle contraction, when measured electomyographically, or as spontaneous motor unit activity *(Travell, Simons, 1983)*. Some authors use the term without defining it *(Thomson et al., 1991)*, some use alternative terms such as muscle guarding *(Hertling, Kessler, 1990)*, while others, perhaps due to the confusion around the term, avoid using it at all *(Buschbacher, 1994)*.

Attempts to define spasm by its causes have been proposed to aid in assessment and treatment *(Janda, 1991)*. **Reflex muscle guarding** describes a muscle spasm in response to pain. This painful stimulus is due to local tissue injury and is present in the acute stages of a condition. The muscle spasm acts to functionally splint the injured structures, reducing movement and preventing further injury. Muscle guarding may also result from referred pain. In both cases, the guarding stops when the pain is relieved *(Kisner, Colby, 1990; Janda, 1991)*. However, the idea that muscle spasm protects the injured tissue has resulted in over-reliance on immobilization, such as bedrest or splinting to treat spasms, especially spasms associated with trauma. Recent studies have shown the benefits of pain-free

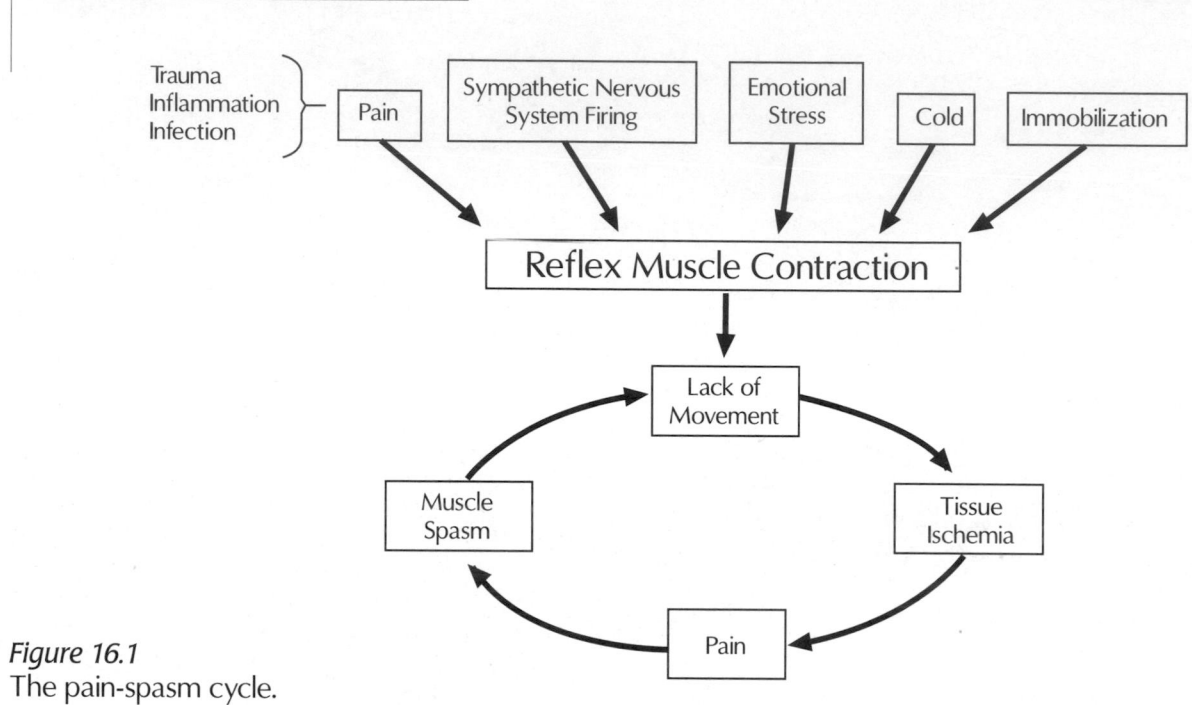

Figure 16.1
The pain-spasm cycle.

controlled mobilization in the recovery from trauma *(Kraus, 1988).*

An **intrinsic muscle spasm** is part of a self-perpetuating pain-spasm cycle *(Figure 16.1).* Pain resulting from direct or indirect trauma, inflammation or infection can initiate a reflex muscle contraction. An increase in sympathetic nervous system firing, emotional stresses, cold or chilling of the tissue and immobilization also lead to reflex muscle contraction. This contraction restricts movement of the joint crossed by the muscle. The lack of movement allows for tissue ischemia or circulatory stasis and metabolite retention, which in turn irritate the nerve endings, registering as pain. The muscle responds to the pain by staying in spasm. This intrinsic spasm will remain, even when the tissue injury that caused the initial reflex muscle guarding is no longer acute *(Kisner, Colby, 1990; Cailliet, 1993; Rachlin, 1994).*

Muscle **tone** has been described as the resistance of a relaxed muscle to passive stretch or elongation *(Taber's Cyclopedic Medical Dictionary, 1981; Vander et al., 1994).* Yet, while palpating a relaxed muscle, the therapist notices a certain resistance of the tissue to direct compression. Therefore, a more complete definition of muscle tone also includes both the resistance of the muscles and connective tissue to palpation and the active, but not continuous, contraction of muscle in response to the stimulation of the nervous system *(Basmajian, 1985).*

A therapist wishing to report the increase in tone palpated in a client's upper trapezius muscle following a whiplash injury may choose either "tension" or "hypertonicity". One explanation of **tension** is muscle fibres that tend to shorten, causing them to perform work *(Thomas, 1981).* While some shortening of the muscle fibres may be noted with a length test of the muscle, the client with the whiplash injury may be incapable of normally working the injured trapezius due to pain. A more applicable definition of muscular tension is a muscle held in a sustained contraction *(Travell, Simons, 1983).*

Neurologists interpret **hypertonicity** as the abnormally high tone usually seen with upper motor neuron disorders. They classify spasticity (increased tone in response to stretch), rigidity (continuous contraction) and spasms as forms of hypertonia *(Vander et al., 1994)*. Some physiotherapists *(Janda, 1991; Rachlin, 1994)* and osteopaths *(Greenman, 1989)*, on the other hand, define hypertonicity as an increase in tone that is present with painful, dysfunctional muscles, making no mention of neuronal disorders at all. The neurological definition of hypertonicity is perhaps confusing in that it includes spasm (a response to pain or metabolic changes) in a category with the increased tone of upper motor neuron disorders. Therefore, this text uses the osteopathic definition for hypertonicity. Spasticity and rigidity are used to describe the tone associated with neuronal disorders.

To understand a muscle in spasm, it is necessary to understand how a muscle contracts normally. Muscles are largely composed of contractile tissue, which has the ability to contract and relax. A skeletal muscle is a bundle of fascicles; each fascicle is a grouping of muscle fibres. The muscle fibres, or muscle cells, themselves are made up of thousands of fine strands called myofibrils. Finally, each myofibril contains thick and thin filaments arranged in units that repeat along the myofibril. These units are called sarcomeres and they are the basic contractile units of muscle fibres *(Figure 16.2)*.

The thick filaments (myosin) and the thin filaments (actin) overlap each other and their interaction produces contractile force. The myosin filaments have protruding heads which are potential cross-bridges between the actin and myosin. These heads can chemically bond to the actin filaments. They act like oars in a boat to move the filaments past each other, alternately bonding, pulling on the actin in a power "stroke", releasing and rebonding. Numerous power strokes are required for the myosin and actin filaments to slide past each other and shorten the sarcomere. Eventually, these repeated actions produce a muscular contraction.

Calcium initiates bonding and adenosine triphosphate (ATP) provides the energy for the contraction. The control over muscular contraction occurs in the following manner. The calcium is stored in and released from a network of sacs that surround each myofibril. This network is called the sarcoplasmic reticulum. When a muscle cell is stimulated by its motor neuron, a minute electrical charge (an action potential) moves from the neuron to the surface of the muscle cell. The action potential is transmitted by numerous transverse tubules to the interior of the cell and to the network of sarcoplasmic reticulum. The action potential stimulates the release of the calcium, initiating muscular contraction. When the action potential stops, the calcium is quickly recovered by the sarcoplasmic reticulum and muscular contraction ceases. In a spasmodic muscle, this contraction continues.

Two structures, the muscle spindle and the Golgi tendon organ, transmit proprioceptive information from muscles to the central nervous system to allow the muscles' proper functioning. The massage techniques of muscle approximation and Golgi

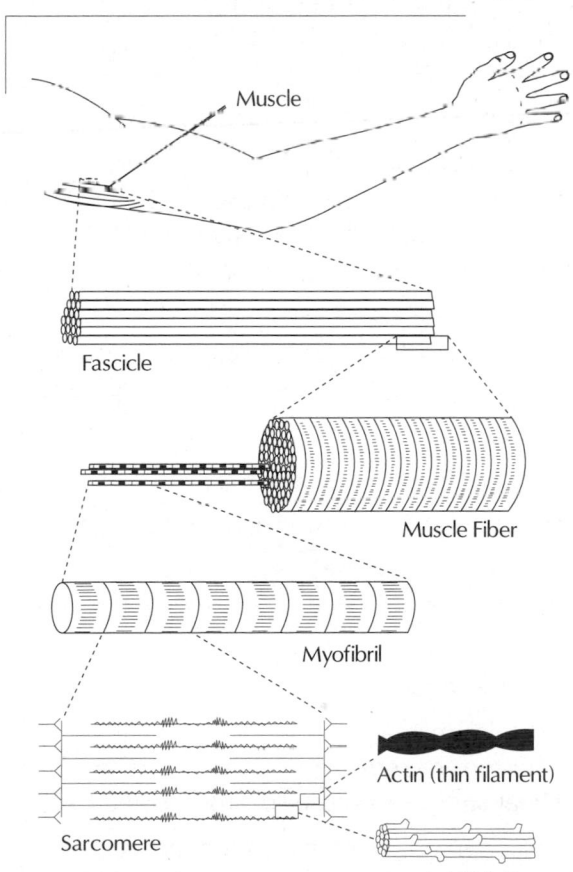

Figure 16.2
Skeletal muscle composition.

195

tendon organ release use the functions of these structures to be effective.

Muscle spindles are the major sensory organs of muscles and aid in the control of muscle movements. The spindles contain nerve filaments coiled around small specialized muscle fibres. They measure both the degree to which a muscle is stretched as it is moving through range and the speed with which this happens. For example, with flexion at the elbow, triceps is stretched. When a muscle is stretched, the spindle is also stretched. This increases the firing of the afferent spindle fibres, sending a sensory signal to the spinal cord. Here the afferent or Ia neuron synapses with the lower motor neuron, or alpha motor neuron. The alpha motor neuron in turn fires and causes the skeletal muscle surrounding the muscle spindle to contract. A reflex contraction of the muscle therefore occurs in response to a stretch of the same muscle, modifying changes in muscle length. This is called the stretch reflex *(Vander, et al., 1994; Guyton, 1986)*. In the example of elbow flexion, the stretch reflex controls the length of triceps, allowing for smooth flexion.

This process can be turned on or off by stimulation or inhibition of the gamma efferent fibres that are part of the muscle spindle. Gamma fibres control the length of the small specialized muscle fibres or intrafusil fibres within the spindle itself. When gamma efferent fibres fire, the two end portions of the spindle contract, causing the spindle to react strongly and rapidly to any degree of stretch. Through the stretch reflex described above, the tension in the skeletal muscle is increased. When gamma efferent fibres are silent, the muscle spindle relaxes and does not react to stretch. The gamma efferent neurons are strongly influenced by the descending output of the reticular system of the brain stem and the sympathetic nervous system *(Porth, 1990; Cailliet, 1993)*. Therefore, a client who is under stress is more likely to have increased muscle tension and spasm *(Porth, 1990; Kisner, Colby, 1990)*.

Golgi tendon organs (GTOs) are nerve receptors located in the tendons near their muscular attachments. These receptors are sensitive to tension in the muscle, whether due to active contraction or passive stretch. When they fire, they inhibit contraction of the muscle attached to the tendon containing them and protect the muscle from an overstretch injury.

✦ Muscles that commonly go into spasm are gastrocnemius, soleus, hamstrings, quadratus lumborum, the intrinsic muscles of the back, the intercostals and sternocleidomastoid.

The causes of muscle spasm and cramps include:

➤ **pain** resulting from inflammation, direct or indirect trauma or infection;

➤ **circulatory stasis** due to reflex muscle guarding, restricted movement and decreased circulation;

➤ **increased gamma neuron firing** due to stress, anxiety, fatigue or an overstretch injury to nearby tissue;

➤ **chilling of the muscle** leading to reflex muscle contraction;

➤ **an impaired nutritional supply.** Decreased calcium intake or loss of sodium through excess perspiration, dehydration, electrolyte disturbance from persistent vomiting, hypocalcemia from persistent diarrhea and heat stress can cause spasms *(Porth, 1990)*;

➤ **a lack of vitamin D**, because the vitamin helps synthesize enzymes that actively transport calcium, which is necessary for normal muscular contraction *(Dunne, 1990)*.

Calf Cramps

✦ Cramps in gastrocnemius are associated with pregnancy, although the exact cause is not known *(Travell, Simons, 1992)*. However, vitamin E deficiency has been associated with gastrocnemius cramps and a lack of vitamin B2 with calf cramps during pregnancy.

✦ Calf cramps have been noted with superior tibiofibular joint hypomobility and associated with trigger points in gastrocnemius *(Travell, Simons, 1992)*.

✦ Nocturnal calf cramps may occur when the ankle is plantarflexed by the weight of heavy bed covers. The plantarflexion shortens gastrocnemius and may cause spasms, waking the client from sleep *(Travell, Simons, 1992)*.

Calf Cramps and Pathologies

The therapist must also be aware that spasms and cramps can be caused by pathologies and medication. In these cases, treatment modifications or referral to a physician may be indicated. For example, calf muscle cramps may occur with **arterial disorders**, such as: acute arterial occlusion due to a thrombus or embolism; chronic arteriosclerotic vascular disorder due to arterial narrowing and fibrosing, which is frequently associated with diabetes mellitus and with the aging process; thromboangiitis obliterans or Buerger's disease, an inflammatory reaction of the arteries to nicotine, found in smokers; and Raynaud's syndrome, an arterial spasm due to abnormal sympathetic nervous system firing, which is most commonly found in the fingers and, occasionally, the feet.

Any of the above conditions may give rise to **intermittent claudication** or pain and cramping in the calf muscles with exercise. Intermittent claudication is due to ischemia. Pain and cramping are often noted when the client is walking. They diminish slowly with rest. Pain increases as the arterial disorder progresses and the client's tolerance for exercise diminishes *(Kisner, Colby, 1990)*.

Deep vein thrombosis can lead to feelings of tightness or "charley horse" in the calf *(Alexander, 1992)*. Deep vein thrombosis (DVT) can result from fracture, surgery, pregnancy and prolonged bedrest, especially in the elderly.

Lumbar degenerative disc disease can cause nocturnal spasm in the muscles supplied by the compressed nerve root.

Calf cramps as neurological symptoms of cancer have also been noted.

Medication such as lithium can cause spasm *(Travell, Simons, 1992)*.

Symptom Picture

✦ There is pain within the muscle due to ischemia and retention of metabolites. Acute trauma and referred pain may also cause the spasm.

✦ Spasm and hypertonicity are present.

✦ There is decreased range of motion of the joint crossed by the shortened affected muscle, whether the spasm is reflex muscle guarding or intrinsic muscle spasm.

♦ Antagonist and synergist muscles are affected. Trigger points in other muscles may refer pain to the spasmodic muscle.

Subjective Information

HEALTH HISTORY QUESTIONS

♦ How is the client's general health? Are there any contributing factors, such as diabetes mellitus, vascular disease or pregnancy? Does the client have any alterations in electrolyte balance due to diarrhea, vomiting or excessive sweating?

♦ Has there been any previous injury to the area?

♦ Is there pain? Where is it located? What is the quality of the pain?

♦ Were there any precipitating factors, such as a change in sleeping or eating patterns, an increase in stress or overall high levels of stress for the client?

♦ Is the client feeling chilled?

♦ When was the onset of the spasm?

♦ Has the client consulted a physician about this? Is the client taking any medication or nutritional supplements for the condition?

Objective Information

Observations

✍ Antalgic gait may be present if the spasm is located in the lower torso or limb.

✍ Antalgic posture may be present with spasm of the postural muscles or muscles of the lower limb, back and neck.

✍ The client may have a pained facial expression.

Palpation

✍ The affected muscle may be hot, due to acute congestion, or cool, due to ischemia.

✍ The affected muscle is point tender due to ischemia.

✍ The texture of an acutely spasmodic muscle is firm, dense and congested. The texture of a muscle with an intrinsic muscle spasm is hard and fibrous.

✍ The affected muscle is hypertonic. The synergists and antagonists may also be hypertonic.

Contraindications

✦ **Do not** attempt to completely eliminate reflex muscle guarding that is splinting an acute injury.

✦ **Avoid passively stretching an acutely spasmodic muscle** because this may tear fibres of the muscle and further injure the client. This is especially true when inflammation is present, as stretching will increase the pain and muscle guarding, resulting in greater tissue damage (Kisner, Colby, 1990).

✦ Hot hydrotherapy applications are contraindicated with a muscle spasm resulting from an acute injury.

✦ Massage is locally contraindicated with deep vein thrombosis or thrombophlebitis of the calf. A medical referral is indicated. With venous thrombosis, the client may complain of calf cramping or tightness, exhibit local tenderness, heat, pallor, swelling and have a diminished or absent dorsalis pedis pulse (Alexander, 1992). This is an important consideration for clients who have had a recent fracture or surgery, for clients who are pregnant or for clients over 50 years of age.

Testing

✍ The **AF ROM** of the joint crossed by the affected muscle is reduced. There is pain on active movement, especially at the end ranges when the affected muscle is being stretched or shortened.

✍ **PR ROM** that lengthens the affected muscle reveals a muscle spasm end feel with pain and decreased range.

✍ **AR submaximal isometric testing** reveals decreased strength with pain on contraction with an intrinsic muscle spasm. Strength testing of an acutely spasmodic muscle is contraindicated.

Special Tests

✍ **Ramirez's test** is positive with deep vein thrombosis. **Homan's sign** is also positive, but may not always detect DVT. Either positive test contraindicates local massage.

Treatment Goals

Break the pain-spasm cycle and decrease the spasm.

Treatment Plan

✋ **Positioning** of the client depends on the location of the affected muscle and the client's comfort.

✋ The therapist can intervene in the pain-spasm cycle in several ways. The task is to choose the appropriate modality or combination of modalities to break this cycle and decrease the spasm. Encouraging **diaphragmatic breathing** and relaxation decreases the sympathetic nervous system firing. **Hydrotherapy** applications depend on the type of spasm that is present. With reflex muscle guarding in response to acute injury, local **cold** applications, such as an ice pack or ice massage, are used for an analgesic effect to break the cycle (Kraus, 1988). With an intrinsic muscle spasm that is occurring in chronically

199

Treatment Goals

Treatment Plan

hypertonic tissue and where the muscles are tight and fibrous, **heat** increases local circulation and flushes out metabolites *(Cailliet, 1993)*. **Contrast** applications may also be useful with an intrinsic spasm.

If the spasm is reflex muscle guarding in response to an acute injury, do nothing to disturb the healing process and decrease only a portion of the spasm present.

In terms of massage techniques, especially with a first-time client where the therapist is unfamiliar with how the client's tissues respond to treatment, it is important not to overwork the affected muscle. While a protective spasm may be reduced when the client is stationary on the massage table, the act of turning over or getting up can cause the protective spasm to return with a vengeance. If this occurs, an application of ice to the muscle is appropriate.

General Treatment

Decrease the pain and sympathetic nervous system firing.

The therapist begins with a full-body massage with a focus on relaxation to decrease the gamma firing and spasm. Any compensatory structures, and the unaffected limb or side of the body, are also treated.

Increase local circulation.

Proximal to the affected muscle, the local circulation is increased to reduce ischemia and metabolic retention using effleurage and petrissage.

Decrease the hypertonicity.

Hypertonicity is reduced with petrissage.

Treat the antagonists and synergists.

Trigger points that refer into the affected muscle are treated using muscle stripping.

Specific Treatment

Decrease the spasm.

At first, techniques that use direct pressure may be too painful for a muscle that is acutely spasmodic. Indirect techniques that employ spinal reflexes, such as agonist contraction *by the client*, Golgi tendon organ release, the origin and insertion technique and muscle approximation by the therapist are used instead. These are described in detail in the remedial exercise and Swedish techniques chapters.

Several applications of the same technique or combinations of different techniques may be necessary to reduce a spasm. The therapist should not focus only on the spasm but should treat the affected muscle, then move to the surrounding tissue and synergists and then return to the spasm.

Once the spasm has decreased or is less painful for on-site work, direct techniques, such as vibrations, shaking, muscle squeezing, petrissage, and joint play, may be used. Repetitive effleurage and petrissage applied to the affected muscle and surrounding tissue are used to flush out metabolites and decrease pain.

Muscles that have an intrinsic spasm will be experiencing ischemia,

Treatment Goals

Once the spasm has been reduced, increase the range of motion.

Treatment Plan

decreased tissue health and possible fibrosing, indicating petrissage techniques.

☝ Joint play to the joint crossed by the affected muscle, or to the proximal and distal joints, may be helpful to maintain muscle length and joint health.

☝ In terms of **remedial exercise** within the treatment, the therapist must significantly decrease the tone in the acutely spasmodic muscle before applying a slow passive stretch. PIR and contract-relax techniques are also indicated and are described in the chapter on remedial exercise. Remedial exercise may be interspersed with massage techniques. The treatment is finished with soothing stroking and muscle squeezing.

☝ For an intrinsic muscle spasm, the muscle energy technique may be used to increase range of motion. This is described in the chapter on non-Swedish techniques.

Self-care Goals

Prevent recurrence and educate the client on reducing muscle imbalances and on correct posture.

Self-care Plan

✍ The same **hydrotherapy** concepts are followed for self-care. Ice packs wrapped in a towel may be applied to reflex muscle guarding sites for an analgesic effect. The client should take care not to chill the tissue; the ice pack should not be left on for more than 20 minutes at a time. Deep moist heat or contrast applications are recommended for an intrinsic muscle spasm.

✍ After the spasm decreases, especially with reflex muscle guarding, **pain-free active free range of motion** of the affected joint is very important (*Kraus, 1988*). The client should also do this before a slow, complete stretch to the muscle (*Kraus, 1988*). For the muscle to completely lengthen, the stretch should be held for up to 30 seconds without bouncing.

✍ Following stretches, active resisted exercises are useful to increase the strength of the antagonist. For example, tibialis anterior can be strengthened with a gastrocnemius spasm.

✍ The client may use diaphragmatic breathing and relaxation techniques to help decrease stress levels.

✍ To reduce nocturnal calf cramps, agonist contraction techniques are important when the cramp is experienced and are most effective when followed by a slow passive stretch. The client will naturally perform what is commonly described as "stretching out" a calf spasm by dorsiflexing the ankle. In fact, this is an excellent example of agonist contraction, because gastrocnemius spasm is inhibited to allow tibialis anterior to dorsiflex the ankle. To perform passive dorsiflexion the client stands with the affected knee extended and slowly leans the torso forward while the heel stays on the floor. This passive stretch is safe for the client to perform because he is in control of the stretch. The client should also avoid using heavy bed covers to prevent the plantarflexion associated with nocturnal calf cramps. A large, firm blanket roll placed at the client's feet under the covers holds the feet in a neutral position and prevents the covers from compressing the feet into plantarflexion (*Travell, Simons, 1992*).

Refer the client.

✍ The client is referred to a physician for suspected vascular diseases or a naturopath for suspected nutritional imbalances.

Treatment Frequency and Expected Outcome

Treatments may be given twice a week if reflex muscle guarding is the cause of the spasm. This frequency can be maintained until the spasm has decreased.

See also stress reduction and relaxation, trigger points, torticollis, all of the musculoskeletal traumas, pregnancy, other circulatory concerns and degenerative disc disease chapters for related conditions.

Treatments may be twice a week for three weeks for an intrinsic muscle spasm.

The outcome depends on whether the spasm is reflex muscle guarding or intrinsic in nature and whether the contributing factors have been eliminated. An acute protective spasm will decrease as the injury resolves, whereas a self-perpetuating intrinsic spasm may require repeated treatments.

17

MYOFASCIAL TRIGGER POINTS

Fiona Rattray

> *A trigger point (TrP) is a hyperirritable spot, usually within a taut band of skeletal muscle or its fascia (Travell, Simons, 1983). It is point tender on site, often exhibits a predictable pain referral pattern and causes a shortening of the affected muscle.*

Medical literature contains numerous terms to describe pain of muscular origins, as well as numerous theories about causes of the pain. Tender or painful palpable nodules, lumps and cords in affected muscles are called many names. These include "muscle callouses", "muscular rheumatism", "chronic rheumatism" and "myogelosis" (muscle hardening). Some of these terms have multiple meanings, depending on the person who wrote the paper. Some authors have used different terms in papers published over several years to describe what may be the same condition. This confusion over terminology has hampered a medical understanding of muscular pain disorders *(Travell, Simons, 1983).*

At the turn of the century, the term "fibrositis" was used to describe local tenderness and regions of hardness in muscles. Pain and hardness were originally attributed to an inflammation of fibrous tissue. However, subsequent research failed to prove that an inflammatory pathology of the connective tissue was present in most cases of what was called fibrositis. The term has become ambiguous and broadly applied to muscle pain of non-organic origin.

In the late 1930s, Kellgren, Gutstein and others contributed to the initial body of knowledge by investigating muscle pain syndromes and pain referral patterns. Also at this time, Kraus advocated treatment of these syndromes using vapocoolant spray. Travell's first paper on trigger points was published in 1942 *(Travell, Simons, 1983).* Travell and Simons have been on the forefront of myofascial trigger point research and treatment.

Trigger points have been documented as a source of muscular pain in people's lives from as early as infancy and childhood. Travell theorized that active trigger points develop in the most physically active years of a person's life, while the restricted range of motion and stiffness of latent trigger points occur in the more sedentary, or later, years. Other researchers found that active trigger points are more likely to develop in people with sedentary lifestyles who do occasional bouts of extremely vigorous exercise than in people who exercise their muscles daily.

A healthy muscle does not contain trigger points. Taut bands of muscle fibres and tenderness are not present. Referred pain cannot be elicited and the local twitch response is absent.

The exact physiological mechanism of palpable taut bands in muscle containing a trigger point is not fully understood. However, the bands have been observed to persist in muscles even after death.

Travell believed a taut band may be a contracture of muscle fibres that were damaged in the trauma that initiated the trigger point. Muscle contraction is normally controlled by the rapid release and reabsorption of calcium by the sarcoplasmic reticulum of individual muscle fibres. Adenosine triphosphate (ATP) provides the energy for contraction of the sarcomeres, which are the contractile units of muscle fibres. The combination of calcium and ATP causes the sarcomeres to shorten. When the calcium is reabsorbed, contraction stops. A damaged sarcoplasmic reticulum would allow calcium to spill onto the sarcomeres. This would set up an uncontrolled, sustained contraction (called a contracture) of the affected sarcomeres for as long as their ATP energy supply lasted. The theory, however, only partially explains the physiology of trigger points, since the calcium would eventually disperse throughout the tissue.

Various studies have revealed the trigger point to be an area of both increased metabolism and decreased circulation. This local vasoconstriction or ischemia is likely a reflexive attempt by the body to contain the uncontrolled metabolic processes occurring at the site of the sustained sarcomere contraction. Both the contracture and the runaway metabolism will stop if the muscle is slowly stretched, disengaging the interlocked contractile components of the sarcomeres (actin and myosin).

Trigger points can occur in ligaments, joint capsules, periosteum and fascia, although these referral patterns are not extensively documented. The symptoms of trigger points may mimic the pain of other conditions, such as osteoarthritis, tendinitis, cardiac pain and radiculopathies. Unrecognized symptoms of trigger points may also be misdiagnosed as psychosomatic, which can be frustrating for the client.

Types of Trigger Points

Trigger points are classified into several types depending on their symptoms and location (*Travell, Simons, 1983*).

✦ An **active trigger point** is painful at rest and with movement of the muscle containing it. The trigger point in the taut band prevents the muscle from fully lengthening and reduces its strength. Tissue local to the trigger point exhibits ischemia. The trigger point within the taut band is tender. When it is compressed, it refers pain in a pattern that is usually specific and predictable for that muscle, although referrals do not always follow the researched patterns. The pain may be referred locally or distant to the affected muscle.

Pain is felt if the muscle containing the active trigger point is passively or actively stretched. As the muscle is lengthened to the point of pain, a protective muscle spasm

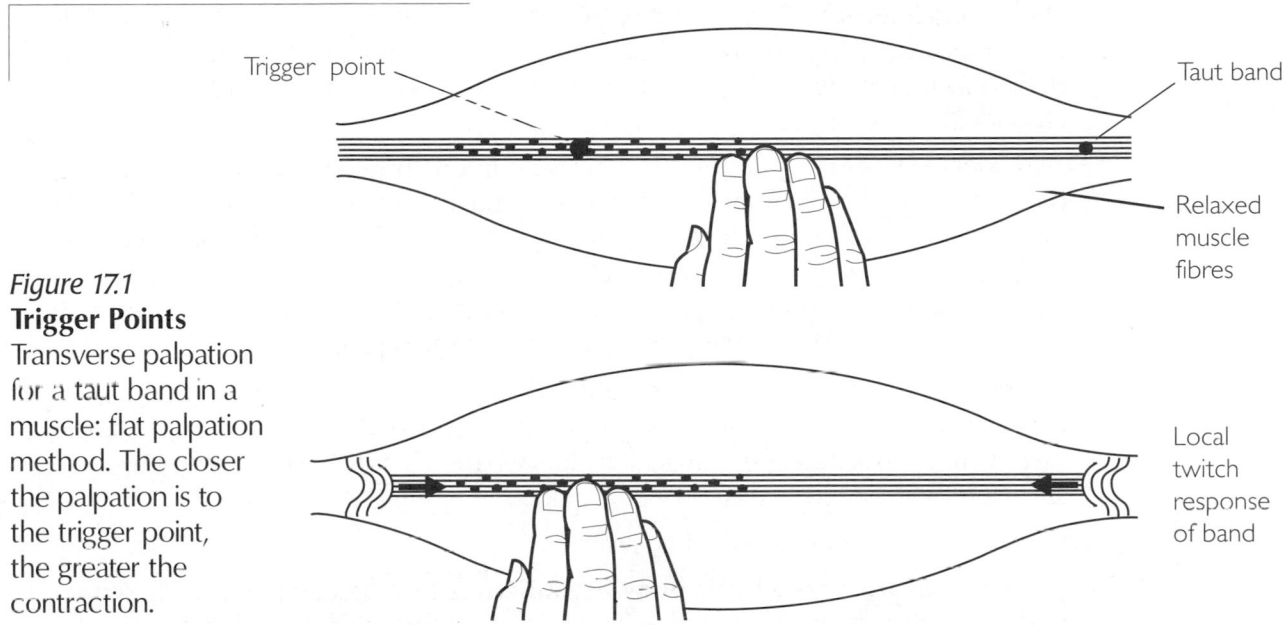

Figure 17.1
Trigger Points
Transverse palpation for a taut band in a muscle: flat palpation method. The closer the palpation is to the trigger point, the greater the contraction.

sets in that painfully prevents further lengthening. However, when the muscle is at rest there is no spasm in the muscle containing the trigger point or in the taut band itself (*Travell, Simons, 1983*). Palpation produces a **local twitch response** and possible **referred autonomic phenomena**. A local twitch response is a transient contraction of the taut band in the muscle containing the trigger point. This response occurs when the taut band is palpated transversely, like strumming over a guitar string. The taut band responds to **pressure** by visibly and palpably contracting or twitching (*Figure 17.1*). The closer the transverse palpation is to the trigger point location in the taut band, the greater the contraction. Autonomic phenomena include vasomotor changes (local pallor with compression of the trigger point and hyperemia with inactivation of the trigger point), increased sudomotor activity (sweating), pilomotor response (gooseflesh), proprioceptive distortions, lacrimation (tearing) and nasal irritation and discharge.

✦ A **latent trigger point** produces pain only when palpated. All the other characteristics of an active trigger point may occur with a latent trigger point, including prevention of full muscle lengthening. Latent trigger points are more common than active ones and may persist for years after the initial injury. A latent trigger point may be reverted to an active state by any referred pain (including pain from active trigger points, visceral pain or osteoarthritic pain), overuse, overstretching or chilling of the muscle containing it.

✦ A **primary trigger point** is directly activated by acute or chronic mechanical strain or overload of the affected muscle.

✦ A **secondary trigger point** is activated in the overworked synergist or antagonist muscles.

✦ A **satellite trigger point** is found in muscle that lies within the referral pattern of another trigger point.

Trigger points are idiopathic in nature.

➤ Travell's theory is that an **initial trauma** to the muscle, such as an acute strain, overloads some of the muscle fibres, giving rise to the trigger point.

➤ **Direct** and **indirect stimuli** can then activate the trigger point. Direct stimuli include trauma, acute muscle overload, overwork fatigue and chilling of the muscle. Indirect stimuli include referred pain from other trigger points, referred visceral pain and emotional stress.

➤ Two additional **specific factors that activate latent trigger points** include leaving the muscle in a shortened position for several hours — for example, during sleep. The other factor is shortening activation during treatment. Shortening activation occurs with the post-treatment stretch of the muscle containing the primary trigger point. If this stretch is performed suddenly, the antagonist muscle is shortened suddenly. This may activate any secondary trigger points present in the antagonist.

➤ The number and severity of **perpetuating factors** increase the likelihood of a latent trigger point becoming active when it is directly or indirectly stimulated. For example, a client with two or three perpetuating factors will more easily have trigger points activated than someone with only one factor.

Perpetuating factors include the following:

➤ **mechanical stresses** including **bony asymmetries** that directly or indirectly shorten muscles, such as a longer second metatarsal bone (Morton's foot), a leg length inequality and a small hemipelvis;

➤ **postural stresses** such as poor posture, improperly fitted furniture (chairs and desks), sustained isometric contraction (working at a keyboard), muscle immobility (sleeping with a muscle in a shortened position) and poor body mechanics (improperly bending and lifting);

➤ **muscle constriction** caused by the straps of a backpack or purse compressing the upper trapezius, for example;

➤ **nutritional inadequacies** such as vitamin B, vitamin C or folic acid deficiency;

➤ **metabolic imbalances** such as hypothyroidism, hypoglycemia and gout;

➤ **psychological factors** such as depression and anxiety;

➤ **chronic infection** including viral disease (herpes simplex and influenza) and bacterial infection (sinusitis, tooth abscess and urinary tract infection);

➤ **impaired sleep** leading to anxiety and increased muscle tension.

Symptom Picture

✦ Pain or tenderness is continuous with an active trigger point and occurs upon compression of a latent trigger point. The pain may be local to the trigger point or may be present in the muscle's referral zone. Referral pain can also occur outside Travell's documented patterns.

✦ The sensitivity of an active trigger point can change over several hours or days.

✦ Passive stretching of the affected muscle is painful.

✦ Contraction of the affected muscle is painful, especially within the inner range of the muscle.

- Possible autonomic symptoms noted in the referral zone include pilomotor response, local vasoconstriction and sweating.

- With sternocleidomastoid muscle trigger points, proprioceptive symptoms include vertigo, distortion of weight perception, tearing, nasal discharge and tinnitus.

- A palpable taut band containing the trigger point is present in the affected muscle. The trigger point is located at the most painful spot in the taut band. Upon palpation, a **local twitch response** is present in the muscle fibres of the taut band containing the trigger point. The client may exhibit the **jump sign** by wincing or abruptly moving the body part away from the palpating fingers.

- There is decreased circulation in the muscle local to the trigger point. There is also reduced blood flow in the tissue that lies within a trigger point's referral zone (*Travell, Simons, 1983*).

- Shortening and hypertonicity of the affected muscle occurs, resulting in a decreased range of motion.

- The synergists and antagonists of the affected muscle may develop secondary trigger points.

- Muscle weakness is present without muscle atrophy or neurological deficit.

- Perpetuating factors such as a leg length inequality, chilling of the muscle and postural stresses may be present.

Subjective Information

HEALTH HISTORY QUESTIONS

- How is the client's general health? Is there a history of metabolic disorders, such as hypothyroidism, or chronic infection, such as sinusitis? These factors may perpetuate the trigger point pain.

- Has there been any previous acute or overuse injury to the affected muscle?

- When was the onset of pain?

- Where is the pain located? Does the pain refer anywhere else? The client can mark this referred pain on the health history form or show the location on a trigger point chart or point to the referral pattern on her body. The therapist records the referred pain on the health history form.

- What is the quality of the pain? Trigger point pain is aching, deep and steady. It is described as **referred** pain. This is distinguished from the pain of nerve root irritation or peripheral nerve compression syndromes, which is described as radiating pain. Nerve pain is prickly and often accompanied by numbness.

- Are any autonomic symptoms present, such as sweating or gooseflesh? Where are they located? For example, an involved limb may feel cool, due to ischemia, in comparison to the unaffected limb.

- What aggravates or alleviates the trigger point? For example, the trigger point is aggravated by use of the muscle, increased stress, compression of the trigger point and cold; it is alleviated by rest, slow stretching and heat.

◆ Was the involved muscle placed in a shortened position for a long period of time? For example, the client may have fallen asleep in a fetal position that aggravated iliopsoas trigger points.

◆ Is muscle stiffness, limitation of movement or weakness present?

◆ Are there any known perpetuating factors? Examples are pain made worse by overusing a muscle, a headache that occurs at the end of a work day due to repetitive actions or shoulder pain that is made worse by standing outside in cold weather.

◆ If the client is returning for subsequent treatment of trigger point pain, has the pattern of referral changed or stayed the same? A **changed referral pattern** indicates that, while the initial trigger point has been successfully eliminated, secondary trigger points need to be treated. An **unchanged pattern** indicates that perpetuating factors need to be addressed before the trigger point can be eradicated.

Objective Information

Observations

✍ Antalgic gait may be present if an active trigger point is located in the lower torso or limb.

✍ Antalgic posture may also be present with an active trigger point. For example, the client with an active trigger point in upper trapezius may elevate the affected shoulder.

✍ The client with active trigger points may have a pained facial expression.

✍ A postural assessment may indicate structural imbalances that are perpetuating factors — for example, an apparent leg length inequality or a scoliosis.

Palpation

✍ Since a referral pattern is often specific for a given muscle, the therapist can use this information to locate the affected muscle and begin palpation assessment there.

✍ The trigger point is located in a palpable taut band of fibres in the affected muscle. The texture of this taut band is distinctly ropy. The tone of the muscle containing the trigger point is increased.

✍ To clearly palpate a taut band and its trigger point, the muscle must be relaxed. It is placed in a comfortably lengthened position that does not produce pain.

✍ There are two approaches to palpating for trigger points: **flat palpation** and **pincer grasp palpation.** Flat palpation is used on muscles that can be approached from one side only, such as infraspinatus and rhomboids. The fingertips are slowly and repeatedly moved across the muscle at right angles to the direction of the individual muscle fibres; the taut band that is associated with the trigger point becomes apparent. Once the taut band is located, the therapist palpates along the length of it, assessing for the most tender spot, which is the trigger point. Travell notes that this maximum tenderness is in response to the therapist's use of minimum pressure while palpating.

✍ Pincer grasp palpation is used on muscles that can be picked up between thumb and fingers, such as sternocleidomastoid, upper trapezius and pectoralis major. The muscle belly is grasped and the tissue is slowly compressed then rolled between the fingers and thumb. The palpation is performed across the fibres of the muscle. The taut band is palpable as a hard strand running the length of the muscle.

✍ **Panniculosis** may be palpated in the skin over trigger points located in superficial muscles. Panniculosis is a thickening of the subcutaneous tissue, often with a granular feel. There is no inflammation present. Skin rolling will reveal the characteristic skin hypersensitivity and subcutaneous tissue resistance associated with panniculosis, over the site of the trigger point. Panniculosis in connection with trigger points is most frequently found in the posterior thoracic and lumbar areas. The thickening can, however, exist independent of trigger points.

✍ The trigger point itself is locally tender or even painful upon direct compression. The pain may be intense enough to cause the client to wince, jump or cry out. This is the **jump sign**.

✍ When a trigger point is accurately located and compressed it will refer pain or autonomic phenomena in its referral zone which is often distant from the trigger point itself. Referred pain may develop immediately or after about 10 seconds of palpating compression.

✍ The client may comment that this pain is very similar to the discomfort that is regularly felt with the presenting condition, whether it be shoulder pain or headache. This indicates the accurate location of the trigger point.

✍ A local twitch response may be noted with cross-fibre palpation in superficial muscles such as the upper trapezius fibres, sternocleidomastoid and gluteus maximus.

✍ While an individual trigger point is a few millimetres in diameter, a cluster of trigger points can seem to be a centimetre in size (*Travell, Simons, 1983*). The trigger point may feel like a tiny "nodule".

✍ There is no inflammation or edema present with a trigger point. However, thermographic studies have shown there to be a "hot spot" two centimetres in diameter over the trigger point. The areas of referral patterns have been variously reported to be hot or cold (*Travell, Simons, 1992*).

✍ When a trigger point is accurately located and compressed it will refer pain or autonomic phenomena in its referral zone.

✍ To prevent the client from having a day or two of discomfort following palpation, Travell advised palpating for trigger points only in the muscles that can be treated during the same appointment.

✍ Once it is found, the trigger point location is noted on the health history form. The record of pain patterns and trigger point location serves as a baseline for subsequent treatments.

Testing

✍ **AF ROM** of a joint crossed by a muscle containing an active trigger point is reduced. Movement that increases the tension of a muscle harbouring an active trigger point, especially a quick movement, causes pain.

✍ **PR ROM** of a joint crossed by a muscle containing an active trigger point is also reduced. The muscle is unable to fully lengthen because of pain and muscle spasm end feel.

✍ **AR testing** of a muscle containing an active trigger point reveals weakness. When the muscle is placed in a shortened position, a maximum contraction is painful.

✍ Specific **length tests** of the affected muscle(s) will show reduced muscle length.

Special Tests

✍ The **trigger point compression test**, the **three-knuckle test**, the **swallowing test** and the **scalene cramp,** the **scalene relief** and the **finger flexion tests** will be positive if active trigger points exist in specific muscles.

Contraindications

✦ Avoid vigorous techniques or deep pressure when treating hyperirritable trigger points, since "kick-back" pain may result. Kick-back pain is a recurrence of the client's symptoms hours or days after treatment. This is especially true if ischemic compressions are applied too quickly and deeply, released too quickly and not followed by either a passive stretch and heat or slow, full active free range of motion and heat.

✦ In treating trigger points that are proximal to an area of acute inflammation, the usual use of heat as post-treatment hydrotherapy is contraindicated. In this situation, repetitive proximal effleurage to increase drainage is indicated following treatment of the trigger point.

✦ In the case of acute or early subacute overstretch injuries, such as strains or sprains, treatment of trigger points **local** to the injury is contraindicated. Trauma and the inflammatory process preclude the use of local muscle stripping and ischemic compressions, as well as post-treatment stretching and heat applications.

✦ Percussion and stretch are contraindicated on the anterior or posterior leg compartments. A possible compartment syndrome could result if a hematoma were created by an overly vigorous application of the technique *(Travell, Simons, 1992).*

✦ Avoid prolonged chilling of a muscle containing a trigger point, as this may activate it.

✦ Avoid combining prolonged ischemic compressions (an aggressive technique) and frictions (another aggressive technique) to the same muscle at the same appointment, since this can overtreat the tissue. In this case, work is arranged so less aggressive techniques, such as muscle stripping, are used for the trigger points.

✦ Although a full stretch usually follows the treatment of a trigger point, it is contraindicated to fully stretch muscles that cross a hypermobile joint. Instead, ischemic compression is followed with repetitive muscle stripping and heat only *(Travell, Simons, 1992).*

Treatment Goals

Decrease sympathetic nervous system firing.

Increase circulation to improve tissue health.

Position and palpate.

Treatment Plan

General Treatment

✋ If indicated, trigger points can be worked on within any treatment. Elements of a stress reduction treatment are included to decrease the client's overall muscle tone. This makes finding the taut band and the trigger point easier. Fully relaxed muscles allow for full lengthening of the affected tissue following treatment. To promote relaxation, both the treatment room and the client should be warm. If the client is hypoglycemic, she should be encouraged to eat a small snack such as fruit or soup before the treatment *(Travell, Simons, 1983)*.

✋ It seems to be common for massage therapists to think only of prolonged ischemic compression when thinking of treating trigger points. However, prolonged ischemic compression by itself can be painful, which increases the client's sympathetic response. Instead, if the principles of massage are followed — for example, using techniques that are general and superficial first, followed by techniques that are specific and deep if needed — the amount of time spent on a potentially painful technique is reduced.

✋ However, there is some degree of discomfort or pain possible with the treatment of trigger points. This is clearly stated by the therapist in the consent to treat statement, so the client may alter or stop the treatment if she wishes. The therapist must ensure that the discomfort or pain is tolerable for the client at all times, working with the client rather than pushing her past her pain limits. The "pain scale" described in the consent to treat chapter is useful. If the client experiences pain sufficient to tense the muscle being worked on, the treatment will be ineffective because the muscle must be relaxed to completely eliminate the trigger point. As breathing increases the relaxation of muscles, the client is directed to perform diaphragmatic breathing during the treatment.

✋ Muscles **proximal** to the trigger point are treated with effleurage and petrissage to increase local circulation.

Specific Treatment

✋ Place the affected muscle in a **pain free comfortably lengthened position.**

✋ **Palpate** and accurately **locate** the taut band and trigger point using skin rolling or flat or pincer grasp palpation.

Common Techniques

✋ Treat using one or several of the following techniques.

Treatment Goals

Treat trigger point.
Reduce pain.
Decrease autonomic
and proprioceptive
symptoms if present.

Treatment Plan

🖐 **Slow skin rolling,** performed in multiple directions, is used to reduce panniculosis over a trigger point and increase local circulation.

🖐 **Slow repetitive muscle stripping** is performed along the entire length of the taut band within the muscle. The ulnar border, fingers or reinforced thumbs are used for this technique, staying within the client's pain tolerance. The pressure is initially light and is gradually increased with successive strokes. The trigger point may be palpated as a small nodule within the muscle tissue.

- Muscle stripping causes a temporary local ischemia, followed by a reactive hyperemia as pressure is released, flushing metabolites out of the tissue. The client indicates when local and referred pain from the trigger point decrease as the technique is repeated. The palpable nodule disappears as the trigger point is inactivated. This technique may be all that is required to reduce a trigger point or it may be followed by ischemic compressions. In one study, 10 separate treatments of repetitive muscle stripping were effective in eradicating trigger points (*Travell, Simons, 1992*).

🖐 **Alternating ischemic compressions** are applied to the trigger point using the therapist's reinforced fingers or thumbs. Pressure within the client's pain tolerance is applied for seven to 10 seconds at a time and then released, creating ischemia and then hyperemia. The pressure is reapplied for seven to 10 seconds and released again.

- Pain from the trigger point should diminish with each application, eventually disappearing as the trigger point is reduced. Repetitive petrissage is interspersed with compressions. This technique is useful in treating hyperirritable trigger points that are too painful for prolonged compression. Full eradication of the active trigger point may take place over several appointments (*Prudden, 1980*).

🖐 **Prolonged ischemic compression** is the most specific massage technique. For superficial muscles, reinforced finger or thumb pressure is slowly applied to the trigger point, maintaining pressure at the client's pain tolerance level. For deeper muscles, such as piriformis or quadratus lumborum, the olecranon may be used if pressure is carefully and gradually applied. Pressure that is applied too quickly may cause excessive pain and the client may tense the muscle. Appropriate pressure is maintained until the trigger point reduces. Ideally, this takes between 20 seconds and one minute (*Travell, Simons, 1992*). As it reduces, the trigger point feels as though it is softening or melting. The client feels pain diminish. The client is instructed to let the therapist know when this is happening. The therapist then slowly releases the compression. Repetitive petrissage is next used to flush the metabolites from the muscle, followed by heat and a slow stretch.

- If pain does not completely diminish, the therapist may need to

Treatment Goals   Treatment Plan

Treat trigger point.
Reduce pain.
Decrease autonomic and proprioceptive symptoms if present.

slowly increase pressure until the client's pain tolerance is reached again, holding until the pain diminishes. To the therapist, it may feel like the trigger point is moving away from under the finger or thumb. The therapist should follow the trigger point, maintaining tolerable pressure until the trigger point is eradicated. Close communication must be maintained with the client so the therapist knows as the tolerable pain levels rise then diminish, rise then diminish, then finally disappear. This technique is useful in treating recent, moderately active trigger points (*Travell, Simons, 1983*).

🖐 If the trigger point is not eradicated after a minute of ischemic compression, the therapist should apply repetitive petrissage, use a slow stretch and heat, and leave the trigger point until a subsequent appointment. This is especially important when treating a client for the first time, when the client's post-treatment reactions, if any, are not yet known.

🖐 Restore range of motion and muscle length.

🖐 Use appropriate hydrotherapy.

Other Techniques

🖐 After applying one of the techniques listed above, the therapist returns the muscle to its normal length by a slow, full passive stretch or post-isometric relaxation (PIR). These techniques are described in the chapter on remedial exercise. If possible, the client may also take the muscle slowly through active free range, moving from the entirely shortened to the entirely lengthened position.

Increase local circulation.

🖐 Post-treatment hydrotherapy of local deep moist heat is usually indicated for the affected muscle after trigger point treatment (*Travell, Simons, 1992*). This will increase local circulation, encouraging the removal of irritating metabolites and increasing tissue health.

🖐 Trigger points that are particularly stubborn and located in fibrosed tissue may benefit from additional pre-treatment deep moist heat.

🖐 In the case of a fibrositic headache caused by trigger points, a cool cloth applied to the referral pattern only may be indicated for an analgesic effect. Again, care is taken to avoid chilling the muscle containing the trigger point, which will activate it and increase the client's symptoms.

🖐 **Percussion and stretch** uses a rubber reflex hammer. The trigger point is slowly, directly tapped about 10 times to deactivate it. The frequency of each percussion is ideally one impact every five seconds. The force is equal to that used to elicit a tendon reflex jerk, again within the client's pain tolerance. Trigger points in brachioradialis,

Treatment Goals

**Treat trigger point.
Reduce pain.
Decrease autonomic
and proprioceptive
symptoms if present.**

Treatment Plan

the long finger extensors and the peroneals are reported to respond to this approach *(Travell, Simons, 1992).*

Intermittent cold distraction and stretch is a technique that relies on the temporary sensory and reflex effects of cold on the skin to inhibit pain perception. A trigger point can be fully inactivated by passively stretching the affected muscle to its full length. However, this becomes difficult as stretching by itself is painful and causes a protective muscle spasm, restricting any further lengthening of the muscle. Intermittent cold provides the distraction to temporarily block pain transmission at the level of the spinal cord and allow the stretch.

- The relaxed muscle is placed in a comfortably lengthened position. The client is instructed to breathe throughout the technique to maintain relaxation. One end of the muscle is anchored or stabilized so the therapist can place a stretch on it from the other end. A preliminary sweep of cold is applied before the stretch occurs. The cold is unidirectionally applied in parallel lines over the entire affected muscle. The speed of each sweep is 10 centimetres per second. The therapist then slowly, steadily, passively stretches the muscle to just before the onset of pain and holds it there. The cold application is continued in parallel sweeps over the referral pattern and the muscle is slowly passively stretched to a new pain-free position. The cold and stretch are continued until the muscle is fully lengthened.

- The therapist must take care not to stretch the muscle too quickly or in a jerky fashion since this may cause pain and protective spasms. The cold and stretch applications can be repeated two or three times on one area of skin. However, care should be taken not to chill the muscle. The tissue can be rewarmed using deep moist heat if this occurs.

- Two methods of cold application are ice and vapocoolant spray. The ice is prepared by filling a paper cup with water and then freezing it. The edges of the cup are torn back, exposing the ice. The client's skin must remain dry to prevent chilling of the tissue, so the exposed ice is covered in plastic film.

- The vapocoolant spray that Travell originally used is fluori-methane. Since this chlorofluorocarbon (CFC) contributes to the destruction of the atmospheric ozone layer, Travell subsequently discouraged its use *(Travell, Simons, 1992).* Vapocoolant sprays that do not contain CFCs should be used.

- Intermittent cold and stretch is effective for treating trigger points in many muscles in one region of the body, such as the shoulder.

214

Treatment Goals

Treat the synergist and antagonist muscles.

Treatment Plan

Other Considerations

✋ The therapist should reassess the muscle length after treating the trigger point. It is important to treat any secondary trigger points in the antagonist and synergists that may also refer pain into the same region, making the referral zone larger and more painful. However, in one massage appointment the therapist should maintain a balance between the desire to thoroughly inactivate all trigger points and overtreatment. For example, if trigger points are found in the client's shoulders, neck and gluteals, the therapist should choose to treat the trigger points that address the client's primary complaint. The remaining trigger points are treated in subsequent visits.

Self-care Goals

Educate the client.

Self-care Plan

✍ The client should rest from activity following the treatment of trigger points. This includes avoiding sports and general overuse of the muscle.

✍ A hot bath is also indicated.

✍ Self-massage consisting of muscle stripping and alternating ischemic compressions and stretch is recommended. Percussion and stretch may also be useful, especially for quadratus lumborum trigger points (*Travell, Simons, 1992*). For trigger points in the back and neck, the client may lie on a tennis ball to provide ischemic compressions.

Stretch short muscles.

✍ The client should repeat slow, full, pain-free stretches to the affected muscle frequently. Slow stretching should also be performed before and after any activity.

Strengthen weak muscles.

✍ A program of gradual strengthening is used.

Reduce or eliminate any perpetuating factors.

✍ Perpetuating factors should be reduced or eliminated, such as a prolonged chilling of the affected muscle.

✍ Postural imbalances should be corrected. Adjusting the height of a chair or the position of a computer monitor and keyboard will help prevent shortening of the muscle for a prolonged time.

✍ The client can be referred to a physician if metabolic imbalances may be present, to a naturopath or nutritionist if nutritional inadequacies are suspected or for orthotics if structural imbalances are perpetuating factors.

Treatment Frequency and Expected Outcome

Reducing trigger points is often incorporated into the treatment of a specific condition, from postural dysfunctions to trauma-related injuries. The reduction of one or two trigger points may also be incorporated into a general stress reduction treatment. If many trigger points are present, or if the trigger points are hyperirritable, half-hour sessions two to three times per week are indicated.

See fibrositic headache, torticollis, tendinitis, bursitis, osteoarthritis and inflammatory arthritides for a few of the many conditions that are associated with trigger points. Also see the stress reduction chapter.

The outcome depends largely on the elimination of all the perpetuating factors. Trigger point symptoms are more likely to resolve if treatment occurs shortly after initial onset. A trigger point that is months or years old may take several treatments to eradicate, especially if the muscle has fibrosed. Full lengthening of the affected muscle is a key factor. The client's compliance in a self-care program is also important to the outcome.

18

EDEMA

Fiona Rattray

> **Edema is a local or general accumulation of fluid in the interstitial tissue spaces.**

Edema is the result of altered physiological function in the body. It is not in itself a disease. Edema may result from a local release of histamine following an injury. It may be a result of a systemic disease such as heart failure or it may occur after an obstruction of the lymphatic vessels. It is, therefore, important to determine the cause of edema before developing a treatment plan *(Harris, 1994)*, since it may not be appropriate to reduce the edema.

In order to understand how to treat edema, it is necessary to understand the function and anatomy of the lymphatic system. Blood is largely composed of red and white blood cells and various proteins suspended in fluid. In the circulatory capillaries, slightly more fluid is pumped through the arterial ends into the interstitial spaces than is absorbed at the venous ends. The excess clear, watery interstitial fluid is collected, filtered and returned to the circulation by the lymphatic system. Once in the lymphatic system, the fluid is called lymph. The lymphatic system returns between one per cent and 10 per cent *(Guyton, 1986)* of the total interstitial fluid to circulation. The average volume of lymphatic fluid returned to the circulatory system is 2.4 litres per day *(Guyton, 1986)*. The lymph also contains white blood cells, plasma proteins, fats and debris such as cell fragments, bacteria and viruses. An equilibrium is maintained as long as the fluid entering the interstitial tissues via the arterioles equals the fluid leaving through the venules and the lymphatics. Edema results if this equilibrium is upset.

Although the lymphatic system is often called passive compared to the circulatory system, the lymphatic vessels have a minor contractile capability and a pulse of one to 30 beats per minute *(Wittlinger, Wittlinger, 1990; Immen, 1995)*. This minor contraction is stimulated by stretching the vessels, either internally, by the vessels filling, or externally, by light massage.

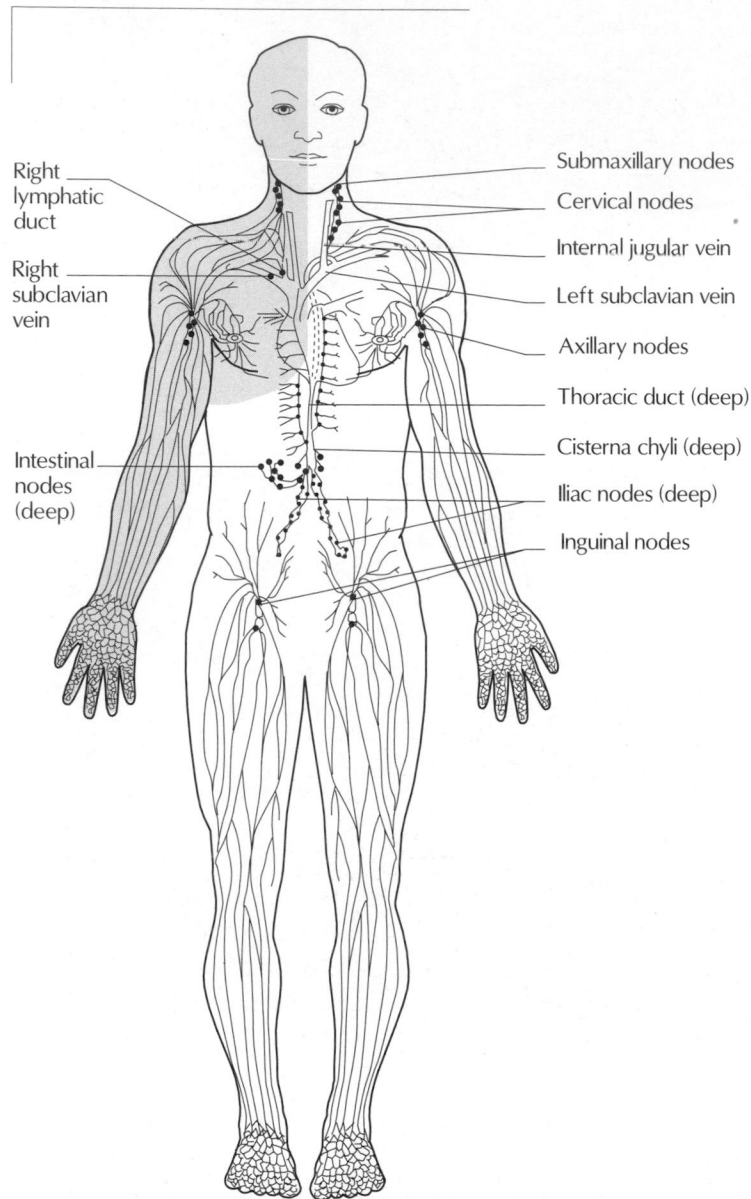

Right lymphatic duct

Right subclavian vein

Intestinal nodes (deep)

Submaxillary nodes

Cervical nodes

Internal jugular vein

Left subclavian vein

Axillary nodes

Thoracic duct (deep)

Cisterna chyli (deep)

Iliac nodes (deep)

Inguinal nodes

Figure 18.1
Superficial and deep lymphatic drainage system. The shaded area drains into the right lymphatic duct, while the rest of the body drains into the thoracic duct.

However, the majority of lymphatic flow is stimulated by the movement of skeletal muscles, the diaphragm when breathing, peristalsis and contraction of arteries where they are in contact with lymphatic vessels. The lymphatic flow is unidirectional towards the heart.

Lymphatic vessels begin in the tissue as tiny, delicate capillaries, gradually increasing to about the diameter of a silk thread *(Wittlinger, Wittlinger, 1990)*. These initial vessels connect subcutaneously to deeper vessels in the limbs and trunk, called precollectors. Larger vessels are called collectors. These group into distinct lymphatic bundles *(Bollinger et al., 1985)*. The largest lymph vessels, called ducts, drain into the venous system at the subclavian veins, just before the vena cava *(Netter, 1989)*. The initial vessels lack valves. The precollectors and the larger collector vessels have valves to prevent backflow. Interspersed along the lymphatic vessels are lymph nodes which filter the fluid. The nodes contain lymphocytes and are a part of the body's immune system *(Figure 18.1)*.

Initial, superficial lymphatic vessels form a dense, overlapping network in the skin for maximum drainage *(Wittlinger, Wittlinger, 1990)*. They follow specific drainage patterns or territories *(Figure 18.2)* before they run to the deeper lymphatic ducts in the abdomen. The drainage territories are separated by watersheds. There are minor anastomoses of the initial lymphatics and the precollector vessels between these watersheds to allow lymph to flow through alternate routes if normal drainage is blocked *(Casley-Smith, Casley-Smith, 1986)*. Nearby lymphatic collectors also attempt to take over the lymphatic load of a traumatically or surgically damaged collector *(Bollinger et al., 1985)*. However, in normal drainage, the superficial lymph generally flows along the course of least resistance through a given drainage territory and does not cross the watershed *(Kurz, 1989)*. It is important to note that the lymphatics of the right arm, the anterior and posterior right shoulder and the right side of the head drain through the right lymphatic duct. The lymphatics of the rest of the body drain through the thoracic duct *(Tortora, Anagnostakos, 1981)*.

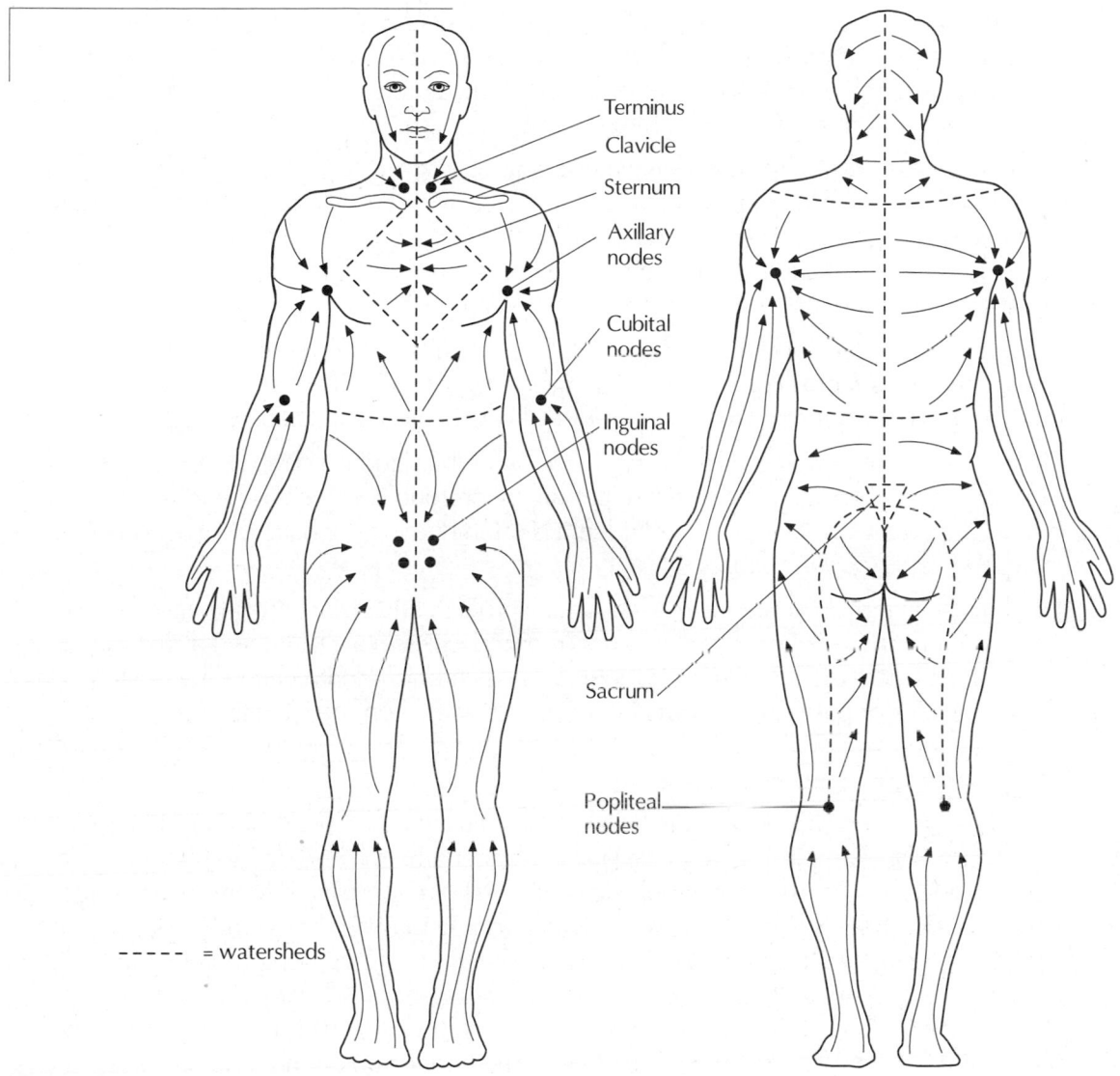

Terminus
Clavicle
Sternum
Axillary nodes
Cubital nodes
Inguinal nodes
Sacrum
Popliteal nodes

- - - - - = watersheds

Figure 18.2
Superficial lymphatic drainage patterns of the body showing watersheds.

Causes of edema are:

➤ **increased permeability of the capillaries** resulting from inflammation, tissue trauma, immune response or burns *(Porth, 1990);*

➤ **obstruction of the lymphatic flow** due to infection, parasites in the lymphatic system, lymphatic disease, surgical removal of the lymph nodes, radiation treatment, scarring or a congenitally reduced number of lymph vessels. Obstruction of the lymphatics (lymphostasis) leads to a retention of plasma proteins, which, in turn, attracts more fluid. This is called a low-flow, high-protein edema *(Casley-Smith, Casley-Smith, 1986);*

➤ **increased capillary pressure** (or venous pressure) from heart failure, thrombophlebitis, pregnancy or a generalized allergic response such as hives. Edema forms in the extremities in hot weather due to capillary dilation and sodium retention. An increase in sodium retention leads to premenstrual edema *(Cawson et al., 1982; Porth, 1990).* There is also gravity-induced (orthostatic) edema from prolonged standing or sitting

219

(Streetnen, 1987). This affects people using wheelchairs. With a peripheral nerve lesion, edema is present distal to the lesion site due to flaccidity of the affected muscles. In this case, the edema is more pronounced if the autonomics are also affected, since vasomotor control of the vasculature is lost;

➤ **a decrease of plasma protein** accompanying liver and kidney diseases and starvation, and following extensive burns. This, in turn, causes lymphodynamic edema, which is a high-flow, low-protein edema *(Casley-Smith, Casley-Smith, 1986)*. Although there is a normal and functioning lymphatic system, the increasing volume of fluid overwhelms the ability of the lymphatics to remove it.

Whereas causes are listed under discrete categories, in fact, edema may have more than one contributing factor. For example, edema in pregnancy results not only from increased capillary pressure but also from increased fluid volume and orthostatic pressure.

Edema can be generalized throughout the body or localized to a limb or area. Generalized edema is frequently due to a systemic pathology or condition such as heart failure, liver disease or kidney disease. Localized edema is often due to lymphatic obstruction or increased capillary permeability.

Edema resulting from acute trauma is a natural process and is part of the inflammatory response. It usually resolves when tissue has repaired, unless fibrin laid down during the repair process obstructs the lymphatics. Lymphedema is chronic edema caused by obstruction of the lymphatics or pathology. Edema becomes chronic when the interstitial spaces have widened and the initial lymphatic capillaries are dilated *(Casley-Smith, Casley-Smith, 1986)*. The edematous tissue has become stretched and is unable to return to its original shape.

Lymphedema, the chronic accumulation of interstitial fluid in tissues, can be primary or secondary. For example, primary congenital lymphedema may be due to hypoplasia (a small or decreased number of lymphatic collectors) or hyperplasia (incompetent valves leading to distended vessels). Secondary lymphedema may be due to tumours, trauma (including post-operative and post-radiation) and parasitical infections. People who, congenitally, have fewer lymphatic collectors are at a greater risk for developing lymphedema. In the lower limb, this risk increases following surgical incisions at the inguinal area and at the knee *(Bollinger et al., 1985)*. In the upper limbs, lymphedema risk increases following mastectomy *(Brennan, Weitz, 1992)*.

When massage techniques are performed on the superficial lymphatic vessels, a pressure of more than 60 mm Hg will compress and temporarily collapse these vessels. This temporarily prevents the drainage of lymph. An average pressure of 30 mm Hg has been found to have the greatest effect on moving the lymph *(Wittlinger, Wittlinger, 1990; Casley-Smith, Casley-Smith, 1986)*. In one study, the initial lymphatics took five seconds to refill after compression *(Casley-Smith, Bjorlin, 1985)*.

An experiment on chronic human leg edema, which subjects had for up to 10 years, revealed that manual pressures of 100 mm Hg at a rate of 25 strokes per minute (in an area 10 centimetres by "two fingers") was found to damage the lymphatics. After three to five minutes of this pressure, desquamation of the endothelial lining of the initial lymphatics was noted *(Eliska, Eliskova, 1995)*. However, this is much in excess of the 30 mm Hg pressure recommended to treat edema *(Foldi, 1995a)*.

Medical treatment of chronic edema varies from medication, such as diuretics and benzopyrones, to surgery and mechanical compression sleeves. Complex decongestive physiotherapy includes skin hygiene, manual lymph drainage, bandaging and remedial exercise *(Foldi et al., 1985).*

Manual lymphatic drainage techniques have been found more effective in draining chronically edematous limbs than machines designed to reduce edema *(Swedborg, 1985; Casley-Smith, Casley-Smith, 1986).*

Symptom Picture

+ There is increased interstitial fluid in the affected body part. The edema varies in texture and temperature according to the cause. Edema due to trauma is local or sometimes distal to the injury site. It looks taut and firm. The tissue is hot in the acute stage and, as healing progresses, the temperature decreases. In the case of chronic edema, the tissue may be cool due to ischemia.

+ **Lymphedema** due to **general systemic conditions** affects the entire body. The edema frequently results in puffy and congested tissue.

+ **Lymphedema** due to **local lymphatic obstruction** usually involves the whole limb distal to the edema site. It can be taut and firm (with parasitic infection or thrombophlebitis) or puffy and congested (following a lymphectomy) depending on the cause of the obstruction. The temperature may be cool due to ischemia or warm due to congestion.

+ With **lymphedema resulting from surgery**, there may be a latent period following the operation where the tissue appears to return to normal. Weeks or years after the surgery, an apparently insignificant injury – a bruise, a cut, a sprained ankle, the pinprick of a diabetes blood sugar test or even an insect bite *(Brennan, Weitz, 1992)* – may provoke lymphedema distal to the scar.

  • It is possible that, during the latent period, excess fibrin not completely removed during the inflammatory repair process allows a gradual build up of plasma proteins in the distal tissue, leading to a state of "edemic readiness" *(Harris, 1996).* The addition of even a small amount of plasma proteins in the inflammatory response following a bruise or cut may tip the equilibrium towards lymphedema *(Brennan, Weitz, 1992; Casley-Smith, Casley-Smith, 1986).*

+ **Non-pitted edema** is firm and discoloured. It results from coagulation of serum proteins in the interstitial spaces, usually following local trauma or infection *(Porth, 1990).*

+ **Pitted edema** is boggy to the touch. The tissue retains an indentation after pressure is applied. In this type of edema, usually found with a chronic pathology, accumulation of the interstitial fluids exceeds their absorption rate *(Porth, 1990; Wittlinger, Wittlinger, 1990).*

+ Pain or a feeling of discomfort or fullness is present in the affected body part. This may be local, as with a trauma, or diffuse, with chronic edema *(Casley-Smith, Casley-Smith, 1986).*

+ There can be a decreased range of motion of an edematous limb. To the client, the limb may feel stiff or heavy.

+ Local edema due to trauma follows a release of histamines. As part of the inflammatory process and tissue repair, fibrin and then adhesions form in the tissue. With a moderate or severe trauma, a hematoma may be present.

+ An increase in lymphatic return prevents excess scar tissue formation *(Wittlinger, Wittlinger, 1990).*

221

Subjective Information

HEALTH HISTORY QUESTIONS

✦ What is the client's overall health history? Is there a history of cardiac, liver or kidney pathologies that may be causing the edema? Does the client have a local thrombophlebitis?

✦ Is the edema caused by a local or general infection (bacterial, viral, fungal or parasitical)? These conditions necessitate treatment modifications or contraindicate lymphatic drainage and massage, and medical referral if the client has not already seen a physician. Is the client on any medication for the above conditions, such as antibiotics?

✦ Has the client had surgery that may disrupt the lymphatics? Has the client had a portion of the lymphatic nodes removed due to a pathology?

✦ Does the client have a peripheral nerve lesion that may cause edema; for example, a median nerve lesion?

✦ Is the edema due to pregnancy or premenstrual sodium retention?

✦ Is the edema caused by position (standing for long periods of time or using a wheelchair) or by a rise in the temperature outdoors?

✦ Has there been a history of recurrent edema?

✦ How long has the edema been present? There is a greater possibility of fibrosis and hardening of the tissue with resultant tissue dysfunction the longer the edema has been present (Harris, 1994).

✦ If the edema is caused by an injury, when did the injury occur? What was done at the time of injury? Was first aid applied? Was the limb elevated, iced and supported with an elastic bandage?

✦ Is there swelling or edema local or distal to the injury? Edema, if possible, should be differentiated from hematoma or joint effusion. If the swelling occurred very soon after the injury — for example, within 20 minutes to one hour — there may be a hematoma. Joint effusion occurs between eight and 24 hours after injury to a joint. The client should be referred for immediate medical treatment with either of these conditions.

✦ Did the client see any other health care practitioner — a physician or physiotherapist? What treatment was given? Is the client still receiving this treatment?

✦ If the edema is trauma related, is the client taking any medication for the injury, such as anti-inflammatories? This includes self-medication such as Aspirin or other over-the-counter products.

✦ Is the client taking any medication specifically for edema, such as diuretics?

✦ Is the client using any elastic bandages or stockings to reduce the edema?

✦ Does the edema interfere with activities of daily living?

✦ What aggravates or relieves the edema? For example, standing and heat worsen an ankle edema following a sprain, while elevation and cold reduce it.

Objective Information

Observations

✍ Edema due to trauma is local and sometimes distal to the injury site. The area looks taut and firm. The edema usually increases with the severity of the injury. The amount of edema present in the acute stage diminishes as healing progresses through the early and late subacute stages. It is usually absent in the chronic stage but, with repeated injuries, edema may remain local to the lesion site.

✍ Edema due to local lymphatic obstruction involves the whole limb distal to the lesion site. The limb can be taut and firm or puffy and congested depending on the cause of the obstruction.

✍ Edema due to general systemic conditions affects the entire body. It is usually noted in all the extremities and may also appear on the face and around the eyes. Swollen areas appear puffy and congested. This edema may be mild, as with pregnancy or premenstrual sodium retention, or severe, as with chronic congestive heart failure or advanced kidney pathologies.

✍ Reddening of the skin in the edematous area may indicate infection, either bacterial (streptococcus) or fungal (mycosis) *(Kurz, 1990)*.

Palpation

✍ Edema due to trauma is tender, hot, firm and local to the injury in the acute stage. These signs diminish as the healing progresses through the subacute and chronic stages. See the appropriate musculoskeletal chapter for more details.

✍ In the case of local or general chronic edema that is not trauma related, the tissue may be cool due to ischemia or warm due to congestion. It may be boggy or taut in texture. Tenderness may or may not be present.

Testing

✍ **AF** and **PR ROM** of the edematous limb are reduced. The amount of limitation increases with the severity of the edema.

Special Tests

✍ The extent of the edema is assessed with the **swelling or edema girth measurement**. A bilateral comparison is made with the unaffected limb.

• With an acute injury, if a swelling occurs rapidly, a hematoma is indicated and the client should be referred for emergency medical attention.

✍ A **pitted edema** test is positive if chronic pitted edema resulting from a pathology is present.

Contraindications

♦ Avoid full-body lymphatic drainage techniques or elevation of the limbs above the level of the heart with chronic congestive heart failure. A sudden increase in the volume of lymphatic fluid or venous return through compromised tissues and organs has potentially serious results, such as pulmonary edema *(Wittlinger, Wittlinger, 1990)*.

♦ Local or distal techniques are contraindicated with edema that is due to thrombophlebitis or deep vein thrombosis, since there is a danger of embolism.

♦ Lymphatic drainage techniques are contraindicated with untreated or metastasizing neoplasms, including melanomas *(Wittlinger, Wittlinger, 1990; Kurz, 1990)*. However, with edema that is a result of medical treatment (for example, following lymph node removal or radiation therapy), lymphatic drainage and massage techniques may proceed with a physician's approval.

♦ Local lymphatic drainage and hydrotherapy are contraindicated if the edema results from bacterial, viral or fungal infection. In the acute or subacute stage, these modalities will promote the spread of toxins and are to be avoided. Hot hydrotherapy is also contraindicated with lymphedema where the tissue is already congested *(Kurz, 1990)*.

♦ In the case of chronic inflammation, such as sinusitis or bronchitis, lymphatic drainage should initially be performed for shorter periods of time and not on site. In the case of sinusitis, work is done only on the neck, not the face. The client is monitored for signs of a flare-up of the condition. If this occurs, lymphatic drainage is discontinued. If no flare-up occurs, the time spent performing drainage work is slowly increased and the site of the infection is gradually included *(Kurz, 1990)*.

♦ Lymphatic obstruction due to parasites (filarium) contraindicates lymphatic techniques and Swedish techniques which increase the circulation *(Kurz, 1990)*.

♦ With acute tuberculosis, any lymphatic drainage is contraindicated. If the client has had tuberculosis affecting the lymphatic nodes, **local** lymphatic techniques are contraindicated because the techniques may activate the encapsulated tuberculosis bacteria *(Kurz, 1990)*.

♦ Lymphatic drainage is contraindicated with toxoplasmosis, a lung infection that can be associated with AIDS, since it may cause a flare-up of the infection *(Kurz, 1990)*.

♦ Lymphatic drainage performed on low-protein edemas such as those accompanying liver and kidney pathologies or starvation will have no effect, because the forces causing the edema will overwhelm the effects of the techniques *(Wittlinger, Wittlinger, 1990)*.

♦ **On-site** lymphatic drainage techniques are contraindicated in the acute and early subacute stages of trauma. They are used proximally only.

♦ **Distal** to the lesion site, lymphatic techniques and Swedish circulatory techniques are contraindicated in the acute or early subacute stage. The edema can function as a bottleneck *(Casley- Smith, Casley-Smith, 1986)*, painfully congesting the distal limb if the therapist attempts to move the circulation through the lesion site. These techniques are only used once the edema has been reduced sufficiently to allow the lymph and blood to flow through local vessels.

♦ In the case of edema arising from trauma, avoid using hot or warm hydrotherapy immediately proximal to inflamed tissue, as this can draw the distal circulation towards the heart, congesting the lesion site.

♦ See the chapter on contraindications for specific conditions and medications for more information.

Treatment Goals   Treatment Plan

✋ Specific lymphatic drainage techniques are described in the chapter on non-Swedish techniques. The therapist spends 15 to 20 minutes on lymphatic techniques to treat an edematous limb.

Acute

Reduce the edema if safe to do so. Decrease pain or discomfort.

✋ If the initial treatment goal is to decrease the edema, lymphatic drainage is performed first, before any general work to compensating structures or specific local massage. This greatly reduces the pain and congestion.

Decrease sympathetic nervous system firing.

✋ If the initial goal is to accustom the client to the therapist's touch, to decrease the sympathetic nervous system firing and to treat compensatory structures, Swedish massage begins on the trunk or the contralateral limb, followed by lymphatic drainage of the edematous limb and Swedish massage treatment for the specific condition.

✋ In the case of edema resulting from an acute trauma, the positioning of the client depends on the location of the edema and the client's comfort. If the edema is in a limb, the affected limb is elevated **in a pain-free range** and pillowed securely. If the edema is in the trunk, the client is positioned so the edema is uppermost. In all cases, a **cold hydrotherapy** application such as an ice pack or a gel pack is applied to the edematous area.

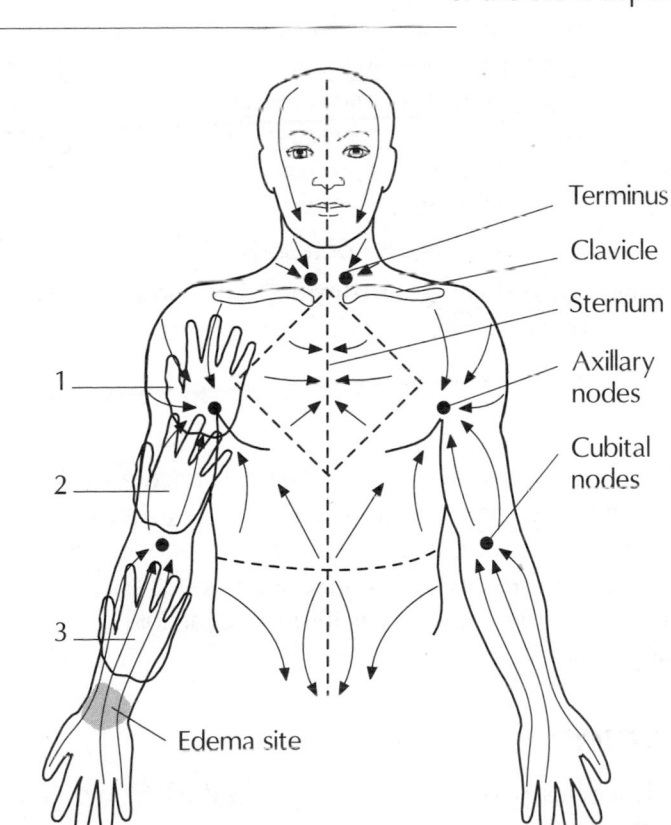

Terminus

Clavicle

Sternum

Axillary nodes

Cubital nodes

1

2

3

Edema site

Figure 18.3
Sequence of hand positions for lymphatic drainage, starting proximally and working distally towards the edema.

Specific Treatment

✋ The client is directed to do **diaphragmatic breathing** throughout the treatment to facilitate lymphatic return. All work is performed in a slow, soothing manner to reduce pain perception.

✋ Assuming that the initial treatment goal is to reduce edema, the therapist begins with nodal pumping at the terminus, then the proximal lymph nodes of the injured limb *(Kurz, 1989; Casley-Smith, Casley-Smith, 1986)*. Following the drainage patterns of the lymphatic vessels, stationary circles and the local lymphatic technique are used proximal to the edema *(Figure 18.3)*.

✋ Starting proximal to the edema, light

Treatment Goals   Treatment Plan

unidirectional effleurage and stroking are also used in a distal to proximal direction.

Do not disturb a hematoma if present.

✍ On-site work is contraindicated. Distal lymphatic drainage is contraindicated due to congestion at the edema site.

Maintain the range of motion.

✍ **Passive relaxed range of motion** of the proximal and distal joints is performed **only to the onset of pain.** This helps to increase lymphatic drainage.

Early Subacute

✍ The treatment approach outlined for general acute work is indicated in this stage also, including reducing pain perception and encouraging **diaphragmatic breathing.** The edematous area is once again elevated. **Hydrotherapy applications** on site are cold to cool.

Specific Treatment

Prevent adhesion formation where appropriate.

✍ Proximally, lymphatic drainage techniques, including terminus proximal nodal pumping and stationary circles, and unidirectional effleurage and stroking are used. The local lymphatic drainage technique is used right up to the proximal border of the edema. Lymphatic drainage will reduce the build up and organization of excess fibrin which leads to scar tissue *(Casley-Smith, Casley-Smith, 1986; Kurz, 1990).*

✍ On-site and distal lymphatic drainage is contraindicated.

✍ **Mid-range passive relaxed range of motion** to the onset of pain only, is used on the joints proximal and distal to the edema.

Late Subacute

✍ The treatment approach outlined for general early subacute work is indicated in this stage also. The edematous area is once again comfortably elevated. **Diaphragmatic breathing** is encouraged. **Hydrotherapy applications** on site are cold-warm contrast. If acute inflammation recurs, the therapist returns to using local cold hydrotherapy applications.

Specific Treatment

✍ As the edema diminishes in the late subacute stage, the length of time spent on drainage techniques decreases.

✍ The proximal limb is treated with lymphatic techniques, unidirectional effleurage and stroking.

✍ As the edema diminishes, the bottleneck effect is reduced. Therefore,

226

Treatment Goals Treatment Plan

the local lymphatic drainage technique is now used through the edema site itself, covering the proximal border of the edema through the centre area, to the distal border. The direction of pressure is towards the heart.

✋ Unidirectional effleurage is now introduced through the edema site and distally. At this stage, the possibility of causing further congestion local to the edema has diminished.

If safe, increase the range of motion.

✋ **Mid- to full-range passive relaxed range of motion** is used by the therapist on the joints proximal and distal to the edema. This is performed to the onset of pain only.

Chronic

✋ The client's position is chosen for comfort. The edematous area is elevated and **diaphragmatic breathing** is encouraged.

Specific Treatment

✋ **Hydrotherapy applications** will depend on the tissue health and the temperature of the tissue. For example, with a local cool, firm edematous pocket following a lateral ankle sprain, a warm application can be used to increase local circulation or a contrast application can be used to flush out the tissues. With a hot and congested extremity, a cool application is indicated.

✋ Chronic edema can result from trauma, such as repeated ankle sprains, where scar tissue or fascial restrictions interrupt or restrict the superficial lymphatic flow. This results in a local area of chronic edema distal to the scar tissue. Lighter pressure connective tissue techniques may be indicated *(Kurz, 1990)*. The therapist assesses for restrictions using fascial glide and gentle skin rolling. Light pressure fascial techniques and skin rolling are then applied to the restrictions. Petrissage may be used on the proximal muscles if these are hypertonic *(Kurz, 1990)*. Once the restrictions are reduced, lymphatic drainage techniques, unidirectional effleurage and stroking mentioned in the subacute treatment are used.

✋ Chronic edema resulting from pregnancy, peripheral nerve lesions, prolonged sitting or standing, or sodium retention during the menstrual cycle is treated using Swedish massage techniques followed by lymphatic drainage techniques, unidirectional effleurage and stroking. These are started proximally and finished distally, as previously described.

✋ With **lymphedema**, deeper pressure Swedish techniques (above 40 mm Hg) and frictions are avoided local to the edema.

227

Treatment Goals Treatment Plan

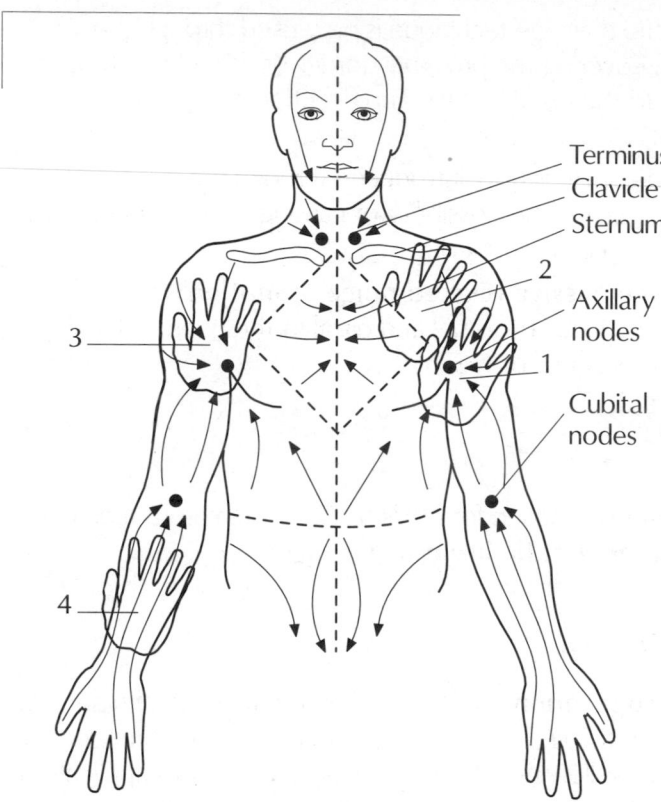

Terminus
Clavicle
Sternum
Axillary nodes
Cubital nodes

Figure 18.4
Treating right arm lymphedema following surgery: Begin on the contralateral quadrant at 1 and 2; then progresses to the proximal affected arm at 3, working distally to 4.

- Lymphatic drainage is used to prepare the healthy, unaffected neighbouring watersheds to take an increased lymph load before draining the affected lymphedematous watersheds. Otherwise, a sudden increase in the lymphatic load in these watersheds can cause a local proximal low-protein edema, potentially trapping the edema in the limb (*Foldi, 1995a*).

- Hot hydrotherapy applications are contraindicated with lymphedema (*Wittlinger, Wittlinger, 1990*).

- It is possible that, in the clinically latent period (weeks or years) following surgery, especially where the lymphatics have been removed, the distal limb may be in a state of "edemic readiness" (*Harris, 1996*). The heavy pressure technique of frictions, which relies on the inflammatory process, should, therefore, be avoided at the scar or in the distal limb, so as not to provoke a lymphedema.

- With full limb lymphedema resulting from surgery, such as mastectomy, removal of the lymph nodes, radiation, peripheral nerve lesions or spinal cord lesions, there is either an interruption of the lymphatics or no muscular pump to promote the lymph flow. The tissue feels waterlogged, soft, spongy and congested. As a result, only lymphatic drainage techniques, unidirectional effleurage and stroking are used. The techniques are started in the contralateral quadrant (*Figure 18.4*). For example, with a right arm lymphedema, the left axillary nodes and skin over the pectorals are treated first. This allows the functioning lymphatics of the healthy quadrant to begin draining the edematous quadrant through the anastomoses across the watershed. The edematous limb is then treated, again starting proximally and working distally (*Foldi et al., 1985; Casley-Smith, Casley-Smith, 1986*).

- **Mid- to full-range passive relaxed range of motion** is used by the therapist on the joints proximal and distal to the edema.

Self-care Goals

Self-care Plan

Educate the client about proper self-care and preventative edema strategies where appropriate.

✍ Hydrotherapy is chosen that is appropriate for the stage of healing.

✍ Self-massage is very helpful. The client is instructed to comfortably elevate the affected area and to use nodal pumping, light unidirectional effleurage and stroking. The client should clearly understand that pressure is light, unidirectional and towards the heart, starting proximally and working distally. The client is also made aware that only the limb proximal to the edema is treated to avoid the bottleneck effect.

✍ If the edema is local and chronic and is due to proximal scarring and fascial restrictions, careful skin rolling over the scar tissue can be done prior to elevation and drainage.

✍ Diaphragmatic breathing is encouraged to aid in lymphatic return.

✍ Remedial exercise is dependent on the stage of healing and the severity of the injury.

✍ In the acute and subacute stages, the client is asked to perform pain-free active free range of motion with the distal and proximal joints, and pain-free isometrics in the edematous tissue.

✍ In addition to the above, in the late subacute and chronic stage for lower limb edema, **Buerger's exercise** may help to temporarily increase circulation and lymphatic return in the lower limbs. The client lies supine in bed with the legs flexed at the hips to 45 degrees and supported in this position with pillows until the skin blanches. This may take up to two minutes. The client then sits up and allows the feet to hang over the edge of the bed for three minutes or until the skin congests. Next, the client lies flat until circulation in the legs is normal. This cycle is repeated four or five times, three times per day *(Kisner, Colby, 1990)*.

✍ Clients with lymphedema, especially of the upper limb, should be encouraged to perform moderate active free range of motion exercises without overexercising. Isometric resisted exercises are also indicated *(Stillwell, 1969)*.

✍ Clients with lymphedema may also be referred to a manual lymphatic drainage specialist for treatment such as someone trained and certified in Vodder's Manual Lymph Drainage and Combined Decongestive Therapy.

Treatment Frequency and Expected Outcome

More frequent treatments — for example, a half hour three times a week — will address the inflammatory process in the acute and subacute stages.

See stress reduction, musculoskeletal concerns, scars, pregnancy, deep vein thrombosis, conditions of the peripheral nervous system and spinal cord injuries in this text for related treatments.

Ongoing treatments are required with chronic edema, especially following lymph node removal and with peripheral nerve lesions.

The outcome is variable, depending on the nature of the underlying cause of the edema (for example, edema following a trauma, as opposed to edema due to surgical removal of lymph nodes). Outcome will also depend on the client's age, general health and compliance with the self-care program.

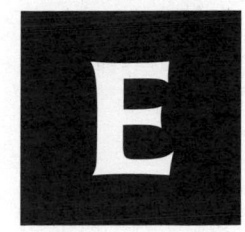

MUSCULOSKELETAL INJURIES

19

STRATEGIES:
Massage and the
Inflammatory Process

Linda Ludwig, Fiona Rattray

> *The inflammatory process is a necessary step towards the healing of injured tissue.*

The inflammatory process and its implications for massage must be understood so safe and effective modalities are chosen for the treatment. The inflammatory process and the subsequent healing process consist of several stages. These are divided in different ways depending on the author. In this text, acute, early and late subacute and chronic are the names given to the various stages of the healing process.

Healing time is variable. The therapist must rely on his observation and palpation skills, treating the tissue as it is presenting and *not* strictly according to the time that has elapsed since the injury.

The ultimate goal of treating an injury is to promote a strong, mobile scar and, as much as possible, full, pain-free movement of the affected structures and full strength. This chapter includes a general treatment plan overview. However, individual chapters should be consulted for the specifics of each condition.

Inflammation is an immediate, local response to injury and tissue damage. The acute inflammatory response enables wounds and other soft tissue injuries to heal and infections to resolve with the assistance of the body's immune system. The tissue moves through the subacute stage and by the chronic stage is fully healed. In some cases, chronic inflammation can develop if an irritant remains.

> ➤ **The cause of tissue damage** can be **internal** or **external**. Common causes are trauma, infection, surgery, immune responses, extremes of heat and cold, ischemic damage and chemical or radiation damage *(Porth, 1990)*.

233

Types of Healing

A few types of healing can occur following injury and inflammation depending on the type and extent of tissue damage. The point of the healing process is to restore the integrity of the tissue. Where possible, there is simply replication of the missing cells. However, this is impossible with most types of tissue and, instead, structure is created using scar tissue.

If the damage is superficial involving only the epithelial layer of tissue, healing will occur through regeneration of this tissue. This is referred to as re-epithelialization. There is no scar tissue — instead, normal tissue structure results. Regeneration is possible with epithelial cells as well as nerve and hepatic cells *(Flanagan, 1997)*. If excessive exudate occurs, some fibrosis in the tissue will result.

When there is an increased loss of epidermal and dermal tissue layers, or damage to other types of tissue such as muscle, tendon and ligament, healing results from the *synthesis of new tissue*. The repair process requires the production of connective tissue consisting of collagen fibres to replace the area where tissue loss or injury has occurred. This restores the continuity of the affected structure but with tissue different from the original. The matured collagen repair is commonly called **scar tissue**. Two types of healing can occur in this case. **Primary or first intention** healing occurs when there is some tissue loss and the wound edges are approximated. Approximation may be done with the use of tape, sutures or staples. Healing is efficient, with only small amounts of collagen produced to repair the tissue. **Secondary or second intention** healing results when there is extensive tissue loss or a large surface area affected. The wound edges cannot be brought together easily. Healing takes longer through extensive re-epithelialization, when the skin is damaged, and wound contraction as well as the production of large amounts of granulation tissue.

Tissue Healing and the Inflammatory Process

The following is a simplified version of the inflammatory process and tissue healing. There is overlap between these stages and the time frames are only guidelines. If the therapist notices that the healing seems to be taking longer than average, he should consider the factors that could be delaying the process. Referral to a physician or other appropriate practitioner is made.

Acute Stage

✦ Time frame: This is a short stage starting at the moment of injury. It lasts up to three to four days post-injury. This is the beginning of healing.

✦ Symptom picture: Redness, swelling (edema), heat, pain and, often, loss of function occur, accompanied by muscle spasm and guarding. If bruising is present, it is black, blue, red or purple.

When an injury occurs, vascular changes ensue. An initial vasoconstriction is followed by vasodilation. Observable redness and palpable heat are due to this dilation of local blood vessels. Swelling is caused by fluid leaking into the interstitium due to increased permeability of the blood vessels. This permeability is due to the release of histamine, a chemical mediator of the inflammatory process.

Pain is secondary to muscle spasm as well as irritation and compression — from swelling — of local nociceptors. Loss of function can follow if the injury and swelling are severe. In addition, muscle spasms and guarding contribute to a loss of function, as the body attempts to immobilize the injured area.

On a cellular level, platelets play several roles. They cause coagulation of the blood which reduces blood loss, isolates the injury and prevents or reduces bacterial infiltration. Platelets combined with fibrin and other cells form a strong clot to occlude the damaged site. These cells also release chemotactic agents for the attraction of leucocytes.

Several types of leucocytes migrate to the injured site. They clean the area of bacteria and foreign debris, indirectly attract fibroblasts, stimulate the proliferation of fibroblasts and regulate collagen synthesis *(Oloff, 1994)*.

The inflammatory process begins to resolve at the end of the acute stage. However, if the tissue damage is severe or the body's inflammatory response is excessive or the causal agent is not eliminated, the inflammatory process will continue. This causes an increase in fibroblastic activity which increases collagen formation and leads to additional adhesions.

Treatment Considerations at the Acute Stage

The appropriate testing protocol, listed in each chapter, is used to assess the injury.

The **treatment goals** are to limit the inflammatory process, reduce pain and swelling, decrease sympathetic nervous system firing and prevent reinjury. Protective spasms are reduced but not removed. Compensatory structures are also treated.

Positioning of the client should be comfortable and should not stress the injury site. If uncertain of an appropriate position, the therapist asks the client what her sleeping position is.

Hydrotherapy is a cold application, such as an ice pack, placed on the injury to reduce pain and swelling.

First aid for an acute injury is termed "RICE" — rest, ice, compress, elevate.

Massage at the Acute Stage

🖑 Pain is reduced and the client's comfort is increased through the performance of a relaxation massage on the unaffected parts of the body. This also accustoms the client to the therapist's touch and treats any compensating areas. Passive movement is performed on unaffected joints in order to maintain range of motion.

🖑 First, the swelling which contributes to pain and reduced movement is addressed *(Cyriax in Basmajian, 1985)*. The affected area is pillowed in elevation and cool hydrotherapy is applied. Pumping of the relevant lymph nodes is followed by lymphatic drainage techniques proximal to the injury site.

🖑 On the site of the lesion and distal to this site, no lymphatic or circulatory strokes are performed. The injured tissue is not able to accommodate the increased flow of fluid. Painful congestion could result.

🖑 With some injuries, for the first 24 to 48 hours, passive movement is not tolerated on the affected tissue or the joints this tissue crosses. In cases where passive movement is possible, even a few degrees of carefully applied passive motion are beneficial — provided the actions do not elicit pain or increase inflammation *(Kisner, Colby, 1996)*. Protective muscle spasms that occur local to the injury site are not directly treated at this time, but rather in the subacute stage.

👋 All modalities used are applied with care so as not to further compromise the injured tissue.

Self-care at the Acute Stage

✎ The client generally limits active movement due to local pain, swelling and muscle guarding. With moderate and severe acute injuries, immobilization may be insured through wrapping, splinting or casting.

✎ In cases where injuries are not severe, limited pain-free active movement is encouraged. Active movement is appropriate in the uninjured tissue.

✎ See also the contraindications chapter for specific local contraindications.

Subacute Stage

✦ Time frame: This stage occurs within two days and continues for up to three weeks after the injury *(Oloff, 1994)* and occasionally for as long as six weeks *(Kisner, Colby, 1996)*. The signs of inflammation diminish over this time. Wound closure takes an average of five to eight days with muscle and skin injuries, and three to five weeks with tendon and ligament injuries.

✦ During the subacute stage, there is a gradual restoration of the damaged structure. To better understand the diverse processes during this dynamic stage and how these affect the treatment goals, early and late designations are used.

Early Subacute Stage

✦ Time frame: This stage occurs within two days and may continue for up to a few weeks.

✦ Symptom picture: The affected area shows diminishing signs of inflammation, with pink, warm, slightly edematous and somewhat less painful tissue. Muscle spasm diminishes. If bruising is present, it is relatively unchanged from the acute stage. With range of motion, pain is experienced when tissue resistance is encountered.

The primary process of this stage is the filling of the damaged area with new tissue. During the acute stage, all the cells and material necessary for this task have been brought to the site.

Re-epithelialization: This stage only applies if the skin is damaged. If epithelial tissue was lost in the injury, it begins to regenerate during this stage. First the cells of the epidermis migrate to the edges of the wound. This is followed a few days later by proliferation of epithelial cells at the wound's edges or within the wound from intact hair follicles or sebaceous or sweat glands. The length of time for completion of this process is variable. For example, when healing by second intention, re-epithelialization will occur only after granulation tissue has filled the injury site *(Flanagan, 1997)*. In cases of deep and large injuries, re-epithelialization is not possible and skin grafts may be necessary to cover the wound site.

Granulation tissue: Unlike re-epithelialization, the formation of granulation tissue is part of any tissue repair where there is first or second intention healing. To support the process of restoring structure, an adequate blood supply and nutrients must be present. New blood vessels develop from venules at the edge of the injury in a process called "neoangiogenesis". They provide nutrients for the ensuing cellular activity and then retract during the late subacute stage. Fibroblasts are important cells during this stage. They synthesize collagen fibres that form a loose connective tissue matrix in the area of tissue loss. This matrix replaces the clot which developed in the acute stage. The resultant vascular connective tissue is referred to as granulation tissue.

Local lactic acid levels increase after an injury due to hypoxia and secondary to macrophage activity. Initially, this rise can lead to increases in collagen production *(Oloff, 1994)*. This could result in excessive scar tissue development; it reinforces the necessity of reducing edema and promoting the removal of local cellular debris.

Until the collagen is well organized, granulation tissue is very fragile and most susceptible to reinjury with overstretch *(Krasner, 1990)*.

Treatment Considerations at the Early Subacute Stage

The appropriate testing listed in each chapter is again performed before the treatment.

The **treatment goals** are to continue to decrease the effects of inflammation, pain, swelling and spasms, while maintaining the available range of motion and strength.

The general treatment remains the same as in the acute stage, though now the therapist may also begin to treat the tissue peripheral but not distal to the lesion site.

Hydrotherapy includes cool applications and the introduction of mild contrast applications.

Massage at the Early Subacute Stage

- The treatment is started with elevation of the affected area. Cool hydrotherapy is used, followed by the performance of lymphatic drainage techniques *(Cyriax in Basmajian, 1985)*. These techniques address edema not only proximal to the injury but at the edges of the injury site.

- Swedish massage techniques are used on the proximal tissue. Trigger points in muscles that refer to the injury site can be treated. Techniques to reduce spasm are used. As the injury site is approached, the pressure of massage techniques directed towards the injury site will avoid placing excessive drag on the healing tissue. For strokes with pressure directed away from the site, the therapist must be vigilant for drag on the fragile granulation tissue. A hand can be placed just proximal to the injury site to monitor the amount of pull the techniques create. Techniques are modified accordingly. Slightly more vigorous techniques are used than in the acute stage.

- With injuries that break the skin, it is only once the wound site is closed and re-epithelialized that peripheral and on-site treatment is started. Initially, stroking is used, then gentle petrissage such as fingertip kneading. The therapist must take care to avoid reinjuring and reinflaming the healing tissue, since the granulation tissue present at this stage is fragile.

- Distal to the injury, only gentle stroking and muscle squeezing are performed to avoid congestion at the lesion site.

- Passive movement in full range is applied to the unaffected joints. The affected joints are slowly moved a few degrees and up to mid-range of pain-free motion to maintain joint health and joint range.

Self-care at the Early Subacute Stage

✍ The client often returns to activity too soon and reinjures the site. As swelling begins to diminish and pain is less constant, pain-free active movement in a variety of ranges is encouraged.

✍ Strength must be maintained through submaximal isometric contractions. The affected tissue is in a shortened or relaxed position during this exercise in order not to stress the granulation tissue. With a joint injury, any comfortable position is used. The intensity of the muscle contraction is determined by the client; she should use as much strength as possible while remaining pain free. Initially, it may be only 20 or 30 per cent of the muscle's capability.

✍ If inflammation increases as a result of overdoing the exercises, there will be pain at rest, a decrease in the range of motion and possible spasm. In this case, the exercises should be made less vigorous.

Late Subacute Stage

✦ Time frame: This stage begins in approximately the second to third week of the subacute stage.

✦ Symptom picture: There may or may not be a pocket of residual swelling. Minimal discomfort is experienced but with potential loss of range of movement due to adhesions and muscle weakness. The blood vessels that developed with neoangiogenesis retract during this stage. If bruising is present, it changes to yellow, brown or green, then disappears. Pain is encountered with overpressure to the affected tissue.

Wound contraction: Myofibroblasts, cells found within the wound matrix, contain contractile fibres. They may generate isometric contractions or isotonic contractions or both *(Oloff, 1994)*. The purpose of wound contraction through myofibroblastic activity is to speed the healing process because less scar tissue is needed to fill the smaller damaged site. This process peaks at about two weeks after injury but continues into the late subacute stage *(Kloth et al., 1990)*. Unfortunately, wound contraction can result in deformation of the tissue and possible dysfunction. In places of tissue tension, such as over bony prominences like the greater trochanter or the malleolus, wound contraction is difficult; often an increased amount of granulation tissue is required to heal these injuries adequately, resulting in excessive scar tissue *(Flanagan, 1997)*.

Scar remodelling: Reshaping and reorganizing of the healing area begin as existing collagen is broken down, new collagen is synthesized and cross links develop among the collagen fibres. Strength of the site begins to increase during this time. It is dependent on the amount and type of collagen, the number of cross links between these fibres and the balance between collagen synthesis and breakdown.

If an abnormal amount of connective tissue fibres is laid down following the trauma or during immobilization, adhesions begin to form. As a result, the tissue layers stick together and the range of motion is reduced *(Kisner, Colby, 1990)*.

Treatment Considerations in the Late Subacute Stage

The appropriate testing protocol, listed in each chapter, is used to assess the injury.

The **treatment goals** include decreasing any remaining edema, reducing trigger points,

238

pain and adhesions and improving range of motion and muscle strength. Adhesions are successfully reduced through treatment during this stage and into the chronic stage — that is, in the few weeks after the injury and during the following two to three months (*Kisner, Colby, 1996*).

As with previous stages, a relaxation massage is performed, including attention to compensating structures.

Hydrotherapy applications of hot and cold contrast are indicated.

Massage in the Late Subacute Stage

✋ Any pockets of edema that may be present are treated as in the early subacute stage. Swedish massage techniques are performed over the entire affected limb, both proximal and distal to the injury site. Trigger points in proximal and local tissue are treated.

✋ Massage to the injury site begins peripherally and proceeds, in a systematic manner, centrally. Techniques to break down adhesions include any that place a stress, or torque, on the site. S-bowing, C-bowing, skin rolling and muscle stripping are performed slowly, with a focus on picking up the affected tissue and applying counterpressure. Hyperemia should result if the techniques are effectively applied. The client will likely feel a burning sensation or some discomfort. Gentle frictions are performed on specific adhesions. The application of these techniques is modified to the client's tolerance.

✋ A prolonged stretch is applied to the scar tissue that has been treated so the collagen fibres will align more functionally. After frictions and with any other techniques that create lasting hyperemia and warmth, cool or cold hydrotherapy applications are used. During and following these more vigorous techniques, circulatory strokes such as effleurage promote the removal of debris from the inflammatory process and the breakdown of adhesions.

✋ Passive range of motion is applied in mid-range, working towards achieving full range of the affected joints. Joint play is used to prevent adhesions within the affected joints and to mobilize hypomobile joints.

Self-care in the Late Subacute Stage

✍ Remedial exercise includes stretching and strengthening. Passive stretches or PIR, if possible, are used by the client to encourage proper alignment of the scar tissue. Strengthening may progress from full-strength isometric contractions to isokinetic exercises.

✍ If discomfort lasts for more than four hours after exercising or if swelling results, the exercise program is too vigorous or is progressing too quickly (*Kisner, Colby, 1996*).

Chronic Stage

✦ Time frame: This stage overlaps with the latter part of the late subacute stage at about two to three weeks post-injury and continues for up to one to two years.

✦ Symptom picture: The inflammatory process is resolved. There is likely no edema but there is a loss of full range of motion; a subsequent decrease in function is possible. Pain may occur in the affected tissue with overpressure or secondary to stress placed on contractured tissue.

The scar tissue continues to remodel and reorient in response to stress. Functional organization through proper alignment of the collagen fibres can be influenced by activity and stretching. Increased amounts of collagen result in a longer remodelling stage. The process is quite rapid in the first few months but slows as this remodelling continues for many more months. It is during the chronic stage that scar tissue strengthens dramatically, yet even at maturity is only 70 to 80 per cent as strong as the tissue it has replaced.

✦ **Chronic inflammation** may result as part of a self-perpetuating cycle if an irritating agent persists, such as an inflammatory arthritide, or inflammation may develop following repeated microtrauma, such as with tendinitis.

- Time frame: Chronic inflammation can last for weeks or years.

- Symptom picture: It is not characterized by the cardinal signs of inflammation, though pain, swelling and muscle guarding may occur after activity. Stiffness may be experienced after rest.

With chronic inflammation there is a proliferation of fibroblasts and new, immature collagen fibres. This leads to an increased risk of excessive scarring and loss of motion as well as general weakness in the affected tissue *(Kisner, Colby, 1996)*.

Treatment Considerations in the Chronic Stage

The appropriate testing protocol, listed in each chapter, is used to assess the injury.

The **treatment goals** are to reduce restrictive adhesions and trigger points, and to restore range of motion and strength to the affected areas. Those areas compensating for the injury are also treated.

Hydrotherapy includes contrast or hot applications.

Massage in the Chronic Stage

 The techniques used to reduce adhesions are the same as in the late subacute stage. They are now applied with increasing vigour, but always within the client's pain tolerance. It is essential to intersperse this work with soothing circulatory techniques.

 A prolonged stretch is applied to the scar tissue that has been treated. After frictions and with any other techniques that create lasting hyperemia and warmth, cool or cold hydrotherapy applications are used.

 Trigger points, hypertonicity and fascial restrictions are addressed. Joint play is applied to hypomobile joints to increase mobility.

Self-care in the Chronic Stage

 Generally, an appropriate remedial exercise program of stretching and strengthening is designed. Endurance and cardiovascular exercises are also encouraged.

The general treatment and self-care principles for chronic inflammation are discussed in the Strategies: Overuse Injuries chapter.

Factors that Affect the Healing Process

✦ **Severity of the injury.** A severe injury where more tissue is damaged will take longer to heal than a mild injury where there is little tissue damage.

✦ **Age.** Both extreme youth and increasing age can affect healing. In older people, there is a slowing of fibroblast production and wound contraction. Characteristics of collagen and elastin fibres change with aging. The skin loses its ability to hold water and becomes thinner. This increases the risk of injury.

  • When people are very young, there is increased fibroblast and collagen production. While healing itself is faster, unfortunately once the scar tissue is developed, it does not grow as the body does. Over time, contractures may form and tension is experienced in the affected structures. In some cases, several surgical releases are necessary over the course of a child's growth cycle.

✦ **Infection.** An infection results in poor healing because it causes an increased inflammatory response and increased local tissue necrosis and will impair wound contraction.

✦ **The presence of foreign material.** A piece of glass, wood or steel imbedded in the wound will prolong healing and increase the risk of infection.

✦ **Nutritional support.** Nutrients are required for the healing process. Vitamin C is necessary for collagen synthesis, vitamin A supports the fibroblasts and increases collagen synthesis and vitamin E promotes tissue healing and prevents scarring. Zinc is required for many enzyme reactions as well as for the production of many of the cells involved in the repair process. Iron facilitates bonding between the collagen fibres. Increased protein and caloric intake is needed during the time of tissue repair to promote the cellular processes (*Balch, Balch, 1997*).

✦ **Existing conditions.** A condition such as diabetes has associated vascular problems as well as causing an increased susceptibility to infection. These contribute to poor healing. Chronic liver and renal conditions, lymphedema or carcinomas may also impair healing of wounds (*Richard, Staley, 1994; Oloff, 1994*).

✦ **An adequate blood supply.** Inadequate blood flow interferes with the local nutritional needs of the tissue as well as with the removal of toxins, bacteria and debris. Inadequate blood supply may be the result of edema, pre-existing circulatory pathologies or mechanical compression of soft tissue over bone.

✦ **Wound separation.** Approximation of wound edges according to the nature of the injury or from sutures facilitates the healing process. Open wounds with a large gap are unable to heal effectively over the area.

✦ **Effects of some drugs.** Steroids inhibit the inflammatory process, collagen synthesis and, in turn, the healing process. Drugs used to suppress the immune system also affect the healing process.

✦ **Smoking.** Cigarette smoking delays healing and interferes with the actions of certain drugs (*Balch, Balch, 1997*).

If an injury is not healing within a reasonable time frame, the therapist should consider the presence of some of these factors. A referral to a physician may be necessary. If nutrition is a concern, a referral to a naturopath or nutritionist is suggested.

SCAR TISSUE

Linda Ludwig

Scar tissue is a collagen-based tissue that develops as a result of the inflammatory process.

The inflammatory process and the production of scar tissue are necessary for healing damaged tissue — skin, muscle, tendon, ligament, fascia or nerve. Depending on the amount of tissue loss, the body will heal with first or second intention healing (see Strategies: Massage and Inflammatory Process chapter). More collagen is required with healing by second intention. When the collagen used to mend the injury matures, it is referred to as scar tissue. The scar is weaker than the tissue it is replacing. For example, scar tissue replacing damaged dermis will only reach about 80 per cent of the strength of the original tissue *(Richard, Staley, 1994)*.

Causes of scar tissue are:

➤ the **inflammatory response** that results from wounds, burns, musculoskeletal trauma, inflammatory arthritides or the late stage of osteoarthritis (after cartilage is destroyed);

➤ **prolonged immobilization** of a structure;

➤ **paralysis** or **paresis** of a structure due to a peripheral or central nervous system lesion.

Types of Scar Tissue

✦ A **contracture** is the shortening of connective tissue supporting structures over or around a joint. These structures include muscles and other soft tissue such as tendons and joint capsules. A contractured muscle, or other soft tissue, cannot fully lengthen and results in a reduced range of motion in the joint. Soft tissue contractures include adhesions and irreversible contractures.

• A contracture should not be confused with a muscular contraction. In a contraction, the muscle develops tension as it shortens (concentric contraction) or lengthens (eccentric contraction). When a contracting muscle relaxes, it is able to lengthen and allow for full range of motion of the joints that it crosses *(Kisner, Colby, 1990)*.

✦ An **adhesion** occurs when reduced motion at a joint allows cross-links to form among the collagen fibres, further reducing the range of motion. This is most evident when tissue is left in a shortened position for prolonged periods of time, as in postural dysfunctions or immobilization of a limb.

✦ A **scar tissue adhesion** occurs with an injury or an acute inflammatory process. Collagen fibre formation during the tissue repair process allows adhesions and contractures to form in a random pattern. These adhesions within and between skin, muscles, tendons, groups of muscles and joint capsules reduce range of motion. Adhesions can also form within the joint itself *(Apley, Solomon, 1993)*. The effects of the adhesions can usually be reduced with fascial techniques, cross-fibre frictions, joint play techniques and stretching.

✦ **Fibrotic adhesions** occurring with ongoing chronic inflammation can cause moderate to severe restrictions in range of motion. Such adhesions are difficult to eradicate.

✦ An **irreversible contracture** occurs when fibrotic tissue or bone replaces muscle and connective tissue. There is a permanent loss of range of motion that can only be restored by surgical means *(Kisner, Colby, 1990)*.

✦ **Proud flesh** is a term used to refer to the thick dermal granulation tissue that results from an abnormal healing process. When a wound does not re-epithelialize, there is chronic inflammation. The resulting granulation tissue is composed of disorganized collagen and capillaries. This gives a raised, red structure that is susceptible to damage *(Richard, Staley, 1994)*. Re-epithelialization is difficult over these raised areas; however, they can be surgically cut back to the epithelial tissue level.

✦ **Hypertrophic scarring** is an overgrowth of dermal tissue that remains within the boundaries of the wound *(Richard, Staley, 1994)*. With this type of scar, the collagen fibres are randomly organized in nodular or whirl (circular) patterns rather than the normal loose, wavy pattern found in the dermis *(DeLisa, Gans, 1993)*. This scar is associated with deep partial- or full-thickness burns (severe second degree and third degree burns) that have healed through second intention healing, or with healing at the edges of skin grafts. Likewise, hypertrophic scarring can develop at skin graft donor sites that have been harvested too deeply or too often, or which have delayed healing due to infection or trauma. Small hypertrophic scars may be surgically excised and sutured to close the site. In larger scars, only portions of the scar tissue are removed and these sites are sutured. This process must be performed repeatedly until the scar tissue is completely removed. Once it is removed, the area may be covered by a skin graft.

✦ A **keloid** is dermal scar tissue that extends beyond the boundaries of the original wound, in a tumour-like growth *(Settle, 1996)*. A keloid is thought to contain increased amounts of collagen in a more random pattern compared to a hypertrophic scar. It may continue to grow for many years. Both hypertrophic and keloid scars seem to result from an imbalance between collagen synthesis and collagen breakdown within the wound. However, the term hypertrophic scar is sometimes used incorrectly to describe a keloid scar. Keloids do not respond well to surgical excision and they frequently recur *(Richard, Staley, 1994)*. Steroids, such as the corticosteroid triamcinolone, are commonly used and more effective than surgery in preventing or reducing keloids.

Several factors influence the excessive production of scar tissue. The prolific scar formation found with hypertrophic and keloid scars is more prominent in darker pigmented people such as those from Asian or Black ancestry.

Increased amounts of scar tissue are produced by younger people due to a greater rate of collagen synthesis — 88 per cent of hypertrophic and keloid scars are present in people under 30 years of age *(Richard, Staley, 1994)*.

Certain areas of the body tend to produce more scar tissue. Hypertrophic scar tissue is more likely to develop on the sternum, upper back and shoulder-deltoid area as well as the buttocks and dorsal surface of the foot. Keloid scars are more likely to appear from ear level to the waist and from the shoulder to the elbow.

Anything that prolongs healing can result in excessive scar tissue production — for example, increased tension on a healing site such as occurs with tissue over a joint. This is likely due to ongoing microtrauma creating chronic inflammation. Deeper burns tend to produce more scar tissue due to excessive edema and increased amounts of granulation tissue.

Effects of Massage on Scar Tissue

Before scar tissue develops, massage techniques to decrease edema are important. Because collagen fibres form in edema, removal of this excess extracellular fluid can ultimately reduce the amount of scar tissue that develops *(Wittlinger, Wittlinger, 1990; Kurz, 1990)*. Massage has been found to soften scar tissue by freeing restrictive fibrous bands and increasing circulation. The therapist needs to apply enough pressure to create blanching followed by hyperemia *(Richard, Staley, 1994)*. Stretching the scar tissue, especially after massage treatment, is essential.

Contraindications

+ Frictions are contraindicated if the client is taking anti-inflammatory medication.

+ Frictions are not recommended for proud flesh or keloid scars.

Massage helps to desensitize hypersensitive scars through tactile stimulation. It assists in relaxing the client and decreasing pain, which often results in better compliance with any uncomfortable techniques or modalities used during the treatment. Massage performed before the collagen matures can prevent hypertrophic scarring, especially in the case of burns *(Richard, Staley, 1994)*.

Treatment Considerations

Assessment

✍ **Observations:**

* Edema is present in the early stages of scar tissue development. Edema may persist into the maturation stage.

* Initially with a wound, the scar is red and raised, but it becomes increasing flat and pale with maturation. The entire healing process may be a few weeks with minor injuries or it may last up to two years. There is a loss of normal pigmentation;

discolouration may result in hyperpigmentation or hypopigmentation.

- Scar tissue may be aneural or partially innervated.

- Scar tissue is avascular and has no hair, sebaceous or sweat glands *(Flanagan, 1997)*. These structures are unable to penetrate the mature collagen fibres of the scar tissue or they were damaged with the injury.

- Excessive scar tissue may be observed, such as a hypertrophic scar or keloid scar.

- Postural dysfunction can result from the presence of scar tissue. This can be directly due to adhesions, which inhibit the full lengthening of affected structures, or secondary to compensatory changes.

✍ **Palpation:**

- Scar tissue and adhesions are thick, hard areas. The elasticity of normal tissue is lost, since scar tissue consists primarily of collagen. Puckering may occur due to the contracting ability of myofibroblasts within the developing scar tissue.

- The scar tissue may be cool due to ischemia.

- Disuse atrophy may be present in affected muscles with long-term loss of range of motion.

✍ **Testing:**

- **AF** and **PR ROM testing** will likely reveal a reduced range of motion and possible pain in the joints and muscles affected by the injury. The flexors and adductors have a tendency to develop contractures. In the chronic stage, once the scar has matured, overpressure will result in pain, if the area is not painful within the normal range of passive movement.

- **AR testing** reveals weakness in the muscles affected by the injury or from immobilization.

Massage

The following treatment is for remodelling scar tissue or addressing mature scar tissue in the late subacute to chronic stages.

✋ **Pre-treatment hydrotherapy** applications of heat, such as paraffin wax or a hydrocollator, are used with maturing scar tissue.

✋ **Positioning** is for client comfort and accessibility of the tissue to be treated.

✋ Rigid and restricted sections at the periphery of the scar are treated first, with the goal being to form a mobile, functional scar. The techniques should create torsion in a specific area of the restricted tissue. Fascial techniques such as skin rolling, connective tissue cutting, fascial spreading, S-bowing and C-bowing are employed. Cross-fibre frictions are used on remaining adhesions. Depending on the density of scar tissue or the size of the affected area, techniques are applied gradually from least adhered to most adhered areas. This is a slow process done within the client's pain tolerance, over a series of treatments.

✋ Massage to scar tissue is always followed by passive stretch. This promotes the alignment of the collagen fibres laid down during the healing process. It also promotes the development of loose or areolar scar tissue rather than a dense connective-tissue scar. The former type of scar is supple, allowing for movement

🖐 Post-treatment hydrotherapy of cold applications is appropriate after frictions and any other techniques where extreme hyperemia and heat persist.

Self-care

✍ As the scar is remodelling and maturing, techniques can be applied up to six times daily for 10 to 15 minutes at a time *(Richard, Staley, 1994)*.

✍ Pain free movement is performed as soon as possible after the injury. In as little as four days after immobilization, fibrosis can occur *(Kottke et al., 1982)*.

✍ In early stages of healing, only partial ranges are performed by the client so the healing process is not disrupted and no excessive stress is placed on sutures. Movement is passive or active assisted, with available active movement encouraged. Initially, pain-free range of motion is practised in the acute and early subacute stages. The ranges are gradually increased as collagen matures through the late subacute and chronic stages. These movements are to pain tolerance.

✍ Prolonged passive self-stretching is introduced after the granulation stage, in the late subacute stage. Areolar scar tissue responds well to this exercise.

✍ Strengthening exercises begin with submaximal isometric contractions in the early subacute stage, increasing in force of contraction as the scar tissue matures during the late subacute stage. Finally, isotonic exercises are used. These are important not only to maintain strength but to build strength in the injured or formerly immobilized muscles.

See also musculoskeletal and peripheral nerve injuries and edema chapters.

✍ Strengthening of the antagonist muscles will help prevent contractures from developing in the agonists. For example, if the soft tissue of the flexor surface of the forearm is affected in an injury, the extensors are strengthened to counteract the tendency of the wrist to be drawn into flexion as scar tissue contracts.

WOUNDS AND BURNS:
Injuries That Break the Skin

Linda Ludwig

An injury is the disruption of the continuity of any tissue.

For the purpose of massage therapy, it is important to understand the process of tissue healing where there is a disruption of the continuity of the skin and of the underlying tissue by a wound or, specifically, a burn.

The Anatomy of Skin

The body is covered by skin, which is its largest protective organ, forming a barrier between the body and the external environment. Skin is comprised of three different layers (*Figure 21.1*).

The **epidermis** is the outer layer. The cells of the epidermis have a short lifespan of 28 to 30 days, which results in a continuous sloughing off and renewal of this layer.

Below this lies the **dermis**. It anchors and nutritionally supports the epidermis. This layer is composed of elastin and collagen which give the tissue flexibility and strength. The dermis contains sebaceous (oil) and sweat glands, hair follicles, nerve receptors, blood vessels and lymphatic vessels.

The **subdermal** layer is also called the **subcutaneous** layer. It contains adipose tissue, larger blood vessels and deep hair follicles. Below this layer are the muscles and bone.

The Function of Skin

Skin prevents the invasion of infective organisms and protects the underlying tissue from injury. Nerve endings in the skin inform the body of various sensory stimuli such as temperature, pressure, touch and pain. The ability to detect all these stimuli can play a role

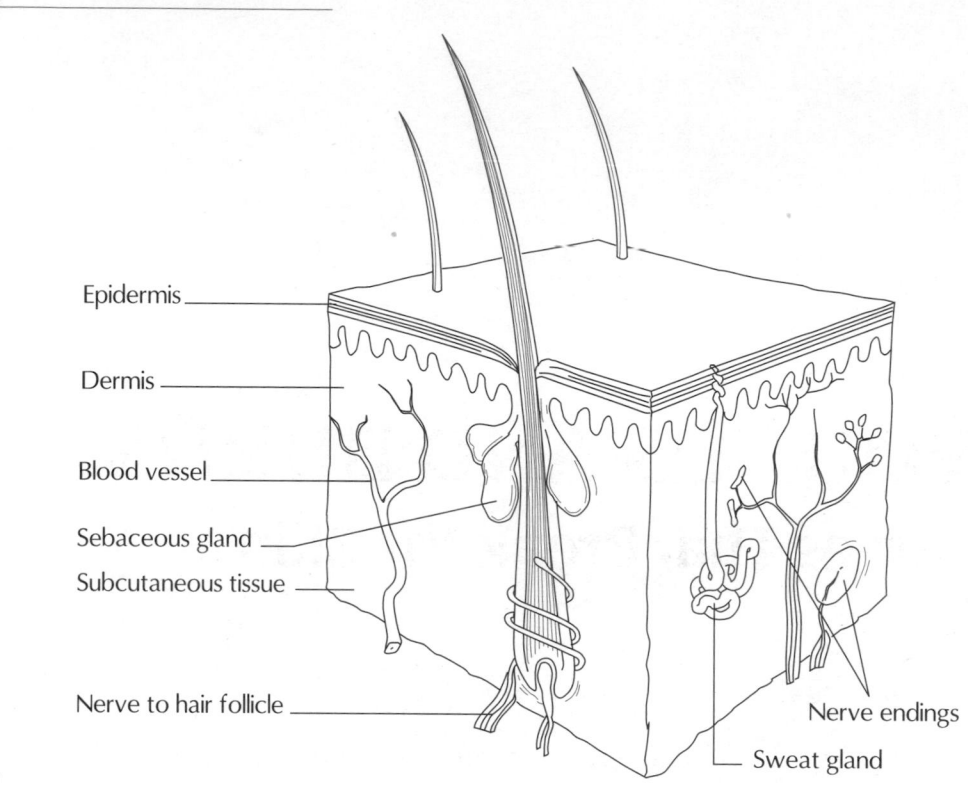

Figure 21.1
A cross-section of skin.

in protecting the skin and underlying tissue from injury.

The skin controls body temperature through sweating or shivering as well as through constriction and dilation of blood vessels. It allows gas exchange through the pores and keeps the body systems' fluids and electrolytes balanced. Absorption of sunlight by the skin aids in the synthesis of vitamin D. The subcutaneous layer stores water and fat which act as a layer of insulation and protection of underlying tissue.

Wounds

A wound is a disruption of the continuity of the skin.

Depending on the severity of the injury, skin is split, muscles and ligaments torn, nerves and blood vessels damaged or bones broken.

Causes of wounds are:

➤ **thermal sources**, such as extreme temperatures, and **chemical** and **electrical sources**, all of which result in a burn;

➤ **mechanical forces** such as direct **trauma** or **pressure**; **shear or friction forces** that result in an impact between the body and an object, or within the body — as can occur with the development of a decubitus ulcer.

Types of Wounds

An abrasion is a superficial wound with ragged edges. It is usually the result of a scrape or tear causing loss of skin, as with a fall on a gravel surface. It is often extremely painful. After careful cleaning, a dressing is applied to the wound to keep it moist. Pain is reduced if the nerve endings do not dry out.

A laceration has increased tissue loss with ragged wound edges. Once cleaned to facilitate healing by first intention, sutures or tape may be used to bring the edges together. If it is impossible to remove all the dirt and debris, closure of the wound with sutures could result in infection. In such cases, the area is left open but covered by a dressing.

An incision has clean, approximated wound edges and results from a sharp-edged object such as a scalpel in surgery or a piece of glass. Sutures or tape are used to secure the edges together.

A puncture has clean edges with a small entry. It can penetrate deeply, such as a bullet wound or an injury from stepping on a nail. This type of wound can close over at the entry into the body before the rest of the damage heals and result in an increased risk of infection.

An animal bite is often a combination of crush, laceration and puncture wounds.

For a burn see the Burns section in this chapter.

History of the Treatment of Wounds

For centuries, wound management has included the control of bleeding through pressure and the application of a topical ointment and a dressing. Prehistorically, there is evidence of dressings made of leaves, mud and lichen. Dating back to 3000 to 2500 BC, records indicate papyrus was used as a dressing and gum-coated strips of linen were used as adhesive bandages *(Dealey, 1994)*. Grease, honey and fresh meat were applied topically; frankincense and myrrh deodorized wounds, while mercury was used as an antibacterial agent *(Flanagan, 1997)*.

Many of the principles that governed wound care in the time of Hippocrates, 460 to 377 BC, are still used today. At that time, care included keeping the wound clean by washing it with warm water, wine or vinegar, then bringing the wound edges together and covering the injury with a clean dressing. It was Hippocrates who gave the definition of first and second intention healing based on wound-edge approximation. While he did not entirely understand why, he also believed that the physician must keep his hands clean while treating such injuries *(Flanagan, 1997)*.

In Roman times, 200 to 25 BC, the physician Celsus described the cardinal signs of inflammation and agreed that a non-aggressive approach to wound management was optimal. Years later, Galen, a Roman physician whose prolific writings spread to many countries, provided an aggressive model for wound management that would persist for many centuries. He was responsible for the concept of "laudable pus" — that is, fluid seepage — referred to as pus — which was thought to be a necessary part of the healing process and one that should be encouraged. If the wound did not show signs of pus, foreign bodies such as hot oil, pigeon blood or turpentine would be forced into the site. This would result in infection and the desired laudable pus. His theory likely resulted from his observations of the many infected wounds of the gladiators he treated. Through the years, some physicians challenged the theory, finding the practice of clean dressings and good nutrition allowed better healing than hot irons and boiling oil. Unfortunately, the encouragement of infection to promote healing, and the resulting death of patients from sepsis, continued well into the nineteenth century. It was during that century that the Scottish surgeon Lister introduced the use of antiseptics combined with the practice of frequent hand washing and application of clean dressings to dramatically reduce surgical infection. For years, there was resistance to these ideas, as Galen's theories prevailed. During the First World War, antiseptics were finally widely and successfully used to prevent sepsis and gas gangrene in wounds. The antibiotic penicillin was discovered in 1928 and was commercially available by the mid-forties. This led to more successful treatment of wounds with an increasing ability to prevent infection. Wound care gradually evolved to the more current practices — and came full circle, back to Hippocrates's original ideas.

Healing of Wounds

Disruptions in the continuity of the skin heal through the inflammatory response (see Massage and the Inflammatory Process). Depending on the type of wound and the amount of tissue loss, healing can occur with simple regeneration or by first or second intention healing (see Types of Healing in the Strategies: Massage and the Inflammatory Process chapter).

First Intention Healing and Sutures

First intention healing is likely when there is minimal tissue loss and the edges of the wound are approximated. An example is an incision-type injury. If necessary, stitches are used to further approximate the wound edges to facilitate healing and protect the site from infection. Within a short time, a thin layer of fibrin, the basis for a clot, is laid down under the incision site. Re-epithelialization is completed in two to three days (Krasner, 1990). While the site is not strong enough to withstand a substantial impact, it is, in fact, closed to external intruders such as bacteria. Sutures are usually treated topically with an antibiotic cream and covered by gauze and an elastic bandage for the first 48 hours after injury. After this time, it is recommended that the site remain covered to protect the area from trauma or from snagging the sutures.

Gradually, over 10 to 14 days, fibroblasts and the deposition of collagen add strength to the site, so the sutures may be removed. If infection does occur beneath the skin surface, redness, swelling or pus are evident and a physician is seen as soon as possible. The physician should be consulted as to the optimal time to begin gentle range of motion exercises. In some cases, this may be as soon as a few days after wound closure (Richard, Staley, 1994). The importance of active movement to optimally align collagen fibres and prevent excessive contracture cannot be overemphasized.

Second Intention Healing

Second intention healing is necessary if a wound penetrates the dermis, with increased tissue loss and poor approximation of wound edges. Initially, after ice or a cold application, the wound is cleaned to prevent infection. An antibiotic cream such as silver sulfadiazine, bacitracin zinc or a triple antibiotic ointment is applied (Uloff, 1994). If the wound is not infected, a dressing is applied to provide protection from infection and trauma as well as to keep the site moist.

Moisture allows better re-epithelialization compared to wounds left exposed to air. The dressing Second Skin is a gel sheeting that is primarily water with four per cent polyethylene oxide. This dressing reduces friction on the wound site. It also has the ability to absorb exudate into the gel and keep the area moist. It is particularly good for abrasions or burns, providing a cooling effect and reducing itching *(Pedretti, Zoltan, 1990)*. In one study, a moist, covered wound was re-epithelialized in 12 to 15 days versus 25 to 30 days for an air-exposed wound. Air exposure causes the site to dry out and develop a scab; the epithelial cells must migrate from the wound edges under this crust *(Ulott, 1994)*. Re-epithelialization also takes longer with deeper and larger wounds.

Burns

A burn is a specific type of wound caused by an external thermal agent.

The severity of a burn may range from mild redness to full-thickness tissue destruction of the dermis and deeper tissues. Many factors are taken into consideration when assessing the severity of a burn: depth; amount of body tissue burned; the specific area burned; the cause of the burn; the age of the person; pre-existing illness; and associated injuries such as smoke inhalation and fractures. These will influence the type of therapy the person receives and the functional difficulties that may result.

Types of Burns Based on Depth of Damage

✦ A **superficial burn** (first degree burn) affects the epidermis. It is usually the result of prolonged exposure to low intensity heat or quick exposure to high intensity heat. It results in redness and pain. Some mild localized edema is present in the superficial tissue (though it is not observable). Within a week, the epithelium sloughs off, as with a sunburn. Healing is rapid and without scar tissue, though in some cases there may be discolouration of the skin.

✦ A **partial-thickness burn** (second degree burn) is an injury that extends to the dermis. Along with redness, pain and some localized edema, the most distinguishing feature is the presence of blistering. Partial-thickness burns are classified as *superficial* or *deep*. The increased depth of the burn results in increased edema, increased risk of infection and often decreased pain due to some nerve damage. With a superficial partial-thickness burn, a new skin layer that can actively regulate temperature and act as a barrier to bacteria develops within 14 to 21 days, whereas a deeper burn will require 21 to 35 days to develop this layer *(Richard, Staley, 1994)*. A more superficial second degree burn will re-epithelialize with good functional return and minimal scar tissue, though with some pigment changes. Deeper second degree burns epithelialize with difficulty and result in fibrosis, contracture and joint mobility restrictions.

✦ A **full-thickness burn** (third degree burn) causes damage that affects all tissue layers including the epidermis, the dermis and the subcutaneous tissue.

253

- A *fourth degree burn* (also considered a full-thickness burn) is used to describe a burn that damages all the skin layers as well as fascia, muscles and even bone that is immediately under the skin. With full-thickness burns, substantial damage occurs to structures in the tissue layers, such as hair follicles, sweat glands and nerves. These burns appear dry and inelastic, white and waxy or charred in colour; they are painless because of nerve damage. Re-epithelialization over the wound is not possible because of the extensive tissue damage, though it may occur at the wound edges after many weeks *(Achauer, 1987)*. Skin grafts are required to cover the wound and facilitate healing of the affected area.

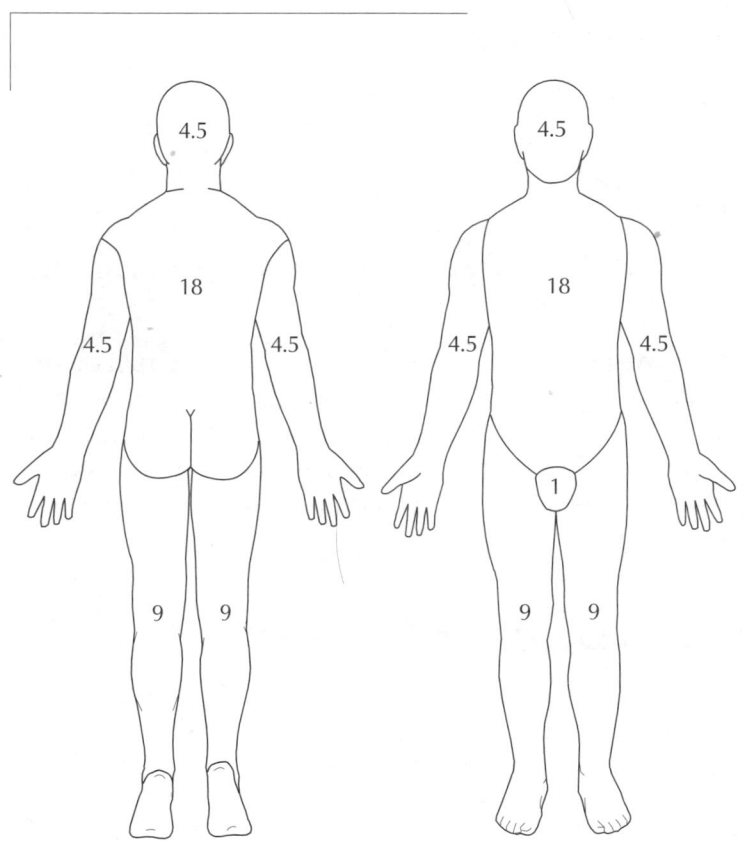

Figure 21.2
Rule of nines to calculate percentage of body area damaged.

The percentage of the body surface damaged by the burn is calculated using "the rule of nines" *(Figure 21.2)*. The head equals nine per cent of the body surface area, each arm equals nine per cent, each leg equals 18 per cent, the anterior trunk and the posterior trunk each equal 18 per cent and the perineum equals one per cent *(DeLisa, Gans, 1993)*. In children, the head represents 18 per cent of the body surface area with each limb equalling about 13 per cent *(Kottke et al., 1982)*.

Burns are caused by:

➤ **thermal damage** from heat, such as an open flame or scalding from a hot liquid, as well as from cold — a severe example is frostbite. Common causes of deep partial-thickness burns are grease burns, scalding from liquids over 71 degrees Celsius (160 degrees Fahrenheit) and flame burns *(Kottke et al., 1982)*;

➤ **chemical substances** such as acids and alkalines. These must be deactivated through the removal of contaminated clothing and cleansing of the skin to prevent continuation of the injury. Depending on the type and concentration of the chemical, injury can result from skin contact or inhalation. Secondary injuries can occur. For example, phenol depresses the central nervous system and causes kidney damage. It appears that chemical burns heal more slowly than other types of burns *(Achauer, 1987)*.

➤ **electrical sources**. Thin, wet or sweaty skin is the most susceptible to electrical burns. The superficial damage caused by an electrical burn can be misleading. The entry site appears black at its centre surrounded by a ring of white necrotic tissue and an outer ring that is hyperemic. Internally, along the path of the current, substantial damage results to the muscle, bone and nerves. Cardiac arrhythmias often occur. The greatest numbers of amputations occur with this type of burn *(DeLisa, Gans, 1993)*. Central nervous system damage may result. Memory loss, headaches, personality changes, deafness, visual disturbances, weakness, paralysis and convulsions may occur temporarily or become permanent;

➤ **radiation** including burns from ultraviolet sources such as sunburn.

Burns Requiring Hospitalization

Many burns do not require medical attention, but hospitalization and specialized treatment are required with:

✦ moderate partial-thickness (second degree) burns on 15 to 25 per cent or greater of the total surface area of the body in adults (10 to 20 per cent in children);

✦ full-thickness (third degree) burns on 10 per cent or greater of the total surface area of the body in adults;

✦ burns on specific areas such as the face, eyes, ears, perineum, hands or feet;

✦ burns complicated by smoke inhalation or other major trauma such as a fracture;

✦ high voltage electrical burns;

✦ burns on people with compromised health, under two years of age and of advanced age. Those very young and over 65 often sustain severe injuries from relatively minor traumas. This is in part due to the thinner consistency of the skin.

With advances in medical treatment, the survival rate from severe burns has increased, with additional attention being given to restoring function and improving quality of life.

Burns: Acute and Early Subacute Stage Concerns

In the case of smaller burns, the wound should be cooled after a thermal injury to prevent further tissue necrosis. Immersion of the affected area for 10 minutes in cold water has proven helpful in stabilizing the tissue and improving healing time. With burns over a very large surface area, this application is not used due to the risk of hypothermia *(Achauer, 1987)*.

Destruction of the skin causes an inflammatory response locally. The most significant aspect of this process is the increased permeability of the capillaries, in combination with a loss of integrity of many of these capillaries with partial- and full-thickness burns. This results in **massive edema and loss of fluids**, including water and electrolytes, in the burned tissue and distal to it. If the burn is large enough — covering 25 to 30 per cent of the body — systemic circulation is affected which causes generalized edema *(Achauer, 1987)*. Intravenous fluids are given immediately post-trauma and over a 48-hour period to prevent shock and to stabilize the fluid levels in the body.

Although local nerves may be damaged, spasm and muscle splinting in the surrounding area can cause pain and create additional edema. Collagen fibres form in this protein-rich fluid which accumulates in the extracellular compartments. These fibres restrict blood flow and further restrict lymphatic flow.

Excessive edema can cause destructive pressure on local and distal nerves and blood vessels. Further, the burned tissue itself, which is inelastic, can act as a tourniquet and exacerbate edema, as well as being a damaging force in itself. In such a case, an *escharotomy* — an incision made through the burned tissue — is performed to relieve pressure on susceptible structures.

Sepsis is the most common cause of death among those experiencing burns *(Richard, Staley, 1994)*. This increased risk of infection is due to the loss of the protective skin barrier, accompanied by depressed immune function as a result of deeper burns. Prevention of sepsis is an early concern. The wound is treated with a topical antibiotic such as silver sulfadiazine (Silvedene) and covered with a synthetic or biological dressing. The biological dressing is produced from pigs, cadavers or human amniotic membranes. The dressings are temporary and used not only to prevent bacterial growth but also to prevent fluid loss, to decrease pain and to encourage granulation tissue formation. They are changed regularly, until the tissue is healed or ready for a skin graft.

To promote further healing and to prevent bacteria growth, **debridement** of the tissue is performed. Debriding involves the removal of dead tissue layers until living, viable tissue is reached, indicated by local pain and bleeding. Debridement is performed using a variety of methods. Mechanical debridement, using scissors and forceps, is usually performed during hydrotherapy. Immersion in a whirlpool or Hubbard tank decreases pain during debridement, removal of dressings and cleansing the body. A wet dressing may also be applied to the burned tissue and left to dry. The dead tissue softens and sticks to the dressing. Debridement occurs when the dressing is removed. Enzymatic debridement uses agents that selectively digest the dead tissue. Surgical techniques may be used to debride deep burns.

Skin grafting is necessary with all but the smallest full-thickness burns and deep partial-thickness burns. Grafting is also necessary if, after three weeks, a partial-thickness burn has not shown signs of significant healing. Once debridement has successfully removed burned tissue, the area is ready for a skin graft. Autografting is the harvest of skin from one area of the body for transfer to another part. Thin layers of skin are shaved from an unburned area of the body *(Richard, Staley, 1994)*. As a result, the donor site is painful and may result in reduced mobility. Grafts are used over the neck and face because skin grafts inhibit or limit wound contraction, enabling good cosmetic effects *(Oloff, 1994)*.

The harvested skin may also be processed in a variety of ways, which often include expanding the tissue to allow coverage of large areas. Called a "mesh graft", it leaves a lined pattern after healing, showing where each piece was placed. Therefore, this type of graft is better used on less visible areas of the body. The grafts are fixed to the surrounding skin with sutures, staples or steri-strips. The area is generally immobilized from five to 10 days *(Richard, Staley, 1994)*. The surgeon is consulted before gentle, active movement is encouraged — usually five to seven days post-graft. Active assisted movement and passive movement are introduced after 10 days, to increase range of motion as needed *(Achauer, 1987)*.

Splints and positioning are used to prevent contracturing of healing tissue. It is natural for the burn patient to hold the burned limb in a shortened and relaxed position to relieve any stretch on the damaged tissue. The limb is commonly held in flexion and adduction, which, unfortunately, encourages contractures that decrease functional ability. Therefore, the person is encouraged to place the affected limbs into extension and abduction. Splints and specialized frames are used to assist in optimal positioning *(Figure 21.3)*. Ankle splints

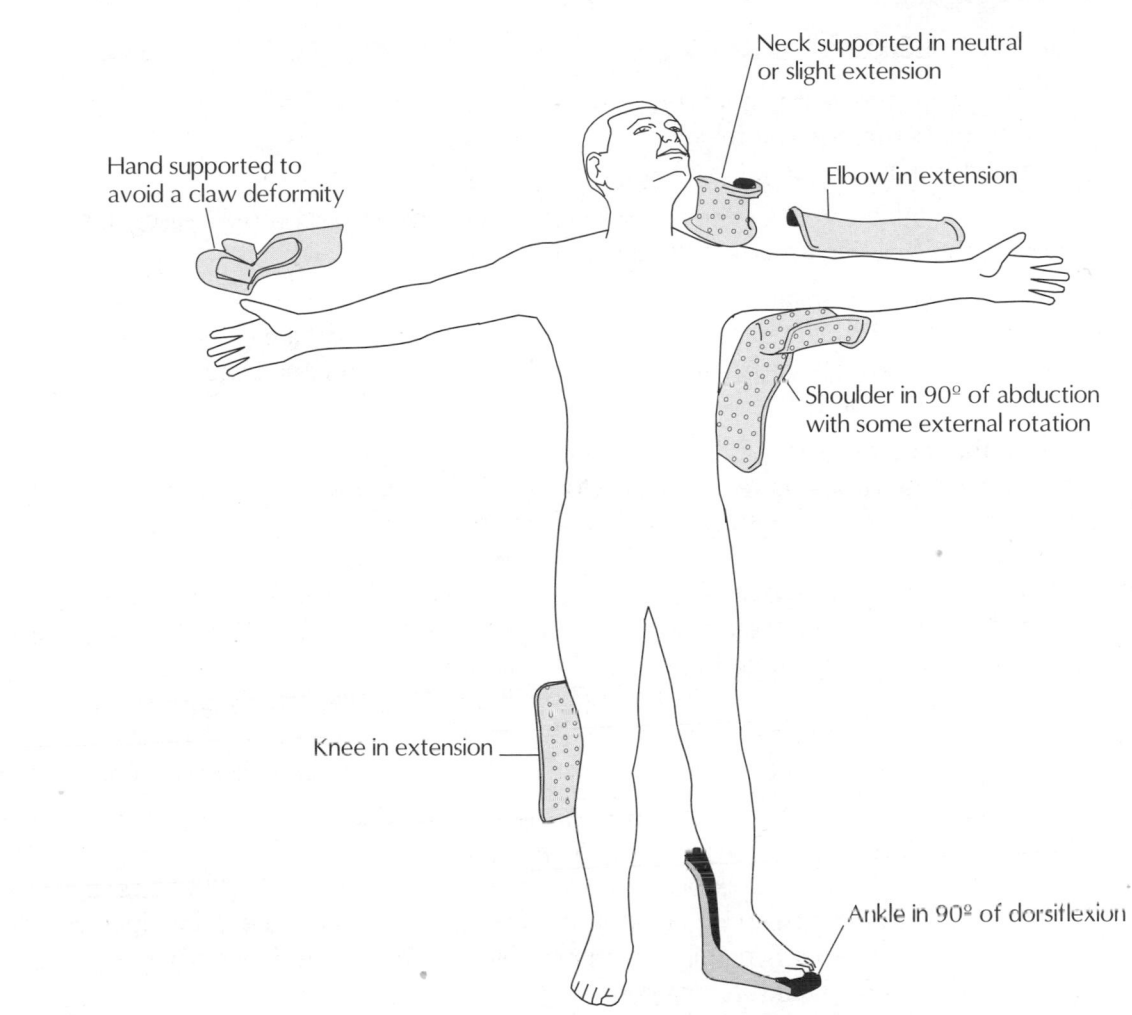

Neck supported in neutral
or slight extension

Elbow in extension

Hand supported to
avoid a claw deformity

Shoulder in 90° of abduction
with some external rotation

Knee in extension

Ankle in 90° of dorsiflexion

Figure 21.3
Splints are used to minimize contracturing as the burned tissue heals.

prevent plantarflexion by supporting the ankle in 90 degrees of dorsiflexion. Knee splints prevent excessive knee flexion by supporting knee extension. Contractures of the neck in forward or lateral flexion are prevented using a splint that conforms to the contours of the anterior neck. This supports the neck in a neutral or slightly extended position. Elbow splints prevent excessive elbow flexion by supporting the elbow in extension. Shoulder splints support the shoulder in 90 degrees of abduction with external rotation *(DeLisa, Gans, 1993)*. A claw hand deformity is avoided by using splints to support the wrist in 30 to 45 degrees of extension; the metacarpophalangeal joints are positioned in 70 to 90 degrees of flexion. Both the proximal and distal interphalangeal joints are positioned in extension with the thumb supported in a slightly abducted position with interphalangeal extension. This provides a functional position as well as maintaining the thumb-index-finger web space *(Achauer, 1987)*.

Pain control allows a more positive attitude to recovery *(Achauer, 1987)*. Analgesics are given during and after debridement procedures.

Burns: Late Subacute and Chronic Stage Concerns

The later stages of healing burns bring many physical and emotional changes for the person and her family. The full impact of the burn injury becomes apparent over the course of the hospital stay.

Physically, wound care, exercise and splinting are continued to promote healing and improve the functional ability of the person.

Upon leaving the hospital, the person's wound and skin graft donor sites are not completely healed. Debridement and cleaning are still required. Newly formed skin is fragile and susceptible to damage from stretching, splints or trauma. Affected areas are moved with care and observed for any new injuries.

During the time that the scar is developing, there is ongoing deposition and destruction of collagen. Gradually, the fibres organize into unyielding adhesions with reduced elasticity. This process, combined with contraction of the myofibroblasts, causes a "heaped up" appearance to the scar, referred to as **hypertrophic scar tissue**. During the healing process, hyperemia of the affected area suggests ongoing changes in the scar tissue and the likelihood of hypertrophic scarring. These changes peak at about three to six months post-burn and continue until the scar is fully matured, often many months after the initial trauma. Pressure is applied to the susceptible area to flatten the scar. Pressure is thought to prevent the development of hypertrophic scar tissue by restricting nutritional support to the various aspects of scar tissue production and causing scar tissue hypoxia *(Oloff, 1994)*.

Bandages or elastic cloth garments that are tailored individually, known as *pressure garments*, provide at least 25 mm Hg or more of pressure and must be worn for most of each day over a prolonged period of time until the scar is no longer red and begins to soften. This signals the maturing of the scar. After the scar has matured, discolouration of the area results in either hyperpigmentation or hypopigmentation depending on the amount of melanin in the surviving skin.

Range of motion of joints must be maintained, though this becomes increasingly difficult as the scar contracts and thickens. The six-month to two-year period during which the collagen is synthesized and degraded is the time when the scar is most plastic and susceptible to change and stretching. After the scar has matured, the impact of stretching is less profound. Splints, including dynamic splints, continue to be used to prevent contractures.

Emotionally, the person attempts to come to terms with alterations in appearance and function. The stress of the incident itself and the painful recovery process can lead to depression or **post-traumatic stress disorder**. With the stress disorder, the person vividly re-experiences the trauma, has difficulty with memory and concentrating, has an exaggerated startle response and experiences intensified distress when reminded of the burn. Counselling is usually required along with relaxation strategies to reduce stress and pain. It has been proven that when people establish, early on, some forms of control, such as techniques for coping with stress and pain, and decision-making about treatment, such as requesting additional medication before painful procedures, they have an enhanced sense of well being and they cope better with the recovery process. The supportive touch of massage is helpful in promoting a positive self-image with a person who has experienced disfiguring burns *(Settle, 1996)*.

Complications of Burns

Breathing is affected by thoracic burns. These burns interfere with lung expansion, which increases susceptibility to respiratory pathologies such as pneumonia.

Inhalation injuries occur by inhaling extremely heated air or noxious chemicals. Respiratory failure can result up to two days after the injury; combined with a thermal injury, the mortality rate is from 25 to 65 per cent *(Richard, Staley, 1994)*. Secondary to an inhalation injury is airway obstruction from edema accompanied by bronchospasm, which results with burns to more than 25 to 30 per cent of the body. Over the long term, pulmonary edema and pneumonia continue to be risks.

Gastrointestinal complications are common with severe burns, with up to 66 per cent of burn victims having gastric and duodenal ulcerations *(Achauer, 1897)*.

Contraindications

- Infection risk is a concern with any wound or burn severe enough to cause a disruption of the continuity of the skin. This requires that the therapist take appropriate precautions. Hand washing is necessary. Gloves may be worn and oil is not used around the site of the wound. In a hospital setting in the early stages of burn treatment, a mask is often worn by those treating the client.

- Avoid direct contact with burns that produce blisters to prevent accidentally rupturing them. Once a blister ruptures, an avenue for bacterial infection is present and local massage continues to be contraindicated.

- Modifications of hydrotherapy are required when applied to the affected area. As the tissue heals, there is often a hypersensitivity to temperature extremes. With burns, there is also an inability to dissipate heat.

- Direction of the pressure of techniques must be modified in the early healing stages. Due to the fragility of granulation tissue, drag and torquing of the tissue are avoided. The pressure of techniques is directed towards the injury site.

- With burns, active resisted exercise may be contraindicated in the acute stage if a large area is affected and if other complications are present, such as respiratory or heart problems.

Renal complications may result if there is insufficient fluid replacement or the person goes into shock. This is less common due to better emergency care which focuses attention on fluid losses in the first hours after a burn injury.

Heterotopic calcification may occur at joints in burned or unburned areas. This occurs at the end of the wound healing process. There is increased difficulty in performing exercises, pain in the joint and limited range of movement.

Burned skin has lost its protective pigment, melatonin, and is very sensitive to ultraviolet light. Usually, a few years after the burn, the skin becomes less sensitive.

Thermoregulation is impaired with deep partial- and full-thickness burns. The diminished vascularity and damaged sweat glands in scar tissue impair the ability to dissipate heat. In addition, severe burns often lead to an increased sensitivity to cold even 10 years after the burn.

Peripheral nerve damage is possible, especially with electrical burns, but is difficult to diagnose due to the complicating symptoms present with a burn. However, the person usually recovers partial or full function. Compartment syndromes may result due to compression on nerves, initially from edema and eventually from

from edema and eventually from restricted fascia and scar tissue.

Sensory impairment or loss may occur at the site of the burn, primarily on those sites that were grafted. In some cases, sensory fibres may be unable to penetrate thick scar tissue. In other cases, there may be nerve damage. After skin grafting, 99 per cent of those tested for sensory impairment demonstrated a loss of all but deep touch over the affected area *(Richard, Staley, 1994)*. Sensory perception may remain intact but be altered. The person may experience itching, pain, sensitivity to temperatures, a feeling of tightness, tingling or burning.

Subluxation and dislocation of the joints of the hands and feet, particularly at the metacarpophalangeal joints and metatarsophalangeal joints, are often present. A burn on the dorsal surface pulls the joint into hyperextension as the wound contracts and subluxation can occur. Splinting and exercise in the acute stages are key components of treatment for this problem.

Amputation may be necessary in limbs that suffer severe infection and ischemia, particularly with electrical burns.

Treatment Considerations For Wounds and Burns

Assessment

✍ **Observations and Palpation:** See Strategies: Massage and the Inflammatory Process.

✍ **Testing** is **AF,** then **PR ROM** of the affected area. Range is reduced due to pain, edema and fear, especially in the acute stage. Ranges which could pull the damaged tissue are most affected. **AR isometric testing** begins in the early subacute stage and may reveal weakness in the affected muscles. As healing progresses, ranges and strength usually improve unless adhesions or contractures remain.

Massage

✋ The therapist must establish clear treatment goals with the client. A supportive environment is created. A signal is established so the client can easily indicate to the therapist when she has had enough, especially when treating the wound or burn site. The therapist must respect the request to stop or modify immediately — not a few minutes later after several more strokes have been applied.

Acute and Early Subacute

✋ The essential components of the treatment are to promote relaxation, reduce pain, reduce edema, prevent infection and encourage any activity that the person can perform without reinjury to the healing wound.

✋ Currently, therapists are less likely to treat acute moderate and severe burns of hospitalized patients. But in such cases, the same treatment goals apply. The treatment is performed in consultation with the burn unit team.

260

- Slow diaphragmatic breathing is encouraged throughout the treatment.

- Massage of uninjured areas of the body provides comfort and stress reduction for the client. It will also reduce some of the pain. In the early stages of healing, before re-epithelialization and when enriched oils are not appropriate to use, a diffuser containing a relaxing essential oil, such as lavender, can scent the air to be inhaled.

- The affected limb is elevated, the appropriate lymphatic nodes are pumped and lymphatic drainage techniques are applied proximally up to the injury site (*DiGregorio, 1984*). No on-site massage is performed.

- Distally, only techniques that do not increase circulation through the injury site are performed, such as muscle squeezing or stroking.

- Movement therapy within 48 hours of injury is used to minimize edema and prevent dense fibrosis — even in moderate to severe burns. Pain-free movement to both the affected and unaffected joints also maintains joint health. Generally, active movements are encouraged, though active assisted and passive movements are also indicated, especially when the person has difficulty moving the affected joints. To prevent contractures, the movements that take the joint in the direction opposite to common contracturing positions are encouraged. For example, extension of the elbow is a focus because of its tendency to flexion contracture

- **With sutures**, the incision usually closes within a few days. The skin will hold together under normal stress and movement after a week.

- **After skin grafting**, passive and active movement is performed to the affected area within five to 10 days.

- All remedial exercises are performed within the person's pain tolerance and initially performed in reduced ranges so as not to disrupt the healing process (*Kottke et al., 1982*).

- **After re-epithelialization** or after any sutures have been removed from the affected area, the risk of infection diminishes. Introduction of a lavender-enriched oil — 25 drops of pure essential oil in 50 ml. of carrier oil — helps in the growth of healthy tissue, especially with burns (*Smith, 1994*). Lubricants such as vitamin E oil and aloe vera moisturizers are also appropriate at this stage. They improve pliability of the healing tissue, decrease skin hypersensitivity and ease itching (*Settle, 1996*). Without a lubricant, massage and stretching techniques can increase pain and pull the skin of larger wounds. Mineral oil is not recommended because it may irritate the skin (*DeLisa, Gans, 1993*).

- Before the scar has matured, in the early subacute stage, massage to reduce edema is still appropriate. Additional Swedish techniques may be performed. Since granulation tissue is present, the therapist takes care when massaging the tissue both near the injury site and over the wound site. The tissue just proximal to the wound can be stabilized with one hand. This hand monitors the drag placed on the injury site and senses if the proximally applied techniques should be modified. Initially, techniques that do not have a shear force are used, the pressure being directed towards the injury site. On site, the effect of the massage techniques is monitored so the relatively fragile skin is not overworked. Again, techniques that do not have a shear force are used, such as gentle stroking or scooping. They are applied peripherally then centrally to the injury site. Distal massage is continued as before.

Late Subacute and Chronic

- The goals at the late subacute and chronic stages are to reduce any remaining edema, decrease sympathetic nervous system firing, decrease pain, increase local circulation, reduce adhesions and improve range of motion.

- Promoting relaxation of the client decreases pain perception and improves client compliance. All techniques are applied within the client's pain tolerance. Slow diaphragmatic breathing is encouraged throughout the treatment but especially if techniques become painful.

- Edema is treated for as long as it is observed. General Swedish techniques are used proximal to the injury.

- The massage techniques are applied cautiously nearby and on site with increased vigour and torquing forces. Over a series of treatments, gentle bowing and picking up techniques are introduced to prevent restrictions and to promote elasticity of the scar tissue *(Masellis, Gunn, 1995)*. Massage at this stage is also part of the preventative treatment for hypertrophic and hypersensitive scar tissue. With burns, depending on the time it takes for the area to re-epithelialize, preventative techniques are performed as early as one month and for as long as 18 months post-injury *(Achauer, 1987)*.

- Eventually, as the scar matures, deeper specific C-bowing, S-bowing, skin rolling and, finally, cross-fibre frictions are performed on the periphery of the scar tissue. These are slowly and gradually applied to restrictions found towards the central area of burned tissue. Aggressive techniques are interspersed with effleurage and stroking.

- PIR or slow sustained stretching is then applied to stress the treated scar tissue. There will be blanching of the scar. It is essential to position the limb so the stretch is applied along the entire line of the restriction. Optimally, the stretch is maintained until the area becomes more pliable or the colour returns to normal.

- Hydrotherapy such as wax is useful before stretching because the oil in paraffin lubricates the tissue. The local heat also increases local circulation and helps to relax the client. For burns, the temperature of the wax is lowered to between 116 degrees and 118 degrees Fahrenheit (45 to 46 degrees Celsius) for hypersensitive skin.

- Ice is useful for decreasing pain in hypertrophic scar tissue, after cross-fibre frictions are performed or if the treated area remains hyperemic and warm. The application time or type of cold modality may need to be modified if the client is hypersensitive to cold. With burns, painful scarring often occurs over the lateral chest wall, medial arm and flexor surface of the wrist.

- Joint play is performed on the affected joints. With burns, it is introduced only when the tissue has healed sufficiently to accommodate the forces that must be applied to perform this technique.

Self-care

- Biofeedback, relaxation exercises and diaphragmatic breathing are used to decrease pain and stress. Tai Chi improves coordination, provides stretching and increases relaxation. Essential oils can be used to enhance relaxation. See the stress reduction chapter.

✍ Self-massage to the scar tissue is encouraged to desensitize the scar and reduce restrictions during its development. An enriched oil is used after the risk of infection is gone. Due to the longer healing time of burns, it is suggested that massage be taught to family members or friends. This helps them to participate in a gentler part of the burn injury care.

✍ A stretch and strengthen program is promoted. Generally, heat is applied first; with a burn injury, an enriched lubricant is applied first.

✍ From the first days after the injury, activities of daily living are encouraged. After massage treatment of the scar, active movements that will stress this tissue should be performed. A thorough stretching routine is suggested for all the restricted areas once the granulation tissue is no longer fragile. Movement prevents contractures and promotes optimal alignment of the scar's collagen fibres.

✍ A strengthening program using submaximal isometric contractions is started in the early subacute stage after the injury. This maintains and improves the strength of muscles subjected to prolonged inactivity or immobilization. After wound closure, isometric contractions of greater force are used to strengthen the antagonists and counteract the pull of contractured tissue. In conjunction with obtaining full range of motion, isotonic exercises can be gradually introduced

See also strategies for the inflammatory process, stress reduction, edema, scar tissue, peripheral nerve lesions, dislocations and fractures for related treatment.

✍ With burn injuries, endurance and coordination are enhanced through the performance of more difficult activities of daily living as well as through organized exercise such as swimming.

✍ Cool to cold hydrotherapy applications are recommended in the early stages of wound healing and after activity. In late subacute and chronic stages, heat is used before self-massage with cool applied afterwards.

22

CONTUSIONS

Fiona Rattray

> *A contusion is a crush injury to a muscle.*

With a contusion there is damage to the muscle fibres and resultant bleeding into the subcutaneous tissue and skin. This bruising or ecchymosis ranges from a local, minor discolouration to large, debilitating areas. The bruising may track inferiorly along fascial planes to appear at a distance from the injury site *(Thomson et al., 1991)*. The skin overlying the contusion is intact *(Porth, 1990)*. It is also possible for the periosteum to be contused *(Hartley, 1995b)*.

A hematoma is a large area of local hemorrhage following a trauma. The pooling blood causes swelling and pain as it compresses nearby nerve endings. Since blood is being continuously supplied under pressure by the arterial system, the swelling of a hematoma is more rapid than the swelling of edema. The hematoma may be contained within a fascial compartment. Pain increases on movement or if pressure is applied to the injury site. Fibroblasts lay down fibrin and the hematoma then becomes "organized" or filled in by collagen fibres. A hematoma may be treated medically by aspirating the blood *(Kurz, 1990)*.

Myositis ossificans is an occasional complication following a hematoma, where the blood within the muscle calcifies. It is not known why some contusions result in calcification. Fibroblasts are replaced by osteoblasts, which begin to lay down new bone over a period of approximately six weeks. An X-ray taken 10 days to three weeks after a contusion may reveal the ossification *(Brukner, Khan, 1993)*. Although some of the bone may be slowly resorbed, a portion of it remains. Myositis ossificans may form within a muscle or may have an attachment to an existing bone, such as the femur. Spasms and local inflammation may occur in muscle tissue containing myositis ossificans. The strength of the muscle decreases. The more severe or more frequent the contusion, the higher the risk of myositis ossificans formation. An athlete's participation in a sport may be severely limited by myositis ossificans

(*Buschbacher, 1994*). If the ossification is within the muscle and not attached to the bone, surgical excision may be performed (*Thomson et al., 1991*). If the myositis ossificans is attached to a bone, surgery is not usually an option since the surgery itself is a form of trauma that stimulates the periosteum, resulting in more bone growth.

The cause of a contusion is a direct blow to the muscle:

➤ in **contact sports**, this may be from a collision with another athlete or with a piece of equipment, such as a hockey stick, a goal post, a ball or a puck;

➤ **motor vehicle accidents** also produce this kind of injury, often at the shoulder or abdomen from seatbelt use or at the knees from hitting the dashboard;

➤ a **fall** may result in a contusion, as may a **fracture** or **dislocation** (*Hertling, Kessler, 1990*).

Other soft tissue injuries such as strains, sprains and dislocations may occur with a contusion.

✦ Contusions are classified according to **three levels of severity** (*Booher, Thibodeau, 1989*).

• **Mild Contusion**: This is a minor crush to the muscle with minimal bleeding. There is minimal or no loss of strength and minimal loss of range. The person can continue the activity with mild discomfort.

• **Moderate Contusion**: There is a moderate crushing of the muscle with bleeding and swelling. The person has difficulty continuing the activity due to pain and muscle weakness.

• **Severe Contusion**: There is a severe crushing of the tissue with rapid bleeding and swelling. The person cannot continue the activity due to significant pain and muscle weakness.

The first 24 hours after the injury are the most critical to treatment. The primary goal is to control bleeding. At the time of injury and shortly afterwards, several factors may increase the bleeding and these are to be avoided. They include stretching, exercise, heat, alcohol consumption and vigorous massage (*Brukner, Khan, 1993*). In the acute stage, the client should be referred to a physician if the health history reveals rapid swelling, significant muscle weakness or loss of function following the injury. It is important to accurately assess a contusion for the severity and the specific muscle tissue involved, although it may take up to a 24 hours for the full extent of the injury and the amount of bleeding to become apparent (*Booher, Thibodeau, 1989*).

While a contusion may occur to any muscle, it most frequently affects the quadriceps muscles (*Figure 22.1*). This injury is commonly called a "charley horse" or "cork thigh". The magnitude of a quadriceps contusion may not be known for a full day, because bleeding may continue over this time period (*Booher, Thibodeau, 1989*). Other common injury sites include the dorsum of the foot, the periosteum of

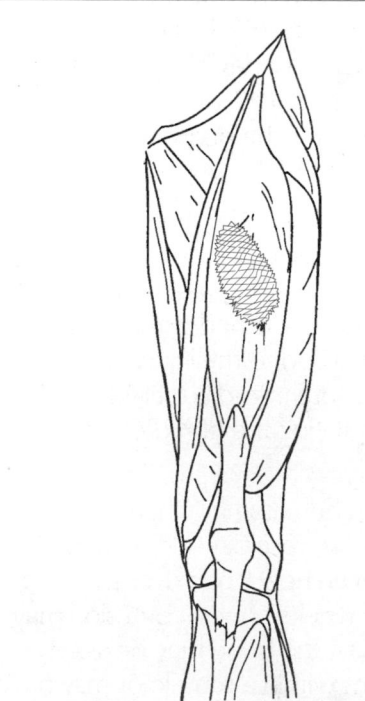

Figure 22.1
A common location for a contusion is the quadriceps muscle.

the anterior tibia, the sacrum, the iliac crest (also called a "hip pointer"), the greater trochanter, the acromion (known as a "shoulder pointer"), the olecranon and the dorsum of the hand. The gluteal, deltoid, biceps and triceps muscles are also common injury locations. The brachialis muscle may be contused by a fracture of the humerus or dislocation of the ulna (*Hertling, Kessler, 1990*). Palmar surface contusions, especially to muscles overlying the hamate or pisiform bones, can cause swelling that compresses the ulnar nerve (*Hartley, 1995b*).

Symptom Picture

Acute

✦ **Mild:** There is a minor crush to the muscle.

- Minimal local edema, heat and bruising are present.
- There is tenderness at the lesion site.
- There is minor discomfort local to the injury site with activity that contracts or stretches the muscle.
- There is five to 20 per cent loss of range of motion and minimal or no loss of strength.
- The client can usually continue the activity

✦ **Moderate:** There is crushing of several or many fibres of the muscle.

- Moderate local swelling due to hematoma, heat and bruising is present.
- There is moderate tenderness at the lesion site.
- There is 20 to 50 per cent loss of range of motion and moderate loss of strength.
- The pain is moderate with activities that contract or stretch the muscle.
- The client has difficulty in continuing the activity due to pain and experiences disability the next day.

✦ **Severe:** There is crushing of many of the muscle fibres.

- Marked, rapid local swelling is present due to hematoma, edema, heat and bruising.
- There is severe pain at the lesion site.
- There is more than 50 per cent loss of range of motion and functional loss of strength.
- The client cannot continue the activity.

✦ With all contusions, the bruising is red, black and blue.

✦ With moderate and severe contusions, swelling and hematoma formation occur. The swelling of a hematoma occurs much more rapidly than the swelling of edema, since arterial pressure forces blood through the damaged blood vessels into the injury site. There is a risk of rebleeding in the first 10 days (*Brukner, Khan, 1993*).

✦ There is decreased range of motion of the joints crossed by the affected muscle as swelling and protective muscle spasms limit movement. The contusion is often bandaged to prevent further swelling (*Brukner, Khan, 1993*).

Early Subacute

✦ A **mild** contusion has little or no pain or reduced strength, a **moderate** contusion has pain and moderately reduced strength and a **severe** contusion has pain and markedly reduced strength with active resisted strength testing.

✦ The bruising is black and blue.

✦ With a moderate or severe contusion, the hematoma is still present but reduced from the acute stage.

✦ The pain, edema and inflammation are still present but reduced from the acute stage.

✦ Adhesions are developing around the injury.

✦ The protective muscle spasm diminishes. Trigger points occur in the affected muscle, its synergists and its antagonists.

✦ With moderate and severe contusions, the injury may still be bandaged to prevent further swelling.

✦ The client is still using crutches or a cane with a contusion to a lower limb or a sling with an upper limb contusion.

✦ The range of motion is reduced.

Late Subacute

✦ The bruising is yellow, green and brown.

✦ The pain, edema and heat are diminishing.

✦ Adhesions are maturing around the injury.

✦ The protective muscle spasm is replaced by increased tone in the affected muscle, its synergists and antagonists. Trigger points occur in the affected muscle and in compensatory muscles.

✦ With a moderate or severe contusion, the hematoma diminishes.

✦ The range of motion and strength are reduced.

✦ Peripheral nerves may be compressed by the edema and swelling that result from a contusion.

Chronic

✦ The bruising is gone.

✦ Adhesions have matured around the injury.

✦ Hypertonicity and trigger points are present in the affected muscle and in any compensating structures, especially from crutch use.

✦ The tissue may be cool due to ischemia.

✦ With a moderate or severe contusion, there is discomfort local to the lesion site only if the muscle is stretched. The full range of motion and strength of the affected muscle may be reduced.

✦ Some hematomas calcify into myositis ossificans within three to six weeks after the injury. With myositis ossificans formation, there is reduced strength and local inflammation. If bone formation is within the muscle belly, it may be surgically removed.

Subjective Information

HEALTH HISTORY QUESTIONS

✦ What is the client's overall health history? Is the client on any medication for unrelated conditions that indicate treatment modifications? For example, blood thinners contraindicate the use of specific cross-fibre frictions.

✦ Has there been a history of injury or recurrent contusions of this muscle? For an athlete, these may add up over the game or the season, possibly contributing to myositis ossificans formation.

✦ In terms of the presenting complaint, when did the injury occur?

✦ How did it happen?

✦ What was done at the time of injury? Was first aid applied? Was the contusion supported with an elastic bandage?

✦ Was the client able to continue with the activity after the contusion? With a **mild** contusion, the client would have continued the activity with minor discomfort. With a **moderate** injury, the client would have continued the activity with pain and some swelling and weakness, but would have experienced disability either later that day or the next one. With a **severe** contusion, the client would have been unable to continue the activity, suffering immediate swelling, weakness and pain (Booher, Thibodeau, 1989).

✦ Did the limb "give way" at the time of injury? This indicates the loss of function of a severe contusion.

✦ Is any swelling or any edema present local or distal to the injury? If the swelling occurred rapidly after the injury — for example, within 20 minutes — this may indicate a hematoma. The client should be referred for medical treatment.

✦ Did the client see any other health care practitioner for this injury, such as a physician, physiotherapist, chiropractor or sports therapist? What treatment was given? Is the client still receiving this treatment?

✦ Is the client taking any medication for the contusion, such as analgesics, muscle relaxants or anti-inflammatories? This includes self-medication such as Aspirin, or other over-the-counter products.

✦ Is the client using any elastic bandages, supports or crutches for the affected limb? This is expected with an acute contusion of any severity and with a subacute contusion that is moderate or severe.

✦ What symptoms is the client currently experiencing? Does the client have pain now? Where exactly is the pain? Is the pain sharp or diffuse? Sharp, hot pain indicates an acute injury, while achy pain is associated with a chronic injury. A client with a severe contusion may be unable to sleep due to the pain (Brukner, Khan, 1993).

✦ What aggravates or relieves the pain? What activities are difficult or painful to complete?

✦ What are the client's activities of daily living? Does the client's occupation or recreational activity place stress on the muscle?

✦ Were there any complications other than a local hematoma, such as myositis ossificans or nerve damage? If myositis ossificans is suspected, was a diagnosis made using X-rays?

Objective Information

Observations

Acute

✍ Antalgic gait occurs if the contusion is in a lower limb. The more severe the injury, the less the client is able to weight bear. For example, in terms of a quadriceps contusion, the client with a mild injury has a slight limp or none at all. With a moderate contusion the client has a more pronounced limp. With a severe contusion, the client has complete disability (Booher, Thibodeau, 1989).

✍ The affected muscle is likely supported by elastic bandages to control and prevent swelling. With more severe contusions of the lower limb, the client will use crutches.

✍ Antalgic posture may be present. For example, with a moderate quadriceps contusion, the limb is held in a position of non-weight-bearing with the knee slightly flexed.

✍ The client may have a pained or medicated facial expression.

✍ Edema is present at the lesion site. There is minimal edema with a mild contusion, limited edema with a moderate contusion and marked edema with a severe contusion. There may be distal edema.

✍ With a moderate or severe contusion, the swelling of a hematoma is present at the lesion site (Brukner, Khan, 1993). With a severe contusion, the swelling is rapid.

✍ Red, black or purple bruising over the injury site is visible.

✍ Some redness may be present local to the injury.

Early and Late Subacute

✍ Antalgic gait has diminished from the presentation in the acute stage.

✍ The affected muscle is likely supported by elastic bandages. In moderate or severe contusions in the lower limb, the client may use crutches.

✍ Antalgic posture may also occur.

✍ Edema diminishes from the early to late subacute stage, both on site and distally.

✍ With a moderate or severe contusion, the swelling of a hematoma is present at the lesion site.

✍ Bruising over the injury site changes from purple and black in the early subacute stage to brown, yellow and green in the late subacute stage, and then disappears. There may be distal bruising. Contusions that occur in the distal thigh may drain down to the knee and produce local irritation (Brukner, Khan, 1993).

Chronic

✍ Possible habituated antalgic gait and posture may be present with a contusion in a weight bearing limb. A postural assessment is indicated in this case.

✍ With severe contusions, the affected muscle may be supported during activities that stress the tissue.

✍ With a severe contusion, there may be an alteration in the contour of the muscle. The tissue may be indented due to adhesions. With a more superficial myositis ossificans deposit, the area may be raised and locally inflamed.

Palpation
Acute

✍ Heat is present over the injured muscle and possibly in the surrounding tissue.

✍ Tenderness is present local to the lesion site and refers into the nearby tissue.

✍ The texture of the edema is firm. With moderate or severe contusions, a hematoma is palpable as a clearly demarcated lump.

✍ Protective muscle spasm is present in the affected muscle, the synergists and the antagonists.

Early and Late Subacute

✍ The temperature over the injury site diminishes from the early subacute to late subacute stage.

✍ Tenderness is present local to the injury.

✍ The texture of the edema is less firm. Adhesions are present as the healing progresses from the early to late subacute stage. The swelling of the hematoma diminishes.

✍ The tone of the affected muscle and the synergists and antagonists changes from spasm in the early subacute stage to tightness and hypertonicity in late subacute. There may be trigger points in these muscles.

Chronic

✍ The injury site may be cool due to ischemia.

✍ Point tenderness occurs local to the lesion site.

✍ Adhesions and fascial restrictions are present local to the injury site.

✍ Hypertonicity and trigger points are present local to the injury and in the compensating muscles.

✍ If myositis ossificans is present, there is local inflammation and the bony island is palpable as a hard, unyielding nodule.

Testing
Acute

✍ **AF ROM** of the joints crossed by the affected muscle is reduced. With a mild contusion, there is mild local pain when the muscle is contracted or stretched; range is reduced by up to 20 per cent. With a moderate contusion, the pain is moderate and range is reduced by 20 to 50 per cent. With a severe contusion, the pain is severe and range is reduced by more than 50 per cent *(Brukner, Khan, 1993)*.

- If a moderate or severe contusion is suspected, other testing is contraindicated in the acute stage. This is indicated by:

  (1) marked swelling,

  (2) the client having difficulty continuing the activity or being unable to continue the activity and

  (3) by the AF ROM results.

  - The client should seek medical attention *(Booher, Thibodeau, 1989)*.

- **PR ROM** for a mild contusion only is performed on the cardinal planes of motion, with the range that stretches the affected muscle tested **last**. A painful, muscle spasm end feel is present before the affected muscle reaches its full length. Pain may also be encountered with tissue approximation. For example, full elbow flexion could compress a contused brachialis muscle *(Magee, 1992)*.

- **AR isometric testing** of the affected muscle with a mild contusion reveals minor to no loss of strength and some discomfort.

Acute Special Tests

- With a moderate or severe contusion, a **girth measurement test** is positive with a hematoma and the client should be referred for emergency medical attention.

Early and Late Subacute

- **AF ROM** of the joints crossed by the affected muscle is reduced. The range is limited due to pain but less so than in the acute stage. Again, the degree of limitation increases with the severity of the injury.

- **PR ROM** is performed on the cardinal planes of motion, with the range that stretches the affected muscle tested **last**. A painful, tissue-stretch end feel is present before the affected muscle reaches its full length. Pain may also be encountered with tissue approximation *(Magee, 1992)*.

- **AR isometric testing** of the affected muscle will reveal pain at the injury site. The contraction of the muscle is held to the onset of pain only. The severity of the contusion is graded in the following manner *(Brukner, Khan, 1993; Booher, Thibodeau, 1989)*:

  - a **mild** contusion reveals minor to insignificant loss of strength and some discomfort;

  - a **moderate** contusion reveals moderate loss of strength and pain;

  - a **severe** contusion reveals significant loss of strength and pain. AR strength tests for a *quadriceps* contusion have the following results. A client with a mild quadriceps contusion can perform a stand-to-squat-to-stand knee bend with some pain. With a moderate quadriceps contusion the client cannot rise easily from a knee bend and may use the table or wall for support. A client with a severe quadriceps contusion is unable to complete the knee bend or may not even try to perform it.

Chronic

✍ **AF ROM** of joints crossed by the affected muscle may be limited by any remaining pain at the end ranges of motion.

✍ **PR ROM** may reveal a mildly painful, tissue stretch end feel on fully stretching the affected muscle.

✍ **AR testing** of the affected muscle may reveal decreased muscle strength, especially with severe contusions.

Chronic Special Tests

✍ **Length tests** for rectus femoris (Thomas and Ely's tests), gastrocnemius, soleus, adductors or hamstrings with a moderate or severe contusion reveals shortness of these muscles.

Contraindications

✦ In the acute stage, testing of a moderate or severe contusion other than pain-free active free range of motion is contraindicated to prevent further tissue damage.

✦ In the acute stage of a mild contusion, on-site work is contraindicated.

✦ In the acute and early subacute stages of a moderate to severe contusion, local and on site Swedish massage is contraindicated so as not to disturb the hematoma. However, proximal lymphatic drainage is indicated (Kurz, 1990).

✦ Avoid removing the protective muscle splinting of acute contusions.

✦ In the first week to 10 days with a moderate to severe contusion, take care with stretching and avoid vigorous massage since there is a risk of rebleeding. Any applications of heat or contrast hydrotherapy are contraindicated for the same reason (Brukner, Khan, 1993).

✦ Distal circulation techniques are contraindicated in the acute and early subacute stages to avoid increasing congestion through the injury site.

✦ With moderate or severe contusions in the acute or early subacute stages it is contraindicated to take range of motion or passive stretch beyond the onset of discomfort or pain.

✦ Frictions are contraindicated if the client is taking anti-inflammatories or blood thinners.

✦ There is a possibility of complications such as hematoma, myositis ossificans or nerve compression.

Treatment Goals Treatment Plan

Acute

Assess the severity of the injury and refer for medical attention if moderate or severe.

Reduce inflammation.

☝ **The muscle is treated with RICE:** Rest, Ice, Compression and Elevation. The muscle is placed in a pain-free position while the ice is applied.

☝ **Positioning** depends on the location of the contusion and the client's comfort. If the contusion is to a limb, the affected limb is elevated *without placing a stretch on the muscle* and is pillowed securely. If the contusion is to the sacrum or gluteals, the client is prone with a pillow under the abdomen to reduce the stretch on the injured tissue; the client is not turned supine.

☝ **Hydrotherapy** in acute is cold, such as an ice pack or a gel pack, applied to the injured area.

General Treatment

☝ If the initial treatment goal is to decrease the edema, lymphatic drainage is performed first, before any general compensatory work begins.

Reduce pain. Decrease sympathetic nervous system firing.

☝ If the initial goal is to accustom the client to the therapist's touch and to decrease sympathetic nervous system firing, the treatment begins on the trunk or the contralateral limb in the context of a relaxation massage. The client is directed to do **diaphragmatic breathing** throughout the treatment.

Treat any compensating structures.

☝ With a contusion of a limb, the trunk and uninjured limb are treated using effleurage and slow petrissage, such as palmar kneading, fingertip kneading and C-scooping. The focus of the work depends on the muscles that are compensating. For example, the shoulders and back are treated if crutches are used. With a contusion of the gluteals, the low back and thoracic muscles are the focus of the compensatory work.

Specific Treatment

Reduce edema.

☝ Assuming that the initial treatment goal is to reduce edema, lymphatic drainage techniques are used on the injured limb, beginning with nodal pumping at the proximal lymph nodes. Unidirectional effleurage, stationary circles and the local technique are used proximal to the injury to reduce the edema. For lymphatic drainage of the trunk, see the chapter on edema.

Maintain local circulation proximal to the injury only.

☝ If the contusion is to a limb, the proximal limb is treated to reduce pain and hypertonicity as well as to increase drainage and venous return. Techniques include effleurage and repetitive petrissage, such as the origin and insertion technique and palmar kneading

Treatment Goals

Reduce but do not remove the protective spasm.

Do not disturb the hematoma.

Maintain range of motion.

Treat other conditions.

Reduce inflammation.

Reduce pain. Decrease sympathetic nervous system firing. Treat any compensatory structures.

Reduce edema. Prevent adhesion formation.

Maintain local circulation proximal to the injury only.

Reduce spasm.

Treatment Plan

✋ The therapist should take care not to significantly reduce any protective muscle spasm in the synergists and antagonists of the injured muscle by overtreating these tissues. If the contusion is to the trunk, the synergists and antagonists are treated.

✋ On-site work is contraindicated.

✋ Careful muscle squeezing and light stroking are used distally.

✋ **Passive relaxed range of motion** of the proximal and distal joints, to the onset of pain only, is used for **mild** contusions. This will maintain the successive action and help increase lymphatic drainage.

✋ Any other injuries, such as sprains or dislocations, are also treated. See the appropriate chapters for details.

Early Subacute

✋ Do not interfere with the healing process of a moderate to severe contusion. The healing tissue is still fragile. Therefore, the treatment goals are achieved with care.

✋ The limb is once again elevated if the contusion is in a limb.

✋ **Hydrotherapy applications** on site are cold/cool.

General Treatment

✋ The treatment approach outlined for acute general work is indicated at this stage also, including reducing pain perception, treating compensatory structures and encouraging **diaphragmatic breathing.**

Specific Treatment

✋ Proximal lymphatic drainage techniques to reduce any edema are indicated for an injured limb. These include proximal nodal pumping, unidirectional effleurage, stationary circles and the local technique. The work is performed proximal to the lesion site to prevent congestion through the injury.

✋ The proximal limb is treated to reduce hypertonicity and maintain drainage and venous return. In the early subacute stage of a **moderate** or **severe** contusion, this is performed carefully so as not to disturb the hematoma. Techniques include effleurage and petrissage such as palmar kneading, C-scooping, fingertip kneading and the origin and insertion technique.

✋ Because protective muscle spasming is no longer as important to stabilize the injured tissue, Golgi tendon organ release is used on the

Treatment Goals   Treatment Plan

proximal tendons of the affected muscle and on its synergists or antagonists. Agonist contraction may also be used.

Reduce trigger points without disturbing the injury site.

Trigger points in proximal muscles that refer to the injured limb and the injury site itself are now treated. Trigger points that are in the injured muscle are only treated if they are well proximal to the injury site and the techniques used pose no risk to tissue healing. Careful intermittent ischemic compression is used for this in the early subacute stage.

On-site work is now indicated with a **mild** contusion only. Vibrations and stroking to the client's pain tolerance are used on the site of the contusion.

Do not disturb the hematoma.

Due to the presence of the hematoma with a **moderate** to **severe** contusion, on-site work is delayed until the late subacute stage.

Maintain range of motion.

Inner to mid-range passive relaxed range of motion is used with **mild** contusions on the joints proximal and distal to the contusion. This maintains the successive action and helps promote lymphatic drainage. The range that stretches the injured muscle is introduced **last.**

In a limb, distal techniques for all contusions in the early subacute stage include stroking and muscle squeezing only. This reduces the possibility of causing congestion through the lesion site.

The same principles are followed for a contused muscle in the gluteals or low back.

Late Subacute

The healing tissue is less fragile. Therefore, the treatment goals can be achieved using more vigorous techniques.

Positioning may be prone or supine as long as it is comfortable. The limb is once again **elevated** without placing a stretch on the muscle.

Hydrotherapy applications on site are cold/warm. If acute inflammation recurs, local cold hydrotherapy applications are used.

General Treatment

Reduce pain. Decrease sympathetic nervous system firing. Treat any compensating structures.

The treatment approach outlined for early subacute general work is indicated in this stage also.

Treatment Goals Treatment Plan

Specific Treatment

Reduce edema.

🖐 As the edema diminishes in the late subacute stage, the length of time spent on drainage techniques decreases.

Reduce hypertonicity and trigger points.

🖐 The proximal limb is treated to reduce hypertonicity and increase drainage and venous return. Trigger points in muscles that refer to the injured limb and the injury site itself are treated using muscle stripping and ischemic compressions to the client's pain tolerance. If ischemic compressions are used to treat the injured muscle, repetitive petrissage is used to flush circulation through the muscle. Heat and a full stretch are not used as they may compromise the contused tissue.

Reduce adhesions.

🖐 On-site work includes vibrations, stroking and fingertip kneading, working from the periphery to the centre and back to the periphery. As inflammation subsides in the late subacute stage, the focus shifts to reducing adhesions within the muscle. It is also important to realign the developing connective tissue so it forms a functional scar *(Figure 22.2)*. It is essential to accurately palpate the lesion site and any restricting adhesions before attempting to reduce them. Slow skin rolling followed by specific petrissage, such as longitudinal muscle stripping and short cross-fibre strokes *(Brukner, Khan, 1993)*, are used on the lesion site. Any remaining adhesions are treated with gentle cross-fibre frictions. All this work is performed within the client's pain tolerance.

🖐 After the adhesions have been frictioned, the specific stretch that lengthens the muscle is used to realign the fibres. The stretch is performed cautiously, gently and to the onset of pain only to avoid overstretching the injured tissue. Ice is applied to the frictioned tissue to inhibit the inflammatory process.

🖐 Joint play techniques to the proximal and distal joints are introduced in the late subacute stage if these joints are hypomobile due to compensation.

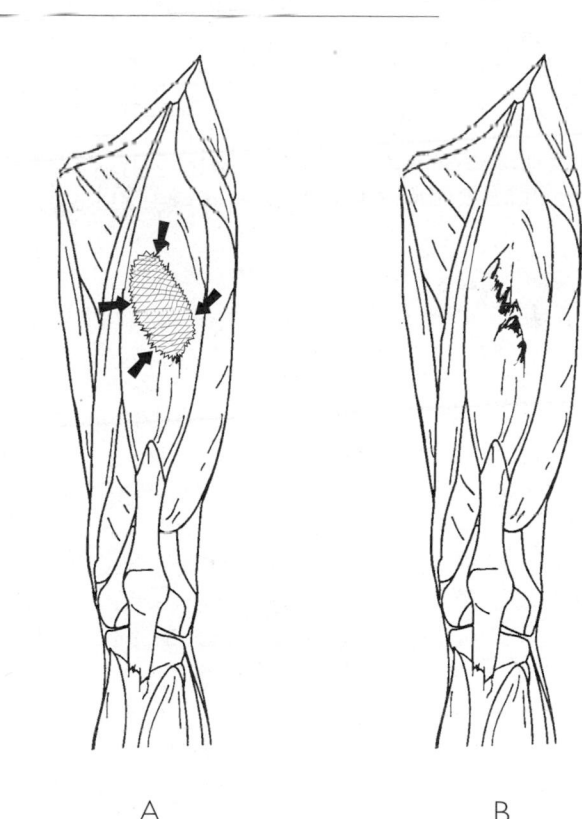

A   B

Figure 22.2
(A) Cross-fibre frictions applied across the fibres of the adhesions in late subacute to create a (B) functional scar in the muscle.

Treatment Goals Treatment Plan

Increase the range of motion.

✋ **Mid- to full-range passive relaxed range of motion** is used by the therapist on the joints proximal and distal to the contusion to the onset of pain only. The range that stretches the injured muscle is introduced **last.**

Increase local circulation.

✋ In the late subacute stage with any severity of contusion, the risk of causing congestion local to the injury or disturbing the hematoma diminishes. Effleurage and petrissage are now introduced distally to increase circulation and promote tissue health.

Chronic

✋ **Positioning** is now chosen for comfort and for accessibility to the structures that the therapist is treating.

✋ **Hydrotherapy applications** proximal to the contusion and on the lesion site itself include deep moist heat, such as a hydrocollator or a wax application, to soften any remaining adhesions and increase local circulation.

General Treatment

Reduce sympathetic nervous system firing. Treat compensatory structures.

✋ The client's trunk and compensating structures are massaged as before. Rhythmic techniques to the trunk and unaffected limb are indicated.

Specific Treatment

Reduce hypertonicity and trigger points.

✋ The proximal limb is treated to reduce any remaining hypertonicity or trigger points and to increase the local circulation. Rhythmic techniques, effleurage, repetitive petrissage and ischemic compressions are indicated. For a trunk contusion, the synergists and antagonists are treated.

Reduce adhesions.

✋ If the therapist has been treating the client's injury throughout the healing process, the focus is on reducing the remaining restricting adhesions and scar tissue. Specific kneading, muscle stripping and fascial techniques are used.

✋ Cross-fibre frictions are performed to any remaining adhesions. These are followed by a passive stretch or post-isometric relaxation of the muscle to realign the fibres. An application of ice follows this work.

✋ Joint play techniques to the proximal and distal joints are used if these structures are restricted due to compensation.

Restore the range of motion.

✋ **Passive relaxed range of motion** to full range of motion is used on the proximal and distal joints to maintain joint health.

Treatment Goals

Increase local circulation.

Self-care Goals

Educate the client.

Maintain range of motion.

Maintain strength of the affected muscle in a pain-free manner.

Increase the strength.

Treatment Plan

- The distal limb is treated with effleurage and petrissage to increase local venous return.
- If treatments are started when the client is in the chronic stage, one approach is to focus on reducing the hypertonicity and trigger points that have developed from the client's compensation patterns, before addressing any adhesions.
- The same principles are followed for a contusion to the trunk.

Self-care Plan

- **Hydrotherapy** is chosen that is appropriate for the stage of healing. As soon as the early subacute stage has passed, contrast hydrotherapy is used.
- **Self-massage** is useful for the affected muscle in the late subacute and chronic stages. This includes skin rolling, muscle stripping and gentle frictions with the client working within his pain tolerance.
- **Remedial exercise** that is given depends on the stage of healing and the severity of the injury.
- In the **acute** stage, with a mild contusion, the client is asked to perform pain-free active free range of motion of the distal and proximal joints. A gentle stretch **only to the onset of pain** is indicated with a mild contusion (Brukner, Khan, 1993). Pain-free active resisted isometrics for the antagonists are also performed. Further remedial exercise is contraindicated in the acute stage with moderate and severe contusions.
- In the **early subacute** stage, with mild or moderate contusions, the client can perform pain-free active free range of motion of the proximal and distal joints. As soon as possible, the client begins to increase the range, again to the onset of pain only. With moderate contusions, the isometric contractions are gradually increased and performed from inner to mid-ranges. These are progressed to active resisted isotonic concentric and eccentric exercises, once activities that stretch or contract the muscle are pain free both during and after the exercise (Brukner, Khan, 1993).
- In the **late subacute** stage, all stretching and strengthening exercises are gradually increased in duration and repetition. With repeated contusions, the client can resume stretching and activity gradually **once the symptoms of inflammation and pain have ceased** (Booher, Thibodeau, 1989; Brukner, Khan, 1993). It is important that the exercises progress gradually to avoid reinjury.

Self-care Goals

Self-care Plan

Increase the strength.

✍ In the **chronic** stage, the focus continues to be active resisted isotonic concentric and eccentric exercise to gradually strengthen the affected muscle.

Encourage activity.

✍ The client is encouraged to return to the activities that caused the injury once the range of motion is almost completely recovered and performed **without a significant increase in pain** *(Booher, Thibodeau, 1989).*

✍ The client may need to use an elastic bandage or other support to protect the contusion on activity, especially in a weight bearing limb. In sports activities, a lack of protective equipment may lead to repeated contusions.

Treatment Frequency and Expected Outcome

Shorter, more frequent treatments will address the inflammatory process in the acute and subacute stages. Treatment may progress to once a week for chronic stages, then the client is reassessed.

The outcome is variable, depending on the severity of the injury, the treatment approach used (initially RICE, then stretching and soft tissue work) and the client's age, general health and compliance with the self-care program.

See stress reduction, edema, spasm, sprains, dislocations, fractures, scars, whiplash and conditions of the peripheral nervous system for related treatments.

✦ **Return to activity** (the following are guidelines only):

- Mild contusion — The client can return to the activity after two to three days with support such as an elastic bandage;

- Moderate and severe contusion — the client can return to activity one week to several weeks once activity is pain free *(Thomson et al., 1991; Brukner, Khan, 1993).*

Sample Treatment: Moderate Distal Quadriceps Contusion

Acute

- The client is in a comfortable position, likely supine, with the injured leg elevated by slight flexion of the knee and hip so there is no stretch placed on the quadriceps. Ice is placed over the injury site and the client is instructed to breathe diaphragmatically. The therapist uses lymphatic drainage techniques on the affected leg, starting with inguinal pumping and treating the proximal leg. Lymphatic drainage is stopped just proximal to the edema.

- Swedish techniques are used on the uninjured limb to treat the compensating structures and decrease sympathetic nervous system firing and pain. The injured thigh, including the tensor fascia lata, is treated with gentle Swedish techniques proximal to the injury site only. Care is taken not to disturb the hematoma or completely reduce protective muscle spasm. If the treatment is half an hour in length, the shoulders, neck and head can be included, especially if the client is using crutches.

- For **self-care**, the client is instructed to rest (no weight bearing), ice and elevate the limb in a position that does not stretch the muscle. The ice should be applied at frequent intervals for 15 to 20 minutes. Pain-free isometric resisted exercises for the hamstrings, gluteals and iliopsoas are performed to maintain strength.

Early Subacute

- The treatment plan for the early subacute stage is much the same as for the acute stage in terms of positioning and lymphatic drainage. If it is comfortable, the client can be turned onto the uninjured side to treat the compensating hamstrings and gluteals.

- Cold hydrotherapy can be applied to the contusion while the uninjured leg is treated. Swedish techniques for the unaffected and affected leg are similar to those used in the acute stage, except that the focus is placed on reducing spasms using Golgi tendon organ release for rectus femoris at the anterior superior iliac spine. Care is taken not to disturb the hematoma with the proximal techniques.

- Hypertonicity and trigger points are treated, specifically those in the tensor fascia lata, vastus intermedius, vastus medius, vastus lateralis and iliopsoas, that may refer into the anterior thigh. This work is performed well proximal to the contusion site.

- On-site work is contraindicated. Vibrations, stroking and muscle squeezing are performed on the distal leg.

- For **self-care**, active resisted isometric exercises are continued from the acute stage. The client can now begin to stretch the muscle, carefully and to the onset of pain only. Cold hydrotherapy applications are continued as needed.

Late Subacute

- The positioning for the early subacute stage is used. If it is comfortable, the client can be placed in sidelying on the uninjured side, or even prone, to treat the compensating hamstrings and gluteals. Less time is spent on lymphatic drainage. Contrast hydrotherapy is introduced. Circulation techniques are also used on the proximal affected thigh.

🖐 An injury to the quadriceps may also affect the sacroiliac joint. If this joint is hypomobile, joint play techniques are used. The hands are first placed on the lateral borders of both anterior superior iliac spines (ASIS) and both hands compress towards midline and slightly posteriorly, stretching the posterior sacroiliac ligaments. The therapist next places one hand palm up between the table and the client's sacrum, with the sacrum resting on the fingertips and the posterior superior iliac spine (PSIS) resting on the proximal interphalangeal joints. The therapist's other hand is cupped and the heel of the hand is placed over the anterior superior iliac spine, with the fingers resting on the lateral surface of the client's hip. The joint is mobilized in a posterior-anterior direction by the therapist rhythmically compressing the ASIS down into the table and then releasing, followed by pressure on the PSIS upwards.

🖐 Pain-free passive relaxed range of motion in the supine position is done in the following order: internal and external rotation of the hip, followed by hip flexion and, finally, knee flexion with hip flexion.

🖐 Hypertonicity and trigger points that may refer into the anterior thigh are treated using ischemic compressions.

🖐 Specific work to the contused quadriceps is done with palmar kneading. Gentle on-site vibrations, stroking and fingertip kneading are also used. Skin rolling, longitudinal muscle stripping, short cross-fibre strokes and gentle frictions are used on the adhesions. The techniques are applied from the periphery towards the centre of the contusion. All work is done within the client's pain tolerance. Repetitive effleurage is used to flush out the tissue after this deeper work.

🖐 Swedish techniques to increase circulation are used on the distal leg.

🖐 After the anterior leg is treated, the quadriceps muscle requires stretching to align the fibres following frictioning. The client is turned prone and the knee is flexed, bringing the heel to the gluteals in a slow, passive stretch to the onset of pain only. Post-isometric relaxation is also used to gently stretch the muscle. This is followed with an application of ice.

✍ In terms of **self-care**, the client is shown a standing stretch where the affected knee is flexed and the hip is in a neutral position. The client pulls the heel of the foot towards the buttock. This is performed to the onset of pain only *(Brukner, Khan, 1993)*.

Chronic

🖐 The client may be started in a prone position to provide access to the low back, gluteals and posterior legs. Hypertonicity and compensatory changes are treated as in the previous stages. Passive relaxed ranges of the hip and knee are performed, with knee flexion done last. When the client is turned supine, Swedish techniques are used on the anterior legs to increase local circulation. Trigger points in the quadriceps and iliopsoas referring into the anterior thigh are addressed.

🖐 Fascial techniques and frictions are performed on the lesion site.

🖐 A combination of fascial release and range of motion is also used. The hip and knee of the unaffected leg are flexed so the foot is flat on the table. This takes the pressure off the sacroiliac joints. The client's affected thigh is slightly abducted so that the knee is over the edge of the table and the lower leg is able to drop into flexion. The therapist holds the client's ankle with the knee in extension while placing the ulnar border of the other arm over the distal quadriceps. As the client's knee is slowly brought into flexion, the therapist muscle strips in a proximal direction over the lesion site. This stretches and mobilizes the tissue at the same time *(Brukner, Khan, 1993)*. The therapist will need to watch her posture while performing this technique. Care is taken not to bend at the waist but rather use the "lunge" position — one leg is forward and flexed at the knee, the other leg is extended behind her. This allows the therapist to move forward as the forearm strips the muscle.

✋ Joint play to the sacroiliac joint and knee, as well as fascial techniques for other restrictions, are used if indicated.

✋ The client's gait patterns are reassessed and corrected, if necessary, to prevent reinjury.

✍ For **self-care**, once length and strength have been regained in the quadriceps, stretching of the quadriceps, hamstrings, adductors, gluteals and iliopsoas is important. Gradually the client will return to his regular activities or sport. The client may need to use taping that covers the thigh when exercising to prevent reinjury.

23

STRAINS

Fiona Rattray

A strain is an overstretch injury to a musculotendinous unit (Booher, Thibodeau, 1989).

A musculotendinous unit is the muscle, its tendons, their osseous attachments and the musculotendinous junction.

There are two types of muscle contraction: concentric and eccentric. In a **concentric** muscle contraction, as the origin and insertion of the muscle come closer together, the muscle fibres shorten. In an **eccentric** muscle contraction, as the origin and insertion move farther apart, the muscle fibres lengthen. Eccentric contraction can produce greater forces within the muscle than concentric contraction, predisposing the muscle to injury at this time. For example, during the gait cycle, the hamstrings produce the greatest eccentric force to decelerate the leg during the terminal swing phase and heel strike. This is frequently when hamstring strains occur *(Brukner, Khan, 1993)*. Single, explosive muscle contractions, either eccentric or concentric, can also result in a strain *(Hartley, 1995b)*.

The weakest link in the musculotendinous unit at the time of injury is the structure that is damaged. For example, with older adults, chronic muscle overuse frequently causes damage to the musculotendinous junction or the tendon itself. Also, the hypovascular nature of tendons contributes to decreased tissue health, allowing the tendon itself to rupture. With younger people where the epiphyseal (or growth) plate in the bone has not yet ossified, the muscles and tendons are stronger than the bone. The tendon may avulse or the bone may fracture along the epiphyseal line *(Booher, Thibodeau, 1989; Hartley, 1995b)*.

Because tendons are moderately vascularized, they are prone to partial or complete rupture at the area of least blood supply. This is usually either in the middle of the tendon or at the musculotendinous junction *(Brukner, Khan, 1993)*.

The causes of a strain are:

➤ **a sudden overstretching** of the muscle;

➤ **an extreme contraction** of the muscle against heavy resistance.

Contributing factors include inadequate warm-up before an activity, limited flexibility, fatigue, repetitive overuse or overstressing of the muscle, a strength imbalance between the muscle and its antagonists, a history of previous strains to that muscle and altered biomechanics that place stress on the muscle.

Other soft tissue injuries such as a sprain, a contusion or a dislocation may occur with a strain.

✦ Strains are classified according to **three levels of severity** *(Booher, Thibodeau, 1989)*.

• **Grade 1, Mild or First Degree Strain:** This is a minor stretch and tear to the musculotendinous unit. There is minimal loss of strength. The person can continue with the activity with mild discomfort.

• **Grade 2, Moderate or Second Degree Strain:** Tearing of the musculotendinous fibres occurs. The degree of tear is quite variable, from several fibres to the majority of the fibres. There may be a snapping sensation or sound at the time of injury. A palpable gap may appear at the injury site. The person has difficulty continuing the activity due to pain and muscle weakness.

• **Grade 3, Severe or Third Degree Strain:** This is a complete rupture of the musculotendinous unit or an avulsion fracture as the bony attachment of the tendon is torn off while the unit remains intact. There is a snapping sensation or sound at the time of rupture. A palpable and often visible gap appears at the injury site. Often, the muscle shortens and bunches up. The person cannot continue the activity due to significant pain and muscle weakness.

In the acute stage, the client should be referred to a physician if the health history reveals that there is significant muscle weakness, loss of function or a palpable gap in the tissue *(Booher, Thibodeau, 1989)*.

Muscles and tendons in acute Grade 3 strains may be surgically repaired. If the injury is left to the chronic stage, the ends of the tissue fibrose and make surgical repair difficult.

With a Grade 1 or 2 strain, after the acute stage has passed, it is important to first maintain and then increase the range of motion of the joints crossed by the affected muscle. It is also important to maintain and then progressively increase the strength of the muscle itself. A period of total inactivity following a strain allows the injured musculotendinous unit to shorten and disuse atrophy to occur *(Edwardson, 1995)*. If the injury is not treated to reduce adhesions, scar tissue develops within the muscle or tendon, limiting its ability to fully lengthen *(Buschbacher, 1994)*. It may then be difficult to stretch and strengthen the tissue. As the person attempts to use the muscle, repeated microtearing occurs between the scar tissue and the nearby healthy muscle tissue, contributing to chronic inflammation.

In contrast, if the person continues to overuse the injured muscle or tendon without allowing healing to occur in the acute and early subacute stages, a cycle of repeated strains occurs. Chronic inflammation at the lesion site may also result if the person's training program is too intense or the person performs repetitive specific movements.

While a strain may occur to any muscle, it most frequently affects the muscles of the lower limbs. The hamstrings, quadriceps and gastrocnemius muscles all cross two joints and

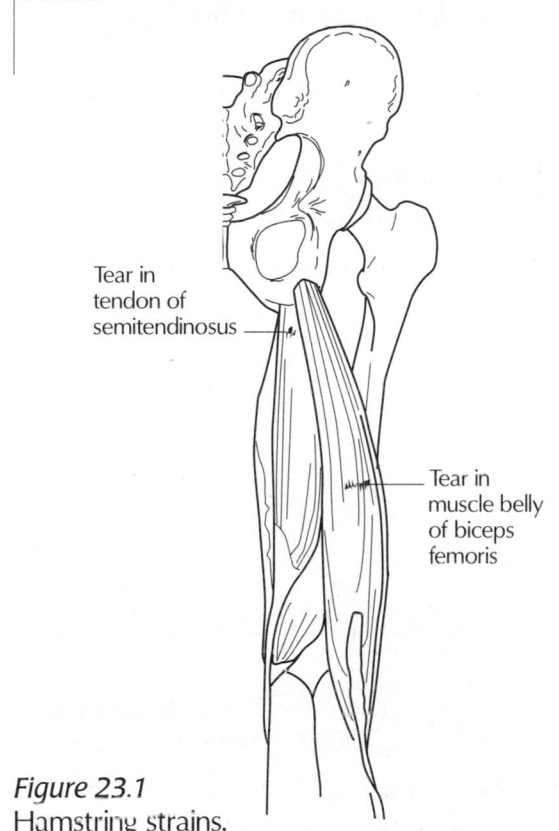

Tear in
tendon of
semitendinosus

Tear in
muscle belly
of biceps
femoris

Figure 23.1
Hamstring strains.

are, therefore, subject to increased stress *(Brukner, Khan, 1993)*. A strain of the gastrocnemius usually occurs at the musculotendinous junction or at the attachment of the Achilles tendon to the calcaneus. Hamstrings *(Figure 23.1)* often sustain damage in the middle of the muscle belly or at the musculotendinous junction close to the ischial tuberosity *(Booher, Thibodeau, 1989)*. The adductors, quadriceps (especially rectus femoris), gracilis and erector spinae are prone to injury. Iliopsoas may be injured at the attachment of iliacus in the pelvis or at the combined tendon attachment to the femur.

The rotator cuff muscles are also frequent sites of strains or ruptures, with the supraspinatus tendon being the most frequently affected. A pectoralis major rupture usually occurs at the insertion on the humerus. The long head of biceps brachialis or the transverse humeral ligament that holds the biceps tendon into the bicipital groove may also rupture. With an acute whiplash, the muscles of the neck including the scalenes, levator scapulae, the posterior cervical muscles, the infrahyoids, the suprahyoids and longus colli may suffer strain.

Symptom Picture

Acute

✦ **Grade 1:** With a minor stretch to the musculotendinous unit, there is minor discomfort local to the injury site on activity that contracts or stretches the muscle.

- Local edema, heat and bruising are minimal or not present.
- There is tenderness at the lesion site.
- There is little or no loss of strength or range of motion.
- The client can continue the activity.

✦ **Grade 2:** There is tearing of several or many fibres of the musculotendinous unit.

- There is a snapping noise or sensation at the time of injury.
- Moderate local edema, heat, hematoma and bruising are present.
- A gap may be palpated in the tissue.
- There is moderate tenderness at the lesion site.
- There is moderate pain with activities that contract or stretch the musculotendinous unit.
- There is a moderate loss of strength and range of motion.

- The client has difficulty in continuing the activity due to pain and experiences disability the next day.
- ✦ **Grade 3:** There is a complete rupture of the muscle or an avulsion fracture of the tendinous attachment.
  - There is a snapping noise or sensation at the time of the injury.
  - Marked local edema, heat, hematoma and bruising are present.
  - A gap is palpated in the tissue. The muscle will likely bunch up due to spasmodic contractions.
  - There is severe pain at the lesion site.
  - There is immediate loss of strength and range of motion.
  - The client cannot continue the activity.
- ✦ In **Grade 2 and 3** strains the following occurs:
  - The bruising is red, black and blue.
  - A hematoma is present at the lesion site.
  - There is decreased range of motion of the joints crossed by the affected muscle as protective muscle spasm limits movement.
  - Depending on the severity, there is little, moderate or severe loss of function of the affected limb. Other structures compensate for this, especially if supports are used.
  - The muscle may be bandaged to prevent further injury. The client may be using crutches or a cane with a strain in a lower limb or a sling with an upper limb injury.
  - With a Grade 3 strain of the lower limb, the ruptured muscle is usually surgically repaired and then immobilized in a cast for four to eight weeks. However, it is possible that a Grade 3 strain in the upper limb occurs and the client does not seek immediate medical attention. In such cases, it is possible that surgical repair has not been performed (Brukner, Khan, 1993).

Early Subacute

- ✦ A **Grade 1** strain has little or no pain and reduced strength, a **Grade 2** strain has pain and moderately reduced strength and a **Grade 3** strain has pain and markedly reduced strength with active resisted strength testing.
- ✦ With a Grade 2 or 3 strain, the bruising is black and blue and a hematoma is present.
- ✦ With a Grade 2 strain, there is an alteration in the contour of the muscle. With a Grade 3 strain, there is a gap in the tissue and the muscle may bunch up, unless it was surgically repaired.
- ✦ The pain, edema and inflammation are still present but reduced from the acute stage.
- ✦ Adhesions are developing around the injury site.
- ✦ Since tendons are hypovascular, they heal relatively slowly.
- ✦ The protective muscle spasm diminishes. Trigger points occur in the affected muscle, its synergists and its antagonists.
- ✦ With Grade 2 and 3 strains, the muscle is still bandaged or casted to prevent further

injury. The client is still using crutches or a cane with a strain in a lower limb or may still use a sling with an upper limb injury.

✦ The range of motion is reduced.

Late Subacute

✦ With a Grade 2 or 3 strain, the bruising is yellow, green and brown. The hematoma diminishes. A gap is still palpable in the tissue.

✦ With all strains, the pain, edema and inflammation are diminishing.

✦ The protective muscle spasm is replaced by increased tone in the affected muscle, its synergists and its antagonists. Trigger points occur in the affected muscle and in compensatory muscles.

✦ Adhesions are maturing around the injury.

✦ The range of motion is reduced.

Chronic

✦ The bruising is gone.

✦ Hypertonicity and trigger points are present in the affected muscle and in any compensating structures.

✦ Adhesions have matured around the injury.

✦ The tissue may be cool due to ischemia.

✦ There is discomfort local to the lesion site only if the muscle is stretched.

✦ With Grade 2 and 3 strains, the full range of motion of the joint crossed by the affected muscle may be reduced.

✦ With a Grade 3 strain, if surgery was performed and the limb casted, see the chapter on fractures for the symptom picture of tissue that was under the cast. If the ruptured muscle was not surgically repaired, there is reduced strength since only the synergists of the affected muscle can function.

✦ Repeated strains result from overuse, usually from workloads that are too stressful for the muscle. Chronic inflammation results from overuse or from continuing to work an injured muscle. With repeated strains, a pocket of chronic edema may remain local to the injury site.

✦ There is reduced strength of the affected musculotendinous unit and possible disuse atrophy.

Subjective Information

HEALTH HISTORY QUESTIONS

✦ What is the client's overall health history? Is the client on any medication for unrelated conditions that indicate treatment modifications?

✦ Has this muscle been injured before? If yes, what was the injury and when did it happen? Has there been a history of recurrent strains of this muscle?

✦ In terms of the presenting complaint, when did the injury occur?

✦ Does the client know the mechanism of injury — for example, a sprinter "pulling" a hamstring muscle when explosively leaping out of the starting blocks; or a person who while weight training "feels something go" in a biceps muscle while using a greater weight than usual?

✦ Did the client hear any noise or feel any sensation at the time of the injury? For example, with a Grade 2 or 3 strain, a snapping noise or sensation may be noticed *(Booher, Thibodeau, 1989)*. A rotator cuff strain may present with a "twinge", or sudden pain at the shoulder.

✦ What was done at the time of injury? Was first aid applied?

✦ Was the client able to continue with the activity after the strain? With a Grade 1 strain, the client would have continued the activity with minor or no discomfort. There would have been little or no disability experienced. With a Grade 2 injury, the client would have continued the activity with pain and some weakness, but experienced disability either later that day or the next one. With a Grade 3 strain, the client would have been unable to continue the activity, suffering immediate disability, weakness and pain *(Booher, Thibodeau, 1989)*.

✦ Did the client see any other health care practitioner for this injury, such as a physician, physiotherapist, chiropractor or sports therapist? If so, was a diagnosis made using ultrasound or magnetic resonance imaging (MRI)? What treatment was given? Is the client still receiving this treatment?

✦ Is the client taking any medication for the strain, such as analgesics, muscle relaxants or anti-inflammatories? This includes self-medication such as Aspirin or other over-the-counter products. Commonly, with a rotator cuff injury, local corticosteroid injections are administered *(Hertling, Kessler, 1990)*.

✦ Were there any complications, such as a local hematoma, nerve damage or an avulsion at the tendon's attachment?

✦ Is the client using any supports or crutches for the affected limb? This is expected with an acute or subacute Grade 2 or 3 strain. A Grade 3 strain of a leg muscle is usually surgically repaired, then immobilized. A weight bearing limb that had previously experienced a Grade 2 or 3 strain, or one that repeatedly strains, may require an elastic bandage or other support when the client is performing an activity that stresses the muscle.

✦ What symptoms is the client currently experiencing? Does the client have pain now? Where exactly is the pain? Is the pain sharp or diffuse? Sharp, hot pain indicates an acute injury, while an ache is associated with a chronic injury.

✦ What aggravates or relieves the pain?

✦ Is any swelling or any edema present local or distal to the injury? Swelling that occurred rapidly after the injury — for example within 20 minutes — may indicate a hematoma. The client should be referred for medical treatment.

✦ With a strain of a weight bearing limb, did the limb "give way" at the time of injury? This indicates the loss of function of a Grade 3 strain.

✦ What activities are difficult or painful to complete?

✦ What are the client's activities of daily living? Does the client's occupation or recreational activity place stress on the muscle?

Objective Information

Observations
Acute

✍ Antalgic gait occurs if the strain is in a lower limb. The more severe the injury, the less the client is able to weight bear. For example, with a Grade 1 hamstring strain, the client has a slight limp or no limp at all. With a Grade 2 strain, the client has a more pronounced limp. With a Grade 3 strain, the client has complete disability (Booher, Thibodeau, 1989).

✍ The affected muscle may be supported by taping, elastic bandages or splints. With more severe strains of the lower limb, the client will use crutches. A Grade 3 strain is immobilized in a cast.

✍ Antalgic posture may be present. For example, with a Grade 2 hamstring strain, the limb is held in a position of non-weight-bearing with the knee slightly flexed (Brukner, Khan, 1993).

✍ The client may have a pained or medicated facial expression.

✍ Edema is present at the lesion site. There is minimal or no edema at all with a Grade 1 strain, moderate edema with a Grade 2 strain and marked edema with a Grade 3 strain. There may be distal edema.

✍ With a Grade 2 or 3 strain, a hematoma is present at the lesion site (Brukner, Khan, 1993).

✍ Some redness may be present local to the injury.

✍ Red, black or purple bruising may be visible over the injury site.

✍ With Grade 2 strains, a gap in the tissue or an alteration in the contour of the muscle may be noted. With a Grade 3 strain, there is a visible gap at the lesion site and the muscle may bunch up.

Early and Late Subacute

✍ Antalgic gait is present with a strain in a weight bearing limb. It has diminished from the presentation in the acute stage.

✍ The affected muscle may be supported by taping or ace bandages. With Grade 3 strains in the lower limb, the client may use crutches.

✍ Antalgic posture may also occur.

✍ Edema diminishes from the early to late subacute stage, both on site and distally.

✍ With a Grade 2 or 3 strain, a hematoma is resolving at the lesion site.

✍ Bruising over the injury site changes from purple and black in early subacute to brown, yellow and green in late subacute and then disappears. Distal bruising may be present.

✍ With Grade 2 strains, an alteration in the contour of the muscle is still apparent. With a Grade 3 strain, there is still a visible gap at the lesion site and the muscle may remain bunched up if it was not surgically repaired.

✍ Scars are present if the musculotendinous unit was surgically reduced.

Chronic

✍ Habituated antalgic gait and posture may be observed with a strain in a weight bearing limb. A postural assessment is indicated in this case.

✍ With a Grade 2 or 3 strain, the affected muscle may be supported during activities that stress the tissue.

✍ There may be some residual chronic edema present local to the injury site with repeated strains of the same muscle.

✍ With a Grade 2 strain, an alteration in the contour of the muscle is still present. With a Grade 3 strain, the visible gap at the lesion site remains and the muscle may be bunched up if it was not surgically repaired. Fascial distortions may be noted around the injury site.

✍ If the musculotendinous unit was surgically reduced, the site should be assessed for scars.

Palpation

Acute

✍ Heat is present over the injured muscle and possibly in the surrounding tissue.

✍ Tenderness is present local to the lesion site and refers into the nearby tissue.

✍ The texture of the edema is firm. With a Grade 2 or 3 strain a hematoma may be palpable.

✍ A palpable gap or alteration in the muscle's contour is present with a Grade 2 or 3 strain.

✍ Protective muscle spasm is present in the affected muscle, the synergists and the antagonists.

Early and Late Subacute

✍ The temperature over the injury site diminishes from the early subacute to late subacute stage.

✍ Tenderness is present local to the injury.

✍ The texture of the edema is less firm. Adhesions are present as healing progresses from the early to late subacute stages. The hematoma diminishes.

✍ A palpable gap or alteration in the muscle's contour or fascial distortions may be present with a Grade 2 or 3 strain.

✍ The tone of the affected muscle and the synergists and antagonists changes from spasm in the early subacute stage to tightness and hypertonicity in the late subacute stage. Trigger points are present in these muscles.

Chronic

✍ The injury site may be cool due to ischemia.

✍ Point tenderness occurs local to the lesion site. With a rotator cuff tear, the client may be unable to sleep on the affected shoulder due to pain.

✍ Adhesions are present local to the injury site. With a rotator cuff injury, thickening and scarring of the musculotendinous tissue occur and crepitus may be present (Brukner, Khan, 1993).

✍ A palpable gap may be present with a Grade 2 or 3 strain.

✍ Hypertonicity and trigger points may be present local to the injured musculotendinous unit and in the compensating muscles. Disuse atrophy may be present in the affected muscle or the synergists if full range of motion is not present, or with a Grade 3 strain following immobilization.

Testing

The term "muscle" implies that the musculotendinous unit is being affected.

Acute

✍ **AF ROM** of the joints crossed by the affected muscle is reduced. The degree of limitation increases with the severity of the injury. With a Grade 1 strain, there is mild local pain when the muscle is contracted or stretched; the range is normal or near normal. With a Grade 2 strain, the pain is moderate and only mid ranges of movement are possible. With a Grade 3 strain, the pain is severe and there is loss of function (Booher, Thibodeau, 1989).

✍ Other testing is **contraindicated** in the acute stage if a Grade 2 or 3 strain is suspected. This is indicated by:

(1) the client hearing or feeling a snapping sensation at the time of injury,

(2) the client having difficulty continuing the activity or being unable to continue the activity,

(3)   the presence of a palpable gap in the tissue and

(4)   the AF ROM results. The client should seek medical attention *(Booher, Thibodeau, 1989).*

✐ **PR ROM** for a Grade 1 strain is performed on the cardinal planes of motion, with the range that stretches the affected muscle tested **last**. A painful, muscle spasm end feel is present before the affected muscle reaches its full length. Pain may also be encountered with tissue approximation. For example, full knee flexion could compress a strained hamstring muscle *(Magee, 1992).*

✐ **AR isometric testing** of the affected muscle with a Grade 1 strain reveals minor to insignificant loss of strength and some discomfort.

Early and Late Subacute

✐ **AF ROM** of the joints crossed by the affected muscle is reduced. The range is limited due to pain but less so than in the acute stage. Again, the degree of limitation increases with the severity of the injury.

✐ **PR ROM** is performed on the cardinal planes of motion, with the range that stretches the affected muscle tested **last**. A painful, tissue-stretch end feel is present before the affected muscle reaches its full length due to adhesions. Pain may also be encountered with tissue approximation. For example, full knee flexion could compress a strained hamstring muscle *(Magee, 1992).*

✐ **AR isometric testing** of the affected muscle is the differential assessment for a strain. To avoid further injury to the muscle, it is important that the strength of the client's contraction is gradually increased to the maximum strength and that the therapist applies gradually increased counterpressure *(Kendall et al., 1993).* The contraction is increased to the **onset of pain only.** Pain is experienced **at the injury site** itself which is, in this case, either the muscle, the musculotendinous junction or the attachment of the tendon to the bone. The severity of the strain is graded in the following manner *(Brukner, Khan, 1993; Booher, Thibodeau, 1989):*

• a **Grade 1** strain reveals minor to insignificant loss of strength and some discomfort;

• a **Grade 2** strain reveals moderate loss of strength and pain;

• a **Grade 3** strain reveals significant loss of strength and pain.

✐ **AR strength tests** are weak with a strain of the following muscles: tibialis posterior, tibialis anterior, peroneals, gluteus maximus, gluteus medius (Trendelenburg's sign), piriformis, iliopsoas, rhomboids, middle trapezius, anterior neck flexors, anterolateral neck flexors and posterolateral neck flexors.

✐ Pinpointing the location of the pain may help when attempting to differentiate strains of synergists with similar functions. By altering the position of the limbs for AR testing, specific injured muscles can be assessed.

• A strain of the following muscles may be differentiated: **gastrocnemius** and **soleus**; **medial** and **lateral hamstrings;** and the **adductors.** See Appendix C for details.

Chronic

- ✍ **AF ROM** of joints crossed by the affected muscle may be limited by any remaining pain at the end ranges of motion.

- ✍ **PR ROM** is performed on the cardinal planes of motion, with the range that stretches the affected muscle tested **last**. A mildly painful, tissue-stretch end feel may be present on fully stretching the affected muscle.

- ✍ **AR strength testing** of the affected muscle may reveal decreased muscle strength, especially with disuse atrophy or Grade 3 strains.

Contraindications

- ✦ In the acute stage, testing of a Grade 2 or 3 strain other than pain-free active free range of motion is contraindicated to prevent further tissue damage.

- ✦ Avoid removing the protective muscle splinting of acute strains.

- ✦ Distal circulation techniques are contraindicated in the acute and early subacute stages to avoid increasing congestion through the injury site.

- ✦ With Grade 3 strains that are casted, hot hydrotherapy applications should not be applied to the tissue immediately proximal to the cast to prevent congestion under the cast.

- ✦ Frictions are contraindicated if the client is taking anti-inflammatories or blood thinners.

- ✦ There is a possibility of a complication such as hematoma formation.

Special Tests

- ✍ With a Grade 3 gastrocnemius strain, a **Thompson's test** is positive. With a Grade 3 supraspinatus strain, a **drop arm test** is positive. A **Yergason's test** is positive when there is a rupture of the transverse humeral ligament which results in the subluxation of the long head of the biceps tendon. **Length tests** may reveal shortness due to the scar tissue within the musculotendinous unit following Grade 2 and 3 strains. Adductors, rectus femoris (Thomas and Ely's tests), piriformis, hamstrings (straight leg raise), iliopsoas (Thomas and Fabere tests), pectoralis minor, pectoralis major and the muscles of the rotator cuff (Apley's scratch test) may be short.

Treatment Goals   Treatment Plan

Acute

Assess the severity of the injury and refer for medical attention if moderate or severe.

Reduce inflammation.

🖑 **The muscle is treated with RICE:** Rest, Ice, Compression and Elevation. The muscle is placed in a pain-free position while the ice is applied.

🖑 **Positioning** depends on the location of the strained musculotendinous unit and the client's comfort. If the strain is in a limb, the affected limb is elevated and pillowed securely. If the strain is in the low back, a

Treatment Goals   Treatment Plan

pillow is placed under the client's abdomen while the client is prone. One or two pillows are placed under the knees while the client is supine to prevent hyperextension of the lumbar spine and aggravation of symptoms. If the strain is in the neck, a face cradle is used while the client is prone, to prevent rotation of the cervical spine.

🖐 **Hydrotherapy** in acute is cold such as an ice pack or a gel pack to the injured area.

General Treatment

🖐 If the initial treatment goal is to decrease the edema, lymphatic drainage is performed first, before any general compensatory work.

Reduce pain. Decrease sympathetic nervous system firing.

🖐 If the initial goal is to accustom the client to the therapist's touch and to decrease the sympathetic nervous system firing in the context of a relaxation massage, the treatment begins on the trunk, away from the lesion, or on the contralateral limb. The client is directed to do **diaphragmatic breathing** throughout the treatment.

Treat any compensating structures.

🖐 With a strain to a limb, the trunk and uninjured limb are treated using effleurage and slow petrissage such as palmar kneading, fingertip kneading and C-scooping. For example, the shoulders and back are treated if crutches are used. With a strain of the low back, the gluteals, leg muscles and thoracic muscles are addressed first. With a neck strain, the low back and thoracic muscles are the focus of the compensatory work.

Specific Treatment

Reduce edema.

🖐 Assuming that the initial treatment goal is to reduce the edema, lymphatic drainage techniques are used on the injured limb, beginning with nodal pumping at the proximal lymph nodes. Unidirectional effleurage, stationary circles and the local technique are used proximal to the injury to reduce edema. For lymphatic drainage of the neck and trunk, see the chapter on edema.

Maintain local circulation proximal to the injury.

🖐 If the strain is in a limb, the proximal limb is treated to reduce pain and hypertonicity as well as increase drainage and venous return. If the strain is in the trunk or neck, the synergists and antagonists are treated. Techniques include effleurage and repetitive petrissage, such as the origin and insertion technique and palmar kneading.

Reduce but do not remove protective muscle spasm.

🖐 Care is taken not to significantly reduce any protective muscle spasm in the synergists and antagonists of the injured muscle by overtreating the tissue.

Do not disturb the hematoma.

🖐 On-site work is contraindicated at this time.

🖐 Stroking and muscle squeezing are used distally for all grades of strains.

Treatment Goals   Treatment Plan

Maintain range of motion.

- Careful **mid-range passive relaxed range of motion** is used by the therapist on the proximal joints to maintain the successive action and help increase lymphatic drainage. This is only performed on joints that are not crossed by the injured muscle.

Treat other conditions.

- Any other injuries such as sprains or contusions are also treated. See the appropriate chapters for details.

Early Subacute

- The healing tissue is still fragile. Therefore, the treatment goals are achieved with care.
- The limb is once again elevated if edema is present.

Reduce inflammation.

- **Hydrotherapy applications** on site are cold/warm contrast.

General Treatment

Reduce pain. Decrease sympathetic nervous system firing. Treat compensatory structures.

- The treatment approach outlined for acute general work is indicated in this stage also, including reducing pain perception and encouraging **diaphragmatic breathing.** Rhythmic techniques to the trunk and unaffected limb are indicated if the client is comfortable with this type of work.

Specific Treatment

Reduce edema. Prevent adhesion formation.

- Proximal lymphatic drainage techniques to reduce any edema are indicated for an injured limb. These include proximal nodal pumping, unidirectional effleurage, stationary circles and the local technique. The work is performed proximal to the lesion site to prevent congestion through the injury.

Maintain local circulation proximal to the injury only.

- The proximal limb is treated to reduce hypertonicity and maintain drainage and venous return. Techniques include effleurage and repetitive petrissage, such as palmar kneading, C-scooping, fingertip kneading and the origin and insertion technique.

Reduce spasm.

- Since protective muscle spasm is no longer as important in stabilizing the injured tissue, Golgi tendon organ release is used on the tendons of the affected muscle, its synergists or its antagonists. Agonist contraction may also be used.

Reduce trigger points without disturbing the injury site.

- Trigger points in muscles that refer to the injured limb and the injury site itself are now treated using muscle stripping.
- With Grade 1 strains, on-site work consists of palmar and fingertip kneading to the client's pain tolerance. With Grade 2 and 3 strains, on-site work is restricted to light stroking and vibrations, to the client's pain tolerance.

Treatment Goals   Treatment Plan

Do not disturb the hematoma.

🖐 If a hematoma is present with a Grade 2 or 3 strain, on-site work is delayed until the late subacute stage.

Maintain range of motion.

🖐 **Mid-range passive relaxed range of motion** to the onset of pain only is used on the joints proximal and distal to the strain. This maintains the successive action and helps increase lymphatic drainage. The range that stretches the injured muscle is introduced **last.**

🖐 In a limb, distal techniques are restricted to stroking and muscle squeezing. As in the acute stage, this reduces the possibility of congesting the injury site.

Late Subacute

🖐 The healing tissue is less fragile. Therefore, the treatment goals can be achieved using more vigorous techniques.

🖐 The limb is once again elevated if edema is present.

🖐 **Hydrotherapy applications** are cold/hot contrast local to the injury. If acute inflammation recurs, the therapist returns to using local cold hydrotherapy applications.

General Treatment

🖐 The treatment approach outlined for early subacute general work is indicated in this stage also. Rhythmic techniques to the trunk and unaffected limb are indicated if the client is comfortable with this type of work.

Reduce pain. Decrease sympathetic nervous system firing. Treat any compensating structures.

Specific Treatment

Reduce edema.

🖐 As the edema diminishes in the late subacute stage, the length of time spent on lymphatic drainage techniques decreases.

Reduce hypertonicity and trigger points.

🖐 The proximal limb is treated to reduce hypertonicity and increase drainage and venous return. Trigger points in muscles that refer to the injured limb and the injury site itself are now treated directly using muscle stripping and ischemic compressions according to the client's pain tolerance. With a grade 3 strain, if ischemic compressions are used to treat the injured muscle, repetitive petrissage is used to flush circulation through the muscle instead of heat and a stretch, since this may compromise the strained tissue.

Reduce adhesions.

🖐 As the inflammation subsides with Grade 1 and 2 strains, the on-site focus shifts to reducing adhesions within the muscle. It is also important to encourage the formation of a functional scar by realigning the developing connective tissue. It is essential to accurately palpate the lesion site and any restricting adhesions before attempting

Treatment Goals   Treatment Plan

to reduce these adhesions. Myofascial release techniques, slow skin rolling and longitudinal muscle stripping are used. These are followed by specific petrissage, such as short cross-fibre strokes and frictions to the adhesions (*Hertling, Kessler, 1990; Thomson et al., 1991; Brukner, Khan, 1993*). All this work is performed within the client's pain tolerance.

- After the adhesions have been frictioned, the specific stretch that lengthens the muscle is used to realign the fibres. A **passive stretch** is performed cautiously, gently and in a pain-free manner to avoid overstretching the injured tissue. **Ice** is applied to the frictioned tissue to restrict the inflammatory process.

- Joint play techniques to the proximal and distal joints are introduced in the late subacute stage if these structures are hypomobile due to compensation.

Increase the range of motion.

- **Mid- to full range passive relaxed range of motion** to the onset of pain is used by the therapist on the joints proximal and distal to the strain. The range that stretches the injured muscle is introduced **last**.

Increase local circulation.

- The risk of causing congestion local to the strain is diminished. Effleurage and petrissage are now introduced distally to increase circulation and promote tissue health.

- With a Grade 3 strain that is immobilized, see the chapter on fractures for more details on treating the tissue proximal and distal to the cast.

- The same principles are followed for a strained muscle in the low back or neck, with an additional focus on the antagonists.

Chronic

- **Positioning** is now chosen for comfort and for accessibility to the structures that are treated. An affected limb is only elevated if chronic edema remains, otherwise it is positioned comfortably.

- **Hydrotherapy** proximal to the strain and on the lesion site itself includes deep moist heat, such as a hydrocollator or a wax application, to soften any remaining adhesions and increase local circulation.

General Treatment

Reduce sympathetic nervous system firing. Treat compensatory structures.

- The client's trunk and compensating structures are massaged as before. Rhythmic techniques to the trunk and unaffected limb are indicated.

Specific Treatment

Reduce any chronic edema.

- A pocket of chronic edema remaining local to the injury may be caused by proximal connective tissue restrictions. Fascial glide is used first to assess the restrictions. Fascial techniques used to treat the

Treatment Goals

Treatment Plan

restrictions include crossed-hands or ulnar border spreading. Proximal lymphatic drainage is also indicated once the restrictions are reduced. A **contrast hydrotherapy** application of alternating hot and cold towels is useful to flush out the edema.

Reduce hypertonicity and trigger points.

The proximal limb is treated to reduce any remaining hypertonicity or trigger points and to increase local circulation. Rhythmic techniques, effleurage, repetitive petrissage and ischemic compressions are indicated. For a trunk or neck muscle strain, the synergists and antagonists are treated.

Reduce adhesions.

If the therapist has been treating the client's injury throughout the healing process, the focus is on reducing the remaining adhesions and scar tissue. Preparatory work includes specific kneading, muscle stripping and fascial techniques. With a Grade 1 or 2 strain, cross-fibre frictions are performed on any remaining adhesions. These are followed by a passive stretch or post-isometric relaxation to the muscle to realign the fibres. An application of **ice** follows this work.

Joint play techniques to the proximal and distal joints are used if these structures are restricted due to compensation.

Restore the range of motion.

Passive relaxed range of motion is used by the therapist on the proximal, distal and affected joints to maintain joint health.

Increase local circulation.

The distal limb is treated with effleurage and petrissage to increase local venous return.

If the therapist starts treating the client in the chronic stage, one approach is to focus on reducing the hypertonicity and trigger points that have developed from the client's compensation patterns. This would be done before addressing any adhesions.

The same principles are followed for a strain in the trunk or neck.

Treat the scar if the muscle was surgically repaired.

To treat the limb during immobilization of a Grade 3 strain and for the first week after the cast is removed (when tissue health may be decreased), the therapist should refer to the chapter on fractures. When tissue health has improved, the adhesions and the scar itself are treated as described above. Joint play and passive stretching are also indicated to increase mobility.

Self-care Goals

Self-care Plan

Educate the client.

Hydrotherapy is chosen that is appropriate for the stage of healing. Because tendons are hypovascular, it is important to introduce contrast hydrotherapy to help increase local circulation as soon as the acute stage has passed.

Self-massage is useful for the affected muscle in the late subacute and chronic stages. This includes skin rolling, muscle stripping and

Self-care Goals

Self-care Plan

gentle frictions to the client's pain tolerance. Frictions are useful with Grade 3 strains once the tone has returned to the tissues that were under the cast.

Maintain strength of the affected muscle in a pain-free manner.

✍ **Remedial exercise** that is given is dependent on the stage of healing and the severity of the injury. To avoid a repeated strain or tendon rupture, training programs for fitness or strength should be designed to **gradually** strengthen the muscles and tendons. This gradual approach also applies to stretching. It is, therefore, important in any of the acute and subacute exercises to work to the onset of pain only. In this way, contractile tissue can withstand incrementally heavier workloads or increasing stretches without reinjury.

✍ In the **acute** stage, with a Grade 1 strain, the client is asked to perform pain-free active free range of motion of the distal and proximal joints. With a Grade 2 strain, submaximal pain-free isometric contractions of the muscle are performed in **inner** ranges (Brukner, Khan, 1993). With a Grade 3 strain, the client's physician will indicate when isometric exercises and stretching can begin. A gentle stretch to the onset of pain only is indicated with Grade 1 and 2 strains (Brukner, Khan, 1993). Further remedial exercise is contraindicated in the acute stage with Grade 2 and 3 strains.

Stretch shortened muscles.

✍ In the **early subacute** stage, with Grade 1 and 2 strains, the client can perform pain-free active free range of motion of the proximal and distal joints. As soon as possible, the client begins to increase the stretch, again to the onset of pain only. With Grade 2 strains, the submaximal isometric contractions are gradually progressed and performed from inner to mid-ranges.

Gradually increase strength.

✍ In the **late subacute** stage, all stretches and strengthening exercises are gradually increased in duration and repetitions. These are progressed to active resisted isotonic concentric and eccentric exercises once activities that stretch or contract the musculotendinous unit are pain free both during and after the exercise (Brukner, Khan, 1993).

✍ In the **chronic** stage, the focus continues to be on active resisted isotonic concentric and eccentric exercise. With a Grade 3 strain that was immobilized, once the cast is removed and tone has returned to the tissues, stretching and strengthening of the affected muscles begin. With a Grade 3 strain that was not surgically repaired, the synergists are strengthened.

Encourage activity.

✍ The client is encouraged to return to the activities that caused the injury on a gradual basis to avoid reinjury. With repeated strains, the client can resume stretching and activity gradually **once the symptoms and pain have ceased** (Booher, Thibodeau, 1989; Brukner, Khan, 1993).

301

Self-care Goals

Self-care Plan

✍ The client may need to use tape, a brace or other supports to protect a Grade 2 or 3 strain on activity, especially in a weight bearing limb.

Treatment Frequency and Expected Outcome

Shorter, more frequent treatments will address the inflammatory process in the acute stages. Treatment should progress to once a week for chronic stages, then the client is reassessed.

The outcome is variable, depending on the severity of the injury, the treatment approach used (strengthening exercises and soft tissue work, immobilization or surgery) and the client's age, general health and compliance with the self-care program.

See stress reduction, edema, spasm, contusions, sprains, dislocations, fractures, tendinitis, scars and whiplash for related treatments.

✦ **Return to activity** (the following are guidelines only):

• Grade 1 strain – the client can return to the activity with support such as an elastic bandage after two days;

• Grade 2 strain – the client can resume activity several days to several weeks after injury (*Booher, Thibodeau, 1989; Hertling, Kessler, 1990*);

• Grade 3 strain – immobilization is generally removed at four to eight weeks (*Brukner, Khan, 1993*). Return to activity follows this and may be delayed for up to several weeks due to disuse atrophy.

Sample Treatment: Grade 2 Biceps Femoris Strain

Acute

✋ The client is in a comfortable position, likely prone, with the injured leg pillowed so the knee is flexed and no stretch is placed on the hamstring. An ice pack is placed over the injury site and the client is instructed to breathe diaphragmatically. Lymphatic drainage techniques are used on the affected leg, starting with sacral pumping and treating the gluteals and proximal leg. Lymphatic drainage is stopped just proximal to the edema. Swedish techniques are used on the uninjured limb to treat the compensating structures and decrease sympathetic nervous system firing and pain. The gluteals on the injured side and the upper thigh are treated with Swedish techniques, working proximal to the injury site only and being careful not to completely reduce the protective muscle spasm. If the treatment duration is 45 minutes to one hour, the low back, shoulders, neck and head can be included, especially if the client is using crutches.

✍ For **self-care**, the client is instructed to rest (no weight bearing) and ice and elevate the limb in a position that does not stretch the muscle. Pain-free isometric exercises for the quadriceps, gluteals, iliopsoas, gastrocnemius, soleus and tibialis anterior are performed. A gentle stretch of the hamstrings to the onset of pain **only** may be performed. Submaximal isometrics of the hamstrings in the **inner** range may be used.

Early Subacute

✋ The treatment plan for the early subacute stage is much the same as for the acute stage in terms of positioning and lymphatic drainage. Contrast hydrotherapy can be applied to the strained muscle. Then the uninjured leg is treated. Swedish techniques for the unaffected and affected leg are similar to the acute stage, except the focus is on reducing spasms using Golgi tendon organ release at the ischial tuberosity. Trigger points are treated, specifically those in the gluteus minimus, piriformis and vastus lateralis that may refer into the posterolateral thigh. Pain-free passive relaxed range of motion is done in the following order: external and internal rotation of the hip; knee and hip flexion. Gentle on-site vibrations, stroking and muscle squeezing are indicated as long as no hematoma is present.

✋ Distal Swedish techniques include stroking and muscle squeezing of the leg.

✍ **Self-care** isometrics are performed in the inner to mid-ranges or with the knee in some flexion. In terms of self-stretch, the client is shown a seated stretch with the knee in extension and the torso flexed forward at the hips. Once again, the stretch is to the onset of pain only to prevent reinjury. The client can include varying amounts of internal and external rotation of the femur to make the stretch the most effective. The upper hamstrings are stretched in the standing position by the client putting the heel of the injured leg up on a chair with the knee flexed. The client then leans the torso forward from the hips *(Brukner, Khan, 1993)*.

Late Subacute

✋ The treatment plan for the early subacute stage is also followed in regard to positioning. Less time is spent on lymphatic drainage. Proximal techniques include petrissage and trigger point work. Specific work to the strained hamstring includes a myofascial release. The client's knee is passively flexed in mid-range and then slowly extended as the therapist muscle strips distally to proximally over the lesion site using his ulnar border *(Brukner, Khan, 1993)*. Skin rolling, longitudinal muscle stripping and short cross-fibre strokes to the adhesions are performed next. All this work is done within the client's pain tolerance. Circulation techniques are introduced to the distal affected leg.

In supine position the anterior legs are treated. A passive stretch is used to lengthen the hamstrings after frictions. Again, this is performed to the client's pain tolerance. This is followed with an application of ice. Passive relaxed range of motion of the knee and hip are performed.

If it is comfortable for the client, the quadriceps, tensor fascia lata and iliopsoas muscles are treated to reduce hypertonicity and any trigger points. An injury to the hamstring may also affect the sacroiliac joint. If this structure is hypomobile, joint play techniques are used.

The client continues with the isometric exercises and **self-stretches**, gradually increasing them.

Chronic

The client is started in a prone position to treat the low back, gluteals and posterior legs. Hypertonicity and compensatory changes are treated as in the previous stages. Trigger points in the vastus lateralis referring into the lateral leg and trigger points in the piriformis and gluteus medius referring into the hamstrings are addressed. Fascial techniques and frictions are performed on the lesion site. When the client is turned supine, Swedish techniques are used on the anterior legs to increase local circulation. Joint play on the sacroiliac joint and knee, as well as fascial techniques for restrictions, are used if indicated. Passive relaxed ranges of the affected hip and knee are performed, with a straight leg raise done last.

The client's gait patterns are reassessed and corrected if necessary to prevent reinjury.

For **self-care**, once length and strength have been regained in the hamstrings, stretching of the quadriceps, adductors, gluteals and iliopsoas is important. Gradually, the client will return to activities such as running or cycling. The client may need to tape the thigh when exercising to prevent reinjury.

24

SPRAINS

Fiona Rattray

A sprain is an overstretch injury to a ligament.

Ligaments are composed of flexible, noncontractile connective tissue. They occur in bands around a synovial joint, blending into the periosteum and joining bones together *(Thomson et al., 1991)*. Ligaments add stability to the connective tissue joint capsule. They are named according to the bones they attach to and their anatomical position. For example, the anterior talofibular ligament joins the talus to the fibula at the front of the ankle. Ligaments limit and control the range of motion at a joint, while allowing the motion to occur. A ligament is taut at the end range of the motion it prevents and is slack both in mid-range and at the end range of the motion opposite that which it prevents.

➤ **The cause of a sprain is a trauma-related sudden twist or wrench of the joint beyond its normal range of motion.**

➤ **Contributing factors** include congenital ligamentous laxity (hypermobility), a history of previous sprains to that joint, altered biomechanics that place stress on the ligament and joint, and connective tissue pathologies, such as rheumatoid arthritis.

Other soft tissue injuries such as strains and contusions may occur with a sprain. Also, an osteochondral fracture to the articular cartilage may be present in conjunction with a sprain.

✦ Sprains are classified into **three levels of severity** *(Booher, Thibodeau, 1989)*.

• **Grade 1, Mild or First Degree Sprain:** This is a minor stretch and tear to the ligament. There is no instability on passive relaxed testing. The person can continue with the activity with some discomfort.

• **Grade 2, Moderate or Second Degree Sprain:** Tearing of the ligament fibres occurs. The degree of tear is quite variable, from several fibres to the majority of the fibres. There is a snapping sound at the time of injury and the joint gives way. The joint is hypermobile yet stable on passive relaxed testing. The person has difficulty continuing the activity due to pain.

- **Grade 3, Severe or Third Degree Sprain:** This is either a complete rupture of the ligament itself, or an avulsion fracture as the bony attachment of the ligament is torn off while the ligament remains intact. There is a snapping sound and the joint gives way. There is significant instability with no end point on passive relaxed testing. The person cannot continue the activity due to pain and instability. Pain is present in the acute stage, while a chronic sprain may be painlessly hypermobile in the direction the ligament is intended to check *(Hertling, Kessler, 1990)*.

In the acute stage, the client should be referred to a physician if the health history reveals that there is significant instability at the joint (the joint "gave way with a snapping sound") or if there is significant joint effusion — for example, at the knee *(Booher, Thibodeau, 1989)*.

Joint effusion occurs when the injury is severe enough to inflame the synovium, increasing the production of synovial fluid and causing the joint capsule to swell. Effusion is primarily composed of synovial fluid and is intracapsular. Hemarthrosis, or bleeding into the synovial space, may also happen. In contrast, edema occurs in the extracapsular interstitial spaces, as a result of the inflammatory process. Unlike joint effusion, edema is composed of inflammatory exudate.

Ligaments are moderately vascularized and, consequently, heal slowly. Adhesions form between the sprained ligament and nearby structures, painfully limiting the range of motion controlled by the ligament and predisposing the joint to further injury *(Thomson et al., 1991)*. Especially in the ankle, adhesions can form *within* the joint itself, even with a Grade 1 sprain *(Brillhart, 1994; Apley, Solomon, 1993)*. With Grade 2 sprains, new collagen is laid down in the first one to two weeks after injury *(Hertling, Kessler, 1990)*. Scar tissue in the ligaments takes six weeks to develop. However, it takes a full six months for scar tissue to completely mature and provide maximum strength at the affected joint *(Booher, Thibodeau, 1989)*.

Ligaments in Grade 3 sprains may be surgically repaired or treated by the medically conservative approach of immobilizing the joint in a cast or strapping. At the knee, the medial collateral ligament may be repaired using sutures or a portion of the semitendinosus muscle *(Siliski, 1994)*. In either case, the knee is immobilized for up to 10 weeks in a hinged cast or brace to minimize muscular atrophy *(Brukner, Khan, 1993)*. One source notes that while surgically repaired ankle ligaments do give a more stable joint, the patients suffers more residual pain and swelling in the months following the surgery than those patients treated by the conservative approach of casting only. Of those patients treated conservatively, there appeared to be little difference in joint stability between those casted for six weeks and patients who had strapping to immobilize and support the joint *(Hertling, Kessler, 1990)*.

Common Sprains

While a sprain may occur at any joint, three joints that are commonly sprained are the ankle, knee and wrist. Other joints that are prone to sprains include the acromioclavicular joint ("shoulder separation"), the humeroulnar joint and all the joints in the digits.

Numerous **ankle** ligaments can be injured, such as the anterior talofibular ligament, the

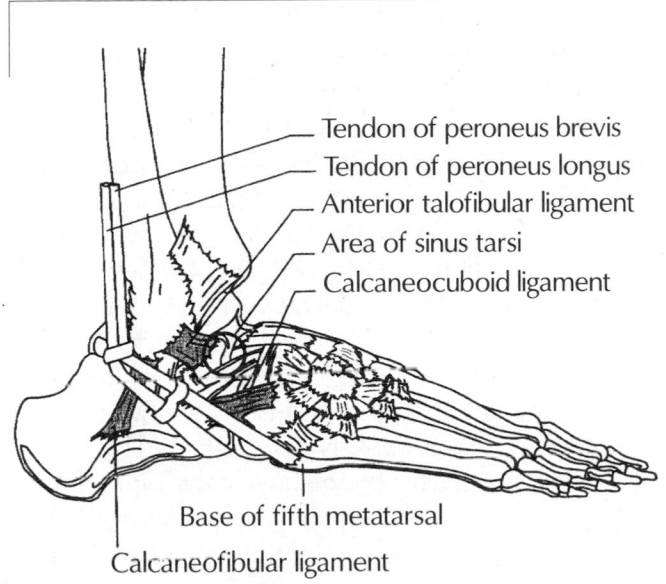

- Tendon of peroneus brevis
- Tendon of peroneus longus
- Anterior talofibular ligament
- Area of sinus tarsi
- Calcaneocuboid ligament

Base of fifth metatarsal

Calcaneofibular ligament

Figure 24.1
Ankle ligaments, lateral view.

calcaneofibular ligament and the calcaneocuboid ligament *(Figure 24.1)*. The most common mechanism of injury is an inversion sprain, where the ankle is forcefully inverted, damaging ligaments on the lateral side of the joint. The person may describe this as "going over on" the ankle. Most frequently sprained is the anterior talofibular ligament. The calcaneofibular ligament is the second most commonly sprained lateral ankle ligament, often injured in conjunction with the anterior talofibular ligament. The calcaneocuboid ligament is less frequently injured.

An eversion sprain, where the ankle is forced into eversion, is less usual. Here, the deltoid ligament on the medial side of the ankle is at risk. Since the deltoid is quite strong, it is more common for the attachment at the tibia to avulse than for the ligament itself to rupture.

However, occasionally, the superficial anterior deltoid fibres are partially torn *(Rockwood et al., 1991)*.

An ankle sprain that does not resolve in the expected time frame and that remains swollen and painful may have an associated osteochondral fracture. The client should be referred for medical assessment *(Brukner, Khan, 1993)*.

In terms of the **knee**, the medial and lateral collateral ligaments as well as the anterior and posterior cruciate ligaments can be sprained *(Figure 24.2)*. Of the two collateral ligaments, the medial collateral is the most frequently injured, often when the foot is fixed to the ground and the knee is struck by a medially directed or valgus force. A laterally directed or varus force to the knee causes a lateral collateral sprain, although this is uncommon. The anterior cruciate is injured when the tibia is forced anteriorly, usually when the person is weight bearing through the leg. If the tibia is pushed posteriorly, the posterior cruciate ligament is injured.

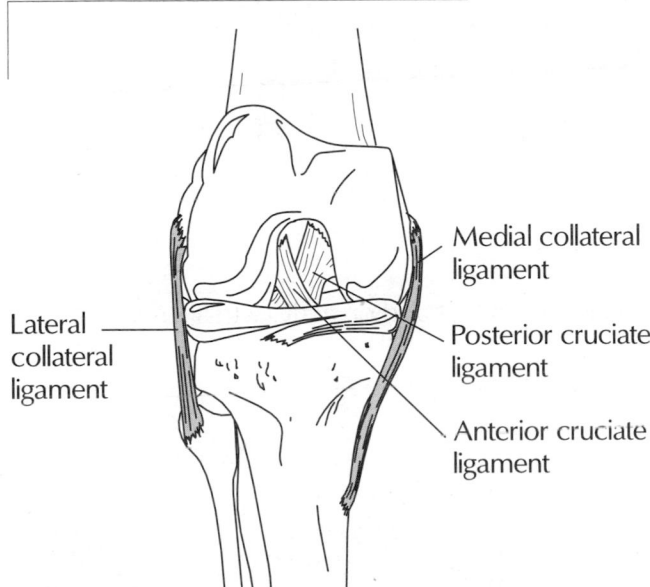

Lateral collateral ligament

Medial collateral ligament

Posterior cruciate ligament

Anterior cruciate ligament

Figure 24.2
Knee ligaments, anterior view.

Since the collateral ligaments are extracapsular, massage therapy can directly treat them, using the techniques outlined in this chapter. The cruciates are deep within the joint and are not directly accessible to massage techniques. These ligaments are often surgically repaired. Massage for these injuries entails treating the edema as well as the scar tissue resulting from the surgery. Self-care includes a strengthening program for

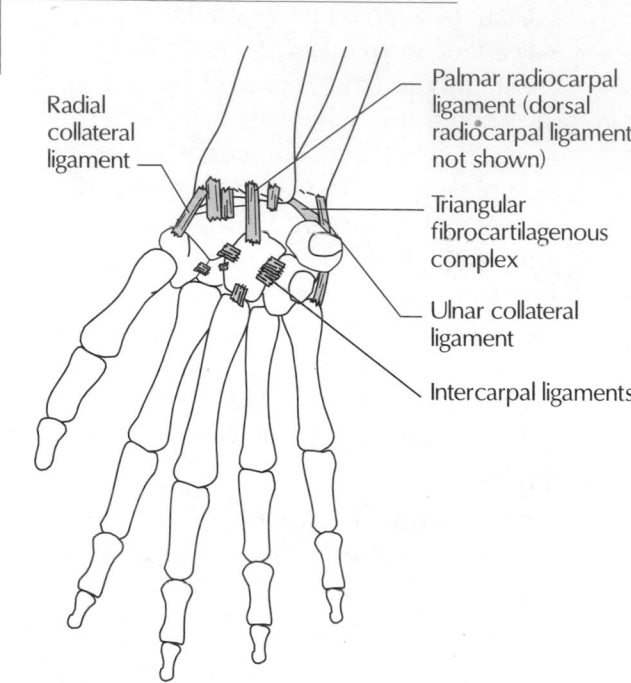

Figure 24.3
Wrist ligaments, palmar view.

Radial collateral ligament

Palmar radiocarpal ligament (dorsal radiocarpal ligament not shown)

Triangular fibrocartilagenous complex

Ulnar collateral ligament

Intercarpal ligaments

muscles crossing the knee. (Refer to the following chapter on meniscal and cruciate injuries for more information.)

There are numerous **wrist** ligaments that can be sprained *(Figure 24.3)*. These include the palmar radiocarpal, dorsal radiocarpal, ulnar and radial collateral and intercarpal ligaments as well as the triangular fibrocartilaginous complex between the ulna and the medial carpal bones *(Brukner, Khan, 1993)*. The most common mechanism of injury to the wrist is forced hyperextension. Since the palmar radiocarpal ligaments are quite strong, they are unlikely to be sprained in isolation. Usually accompanying this type of sprain is damage to the flexor muscles and tendons and the bones of the wrist. The weaker dorsal radiocarpal ligaments may be damaged with a forced hyperflexion injury, possibly in association with injury to the extensor tendons and wrist bones. Since there is a possibility of fracture, a person with an acute wrist sprain should be referred for medical attention *(Booher, Thibodeau, 1989)*.

It should be noted that, at the **shoulder**, a Grade 1 acromioclavicular sprain involves tearing of the joint capsule. A Grade 2 sprain is classified as a tear of the joint capsule and the acromioclavicular ligament, while a Grade 3 sprain involves a tear of the joint capsule, the acromioclavicular ligament and the conoid and trapezoid ligaments. A fracture may also be present. The mechanism of injury is usually falling onto the shoulder itself *(Brukner, Khan, 1993)*.

Symptom Picture

Acute

✦ **Grade 1:** There is a minor stretch to the ligament.

• The pain is mild and is local to the injury site at rest and on activity that stresses the ligament.

• Minimum local edema, heat and bruising are present.

• The joint is stable.

• The client can continue the activity.

✦ **Grade 2:** There is tearing of some or many fibres of the ligament.

• There is a snapping noise and the joint gives way.

• The pain is moderate at rest and with activities that stress the ligament.

- Moderate local edema, heat and bruising are present.
- Joint instability, if present, is slight.
- The client has difficulty continuing the activity due to pain.

✦ **Grade 3:** There is a complete rupture of the ligament or an avulsion fracture of the ligament attachment.
  - There is a snapping noise.
  - The pain may be intense or mild at rest.
  - Marked local edema, heat and bruising are present.
  - A hematoma may be present. Joint effusion may occur if the joint capsule is damaged. If blood goes into the joint space, a hemarthrosis occurs.
  - The joint is unstable.
  - The client cannot continue the activity.

✦ In **all grades of sprain** the following occur:
  - The bruising is red, black and blue.
  - There is decreased range of motion local to the joint as protective muscle spasm, edema and pain limit movement.
  - Depending on the severity, there is little, moderate or severe loss of function of the affected joint. The joint may be taped, splinted or otherwise supported. With a lower limb sprain, the client may use crutches. With a Grade 3 sprain, the ruptured ligament may be surgically repaired, then immobilized. Other structures compensate for this.
  - A strain or contusion of the muscles crossing the joint, vascular damage or nerve complications are possible with Grade 2 and 3 sprains.

Early Subacute

✦ A **Grade 1** sprain is stable, a **Grade 2** sprain is hypermobile yet stable and a **Grade 3** sprain is hypermobile and unstable with ligamentous stress testing.

✦ The bruising is black and blue.

✦ The pain, edema and inflammation are still present but reduced from the acute stage.

✦ Adhesions are developing around the injury. In the ankle, intra-articular adhesions range from a single band to multiple tissue bands which form a dense network of connective tissue. Even a Grade 1 sprain can form adhesions (*Brillhart, 1994*).

✦ Since ligaments are hypovascular, they heal relatively slowly. The protective muscle spasm diminishes. Trigger points occur in the muscles crossing the joint and in compensatory muscles.

✦ Depending on the severity, the injured joint may be taped, splinted or immobilized. The client may still be using crutches or a cane in a lower limb sprain or a sling with an upper limb sprain.

✦ The range of motion is reduced.

✦ There is a loss of proprioception at the joint.

Late Subacute

✦ The bruising changes to yellow, green and brown.

✦ The pain, edema and inflammation are diminishing.

✦ Adhesions are maturing around the injury.

✦ The protective muscle spasm is replaced by increased tone of the muscles crossing the joint.

✦ The affected joint may still be supported. The client may still use crutches or a cane.

✦ The range of motion is reduced.

✦ There is a loss of proprioception at the joint.

Chronic

✦ There is pain local to the ligament only if the ligament is stressed.

✦ The bruising is gone.

✦ Adhesions have matured around the injury.

✦ Hypertonicity and trigger points are present in muscles crossing the joint and in compensating structures.

✦ Full range of motion of the joint is restricted.

✦ A pocket of chronic edema may remain local to the ligament.

✦ The tissue may be cool due to ischemia.

✦ There is a loss of proprioception at the joint.

✦ The joint is unstable with a Grade 3 sprain unless it is surgically repaired. The joint may be immobilized for up to 10 weeks after surgery.

✦ Muscle weakness or disuse atrophy may be present in muscles crossing the affected joint, particularly with immobilization.

✦ The client may need taping or elastic bandages for activities that stress the joint.

Subjective Information

HEALTH HISTORY QUESTIONS

✦ What is the client's overall health history? Is the client on any medication for unrelated conditions that indicate treatment modifications?

✦ Does the client have any contributing conditions or pathologies that predispose him to ligament injuries, such as rheumatoid arthritis or congenital ligamentous laxity?

✦ Has there been a history of injury or recurrent sprains of this joint? If yes, is osteoarthritis present?

◆ In terms of the presenting complaint, when did the injury occur?

◆ Does the client know the mechanism of injury — for example, "going over" on an ankle with an ankle sprain; being struck from the side when the foot is planted and the knee is flexed with a knee sprain; or falling on an outstretched hand with a wrist sprain?

◆ Did the client hear any noise at the time of the injury? For example, *a popping sound in the knee indicates a cruciate injury, not a collateral ligament injury*. A snapping noise in the ankle may occur with a Grade 2 or 3 sprain.

◆ What was done at the time of injury? Was first aid applied?

◆ Was the client able to continue with the activity after the sprain? With a Grade 1 sprain, the client could continue the activity but had pain on stressing the joint. With a Grade 2 injury, the client had difficulty continuing the activity. With a Grade 3 injury, the client was unable to continue the activity *(Edwardson, 1995)*.

◆ Did the client see any other health care practitioner for this injury, such as a physician, physiotherapist, chiropractor or sports therapist? If so, what treatment was given? Is the client still receiving this treatment?

◆ Is the client taking any medication for the sprain, such as analgesics or anti-inflammatories? This includes self-medication such as Aspirin or other over-the-counter products.

◆ With a Grade 3 sprain, was the joint immobilized or was the ligament surgically reduced? If the joint was immobilized, how long was this for? With immobilization, disuse atrophy and adhesions may be present.

◆ Were there any complications, such as nerve damage or an avulsion at the ligament's attachment?

◆ Is the client using any supports or crutches for the affected joint? This is expected with an acute or subacute sprain of any severity. A weight bearing joint that repeatedly sprains may require an elastic bandage or other support when the client is performing an activity that stresses the joint.

◆ What symptoms is the client currently experiencing? Does the client have pain now? Where exactly is the pain? Is the pain sharp or diffuse? Sharp, hot pain indicates an acute injury, while an ache is associated with a chronic injury.

◆ What aggravates or relieves the pain?

◆ Is any swelling or any edema present local or distal to the injury? Swelling that occurred rapidly after the injury — for example, within 20 minutes to one hour — may indicate a hemarthrosis (blood within the synovial cavity) or a hematoma.

  • The client should be referred for medical treatment which usually involves aspiration of the joint since hemarthrosis causes erosion of the cartilage. Swelling that occurred within eight to 24 hours likely indicates synovial effusion *(Magee, 1992)*.

  • However, the amount of swelling does not necessarily indicate the degree of the injury. With a severe sprain of the medial collateral ligament of the knee which ruptures the joint capsule, it is possible for the synovial fluid to leak out of the joint slowly *(Hertling, Kessler, 1990)*.

◆ With a sprain of a weight bearing joint, does the joint "give way"? This indicates altered proprioception due to adhesions within the joint capsule. Does the joint lock in one position? This indicates a loose body within the joint capsule. In the ankle, the loose body may be intra-articular adhesions with any grade of sprain or a portion of a ruptured ligament with a Grade 3 sprain. In the knee, locking indicates meniscal damage rather than collateral ligament damage.

◆ What activities are difficult or painful to complete? For example, there is an inability to turn quickly with a medial or lateral collateral knee sprain. The client may be unable to turn a door knob with a wrist sprain.

◆ What are the client's activities of daily living? Does the client's occupation or recreational activity place stress on the joint?

Objective Information

Observations

Acute

✍ Antalgic gait occurs if the sprain is in a weight bearing joint. The more severe the injury, the less the client is able to weight bear. For example, in terms of an ankle sprain, the client with a Grade 1 sprain may limp but can bear weight. With a Grade 2 sprain, there is a "foot flat" gait, where heel strike and toe off are lacking. In a Grade 3 sprain, the client is unable to weight bear at all *(Edwardson, 1995)*.

✍ The affected joint may be supported by taping, elastic bandages or splints. With Grade 3 sprains, the joint may be casted. The client will use crutches with more severe sprains of weight bearing joints. A sling may be used with a wrist or elbow sprain.

✍ Antalgic posture may be present. For example, with a Grade 2 collateral ligament knee sprain, the limb is held in a position of non-weight-bearing with the knee slightly flexed *(Brukner, Khan, 1993)*.

✍ The client may have a pained or medicated facial expression.

✍ Edema is present at the affected joint. There is minimal edema with a Grade 1 sprain, moderate edema with a Grade 2 sprain and marked edema with a Grade 3 sprain. There may be distal edema.

✍ Some redness may be present local to the injury.

✍ Red, black or purple bruising may be visible over the injury site. A hematoma may be present with a Grade 2 or 3 sprain.

Early and Late Subacute

✍ Antalgic gait is still present with a sprain of a weight bearing joint. It has diminished from the presentation in the acute stage.

✍ Antalgic posture may also occur.

✍ Supports may still be present. With Grade 3 sprains, the joint may still be casted. The client will still use crutches with more severe sprains of weight bearing joints. A sling may still be used with a wrist or elbow sprain.

✍ Edema diminishes from the early to late subacute stage, both on site and distally.

✍ Bruising over the injury site changes from purple and black in the early subacute stage to brown, yellow and green in the late subacute stage and then disappears. There may be distal bruising. If present, the hematoma is diminishing.

✍ If the ligament was surgically reduced, scars are present. These range from half a centimetre long following arthroscopic surgery to several centimetres in length with open reductions.

Chronic

✍ Habituated antalgic gait and posture may be observed with a sprain of a weight bearing joint. A postural assessment is indicated in this case.

✍ Taping or other supports may be used during activities that stress the joint. Following surgery, a Grade 3 sprain may still be immobilized. The client may use crutches or a cane.

✍ There may be some residual chronic edema present local to the ligament. This usually occurs with repeated sprains of the same joint.

✍ If the ligament was surgically reduced, scars are present.

Palpation
Acute

✍ Heat is present over the injured ligament and possibly in the surrounding tissue.

✍ Tenderness is present local to the lesion site and refers into the nearby tissue.

✍ The texture of the edema is firm.

✍ Protective muscle spasm is present in muscles crossing the affected joint.

Early and Late Subacute

✍ The temperature over the injury site diminishes from the early subacute to late subacute stage.

✍ Tenderness is present local to the injury.

✍ The texture of the edema is less firm and adhesions are present as healing progresses from the early to late subacute stage.

✍ The tone of the muscles crossing the joint changes from spasm in the early subacute stage to tightness and hypertonicity in late subacute. Trigger points are present in these muscles.

Chronic

✍ The injury site may be cool due to ischemia.

✍ Point tenderness occurs local to the lesion site.

✍ Any remaining chronic edema has a boggy, possibly jelly-like feel. There are adhesions local to the ligament. Crepitus may be present.

✍ Hypertonicity and trigger points are local to the injured joint and in the compensating muscles. Disuse atrophy may be present in muscles crossing the affected joint if full range of motion is not present or if the sprain was severe enough to be immobilized.

Testing
Acute

✍ **AF ROM** of the proximal, affected and distal joints is performed. The range of the affected joint is limited due to pain. The degree of limitation increases with an increased severity of injury. For example, the range of motion is less limited with a Grade 1 sprain than with a Grade 2 sprain. The range of motion is severely limited with a Grade 3 sprain due to the protective muscle spasm and edema.

Acute Special Tests

✍ The **ballottable patella** and **minor effusion tests** may be performed at the knee, if there is swelling, to rule out severe injuries. Other testing is **contraindicated** in the acute stage.

Early and Late Subacute

✍ **AF ROM** of the proximal, affected and distal joints is performed. The range of the affected joint is limited due to pain but less so than in the acute stage. Again, the degree of limitation increases with the severity of the injury.

✍ **PR ROM** is performed slowly on the cardinal planes of motion of the affected joint, with the range that the injury occurred in tested **last**. The pain is perceived by the client in the range that stresses the injured ligament. There is reduced range of motion. A muscle-spasm end feel or an empty end feel may be present.

✍ **AR isometric testing** reveals that the muscles crossing the affected joint are strong and painless with a strictly ligamentous injury. If muscles or tendons are also involved, there is pain at the lesion site in the contractile tissue.

Early and Late Subacute Special Tests

✍ To determine if a specific ligament has been injured, the affected joint is taken through the range that moves the two bony attachments of the ligament farther apart. This procedure is called a **ligamentous stress test.** A slow and careful overpressure is applied at the end of the passive movement, which stresses the ligament. The amount of pressure used is sufficient to stress the ligament without damaging it.

✍ Physicians use overpressure to determine the severity of an acute sprain, often in an emergency room. However, it is contraindicated for massage therapists to use overpressure in the acute stage of any sprain in order to avoid further damaging the injured ligament. Careful overpressure is only introduced in the **subacute** and **chronic** stages to assess the sprain.

✍ The severity of the sprain is graded in the following manner *(Brukner, Khan, 1993; Buschbacher, 1994; Cailliet, 1988):*

- a **Grade 1** sprain is painful local to the ligament on overpressure at the end of passive range. The joint end feel is stable;

- a **Grade 2** sprain is painful local to the ligament on overpressure at the end of passive range. The joint end feel is **hypermobile but stable.** This may also be described as joint laxity with a firm end feel;

- a **Grade 3** sprain may or may not be painful local to the ligament on overpressure at the end of passive range. The joint end feel is **hypermobile and unstable.** This may also be described as joint laxity without a firm end feel. With a Grade 3 sprain, the ligament is ruptured. Therefore, the nerve receptors that register pain are not stretched by the testing procedure and the joint is painlessly hypermobile.

✍ As the injury resolves from acute through to chronic, the severity of the pain elicited by stressing the ligament will diminish.

✍ With an ankle sprain, depending on the ligament involved, one of **anterior drawer ankle, anterior talofibular, calcaneofibular, calcaneocuboid** or **deltoid ligament tests** is positive.

✍ With collateral ligament knee sprains, depending on the ligament involved, **valgus** or **varus** and **Apley's distraction tests** are positive. The **ballottable patella** and **brush tests** which assess for intracapsular joint effusion in the acute stage are negative with a simple collateral knee sprain. The **anterior-posterior drawer, Lachman's, McMurray's, Bragard's Sign** and **Apley's compression tests**, which check the cruciate ligaments and the menisci, are also negative with a simple collateral ligament knee sprain.

✍ With wrist sprains, depending on the ligament involved, one of **radial stress, PR wrist extension, PR wrist flexion** or **ulnar stress tests** is positive.

✍ Other stress tests for specific ligaments include **acromioclavicular shear test** for the acromioclavicular joint and **sacroiliac joint gapping, sacroiliac joint "squish"** and **Gaenslen's tests** for the sacroiliac joint.

Chronic

✍ **AF ROM** of the affected joint may be limited by any remaining pain at the end ranges of motion.

✍ **PR ROM** is performed on the cardinal planes of motion, with the range that the injury occurred in tested **last.** A painful, possibly hypermobile end feel is present on fully stressing the affected ligament.

✍ **AR testing** of muscles crossing the affected joint is done, checking for possible decreased muscle strength with disuse atrophy or with associated injury to muscles or tendons.

Chronic Special Tests

✍ A **ligamentous stress test** for the injured ligament is positive with a hypermobile end feel in Grade 2 and 3 sprains.

Contraindications

✦ In the acute stage, testing other than pain-free AF range of motion is contraindicated to prevent further tissue damage.

✦ Avoid removing the protective muscle splinting of acute sprains.

✦ Distal circulation techniques are contraindicated in the acute and early subacute stages to avoid increasing congestion through the injury site.

✦ With Grade 3 sprains that are casted, avoid hot hydrotherapy applications to the tissue immediately proximal to the cast to prevent congestion under the cast.

✦ With Grade 3 sprains where the ligaments have been surgically repaired, do not restore full range of motion of the affected joint in the direction that will stretch the repaired ligament. Where the ligaments have not been surgically reduced, joint play of the unstable joint is contraindicated.

✦ Frictions are contraindicated if the client is taking anti-inflammatories or blood thinners.

Treatment Goals

Treatment Plan

Acute

Assess the severity of the injury and refer for medical attention if moderate or severe.

Reduce inflammation.

🖐 **The injury is treated with RICE:** Rest, Ice, Compression and Elevation.

🖐 **Positioning** depends on the location of the sprain and the client's comfort. The limb is elevated and pillowed securely.

🖐 **Hydrotherapy** is cold such as an ice pack or a gel pack applied to the injured area.

General Treatment

🖐 If the initial treatment goal is to decrease the edema, lymphatic drainage on the affected limb is performed first before any compensatory work.

Reduce pain. Decrease sympathetic nervous system firing.

🖐 If the initial goal is to accustom the client to the therapist's touch and to decrease sympathetic nervous system firing in the context of a relaxation massage, the client is directed to do **diaphragmatic breathing** throughout the treatment.

Treat any compensating structures.

🖐 The trunk and uninjured limb are treated using effleurage and slow petrissage, such as palmar kneading, fingertip kneading and C-scooping. The focus of the work depends on the muscles that are compensating. For example, the shoulders and back are treated if crutches are used.

Treatment Goals Treatment Plan

Specific Treatment

Reduce edema.

ꟷ Lymphatic drainage techniques are used on the injured limb, beginning with nodal pumping at the proximal lymph nodes. Unidirectional effleurage, stationary circles and the local technique are used proximal to the injury to reduce edema.

Maintain local circulation proximal to the injury only.

ꟷ The proximal limb is treated to reduce pain and hypertonicity as well as to increase drainage and venous return. Techniques include effleurage and repetitive petrissage, such as the origin and insertion technique and palmar kneading.

Reduce but do not remove protective muscle spasm.

ꟷ Care is taken not to significantly reduce any protective muscle spasm in muscles that cross the affected joint by overtreating the tissue.

ꟷ On-site work is contraindicated.

ꟷ Distal work is restricted to light stroking and muscle squeezing for all grades of sprains.

Maintain range of motion.

ꟷ Careful **mid-range passive relaxed range of motion** is used on the proximal joints to maintain the successive action and to help increase lymphatic drainage. This is only performed on joints that are not crossed by muscles that also cross the sprained joint.

Treat other conditions.

ꟷ Any secondary injuries, such as strains or contusions, are also treated. See the appropriate chapters for details.

Early Subacute

The healing tissue is still fragile. Therefore, the treatment goals are achieved with care. Reduce inflammation.

ꟷ The limb is once again elevated.

ꟷ **Hydrotherapy applications** on site are cold/warm.

General Treatment

Reduce pain. Decrease sympathetic nervous system firing.

ꟷ The treatment approach outlined for acute general work is indicated at this stage also, including reducing pain perception and encouraging **diaphragmatic breathing**. Rhythmic techniques to the trunk and unaffected limb are indicated if the client is comfortable with this type of work.

Specific Treatment

Reduce edema. Prevent excess adhesion formation.

ꟷ Proximal lymphatic drainage techniques to reduce the edema are indicated for the injured limb. These include proximal nodal pumping, unidirectional effleurage, stationary circles and the local technique.

Treatment Goals

Treatment Plan

Maintain local circulation proximal to the injury only.

The proximal limb is treated to reduce hypertonicity and to increase drainage and venous return. Techniques include effleurage and repetitive petrissage, such as palmar kneading, C-scooping, fingertip kneading and the origin and insertion technique.

Reduce spasm.

Since protective muscle spasms are no longer so important in stabilizing the injured joint, Golgi tendon organ release is used on the muscles that cross the joint. Agonist contraction may also be used.

Reduce trigger points.

Trigger points in muscles that refer to the injured limb and the injury site itself are now treated directly. Muscle stripping is used for this in the early subacute stage.

On-site work is now indicated. In the early subacute stage, vibrations, gentle stroking and fingertip kneading to the client's pain tolerance are used on the injured joint.

Maintain range of motion.

Mid-range passive relaxed range of motion is used on the proximal and distal joints to maintain the successive action and to help increase lymphatic drainage.

Distal techniques for the early subacute stage include stroking and muscle squeezing only.

Late Subacute

The healing tissue is less fragile. Therefore, the treatment goals can be achieved using more vigorous techniques.

The limb is once again elevated.

Hydrotherapy applications local to the injury are cold/hot. If acute inflammation recurs, the therapist returns to using local cold hydrotherapy applications.

General Treatment

Reduce pain. Decrease sympathetic nervous system firing. Treat any compensating structures.

The treatment approach outlined for early subacute general work is indicated at this stage also.

Specific Treatment

Reduce edema.

As edema diminishes in the late subacute stage, the length of time spent on the drainage techniques decreases.

The proximal limb is treated to reduce hypertonicity and maintain drainage and venous return.

Reduce hypertonicity and trigger points.

Trigger points in muscles that refer to the injured limb and the injury site itself are treated using muscle stripping and ischemic compressions according to the client's pain tolerance. If ischemic compressions are

318

Treatment Goals   Treatment Plan

used to treat a muscle that crosses the joint, repetitive petrissage is used to flush circulation through the muscle instead of heat and a stretch which may compromise the sprained joint.

Reduce adhesions.

With Grade 1 and 2 sprains, as the inflammation subsides, the on-site focus shifts to preventing the formation of restricting adhesions between the ligament and the surrounding structures. Realigning the developing connective tissue to form a functional scar is also important. It is essential to accurately palpate the ligament and any restricting adhesions before attempting to reduce the adhesions. Longitudinal muscle stripping, followed by specific petrissage, such as short cross-fibre strokes and frictions to the ligament, are indicated (Hertling, Kessler, 1990; Thomson et al., 1991). All this work is performed within the client's pain tolerance.

After the ligament has been frictioned, the specific joint play technique that stresses the ligament is used to realign the fibres. This technique also reduces restrictions in the joint capsule. Instead of a passive stretch, joint play is used after frictions to avoid overstretching the sprained ligament. It is performed cautiously, gently and in a **pain-free** manner. **Ice** is applied to the frictioned tissue to reduce the inflammatory process.

Joint play techniques to the proximal and distal joints are introduced in the late subacute stage if these structure are hypomobile due to compensation.

Gradually increase the range of motion.

In treating a Grade 1 or 2 sprain in the late subacute stage, **pain-free mid-range passive relaxed range of motion** is used on the affected joint, with the range that was injured introduced **last.**

Increase local circulation.

In the late subacute stage, the risk of causing congestion local to the sprain diminishes. Effleurage and petrissage are now introduced distally to encourage the healing process.

Chronic

Positioning is chosen for comfort and for accessibility of the structures that are treated. The limb is only elevated if chronic edema remains. Otherwise, it is positioned comfortably.

Hydrotherapy applications proximal to the sprain and on the lesion site itself include deep moist heat, such as a hydrocollator or a wax application to soften adhesions and increase local circulation.

General Treatment

Decrease sympathetic nervous system firing.
Treat compensatory structures.

The client's trunk and compensating structures are massaged as before. Rhythmic techniques to the trunk and unaffected limb are indicated.

319

Treatment Goals

Treatment Plan

Specific Treatment

Reduce any chronic edema.

✋ A pocket of chronic edema remaining in the hollows around the sprained joint may be trapped by proximal and local connective tissue restrictions. Fascial glide is used to assess, then fascial techniques are used to treat the restrictions. These include crossed-hands or ulnar border spreading. Proximal lymphatic drainage is also indicated. A **contrast hydrotherapy** application of alternating hot and cold towels is useful to flush out the edema.

Reduce hypertonicity and trigger points.

✋ The proximal limb is treated to reduce any remaining hypertonicity or trigger points and to increase local circulation. Rhythmic techniques, effleurage, repetitive petrissage and ischemic compressions are indicated.

Reduce adhesions.

✋ If the therapist has been treating the client's injury throughout the healing process, the focus is on reducing the remaining painfully restricting adhesions and scar tissue. Preparatory techniques include specific kneading and muscle stripping. Then, if the limb has not been immobilized as is likely with a Grade 1 or 2 sprain, cross-fibre frictions to the ligament are performed. These are followed by gentle joint play to the ligament to realign the fibres. This should normalize the range of the joint without overstretching the sprained ligament. An application of **ice** follows this work.

✋ Joint play techniques to the proximal and distal joints are used if these joints are restricted due to compensation. On site, joint play is used to stretch the fibrous joint capsule and maintain the range of motion, again without overstretching the ligament that was sprained.

Restore the range of motion.

✋ **Passive relaxed range of motion** is used on the proximal, affected and distal joints to maintain joint health.

Increase local circulation.

✋ The distal limb is treated with effleurage and petrissage to increase local venous return.

✋ If the therapist starts treating the client in the chronic stage, one approach is to focus on reducing the hypertonicity and trigger points that have developed from the client's compensation patterns. This is done before addressing any adhesions.

If the Limb Is Immobilized

✋ With a Grade 3 (and occasionally a severe Grade 2) sprain, the joint is immobilized. The injury can be immobilized with or without surgical reduction of the sprained ligament. To treat the limb during immobilization, the therapist should refer to the chapter on fractures.

Strengthen muscles that cross the injured ligaments.

✋ Once the immobilization is removed and if the sprain was medically treated using the conservative approach of strapping or casting only, the joint is likely unstable in the direction the sprain occurred. Because

320

Treatment Goals

Treatment Plan

the ligament was not surgically repaired, there is little to prevent hypermobility, other than the support given by the muscles that cross the joint. In this case, mobilizing techniques are contraindicated. Instead, a remedial exercise program to strengthen the muscles that cross the injured ligament is important.

Do not overmobilize a surgically reduced lligament.

☞ If the ligament was surgically reduced, rendering the joint stable, the ligament has been repaired in a shortened position. Because ligaments are not contractile, this repair is done to allow the client to stretch the joint capsule to a functional range without allowing hypermobility to occur. Full range of motion in all ranges of the injured joint is not desired *(Kisner, Colby, 1990)*. It is important for the therapist not to overmobilize the repaired ligament once tone has returned to the muscles that were under the cast.

Self-care Goals

Self-care Plan

Educate the client.

✍ **Hydrotherapy** is chosen that is appropriate for the stage of healing. Since ligaments are hypovascular, it is important to introduce contrast hydrotherapy to help increase local circulation as soon as the acute stage has passed.

✍ **Self-massage** is useful for the muscles that cross the sprained joint in the subacute and chronic stages. This includes skin rolling, muscle stripping and gentle frictions within the client's pain tolerance.

✍ **Remedial exercise** that is given is also dependent on the stage of healing.

Maintain range of motion.

✍ In the **acute** stage, the client is asked to perform pain-free active free range of motion of the proximal and distal joints to maintain the range of motion. With a Grade 1 or 2 sprain, if there is no secondary muscle strain present, or if there is a Grade 1 or 2 muscle strain only, the client can be shown how to do submaximal, pain-free isometric exercises to strengthen the muscles that cross the sprained joint. Further remedial exercise is contraindicated at the acute stage, especially with a Grade 3 sprain *(Thomson et al., 1991)*.

Maintain the strength.

✍ At the **early subacute** stage, the client can perform pain-free active free range of motion of the affected and distal joints to maintain range of motion. If the client does the exercises with both the affected and unaffected limbs, a comparison can be made of the available ranges of motion *(Thomson et al., 1991)*. Submaximal pain-free active resisted isometric exercises for the muscles crossing the joint may be introduced for a Grade 3 sprain.

Re-educate proprioception.

✍ Especially with a weight bearing joint, the client is encouraged to regain proprioception at the joint as soon as possible *(Brukner, Khan,*

Self-care Goals   Self-care Plan

1993). For example, the client is shown the following exercises, which he gradually progresses through. Initially, the client stands on the affected limb only, if necessary supporting himself against the wall or the massage table. It is likely with a Grade 1 or 2 sprain that the client will be able to perform this exercise in the early subacute stage. How quickly the client progresses to the next exercise in this series depends on the severity of the injury and the client's individual healing time. The client progresses to standing on the affected leg with the arms outstretched and the uninjured leg held behind in extension. The client then moves from this stance to swinging the uninjured leg from extension to flexion. Gradually, the client swings the leg in a semicircle in front and behind the weight bearing injured leg.

Gradually increase range of motion. Increase strength and proprioception.

✍ In the **late subacute** stage, the range of motion is gradually increased. Pain-free active resisted isometric exercise is used to maintain the strength of muscles that cross the sprained joint. The client may gradually progress to isotonic active resisted exercise. The proprioception exercises are continued.

Increase the strength.

✍ In the **chronic** stage, the focus continues to be on active resisted isotonic exercises to strengthen the muscles that cross the affected joint.

Re-educate proprioception.

✍ With a weight bearing joint, the client can progress to using a balance board for regaining proprioception *(Brukner, Khan, 1993).*

Increase range of motion.

✍ If tight muscles prevent normal range of motion at the affected joint, stretching is carefully performed to maintain these ranges. The client should take care not to overstretch the muscles and destabilize the joint.

Encourage activity.

✍ The client is encouraged to return to the activities of daily living on a gradual basis, especially with a sprain to a weight bearing joint. Return to regular sports or other activities that stress the joint can occur once functional exercises are pain-free both during and after the exercise *(Brukner, Khan, 1993).*

✍ The client may need to use tape, a brace or other supports to protect an unstable joint on activity, especially a weight bearing joint.

Treatment Frequency and Expected Outcome

Shorter, more frequent treatments will address the inflammatory process in the acute stages. Treatment may progress to once a week for chronic stages, then the client is reassessed.

The outcome is variable, depending on the severity of the injury, the treatment approach used (strengthening exercises and soft tissue work, immobilization or surgery) the client's age, general health and compliance with the self-care program.

Sprains can create joint laxity, leading to a cycle of repeated sprains and further stretching of the ligaments. If this is not corrected, the client may require surgery to stabilize the joint.

See stress reduction, edema, spasm, contusions, strains, dislocations, hypermobility and hypomobility, fractures, scars, whiplash and osteoarthritis in this text for related treatments.

Return to activity (the following are guidelines only):

- Grade 1 sprain – four to five days;

- Grade 2 sprain – seven to 14 days *(Hertling, Kessler, 1990)*;

- Grade 3 sprain – immobilization generally removed at six to eight weeks *(Thomson et al., 1991)*.

- **Total healing** of a sprained ligament may take up to six months for full maturation of the collagen fibres *(Hertling, Kessler, 1990; Booher, Thibodeau, 1989)*.

Sample Treatment: Grade 2 Anterior Talofibular Sprain

Acute

✋ The client is in a comfortable position, likely supine, with the injured leg elevated. An ice pack is placed over the ankle and the client is instructed to breathe diaphragmatically. The therapist uses lymphatic drainage techniques on the affected leg, starting with inguinal pumping and treating the distal leg. Lymphatic drainage is stopped just proximal to the edema. Swedish techniques are used on the uninjured leg to treat the compensating structures and decrease sympathetic nervous system firing and pain. The injured leg is treated with Swedish techniques proximal to the injury site only, with care taken not to completely reduce the protective muscle spasms. The client can then be placed either prone or sidelying on the uninjured side and the gluteals and low back are also treated. If the treatment duration is 45 minutes to one hour, the shoulders, neck and head can be included, especially if the client is using crutches.

✎ For self-care, the client is instructed to rest (no weight bearing) ice and elevate the sprained ankle. Pain-free isometric exercises for tibialis anterior, gastrocnemius, soleus and the peroneals are performed to maintain muscle strength as long as a Grade 3 strain is not present in these muscles.

Early Subacute

✋ The treatment plan for the early subacute stage is much the same as for the acute stage in terms of positioning and lymphatic drainage. Contrast hydrotherapy can be applied to the sprained ankle. Then the uninjured leg is treated. Swedish techniques for the unaffected and affected legs are similar to the acute stage. However, the focus is placed on treating trigger points with muscle stripping, specifically those in the peroneals that may refer into the lateral ankle. Gentle on-site vibrations, stroking, muscle squeezing and fingertip kneading are indicated. The order of pain-free passive relaxed range of motion for an inversion sprain is dorsiflexion, eversion, plantarflexion and, finally, inversion.

- Distal Swedish techniques are stroking and muscle squeezing of the foot.

- For **self-care** exercises, the client can begin in the early subacute stage with active free dorsiflexion and pain-free plantarflexion. Proprioception exercises are performed to the client's ability (*Kisner, Colby, 1990*).

Late Subacute

- The treatment plan is much the same as for the early subacute stage in terms of positioning and proximal work. Less time is spent on lymphatic drainage. Circulation techniques are introduced to the affected leg and trigger points are treated with ischemic compressions. Specific work to the sprained ankle includes frictioning the anterior talofibular ligament followed by passive stress of that ligament. In this case, the tibia is stabilized and the calcaneus and talus are drawn inferiorly then anteriorly. This is followed with an application of **ice.**

- An injury to the ankle may also affect the superior talofibular joint. If this joint is hypomobile, joint play techniques are used. With the client's knee and hip in flexion, the therapist stabilizes the tibia. The fibular head is mobilized anteriorly and posteriorly (*Mennell, 1964*).

- Distal work includes effleurage and petrissage to the foot.

- If comfortable, the client may be treated prone to work the compensating gluteals and posterior leg using Swedish techniques.

- In terms of **self-care,** an easy exercise for all ranges of motion is the "ankle alphabet". The client writes out the letters of the alphabet in the air with the big toe of the injured foot. A special focus on strengthening the peroneals is included. Active resisted eversion is performed. The client is seated, using an elasticized loop that is hooked around both feet at the level of the metatarsal heads. The feet are then repeatedly moved from midline to an everted position, stretching the loop. The proprioception exercises can progress as the client is able (*Kisner, Colby, 1990*).

Chronic

- The client may be started in a prone position to create access to the low back, gluteals and posterior legs. Hypertonicity and compensatory changes are treated as in the previous stages. When the client is turned supine, any remaining chronic edema in the sinus tarsi region is treated. Swedish techniques are used on both anterior legs to increase local circulation. Trigger points in the vastus lateralis, referring into the lateral leg, and trigger points in the peroneals, referring into the ankle, are addressed. Passive relaxed ranges of the ankle are performed, with inversion done last. Frictions are performed to the anterior talofibular ligament. Joint play to the ankle, foot and knee and fascial techniques for restrictions are used if indicated. Joint play will also reduce intra-articular adhesions (*Apley, Solomon, 1993*).

- Hypomobility of the subtalar joint can result from ankle and foot injuries and add to proprioception difficulties at the ankle. To mobilize this joint, the client lies supine with the affected foot over the end of the table. The therapist stands at the end of table, with her back to the client. The therapist's hands are placed around the affected ankle, with the web of the hand on the dorsal surface contacting the talus and the web of the other hand contacting the posterior calcaneus. Both thumbs are on the medial anterior aspect of the calcaneus. A long axis traction is applied to the talus and calcaneus, pulling these bones inferiorly. Once the slack is taken out of the subtalar joint capsule, the calcaneus is rocked anteriorly and then posteriorly on the talus. A further medial and lateral glide can then be placed on the subtalar joint by rocking the calcaneus in these directions.

- The client's gait patterns are reassessed and corrected if necessary. This helps to prevent reinjury.

- For **self-care,** once strength has been regained in the peroneals, stretching of the gastrocnemius and soleus is important, so the ankle has sufficient ability to go into dorsiflexion *(Kisner, Colby, 1990).* Proprioception exercises are continued, with functional activities added, such as bouncing and catching a ball while balancing on the affected leg. Gradually the client will return to activities such as running or cycling. The client may need to use taping or supportive footwear that covers the ankle when exercising, to prevent reinjury.

CRUCIATE AND MENISCAL INJURIES

Fiona Rattray

> *The knee is a frequently injured joint. In addition to the more superficial medial and lateral collateral ligaments which are covered in the chapter on sprains, the deeper anterior and posterior cruciate ligaments present clinical concerns, as do the two menisci.*

With regard to treatment approaches, it is important for the therapist to distinguish between cruciate or meniscal injuries and collateral ligament injuries. Massage techniques have a direct effect on the superficial collateral ligaments. However, the anterior and posterior cruciates and menisci are not directly treatable using massage therapy because they are located deep within the knee *(Figure 25.1)*. Clients with cruciate or meniscal injuries should be initially referred to a physician, especially in the acute stage when a hemarthrosis may be present.

The therapist will likely be part of a rehabilitation team in treating either cruciate or meniscal injuries. This team includes a physician and a physiotherapist. The therapist should contact these practitioners, with the client's permission, to coordinate the rehabilitation plan.

Cruciate Ligaments

The **cruciate ligaments** check motion at the knee and are most taut when the knee is in extension. They cross each other, forming an X shape. Although the cruciates are within the joint capsule, they are not within the synovium *(Hertling, Kessler, 1990; Booher, Thibodeau, 1989)*.

The cruciates are named according to their position on the tibia.

✦ The **anterior cruciate ligament** runs from the anterior portion of the tibial intercondylar area to the medial aspect of the lateral femoral condyle, in the

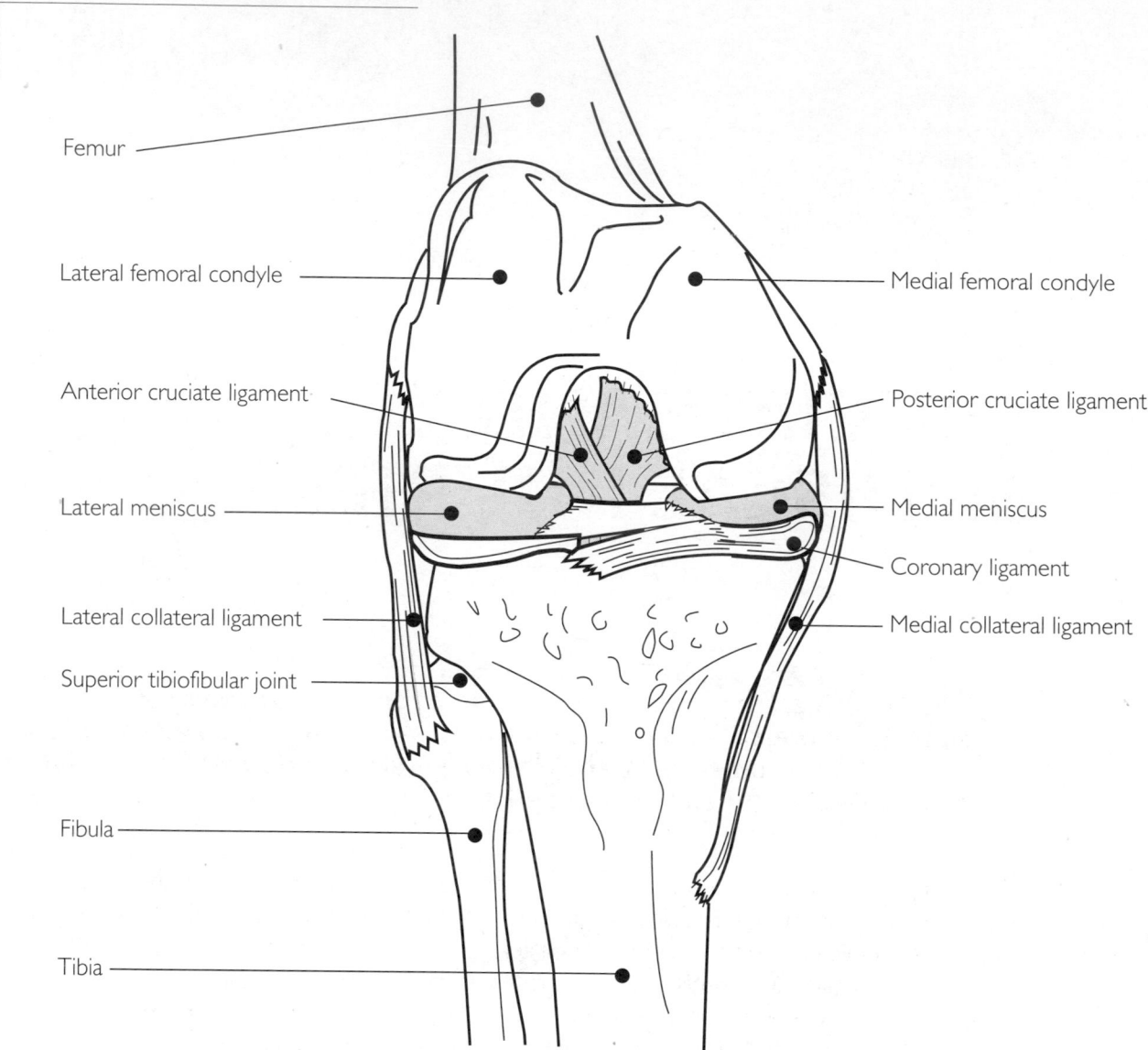

Figure 25.1
Right knee in slight flexion, anterior view, showing cruciate ligaments and menisci.

intercondylar notch. The direction of the fibres from the tibia to the femur is obliquely superior, posterior and lateral. The anterior cruciate functions to prevent knee extension, anterior movement (or translation) of the tibia on the femur and internal tibial rotation. The quadriceps muscles are antagonists in function to the anterior cruciate. In other words, the anterior cruciate, along with the hamstrings, resists the pull of the quadriceps muscles at the knee *(Siliski, 1994; Larson, Grana, 1993).*

✦ The **posterior cruciate ligament** runs from the posterior portion of the tibial intercondylar area to the lateral aspect of the medial femoral condyle, also in the intercondylar notch. The direction of the fibres from the tibia to the femur is obliquely superior, anterior and medial. The posterior cruciate functions to prevent posterior translation of the tibia on the femur and internal tibial rotation. The posterior cruciate, along with the quadriceps, resists the pull of the hamstrings at the knee. The posterior cruciate is stronger than the anterior cruciate and is injured less frequently.

Causes of anterior cruciate ligament injury are:

➤ a blow to the lateral knee;

➤ forced hyperextension with internal rotation of the tibia;

➤ a blow to the posterior tibia.

The client may experience the injury when pivoting, decelerating or landing from a jump *(Brukner, Khan, 1993)*. The anterior cruciate is often injured along with the medial collateral ligament. Ninety per cent of knees with a chronic anterior cruciate ligament instability have additional meniscal disorders *(Larson, Grana, 1993)*.

Causes of posterior cruciate ligament injury are:

➤ a blow to the anterior tibia;

➤ excessive hyperextension, or in a motor vehicle accident "dashboard injury" where the tibia is forced posteriorly during the accident.

The Medical Treatment of Cruciate Injuries

The medical approach to cruciate injuries depends on the degree of instability, any associated injuries, such as collateral ligament or meniscal damage, the demands the client places on the knee and the time and cost involved in the treatment procedure. The conservative medical approach to a cruciate injury includes initial rest, anti-inflammatories, a splint or other support and a remedial exercise program. Surgery is either open or arthroscopic, with arthroscopic procedures requiring less recovery time. The first recorded anterior cruciate ligament reconstruction was in 1917, while an early arthroscope was used to visualize the joint as early as 1931 *(Larson, Grana, 1993)*. Arthroscopic examination may be used to determine whether sprains are partial or complete. Small hematomas are noted even with Grade 1 sprains *(Glinz, 1987)*.

Today, there are numerous approaches to reconstruction of the anterior cruciate ligament following a complete rupture. These include using a portion of the patellar tendon, the iliotibial band or gracilis and semitendinosus tendons. Due to their high failure rate, synthetic ligament replacements are no longer in favour *(Brukner, Khan, 1993; Larson, Grana, 1993)*. Surgery for the anterior cruciate is more commonly performed than for the posterior cruciate. Cruciate reconstruction is usually considered with chronic joint instability.

Traditional rehabilitation for cruciate reconstruction used to include lengthy knee immobilization and non-weight-bearing. This resulted in knee stiffness, muscle weakness and poor proprioception. The health of the articular cartilage within the joint also suffered with immobilization. Another complication with inflammation were adhesions between the proximal patella, the quadriceps tendon and the femur. This resulted in **capsulitis (infrapatellar contracture syndrome)**, with the client experiencing pain, flexion contracture, quadriceps weakness and effusion *(Siliski, 1994)*. Recent concepts for knee rehabilitation have shifted to controlled mobilization, where the client is allowed to move about with the knee protected by braces, or where movement is performed by a continuous passive motion machine.

Management of the inflammation, swelling and pain begins immediately after the injury,

329

resulting in fewer adhesions forming within the joint and a maintenance of the range of motion of the knee. This approach is very helpful if surgery is delayed for weeks or months. Strengthening programs are also begun earlier in the healing process. This change in thinking has led to a marked decrease in joint stiffness and an increase in the range of motion people experience *(Brukner, Khan, 1993)*. However, since a reconstructed anterior cruciate ligament still develops no more than 50 per cent of normal strength, a cautious return to functional activity is suggested. Functional knee braces may be worn for up to 18 months after a cruciate injury, whether or not surgery is performed *(Larson, Grana, 1993)*.

Menisci

The **menisci** are designed to provide shock absorption and to add increased gliding potential between the femur and the tibia. The menisci transmit between 30 and 55 per cent of the load at the knee *(Larson, Grana, 1993)*. They are slightly more mobile anteriorly than posteriorly, moving with knee action. For example, during knee extension the anterior portions of the menisci glide anteriorly, while during extension they glide posteriorly.

In cross section, the menisci are somewhat triangular, with the thicker convex outer edge attaching to the joint capsule and the thinner concave edge being unattached *(Figure 25.2)*. The middle and inner portions of the menisci are avascular, with only the very outer portion where the menisci attach to the joint capsule vascularized. As a result, the menisci heal relatively slowly *(Siliski, 1994)*.

The **medial meniscus** forms a semicircle. It is attached at its periphery to the joint capsule as well as to the outer margin of the medial tibial condyle by the coronary ligament. It is also attached to some of the fibres of the medial collateral ligament. This arrangement means that severe damage to the medial collateral ligament can damage the medial

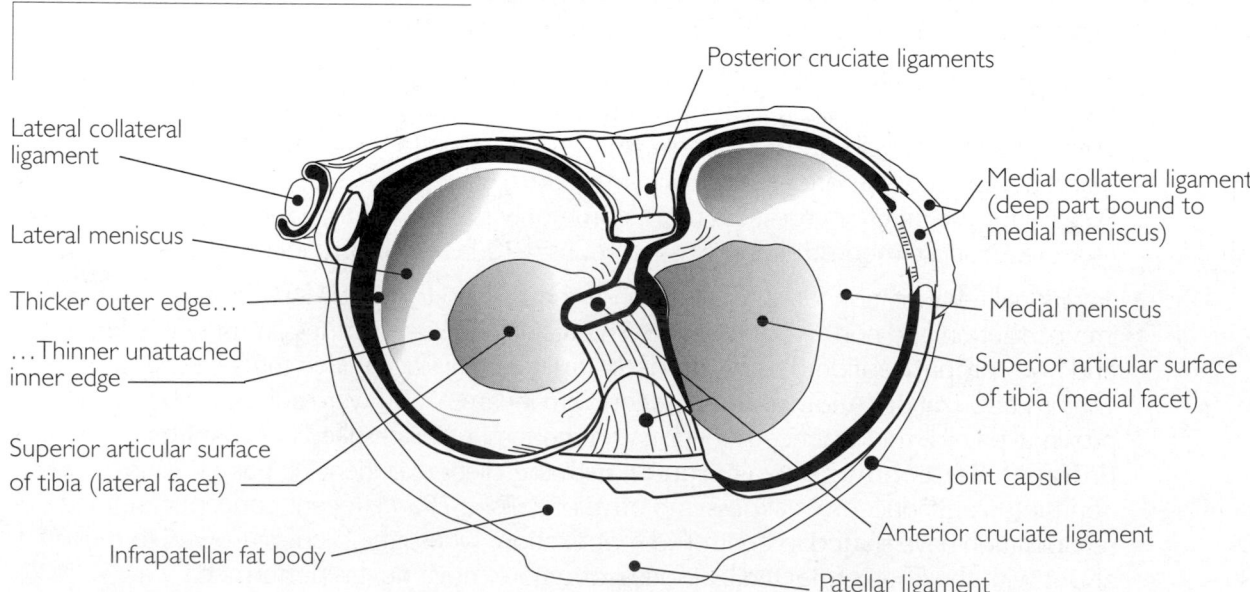

Figure 25.2
Superior view of knee joint showing menisci and tibial attachments of the cruciate ligaments.

meniscus. The posterior aspect of the medial meniscus is the most frequently injured. In younger people, the tear usually runs longitudinally (a "bucket handle tear"). Over time, the tear extends anteriorly and may form a flap which locks the joint. In older people, the injury is often a degenerative horizontal tear, with the upper and lower portions sliding against each other *(Hertling, Kessler, 1990)*.

In contrast, the **lateral meniscus** forms almost a complete circle. It attaches at its periphery to the joint capsule and the tibia but not to the lateral collateral ligament. The lateral meniscus is more mobile than the medial one and is, therefore, less prone to damage. It is moved posteriorly during knee flexion by the tendon of the popliteus muscle *(Hertling, Kessler, 1990)*.

The cause of meniscal injury is:

➤ a twisting injury while the foot is weight bearing and anchored to the ground.

The Medical Treatment of Meniscal Injuries

How the injury is treated depends on several factors. If symptoms develop over 24 to 72 hours, if there is minimal swelling, if the client is able to weight bear and if there is pain only at the end range of motion or at the end range of McMurray's test, the medical approach is likely to be rest, supports and remedial exercises. On the other hand, if the client is unable to continue the activity, if the knee locks, if there is pain on minimal knee flexion, if there is a positive McMurray's test or if the symptoms do not improve after three weeks of conservative treatment, surgery (either open or arthroscopic) is the likely medical choice *(Brukner, Khan, 1993)*. The client will probably wear a knee brace or other support after surgery for activities.

In the past, the surgical approach to meniscal tears was sometimes to remove the entire meniscus. This led to early degenerative changes in the articular surfaces of the joint *(Henche, Holder, 1988)*. Currently, the medical approach is to remove only the torn portion of the meniscus. New techniques in meniscal repair may replace partial meniscectomies as a standard treatment *(Hertling, Kessler, 1990; Siliski, 1994)*. For example, bucket handle tears may be sutured together with a fibrin clot placed in between the torn pieces before the sutures are pulled tight. The clot stimulates the repair process in the avascular menisci *(Larson, Grana, 1993)*.

✦ **Reflex sympathetic dystrophy** is a complication that may occur at the knee following trauma or surgery. Although poorly understood, the syndrome appears to be an exaggerated physiological response to injury. Persisting for months or years, it consists of increased sympathetic response, prolonged, intensely burning pain, a decreased capillary blood flow and vasospasm, edema, stiffness and limited range of motion. In the knee, the pain is located in the patellofemoral joint and femoral condyles *(Fox, Del Pizzo, 1993)*.

✦ Initially, the area is warm and swollen. As the syndrome progresses, the skin over the joint becomes shiny and may be cool and cyanotic. Slight movement of the joint or light touch exacerbates the symptoms *(Buschbacher, 1994)*. The client will have difficulty in weight bearing. Medically, the syndrome is treated with antidepressants, corticosteroids or sympathetic ganglion blocks. Contrast hydrotherapy baths may also be helpful. Gentle active free and active assisted range of motion can be used to reduce disuse atrophy and knee stiffness; however, it is important not to increase the pain during exercise as this worsens the symptoms. The most important factor influencing improvement is early treatment, within six to 12 months following the onset of the symptoms *(Fox, Del Pizzo, 1993)*.

Symptom Picture of Cruciate and Meniscal Injuries

✦ In the **acute** stage of either a cruciate or meniscal injury, depending on the severity, there is pain, swelling and muscle guarding. While there is often significant swelling present, an absence of swelling does not necessarily indicate minor injury. It is possible that an effusion or hemarthrosis may leak posteriorly out of a severely damaged joint capsule *(Hertling, Kessler, 1990)*. Bruising or redness may be noticeable over the knee. The joint is held in a semi-flexed position, usually due to the swelling. The client will have crutches, elastic bandages or splints to support the joint.

✦ The client with an **acute** Grade 1 or 2 **cruciate injury** will be able to continue the activity. The client with a Grade 3 or total rupture of the anterior cruciate ligament reports a popping feeling in the knee at the time of injury. He is unable to continue the activity. A hemarthrosis develops within the first few minutes or hours of the injury. The skin over the joint is taut and hard to the touch. The pain is often sharp. With effusion, the pain is dull and achy *(Hertling, Kessler, 1990)*.

✦ A client with a **chronic** Grade 2 or 3 anterior cruciate sprain is unable to run forward, while the client with chronic posterior cruciate damage is unable to squat, walk downstairs easily or run backward.

Contraindications

✦ With an acute knee injury where effusion is present, massage is contraindicated until a medical assessment has been made.

✦ Do not force extension or flexion with a locked knee, because further damage to the meniscus may result.

✦ Immersion hydrotherapy (baths) should be avoided for two weeks following surgery or arthroscopy at the knee *(Henche, Holder, 1988)*.

✦ If capsulitis is suspected following ligament surgery, the therapist should avoid aggressive stretching, concentrating instead on maintaining pain-free range of motion. If no improvement is noted within three months of the surgery, the client should be referred to the physician *(Siliski, 1994)*.

✦ The symptoms of **meniscal injuries** vary, depending on the severity. With an **acute**, more severe trauma, the client may feel a tearing sensation in the knee. The knee may "give way", buckle or lock. Initially, there is local pain on the side where the injury occurred, especially on knee flexion. There is effusion at the joint and tenderness along the joint line. A small meniscal tear may not show immediate symptoms; however, pain and swelling will increase over the next day or two *(Brukner, Khan, 1993)*.

✦ In the **chronic** stage, there may be a clicking sound in the joint. The knee may lock in a particular position as the torn meniscus prevents knee motion. There may be accompanying quadriceps disuse atrophy and buckling of the knee joint. Acute symptoms may recur with activity *(Kisner, Colby, 1990; Hertling, Kessler, 1990)*.

Treatment Considerations

Assessment

✍ **Testing for Acute Knee Injury with Swelling:**

- **AF ROM** of the knee is limited in extension and flexion due to effusion. The usual resting position of the knee is 25 degrees of flexion *(Kisner, Colby, 1990).*

- **PR ROM** of the knee may reveal a muscle guarding end feel due to muscle spasm or a springy block end feel due to meniscal involvement. Loose bodies within the joint, whether they be portions of the meniscus or cartilage fragments, may also give a springy block end feel.

- **AR strength tests** for muscles crossing the knee should be painless and indicate normal strength. Pain is present if there is accompanying muscular injury.

- If the swelling of an acute injury prevents full knee movement, it may be difficult to determine which structure has been affected. The **ballottable patella** and **minor effusion tests** may both be positive with cruciate or meniscal injuries. The client is referred for immediate medical attention if these tests are positive. A **suprapatellar girth** measurement is positive with synovial effusion.

- Other testing is **contraindicated** with an acute injury.

✍ **Testing for Early and Late Subacute and Chronic Knee Injury:**

- **AF ROM** may be limited in extension with anterior cruciate repair and limited in flexion with posterior cruciate repair. Loss of extension greater than 10 degrees or loss of flexion greater than 125 degrees is considered significant *(Siliski, 1994).*

- **PR ROM** is limited with a meniscal injury where joint locking is present; the knee does not fully extend. There is a springy block end feel on passive extension.

- **AR strength** of quadriceps may be reduced with disuse atrophy.

- It is important to avoid triggering protective muscle guarding in the hamstrings when performing the ligamentous stress tests, as this could produce a false negative test result *(Hertling, Kessler, 1990).*

- With an anterior cruciate injury, **Lachman's** and the anterior part of the **anterior-posterior drawer tests** are positive. With a posterior cruciate injury, the **posterior "sag" sign** and the posterior part of the **anterior-posterior drawer tests** are positive. The coronary ligament may also be sprained. In this case, a positive sign is pain with passive external rotation of the tibia on the femur but no pain on the **valgus stress test.**

- With a meniscal injury, **McMurray's test, Bragard's sign** and **Apley's compression tests** are positive. **Helfet's test** may be positive.

Massage of Cruciate Injuries

Acute, Early and Late Subacute

✋ The client should rest, ice and elevate the limb following the injury. A knee brace or support will be worn and the client will be on crutches for the first three weeks.

The primary focus of massage is the compensating structures, reducing sympathetic nervous system firing, hypertonicity and trigger points. **Positioning** is prone and supine, with the affected leg comfortably elevated. **Hydrotherapy** is cold on the injury site. The low back, shoulders and unaffected leg are treated using Swedish techniques. If necessary, joint play can be used for hypermobile sacroiliac joints. Lymphatic drainage techniques are used on the affected leg proximal to the knee to reduce edema. The gluteals, proximal hamstrings and quadriceps are also treated with Swedish techniques. Patellar mobilization, consisting of lateral and medial slides and tilts, are used to prevent contracture of the patellar retinaculum (*Siliski, 1994*). On-site work is avoided at the incisions following surgical procedures in the acute and early subacute stages. Distally, muscle squeezing and careful joint play for the ankle and foot are indicated.

As the condition progresses to the late subacute stage, Swedish techniques and contrast hydrotherapy can be employed on site and to the distal leg. Trigger points in the quadriceps muscles can refer pain and other symptoms to the knee joint. Vastus medialis trigger points can produce muscle weakness and buckling of the knee while walking. Rectus femoris trigger points give rise to pain and weakness when going down stairs (*Travell, Simons, 1992*). Muscle stripping and gentle ischemic compressions can be used. Pain-free mid-range passive motion of the knee can follow ischemic compressions while knee extension is still restricted to 45 degrees. Passive relaxed pain-free range of motion for the hip and ankle is also indicated.

Chronic

After four to six weeks, the focus of the massage is on the unaffected and affected leg and low back. Swedish techniques are indicated, as well as heat and fascial techniques for any restrictions, especially those that inhibit knee extension. If surgery was performed, skin rolling and cross-fibre frictions can be used on the scar tissue. Joint play for the sacroiliac joints, hips, superior tibiofibular joint and ankles may be indicated.

Self-Care of Cruciate Injuries

Acute, Early and Late Subacute

The self-care program to regain function immediately following a cruciate injury or repair should avoid exercises that stress the involved ligament due to translation of the tibia on the femur. For example, the pull of the quadriceps muscles causes anterior tibial translation. This stresses the anterior cruciate and should initially be avoided with injuries to this ligament. Likewise, the hamstrings cause posterior tibial translation which should be avoided with posterior cruciate injuries (*Siliski, 1994; Larson, Grana, 1993; Hertling, Kessler, 1990*).

For the first few days following injury while the joint is still swollen, the client should rest, elevate and ice the knee. As the swelling diminishes, the remedial exercise program can begin. For an anterior cruciate injury or repair, in the seated position the client can perform a pain-free active assisted knee extension which prevents anterior tibial translation caused by the quadriceps. The ankle of the unaffected leg is placed behind the ankle of the affected leg. The affected knee is actively extended from 90 to 45 degrees, then the unaffected leg assists the affected knee from 45 degrees to full extension *(Siliski, 1994)*. These exercises can be performed for up to six weeks post-surgery with cruciate repair.

✍ Once adequate pain-free active free range of motion has been obtained, the client can begin strengthening the muscles that cross the knee. With an anterior cruciate injury, the initial focus of active resisted strengthening is on the hamstrings, not the quadriceps. Isometrics for the hamstrings (hamstring setting) can be performed with the knee in extension. The supine client gently pushes her heel into the table, holding this for at least six seconds, then relaxes. When possible, the client can progress to hamstring isotonics. The standing client can flex the knee to 90 degrees, first against gravity, then later against resistance in the form of light ankle weights *(Kisner, Colby, 1990)*.

✍ Once sufficient healing of the anterior cruciate ligament has occurred and the client's physician approves the plan, strengthening of the quadriceps muscles can begin. To prevent disuse atrophy, the supine client is given gentle active resisted isometrics for the quadriceps (quadriceps setting) with the knee in full extension. The client is instructed to gently push the back of the knee into the table, again holding for six seconds and then relaxing. This can be progressed to a straight leg raise, where the client first locks the knee in full extension by contracting the quadriceps muscle before beginning the straight leg raise.

✍ Inner range quadriceps extension can be done, with the supine client placing a towel roll under the knee, then extending the lower leg. When possible, the seated client can perform isometric full knee extensions against gravity. The standing client can progress to one quarter squats, where the knees are flexed to 45 degrees while the client holds on to a chair for support if needed. This closed chain kinetic exercise strengthens both the quadriceps and hamstrings, while preventing tibial translation *(Siliski, 1994)*.

✍ Active resisted isotonic hip abduction while the client is sidelying will help to provide lateral knee stability *(Hertling, Kessler, 1990)*. Active resisted isometrics for gastrocnemius and foot muscles, such as toe raises, are also important.

✍ With anterior cruciate ligament damage, where the client is advised to weight bear only partially or not at all for the first four weeks, continuous passive motion (CPM) is effective in promoting the health of the articular cartilage *(Brukner, Khan, 1993)*.

✍ If the client does not have access to a CPM machine, the following heel slide exercise is useful. The client is seated on the floor, with the hip and affected knee comfortably flexed and the heel resting on the floor. The client places one end of a large towel under her heel and grasps the other end of the towel in the hand on the affected side. By pulling the towel slowly towards herself, the client passively slides the heel towards the buttock, flexing the knee. This flexion occurs in a pain-free range. Using her hand, the client can then gently push the knee back into pain-free extension, sliding the heel and towel back along the floor to the starting position. The floor should be smooth — tile or wood, for example, not carpet — so the foot and towel can slide freely. The exercise is repeated. The client is instructed to take care not to contract the quadriceps or hamstrings muscles during the exercise *(Larson, Grana, 1993)*.

Chronic

✍ The client's self-care can progress to active resisted isometrics with rubber tubing for the quadriceps and hamstrings while wearing a knee brace.

✍ The client can also perform hamstring stretches. The standing squats can be progressed to half squats, with the knees at 90 degrees *(Brukner, Khan, 1993)*. To maintain the health of the articular cartilage, swimming (using the flutter kick only) and work on a stationary bike are useful.

✍ After eight weeks, the client can begin proprioception exercises with a rocker board in addition to the strengthening program previously mentioned. The client may still be using knee support as needed during activities.

Massage of Meniscal Injuries

Acute, Early and Late Subacute

✋ The client should rest, ice and elevate the limb following the injury. A knee brace will be worn and the client will be on crutches for between one and eight weeks. If the meniscus was repaired, no weight bearing is allowed for the first four weeks *(Larson, Grana, 1993)*. With a partial meniscectomy, weight bearing may be allowed in the first week following arthroscopic surgery. Weight bearing on a locked knee is to be avoided.

✋ The primary focus of massage is the same as for a cruciate injury, as is **positioning** and **hydrotherapy.** Treatment of compensating structures and proximal lymphatic drainage for the affected leg are indicated.

✋ Patellofemoral joint mobilization and gentle passive relaxed range of motion into pain-free extension are used. The expected range of motion is up to 120 degrees of flexion *(Brukner, Khan, 1993)*.

✋ In the late subacute stage cross-fibre frictions to the lesion along the joint line are indicated *(Hertling, Kessler, 1990)*. If the meniscus was treated surgically, the scars are frictioned.

Chronic

✋ The focus of massage treatment is similar to cruciate injury treatment, with the low back, gluteals and legs being treated for hypertonicity, fascial restrictions and trigger points. If the client remains on crutches for an extended period of time following a meniscal repair, the focus of the treatment includes the shoulder girdle, neck and arms.

✋ Cautious joint play for the tibiofemoral joint can be introduced in the third week if hypomobility is encountered *(Brukner, Khan, 1993)*.

Self-care of Meniscal Injuries

Acute, Early and Late Subacute

✍ The client with a small tear or a partial meniscectomy can begin quadriceps and hamstring setting, straight leg raises, hip adduction and gastrocnemius setting in the first week. The concern for preventing tibial translation is not the same as with a cruciate injury.

Chronic

✍ When the client with a tear or partial menisectomy has full range of motion, self-care isometric exercises are progressed to isotonic exercises for quadriceps and hamstrings as described in the cruciate injury section. Exercises for the hip adductors and gastrocnemius are included.

✍ Later, resistance exercises are added over a three-week period. Half squats are introduced. The client can begin step-up and step-down exercises and stationary bicycle work, eventually progressing to rocker board exercises, hopping and jumping to retrain proprioception at the knee *(Brukner, Khan, 1993)*. The client with a meniscal repair, on the other hand, will follow a more conservative program at the physician's direction. For example, weight-bearing or closed-chain quadriceps squats and isotonic exercises for the hamstrings are begun six weeks post surgery *(Larson, Grana, 1993)*.

✍ Recovery from a Grade 3 cruciate injury takes up to four months. Recovery from a minor meniscal tear takes three to four weeks, while a major tear requires eight to 12 weeks *(Brukner, Khan, 1993)*. If the client returns to the activity that caused the injury too quickly, there may be recurrent pain and effusion. If the injury was severe enough and surgical repair was not elected, the client's knee may be prone to weakness, hypermobility, buckling or locking.

See edema, spasm, scars, strain and sprains for related conditions.

26

DISLOCATIONS

Fiona Rattray

A dislocation is the complete dissociation of the articulating surfaces of a joint.

A subluxation is when the articulating surfaces of a joint remain in partial contact with each other (Thomson et al., 1991).

Although a dislocation may occur at any joint, certain joints in the body are relatively unstable due to their anatomical configuration.

The most frequently dislocated articulation in the body is the glenohumeral joint, where only a portion of the articulating surface of the humeral head comes in contact with the shallow glenoid fossa. The joint relies largely on ligamentous and muscular support and is prone to a dislocation injury. Joints that are also prone to dislocation are the acromioclavicular joints, the metacarpals and the interphalangeals.

Other joints are inherently more secure, such as the deep ball and socket joint of the hip. Relatively stable joints, such as the ankle, knee, hip and elbow, require a greater force to dislocate and they are more likely to have associated fractures and other injuries (*Brukner, Khan, 1993*). The temporomandibular joint occasionally dislocates.

In a dislocation, a portion of the joint capsule and surrounding ligaments are either completely torn or partially ruptured. The nearby tendons, synovial sheaths and articular cartilage may also be damaged. Other soft tissue injuries, such as strains and contusions, occur with a dislocation. Complications may also occur, such as nerve and vascular damage and fracture (including osteochondral fracture). In a subluxation, the joint capsule is stretched. Some subluxation results with a joint sprain (*Booher, Thibodeau, 1989*).

➤ **The cause of a dislocation is a trauma-related sudden twist or wrench of the joint beyond its normal range of motion.** This can be a direct or an indirect trauma. With a direct trauma, there is a direct force on the joint itself, such as a blow to the posterior shoulder when the arm is abducted which produces an anterior glenohumeral dislocation. With an indirect trauma, the joint becomes the weak link in a closed kinetic chain; for example, falling on the extended and outstretched hand results in an anterior glenohumeral dislocation.

Contributing factors:

➤ **pathologies** such as rheumatoid arthritis, paralysis and neuromuscular diseases *(Porth, 1990)*. For example, a subluxed glenohumeral joint may occur, called a "hemiplegic shoulder", following a stroke;

➤ **congenital ligamentous laxity** or joint malformation (often found with the hip, knee or patella);

➤ **previous dislocations** of the joint.

Once injured, the joint may repeatedly dislocate or sublux, leading to **joint instability**. The joint capsule is weakened, allowing the structure to become painfully hypermobile. This is more common in younger people than with older adults.

The Medical Treatment of Dislocations

Medical treatment of a dislocation involves tractioning the bones that comprise the joint to bring the articulating surfaces back into normal contact. This procedure is called joint reduction. The earlier the joint is reduced after the injury, the easier the procedure will be. If protective muscle spasm has set in, an injection of a muscle relaxant or an anaesthetic is used before the joint is reduced. The joint is supported or protected for several weeks to allow the joint capsule and ligaments to heal. Limited pain-free movement and strengthening of the muscles that cross the joint are usually encouraged *(Brukner, Khan, 1993)*.

In the acute stage, it is most likely that the massage therapist is treating the client after the dislocation has been reduced by a physician. If the dislocated joint has not been reduced, the therapist uses first aid to stabilize and support the limb and then applies ice. The client is immediately referred for emergency medical attention.

Surgery may be required to repair the joint capsule or the glenoid labrum after repeated dislocations. The surgery intentionally shortens the portion of the joint capsule that was overstretched and damaged. Another surgical procedure brings a section of a muscle to cross the joint and support it. As a result, the joint has a reduced range of motion in the direction that the dislocation occurred. This creates more stability. With a complicating fracture — for example, at the acromioclavicular joint — pins or screws may be used to intentionally limit the range of motion. Arthroscopic procedures to repair shoulder dislocations include stapling the glenoid labrum in place *(Bunker, Wallace, 1991)*.

In treating an acute or subacute dislocation, the therapist should contact the client's physician (with the client's permission) in case there are any contraindications to massage.

Dislocation of Specific Joints

In terms of the **glenohumeral** joint *(Figure 26.1)*, the most common form of this injury is an **anterior dislocation**, also called a subcoracoid dislocation. The mechanism of injury is often excessive abduction and external rotation of the humerus. For example, a person

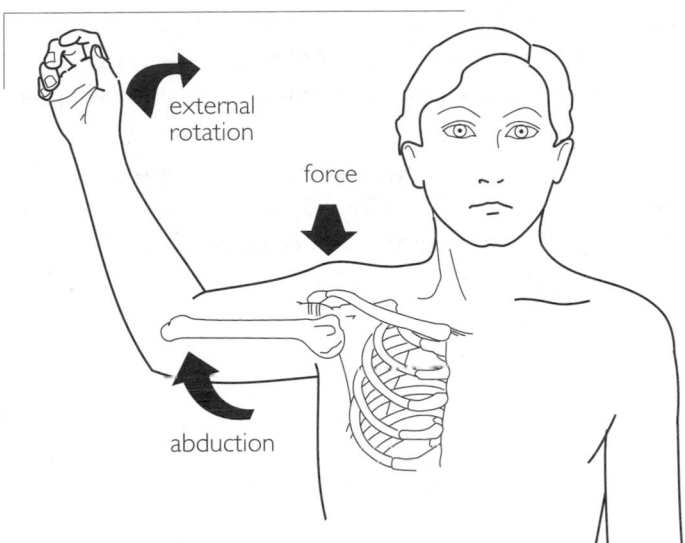

Figure 26.1
Anterior glenohumeral joint dislocation — force from behind.

may be tackled from behind as he is throwing a ball. Another mechanism of injury involves extension of the humerus, where the person falls backwards onto his outstretched hand *(Edwardson, 1995)*. Either of these two mechanisms forces the head of the humerus through the inferior portion of the joint capsule (the foramen of Weitbrecht) where it lodges inferior to the coracoid process. There may be damage to the anterior portion of the glenoid labrum (a Bankart lesion) *(Brukner, Khan, 1993)*. The axillary nerve may also be injured.

Following reduction, the joint is usually stable if it is held in internal rotation. A sling is used to support the arm for between three and six weeks *(Brukner, Khan, 1993; Buschbacher, 1994)*. With a younger person, it may be necessary to bandage the arm to the thorax for two or three weeks to prevent reinjury *(Thomson et al., 1991)*. With an elderly adult where joint capsule stiffness may occur, this immobilization period may be shortened to 10 days *(Buschbacher, 1994)*.

Recurring anterior glenohumeral dislocations may be treated surgically to stabilize the joint. Another indication for surgery is when the joint subluxes easily and the person is able to reduce it himself *(Kisner, Colby, 1990)*. The Putti Platt surgery involves shortening the subscapularis muscle to limit external rotation. The Bankart procedure reattaches the joint capsule to the glenoid fossa using arthroscopy. The shoulder may be immobilized for up to four weeks following surgery *(Thomson et al., 1991)*.

Less frequently, a **posterior dislocation** of the glenohumeral joint occurs. The mechanism of injury is usually flexion, adduction and internal rotation of the humerus *(Edwardson, 1995)*. For example, the person falls forward onto his flexed elbow *(Buschbacher, 1994)*.

The **patella** usually dislocates in a lateral direction. The mechanism of injury involves external rotation of the tibia and foot when the knee is flexed *(Porth, 1990)*. Following reduction, the knee is bandaged for several days. With repeated dislocations, the tibial insertion of the quadriceps may be surgically transposed to a more medial location. This ensures that contraction of the quadriceps will keep the patella tracking more medially. The joint may be immobilized for six to nine weeks with open reduction *(Thomson et al., 1991)*.

The **lunate** is dislocated by a fall on the outstretched hand, forcing the wrist into hyperextension. The radius forces the lunate in a palmar direction, displacing the lunate anteriorly into the wrist between the flexor tendons and the capitate bone. Open reduction may be necessary. After reduction, the wrist is immobilized in 20 degrees of flexion for up to four weeks *(Conwell, 1982)*. Complications include median nerve lesions and possible necrosis of the lunate if the vasculature in the dorsal ligaments connecting the lunate to the radius is torn (called Keinboch disease) *(Booher, Thibodeau, 1989)*.

A dislocation at the **elbow** is usually accompanied by a fracture. This injury occurs after a fall on the outstretched hand or in a motor vehicle accident. The ulna and radius are

341

displaced posteriorly. The brachial artery, the medial nerve or the ulnar nerve may be involved *(Cailliet, 1989)*. The elbow is usually immobilized for three weeks following reduction *(Thomson et al., 1991)*. Myositis ossificans may occasionally result following this injury *(Brukner, Khan, 1993)*.

A **hip dislocation**, although uncommon, may occur following a car or motorcycle accident. If the person is seated, the femur is forced posteriorly by a direct impact to the knee. Complications include fracture of the rim of the acetabulum and compression of the sciatic nerve. Following reduction the limb is tractioned for up to six weeks *(Thomson et al., 1991)*.

Symptom Picture

Acute

+ There is a complete rupture of the joint capsule and supporting ligaments or an avulsion fracture of the capsular attachments.
+ A snapping or popping noise is heard at the time of injury.
+ The pain is intense and sickening at the time of injury.
+ The joint usually appears deformed before reduction.
+ Marked local edema and heat are evident; joint effusion may occur if the joint capsule is damaged. If blood goes into the joint space, a hemarthrosis occurs.
+ The joint is unstable.
+ Complications include strains, contusions, blood vessel and nerve injury and fractures. A hematoma may be present.
+ The bruising is red, black and blue.
+ There is decreased range of motion at the joint as protective muscle spasm, edema and pain limit movement.
+ The client cannot continue the activity.
+ Following reduction, the joint may be taped, splinted, casted or otherwise supported. The ruptured joint capsule and supporting ligaments may be surgically repaired, then immobilized. Other structures compensate for this.

Early Subacute

+ The joint is unstable.
+ The bruising is black and blue.
+ The hematoma is still present but diminished from the acute stage.
+ The pain, edema and inflammation are still present but reduced from the acute stage.
+ Adhesions are developing around the injury.
+ Because the joint capsule and its supporting ligaments are hypovascular, they heal relatively slowly.

- ◆ The protective muscle spasm diminishes. Trigger points occur in the muscles crossing the joint and in compensatory muscles.
- ◆ The muscles crossing the injured joint provide the only stability.
- ◆ The injured joint is taped, splinted or immobilized. The dislocation may have been surgically reduced.
- ◆ The range of motion is reduced. The physician will advise the client on the allowable range.

Late Subacute

- ◆ The bruising changes to yellow, green and brown.
- ◆ The pain, edema and inflammation are diminishing.
- ◆ Adhesions are maturing around the injury.
- ◆ The protective muscle spasm is replaced by an increased tone in the muscles crossing the joint.
- ◆ The muscles crossing the joint still provide the stability.
- ◆ The affected joint is supported or immobilized. The client uses crutches or a cane.
- ◆ The range of motion is reduced.

Chronic

- ◆ There is pain local to the joint capsule when the capsule is stressed.
- ◆ The bruising is gone.
- ◆ Adhesions have matured around the injury.
- ◆ Hypertonicity and trigger points are present in muscles crossing the joint and in compensating structures.
- ◆ Full range of motion of the joint is restricted.
- ◆ A pocket of chronic edema may remain local to the ligament.
- ◆ The tissue may be cool due to ischemia.
- ◆ The joint may be unstable in the direction the injury occurred unless it is surgically repaired. The joint may be immobilized for up to nine weeks after surgery.
- ◆ Muscle weakness or disuse atrophy may be present in muscles crossing the affected joint, particularly with immobilization.
- ◆ There is a loss of proprioception at the joint.
- ◆ The client may need taping or elastic bandages for activities that stress the joint.

Subjective Information

HEALTH HISTORY QUESTIONS

✦ What is the client's overall health history? Is the client on any medication for unrelated conditions that indicate treatment modifications?

✦ Does the client have any contributing conditions or pathologies that predispose the person to ligament injuries, such as congenital ligamentous laxity, rheumatoid arthritis, hemiplegia or cerebral palsy?

✦ Has there been a history of recurrent dislocations or subluxations of that joint? This indicates that the joint is unstable.

✦ In terms of the presenting complaint, when did the injury occur?

✦ Does the client know the mechanism of injury — for example, falling on an outstretched hand? The person may describe feeling the bone "pop out of place" or hearing a snapping or popping noise.

✦ What was done at the time of injury? Was first aid applied?

✦ Did the client see any other health care practitioner for this injury, such as a physician, physiotherapist, chiropractor or sports therapist? If so, what treatment was given? Is the client still receiving this treatment?

✦ Was the joint immobilized or was the joint capsule surgically repaired? Are pins, wires, screws or other appliances present? If the joint was immobilized, how long was this for? With immobilization, disuse atrophy and adhesions may be present.

✦ Is the client using a sling, other supports or crutches for the affected joint? This is expected with an acute or subacute dislocation.

✦ Is the client taking any medication for the dislocation, such as analgesics or anti-inflammatories? This includes self-medication such as Aspirin or other over-the-counter products.

✦ What symptoms is the client currently experiencing? Does the client have pain now? Where exactly is the pain? Is the pain sharp or diffuse? Sharp, hot pain indicates an acute injury, while an ache is associated with a chronic injury.

✦ What aggravates or relieves the pain?

✦ Is there any edema or bruising local or distal to the injury?

✦ Were there any complications, such as nerve or blood vessel damage or fracture?

✦ What activities are difficult or painful to complete? Are any activities impossible to complete? For example, the client may report an inability to place the joint in the position in which the injury occurred. This may be due to the client's apprehension or joint instability. If the capsule was surgically repaired, a reduced range of motion is desired for joint stability.

✦ What are the client's activities of daily living? Does the client's occupation or recreational activity place stress on the joint?

Objective Information

Observations

Acute

✍ Antalgic gait occurs if the dislocation is to a weight bearing joint.

✍ Antalgic posture may be present. For example, with an acromioclavicular or anterior glenohumeral dislocation, the arm is held against the body with the affected shoulder possibly in slight elevation.

✍ The affected joint may be supported by taping, elastic bandages, splints or a cast. The client will use crutches with a dislocation of a weight bearing joint. A sling may be used with a wrist or shoulder dislocation.

✍ The client may have a pained or medicated facial expression.

✍ Edema is observed at the affected joint. There may be distal edema.

✍ Some redness may be present local to the injury.

✍ Red, black or purple bruising over the injury site may be visible. There may be a hematoma.

Early and Late Subacute

✍ Antalgic gait is still present with a dislocation of a weight bearing joint. It has diminished from the presentation in the acute stage.

✍ Antalgic posture will also still occur.

✍ Supports for the limb are still present. The client will continue to use crutches with a dislocation of a weight bearing joint. A sling may still be used with a wrist or shoulder dislocation.

✍ Edema diminishes from the early to late subacute stage, both on site and distally.

✍ Bruising over the injury site changes from purple and black in the early subacute stage to brown, yellow and green in the late subacute stage. It then disappears. There may be distal bruising. The hematoma, if present, is diminishing.

✍ If the joint capsule and ligaments were surgically reduced, scars are present. These range from half a centimetre long following arthroscopic surgery to several centimetres in length with open reductions.

Chronic

✍ Habituated antalgic gait may be observed with a dislocation of a weight bearing joint. Habitual antalgic posture may be present with an upper limb dislocation. A postural assessment is indicated in this case.

✍ Taping or other supports may be used during activities that stress the joint. If surgery was performed to stabilize the joint, the dislocation may still be immobilized. The client may continue to use a sling, crutches or a cane.

✍ There may be some residual chronic edema local to the injury.

✍ There is scarring following surgery.

Palpation

Acute

- Heat is present over the injured joint and possibly in the surrounding tissue.
- Tenderness is present local to the lesion site and refers into the nearby tissue.
- The texture of the edema is firm.
- Protective muscle spasm is present in muscles crossing the affected joint.

Early and Late Subacute

- The temperature over the injury site diminishes from the early subacute to the late subacute stage.
- Tenderness is present local to the injury.
- The texture of the edema is less firm and adhesions are present as healing progresses from the early to the late subacute stage.
- The tone of the muscles crossing the joint changes from spasmodic in the early subacute stage to tightness and hypertonicity in the late subacute stage. Trigger points are present in these muscles.

Chronic

- The injury site may be cool due to ischemia.
- Point tenderness occurs local to the lesion site.
- There are adhesions local to the joint capsule and injured ligaments.
- Hypertonicity and trigger points are present local to the injured joint and in the compensating muscles. Disuse atrophy may be present in muscles crossing the affected joint if full range of motion is not present or with casting.

Testing

Acute, Early and Late Subacute

- **AF ROM** of the proximal and distal joints may be slowly and carefully performed in a pain-free manner.
- **Other testing is contraindicated in the acute or subacute stage.**

Chronic

- This testing protocol is different from any other testing. The main goal in assessing a dislocated joint before treatment is to determine if the joint is stable or unstable (*Figure 26.2*).
- An **AF apprehension test** is used if the mechanism of injury is known. The client

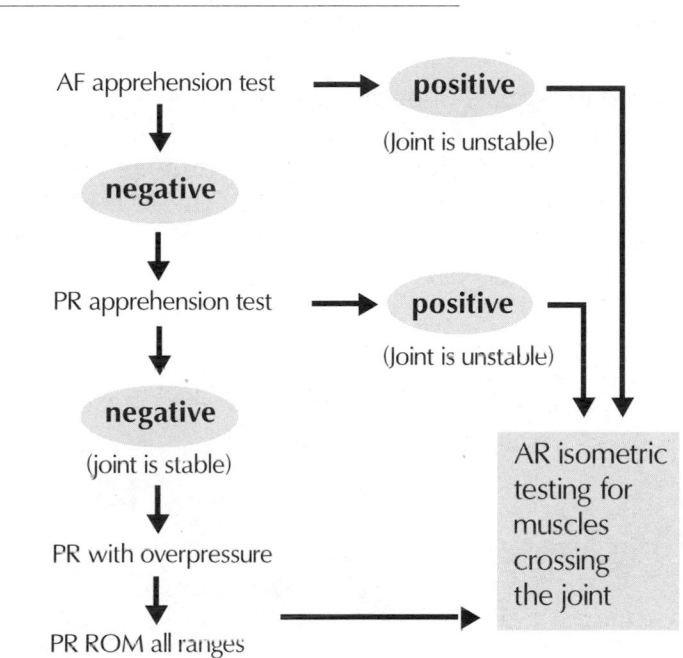

Figure 26.2
Testing protocol for dislocations.

moves the limb **active free** towards the position that the joint was in when it dislocated. If the client is unable to perform this action due to apprehension that the joint will redislocate or sublux, this is considered a **positive** active free apprehension test for joint instability.

✍ **If the active free apprehension test is positive, passive relaxed testing is not performed** because the joint is unstable.

✍ The therapist moves directly into **isometric active resisted testing** of the muscles that cross the joint. This will not harm the joint capsule or cause redislocation because the joint is not moving.

- If the mechanism of injury is unclear for the client, **AF ROM** is performed on the cardinal planes of motion of the affected joint. Range that is limited by any remaining pain or apprehension is noted, because the limb was likely in that position when it was injured.

✍ If the active free apprehension test is **negative**, the therapist performs a **passive relaxed apprehension test**, slowly moving the limb towards the position in which the injury occurred. If the client stops the testing due to apprehension that the joint may redislocate or if the client moves away from the position to relieve the stress on the joint, this is considered a **positive** passive relaxed apprehension test for joint instability. The end feel is empty due to apprehension. The therapist then proceeds to **isometric active resisted testing** of the muscles crossing the joint.

✍ If the passive relaxed apprehension test is **negative**, the therapist applies gentle overpressure to the joint to further assess the joint's stability. The therapist may also perform **PR ROM** on the cardinal planes of motion, with the range that the injury occurred in tested **last**. A painful, possibly hypermobile end feel may be present on stressing the joint capsule and supporting ligaments in the direction that the joint dislocated. With a surgically repaired joint capsule, a capsular end feel is encountered before it would be expected.

✍ **AR testing** of muscles crossing the affected joint is performed, checking for possible decreased muscle strength with associated injury to muscles or tendons, or disuse atrophy.

Special Tests

✍ Following a patellar dislocation, the **patellar apprehension test** is positive.

✍ Combined AF ROM at the glenohumeral joint is assessed using **Apley's scratch test**. The range is reduced, usually in external rotation and abduction.

✍ Both **active free** and **passive relaxed apprehension tests** are positive with a glenohumeral joint dislocation.

✍ **Ligamentous stress tests** are used to assess if a specific portion of any stable joint capsule or its supporting ligaments have been injured. The pressure used is sufficient to stress the joint capsule without damaging it. The end feel is **hypermobile**. A dislocation may or may not be painful local to the joint capsule. If there is a complete rupture, the damaged fibres cannot register the pain of a tissue stretch. If some fibres are intact, they can register pain when stretched. See the sprain chapter for more details.

✍ With a lunate dislocation, a **PR wrist extension test** is positive.

✍ With an acromioclavicular joint dislocation, the **acromioclavicular shear test** is positive.

Contraindications

♦ In the acute and subacute stages, testing other than pain-free AF range of motion is contraindicated to prevent further tissue damage.

♦ Avoid removing the protective muscle splinting of acute and early subacute dislocations.

♦ Distal circulation techniques are contraindicated in the acute and early subacute stages to avoid increasing congestion through the injury site.

♦ If the joint is unstable, do not place the limb in the position that the injury occurred. This position is also avoided when range of motion exercises or rhythmic techniques are performed.

♦ Joint play is contraindicated following dislocations where the capsule has not been surgically reduced and the joint is unstable.

♦ Frictions are contraindicated if the client is taking anti-inflammatories or blood thinners.

♦ Avoid heavy hydrotherapy applications applied to the joint in the acute and subacute stages.

♦ With dislocations that are casted, avoid hot hydrotherapy applications to the tissue immediately proximal to the cast, to prevent congestion under the cast.

♦ Remedial exercise in the acute stage of a dislocation is contraindicated.

♦ Before attempting to restore range in the direction that the dislocation occurred, ensure that the majority of strength is regained in the muscles crossing the joint.

♦ Where the joint capsule and ligaments have been surgically repaired, full range of motion of the affected joint should not be restored in the direction that will stretch the repaired capsule and ligaments.

Treatment Goals

Treatment Plan

Acute

Refer for immediate medical attention if not reduced.

Reduce inflammation.

🖐 **The joint is treated with RICE:** Rest, Ice, Compression and Elevation.

🖐 **Positioning** of the client depends primarily on client comfort and on keeping the limb secure so no stress or torque is placed on the injured joint. The therapist needs to be aware of the possibility of client apprehension and guarding of the injured limb. The limb is elevated and pillowed securely in a position that does not place a stress on the injured joint.

🖐 Hydrotherapy is a cold application, such as an ice pack or a gel pack, applied to the injured area with care taken not to place too much weight on the injury site.

General Treatment

🖐 If the initial treatment goal is to decrease edema, lymphatic drainage on the affected limb is performed first.

Reduce pain. Decrease sympathetic nervous system firing.

Treat any compensating structures.

🖐 If the initial goal is to accustom the client to the therapist's touch in the context of a relaxation massage, the client is directed to do diaphragmatic breathing throughout the treatment.

🖐 The trunk and uninjured limb are treated using effleurage and slow petrissage, such as palmar kneading, fingertip kneading and C-scooping. The focus of the work depends on the muscles that are compensating. For example, the shoulders and back are treated if crutches are used.

Specific Treatment

Reduce edema.

🖐 Lymphatic drainage techniques are used on the injured limb, beginning with nodal pumping at the proximal lymph nodes. Unidirectional effleurage, stationary circles and the local technique are used proximal to the injury to reduce edema.

Maintain local circulation proximal to the injury only.

🖐 The proximal limb is treated to reduce pain and hypertonicity as well as to increase drainage and venous return. Techniques include effleurage and repetitive petrissage, such as the origin and insertion technique and fingertip kneading.

Do not remove protective muscle spasm.

🖐 Care is taken not to significantly reduce any protective muscle spasms in muscles that cross the affected joint by overtreating the proximal tissue.

🖐 On-site work is contraindicated.

🖐 Distal work is restricted to light stroking and muscle squeezing, to the client's pain tolerance.

349

Treatment Goals

Maintain range of motion.

Treat other conditions.

Reduce inflammation.

Reduce pain.
Decrease sympathetic nervous system firing.

Reduce edema.
Prevent excess adhesion formation.

Maintain local circulation proximal to the injury only.

Reduce but do not remove any spasm.
Reduce trigger points.

Treatment Plan

🖐 Careful **mid-range passive relaxed range of motion** is used on the proximal joints to maintain the successive action and to help increase lymphatic drainage. This is only performed on joints that are not crossed by muscles that also cross the dislocated joint.

🖐 Other injuries, such as strains or contusions, are also treated. See the appropriate chapters for details.

Early Subacute

🖐 **The healing tissue is still fragile. Therefore, the treatment goals are achieved with care.**

🖐 The client may still be apprehensive about **positioning** or movement. The limb is once again elevated if this does not compromise the affected joint.

🖐 **Hydrotherapy applications** on site are cold/warm contrast.

General Treatment

🖐 The treatment approach outlined for acute general work is indicated at this stage also, including reducing pain perception and encouraging **diaphragmatic breathing.**

Specific Treatment

🖐 Proximal lymphatic drainage techniques to reduce the edema are indicated for the injured limb. These include proximal nodal pumping, unidirectional effleurage, stationary circles and the local technique. The work is performed proximal to the lesion site to prevent congestion through the injury.

🖐 The proximal limb is treated to reduce hypertonicity and to increase drainage and venous return. Techniques include effleurage and repetitive petrissage, such as the origin and insertion technique, palmar kneading, C-scooping and fingertip kneading.

🖐 Care is taken not to significantly reduce the protective spasm in muscles that cross the affected joint by overtreating the tissue.

🖐 Trigger points in muscles that refer to the injured limb and the injury site itself are now treated directly. Muscle stripping is used for this in the early subacute stage.

🖐 On-site work is now indicated. Vibrations, gentle stroking and gentle fingertip kneading to the client's pain tolerance may be used on the muscles crossing the injured joint.

Treatment Goals

Treatment Plan

Maintain range of motion.

🖐 Careful pain-free mid-range passive relaxed range of motion is used by the therapist on the proximal joints. This is only performed on joints whose muscles do not also cross the dislocated joint.

🖐 Distal techniques for the early subacute stage include stroking and muscle squeezing only. This reduces the possibility of causing congestion through the lesion site.

Late Subacute

🖐 The healing tissue is less fragile. Therefore, the treatment goals can be achieved using slightly more vigorous techniques.

🖐 The limb is elevated without placing a stress on the joint.

🖐 **Hydrotherapy applications** local to the injury are cold/hot contrast. If acute inflammation recurs, the therapist returns to using local cold hydrotherapy applications.

General Treatment

Reduce pain. Decrease sympathetic nervous system firing. Treat any compensating structures.

🖐 The treatment approach outlined for early subacute general work is indicated at this stage also.

Specific Treatment

Reduce edema.

🖐 As the edema diminishes in the late subacute stage, the length of time spent on the drainage techniques decreases.

Reduce hypertonicity and trigger points.

🖐 The proximal limb is treated to reduce hypertonicity and to maintain drainage and venous return.

🖐 Trigger points in muscles that refer to the injured limb and the injury site itself are treated using muscle stripping and ischemic compressions according to the client's pain tolerance. If ischemic compressions are used to treat a muscle that crosses the joint, repetitive petrissage is used to flush circulation through the muscle instead of heat and a stretch which may compromise the dislocated joint.

Prevent excess adhesion formation.

🖐 As inflammation subsides, the on-site focus shifts to preventing the formation of painful and restricting adhesions between the joint capsule, its supporting ligaments and the surrounding structures. Any restricting adhesions are reduced without destabilizing the joint — only a small area of adhesions are addressed in one treatment. Longitudinal muscle stripping followed by specific petrissage, such as short cross-fibre strokes and gentle frictions to the adhesions, are indicated *(Hertling, Kessler, 1990; Thomson et al., 1991)*. Following frictions, **only** a partial stretch is used to prevent overmobilizing the

351

Treatment Goals   Treatment Plan

joint. **Ice** is applied to the frictioned tissue to restrict the inflammatory process. All this work is performed within the client's pain tolerance.

- In subsequent treatments, the range of the joint is reassessed. If necessary, painfully restricting adhesions are further reduced. Again, care is taken to address mobility without destabilizing the joint.

Maintain range of motion.
- To maintain the range of motion and prevent capsular contractures, gentle joint play movements in the direction that the dislocation did not occur are performed *(Kisner, Colby, 1990)*. Joint play is performed cautiously, gently and in a **pain-free** manner.

- Joint play techniques are introduced to the proximal and distal joints in the late subacute stage if these joints are hypomobile due to compensation.

Gradually increase the range of motion.
- **Pain-free active assisted range of motion** and **pain-free mid-range passive relaxed range of motion** are used on the affected joint, avoiding the range that was injured.

Increase local circulation.
- In the late subacute stage, the risk of causing congestion local to the dislocation diminishes. Effleurage and petrissage are now introduced distally to maintain tissue health.

Chronic

- **Positioning** is now chosen for comfort and for accessibility to the structures that the therapist is treating. The limb is only elevated if chronic edema remains. Otherwise it is positioned comfortably and in a way that does not stress the joint.

- **Hydrotherapy applications** proximal to the dislocation and on the lesion site itself include deep moist heat, such as a hydrocollator or a wax application, to soften adhesions and increase local circulation.

General Treatment

Decrease sympathetic nervous system firing. Treat compensatory structures.
- The client's trunk and compensating structures are massaged as before. Rhythmic techniques to the trunk and unaffected limb are indicated as long as the joint is not taken into the position of dislocation.

Specific Treatment

Reduce any chronic edema.
- Proximal and local connective tissue restrictions may be helping to retain a pocket of chronic edema in the hollows around the dislocated joint. Fascial glide is used to assess, then fascial techniques are used to

Treatment Goals   Treatment Plan

✋ treat restrictions. These include crossed-hands or ulnar border spreading techniques.

✋ Proximal lymphatic drainage is also indicated. A **contrast hydrotherapy** application of alternating hot and cold towels is useful to flush out the edema.

Reduce hypertonicity and trigger points.

✋ The proximal limb is treated to reduce any remaining hypertonicity or trigger points and to increase local circulation. Effleurage, repetitive petrissage and ischemic compressions are indicated.

Reduce adhesions.

✋ If the therapist has been treating the client's injury throughout the healing process, the focus is on regaining strength and reducing the remaining restrictive adhesions between the tendons crossing the joint and the capsule itself. This is done without destabilizing the joint. Preparatory techniques include specific kneading and muscle stripping. Then, if the limb is no longer immobilized, cross-fibre frictions to the adhesions are performed. These are followed by a passive relaxed stretch to the muscles to realign the fibres. This should normalize the range of the joint without overstretching the joint capsule and its supporting ligaments. It may not be possible or desirable to regain full range of motion. An application of **ice** follows this work.

Restore range of motion.

✋ Joint play techniques to the proximal and distal joints are used if these structures are restricted due to compensation. If the joint capsule itself is fibrosed, pain-free joint play techniques in all ranges, **except** the one in which the dislocation occurred, are indicated (*Kisner, Colby, 1990*).

✋ Passive relaxed range of motion is used by the therapist on the proximal, affected and distal joints to maintain joint health. With an unstable joint, the range in which the injury occurred is **avoided.**

Increase local circulation.

✋ The distal limb is treated with effleurage and petrissage to increase local venous return.

✋ If the therapist starts treating the client in the chronic stage, one approach is to focus on reducing the hypertonicity and trigger points that have developed from the client's compensation patterns. This is done before addressing any adhesions.

If the Limb Is Immobilized

🖐 The injury may be immobilized with or without surgical reduction of the joint capsule. To treat the limb during immobilization, the therapist should refer to the chapter on fractures.

🖐 Once the immobilization is removed and if the dislocation was medically treated using the conservative approach of strapping or casting only, the joint is likely unstable in the direction the dislocation occurred. Because the joint capsule was not surgically repaired, there is little to prevent hypermobility, other than the support given by the muscles that cross the joint. In this case, mobilizing techniques are contraindicated. Instead, a remedial exercise program to strengthen the muscles that cross the injured ligament is important.

🖐 If the joint capsule was surgically reduced, rendering the joint stable, the capsule and supporting ligaments or muscles have been repaired in a shortened position. Because ligaments are not contractile, this repair is done to give the joint capsule a functional range while preventing hypermobility. Full range of motion of the injured joint is not desired *(Kisner, Colby, 1990; Hertling, Kessler, 1990)*. It is important for the therapist not to overmobilize the repaired joint capsule once tone has returned to the muscles that were under a cast.

Self-care Goals

Educate the client.

Maintain range of motion.

Increase the strength.

Increase the strength.

Self-care Plan

✍ **Hydrotherapy** is chosen according to the stage of healing. Because the joint capsule and supporting ligaments are hypovascular, it is important to introduce contrast hydrotherapy, to help increase local circulation, as soon as the acute stage has passed.

✍ **Self-massage** is useful for the muscles that cross the dislocated joint in the late subacute and chronic stages. This includes fingertip kneading, muscle stripping and gentle frictions within the client's pain tolerance.

✍ **Remedial exercise** that is given is dependent on the stage of healing. It is important to regain the majority of strength of the muscles crossing the dislocated joint (to provide support) before the range is increased in the direction that the injury occurred.

✍ In the **acute** stage, the client is asked to perform pain-free active free range of motion of the proximal and distal joints to maintain range of motion and reduce edema *(Thomson et al., 1991)*. Further remedial exercise is contraindicated in the acute stage.

✍ In the **early subacute** stage, the client can perform pain-free active free range of motion of the proximal and distal joints. If there is no secondary muscle strain present (or if there is a Grade 1 or 2 muscle strain only), the client can be shown submaximal, pain-free isometric exercises to strengthen the muscles that cross the dislocated joint.

✍ In the **late subacute** stage, maximal, pain-free active resisted isometric exercise is used to maintain the strength of the muscles that cross the dislocated joint.

Self-care Goals

Self-care Plan

Gradually increase the range.

✍ The client may gradually progress to isotonic active resisted exercise, still avoiding full range in the direction the injury occurred.

Strengthen muscles.

✍ In the **chronic** stage, the focus is on isotonic active resisted exercises in all ranges to strengthen the muscles that cross the affected joint.

Encourage activity.

✍ The client is encouraged to return to the activities of daily living on a gradual basis. A return to regular activities or sports that stress the joint can occur once functional exercises are **pain-free both during and after the exercise** (Kisner, Colby, 1990).

✍ The client may need to use tape, a brace or other supports to protect an unstable joint on activity, especially a weight bearing joint.

Treatment Frequency and Expected Outcome

Shorter, more frequent treatments will address the inflammatory process in the acute stages. Treatments may progress to once a week for chronic stages, then the client is reassessed.

The outcome is variable, depending on the severity of the injury, the treatment approach used (strengthening exercises and soft tissue work, immobilization or surgery) and the client's age, general health and compliance with the self-care program.

Return to activity (the following are guidelines only):

The client can return to normal activities when an apprehension test is negative and there is no weakness or muscle imbalance. Full rehabilitation may take up to four months (Kisner, Colby, 1990).

See stress reduction, edema, spasm, contusions, strains, sprains, hypermobility and hypomobility, conditions of the peripheral nervous system, fractures, scars, whiplash, osteoarthritis, hemiplegia and cerebral palsy for related treatments.

Complete healing of ligaments may require up to six months for full maturation of the collagen fibres (Hertling, Kessler, 1990; Booher, Thibodeau, 1989).

Dislocations can create joint laxity, leading to a cycle of repeated dislocations or subluxations and further stretching of the ligaments. If joint laxity is not corrected, the client may require surgery to stabilize the joint.

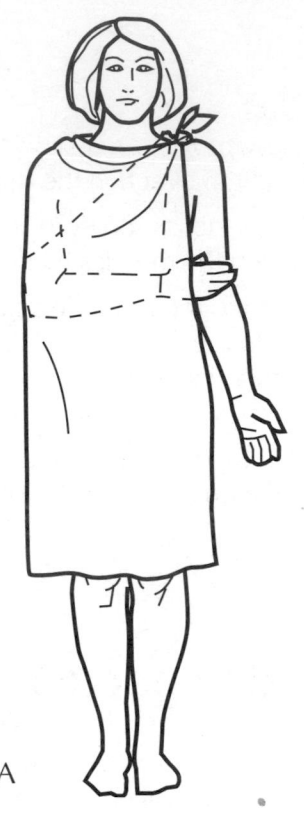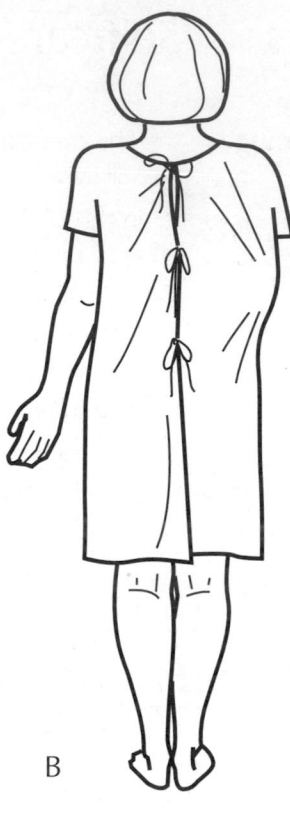

Figure 26.3
A) The client is draped to ensure comfort and privacy. The sheet is tied over the left shoulder leaving the left arm free, the right arm is in a sling underneath the sheet (dotted outline).

A

B

B) A clinic gown is draped over the sling, the right sleeve is empty.

Sample Treatment: Anterior Glenohumeral Joint Dislocation

Acute

🖐 The affected arm is in a sling and should not be moved. Therefore, the client may need help in undressing. The client is draped to ensure comfort and privacy. For example, the client may be draped "toga-style" with a sheet wrapped around the body and over the sling and tied over the unaffected shoulder (*Figure 26.3*). This allows the unaffected arm and unaffected side of the back to be undraped, when the client is seated in front of the massage table. Another option is for the client to put on a clinic gown with the opening at the back. Only the unaffected arm is put into a sleeve of the gown and the rest of the gown is draped around the affected shoulder and over the sling.

🖐 The client is in a seated position. The affected arm is kept in the sling. One or two pillows are placed in the client's lap on which she can rest the elbow of the affected arm. This supports the head of the humerus in the glenoid fossa during the treatment. Several more pillows are placed on the table so the client can comfortably lean forward during treatment and the head is supported. Care is taken to avoid placing stress on the injured shoulder. A towel-wrapped ice or gel pack may be placed on the pillows. The client then leans forward, placing the injured shoulder onto the pack. The client is instructed to breathe diaphragmatically.

🖐 To treat the unaffected arm and shoulder, either the toga drape is untied or the unaffected arm is taken out of the sleeve of the gown. For a female client, appropriate draping is maintained by the client leaning into the pillows which support the anterior chest. She may also use the unaffected arm to secure the draping. Swedish techniques are used on the uninjured shoulder girdle, the neck and the low back to treat the compensating structures and to decrease sympathetic nervous system firing and pain.

🖐 Lymphatic drainage techniques are used on the affected shoulder, starting with pumping at the terminus and treating the pectoral muscles. If necessary, the therapist supports the head of the humerus with one hand while the other hand performs the drainage techniques. Lymphatic drainage is stopped just proximal to the edema.

🖐 The injured shoulder is treated with Swedish techniques proximal to the injury site only. Care is taken not to completely reduce protective muscle spasm. The trapezius and rhomboid muscles are gently kneaded and muscle squeezed, working from the spine laterally to the scapula. No anterior- or inferior-directed pressure is placed on the affected joint without first stabilizing the humeral head with one hand over the anterior deltoid. Proximal passive relaxed range of motion of the cervical spine is not practical with this injury at this time. However, AF or PR ROM of the elbow, wrist and fingers is performed.

🖐 On-site work is contraindicated. Gentle vibrations and stroking may be used on the distal affected arm. The treatment is 30 to 45 minutes in length. At the end of the treatment, the toga drape is re-tied or the client is assisted in slipping the arm back into the sleeve of the gown.

✍ For **self-care**, the client is instructed to rest and ice the dislocated shoulder. Pain-free active free range of motion for the unaffected shoulder and the neck is performed.

Early Subacute

🖐 Positioning for the early subacute stage is much the same as for the acute stage. The client is still wearing a sling. Care is taken not to stress the shoulder. Lymphatic drainage may now include axillary pumping, working over the deltoid and pectoral muscles without moving the humerus or stressing the joint. Mild contrast hydrotherapy can be applied to the injured shoulder while the uninjured shoulder muscles are treated. Swedish techniques for the unaffected and affected shoulder girdle muscles are similar to those in the acute stage, except the focus is on treating trigger points with muscle stripping. Trigger points in the scalenes, pectoralis major, levator scapula and upper trapezius refer into the anterior shoulder.

🖐 Gentle on-site vibrations, stroking and fingertip kneading are indicated.

🖐 Swedish techniques that don't increase circulation are performed on the distal limb, such as stroking and muscle squeezing of the arm and hand.

✍ For **self-care** exercises, the client can begin with submaximal pain-free active resisted strengthening for the deltoids, rotator cuff and pectoral muscles. The client can strengthen the internal rotators of the humerus by pressing the flexor surface of the forearm against her abdomen when the elbow is flexed. Similarly, the adductors can be strengthened by squeezing a small pillow between the elbow and the trunk (Brukner, Khan, 1993). Careful pain-free active free circumduction of the glenohumeral joint and active free range of motion of the neck, elbow and wrist are encouraged.

Late Subacute

🖐 The treatment plan is much the same as for the early subacute stage in terms of positioning and contralateral work. If the client is comfortable, she may be able to be treated lying on the unaffected side. The arm is probably still in a sling and the client is pillowed for security and comfort, with care taken not to place stress on the healing joint capsule. Less time is spent on lymphatic drainage. Circulation techniques are introduced on the affected arm and shoulder. Trigger points are treated with ischemic compressions. Specific work to the deltoid and rotator cuff muscles includes muscle stripping, fingertip kneading and cross-fibre strokes to decrease the tone and trigger points. Gentle frictions may be used on adhesions between muscles and tendons. A gentle, pain-free stretch is used to avoid overmobilizing the joint. This is followed with an application of ice.

An injury to the shoulder may also affect the sternoclavicular joint. If this structure is hypomobile, joint play techniques are used. Without compressing the glenohumeral joint, the therapist grasps the medial portion of the clavicle and mobilizes it anteriorly and posteriorly *(Barral, 1991)*. **Active assisted range of motion** of the glenohumeral joint is performed by supporting the client's wrist and elbow and asking the client to circumduct the humerus in a pain-free manner. Cautious pain-free passive relaxed flexion and extension may be included. Distal work includes effleurage and petrissage to the forearm and hand and passive ROM of the elbow, wrist and fingers.

In terms of **self-care**, an easy exercise for all ranges of motion is the "pendulum". The client circumducts the humerus in small pain-free circles while seated or standing. She can progress to flexion and extension ranges. Maximal isometric active resistance for internal rotation and adduction is continued, adding flexion and extension.

Chronic

The client may be started in a prone position to permit access to the low back and the uninjured and injured shoulders. The therapist should avoid positioning the affected arm in a position of abduction and external rotation if the joint is not stable.

Hypertonicity and compensatory changes are treated as in the previous stages with a focus on the rotator cuff muscles, including subscapularis, pectoralis minor and serratus anterior. When the client is turned supine, any remaining chronic edema in the axillary region is treated. Swedish techniques are used on both anterior shoulder girdles to increase local circulation. Trigger points in the deltoids referring into the lateral shoulder are addressed.

Passive relaxed ranges of the glenohumeral joint are performed, with abduction and external rotation done last. Frictions are performed to any adhesions. Joint play to the sternoclavicular joint is used if the structure is hypermobile. In the case of contracture of the glenohumeral joint where the joint is stable, mobilization is performed in all the restricted ranges **except** anterior glide and extremes of internal rotation and abduction *(Kisner, Colby, 1990)*. Fascial techniques are used for restrictions if indicated.

For **self-care**, the goal is to maintain strength in the deltoids, rotator cuff, trapezius, rhomboids and pectoralis major muscles. The client adds active resisted isometric resistance for mid-ranges of abduction and external rotation of the glenohumeral joint. These exercises are progressed to isotonic ones in all ranges. Gradually, the client will return to activities that involve the shoulder and arm. The client may need to avoid actions that stress the joint capsule.

27

FRACTURES

Fiona Rattray

A fracture is a break in the continuity of a bone.

Fractures are classified into several types according to the nature of the break, its location on the bone and the angle of the broken ends. If the skin is intact, it is termed a **closed,** or **simple,** fracture. If the ends of the bone have broken through the skin or into one of the body cavities, it is called an **open, or compound**, fracture. An open fracture is more prone to infection. Fractures may be **complete**, where the bone is broken into two or more pieces, or **incomplete,** where the bone is bent or cracked and the periosteum remains intact.

Complete fractures are **transverse, oblique, spiral, comminuted, avulsion** and **osteochondral** breaks. Transverse fractures usually stay in place after reduction, which is either tractioning or surgery to bring the separated surfaces of the bone into normal contact, but they take longer to heal. In contrast, while it is more difficult to keep an oblique or spiral fracture in place even when splinted, these type of breaks heal more rapidly. A comminuted fracture is often unstable because it consists of two or more fragments, making healing difficult *(Apley, Solomon, 1993)*. An avulsion fracture occurs when a ligament pulls the portion of bone that it is attached to away from the bone itself. Osteochondral fractures occur when fragments of articular cartilage are sheared from the joint surface, often during a dislocation or sprain *(Brukner, Khan, 1993)*.

Examples of incomplete fractures are **compression, greenstick, perforation** and **stress** fractures. With a compression fracture the bone is crushed. These injuries occur in cancellous bone, such as a vertebral body. With a greenstick fracture, the bone is bent or partially broken, as when breaking a green twig. These fractures are found in children younger than 10 years of age, when the bones are more pliable than those of adults. Perforation fractures are the result of a missile wound, such as a bullet. Stress fractures are cracks in the bone due to overuse or repetitive actions.

In addition to the fractured bone itself, there are associated soft tissue injuries. Ligaments, tendons, muscles, fascia, nerves, blood vessels and skin can all be damaged. As a result of the trauma that caused the fracture, the client may also have associated contusions, strains, sprains and dislocations at the fracture site and at other locations. These other soft tissue injures may be overlooked while the initial medical focus is on reducing the fracture.

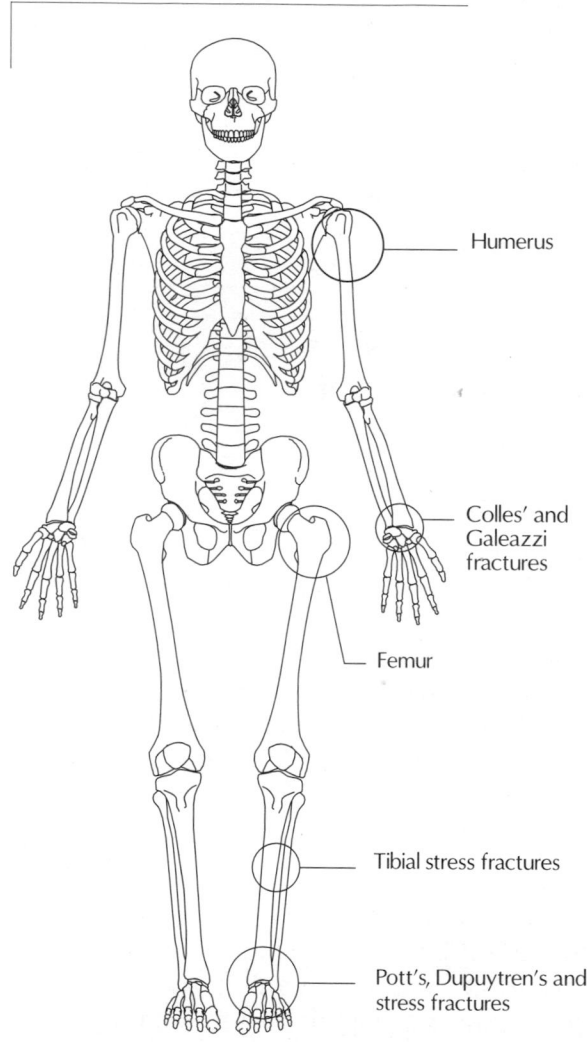

Figure 27.1
Common fracture sites.

Labels on figure:
Humerus
Colles' and Galeazzi fractures
Femur
Tibial stress fractures
Pott's, Dupuytren's and stress fractures

Common Fracture Names

The type and pattern of some fractures are predictable enough for them to acquire names *(Figure 27.1):*

✦ **Colles'** fracture of the wrist was first described by Abraham Colles in 1814. Here, a transverse fracture of the radius just proximal to the wrist allows the fragment to rotate and displace dorsally. This gives the wrist the classic "dinner fork" deformity before it is reduced. It is the most common fracture in older people *(Apley, Solomon, 1993)*. The usual mechanism of injury is a fall onto the outstretched hand. A Colles' fracture can be difficult to reduce successfully. The cast is left in place for four to six weeks *(Morgan, 1989)*. Complications following this fracture can include malunion and reflex sympathetic dystrophy, or shoulder-hand syndrome, where edema and capsular tightening painfully affect the wrist and shoulder *(Hertling, Kessler, 1990)*. Carpal tunnel syndrome may occasionally result.

✦ The **Galeazzi** fracture involves a break of the radial shaft and a dislocation of the inferior radioulnar joint. A fall on the hand with some rotational component is the mechanism of injury. Casting time is approximately six weeks *(Fleetcroft, 1982)*. An ulnar nerve lesion may occur with this injury *(Apley, Solomon, 1993)*.

✦ A **Pott's** ankle fracture affects one or both malleoli. The distal fibula breaks close to the lateral malleolus. The deltoid ligament may also rupture or avulse the medial malleoli.

✦ With a **Dupuytren's** fracture, the fibula fractures higher up, the medial malleoli avulses and the talus is pushed superiorly between the tibia and fibula *(Sammarco, 1995)*. The mechanism of injury in both cases is usually eversion with some external rotation. Screws or wires are often used to reduce and stabilize ankle fractures. The leg is casted for six to 12 weeks. Malunion and joint stiffness are possible complications *(Apley, Solomon, 1993)*.

✦ Common sites of stress fractures include the tibia, the metatarsals, the navicular, the femur and pelvis *(Brukner, Khan, 1993)*.

✦ The humerus and femur often suffer complete fractures to the upper shaft or neck.

Causes of a fracture are:

➤ **a trauma or sudden force which creates more stress than the bone can absorb.** With a **direct force** from an object striking it, a bone breaks at the point of impact. There is associated soft tissue damage. A blow causes a transverse fracture and often minor local soft tissue lesions, while a crushing injury causes a comminuted fracture and considerable soft tissue damage *(Apley, Solomon, 1993)*. With an **indirect force** a bone breaks at a distance from the site of the force. A torquing or twisting force causes a spiral fracture, often with little soft tissue damage;

➤ **overuse or repeated wear** which causes cracks in a bone or a stress fracture;

➤ **pathologies such as osteoporosis, tumours, local infections or bone cysts** which can cause a brittleness or weakening of the bone, so a fracture may occur spontaneously with little apparent force.

Stages of Healing

The physiological process of fracture repair depends on the type of bone that is injured and the amount of movement that occurs at the fracture site. For example, a bone that is tubular and that is not rigidly fixated is thought to follow five healing stages. Sources differ as to the specifics of each stage of healing, perhaps because the exact mechanism of bone healing is not clearly understood and remains controversial *(Apley, Solomon, 1993; Porth, 1990; Leung et al., 1994; Lane, 1987)*.

✦ In the **first stage,** a hematoma forms around the ends of the fractured bone within 72 hours of the initial trauma. A mesh of fibrin forms around the injury site. The ends of the bone die back several millimetres.

✦ In the **second stage,** there is an inflammatory reaction and a proliferation of osteoblasts at the periosteum. These cells create a fibrocartilaginous bridge between the fragment ends.

✦ In the **third stage** of healing, a soft callus or splint is formed from the mass of proliferating osteoblasts. Osteoclasts are also present, cleaning up the dead bone and debris. As the fibrous, immature bone (or woven bone) is gradually calcified, movement at the fracture ends gradually decreases. **Union** of the fracture ends occurs at about four weeks. However, the repair is incomplete, because the callus is merely calcified and not yet mature bone. The unsupported bone cannot safely withstand stress. Clinically, the fracture site is tender.

✦ In the **fourth stage, consolidation** occurs as the immature woven bone is changed into mature lamellar bone. Consolidation is a complete repair, because the callus is now ossified. However, it may be several months before the bone is capable of bearing normal loads. There is no tenderness at the fracture site. Therapists should note that with fractures of the non-weight-bearing upper limb, the cast may be removed before consolidation has occurred.

✦ In the **fifth stage,** remodelling of the irregular outer surface and reshaping of the marrow space inside the bone take place through alternating osteoclastic and osteoblastic activity. This process is governed by Wolff's law, where a bone responds to mechanical stress by becoming stronger and thicker the more strenuous its function *(Apley, Solomon, 1993; Porth, 1990)*.

The physiological process of bone repair does not always follow this format. A callus forms to bridge the bone ends in response to micromovements, not to rigid immobilization. When the bone ends are rigidly immobilized — for example with metal plates and screws — a callus does not form. Instead, bone formation occurs directly as capillaries and then osteoblasts grow into the gap between the bone ends. Healing by callus formation is termed indirect or secondary healing, while direct osteoblastic bone formation is termed gap healing or primary repair *(Apley, Solomon, 1993; Lane, 1987)*. Specific complications can occur with gap healing as a result of plate and screw use. These complications are discussed later in this section.

The Medical Treatment of Fractures

Medically, a fracture may be treated either by **closed** or **open (surgical) reduction,** both of which bring the broken ends into alignment and allow healing to occur. Methods of holding the reduction include **casting, continuous skeletal traction** and **external fixation.**

In a closed reduction, manual traction is applied and the bone ends are realigned. The fracture is then held in place until fracture repair occurs. Casting or fixation allows the bone ends to unite in a good position. It reduces pain and allows early movement and a quick return to function.

Casts may be constructed of plaster of Paris or fibreglass. Plaster casts are easier to apply and less expensive, while fibreglass casts are lighter and do not disintegrate in water. Casts may be bivalved (split in half lengthwise) so they can be partially or completely removed. Functional cast braces allow joint motion while splinting the injury. For example, sections of cast distal and proximal to the elbow are joined by metal hinges *(Morgan, 1989; Wu, 1987)*.

Continuous skeletal traction may be used for the femur or tibia. With this method, pins or wires are inserted through the bone distal to the fractured bone and a pulling force is applied along the axis of the limb. External fixation devices may also be used, such as the Hoffman-Vidal device. Long pins are inserted into the bone above and below the fracture site. The ends of the pins are secured to a metal frame. The frame is adjusted to provide correct alignment and compression of the fractured bone pieces *(Lane, 1987)*.

In an open reduction, the bones or bone fragments are stabilized by devices such as **screws, nails, Kirschner wires, long intermedullary nails** placed inside the bone along its length — for example, in tibial or femoral fractures — and **metal plates** fixed by screws *(Apley, Solomon, 1993; Lane, 1987)*. External fixation devices may also be used, especially with open fractures, because they allow easy care of the wound site. Biodegradable pins, plates and screws are being developed for fracture repair. The most successful appear to be biodegradable polymers, such as Poly L-lactide, that allow bone repair to occur and then, over several years, break down and are slowly resorbed by the body as water and carbon dioxide *(Leung et al., 1994)*.

From the nineteenth century up until the 1980s, the medical management of fractures and joint injuries strongly favoured prolonged immobilization and rest. More recently, medical opinion has come to recognize that prolonged immobilization allows muscle shortening and connective tissue contracture. In addition, the successive action of joints is prevented by immobilization, causing the articular cartilage to degenerate and fibrous adhesions to develop within the joint *(Rockwood et al., 1984)*. Subchondral bone atrophy begins within days of immobilization and can become permanent after eight weeks *(Larson, Grana, 1993)*. Extra-articular adhesions can also form, painfully restricting range of motion. For example, adhesions between the vastus intermedius and the femur can occur in distal femoral fractures, with fibrosis and contracture possible at six weeks post-injury. It has also been noted that prolonged skeletal traction causes knee stiffness *(Siliski, 1994)*. The trend is now towards range of motion and exercise as early as is safely possible. Recent studies have shown that, in the lower limb, exercise combined with weight bearing activities will help to prevent the soft tissue change associated with immobilization *(Larson, Grana, 1993)*.

It is most likely that the massage therapist is treating the client after the fracture has been reduced by a physician. If the fracture has not been reduced, the therapist uses first aid to stabilize and support the limb. The client is then immediately referred for emergency medical attention.

Complications

Complications of fractures can develop **early**, in the first few weeks following the trauma, or **late,** a few weeks to several years after the fracture.

The therapist should be alert for signs of early complications to fracture healing. The client may note a marked increase in pain levels, edema, bruising, paresthesia or temperature local to the fracture. However, the significance of these signs and the need for immediate medical attention may not be apparent to the client.

Early complications include torn muscles and tendons, ligament damage, compartment syndromes, nerve injuries, vascular injuries, joint hemarthrosis, bone and soft tissue infections, deep vein thrombosis and problems caused by poorly fitting casts.

✦ A **compartment syndrome** can occur in the forearm or the leg following a fracture. The swelling that accompanies marked edema, hematoma or inflammation increases the pressure within the fascial compartment. This leads to a cycle of reduced circulation, ischemia of the muscles within the compartment, then more edema, followed by an increase in pressure and more intense ischemia. In less than 12 hours, the muscle and nerve tissue within the compartment necrose. In severe cases, the limb becomes gangrenous. In less severe cases, the necrosed muscle is replaced, over time, by inelastic fibrous tissue and a flexion deformity results (Volkmann's ischemic contracture). A tight cast can also trigger a similar ischemia. A client with a compartment syndrome following a forearm or lower leg fracture complains of a sudden increase in pain levels, muscle stiffness, paresthesia and edema. Cyanotic fingers or toes and sometimes (but not always) a diminished pulse are also present. Immediate medical attention is indicated *(Apley, Solomon, 1993)*.

✦ **Nerve compression** may be indicated by paresthesia in the tissues under the cast. For example, with wrist fractures, numbness may occur in the median or ulnar nerve distribution. The common peroneal nerve can be compressed by a leg cast. A client with paresthesia should be referred to the physician for assessment *(Wu, 1987)*.

✦ Untreated **vascular damage** may be indicated by an increase in observable distal red, black or blue bruising. The client is referred to the physician.

✦ **Bone and soft tissue infections** can occur with external fixation or skeletal traction along the pin tract if proper wound care is not observed. Infections under the cast may also arise with open fractures that have been casted *(Wu, 1987)*. An increase in temperature, pain and edema as well as a foul odour indicate infection. With an open reduction in a plaster cast, seepage of blood may occur through the cast. Either of these indicates immediate medical referral.

✦ **Deep vein thrombosis** may occur after a lower limb fracture, especially in the veins of the calf. Deep vein thrombosis is indicated by pain, an increase in swelling local to the calf and a slight increase in temperature. This is most likely with clients who are confined to bed after trauma or surgery, clients with cardiovascular pathologies and elderly clients. Again, medical referral is indicated *(Apley, Solomon, 1993)*.

✦ A **pressure** or **plaster sore** occurs where the cast ischemically compresses the skin over a bony prominence. The client initially feels a local burning pain under the cast, usually over a bony prominence. The client should be referred for immediate medical attention as skin necrosis can proceed rapidly *(Wu, 1987)*.

✦ **Cast dermatitis** may result from poor ventilation and hygiene of the skin under the cast. Allergic reactions to the chemicals present in fibreglass casts are also possible *(Wu, 1987)*.

✦ **Loose cast syndrome** occurs when a cast that is too loose rubs on bony prominences, causing skin abrasions. If the cast is easily moved around on the limb, the client is referred to the physician.

Late complications include delayed union and non-union of the fracture, malunion, myositis ossificans, nerve compression, nerve entrapment, bone necrosis, Volkmann's ischemic contracture, joint stiffness and disuse atrophy *(Wu, 1987)*. There may also be complications relating to the various external fixators or to the metal plates used in some open reductions. Following a sprain, an osteochondral fracture may be present if the injury does not resolve in the expected time frame and if the joint remains painful and swollen *(Brukner, Khan, 1993)*. The client should be referred to the physician if late complications are suspected.

✦ **Delayed union** occurs if the bone does not unite within the expected time frame. This may be due to inadequate circulation, insufficient splinting, excessive traction or infection. With delayed union, the fracture site is tender and the bone may angulate if subjected to stress.

✦ **Non-union** is the failure of the bone to heal before the repair process finishes. This may be caused by an overly large gap between the bone ends either due to bone destruction, bone loss, excessive tractioning, inadequate fracture reduction, bone infection or soft tissue, such as periosteum or muscle, interposed between the bone ends. The fracture site is not tender and painless movement occurs at the fracture site.

✦ **Malunion** is unacceptable joining of the bone ends, so that a deformity occurs. This may be due to improper alignment of the bone ends when the fracture was reduced or displacement of the bone ends while the limb was casted. Malunion can lead to altered biomechanics and possibly, over time, tendinitis, bursitis and osteoarthritis. The client will complain of an observable deformity and sometimes an altered or painful range of motion.

✦ **Myositis ossificans** is bone formation within a muscle, which occurs weeks after the initial trauma, such as a fracture or a dislocation at the elbow. It may also result from muscle injury, such as contusions to the quadriceps. Heterotopic ossification is bone formation within soft tissue. This occurs without any local injury in people who are unconscious or who are paraplegic. Its causes are not clearly understood *(Apley, Solomon, 1993)*.

+ **Avascular bone necrosis** can occur in areas of bone that are poorly vascularized, such as the proximal scaphoid, the lunate after dislocation, the body of the talus and the neck of the femur. Although ischemia occurs shortly after the fracture or dislocation, the necrosis may not be noticed on X-rays for weeks *(Apley, Solomon, 1993)*.

+ **Volkmann's ischemic contracture** may eventually result after a compartment syndrome or injury to an artery causes ischemic contracture of the affected muscle. While over time the ischemic muscles in the compartment are replaced by inelastic fibrous tissue, the ischemic nerve may be able to recover partial function. Flexion deformity, muscle atrophy, stiffness and paresthesia are present in the affected limb. This condition primarily affects the forearm and hand, although it may also appear in the foot *(Apley, Solomon, 1993)*.

+ **Disuse osteoporosis** may occur with prolonged immobilization. It is reversible once full use of the limb is regained *(Wu, 1987)*.

+ There are several complications relating to **metal plates** at the fracture site. Local inflammation may be caused by the release of metallic ions, necessitating early removal of the plate *(Leung et al., 1994)*. The plate or screws may loosen or break if the limb is not properly casted until the bone heals and a load is placed on the limb. If the ends of the bone are fixed too far apart, non-union may result *(Apley, Solomon, 1993)*. In addition, stress shielding may occur, where load transmission is through the plate itself, instead of through the bone ends. This delays fracture healing and may also lead to osteoporosis. The plate then needs to be removed *(Leung et al., 1994; Lane, 1987)*. External fixators may cause over-distraction of the fracture, leading to non-union and stress shielding. However, the fixators can be dynamized (made more flexible) or removed altogether after six weeks and replaced by a cast or brace which allows for loading of the bone *(Apley, Solomon, 1993)*.

Symptom Picture

+ Immediately after the fracture occurs and before reduction is performed, unnatural mobility and deformity are present at the fracture site. Shock, pain, bleeding, inflammation, swelling, loss of function, muscle splinting and edema are present.

+ The soft tissue is also injured. The periosteum, ligaments, tendons, nerves, blood vessels, muscle, fascia and skin can be damaged.

+ With stress fractures, the fracture is painful upon compression.

During Immobilization

+ Following closed or open reduction, the limb may be casted or otherwise immobilized. Other structures compensate for this. With an open reduction that was not casted or with an external fixation device, there are incisions or pin tracks that are possible sites of infection. A stress fracture is likely not casted. However, there may be crutches, taping or other supports.

+ Pain is present both locally and possibly at a distance from the fracture.

+ Tissue repair and callus formation are occurring at the fracture site. Adhesions are developing around the injury.

+ Due to immobilization, reduced circulation, edema, disuse atrophy and connective tissue contracture occur in the tissues under the cast *(Kisner, Colby, 1990)*. Cartilage health decreases in joints that are immobilized with the lack of succussive action and reduced circulation.

+ Hypertonicity and trigger points are present in compensating structures, such as with crutch use.

+ Short-term complications may occur, such as compartment syndrome, nerve compression, infection, plaster sores, poor cast fit or non-union.

Immobilization Removed

+ The fracture site is healing and remodelling.

+ There is decreased tissue health in the tissue that has been under the cast. For the first few days after the immobilization has been removed, the tissue is somewhat fragile and muscle tone is likely to be decreased.

+ Adhesions have matured around the injury. Connective tissue contractures are likely with immobilization. Initially, pain and stiffness may be present on movement of joints that were immobilized. There may also be a loss of proprioception.

+ With open reduction, scars will be present.

+ Hypertonicity and trigger points are present in muscles crossing the fracture site and in compensating structures.

+ Muscle weakness or disuse atrophy is likely present in muscles crossing the fracture site. Altered posture and gait are possible.

+ Occasionally, a pocket of chronic edema may remain local to the injury.

+ Long-term complications may occur, such as delayed union, non-union, malunion, myositis ossificans, nerve compression and Volkmann's ischemic contracture. Years later, osteoarthritis may occur at the old fracture site.

Subjective Information

HEALTH HISTORY QUESTIONS

✦ What is the client's general health? Are there any pathologies that may have contributed to the fracture, such as osteoporosis or tumour?

✦ When did the fracture occur? Does the client know the mechanism of injury?

With a recent fracture:

✦ Does the client know the type of fracture — for example, spiral or transverse? This may help to estimate the length of time for healing.

✦ What other health care practitioners is the client seeing for this injury, such as a physician, physiotherapist or occupational therapist? What treatment was given? Is the client still receiving this treatment?

✦ What type of immobilization was used, if any? For example, a cast or an external fixation device is used with a complete fracture, while stress fractures are rarely casted (Rockwood et al., 1991).

✦ If there was an open reduction, were implants such as pins, screws, wires or plates used?

✦ Is the client taking any medication for the fracture, such as analgesics or antibiotics? This includes self-medication, such as Aspirin or other over-the-counter products.

✦ Is the client using any supports, slings or crutches for the affected limb?

✦ What symptoms is the client currently experiencing? Does the client have pain now? Where exactly is the pain? What aggravates or relieves the pain? Is swelling, edema or bruising present local or distal to the fracture site?

✦ Are any early complications present, such as a compartment syndrome, infection or plaster sores? If so, the client is referred for immediate medical attention.

✦ What are the client's activities of daily living? What activities are difficult or painful to complete? Are any activities impossible to complete? For example, a runner with a stress fracture of the foot or leg will be unable to "run through" the pain.

With a less recent fracture:

✦ What symptoms is the client currently experiencing? Does the client have pain now? Is muscle weakness or joint stiffness present? Is there any paresthesia?

✦ Were there any late complications? For example, is malunion, delayed union or non-union present?

✦ If open reduction was performed and metal implants such as nails, plates or wires were used, are these still present?

Objective Information

Observations

During Immobilization

✍ Antalgic gait occurs if the fracture is in the lower limb.

✍ The affected limb may be casted or an external fixation device may be used. The size and location of a cast vary according to the fracture. For example, a Colles' fracture cast begins several centimetres distal to the elbow and extends to the metacarpophalangeal joints. In contrast, a distal humerus fracture cast begins approximately at the insertion of the deltoid muscle and often extends to the metacarpophalangeal joints *(Morgan, 1989)*.

✍ The client may have crutches, a cane or possibly a walking cast with a lower limb fracture. A sling may be used with an upper limb fracture.

✍ Antalgic posture may be present. For example, if the client is using a sling with a casted Colles' fracture, the limb may be held in a protective position with the shoulders elevated.

✍ Edema is present at the fracture site and distal edema may also occur. A cast will obscure local edema.

✍ Red, black or purple bruising may be visible at the fracture site or distal to it. A cast will obscure local bruising.

✍ A pained or medicated facial expression may be present.

Immobilization Removed

✍ Habituated antalgic gait and posture may be observed. A postural assessment is indicated in this case.

✍ Chronic edema may remain at the fracture site and distal to it.

✍ When a cast is initially removed, the skin that was under the cast is likely dry, scaly or flaky.

✍ Disuse atrophy may be visible, especially if the limb was casted or the client did not isometrically exercise the immobilized limb.

✍ Bruising should resolve to brown, yellow and green and then disappear.

✍ If surgery was performed, scars will be present. These range from half a centimetre long following external fixation to several centimetres in length with open reductions.

Palpation

During Immobilization

✍ Heat and edema are present at the fracture site, although not palpable due to casting.

✍ Pain is present local to the fracture site and refers into the nearby tissue.

- Protective muscle spasm is present in muscles crossing the fracture site. This diminishes over time.

- Hypertonicity and trigger points are present in compensating muscles. These may be in the neck, affected shoulder and contralateral shoulder with an upper limb fracture. They may occur in the pelvis, contralateral leg, back and shoulders with a lower limb fracture and crutch use.

Immobilization Removed

- The health of the tissues that were under the cast is assessed in the first few days following cast removal. Conditions may include disuse atrophy, dry or flaky skin, local paresthesia, reduced vasomotor control, signs of inflammation, such as heat, or signs of tissue ischemia, such as coolness and boggy edema. There may be point tenderness around the fracture site.

- After one week, as tissue health returns, adhesions associated with the fracture site are palpated.

- Hypertonicity and trigger points are present in the compensating muscles.

Stress Fractures

- With stress fractures, the site of the fracture is painful upon compression. Inflammation may or may not be palpable.

Testing

During Immobilization

- Testing of muscles and joints directly involved in the fracture is **contraindicated.**

- AF ROM of the proximal and distal joints is assessed within **pain-free ranges.** Reduced ranges are likely — for example, in the interphalangeal joints with a forearm fracture.

Immobilization Removed

- **AF ROM** of the proximal and distal joints may be slowly and carefully performed to the onset of pain only. AF ROM ranges are reduced, especially within the first week after immobilization has been removed.

- **PR ROM** is performed with care. With upper limb fractures, immobilization may be removed shortly after union and **before** consolidation. The therapist must not stress the repairing bone during testing. Careful **pain-free** passive relaxed range of motion reveals reduced ranges with a tissue-stretch end feel. Range may also be reduced with malunion.

- **Overpressure** is **contraindicated** before consolidation has occurred. With the client's permission, the therapist may consult with the physician to determine if consolidation has occurred. Once it is safe to proceed with testing, overpressure may reveal leathery or capsular end feels of the joints that were immobilized.

✍ **AR strength testing** is performed, starting submaximally and increasing gradually to the maximum possible pain-free contraction. When immobilization is first removed, disuse atrophy is likely present. The strength and tone of the muscles under the cast are decreased. However, if isometric exercises or electrical muscle stimulation were used during immobilization, the muscle strength and tone may have been partially maintained.

Reduction with No Casting

✍ In the case of a fracture that has been surgically reduced either by external fixation or by pins or plates and where no casting is present, testing follows the above protocol. Disuse atrophy is much less likely to occur. The therapist should be aware that even though the bones are fixed by implants, bony consolidation has to occur **before** overpressure can be performed *(Apley, Solomon, 1993)*.

Special Tests

✍ If a **compartment syndrome** is present in the forearm or leg, especially if the fracture was casted, **passive hyperextension** of the fingers or toes will result in pain in the affected compartment *(Apley, Solomon, 1993)*.

✍ With **stress fractures**, the site of the fracture is painful upon direct compression.

Contraindications

During Immobilization

✦ The limb must not be tractioned before union has occurred.

✦ Hot hydrotherapy applications should not be placed distal or immediately proximal to the cast, as this may cause congestion in the distal limb and under the cast.

✦ If the fracture was at the site of a muscle attachment or if there was laceration or severance of a tendon crossing the fracture site, to avoid further soft tissue damage, AF and AR isometrics should only be performed with the physician's approval.

✦ With open reduction, on-site work is avoided until the skin has healed.

✦ In the case of fractures that have been treated by open reduction and stabilized without a cast (for example, a pin at the femoral neck or an external fixation device), infection is possible. Local techniques are avoided until the skin is fully healed.

✦ With stress fractures, on-site massage is contraindicated while the fracture site is point tender.

Immobilization Removed

✦ Overpressure testing of the involved joints is contraindicated before union has occurred *(Hertling, Kessler, 1990)*.

✦ Hydrotherapy temperature extremes are avoided on the tissues that were under the cast. The client may experience dysesthesia in the limb when the cast first comes off. In addition, the client's perception of heat, cold and pressure may be temporarily altered.

✦ Until tissue health and muscle tone are regained in the muscles that were under the cast, it is contraindicated to use deep longitudinal techniques on these muscles.

✦ Until tissue health and muscle tone are regained, passive stretching should be done carefully and to the onset of pain only to avoid further trauma to the tissues *(Kisner, Colby, 1990)*.

✦ If metal implants such as pins or plates have been used to repair the fracture, avoid local hot hydrotherapy applications.

Treatment Goals

Treatment Plan

During Immobilization

Do not interfere with the healing process. Refer the client to the physician if complications are suspected.

Reduce inflammation.

🖑 The client will be treated by a physician and other health care practitioners, such as a physiotherapist. With the client's permission, it is important that the therapist contact these other practitioners to coordinate the treatment plan.

🖑 **Positioning** depends on the location of the fracture and the client's comfort. The limb is elevated and secured so no stress is placed on the fracture site. The client may be apprehensive and may guard the injured limb.

🖑 **Hydrotherapy** is a cold application such as an ice pack or a gel pack, applied to the limb distal to the cast — for example, to the fingers or toes. Hydrotherapy applications to compensating structures include contrast or heat, but they are not applied immediately proximal to the cast. For example, with an ankle fracture where the cast extends to below the knee, heat may be applied to the low back but not to the knee.

General Treatment

🖑 If the initial treatment goal is to decrease the edema, lymphatic drainage on the affected limb is performed first.

Reduce pain. Reduce sympathetic nervous system firing. Treat any compensating structures.

🖑 If the initial goal is to accustom the client to the therapist's touch and to treat compensatory structures, the treatment begins on the trunk or contralateral limb in the context of a relaxation massage. The client is directed to do **diaphragmatic breathing** throughout the treatment to reduce sympathetic nervous system firing and pain perception. The trunk and uninjured limb are treated using slow gentle rhythmic techniques, effleurage and petrissage, such as palmar kneading, fingertip kneading and C-scooping. The focus of the work depends on the muscles that are compensating. In the above case, the shoulders and back are treated if crutches are used. Trigger points

Treatment Goals   Treatment Plan

in muscles that refer to the injured limb and the fracture site itself are treated using muscle stripping and ischemic compressions according to the client's pain tolerance, followed by effleurage.

Specific Treatment

Reduce edema.

🤚 Lymphatic drainage techniques are used on the injured limb proximal to the cast, beginning with nodal pumping at the proximal lymph nodes. Unidirectional effleurage, stationary circles and the local technique are used proximal to the injury to reduce edema.

Maintain local circulation proximal to the injury only.

🤚 The limb proximal to the cast is treated to reduce pain and hypertonicity as well as to increase drainage and venous return. Techniques include effleurage and repetitive petrissage, such as slow palmar kneading and fingertip kneading.

Do not interfere with the healing process.

🤚 Before union occurs, the therapist should take care not to put traction on the casted limb.

Maintain range of motion.

🤚 Careful, **mid-range pain-free passive relaxed range of motion** to proximal and distal joints is interspersed to promote lymphatic drainage and reduce adhesions.

🤚 Vibrations through the cast over the fracture site may help to decrease sympathetic nervous system firing.

🤚 Work distal to the cast is restricted to light stroking, muscle squeezing and vibrations, performed to the client's pain tolerance. This reduces the possibility of causing congestion through the tissues under the cast.

Treat other conditions.

🤚 Any secondary injuries, such as strains or contusions, are also treated. See the appropriate chapters for details.

Immobilization Removed

🤚 **Positioning** is chosen for comfort and for accessibility to the structures that the therapist is treating.

🤚 If the therapist is treating the client in the days immediately following removal of the cast before soft tissue health has returned, certain hydrotherapy modifications need to be observed.

• **Mild contrast hydrotherapy** (for example, alternating warm and cool towels) is initially used on the tissues that were under the cast. This helps to normalize circulation and vasomotor tone. There may be initial dysesthesia of the skin that was under the cast. The therapist may progress to more extremes of contrast as the client's tolerance improves over the next few days.

• Once muscle tone has returned, **deep moist heat** can be used to

Treatment Goals   Treatment Plan

increase the flexibility of connective tissue contractures and adhesions prior to treatment. Care is taken not to apply heat directly over any metal implants.

General Treatment

Reduce pain. Decrease sympathetic nervous system firing. Treat compensatory structures.

   Diaphragmatic breathing is encouraged. The client's trunk and compensating structures are massaged as before. Rhythmic techniques to the trunk and unaffected limb are indicated. The limb is elevated only if chronic edema remains.

Specific Treatment

Reduce edema.

   Proximal lymphatic drainage is indicated if edema is still present, including nodal pumping and light repetitive effleurage.

Reduce hypertonicity and trigger points.

   The proximal limb is treated to reduce any hypertonicity or trigger points and to increase local circulation. Effleurage, repetitive petrissage and ischemic compressions are indicated.

Improve tissue health.

   At the area that was under the cast, a textured mitten or soft loofah can be used to gently remove any dead, flaky skin and increase local circulation.

   Stimulating, light techniques are used on the muscles suffering disuse atrophy. Gentle petrissage, such as muscle squeezing, shaking and static point kneading, and light tapotement, such as tapping and pincement, are indicated.

   Massage oils or lotions containing emollients, such as vitamin E, or pure essential oils can be used to help nourish the skin that was under the cast. Sandalwood or rose essential oils at a one per cent dilution or 10 drops of the essential oil in 50 ml. of the carrier oil are indicated (*Lawless, 1995*).

Maintain range of motion.

   Pain-free mid-range passive relaxed and active assisted range of motion are interspersed with the massage techniques. Until the tone has improved, stretching the muscles is avoided.

Mobilize hypomobile joints.

   Joint play techniques are performed to joints that are hypomobile due to compensation, such as the sternoclavicular joint with a wrist fracture.

   As tissue health improves and muscle tone returns, fewer modifications need to be made. The on-site focus is on reducing the restricting adhesions and scar tissue so that pain-free range of motion can be regained.

Reduce any chronic edema.

   A pocket of chronic edema remaining around the fracture site may be partially trapped by proximal and local connective tissue restrictions. The therapist first uses fascial glide to assess them. Then

Treatment Goals   Treatment Plan

fascial techniques are used to treat the proximal restrictions. These include skin rolling and crossed-hands or ulnar border spreading techniques. This is followed by proximal lymphatic drainage.

Reduce hypertonicity and trigger points. Increase local circulation and venous return.

🖐 As above, the proximal limb is treated to reduce hypertonicity or trigger points and to increase local circulation.

Reduce adhesions.

🖐 *Once the muscle tone has improved,* or if minimal disuse atrophy is present, more vigorous petrissage and connective tissue techniques may be used near the fracture site. Preparatory techniques include effleurage and specific kneading. This progresses to skin rolling, longitudinal muscle stripping and then gentle cross-fibre frictions to reduce the adhesions surrounding the fracture. The work is followed by a **pain-free passive relaxed stretch** to the muscles to realign the fibres. In subsequent treatments, range of the joint is reassessed. Painfully restricting adhesions, including scars, are further reduced with fascial work and deeper frictions.

🖐 Trigger points in muscles near the fracture site can be treated with muscle stripping and ischemic compressions.

Mobilize hypomobile joints.

🖐 *Once consolidation has occurred,* careful joint play is indicated to mobilize contractured joints that were under the cast and restore the range of motion *(Kisner, Colby, 1990)*. The therapist should contact the physician with the client's permission to determine the appropriateness of joint play after union but before consolidation.

Maintain ROM and joint health.

🖐 With fractures near joints that have been fixed by wires, pins or screws, full range of motion is not possible nor desirable. It may not be possible to regain full range of motion, especially with malunion.

🖐 **Passive relaxed range of motion** is interspersed throughout the treatment on the proximal, affected and distal joints to maintain joint health.

Promote venous return.

🖐 The distal limb is treated with effleurage and petrissage to increase local venous return.

Reduction without Casting

🖐 With a fracture that was medically treated by open reduction without a cast, or by reduction using an external fixation device, care must be taken to avoid interfering with the healing process until union occurs. Until the incisions heal, there is the possibility of infection at the incision or along the pin tracks that occur with external fixation. Therefore, on-site work is contraindicated.

🖐 With a stress fracture that is not casted, on-site massage is contraindicated while the fracture site is tender.

Treatment Goals

Treatment Plan

✋ Proximally, the limb is treated using the techniques described in the immobilization treatment.

✋ Once any external fixation devices are removed and the pin tracks are healed, work is done to decrease adhesion and scar formation.

✋ After union has occurred, techniques that focus on circulation, drainage and reducing adhesions are indicated.

✋ Once consolidation has occurred, passive forced range and joint play as listed in the Immobilization Removed (Treatment Plan) section can be used to increase range of motion.

Self-care Goals

Self-care Plan

During Immobilization

Educate the client.

✍ The limb should be elevated as often as possible to reduce edema.

✍ The client should be alert for signs of early complications, such as increased pain, heat and swelling. If these signs are noted, the client should seek medical attention.

✍ **Hydrotherapy** is chosen according to the presenting symptoms. For example, edema distal to the cast is treated with cold or cool applications.

✍ **Remedial exercise** is developed for two areas: the compensating structures and the muscles under the cast.

✍ Initially, depending on the fracture, the client may be advised by her physician to rest.

Safely maintain range of motion and strength.

✍ As soon as exercise is permitted, strength and flexibility should be maintained in the compensating structures. For example, with a wrist fracture where the client is wearing a sling, active free range of motion of both shoulders and the neck is performed. This can be gradually increased to active resisted exercises. Stretches for the upper trapezius, scalenes and pectoral muscles are indicated.

✍ With respect to the injured limb, as soon as the physician permits, active free range of motion of the joints distal to the cast can begin. For strengthening, submaximal isometric contractions of the muscles under the cast are performed. These exercises, which are initially performed in a pain-free manner, help to reduce the effects of disuse atrophy. For example, the client with a wrist fracture can flex and extend the fingers and thumb. However, fractures that are near muscle attachments or that involve secondary tendon injury may need adequate healing time before exercise is attempted.

Self-care Goals

Self-care Plan

Immobilization Removed

✍ The client can use a textured cloth to gently exfoliate any dry skin. Emollient oils or lotions are applied afterwards to lubricate the skin. Ten drops of pure sandalwood essential oil can be added to 50 ml. of carrier oil *(Lawless, 1995)*.

✍ The limb should be elevated as often as possible to reduce any remaining edema.

✍ **Hydrotherapy** applications when the cast is first removed are cool or mild contrast on site. Gradually increasing the temperature difference between the contrast applications will help to restore vasomotor control.

✍ **Remedial exercise** is continued for the compensating structures as before.

Regain strength.

✍ Active free range of motion for joints that were under the cast is performed to the onset of pain only. If disuse atrophy is minimal, the client can progress to active resisted exercises to gradually regain muscle strength and reduce any muscle imbalances.

Increase range of motion.
Increase proprioception.

✍ Stretches are indicated to regain range of motion once consolidation has occurred, although full range of motion may not occur with malunion. If proprioception is reduced at joints that were under the cast, see the chapter on sprains for proprioception exercises.

✍ **Self-massage** to adhesions is indicated.

Treatment Frequency and Expected Outcome

Treatments may be given once or twice a week until the cast is removed. The client may come twice a week for shorter treatments when the cast is first removed. Treatment may progress to once a week for four weeks, then the client is reassessed.

Some factors that affect fracture healing are the type of fracture (for example, simple or compound), the amount of bone lost, if any, the type of bone that is injured and the degree of immobilization that has been applied. Other factors include the client's age, general health, local circulation, nutrition and systemic diseases such as rheumatoid arthritis or diabetes *(Porth, 1990)*. Some sources indicate that the use of continuous passive motion (CPM) machines may help maintain joint health and prevent connective tissue contractures and joint stiffness that would otherwise arise post-fracture *(Lane, 1987; Rockwood et al., 1984)*. However, other sources feel that CPM machines have a limited usefulness and may in fact disturb fracture and wound healing *(Larson, Grana, 1993)*. Finally, the client's compliance with a self-care plan will shorten the recovery time.

Spiral and oblique fractures heal more rapidly than transverse fractures because there is a greater periosteal surface area involved. There is an increased blood supply and, therefore, a faster repair process.

See stress reduction, edema, spasm, contusions, scars, strains, sprains, dislocations, periostitis and compartment syndromes, frozen shoulder, osteoarthritis, rheumatoid arthritis, conditions of the peripheral nervous system, carpal tunnel syndrome, other circulatory concerns, decubitus ulcers and osteoporosis treatments for related conditions.

Upper limb fractures usually heal more quickly than lower limb fractures.

Stress fractures take six to 10 weeks to heal completely *(Rockwell et al., 1991)*. Other types of fractures may take two to 12 months for complete recovery.

Suggested healing times are shown in the table below *(Apley, Solomon, 1993)*.

	Upper Limb		Lower Limb	
	Union	Consolidation	Union	Consolidation
Spiral	3 weeks	6	+6	12
Transverse	6 weeks	12	12	+24

28

WHIPLASH

Fiona Rattray

> *A whiplash is an acceleration-deceleration injury to the head and neck.*

H. E. Crowe first identified the clinical syndrome which he called "whiplash" in 1928 *(Foreman, Croft, 1995)* as neck injuries were reported by motorists following automobile accidents. It was also found that military pilots who experienced catapult-assisted takeoffs from aircraft carriers suffered this type of injury.

Since Crowe's original description, there has been a lack of consensus on the definition and classification of the condition. For example, whiplash has been used to describe both the injury itself and the mechanism of the injury. The term has also been used to describe the many seemingly unrelated clinical symptoms that appear following the injury, such as headaches, dizziness and temporomandibular joint disorders. A further source of confusion in reporting precise statistics on the subject is that any vector of vehicle collision — rear, side or front impact — may be described as a whiplash. Since rear-impact collisions result in more long-term symptoms than other vectors *(Hertling, Kessler, 1996)*, it becomes important to know and record the direction of impact.

In addition, there are numerous (and confusing) synonyms for the injury. These include cervical sprain (literally ligamentous injury only), cervical strain (literally muscle injury only), headache of cervical origin, cervical herniated disc and sprained cervical facet joints. Two recent terms attempting to clarify definitions are: cervical acceleration/deceleration (CAD) injury *(Foreman, Croft, 1995)*; and whiplash-associated disorders (WAD), used to describe the many clinical symptoms following a whiplash, such as headache *(Spitzer, 1995)*.

> ➤ **The cause of whiplash is an acceleration-deceleration** of the head and neck relative to the body, usually resulting from vehicular collision but also possible in contact or high-speed sports.

➤ A **contributing factor** to the accident itself may be active trigger points in the clavicular division of sternocleidomastoid muscle. These result in dizziness when a person rotates his head quickly, as when making a shoulder check while driving. This dizziness can be dangerous as it may cause the driver to lose control of the vehicle (*Travell, Simons, 1983*).

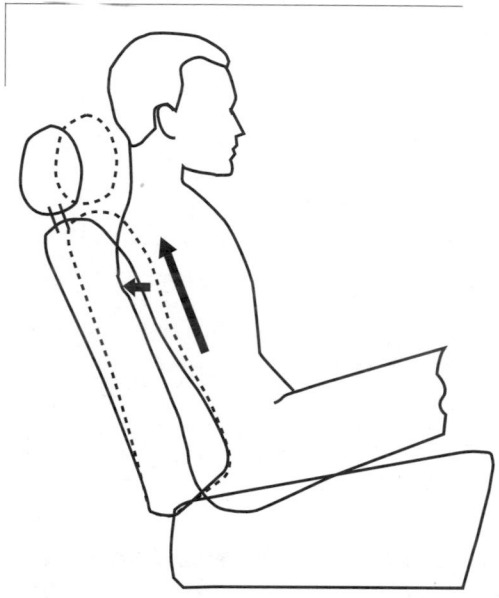

Figure 28.1
Phase 1: Cervical disc injury is possible.

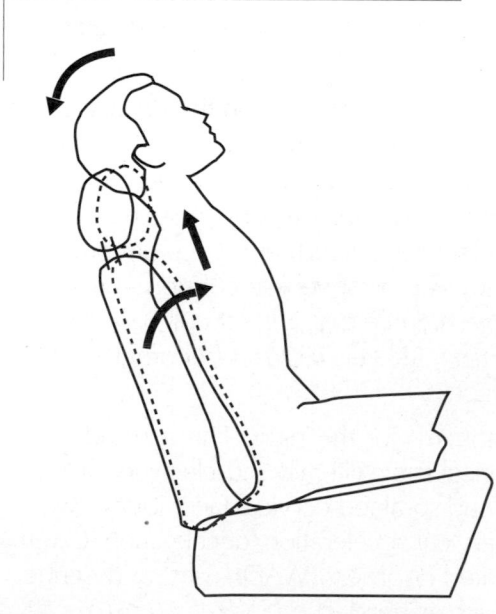

Figure 28.2
Phase 2: Anterior neck muscle and ligament, facet and temporomandibular joint injuries are possible.

Motor Vehicle Accidents, Mechanism of Injury and Direction of Impact

Rear Impact

In a whiplash, the acceleration rate of the victim's head is much greater than that of the vehicle. More severe and long-lasting symptoms result from rear-impact collisions than from front or side impact (*Foreman, Croft, 1995*). Consequently, rear-impact collisions are the most researched. The actual mechanism of injury has been studied using cadavers, rabbits, monkeys, crash test dummies and mathematical models.

The animal studies revealed that different soft tissues could be injured, with varying degrees of severity, depending on the velocity of the impact. These ranged from mild sternocleidomastoid muscle strains to more severe longus colli muscle tears accompanied by retropharyngeal hematoma, to esophageal hemorrhages and even to damage of the cervical sympathetic nervous system. Less common were ruptures of the anterior longitudinal ligament. There were also avulsions of intervertebral discs from the cervical vertebrae, which are only detected by dissection as they do not show on X-rays.

No one model can account for the many variables occurring in whiplash injuries. It is thought, however, that there are four distinct phases to a rear-impact whiplash (*Foreman, Croft, 1995*).

✦ Phase 1 (60 milliseconds)

The vehicle is struck from behind. The back of the seat pushes into the person's torso as the vehicle moves forward. The person's torso initially is compressed into the seat back, then is carried forward along with the vehicle. The head (on the flexible neck) stays fixed in place due to inertia. The torso then moves abruptly upwards, compressing the cervical spine. It is possible that cervical discs are injured at this point (*Figure 28.1*).

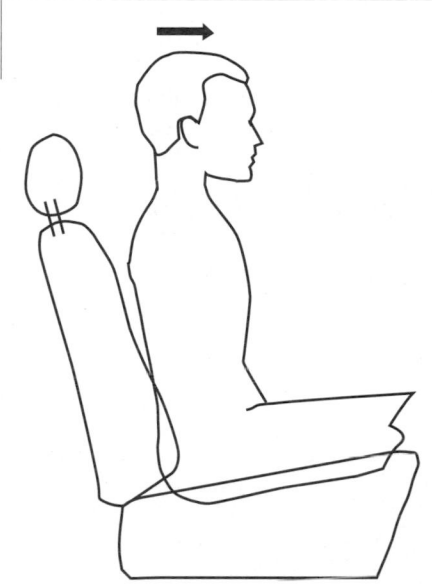

Figure 28.3
Phase 3: Peak acceleration of head and neck

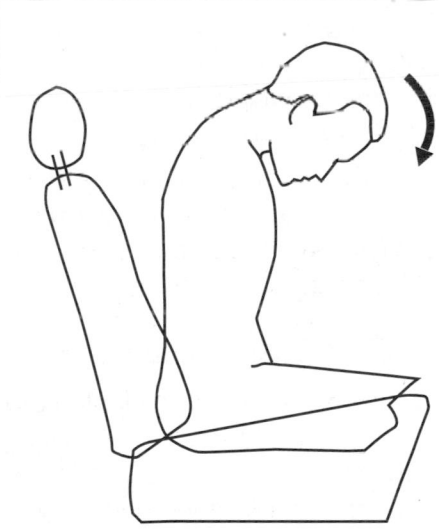

Figure 28.4
Phase 4: Posterior neck muscle and ligament injury is possible.

✦ Phase 2 (120 milliseconds)

The vehicle and torso reach their peak forward acceleration. The seat back begins to recoil to its original position, perhaps adding additional acceleration to the person's torso. The head and neck, however, stay in place as the torso moves forward. The net result is that the neck goes into hyperextension. A shear force occurs between the cervical spine and the thoracic spine. The rising torso creates some slack in the shoulder and lap belt. The anterior neck muscles and ligaments are overstretched and the facet and temporomandibular joints may be injured at this point *(Figure 28.2)*.

✦ Phase 3 (160 milliseconds)

The head and neck are now at their peak forward acceleration while the vehicle and torso are slowing down *(Figure 28.3)*. Slack created in the shoulder and lap belt will increase the forward motion of the torso, neck and head in Phase 4 .

✦ Phase 4 (280 milliseconds)

The head and torso are now at full deceleration *(Figure 28.4)*. The shoulder harness eventually restrains the torso while the head and neck continue to flex forward. In the past, it was thought that the chin would strike the chest, stopping forward motion *(Hertling, Kessler, 1990)*. While this has been proven not to occur, the head does move into hyperflexion. The greatest amount of stress is placed on the muscles, discs and ligaments of the lower cervical and upper thoracic spine, injuring these tissues *(Yeung, 1996)* with C5 to C7 most frequently affected.

Other Factors Affecting Rear-Impact Whiplash

✦ **Head Position:** If a person's head is turned to one side at the time of impact, the cervical spine is biomechanically less able to extend, placing a greater compressive stress on the ipsilateral facet joints. In addition, the ipsilateral intervertebral foramen are reduced in size when the cervical spine is rotated and sidebent *(Figure 28.5)*, potentially compressing the ipsilateral cervical nerve roots *(Edwardson, 1995; Foreman, Croft, 1995)*. Splenius cervicis muscle is also specifically injured with this position *(Travell, Simons, 1983)*. Other studies have found the position of the thoracic spine to be important *(Yeung, 1996)*.

✦ **Seatbelts:** While seatbelts inarguably save lives by preventing the person from being ejected from the vehicle, they can also contribute to neck injuries *(McKinney, 1989)*, especially in low-speed collisions *(Foreman, Croft, 1995)*. Seatbelts also result in injuries

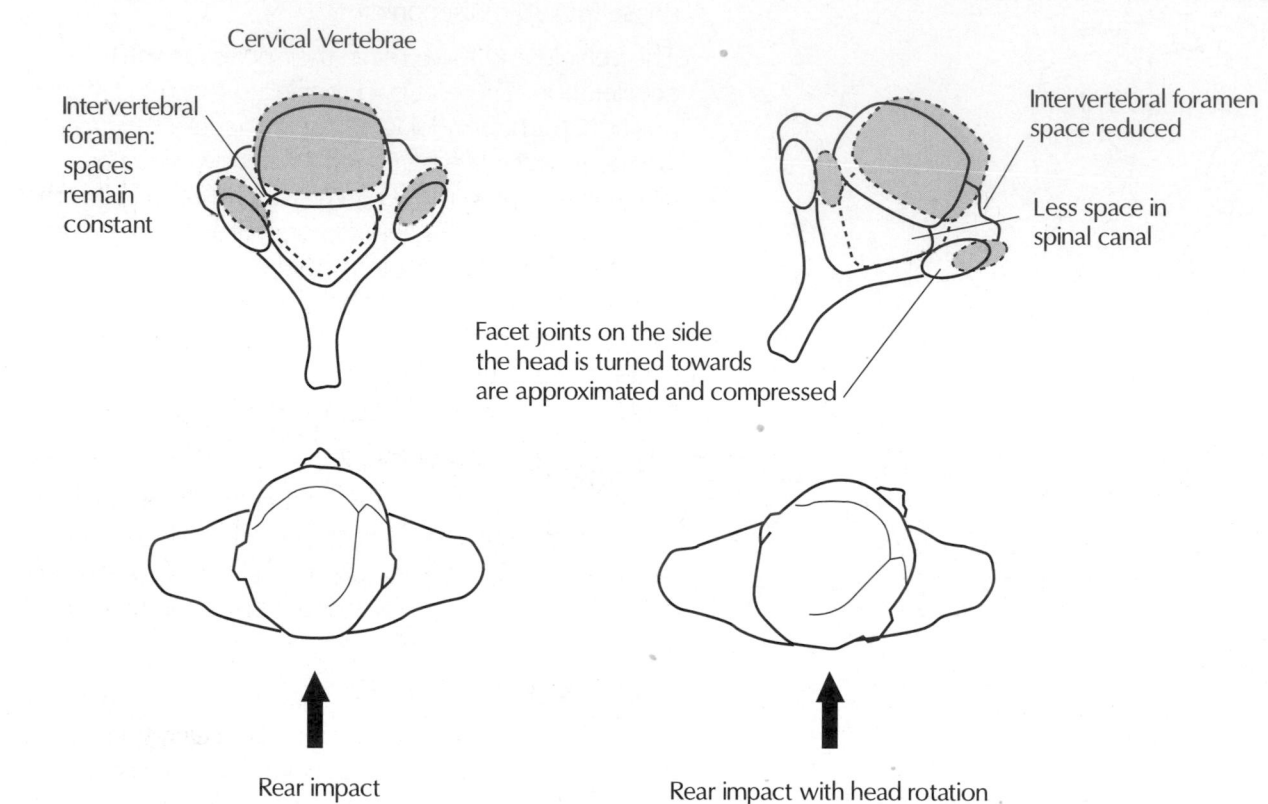

Cervical Vertebrae

Intervertebral foramen: spaces remain constant

Intervertebral foramen space reduced

Less space in spinal canal

Facet joints on the side the head is turned towards are approximated and compressed

Rear impact

Rear impact with head rotation

Figure 28.5
Mechanism for increased severity of symptoms when head is turned in rear-impact whiplash.

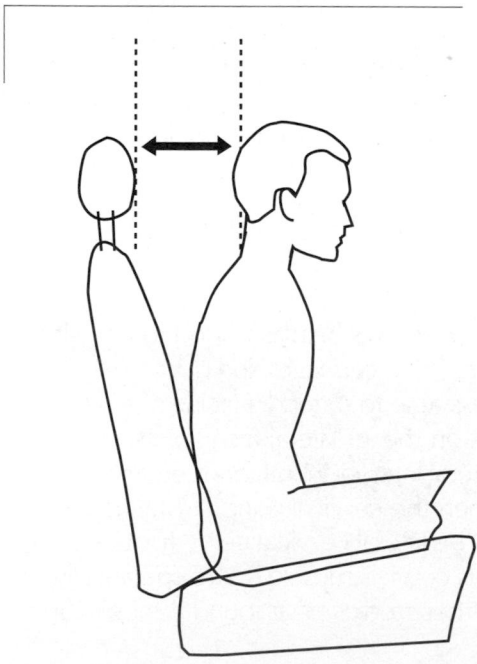

Figure 28.6
Hyperkyphotic posture is a factor in severity of rear-impact whiplash.

to the viscera under the lap belt and bruising to the chest under the shoulder harness. A shoulder belt that is too loose may allow the person's torso and the shoulder that is not under the belt to pivot forward, placing asymmetrical rotational forces on the spine. Low back pain is also a common result.

✦ **Headrest Position:** A headrest that is adjusted too low may act as a fulcrum in Phase 2, intensifying the injury. When the torso rises, the head and neck are allowed to pivot around the low headrest into further extension *(Foreman, Croft, 1995).*

✦ When the **seat back** is inclined too far back the headrest will not reduce injury *(Yeung, 1996).* Similarly, when a person has hyperkyphotic posture the head is positioned too far forward for the headrest to reduce injury *(Figure 28.6).*

✦ **Stature:** Persons shorter than five feet have a 40 per cent lower risk of neck injury than taller persons; however, the risk of cervical vascular injury from shoulder harnesses is greater in shorter persons *(Foreman, Croft, 1995).*

+ **Air Bags:** Air bags are designed to deploy in front-impact collisions, so they provide little protection in rear-impact collisions.

Front Impact

+ The mechanism of injury is the reverse of the rear-impact collision, with the torso accelerating backward as the neck hyperflexes, then hyperextends. The person may be able to see the impending collision and brace for the impact. Seatbelts, air bags, headrests and automobile front-end "crumple zones" all help to reduce injuries.

Side Impact

+ The mechanism of injury is an initial lateral flexion of the neck and torso towards the side of the striking vehicle, then away from it. There is little protection for the person except for the lap belt anchoring the pelvis in place. Since only the pelvis is restrained, the lumbar and thoracic spine may experience severe sidebending movements. The lumbar ligaments, discs and muscles may be injured, as well as the cervical and upper thoracic tissues. Side air bags have been introduced on some European automobile models to reduce these injuries.

Tissues Involved in Any Whiplash

Any of the structures in the neck, upper thorax and head may be injured in a whiplash. This includes the cervical and thoracic vertebrae, intervertebral discs, facet joints, joint capsules and ligaments, temporomandibular joints, anterior and posterior longitudinal ligaments, lymphatics, fascia, blood vessels, cranial, cervical and thoracic nerve roots, the vagus nerve, phrenic nerve, autonomic nervous system (Yeung, 1996) and spinal cord.

Posterior cervical muscles that may be affected include the suboccipitals (rectus capitis posterior major and minor, obliquus capitis inferior and superior), rotatores, multifidi, semispinalis cervicis, longissimus cervicis, upper trapezius and levator scapulae.

Anterior cervical muscles include rectus capitis anterior, longus capitis, longus colli (longus cervicis) responsible for flexing the cervical spine, sternocleidomastoid, mylohyoid, omohyoid, supra- and infrahyoids and platysma.

Lateral cervical muscles include rectus capitis lateralis and anterior, middle and posterior scalenes.

The muscles of mastication and of the thorax, including the intercostals, posterior spinal muscles and diaphragm, may also be affected.

The Expense and Politics of Whiplash

While whiplash could arise from injuries sustained in contact sports and diving accidents, it was the arrival of the automobile and the subsequent motor vehicle accident (MVA) that is responsible for the bulk of whiplash injuries.

The majority of people who suffer whiplash (80 per cent) experience neck pain and stiffness which resolve in less than four weeks (Hertling, Kessler, 1996). However, the symptoms of whiplash include not only neck pain, but also symptoms that cannot be easily explained, such as dizziness, headache, paresthesia, nausea and low back pain.

At first, people reporting these symptoms were thought to be exaggerating their claims for financial gain from third-party (insurance company) payments. However, a study of 266 medico-legal cases found that 45 per cent of the people in the study continued to have symptoms two years after court monetary settlements *(Foreman, Croft, 1995)*.

While only a minority of people who suffer whiplash report chronic symptoms six months after the injury, the cost of treating whiplash-associated disorders is rising. In one study of 4,757 whiplash cases, over 18 million Canadian dollars were paid out in 1987. Of this figure, 70 per cent (13 million) was for the replacement of regular income, while 8.8 per cent (1.6 million) was for physiotherapy and medical and paramedical care *(Weinstein, 1995)*. It has become important (especially for third-party payers) to devise a system to determine the assessment and prognosis of whiplash. For example, if X-rays were recommended to routinely assess the severity of all whiplash injuries, the cost would be enormous. People would be unnecessarily exposed to X-rays if no dislocation or fracture were present. In addition, the majority of damage experienced in a whiplash is to soft tissues which is not usually revealed by X-ray.

Classification of Whiplash

Historically, there was no agreed-upon classification system for whiplash. Two recent efforts have been made to standardize terminology, definition of symptoms, treatment and prognosis.

Stephen Foreman, DC, and Arthur Croft, DC, published a classification system in 1988 based on severity of the injury, stage of healing and type of collision, with a system for determining the client's prognosis based on certain modifying factors. Modifying factors are: size of the spinal canal; pre-existing degenerative changes; loss of the cervical lordotic curve; fixated vertebral segments; and loss of consciousness during the accident *(Foreman, Croft, 1995)*. Foreman and Croft used more than 1,200 references in the scientific literature and their clinical experience to devise their system.

In 1995, the Quebec Task Force (QTF) on Whiplash-Associated Disorders published a classification system based on a clinical/anatomic axis and a time axis, with a standardized health history form for data collection, treatment protocols and research guidelines *(Spitzer, 1995)*. The QTF, a panel of expert clinicians, epidemiologists, engineers and other specialists, was formed after the Quebec Automobile Insurance Society (Société d'assurance automobile du Québec) commissioned a report on the clinical, social and financial factors of "the whiplash problem" *(Weinstein, 1995)*. The QTF based their system on a review of the most recent scientific literature on whiplash. Of more than 10,000 articles on the subject, only 64 met the QTF's criteria *(Spitzer, 1995)*.

Both systems are presented here, as both have useful points of view. The QTF system is the one accepted by the insurance industry in Quebec and is likely to be widely adopted by insurance companies as a requirement for third-party payments in the reporting and treatment of whiplash. However, not all clients coming to massage therapists for treatment of whiplash will be covered by insurance payments, so the therapist may find that Foreman and Croft's classification is just as clinically useful.

Foreman and Croft Classification (F/C)

✦ **Grade 1 or Minimal:**

There is no limitation of motion; no ligamentous injury; no neurological findings.

✦ **Grade 2 or Slight:**

There is limitation of motion; no ligamentous injury; no neurological findings.

✦ **Grade 3 or Moderate:**

There is limitation of motion; some ligamentous injury; neurological findings may be present.

✦ **Grade 4 or Moderate to Severe:**

There is limitation of motion; ligamentous instability; neurological findings are present; fracture or disc derangement is present.

✦ **Grade 5 or Severe:**

The injury requires surgical management or stabilization.

• **Stage 1:** Acute injury, inflammation phase, up to 72 hours post-accident.
• **Stage 2:** Subacute, repair phase, 72 hours to 14 weeks.
• **Stage 3:** Remodelling phase, 14 weeks to 12 months or more.
• **Stage 4:** Chronic, permanent.

• **Type 1 Collision:** Rear impact.
• **Type 2 Collision:** Side impact.
• **Type 3 Collision:** Front impact (*Foreman, Croft, 1995*).

Quebec Task Force Classification (QTF)

✦ **Grade 0**

There is no complaint about the neck; no physical (musculoskeletal or neurological) signs.

✦ **Grade 1**

There is neck complaint of pain, stiffness or tenderness only; there are no physical (musculoskeletal or neurological) signs; microscopic lesions are not serious enough to cause muscle spasm.

✦ **Grade 2**

There is neck complaint of pain, stiffness or tenderness; there are musculoskeletal signs of decreased range of motion and point tenderness; injury to muscles, tendons, ligaments and joint capsules is serious enough to cause muscle spasm.

✦ **Grade 3**

There is neck complaint of pain, stiffness or tenderness; there are neurological signs including decreased or absent deep tendon reflexes, weakness and sensory deficit; injury to the neurological system is due to mechanical injury or secondary to inflammation or bleeding.

✦ **Grade 4**

There is neck complaint and fracture or dislocation.

• **Other Symptoms**

Symptoms and disorders that can appear in all grades include deafness, dizziness, dysphagia, headache, memory loss, temporomandibular joint pain and tinnitus.

• **Time Axis**

People are classified within each grade in terms of days following the injury: less than four days; four to 21 days; 22 to 45 days; 46 to 180 days; and more than six months' duration (*Spitzer, 1995*).

There appear to be shortcomings with both systems. Foreman and Croft's Stage 4 is a chronic permanent category. While this may accurately describe a person who suffers permanent disability following a motor vehicle accident, from a third-party payer viewpoint this potentially allows the person to be treated for a substantial period of time, an expensive proposition.

The QTF uses its time axis to decide the probable progression of the person's symptoms. The time axis is then used to make recommendations for "clinical management" (treatment) of whiplash. This method categorizes whiplash in a manner unlike any other trauma. Normally, an injury is classified and treated according to the client's *presenting symptoms* rather than according to the *length of time since the injury* (*Hertling, Kessler, 1996*). The QTF itself recognizes there is little data on what constitutes a "normal" recuperation period (*Weinstein, 1995; Alexander, 1996*). Not all clients will progress within the limits of the QTF's timeline.

Classifications in all other traumas progress from mild through moderate to severe, indicating the degree of severity. The QTF's classification is again different in that their system does not specify the extent to which the grade reflects the severity of the injury (*Spitzer, 1995*).

If the QTF classification system is mutually exclusive in its categories (*Weinstein, 1995*), there appears to be no provision for a person with an overlap of symptoms from Grades 2 and 3 — that is, no possibility of this system describing someone who has musculoskeletal injuries *and* nerve injuries.

The terminology the QTF uses is unconventional and confusing. For example, the QTF states that whiplash has a "favourable prognosis". This phrase usually means that a condition will resolve without any disability or residual symptoms. The QTF also repeatedly indicates that whiplash is a short-term, "self-limited" disorder. This is in direct contradiction to studies quoted by the QTF itself, which reports that 27 per cent to 66 per cent of people with whiplash are symptomatic six months to two years after the injury — hardly a "favourable prognosis". One source notes that the QTF makes unsupported conclusions and recommendations (*Freeman et al., 1998*).

The Medical Treatment of Whiplash

Those with acute whiplash who have a suspected fracture or dislocation of the cervical spine receive X-ray assessment *(Souza, 1997)*. However, it is possible for these types of injuries to be overlooked, either through improper X-ray techniques or failure to take X-rays due to the seemingly "minor" nature of the whiplash *(Foreman, Croft, 1995)*. Additionally, the QTF recommends that usually only those with Grade 2 or higher symptoms require X-rays for evaluation *(Weinstein, 1995)*.

At one time it was quite common for the acute whiplash patient to be given a cervical support collar, ice applications and medication such as analgesics or muscle relaxants *(Buschbacher, 1994)*. Recent studies have provided little evidence that cervical collars are effective *(Spitzer, 1995)*. Their use beyond 72 hours post-injury may prolong the person's disability, since a period of total inactivity following a strain allows the injured muscles to shorten due to scar tissue formation and allows disuse atrophy to occur *(Edwardson, 1995)*.

Those with subacute and chronic whiplash symptoms that do not resolve are usually referred for physiotherapy. Range of motion exercises, ice or heat, relaxation exercises, isometric strengthening, mobilization techniques, postural retraining and traction are commonly used.

Legal Implications for Massage Therapists Treating Whiplash

In the first 24 hours following the accident the client may feel few, if any, symptoms. If the therapist has any concerns regarding the severity of an acute injury — for example, if there is a suspected dislocation or fracture, radicular symptoms, extreme muscle weakness or difficulty swallowing — the client should be referred to a physician for assessment before massage treatment.

It is important for the therapist to thoroughly document the initial assessment, including all findings, whether *dysfunctional* or *within normal limits*. As with all injuries, every subsequent assessment should also be documented. These are key concepts when the therapist has to create a medico-legal report for third parties.

Pain and functional ability questionnaires, such as the Vernon-Mior Neck Pain and Disability Index *(Chapman-Smith, 1996)*, can be used as well to measure the client's initial symptoms in an accepted manner for both medical and insurance documentation. The results of treatment may also be measured by using a pain questionnaire to record symptoms in a later reassessment, perhaps after six weeks of treatment. Thorough documentation is also important should the therapist be required to go to court.

The therapist may want to request access to records of other health care professionals who are also treating the client. This must be done with *written permission* from the client. Finally, the therapist should not release information about the client — either written or verbal — to anyone except with *written permission* from the client.

Symptom Picture

Acute

✦ With an acute whiplash, in F/C Grade 2 (QTF Grade 2) injuries and higher, the muscles of the neck including sternocleidomastoids, scalenes, levator scapulae, the posterior cervical muscles, the infrahyoids, the suprahyoids and longus colli may suffer spasm, strain and contusion.

✦ Facet joint irritation, cervical ligament sprains and hematomas may occur with higher than F/C Grade 3 (QTF Grade 2) injuries.

✦ Less commonly, with F/C Grades 4 and 5 and QTF Grades 3 and 4 injuries, there may be rupture of the anterior or posterior longitudinal ligaments, ligamentum flavum, cervical disc lesions, vagus and phrenic nerve tractioning, cervical nerve root tractioning, facet dislocations and vertebral fractures. With vagus nerve tractioning the client may experience digestive tract upset. Phrenic nerve tractioning may lead to respiratory difficulties and shortness of breath. Cervical nerve tractioning may lead to peripheral nerve symptoms. If a dislocation or fracture occurred, the vertebrae are surgically treated and immobilized with wires, pins, screws or plates.

✦ Whiplash can result in blunt head trauma, loss of consciousness and post-concussion headache *(Foreman, Croft, 1995)*.

✦ The thoracic and lumbar spine may also be affected. In addition, other injuries may occur to the client's pelvis, limbs, abdomen and viscera during the accident. The shoulder girdle may be affected by a seatbelt injury, while knees may be affected by hitting the dashboard.

✦ Symptoms may recur following aggressive treatment techniques such as extremes of stretching.

✦ The client may develop apprehension with active or passive movement of the cervical spine.

✦ The **direction of impact** influences the structures that are affected. For example, when the head is forced forward, there is strain and sprain of the posterior neck. When the head is forced back, strain and sprain occur to the anterior neck. When the neck is turned and flexed, nerve root compression and facet joint dislocation on the side of head flexion can occur; when the neck is turned and extended, facet joint compression occurs. When the neck is stretched to the side, cervical nerve root and brachial plexus stretch lesions can occur. These lesions often involve transient symptoms of burning pain, numbness into the arm and weakness in shoulder movements on the affected side *(Souza, 1997)*. Cervical nerve root compression or overstretch ("burner" or "stinger") injuries result in sharp, burning or radiating pain on the affected side *(Booher, Thibodeau, 1989)*. Facet joint pain radiates into the neck and shoulder of the affected side *(Gerard, Kleinfield, 1993)*.

✦ In most cases, there is no pain or restriction in range of motion immediately following the injury. Pain and stiffness develop gradually in the larger cervical muscles over 24 to 48 hours *(Hertling, Kessler, 1996)*.

✦ Heat, edema and spasm also develop over this time frame, with more severe injuries producing more severe symptoms.

- Muscle guarding and spasm are likely in sternocleidomastoid and the multifidi at C4 to C6.
- There is tenderness at the injury site.
- A gap may be palpated in the affected muscles.
- Other possible symptoms include deafness, dizziness, dysphagia, headache, memory loss, nausea, temporomandibular joint pain, thoracic outlet syndrome, tinnitus and difficulty swallowing (which may indicate trigger points in sternocleidomastoid or a hematoma between the esophagus and cervical spine or vertebral fracture).
- With neurological involvement, such as peripheral nerve injury, loss of strength and muscle atrophy may appear within 72 hours *(Foreman, Croft, 1995)*.

Early Subacute

- Edema, heat and inflammation are still present but reduced from the acute stage.
- Pain in the injured muscles is diminishing. There are areas of point tenderness in the affected muscles, such as sternocleidomastoid, infra- and suprahyoids, longus colli, scalenes, multifidi, suboccipitals, levator scapulae and upper trapezius.
- With a higher than F/C Grade 2 (QTF Grade 2) whiplash, a hematoma is resolving at the injury site. A gap may be present in the affected muscles.
- Adhesions are developing around the injury site.
- The protective muscle spasm diminishes. Trigger points occur in the affected muscles.
- The range of motion is reduced.
- Since ligaments are hypovascular, they heal relatively slowly.
- Swelling of injured facet joints is too deep to be noticed.
- Neurological signs, such as numbness or tingling in the arms, are present with nerve root tractioning or thoracic outlet syndrome.

Late Subacute

- With all degrees of whiplash, the pain, edema and inflammation are diminishing.
- The original sharp muscle pain is replaced by achy pain which may refer to the head, between the scapulae or into the arm.
- Affected muscles such as sternocleidomastoid and longus colli become progressively less tender.
- Range of motion is improving from the acute stage but is still reduced.
- The protective muscle spasm is replaced by increased tone in the affected muscles and their synergists and antagonists. Trigger points occur in the affected muscles and in compensatory muscles.
- Adhesions are maturing around the injury.
- If present, the hematoma diminishes. A gap is still palpable in the tissue.

Chronic

+ The pain is deep, aching and vague. It may refer to the head, between the scapulae or into the arms.

+ The client may suffer headaches which get worse with activity.

+ Larger cervical muscle groups are shortened and fibrosed.

+ Longus colli is likely in chronic spasm. Over time, this spasm will flatten and reduce the cervical spine lordosis, destabilizing the vertebrae and exerting compression on the cervical discs.

+ Multifidi at C5 to C6 are in chronic spasm in an attempt to stabilize the lower cervical vertebrae.

+ Temporomandibular joint problems and hypertonicity of the muscles of mastication may be present.

+ Hypertonicity and trigger points are present in the affected muscles and in any compensating structures.

+ Adhesions have matured around the injury.

+ The tissue may be cool due to ischemia.

+ The full range of motion is reduced, especially in the upper cervical spine.

+ There is possible hypermobility of C4 to C6 vertebrae *(Hertling, Kessler, 1996)*.

+ There is reduced strength of the affected muscles and possible disuse atrophy.

+ Joint injuries can, over time, lead to degenerative disc disease or osteoarthritis of the cervical spine.

Subjective Information

HEALTH HISTORY QUESTIONS

*These questions reflect some of the Quebec Task Force's minimum data to be collected on the initial visit.

+ What is the client's overall health history? Is the client on any medication, for unrelated conditions, that indicates treatment modifications?

+ *How was the client's health before this collision? Was there any history of headache or pain in the neck, back, shoulder or jaw?

+ *Has the client been injured in a motor vehicle collision in the past? Where and when?

+ *In terms of the current collision, when did it occur?

+ *Was the client the occupant of a car, van or bus? Was the client on a motorcycle or bicycle? Was the client a pedestrian?

◆ *If in a car, van or bus, where was the client seated — for example, in the driver's seat, as a passenger in the front or rear seat?

◆ *Was the vehicle hit from the front, rear, left or right side?

◆ *Was the client's seatbelt fastened? Was it a lap, a shoulder or a lap and shoulder belt? Was there a headrest on the seat?

◆ *Did the client lose consciousness or hit his head?

◆ *What symptoms is the client experiencing now and how severe are they?

◆ Were there any other injuries?

◆ What aggravates or relieves the pain or other symptoms?

◆ *Did the symptoms begin the day of the collision, up to the fourth day after the collision or later than the fourth day?

◆ What was done at the time of injury? Was first aid applied?

◆ Did the client see any other health care practitioner for this injury, such as a physician, physiotherapist or chiropractor? If so, was a diagnosis made using X-ray or magnetic resonance imaging (MRI)? What treatment was given? Is the client still receiving this treatment?

◆ Is the client taking any medication for the whiplash, such as analgesics, muscle relaxants or anti-inflammatories? This includes self-medication such as Aspirin or other over-the-counter products.

◆ Were there any complications, such as a local hematoma, nerve damage or fracture?

◆ Is the client using any supports such as a hard or soft cervical collar?

◆ Is any swelling or any edema present local or distal to the injury? Swelling that occurred rapidly after the injury — for example, within 20 minutes — may indicate a hematoma. In this case, the client should be referred for medical treatment.

◆ What activities are difficult or painful to complete?

◆ What are the client's activities of daily living?

◆ *What is the client's main work activity? Does the client perform heavy or light labour? Does the client sit at a desk, stand, walk or move about? Does the client drive or operate a vehicle?

◆ *Did the collision occur in the course of the client's work?

◆ Is this an insurance claim?

Objective Information

Observations

Acute

✍ Immediately following the injury, there may be little to observe.

✍ Over 24 to 48 hours, antalgic posture may develop. In a **lateral view**, the head may be pulled anteriorly into a head-forward posture; that is, the external auditory meatus is anterior to the plumb line.

✍ The client may have a pained or medicated facial expression.

✍ Edema develops at the lesion site. There is minimal or no edema at all with an F/C Grade 1 (QTF Grades 0-1) whiplash, moderate edema with an F/C Grade 2 (QTF Grade 2) whiplash and marked edema with F/C Grades 3-5 (QTF Grades 3-4) whiplash. There may be edema in other locations, such as the anterior chest on the side of the shoulder harness.

✍ Some redness may be present local to the injury.

✍ Red, black or purple bruising may be visible over the primary injury site or in other locations such as the anterior chest.

✍ With an F/C Grade 2 (QTF Grade 2) whiplash and higher, a gap may be visible in the contour of the sternocleidomastoid muscle, often in the proximal third of the muscle *(Herling, Kessler, 1996)*.

✍ A cervical support collar may be worn.

Early and Late Subacute

✍ In a **lateral view**, an antalgic head-forward posture is present, although it may be less than in the acute stage.

✍ The client may still have a pained or medicated facial expression.

✍ Edema diminishes, then disappears, from the early to late subacute stage, both on site and at other locations.

✍ Bruising, if visible, changes from purple and black in the early subacute stage to brown, yellow and green in the late subacute stage and then disappears.

✍ With an F/C Grade 2 (QTF Grade 2) whiplash and higher, a gap in the contour of the sternocleidomastoid muscle is still apparent.

Chronic

✍ In a **lateral view**, a habituated antalgic head-forward posture may be observed, with an accompanying increase in the cervical lordotic curve.

✍ With a head-forward posture, the sternocleidomastoid muscle assumes a more vertical orientation. In a normal posture, this muscle angles posteriorly from the inferior to superior attachments.

✍ The scapulae may be protracted.

✍ In **anterior** and **posterior views**, an assessment of the levels of the occiput, the mandibular angles and acromioclavicular joints will, with an F/C Grade 2 (QTF Grade 2) whiplash and higher, show an alteration in the contour of the muscle.

Palpation

Acute

✍ Heat is present over the injured tissues in the neck and thorax and possibly in the surrounding tissue.

✍ Tenderness is present local to the lesion site and refers into the nearby tissue.

✍ The texture of the edema is firm. With an F/C Grade 2 (QTF Grade 2) or F/C Grade 3 whiplash a hematoma may be palpable in sternocleidomastoid, although it is more likely to occur in longus colli.

✍ With an F/C Grade 2 (QTF Grade 2) whiplash and higher a palpable gap or alteration in the sternocleidomastoid's contour is present and protective muscle spasm is present in the affected muscles, the synergists and the antagonists.

Early and Late Subacute

✍ The temperature over the injury site drops from the early subacute to late subacute stage.

✍ Point tenderness is present local to the injury.

✍ The texture of the edema is less firm. Adhesions are present as healing progresses from the early to late subacute stage. The hematoma, if present, diminishes.

✍ The tone of the affected muscle and the synergists and antagonists changes from spasm in the early subacute stage to tightness and hypertonicity in the late subacute stage. Trigger points are present in these muscles.

Chronic

✍ The injury site may be cool due to ischemia.

✍ Point tenderness occurs local to the injury and possibly in the muscles of mastication and the thorax.

✍ Adhesions are present local to the injury in, for example, sternocleidomastoid. Thickening and scarring of the muscles occur and crepitus may be present *(Brukner, Khan, 1993)*.

✍ A palpable gap or alteration in the sternocleidomastoid muscle's contour or fascial distortions may be present with an F/C Grade 2 (QTF Grade 2) or higher whiplash.

✍ Hypertonicity and trigger points may be present local to the injured muscles and in the compensating muscles, including the muscles of mastication. Segmental muscle guarding may occur at C5 to C6 multifidi. Disuse atrophy may be present in the affected muscle or the synergists if full range of motion is not present or following the prolonged use of a cervical collar.

Testing

Nerves, joints, ligaments, tendons and muscles should all be assessed. The thoracic and lumbar spine, shoulder and jaw may need to be assessed as well. The test results that follow are primarily for the cervical spine.

Acute

✍ Since the symptoms of whiplash develop gradually over 28 to 48 hours *(Hertling, Kessler, 1996)*, there may be little pain or reduced range of motion immediately after the accident.

✍ **AF ROM** of the neck on the cardinal plane is reduced due to pain. The degree of limitation increases with the severity of the injury.

✍ Testing other than AF ROM, neurological testing (deep tendon reflexes, sensory and motor testing) and the swallowing test are **contraindicated** in the acute stage if an F/C Grade 2 (QTF Grade 2) or higher whiplash is suspected. This is indicated by:

    (1) the presence of a palpable gap in the tissue,

    (2) protective muscle guarding and

    (3) the AF ROM results of severe pain and reduced ROM. The client should seek medical assessment *(Booher, Thibodeau, 1989)* with an F/C Grade 2 (QTF Grade 2) or higher whiplash or if neurological testing is positive.

✍ **PR ROM** for an F/C Grade 1 (QTF Grades 0-1) whiplash is performed on the cardinal planes of motion, with the range that stretches the affected muscles tested **last**. A painful, muscle spasm end feel is present before the affected muscles reach their full length *(Magee, 1992)*. The range is slightly greater than the AF ROM.

✍ **AR isometric testing** of the affected muscles with an F/C Grade 1 (QTF Grade 0-1) whiplash reveals minor to insignificant loss of strength and some discomfort.

Early and Late Subacute

✍ **AF ROM** of the neck is limited due to pain but less so than in the acute stage. Again, the degree of limitation increases with the severity of the injury.

✍ **PR ROM** is performed on the cardinal planes of motion, with the range that stretches the affected muscles tested **last.** A painful, tissue-stretch end feel is present before the affected muscles reach their full length due to adhesions. The range is painfully restricted but less so than in the acute stage. Capsular restriction is present if the facet joints were injured *(Hertling, Kessler, 1996)*.

✍ **AR isometric testing** of the affected muscle is the differential assessment for a strain, which is likely present with a whiplash. To avoid further injury to the muscle, it is important that the force of the client's contraction is gradually increased to the maximum strength and that the therapist applies gradually increased counterpressure *(Kendall et al., 1993)*. The contraction is increased to the **onset of pain only.** Pain is experienced **at the injury site** itself. See the chapter on strains for more details.

    • In terms of AR isometric testing of the anterior neck flexors, one source notes that the facet joints in the lower cervical spine may cause pain even if the joints do not move, since contraction of the muscles of the anterior cervical spine compresses the joints together. By repeating the isometric test in full flexion, the therapist can differentiate pain due to a compressed facet joint from muscular pain. Flexion reduces the compression on the joints; therefore, a reduction in pain means the facet joints, not the muscles, were the source of the pain *(Foreman, Croft, 1995)*.

- **AR strength tests** of an F/C Grade 2 (QTF Grade 2) or higher whiplash show weakness and pain with a strain of the following muscles: rhomboids, middle trapezius and anterior, anterolateral and posterolateral neck flexors.

Chronic

- **AF ROM** of joints crossed by the affected muscles may be painfully limited by as much as 50 per cent *(Hertling, Kessler, 1996)*.

- **PR ROM** is performed on the cardinal planes of motion, with the range that stretches the affected muscles tested **last**. A mildly painful, tissue-stretch end feel may be present on stretching the affected muscles. Active and passive ranges of motion will be approximately the same. Capsular restriction is present in the upper cervical spine if ligaments and facet joints were injured *(Hertling, Kessler, 1996)*.

- **AR strength testing** of the affected muscles may reveal decreased muscle strength, especially with disuse atrophy or an F/C Grade 2 (QTF Grade 2) or higher whiplash.

Special Tests

- The **vertebral artery test** is used to rule out any vertebral artery insufficiency before performing any test that extends, sidebends and rotates the cervical spine, such as Spurling's test.

- The **swallowing test** is used to differentiate between sternocleidomastoid trigger points and other cervical pathologies.

- Various neurological tests are performed to assess the nerve roots and peripheral nerves:

  - **Deep tendon reflexes** are assessed at C5 to C7 and are decreased or absent with certain cervical lesions such as disc herniation. **Sensory testing** is performed for C5 to C8 dermatomes; **touch perception** or **two-point discrimination testing** may be positive with specific lesions.

  - **Strength tests** are used to assess motor weakness. Active resisted isometric testing is performed for deltoids (C5 level), biceps (C6), triceps (C7) and finger flexors (C8). Muscles are checked bilaterally and strength may be reduced with specific lesions *(Hoppenfeld, 1976)*. See muscle strength grading in Appendix C.

  - An **upper limb tension test** is positive with cervical nerve root, brachial plexus or peripheral nerve pathologies.

  - **Spurling's, cervical compression** and **cervical distraction tests** are positive with cervical nerve root compression. Spurling's may also indicate facet joint irritation. With facet joint irritation of C5 to C7, often the client will draw a line of pain down the outer arm to the hand; this arm and hand pain often does not fit a specific dermatome *(Souza, 1997)*.

- Various joint play tests are used:

- Both **motion** and **static palpation** are performed on the cervical and thoracic spine and may reveal areas of hyper- and hypomobility. Motion palpation is more likely to reveal vertebral dysfunction than static palpation *(Foreman, Croft, 1995)*.

- **Passive relaxed atlanto-occipital articulation** may have restrictions. Since 50 to 60 per cent of axial rotation occurs between C1 and C2 *(Souza, 1997)*, the **atlanto-axial articulation test** likely will be restricted with a capsular pattern. **Passive relaxed anterior** and **lateral spinous challenges** are likely to be hypermobile at C4 to C6 levels.

✍ **First rib mobility, rib motion** and **levatores costarum fixation tests** may show areas of hypo- or hypermobility.

✍ The **scalene cramp** and **scalene relief tests** are positive with scalene trigger points.

✍ Any of **Adson's, Travell's variation on Adson's, Wright's hyperabduction, costoclavicular syndrome** and **Eden's tests** may be positive with various thoracic outlet syndromes.

✍ With temporomandibular joint dysfunction temporomandibular joint **AF range of motion** and **three-knuckle tests** will be positive.

✍ **Length tests** may reveal shortness due to the scar tissue within the muscles following an F/C Grade 2 (QTF Grade 2) and higher whiplash. Pectoralis minor and pectoralis major may be short.

Contraindications

♦ In the acute stage, testing of an F/C Grade 2 (QTF Grade 2) or higher whiplash other than pain-free active free range of motion and neurological testing (deep tendon reflexes and sensory and motor testing) is contraindicated to prevent further tissue damage. If the therapist suspects F/C Grades 4-5 (QTF Grade 4) whiplash (dislocation or fracture, or if radicular symptoms, extreme muscle weakness or difficulty swallowing due to a hematoma are present), refer the client to a physician for further assessment.

♦ In the subacute and chronic stages, refer the client for medical attention if the vertebral artery test is positive.

♦ Avoid removing the protective muscle splinting of acute whiplash.

♦ Do not passively stretch a muscle that is in spasm.

♦ Avoid extreme stretches of the cervical muscles, especially to sternocleidomastoid and the larger posterior cervical muscles in the acute to subacute stages *(Hertling, Kessler, 1996)*.

♦ Avoid mobilizing hypermobile vertebrae, usually at C4 to C6 levels.

♦ Joint play for the spine should not be painful.

♦ Avoid overly aggressive techniques in the subacute and chronic stages; these may provoke a flare-up of acute symptoms *(Hertling, Kessler, 1996)*.

♦ Do not compress over the carotid artery or carotid sinuses when treating the anterior neck muscles.

♦ Do not use massage techniques bilaterally on both sternocleidomastoid muscles at the same time, as the carotid arteries may be compressed. The client may also feel choked.

♦ Frictions are contraindicated if the client is taking anti-inflammatories or blood thinners.

Treatment Goals

Treatment Plan

Acute

Assess the severity of the whiplash and refer for medical attention if it is F/C Grades 4-5 (QTF Grade 4). Assess for other injuries.

🖐 **Positioning** depends on the client's comfort and apprehension levels. The seated or supine position is appropriate. In a seated position, pillows are built up on the table in front of the client. The head is well supported so the neck is not rotated to one side. In a supine position the client may need to take care getting on and off the table so as not to stress the neck muscles. Additional pillowing may be needed for elevation of any other injured areas.

🖐 **Hydrotherapy** in the acute stage is cold, such as an ice pack or a gel pack, applied to the injured areas.

General Treatment

🖐 If the initial treatment goal is to decrease the edema, lymphatic drainage is performed first, before any general compensatory work.

Reduce pain. Decrease sympathetic nervous system firing.

🖐 If the initial goal is to accustom the client to the therapist's touch and to decrease the sympathetic nervous system firing in the context of a relaxation massage, the treatment begins on the trunk or on the arms. The client is directed to do **diaphragmatic breathing** throughout the treatment (Alexander, 1996/7).

Treat any compensating structures. Maintain local circulation.

🖐 The trunk, shoulder girdle and uninjured limbs are treated to reduce hypertonicity as well as to increase drainage to and venous return from the affected tissues. Muscles of respiration are treated in clients who are apical breathers. Effleurage and slow petrissage such as palmar kneading, fingertip kneading and C-scooping are used.

Specific Treatment

Reduce inflammation. Reduce edema.

🖐 Assuming that the initial treatment goal is to reduce the edema, lymphatic drainage techniques are used, beginning with nodal pumping at the terminus (just superior to the clavicle, immediately lateral to the sternocleidomastoid muscle), then at the proximal lymph nodes in the neck and axilla. Nodes are found in chains anterior and posterior to sternocleidomastoid, below the angle of the mandible and at the occiput. Unidirectional effleurage, stationary circles and the local technique are used proximal to the injury — whether neck or shoulder — to reduce edema and prevent adhesion formation. For specific lymphatic drainage patterns of the neck and trunk, see the chapter on edema.

Reduce but do not remove protective muscle spasm.

🖐 Care is taken not to significantly reduce any protective muscle spasm in the injured muscles, such as sternocleidomastoid, by overtreating the tissue. In an F/C Grade 1 (QTF Grades 0-1) whiplash, techniques include isometric agonist contraction, gentle vibrations and

Treatment Goals Treatment Plan

effleurage to the antagonists. Golgi tendon organ release and the origin and insertion technique are used on the tendons of affected muscles and their antagonists. In the higher grades, indirect techniques such as isometric agonist contraction may be all the client can tolerate for the affected muscles. Other indirect work such as craniosacral techniques may also be useful.

Do not disturb any hematoma present.

- Other specific on-site work is contraindicated at this time.
- Stroking and muscle squeezing are used on the head, muscles of mastication and distal arms for all grades of whiplash.

Treat other conditions.

- Any other injuries are also treated, such as sprains or contusions to other body parts. See the appropriate chapters for details.

Early Subacute

- The healing tissue is still fragile. Therefore, address treatment goals with care.

Reduce inflammation.

- **Hydrotherapy applications** on site are cold/warm contrast.

General Treatment

Reduce pain. Decrease sympathetic nervous system firing. Treat compensatory structures.

- The treatment approach outlined for acute general work is indicated in this stage also, including reducing pain perception and encouraging **diaphragmatic breathing.** Rhythmic techniques to the trunk and unaffected limbs are indicated if the client is comfortable with this type of work.

Specific Treatment

Reduce edema. Prevent adhesion formation.

- Proximal lymphatic drainage techniques are indicated to reduce any edema. These include pumping at the terminus and proximal nodes, unidirectional effleurage, stationary circles and the local technique. The work is performed proximal to the injured tissues to prevent congestion through the injury.

Maintain local circulation proximal to the injured tissues only.

- The trunk and shoulder girdle muscles are treated to reduce hypertonicity and maintain drainage and venous return. Techniques include effleurage and repetitive petrissage, such as palmar kneading, C-scooping, fingertip kneading and the origin and insertion technique.

Reduce spasm.

- Since protective muscle spasm is no longer as important in stabilizing the injured tissues, Golgi tendon organ release is used on the tendons of the affected muscles, such as sternocleidomastoid, the scalenes, upper trapezius, levator scapulae and the posterior cervical muscles. Agonist contraction and the origin and insertion technique are also useful.

Treatment Goals   Treatment Plan

Reduce trigger points without disturbing the injury site.

Trigger points in muscles that refer to the neck, head and other affected areas such as the arms are now treated using gentle muscle stripping or intermittent ischemic compressions. As it is still important not to overstretch the healing tissues, trigger point work is followed by PIR that only partially lengthens the affected muscle. See Late Subacute for details about specific muscles.

Treat specific injury site.

With an F/C Grade 1 (QTF Grades 0-1) whiplash, on-site work consists of thumb and fingertip kneading to the client's pain tolerance. With an F/C Grade 2 (QTF Grade 2) and higher whiplash, on-site work is restricted to light stroking and vibrations, to the client's pain tolerance.

Do not disturb the hematoma.

If a hematoma is present with an F/C Grade 2 (QTF Grade 2) or higher whiplash, on-site work is delayed until the late subacute stage.

Maintain range of motion.

Careful **pain-free, mid-range passive relaxed range of motion,** to the onset of pain only, is used on the cervical spine and scapulothoracic articulation. This maintains the successive action and helps increase lymphatic drainage. Ranges that stretch injured muscles are introduced **last.**

The head, muscles of mastication and arms are also treated as in the acute stage.

Treat other conditions.

Any other injuries, including temporomandibular joint dysfunction, are also treated.

Late Subacute

The healing tissue is less fragile. Therefore, the treatment goals can be achieved using more vigorous techniques.

Positioning may now include sidelying or the prone position as long as the client's head and neck are securely pillowed and the cervical spine is not rotated or sidebent in sidelying. A face cradle is used in the prone position.

Hydrotherapy applications are cold/hot contrast therapy local to the injury. If acute inflammation recurs, the therapist returns to using local cold hydrotherapy applications.

General Treatment

Reduce pain. Decrease sympathetic nervous system firing. Treat any compensating structures.

The treatment approach outlined for early subacute general work is indicated in this stage also. Rhythmic techniques to the trunk and arms are indicated if the client is comfortable with this type of work.

Treatment Goals   Treatment Plan

Specific Treatment

Reduce edema.

☝ As the edema diminishes in the late subacute stage, the length of time spent on lymphatic techniques decreases.

Reduce hypertonicity and trigger points in the neck and shoulder muscles.

☝ The muscles of the shoulder girdle are treated to reduce hypertonicity and increase drainage and venous return. Trigger points in the affected muscles that refer to the neck and head are now treated directly using muscle stripping and ischemic compressions according to the client's pain tolerance.

- Posteriorly, these muscles include **upper trapezius, levator scapulae, splenius cervicis** and **capitis, semispinalis capitis**, the **suboccipitals, cervical multifidi** and **rotatores.**

- Suboccipital hypertonicity is reduced with the Golgi tendon organ release technique. Specific passive stretching for short suboccipitals is achieved with the client in the prone position by the therapist first stabilizing the spinous process of C2 with the index and middle finger of one hand *(Kisner, Colby, 1990)*. The fingertips of the other hand grasp the occiput and slowly traction the occiput into flexion.

- Anteriolaterally, **sternocleidomastoid** and the **scalenes** also are affected. See the chapter on thoracic outlet syndrome for details of scalene palpation and treatment. Trigger points in the sternal division of sternocleidomastoid refer into the occiput, cheek and around the eye. A trigger point near the sternal attachment refers into the throat; autonomic phenomena from the sternal division include visual disturbances and tearing of the affected eye. Trigger points in the clavicular division of sternocleidomastoid refer to the forehead (frontal headache) and into the ear; autonomic phenomena include dizziness and nausea *(Travell, Simons, 1983)*.

Treat SCM trigger points.

☝ Sternocleidomastoid trigger points are most easily treated with the pincer grasp technique when the muscle is placed in a slightly shortened, slack position. To treat the left muscle, the neck is slightly sidebent to the left and the head is slightly rotated to the right. By curling the index finger into flexion and placing it underneath and behind the muscle, while applying ischemic compression in a slow, controlled manner with the left thumb, the therapist can work the relaxed muscle without causing the client discomfort.

- The therapist should work one sternocleidomastoid at a time and should avoid direct compression over the deep carotid artery, located in the carotid triangle *(Pansky, 1979)*. The area is bordered posteriorly by the upper half of the sternocleidomastoid, superiorly by the posterior digastric muscle and anteriorly by the omohyoid muscle *(Figure 28.7)*. The therapist should also work around the external jugular vein which runs over the sternocleidomastoid *(Travell, Simons, 1983)*.

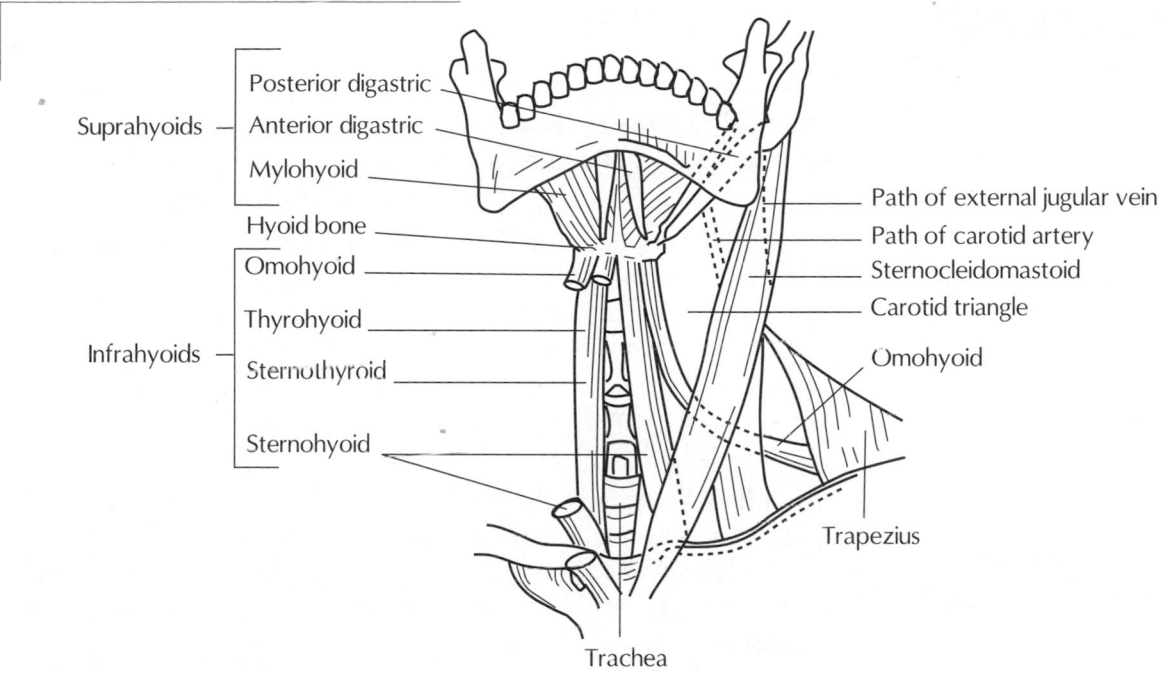

Figure 28.7
Supra- and infrahyoid muscles. The carotid artery is deep to the carotid triangle.

Treatment Goals   Treatment Plan

Reduce hypertonicity and trigger points in the infra- and suprahyoid muscles.

🖐 Clinical experience indicates that trigger points in the **infra- and suprahyoid muscles** seem to refer into the throat. Specific client consent is recommended to treat these muscles that run over the front of the throat. They are frequently injured in a whiplash accident and just as frequently overlooked during treatment. The infra- and suprahyoid muscles are sometimes called the "anterior strap muscles", due to their shape.

• To locate these muscles accurately, the therapist uses the hyoid bone as an initial reference. This delicate horseshoe-shaped bone is found below the angle of the mandible. It is five to six centimetres wide. The therapist stands at the client's shoulder, facing the supine client so his comfort levels are constantly monitored during palpation and treatment.

Treat infra- and suprahyoid trigger points.

• Using the thumb and index *or* second finger of one hand, the therapist gently palpates for the lateral posterior borders of the hyoid. The two **sternohyoid muscles** run inferior from the hyoid to the sternum, just anterior to the trachea. Gentle resisted depression of the mandible makes these muscles palpable.

• To prevent the client from feeling choked, these muscles are treated unilaterally. The therapist's thumb (or finger) stabilizes on the lateral trachea just inferior to the hyoid, applying gentle, medially directed pressure *(St. John, 1991)*. The thumb does not move, it just stabilizes

Treatment Goals Treatment Plan

the trachea. Direct pressure on the *anterior* aspect of the trachea provokes a choked feeling and is avoided.

- The treating finger (or thumb) of the same hand applies gentle *cross-fibre strokes* to the ribbon-like sternohyoid muscle, moving from *lateral to medial,* again to avoid any choking sensation. If a trigger point is found, *gentle* ischemic compression is applied. The therapist then moves the stabilizing thumb (or finger) inferiorly and repeats the cross-fibre strokes, working systematically along the muscle. The therapist avoids the carotid triangle. The other sternohyoid is treated in a similar manner.

- **Mylohyoid** runs from the hyoid to the underside of the mandible. It is also treated using a stabilizing thumb on one side, while short cross-fibre strokes are used to locate trigger points in the other side of the muscle. Gentle ischemic compression is used to treat trigger points.

- Trigger points in **omohyoid** cause this muscle to tighten, compressing the brachial plexus *(Travell, Simons, 1983).* The superior portion of omohyoid runs just lateral to sternohyoid, then continues deep to sternocleidomastoid. It is treated in conjunction with sternohyoid.

- **Longus colli** hypertonicity is treated indirectly using isometric agonist contraction of the cervical multifidi. If left untreated, a hypertonic longus colli (attaching on the anterior aspect of vertebrae C2 to T3) reduces the cervical lordotic curve. With the client in the seated position, the therapist places two fingers on the back of the client's neck at the vertebral level to be treated; for example, at C4. The client *slightly* sidebends and extends the neck over the therapist's fingers. Isometric resistance in the direction of sidebending and flexion is applied by the therapist *(Hertling, Kessler, 1996).* **Multifidi** on the contralateral side of this vertebral level are then treated.

Reduce hypertonicity and trigger points in the anterior and posterior thoracic region.

- Muscles in the anterior thoracic region are treated for hypertonicity and trigger points, including pectoralis major and minor, subclavius, rotator cuff muscles, the intercostals and the diaphragm.

- When the client has head-forward posture, the posterior thoracic muscles are treated after the anterior chest, either in the sidelying or prone position. This includes middle and lower trapezius, rhomboids, latissimus dorsi, thoracic erector spinae and the deeper postural muscles. Levator costarum may be tight with thoracic injury *(Barral, 1991),* as may the intercostals. See the hyperkyphosis and asthma chapters for details of treating these muscles.

Provide post-treatment care for trigger points.

- If ischemic compressions are used to treat the injured muscles, repetitive petrissage and a partial-length PIR are used to flush circulation through the muscle instead of heat and a full stretch, since

Treatment Goals Treatment Plan

this latter technique may compromise the strained tissues.

Reduce adhesions.

As the inflammation subsides in the late subacute stage with F/C Grades 2-3 (QTF Grades 2-3) whiplash, the on-site focus shifts to reducing adhesions within the affected muscles. It is also important to encourage the formation of functional scars by realigning the developing connective tissue. It is essential to accurately palpate the lesion site and any restricting adhesions before attempting to reduce these adhesions. Myofascial release techniques, slow skin rolling and longitudinal muscle stripping are used *(Foreman, Croft, 1995)*. These are followed by specific petrissage, such as short cross-fibre strokes and frictions to the adhesions *(Hertling, Kessler, 1990; Thomson et al., 1991; Brukner, Khan, 1993)*. All this work is performed within the client's pain tolerance. Frictions to the infra- and suprahyoid muscles are avoided.

Provide post-treatment care for adhesions.

After the adhesions have been frictioned, the specific stretch that lengthens the muscle is used to realign the fibres. A **passive stretch** is performed cautiously, gently and in a pain-free manner to avoid overstretching the injured tissues, especially the larger posterior cervical muscles. These muscles need to be strong, not stretched, to balance the tight, short sternocleidomastoid muscles and prevent or reduce head-forward posture *(Hertling, Kessler, 1996)*. **Ice** is applied to the frictioned tissue to restrict the inflammatory process.

It is also important to avoid overstretching the neck due to the possibility of overmobilizing the hypermobile cervical vertebrae C4 to C6. Mobilization or stretching that stresses the facet joints may also contribute to an increase in heat and swelling too deep to be palpated.

Gradually increase the range of motion.

Joint play techniques are used to restore range of motion for the hypomobile vertebrae in the cervical and thoracic spine. Adhesions in the facet joint capsules are also treated with these techniques. Long-axis traction and oscillations on the anterior-posterior and lateral planes are used to mobilize individual segments *(Hertling, Kessler, 1996)*. Any joint mobilization should not be painful or cause pain after treatment.

Careful **mid- to full range passive relaxed range of motion** to the onset of pain only is used on the cervical spine. This maintains the succussive action, mobilizes adhesions and helps increase lymphatic drainage. Ranges that compress the facet joints are avoided, such as extreme extension, rotation and sidebending *(Hertling, Kessler, 1996)*.

Increase local circulation.

The risk of causing congestion local to the injury is diminished. Effleurage and petrissage are now introduced to increase circulation and promote tissue health.

Treat other conditions.

Other possible conditions include temporomandibular joint dysfunction and thoracic outlet syndrome.

403

Treatment Goals   Treatment Plan

Chronic

✋ A gradual approach at this stage of treatment is recommended, as whiplash appears to respond better when rapid increases in the range of motion are avoided *(Hertling, Kessler, 1996)*. This is important especially if the whiplash has not been treated in the earlier stages to reduce adhesions. Attempts at rapid stretching of untreated tissue can cause microtearing and inflammation *(Edwardson, 1995)*.

✋ **Positioning** is now chosen for comfort and for accessibility to the structures that are treated. Prone, sidelying and supine positions are all indicated.

✋ **Hydrotherapy** is deep moist heat, such as a hydrocollator or a wax application, to soften any remaining adhesions and increase local circulation.

General Treatment

Reduce sympathetic nervous system firing. Treat compensatory structures.

✋ The client's thorax and compensating structures are massaged as before. Diaphragmatic breathing is encouraged. Rhythmic techniques to the trunk and unaffected limbs are indicated.

Specific Treatment

Reduce hypertonicity and trigger points in the neck and shoulder muscles.

✋ The shoulder girdle and the muscles mentioned in the late subacute section are treated to reduce any remaining hypertonicity or trigger points and to increase local circulation. Effleurage, repetitive petrissage and ischemic compressions are indicated.

Reduce adhesions and provide appropriate after care.

✋ If the therapist has been treating the client's injury throughout the healing process, the focus is on reducing the remaining adhesions and scar tissue in, for example, sternocleidomastoid. Preparatory work includes specific kneading, muscle stripping and fascial techniques *(Souza, 1997; Edwardson, 1995; Barral, 1991)* to the affected muscles mentioned in the late subacute section. Cross-fibre frictions are performed on any remaining adhesions. These are followed by a **passive stretch** or **PIR** to the muscles to realign the fibres. Again, care is taken not to overstretch the larger posterior cervical muscles such as upper trapezius and splenius cervicis. An application of **ice** follows this work.

✋ If the therapist starts treating the client in the chronic stage, one approach is to focus on reducing the hypertonicity and trigger points that have developed from the client's compensation patterns, such as a head-forward posture. This is done before addressing any adhesions. See the chapter on hyperkyphosis for details.

Treatment Goals

Restore the range of motion.

Increase local circulation.

Treat other conditions.

Self-care Goals

Educate the client.

Maintain range of motion. Maintain strength of the affected muscles in a pain-free manner.

Treatment Plan

✋ Joint play techniques are indicated for hypomobile cervical vertebrae and other joints in the thorax and shoulder. With the client supine, long-axis traction of the upper cervical vertebrae is performed. The client's neck is in *slight* extension so the suboccipital muscles are relaxed. The therapist grasps under the occiput with one hand and on top of the forehead with the other hand. Gentle traction is applied to the neck *(Hertling, Kessler, 1996)*. **Pain-free passive relaxed range of motion** is used by the therapist on the affected joints to maintain joint health.

✋ The shoulder girdle and neck muscles are treated with effleurage and petrissage to increase local venous return.

✋ Head-forward posture, temporomandibular joint dysfunction and thoracic outlet syndrome are treated.

Self-care Plan

✍ Relaxation techniques such as diaphragmatic breathing are encouraged.

✍ **Hydrotherapy** is chosen that is appropriate for the stage of healing. In the acute stage, ice is applied to areas of inflammation. Ice is also used if acute flare-ups occur during the healing process. Because ligaments are hypovascular, it is important to introduce contrast hydrotherapy to help increase local circulation as soon as the acute stage has passed.

✍ **Self-massage** is useful for the affected muscle in the late subacute and chronic stages. This includes skin rolling, muscle stripping and gentle frictions to the client's pain tolerance.

✍ Vehicle headrests should be properly adjusted so, when viewed from the side, the middle of the headrest is at the level of the external auditory meatus. The person's head should be about four centimetres from the headrest and the seat back should not be inclined too far back *(Foreman, Croft, 1995)*. Seatbelts should always be worn.

✍ **Remedial exercise** that is given is dependent on the stage of healing and the severity of the injury. Since both muscles and ligaments can be injured, the therapist must combine principles for treating both tissues into the remedial exercise plan. It is important to **gradually** increase range and strength of the muscles to avoid reinjury and muscle imbalances. Sidebending, rotation, flexion and extension are performed. The range that was most injured — for example, extension — is regained **last.**

✍ In the **acute** and **early subacute stages,** the client is encouraged to

Self-care Goals

Self-care Plan

perform active free range of motion of the neck to the *onset* of pain only *(Hertling, Kessler, 1996)*. In this way, contractile tissue can withstand incrementally heavier workloads or increasing stretches without reinjury. If the shoulder girdle, temporomandibular joint or thoracic or lumbar spine is affected, active free range of motion within limits of pain is performed for the affected area.

Gradually increase range of motion.

✍ In the **late subacute** stage, the active free range of motion is gradually increased.

Gradually increase the strength of the affected muscles in a pain-free manner.

✍ As early as possible in the late subacute stage, submaximal pain-free active resisted isometric exercises for the posterior cervical muscles are introduced. The segmental multifidi strengthening mentioned in the treatment section of this chapter is used. The seated client applies the resistance to a specific vertebral level using the fingers of both hands placed behind the neck *(Hertling, Kessler, 1996)*. This is important to stabilize the hypermobile C4 to C6 levels.

• The same effect can be achieved by the client using a rolled towel behind the neck at the level to be strengthened. The ends are held in both hands and the client isometrically resists neck extension *(Foreman, Croft, 1995)*.

✍ To isometrically strengthen the larger posterior neck muscles, the seated client places both hands behind the head, linking the fingers and resisting neck extension. To isometrically strengthen lateral neck muscles such as the scalenes, the client places one hand on the side of the head and resists sidebending *(Kisner, Colby, 1996)*.

✍ Aerobic activity will also strengthen the neck muscles, since many of the neck muscles are accessory muscles of respiration.

✍ Specific anterior neck muscle strengthening is avoided at this time.

Gradually stretch specific shortened muscles.

✍ If tight sternocleidomastoid and pectoralis major muscles are creating a head-forward posture, for example, and preventing normal range of motion of the neck, gentle stretching is performed to the onset of pain only. Instead of full rotation and extension of the head to stretch sternocleidomastoid, only partial ranges are used. The client can simply move the neck through its range of motion, contracting antagonist muscles to create the stretch instead of using the hands to *pull* the neck into a stretch *(Foreman, Croft, 1995)*. The client should take care not to overstretch the muscles and further injure the facet joints *(Hertling, Kessler, 1996)*.

Strengthen weak muscles.

✍ In the **chronic** stage, the client may gradually progress to isotonic active resisted exercises for the posterior and lateral neck muscles once activities that stretch or contract the muscles are pain free both during and after the exercise *(Brukner, Khan, 1993)*.

✍ Multifidi at C4 to C6 are isometrically, segmentally strengthened.

Self-care Goals

Self-care Plan

✍ Neck and thoracic extensors are strengthened in the prone position using axial extension. The client is lying on the floor, with both arms at the sides, chin tucked in and forehead resting on the floor. The client lifts the head off the floor in a small motion while keeping the chin tucked in and avoiding head extension *(Kisner, Colby, 1996)*.

✍ Rhomboids, middle trapezius and thoracic erector spinae also need to be strengthened. See the hyperkyphosis chapter for details.

✍ Sternocleidomastoid and supra- and infrahyoids may require careful isometric strengthening once the posterior cervical muscles are stronger. The seated client places the palms of both hands on the forehead and isometrically resists neck flexion to strengthen the sternocleidomastoids *(Kisner, Colby, 1996)*. The palms of both hands are placed under the mandible and the client isometrically resists mandibular depression to strengthen supra- and infrahyoids.

Stretch shortened muscles.

✍ In the chronic stage, the client should avoid prolonged stretching of the larger posterior muscles by pulling the head into flexion, since this provides temporary relief only. Over the long term, it allows sternocleidomastoid to pull the neck into a head-forward posture. Instead, the suboccipitals are stretched using the chin-tuck exercise. The seated client places the index finger of one hand on the point of the chin and moves the occiput into extension by tucking the chin in. The movement is very small and correct movement is monitored by the finger on the chin. It is important that the client be instructed not to continue this exercise for more than six weeks, since the cervical lordosis is flattened through this action *(Hertling, Kessler, 1996)*.

✍ Scalenes and upper trapezius may also be stretched.

Encourage activity.

✍ Sources agree that it is important to tell the client that many cases resolve in four to six weeks and that the client should be as active as possible *(Foreman, Croft, 1995; Hertling, Kessler, 1996; Spitzer, 1995)*. Pain-free activities of daily living are encouraged.

Refer the client.

✍ The client may be referred to a chiropractor, physiotherapist or osteopath if his condition is not improving.

✍ Movement therapy, such as the Mitzvah, Feldenkrais or Alexander technique, may be helpful for retraining the client's posture.

Treatment Frequency and Expected Outcome

Shorter, more frequent treatments will address the inflammatory process in the acute and early subacute stages. This could be two half-hour treatments per week for three weeks. The client is reassessed each week. The treatment frequency is decreased if the client is improving, to once a week for the late subacute stage. Then the client and the remedial exercise plan are totally reassessed at six weeks. Clinical experience suggests that a combination of complementary therapies optimizes the client's recovery. The specific combination is individual for each client. Referrals for chiropractic, acupuncture, physiotherapy, among others, should be considered.

The QTF recommends that if the client is not improving, he is referred to another type of therapy at six weeks with a QTF Grade 1 whiplash; QTF Grades 2 and 3 whiplash are referred at 12 weeks *(Spitzer, 1995; Souza, 1997)*.

The outcome is variable, depending on the severity of the injury, pre-existing conditions and the client's age, general health and compliance with the treatment and self-care program. Apical breathers may also have a poorer prognosis *(Alexander, 1996/7)*. Another factor affecting prognosis is a history of four or more episodes of whiplash *(Souza, 1997)*.

Because one of the following outcome scales depends on X-ray findings, the massage therapist may obtain X-ray information (with the client's written consent) from the physician's or chiropractor's report.

The following are guidelines only:

Foreman and Croft Expected Outcome

✦ The client is placed on a prognosis scale with point values awarded depending on the presenting symptoms and X-ray findings. No specific time frame is given for recovery, nor is treatment frequency or duration intended to be extrapolated from the scale. Instead, prognosis is made on the basis of full recovery or long-term dependence on medication or neurological deficit or possible surgery.

- **Major Injury Category (MIC) 1**

   There are symptoms directly relating to the injury such as pain; however, there are no objective findings of loss of motion or neurological deficit with the person's complaints (10 points).

- **Major Injury Category 2**

   There are symptoms directly relating to the injury (MIC 1), plus decreased range of motion. There are no neurological signs (50 points).

- **Major Injury Category 3**

   There are symptoms directly relating to the injury and decreased range of motion (MIC 1 and 2), plus objective neurological signs, either sensory or motor (90 points).

✦ **Modifiers to Prognosis**

- Certain factors can modify the person's recovery and are awarded additional points, which are added to the MIC points. The person may have more than one modifier.

- Factors include:

   — small vertebral canal size: 10 to 12 mm (20 points), 13 to 15 mm (15 points);

   — kyphotic cervical curve (15 points);

   — loss of consciousness (15 points);

   — straight cervical curve (10 points);

   — pre-existing degeneration (10 points).

- **Excellent prognosis:** 10 to 30 points. MIC 1 with muscle pain and occipital headaches which will resolve.

- **Good prognosis:** 35 to 70 points. MIC 1 and 2 with residual problems such as occasional or intermittent neck pain or restricted range of motion.

- **Fair prognosis:** 75 to 100 points. MIC 2 with modifiers and some MIC 3; residual symptoms such as numbness or weakness are possible; symptoms may resolve with conservative care.

- **Poor prognosis:** 105 to 125 points. MIC 2 with many modifiers and MIC 3; likely persistent neurological signs such as muscle weakness, atrophy, radiculitis; long-term dependence on medication; may need surgery.

- **Unstable prognosis:** 130 to 165 points. Persistent neurological signs; improvement not likely with conservative care; long-term medication dependence; surgery often indicated (*Foreman, Croft, 1995*).

Quebec Task Force Prognosis

✦ The QTF relies on pathophysiological studies of animal soft tissue injuries as the basis to predict healing times for whiplash. It is important to note that the QTF's definition of *unresolved* is that the person is unable to resume usual activities; the definition of *resolved* is that the person is able to resume work or other activities, but may still have "residual pain or limitation of range of motion" (*Spitzer, 1995*).

✦ Figures from the QTF show that of those with Grade 1 whiplash, 44 per cent had neck pain, 37 per cent had headaches and 37 per cent had paresthesia *six months* to *two years* after the accident.

✦ Persons with Grade 2 whiplash reported symptoms of neck pain (81 per cent), headache (37 per cent), paresthesia (29 per cent) and auditory (14 per cent) and visual symptoms (10 per cent) within the same time frame. Grade 3 whiplash resulted in symptoms of neck pain (90 per cent), headache (70 per cent), paresthesia (60 per cent) and auditory (20 per cent) and visual symptoms (10 per cent) also within the same time frame.

- **Grade 1 Whiplash Associated Disorder (WAD)**

  Usually resolves in less than three weeks; if unresolved, the client is referred for specialized advice.

See stress reduction, edema, spasm, trigger points, contusions, strains, sprains, dislocations, fractures, tension headache, temporomandibular joint dysfunction, thoracic outlet syndrome, conditions of the peripheral nervous system, torticollis, hyperkyphosis, osteoarthritis and degenerative disc disease for related treatments.

- **Grade 2 WAD**

  Usually resolves in four to six weeks; the client is referred if unresolved.

- **Grade 3 WAD**

  No specific time frame is given; animal studies do not apply because nerve tissue may be injured in Grade 3 WAD and these structures were not included in the studies; the client is referred if unresolved at six weeks.

- **Grade 4 WAD**

  No time frame is given; it is assumed that the client is in surgical care (*Spitzer, 1995*).

F

OVERUSE INJURIES

29

STRATEGIES:
Overuse Injuries

Fiona Rattray

> *Any repeated activity, occupational or recreational, can lead to an overuse injury. This type of injury occurs when repetitive microtrauma overloads a tissue's ability to repair itself.*

Overuse injuries occur to muscles, tendons, ligaments, fascia and bone. Today this type of injury is on the rise, especially in amateur and professional athletes who train more intensely and for longer periods of time.

The inflammatory response initially results in acute inflammation and tissue repair. Continuing the activity perpetuates the microtrauma, tearing the remodelling scar tissue or microadhesions. Over time, chronic inflammation occurs. Immature collagen is continuously laid down at the injury site, reducing the overall tissue strength. This scar tissue painfully reduces the range of motion.

➤ **The causes of overuse injuries** may be grouped according to **extrinsic** and **intrinsic** factors *(Brukner, Khan, 1993)*. Extrinsic factors include: a rapid increase in length or intensity of an activity or sudden change in activity; inadequate rest; shoes or equipment that are inappropriate or worn out; faulty technique or posture; and inadequate nutrition. Intrinsic factors include: postural dysfunctions; bony asymmetries such as knee valgus, tibial torsion, patella alta or a hooked acromion; leg length discrepancy; muscle imbalance; muscle weakness; tight fascia; and lack of flexibility.

Sources differ regarding the naming of the inflammatory stages with overuse injuries. For example, bursitis has either an acute stage and a chronic stage *(Hertling, Kessler, 1996)* or an acute stage and a subacute stage *(Kisner, Colby, 1990)*. In this book, overuse injuries are categorized as acute and chronic. The differences perhaps arise from two meanings attributed to the word "chronic". It describes either the third stage of the healing process after acute and subacute stages or an ongoing condition that does not resolve because the factors causing it have not been addressed.

Symptom Picture

✦ Overuse injuries are usually **progressive** in their manifestation; microscopic damage occurs to the tissue fibres due to overuse. There may be an initial acute stage which settles into chronic inflammation as with tendinitis; or there may be a slow onset with no initial acute stage as with plantar fasciitis. Episodes of acute inflammation may occur if the person does not rest for long enough to allow healing to take place or if activity levels are increased.

✦ In general with overuse injuries, at first, discomfort may be felt after an activity. As the condition progresses, pain occurs during the activity and even after the activity stops.

✦ **Inflammation** is chronic. Heat may be palpated in the affected tissue if it is superficial enough. Chronic edema may or may not be visible.

✦ **Pain and decreased function** are present. The person may be inflexible, with short, tight fascia and muscles. There are increased muscle hypertonicity and progressive, increasing stiffness as long as the irritation persists.

✦ Eventually there is **weakness** in overused muscles. The affected tissue may break down, rupture or crack.

✦ Continued overuse leads to injury of **compensating structures.** The person has to stop the activity or sport, or change occupations.

Treatment Considerations

Assessment

✍ It is important for the therapist to determine the cause of the injury. This may be obvious, such as occupational overuse of a muscle, or be more elusive, such as a leg length discrepancy, postural dysfunction, habitual downhill running or wearing shoes that do not provide arch support.

✍ The testing protocol listed in each chapter of this section is used to assess the specific injured tissue. This includes a postural assessment, described in detail in Appendix B.

Massage

✋ Treatment plans are often a combination of musculoskeletal injury strategies and postural dysfunction approaches. Depending on the client's presentation, an acute treatment approach may be appropriate.

✋ The treatment goals are to limit the inflammatory process, reduce pain and any swelling, decrease sympathetic nervous system firing, reduce adhesions, stretch any shortened structures — including fascia and the antagonist muscles — and prevent reinjury. Compensatory structures are also treated.

✋ Positioning of the client should be comfortable and should not stress the injury site.

✋ Hydrotherapy varies with the presentation of the injury. A cold application is used to reduce pain and inflammation and to follow friction techniques. Heat may be applied to tight, short fascia that is proximal to the overuse injury and, in some cases, to short antagonist structures or to adhesions at the injury site. Contrast applications may be used to increase local circulation following treatment or to flush out chronic edema.

- Pain is reduced and the client's comfort is increased through the performance of a relaxation massage on the unaffected parts of the body.

- Any postural dysfunction or tight fascia is treated. This treatment goal may be extended over multiple sessions.

- Hypertonicity, trigger points and adhesions are reduced. Any hypomobile joints are addressed with joint play techniques.

- Circulation is increased if the injured tissue is hypovascular, such as with a tendon.

- Chronic edema at the injury site may be trapped by proximal and local connective tissue restrictions. Fascial glide is used to assess, then fascial techniques are used to treat the restrictions. Proximal lymphatic drainage is also indicated.

Self-care

- Self-care may be the most challenging aspect of the client's recovery process. An initial period of rest from the aggravating activity is necessary to avoid stress on the affected tissue and to allow healing to take place. This is termed "relative rest", because the client may still perform activities that do not affect the injured tissue. A certain amount of creativity and motivation is required on both the client's and therapist's parts, especially if the client has to modify a sport or occupational activity.

- Hydrotherapy applications are appropriate to the presentation of the injury. For example, the client applies ice after any activity that causes inflammation.

- Once constant pain is no longer experienced by the client, a controlled stress is introduced to the tissue, such as pain-free stretching. This is used on antagonists as well as affected muscles.

> See also the Strategies: Massage and the Inflammatory Process and Strategies: Fascial and Muscle Imbalances chapters for more information.

- Strengthening activities of affected muscles are gradually progressed from isometric to isotonic exercises. Eventually, the tissue becomes more tolerant of the loads placed upon it. Exercises designed to normalize proprioception are included.

- Education of the client is essential to correct poor biomechanics and improper techniques such as poor warm-up or cool-down.

PLANTAR FASCIITIS

Fiona Rattray

Plantar fasciitis is an overuse condition resulting in inflammation of the plantar fascia.

Plantar fasciitis is the most common cause of foot pain in athletes. The condition occurs due to overuse and stress on the plantar fascia, which can result in tissue fatigue and microtearing at the calcaneal attachments. The person with plantar fasciitis is usually over 40 years of age; however, very active athletes may experience symptoms at as early as 20 years of age.

The plantar fascia attaches to the medial process of the calcaneal tuberosity and merges into the plantar surfaces of the metatarsophalangeal joints and flexor tendon sheaths (*Figure 30.1*). It is composed of a large central portion and smaller medial and lateral slips. The plantar fascia functions as a passive bowstring during the midstance phase of the gait cycle, approximating the calcaneus and metatarsals. This shortens and raises the medial longitudinal arch. The same effect occurs when a standing person goes up on her toes, causing weight bearing through the heads of the metatarsals.

The fat pad that covers the plantar surface of the calcaneus is held in place by connective tissue septa, structures which divide the fat pad into

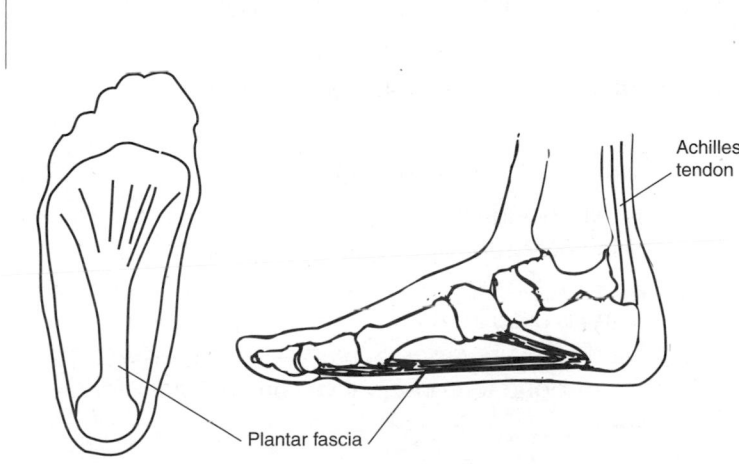

Figure 30.1
Plantar fascia.

compartments. The fat pad is designed to cushion the calcaneus during the initial contact phase of the gait cycle. The muscles of the lower leg, especially the soleus and gastrocnemius, also help to control shock absorption when walking or running.

Excessive pronation stretches the plantar fascia, the supporting ligaments and the intrinsic muscles of the feet. This leads to microtearing near the calcaneal attachments.

With excessive supination due to pes cavus, and with increased body weight, greater than normal compressive forces occur at the heel. Due to its rigidity, the pes cavus foot has decreased shock absorbing qualities. The plantar fascia and the heel fat pad are required to absorb more stress. The soleus muscle compensates by increasing its activity, placing a further stress on the plantar fascia and Achilles tendon.

A bone spur (exostosis) may form on the medial anterior calcaneus. This may be due to traction on the plantar fascia or to compressive forces. There are different theories to explain the formation of bone spurs. One theory states that, over time, repeated microtearing at the periosteum may lead to microhemorrhages, fibroblast activity and new bone formation. Since this inflammatory response is usually painful, it does not explain asymptomatic bone spurs. Another theory states that the body responds to continual stress on the calcaneal attachments by laying down reinforced connective tissue which changes to fibrocartilage and then bone *(Mooney, Maffey-Ward, 1995)*. The presence of bone spurs does not indicate the severity of plantar fasciitis, nor are bone spurs the cause of the condition. In fact, a bone spur can exist independently of plantar fasciitis and severe plantar fasciitis may occur without a bone spur being present *(Hertling, Kessler, 1996)*.

Causes of plantar fasciitis are:

➤ **overuse** due to overtraining, poor technique, running on hard surfaces or prolonged standing and activities that require ankle plantarflexion and simultaneous extension of the metatarsophalangeal joints, such as running and dancing. The symptoms often occur after a major or rapid adjustment to a training program.

Predisposing factors are:

➤ **poor biomechanics** such as excessive pronation or supination of the subtalar joint or excessive external rotation of the hip joint while walking *(Hunt, McPoil, 1995; Brukner, Khan, 1993)*;

➤ **short and tight** gastrocnemius and soleus muscles which predispose the foot to pronation;

➤ **improper footwear** that is worn out, too flexible, too stiff or does not provide adequate arch support;

➤ **weight gain**, including pregnancy, which stresses the plantar fascia.

Medically, treatment of plantar fasciitis may include non-steroidal anti-inflammatories. Corticosteroid injections may be used. However, repeated injections may cause fat pad atrophy and possible plantar fascia rupture *(Richmond, Shahady, 1996)*. Relative rest (the avoidance of the specific causative activity) is used in mild cases, while absolute rest (crutches) and immobilization are indicated in severe cases. Surgery is rarely performed as 95 per cent of those with plantar fasciitis respond to conservative care *(Souza, 1997)*.

Symptom Picture

+ Plantar fasciitis can be unilateral or bilateral.

+ The symptoms range from mild to severe. The pain has an initial slow onset, with no history of injury or trauma.

+ Tension is placed on the plantar fascia with repeated use. Over time, the plantar fascia is unable to repair itself and is partially torn off the calcaneus. After an initial period of acute inflammation, chronic inflammation sets in, accompanied by adhesions and fibrosing of the fascia. The plantar fascia thickens with the chronic inflammation. The healing process can be slow because the fascia is poorly vascularized.

+ Sources conflict on the presence of edema. Some say swelling is rarely present (Oloff, 1994) while others state swelling is present, especially with a pes cavus foot (Richmond, Shahady, 1996).

+ Pain occurs with the first few steps after non-weight-bearing — for example, when getting out of bed in the morning or after periods of sitting. The symptoms are worse during the pre-swing phase of the gait cycle and during stair climbing. The pain lessens after 30 to 45 minutes of activity, then intensifies again two or three hours later with continued activity (Hunt, McPoil, 1995). It is usually relieved by rest.

Contraindications

+ Frictions are avoided if acute inflammation is present, if the client is taking anti-inflammatories or if the client has a history of repeated corticosteroid injections to the plantar fascia.

+ The pain is usually located on the antero-inferior surface of the calcaneus on weight bearing (Mooney, Maffey-Ward, 1995). It may also extend along the medial border of the plantar fascia towards the metatarsal heads (Brukner, Khan, 1993). Paresthesia may be present on compression of the medial longitudinal arch.

+ Pes planus, pes cavus and Achilles tendinitis are often present. With repeated stress, a bone spur may develop on the medial aspect of the calcaneus.

Treatment Considerations

Assessment

✍ **Observations:**

• A postural assessment is performed, noting excessive pronation and signs of swelling in the medial longitudinal arch.

• Gait is observed. Pain is reported as worse during the pre-swing (toe-off) stage of the gait. There may be excessive external rotation of the hip during the gait (abducted gait).

✍ **Palpation** of the anteromedial aspect of the plantar surface of the calcaneus is painful. There may be palpable adhesions near the calcaneal attachment and even into the middle of the foot.

✍ **Testing:**

- **Active and passive extension** of the metatarsophalangeal joints is painful due to stretching of the plantar fascia and the intrinsic foot muscles *(Mooney, Maffey-Ward, 1995)*.

- **Length tests** for gastrocnemius and soleus reveal shortness.

- **Active resisted testing** includes hopping on the affected forefoot to reproduce the pain. Weak intrinsic foot muscles may be present.

✍ **Differentiating Causes of Heel Pain:**

- A **contusion** of the fat pad covering the calcaneus may occur due to overuse, weight gain or footwear that provides poor heel cushioning during the initial contact phase of the gait cycle. Pain is located directly on the plantar surface of the calcaneus and is reproduced by squeezing the fat pad from side to side *(Mooney, Maffey-Ward, 1995)*.

- **Stress fractures** of the calcaneus, due to overuse and poor cushioning of the calcaneus may also cause diffuse heel pain. Pain may be provoked by the stress fracture test or by squeezing the calcaneus from both sides at the same time *(Brukner, Khan, 1993)*. However, the client should be referred to a physician for X-ray or bone scan assessment.

- **Tarsal tunnel syndrome** is an entrapment of the posterior tibial nerve in the tarsal tunnel at the medial malleolus. This may be due to excessive pronation or to trauma such as an inversion sprain. There is sharp pain and possibly paresthesia in the medial arch, heel and occasionally the toes. The symptoms are worse after standing, walking or running. **Tinel's sign** may be positive *(Edwardson, 1995)*. There may be weakness of the intrinsic foot muscles *(Magee, 1997)*.

Massage

✋ The treatment is in the context of a half-hour relaxation massage, including **diaphragmatic breathing**.

Acute

✋ **Positioning** is **prone** at first, to reach the compensating structures. Pillows are placed under the abdomen and ankles.

✋ **Hydrotherapy** is a cold application, usually an ice pack to the affected fascia.

✋ Lymphatic drainage techniques are used on the affected leg to reduce edema, starting with sacral pumping and treating the distal leg. Lymphatic drainage is stopped just proximal to the edema. The techniques are used bilaterally if both feet are affected.

✋ Rhythmic techniques and Swedish techniques, such as effleurage and petrissage, are used on the low back, gluteals, lateral rotators and proximal leg to treat the compensating structures and to decrease sympathetic nervous system firing and pain. Trigger points in the proximal muscles that refer into the feet are treated with muscle stripping and gentle ischemic compressions. Gastrocnemius, soleus, tibialis posterior and flexor digitorum longus muscles can all refer pain into the plantar surface of the foot *(Travell, Simons, 1992)*.

🖐 Stroking and gentle muscle squeezing are used on the foot.

🖐 Treatment in the supine position includes lymphatic drainage, rhythmic techniques and proximal Swedish work similar to the prone position treatment.

Chronic

🖐 **Positioning** is the same as for the acute stage.

🖐 The **hydrotherapy** application is deep moist heat before stretching the fascia of gastrocnemius and soleus. A contrast application is used after treatment to increase local circulation.

🖐 Compensating structures in the low back, gluteals and thighs are treated with Swedish techniques as in the acute stage.

🖐 Fascial techniques to treat the shortened gastrocnemius and soleus include skin rolling, crossed-hands spreading and fingertip spreading. Connective tissue cutting and longitudinal fingertip spreading are also incorporated.

🖐 Effleurage and petrissage, such as wringing and fingertip and palmar kneading, are used on the shortened, hypertonic gastrocnemius, soleus and flexor digitorum longus. Trigger points and taut bands in these muscles are treated with muscle stripping.

🖐 PIR or passive stretching is performed on gastrocnemius and soleus. See the chapter on pes planus for details.

🖐 Joint play for the subtalar joint and navicular bone is indicated with hypomobility (*Hertling, Kessler, 1996*).

🖐 Swedish techniques such as thumb kneading are used on the intrinsic muscles of the foot. Trigger points in abductor hallucis longus, flexor digitorum brevis and abductor digiti minimi cause shortening of these muscles (*Travell, Simons, 1992*).

🖐 Muscle stripping and ischemic compressions are used, working within the client's pain tolerance.

🖐 Cross-fibre frictions are performed on adhesions in the plantar fascia, particularly near the calcaneal attachments (*Oloff, 1994*). Frictions are also appropriate on the Achilles tendon with any associated tendinitis. These are followed by ice and a stretch.

🖐 Repetitive effleurage is used on the posterior leg and foot muscles to increase local circulation and remove metabolites.

🖐 The client is turned **supine** and pillowed appropriately. The anterior thigh and leg are treated with Swedish techniques. Further work to the gastrocnemius may be performed, if necessary, with the client's knee and hip flexed as described in the pes planus chapter.

🖐 Joint play techniques are used on the hypomobile superior tibio-fibular joint and ankle, excluding the hypermobile medial arch. The gastrocnemius and soleus may be stretched again in the supine position.

🖐 The treatment is finished with effleurage to the entire limb.

Self-care

Acute

✍ The client is instructed to rest (no weight bearing if the plantar fasciitis is severe), ice and elevate the affected foot as much as possible.

Chronic

✍ The client should rest from aggravating activities. Return to activity is gradual, beginning with non-weight-bearing activities such as swimming or bicycling.

✍ Ice is applied three or four times per day to control the inflammation and after activities that cause pain.

✍ Heat is applied to the posterior leg compartment before activity. Self-massage is performed to the posterior compartment and plantar fascia. Stretching is encouraged.

✍ To stretch the plantar fascia, the client stands facing a wall. With the heel on the floor, the toes and the heads of the metatarsals rest against the wall. By dorsiflexing the ankle and bringing the knee towards the wall, the toes are extended, stretching the plantar fascia *(Brukner, Khan, 1993)*. Gastrocnemius and soleus should also be stretched.

See also pes planus, iliotibial band contracture, fractures, tendinitis and peripheral nerve lesions for related conditions.

✍ The intrinsic muscles of the feet are strengthened by scrunching up a towel or picking up pencils with the toes.

✍ The client is referred for shoes with adequate support and flexibility and for orthotics or heel cups if needed. Referrals may also be made to a physiotherapist for ultrasound treatments and supportive taping.

31

PERIOSTITIS AND COMPARTMENT SYNDROMES

Fiona Rattray

Periostitis and compartment syndromes produce pain in the lower leg.

These two conditions, as well as tibialis posterior tendinitis and tibial stress fractures are sometimes grouped under the lay term "shin splints", a non-specific phrase that describes pain along the medial border of the tibia with exercise.

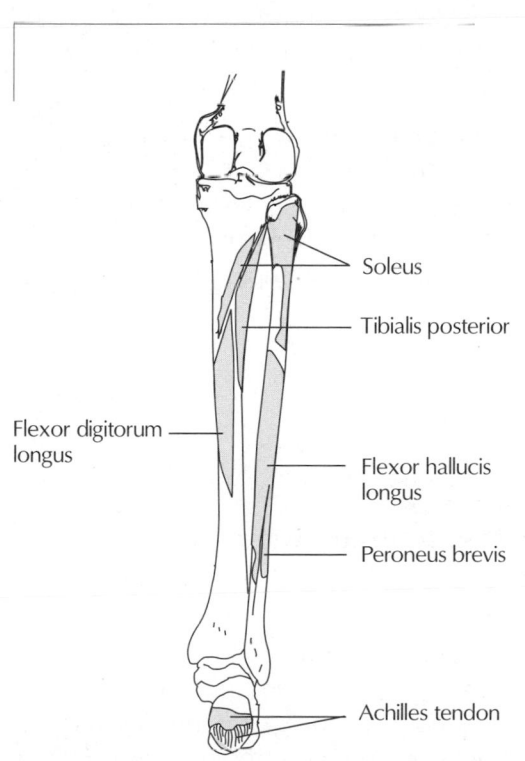

Soleus

Tibialis posterior

Flexor digitorum longus

Flexor hallucis longus

Peroneus brevis

Achilles tendon

Figure 31.1
Muscle attachments on the right posterior leg. Soleus attachments are most commonly affected by periostitis.

Periostitis

Periostitis is inflammation of the periosteum. This inflammation develops at the insertion of the leg muscles on the tibia (*Figure 31.1*). Although it usually occurs in muscles that attach posteromedially to the tibia, periostitis may also affect muscles that attach anteriorly (*Oloff, 1994*). Posteromedial periostitis is also called "medial tibial stress syndrome", "tenoperiostitis" and "soleus syndrome" (*Brukner, Khan, 1993; Travell, Simons, 1992*). Medial tibial stress syndrome comprises up to 18 per cent of running injuries and affects more women than men (*Richmond, Shahady, 1996*). If left untreated, periostitis can progress to a stress fracture (*Hertling, Kessler, 1996*).

Causes of periostitis are:

➤ **overuse** due to overtraining, poor technique, running on hard or uneven surfaces and improper footwear.

423

Predisposing factors are:

➤ **poor biomechanics**: posteromedial periostitis occurs with excessive pronation, varus knee and excessive external rotation of the hip (abducted gait). Anterolateral periostitis occurs with forefoot varus and tight gastrocnemius and soleus muscles *(Brukner, Khan, 1993)*.

Medically, diagnosis is made by a bone scan. The usual conservative treatment is non-steroidal anti-inflammatories (NSAIDS), ice and rest from activity until symptoms subside. Relative rest (the avoidance of the specific causative activity) is recommended in mild cases, while absolute rest (crutches) is indicated in severe cases. Surgery is rarely performed.

Symptom Picture

✦ Excessive pronation is likely present. Tension is placed on the periosteum with repeated muscular contraction. Over time, the periosteum is unable to repair itself and is partially torn off the bone. The symptoms are often bilateral.

✦ After an initial period of acute inflammation, chronic inflammation sets in, accompanied by adhesions and fibrosing of the tissue.

✦ Most commonly, the pain is on the posteromedial border of the tibia at the attachment of tibialis posterior, soleus and flexor digitorum longus muscles. It may extend along the tibia or be localized to an area two or three centimetres long, two-thirds of the way down the tibia.

✦ Initially, achiness is worse on getting up in the morning and with exercise, then decreases after a period of warm-up. It returns towards the end of the exercise period and continues afterwards. The symptoms are worse during the pre-swing phase of the gait cycle. As the condition progresses, the pain may occur throughout the exercise time and during activities of daily living. There is tightness and cramping if the client "runs through" the pain.

Compartment Syndromes

A **compartment syndrome** is the result of an increase in pressure within the compartments of the lower leg. There are four compartments surrounding the tibia and fibula, which are divided by dense, inelastic fascia (*Figure 31.2*).

The *anterior compartment* contains the tibialis anterior, extensor hallucis longus and extensor digitorum muscles as well as the anterior tibial artery and veins and the deep peroneal nerve. The *superficial posterior compartment* contains the gastrocnemius and soleus muscles. The *deep posterior compartment* contains the tibialis posterior, flexor digitorum longus and flexor hallucis longus muscles and the posterior tibial artery and veins, tibial nerve and peroneal artery and veins. The *lateral compartment* contains the peroneus longus and brevis muscles. While any of the compartments can be affected, the anterior

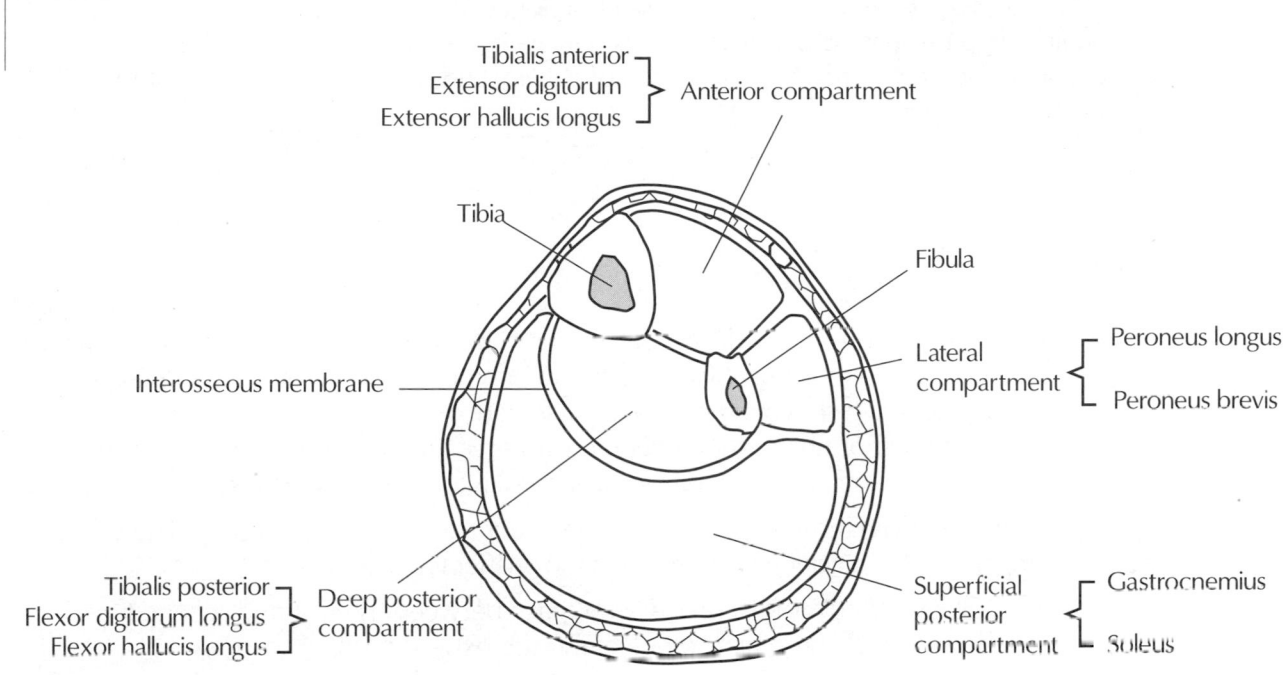

Tibialis anterior ⎤
Extensor digitorum ⎬ Anterior compartment
Extensor hallucis longus ⎦

Tibia

Fibula

Interosseous membrane

Lateral compartment ⎰ Peroneus longus
⎱ Peroneus brevis

Tibialis posterior ⎤
Flexor digitorum longus ⎬ Deep posterior compartment
Flexor hallucis longus ⎦

Superficial posterior compartment ⎰ Gastrocnemius
⎱ Soleus

Figure 31.2
Compartments of the leg.

compartment is most prone at 45 per cent of cases, with the deep posterior compartment affected next at 40 per cent *(Edwards, Myerson, 1996)*. Another term for chronic compartment syndrome is "chronic exertional compartment syndrome". It usually occurs in athletes under 40 years of age.

Causes of compartment syndromes are:

➤ with acute: **trauma** such as a direct blow to the compartment. Although rare, a chronic condition can become acute due to severe overuse *(Richmond, Shahady, 1996)*;

➤ with chronic: **overuse** due to overtraining, poor technique or training on hard surfaces.

Predisposing factors are:

➤ **anatomical configuration** where the affected compartment is smaller than normal;

➤ **muscle imbalance** and **muscle tightness**, especially tight antagonist muscles. With an anterior compartment syndrome, gastrocnemius and soleus are tight, which overloads the anterior compartment muscles;

➤ **improper footwear** that is worn out, too flexible, too stiff or does not provide adequate arch support;

➤ the **muscle type** involved which may create an imbalance. Tibialis anterior is a phasic muscle, responding to stress by fatiguing, while gastrocnemius and soleus are postural muscles, responding to stress by shortening. See Strategies: Fascial and Muscle Imbalances for more details.

Medically, a compartment syndrome is diagnosed with compartment pressure testing. With chronic compartment syndromes, a post-exercise pressure of 15 mm Hg measured

15 minutes after exercise stops is considered diagnostic *(Richmond, Shahady, 1996)*. An acute compartment syndrome is treated with an immediate fasciotomy. In chronic cases, conservative treatment of rest, limitation of activity and stretching is tried first. If this fails, a fasciotomy is performed.

Symptom Picture

+ **Acute compartment syndrome** is a medical emergency. Bleeding and swelling within the unyielding compartment increase the intracompartmental pressure. In the anterior compartment, which is most commonly affected, pressure may increase to the point where the anterior tibial artery and peroneal nerve are compromised. Permanent nerve damage and muscle necrosis may result if a fasciotomy is not performed.

+ The pain is severe and persistent. The skin is taut and shiny from swelling. The affected compartment is harder and hotter than the unaffected side.

+ Sensation may be diminished in the web space between the first and second toes. Paresthesia may be present. Motor loss may be experienced.

+ The dorsalis pedis pulse may be absent, but this is not a reliable indicator of compartment pressure levels *(Brukner, Khan, 1993)*. Active free dorsiflexion and toe extension and inversion are difficult due to pain. Passive stretch of the affected compartment is painful *(Buschbacher, 1994)*.

+ **Chronic compartment syndrome** symptoms are noted with exercise. Pain begins at the same time or distance into the activity and is relieved by rest. Increased blood flow to the muscles during exercise increases their size and, therefore, the intracompartmental pressure. Exercise has been shown to increase muscle volume by 20 per cent *(Richmond, Shahady, 1996)*. Normally, there is sufficient space in the compartment to allow for this hypertrophy and the muscle returns to its original size within five minutes after exercise. However, in symptomatic persons, the space is restricted because of anatomical limitations of the compartment. As the muscles swell and pressure increases in the compartment, smaller capillaries are compressed causing ischemia. As exercise continues, ischemia worsens with the increasing pressure. The pressure may remain high in the compartment for more than 20 minutes after exercise *(Edwards, Myerson, 1996)*.

+ Initially, there is an ache and tightness over the entire compartment. The symptoms increase with exercise and decrease with rest. As the condition progresses, the ischemia causes pain, which limits activity. There may be paresthesia in the leg or foot during exercise *(Buschbacher, 1994)*. Anterior compartment syndrome may be bilateral, but is usually worse on one side. Deep posterior compartment syndrome is often bilateral *(Travell, Simons, 1992)*.

Contraindications

+ Frictions are contraindicated if acute inflammation is present or if the client is taking anti-inflammatory medication.

+ A client with an acute compartment syndrome is referred for emergency medical attention.

Treatment Considerations

Assessment: Periostitis

✍ **Observations** include a postural assessment, noting any pronation and signs of swelling in the lower leg. Excessive external rotation of the hip joint (abducted gait) or knee varus may be present.

✍ **Palpation** along the medial border of the tibia reveals tenderness at the site of the inflammation. Taut bands may be present in the affected muscles. Bony irregularities may be present with chronic periostitis.

✍ **Testing** is the **active resisted test** of hopping on the affected leg to reproduce the pain.

Assessment: Chronic Compartment Syndrome

✍ **Palpation** of the affected compartment may reveal tightness and, occasionally, defects in the fascia from continued pressure.

✍ **Testing:**

- **Range of motion testing** is restricted by pain. With anterior compartment syndrome both active free dorsiflexion and passive relaxed plantarflexion are restricted *(Brukner, Khan, 1993)*.

- **Length tests** for antagonists of the affected compartment reveal shortness. With anterior compartment syndrome, the soleus and gastrocnemius are often short.

✍ **Differentiating Causes of Leg Pain:**

- **Tibialis posterior tendinitis** pain is worse on activity than at rest. The pain is along the course of the tendon, just posterior to the medial malleolus and along the proximal tibia. **AR testing** for tendinitis is positive.

- **Tibial stress fracture** pain is sharp and localized to the fracture site. The medial aspect of the tibia is a common location. There is a two- to three-week onset of symptoms. Initially, the pain is worse on activity and is relieved with rest. With progression, the pain is constant and worse with impact. The person is unable to "run through" the pain. Night pain is experienced. The **stress fracture test** is positive. However, the client is referred to a physician for a bone scan assessment.

- **Deep vein thrombosis** gives a feeling of local tightness and tenderness in the calf. The pain is relatively constant regardless of activity. Warmth and redness are classic indicators; however, these may be absent. Deep vein thrombosis can be caused by fractures, surgery, pregnancy and prolonged bedrest especially in the elderly. **Homan's sign** and **Ramirez's test** are likely positive, but the client should be referred to a physician for diagnosis by contrast venography or doppler ultrasonography *(Travell, Simons, 1992)*.

Massage: Periostitis

🖐 The treatment, whether acute or chronic, is in the context of a half-hour relaxation massage, including **diaphragmatic breathing**. The treatment described below is for posteromedial periostitis.

Acute

- **Positioning** is with the client lying **prone**, to reach the compensating structures. Pillows are placed under the abdomen and ankles.

- **Hydrotherapy** is a cold application, likely an ice pack to the affected leg.

- To reduce inflammation, lymphatic drainage techniques are used on the affected leg, starting with sacral pumping and treating the distal leg. Lymphatic drainage is stopped just proximal to the painful area. The techniques are used bilaterally if both legs are affected.

- Rhythmic techniques and Swedish techniques, such as effleurage and petrissage, are used on the low back, gluteals and proximal legs to treat the compensating structures and to decrease sympathetic nervous system firing and pain. Trigger points are treated with muscle stripping and gentle ischemic compressions. Gluteus medius and semimembranosus muscles can refer pain into the posterior leg *(Travell, Simons, 1992)*. Stroking and gentle muscle squeezing are used on the leg and foot.

- Next, with the client in the **supine** position, treatment includes lymphatic drainage, rhythmic techniques and proximal Swedish work similar to treatment in the prone position.

Chronic

- **Positioning** is the same as for the acute stage.

- The **hydrotherapy** application is deep moist heat before stretching the fascia of gastrocnemius and soleus.

- Compensating structures in the low back, gluteals and thighs are treated with Swedish techniques as in the acute stage.

- Fascial techniques, Swedish massage and passive stretching are used to reduce areas of muscle thickening and shortening which create tension on the periosteum *(Oloff, 1994)*. One source finds deep soft-tissue therapy to be the most effective treatment *(Brukner, Khan, 1993)*.

- Fascial techniques to treat the shortened gastrocnemius and soleus include skin rolling and fingertip spreading. Myofascial release along the affected muscles combined with passive motion is also used. The soleus is treated with longitudinal connective tissue cutting techniques while the therapist dorsiflexes the ankle. Ischemic compressions can be used along soleus and tibialis posterior *(Brukner, Khan, 1993)*. However, the attachments at the periosteum may be too tender for direct work.

- Effleurage and petrissage are used on the shortened, hypertonic gastrocnemius, soleus and flexor digitorum longus. Trigger points and taut bands in these muscles are treated with muscle stripping.

- PIR or passive stretching is performed on gastrocnemius and soleus. See the chapter on pes planus for details.

- Cross-fibre frictions are performed on adhesions in soleus, tibialis posterior and flexor digitorum longus *(Oloff, 1994)*. These are followed by ice and a stretch.

- Joint play for the subtalar joint is indicated with hypomobility *(Hertling, Kessler, 1996)*.

Repetitive effleurage is used on the posterior leg and foot muscles to increase local circulation and remove metabolites.

The client is turned **supine** and pillowed appropriately. The anterior thigh and leg are treated with Swedish techniques.

Joint play techniques are used on the hypomobile superior tibio-fibular joint and ankle, excluding the hypermobile medial arch. The gastrocnemius and soleus may be stretched again in the supine position.

The treatment is finished with effleurage to the entire limb.

Self-care: Periostitis

Acute

Rest from activities and ice applications three to four time per day are used to control the inflammation.

Chronic

Return to activity is gradual, working towards pain-free moderate training levels. The client should correct predisposing training factors such as improper footwear, training on hard, inclined or uneven surfaces and overzealous training.

Pre-activity heat to the posterior compartment muscles, self-massage to the posterior compartment and stretching of gastrocnemius and soleus are indicated (*Richmond, Shahady, 1996*).

Strengthening of the affected muscles occurs only after pain is under control (*Oloff, 1994*). See pes planus and sprains chapters for details.

The client is referred for orthotics if needed. These correct pronation and reduce strain on the periosteum (*Brukner, Khan, 1993*).

Massage: Chronic Compartment Syndromes

The treatment described is for a **chronic anterior compartment syndrome**.

The **positioning and hydrotherapy** are the same as for chronic periostitis, as is the work to the compensating structures.

Fascial techniques, massage and passive stretch are used to elongate the shortened, thickened fascia (*Brukner, Khan, 1993*), starting with the antagonists. Fascial techniques to treat the shortened gastrocnemius and soleus include skin rolling and fingertip spreading. Myofascial release along the affected muscles with combined passive motion is also used. The soleus is treated with longitudinal connective tissue cutting techniques while the therapist dorsiflexes the ankle.

The client is turned supine. The anterior thigh is treated with Swedish techniques. Trigger points that refer into the anterior leg are addressed. These include adductor longus and brevis (*Travell, Simons, 1992*).

Longitudinal fascial techniques such as connective tissue cutting are applied to the borders of the anterior compartment to loosen the fascia and to reduce the compression. Short diagonal strokes are used from the borders to the middle of the compartment to further loosen the fascia. These can be combined with a passive stretch into plantarflexion.

- Cross-fibre frictions are applied to adhesions within tibialis anterior *(Brukner, Khan, 1993)*. These are followed by an application of ice and a stretch.

- Joint play techniques are used on hypomobile joints.

- Effleurage and petrissage to the entire limb, including the foot, complete the treatment.

Self-care: Chronic Compartment Syndromes

- Initially, the client rests from activities that cause pain, with a gradual return to activity. A proper warm-up period may help to reduce the rapid blood flow to the compartment *(Richmond, Shahady, 1996)*.

- Self-massage to the compartment borders and the antagonist muscles is indicated.

- Stretching for the muscles of the lower leg is performed, starting with the antagonists of the affected compartment. In the case of anterior compartment syndrome, the client begins with stretching gastrocnemius and soleus, progressing to stretches for tibialis anterior.

> See Strategies: Fascial and Muscle Imbalances, pes planus, plantar fasciitis, iliotibial band contracture, tendinitis, sprains and fractures for related conditions.

- The client is referred for orthotics if needed. If the condition does not respond to conservative treatment within three months, the client is referred to a physician *(Edwards, Myerson, 1996)*.

32

TENDINITIS

Fiona Rattray

Tendinitis is inflammation of a tendon.

Tendons are made of regularly arranged, dense collagen fibrils. They attach muscle to bone and are part of the musculotendinous unit. Tendons appear in two shapes: cord-like structures; and broad, sheet-like structures called "aponeuroses".

A tendon that moves in a straight line is surrounded by a **paratendon.** Blood vessels are coiled in the loose alveolar tissue of the paratendon, which stretches along with the tendon *(Brukner, Khan, 1993).* A tendon that runs across a bony prominence is surrounded by a **tendon sheath.** This double-layered tubular structure is filled with synovial fluid. The outer layer is attached to surrounding structures, while the inner layer surrounds the tendon itself, allowing the tendon to glide through it easily, almost without friction.

The dense connective tissue of tendons has a limited blood supply originating from muscles and bones. This limited supply is variable. So-called vascular tendons are surrounded by vascularized paratendons, while avascular tendons are surrounded by sheaths. Blood supply to tendons is compromised in areas where the tendon is exposed to compression, friction or torsion. When injuries occur, the limited blood supply reduces tissue repair and prolongs healing time.

Tendons are subject to great tensile stress. When a load is placed on a tendon, the waves of its collagen fibres straighten out. The collagen fibres then temporarily deform. These two actions account for four per cent of tendon lengthening. If this four per cent stretch is not exceeded, the tendon will return to its original length and collagen fibre waves reform. The collagen links begin to fail if the tendon length is exceeded by eight per cent *(Souza, 1994).* Over time, a tendon can experience microtearing, partial tearing or complete rupture, usually at the point of most reduced blood supply. The musculotendinous junction may also suffer microtearing. Acute traumatic tendon ruptures are covered in the chapter on strains.

➤ **The cause of tendinitis is chronic overload of the tendon** leading to microtearing and an inflammatory response in the tendon.

➤ **Contributing factors** include muscle imbalances, poor biomechanics, lack of flexibility, chronic degenerative changes in the tendon, poor blood supply to the tendon, improper equipment and training errors.

Types of Tendon Overuse Injuries

Tendon overuse injuries have all been termed "tendinitis". Several distinct pathologies exist — tendinitis, paratendinitis and tendinosis. To further complicate matters, these injuries may co-exist in the same tendon.

Tendinitis results from microscopic tearing of the tendon fascicles due to overloading of the tendon, with a resulting inflammatory response.

✦ Tendinitis is classified into four grades of severity:

• **Grade 1** tendinitis has pain after activity only;

• **Grade 2** tendinitis has pain at the beginning of activity which disappears during activity then returns after activity;

• **Grade 3** tendinitis has pain at the beginning of activity, during activity and after activity. Pain may restrict activity;

• **Grade 4** tendinitis has pain with activities of daily living. Pain continues to get worse *(Brukner, Khan, 1993).*

Paratendinitis is inflammation of the paratendon or the tendon sheath where these structures are associated with a tendon, either of which may be irritated by the tendon as it rubs over a bony prominence. Paratendinitis is associated with tendon injuries. It is also called "tenosynovitis" or "tenovaginitis" *(Brukner, Khan, 1993).* In the past, a distinction was made between the latter two. Tenosynovitis is irritation of the inner surface of the tendon sheath by the roughened surface of the tendon. Tenovaginitis is irritation and thickening of the sheath itself *(Cyriax, 1991).*

Tendinosis describes *degenerative* changes occurring with chronic overuse tendon injuries, such as with "tennis elbow". Aging and avascularity may be contributing factors to tissue degeneration. With tendinosis, while there are no signs of inflammation in the tendon itself, biopsies have shown angiofibroblastic degenerative changes occurring. This is an invasion of organized vascular tissue and a disorganization of collagen tissue in the tendon *(Buschbacher, 1994).* The granulation tissue is richly supplied with nerve endings, which may explain the painfulness of the lesion. The injury may progress from degeneration to microtearing to a partial or complete tendon rupture.

Tendinosis has been suggested as a more appropriate term than tendinitis, which implies that an inflammatory process is occurring in the tissue *(Andrews, Wilk, 1994).* However, both tendinosis and tendinitis injuries to a tendon may occur *(Souza, 1994),* or tendinosis may start out with an acute inflammatory stage which later disappears *(Pappas, 1995).*

Common Tendinitis Locations and Causes

Supraspinatus Tendon

To palpate the supraspinatus tendon, the arm of the seated client is held behind the back, with the elbow in flexion. The humerus is maximally internally rotated and maximally extended, bringing the humeral attachment of supraspinatus out from under the acromion (Cyriax, Coldham, 1984). The tendon is palpated immediately inferior to the acromioclavicular joint. The therapist palpates through deltoid muscle in the indentation between the anterior and middle fibres (Figure 32.1). A recent cadaver study confirmed that this positioning did allow visual exposure of the tendon (Mattingly, Mackarey, 1998). The musculotendinous junction is palpated with the humerus abducted to 90 degrees. The junction is palpated medial to the acromial arch through the fibres of upper trapezius (Souza, 1994).

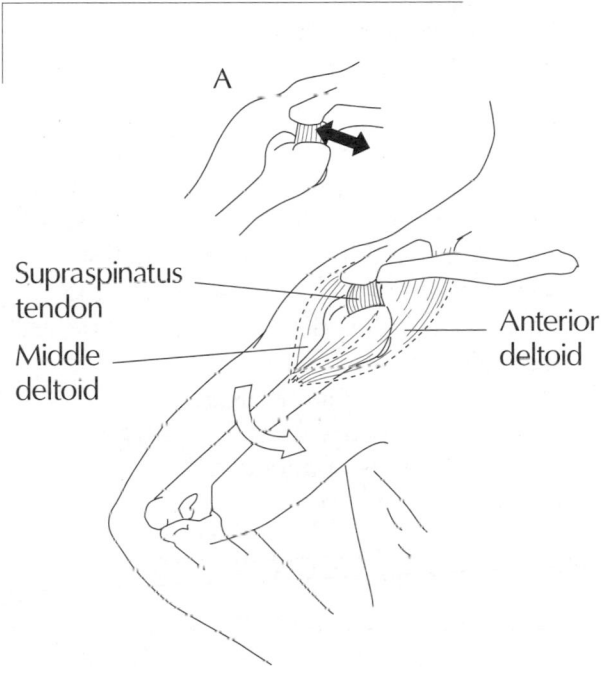

Figure 32.1
Supraspinatus tendon palpation and (A) direction of frictions.

Infraspinatus Tendon

To palpate the infraspinatus and teres minor tendons, the humerus of the seated or prone client is flexed to 90 degrees, adducted 10 degrees and externally rotated 20 degrees (Mattingly, Mackarey, 1998; Souza, 1997). This position brings the tendon out from under the acromion. The tendon is palpated immediately inferior to the acromioclavicular joint and the lateral portion of the spine of the scapula. The therapist palpates the tendon through the posterior fibres of deltoid muscle (Figure 32.2).

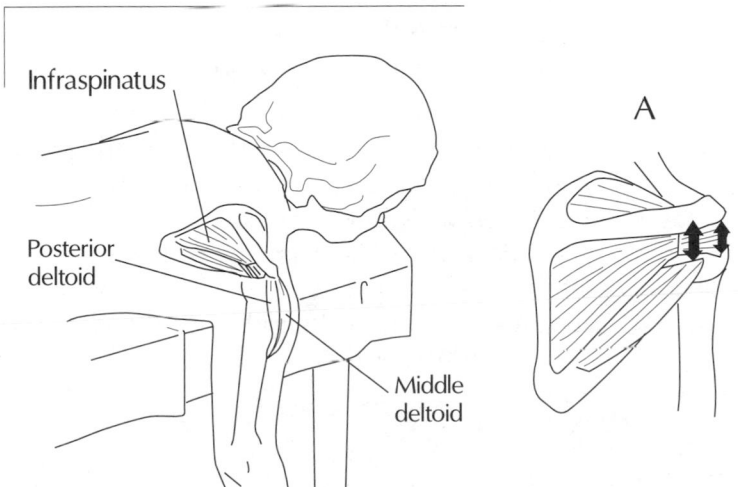

Figure 32.2
Infraspinatus tendon palpation and (A) direction of frictions.

Subscapularis Tendon

To palpate the subscapularis tendon, the seated client keeps the humerus at the side and the elbow is flexed to 90 degrees. The tendon is palpated inferior to the clavicle, lateral to the coracoid process (medial to the anterior deltoid). The humerus can be maximally externally rotated to make the lesser tuberosity prominent as a further landmark (Figure 32.3). The

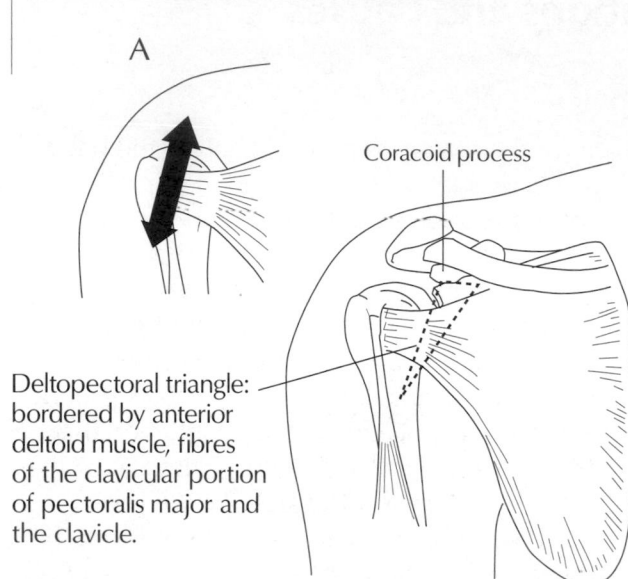

Coracoid process

Deltopectoral triangle: bordered by anterior deltoid muscle, fibres of the clavicular portion of pectoralis major and the clavicle.

Figure 32.3
Subscapularis tendon palpation and (A) direction of frictions.

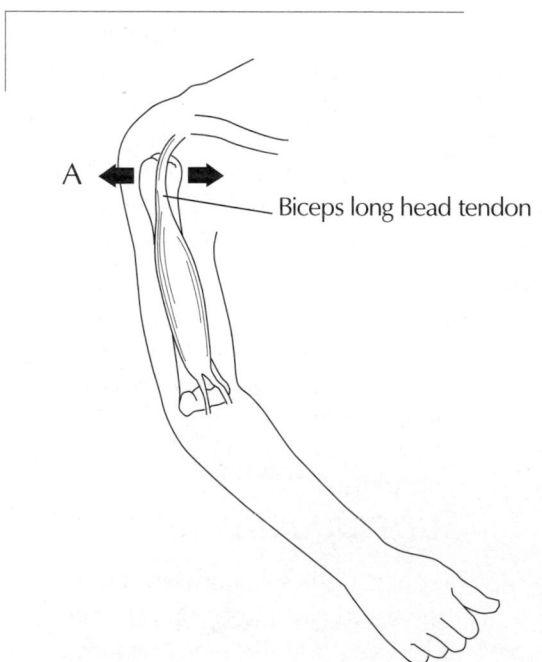

Biceps long head tendon

Figure 32.4
Biceps long head tendon palpation and (A) direction of frictions.

humerus is then medially rotated, returning it to a position midway between external and internal rotation. The tendon is palpated deep in the deltopectoral triangle, between the tendons of the long and short heads of biceps. While the humeral positioning described above is supposed to move the anterior deltoid out of the way *(Mattingly, Mackarey, 1998),* the therapist can also pull the anterior deltoid laterally if it still intervenes *(Cyriax, Coldham, 1984).*

✦ The rotator cuff tendons — supraspinatus, infraspinatus, teres minor and subscapularis — are prone to tendinitis with sports such as swimming, tennis, golf or any throwing sport such as baseball. Occupations or activities that stress the shoulder muscles with the arms in an overhead position, such as drywall installation or assembly line work, may also cause rotator cuff tendinitis. Pain is experienced usually when the arm is in more than 90 degrees of abduction.

Biceps Long Head Tendon

To palpate the long head of the biceps brachialis tendon, the humerus of the seated client is internally rotated 20 degrees, or to a "hands on lap" position *(Mattingly, Mackarey, 1998).* The tendon is palpated inferior to the clavicle, lateral to the coracoid process in the same area as the subscapularis tendon. Internally rotating the humerus brings the biceps tendon out from underneath the anterior deltoid muscle *(Figure 32.4).*

Swimming and throwing sports where the arm is adducted, compressing the tendon, can cause biceps tendinitis. This condition is usually secondary to another shoulder pathology. Inflammation may actually attach the tendon to the groove, reducing the gliding mechanism *(Andrews, Wilk, 1994).*

Common Extensor Tendon

To palpate the common extensor tendon, the elbow of the seated client is placed in slight flexion. The tendon is located distal to the lateral epicondyle *(Figure 32.5).* It may extend over top of the radial head. This can be located by the client pronating and supinating the hand while the therapist palpates for the moving head.

With extensor tendinosis, microtearing occurs in the extensor carpi radialis brevis (ECRB) origin. Extensor carpi radialis longus and extensor digitorum may also become involved.

Repetitive forceful extension, supination and radial deviation are the movements most likely to provoke extensor tendinosis. Racquet sports players, especially novice players with poor backhand technique, are prone to injury. Wheelchair athletes are also susceptible, as are people with occupations such as plumbing and meat cutting. Pain is local to the lateral epicondyle, specifically at the origin of extensor carpi radialis brevis *(Souza, 1997)*.

Sources differ as to whether this is a tendinosis *(Brukner, Khan, 1993)* or a true tendinitis *(Hertling, Kessler, 1996)*. Lateral epicondylitis and tennis elbow are other terms for this condition.

Common Flexor Tendon

To palpate the common flexor tendon, the elbow of the seated client is placed in flexion and the wrist is supinated. The tendon is located distal to the medial epicondyle *(Figure 32.6)*.

With flexor tendinosis, microtearing occurs in the flexor tendon and in the pronator teres tendon *(Brukner, Khan, 1993)*. Repetitive activity such as hammering or using a screwdriver may cause the injury. Sports activities involving wrist flexion and pronation such as golfing and overhead serving in tennis are other causes. Pain is at the medial epicondyle. A weak grip is also a complaint. An ulnar neuropathy may co-exist with flexor tendinosis, as the ulnar nerve passes through a hiatus in the flexor carpi ulnaris muscle *(Souza, 1997)*. There is also disagreement as to whether the pathology is a tendinosis or tendinitis. Medial epicondylitis and golfer's elbow are other terms for this condition.

Abductor Pollicis Longus and Extensor Pollicis Brevis Tendons

DeQuervain's tenosynovitis is inflammation of the abductor pollicis longus and extensor pollicis brevis tendon sheaths *(Figure 32.7)*. The sheaths are palpated at the radial side of the wrist. Activities requiring repetitive thumb use, repetitive

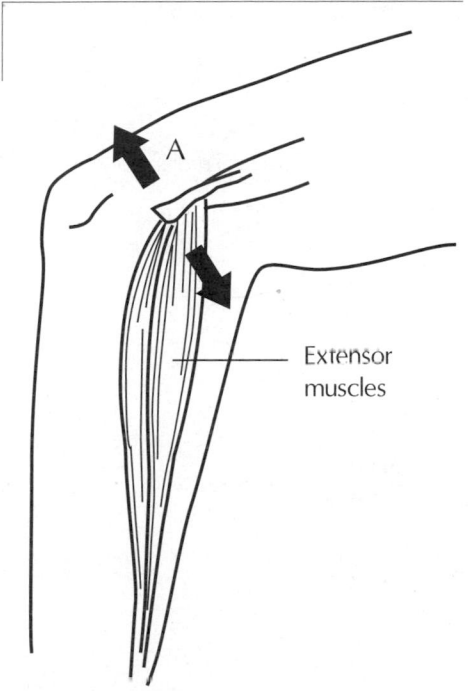

Figure 32.5
Common extensor tendon palpation (lateral view) and (A) direction of frictions.

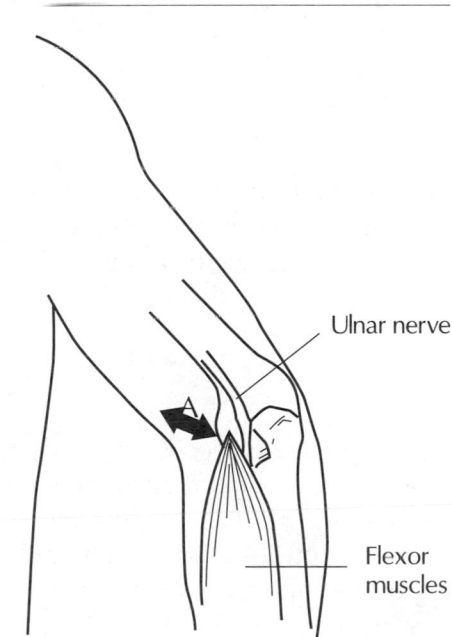

Figure 32.6
Common flexor tendon palpation (posterior view) and (A) direction of frictions.

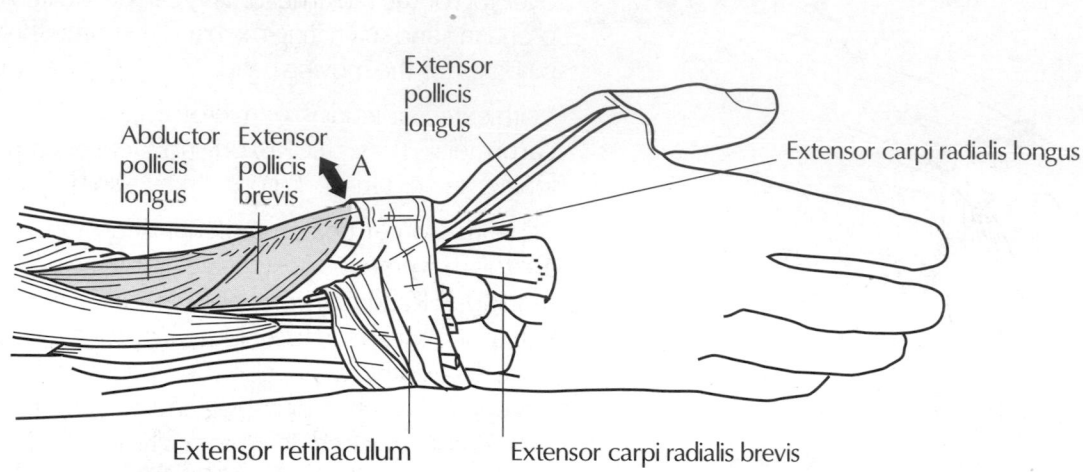

Figure 32.7
DeQuervain's tenosynovitis — palpation of abductor pollicis longus and extensor pollicis brevis tendons and (A) direction of frictions.

radial and ulnar deviation and forceful gripping cause this condition, such as factory work, massage therapy and racquet sports. Pain is located one centimetre proximal to the radial styloid process.

Activities that cause deQuervain's tenosynovitis also cause intersection syndrome *(Pappas, 1995)*. Intersection syndrome is inflammation that occurs where abductor pollicis longus and extensor pollicis brevis tendons cross over the extensor carpi radialis brevis and longus tendons. This is on the radius, about four centimetres proximal to the wrist.

Patellar Tendon

The patellar tendon is palpated immediately inferior to the patella. Pain is localized to the tendon. Activities that include running or jumping, such as track and field, are causes. Iatrogenic tendinitis is possible following knee arthoscopy if a central incision is made *(Fox, Del Pizzo, 1993)*.

Popliteus Tendon

The popliteus tendon is palpated just inferior to the lateral femoral condyle, directly posterior to the lateral collateral ligament and biceps femoris tendon *(Figure 32.8)*. The popliteus tendon is palpated through the lateral gastrocnemius muscle. Pain is at the lateral knee, either in front of or behind the lateral collateral ligament. Activities such as downhill running or downhill walking combined with foot pronation cause this tendinitis. It may be confused with iliotibial band friction syndrome.

Tibialis Posterior Tendon

To palpate the tibialis posterior tendon, the foot is placed in plantarflexion. The tendon in

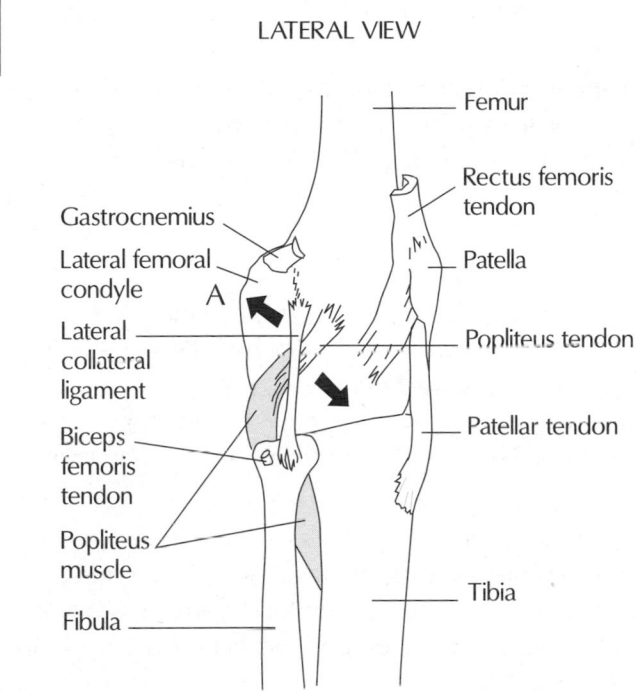

LATERAL VIEW

Femur

Rectus femoris tendon

Gastrocnemius

Lateral femoral condyle

Patella

A

Lateral collateral ligament

Popliteus tendon

Biceps femoris tendon

Patellar tendon

Popliteus muscle

Fibula

Tibia

Figure 32.8
Popliteus tendon palpation and (A) direction of frictions.

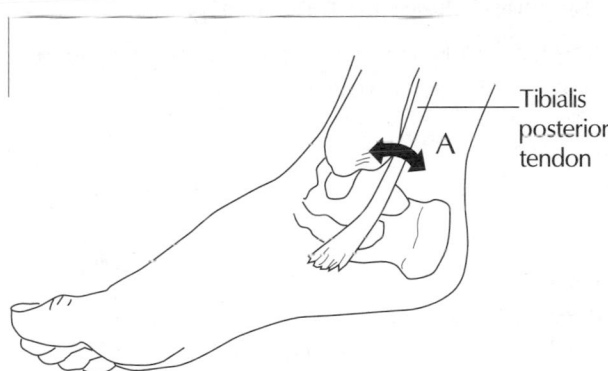

Tibialis posterior tendon

A

Figure 32.9
Tibialis posterior tendon palpation and (A) direction of frictions.

its sheath is palpated just posterior and inferior to the medial malleolus *(Figure 32.9)*. Pain runs along the medial border of the tibia and along the course of the tendon. Activities such as running, using step machines or doing step aerobics combined with excessive pronation can cause this tendinitis.

Achilles Tendon

Tendinitis, paratendinitis and tendinosis can affect the Achilles tendon. This tendon lies between the gastrocnemius-soleus complex and the calcaneus. Pain is felt along the tendon. Activities such as running combined with pronation, poor footwear or tight gastrocnemius-soleus muscles cause this condition.

The Medical Treatment of Tendinitis and Tendon Tears

For acute tendinitis, inflammation is controlled through rest, ice and NSAIDs. Stretching, strengthening and a gradual return to activity are recommended. For flexor and extensor tendinosis of the arm, a support strap may be used around the forearm distal to the tendon. Steroid injections are less favoured today. Surgical repair is necessary with a total tendon rupture, especially in the shoulder. For tenosynovitis, such as deQuervain's tenosynovitis, ultrasound, NSAIDs, stretching and activity modification are suggested. Surgery is rarely needed *(Souza, 1997)*.

Other Tendon Pathologies

Shoulder Tendons

Rotator cuff tendons may suffer **impingement syndrome,** partial or complete **tears** and **calcific tendinitis**. There is clinical overlap of these conditions and tendinitis. Rotator cuff pathologies may be due to *intrinsic factors* such as tendon degeneration and reduced

437

circulation to the supraspinatus tendon or *extrinsic factors* such as impingement of the rotator cuff under the arch of the acromion with resulting mechanical wear.

The normal aging population develops rotator cuff pathologies after 40 years of age, while athletes can develop them at a younger age due to overuse. Athletes with shoulder instability from dislocations or subluxations also appear to develop rotator cuff impingement.

Impingement Syndrome

Impingement syndrome is inflammation, pain and edema in the tissues within the coracoacromial arch and between the acromioclavicular and glenohumeral joints. Painful compression of the tendons, especially supraspinatus, may occur when the humerus is abducted against the acromion. Tendon impingement may also occur against the coracoacromial ligament and coracoid process. The biceps tendon and the subacromial bursa may be affected as well.

The shape of the acromion can influence the wear that the rotator cuff experiences during abduction. A flat or slightly curved acromion provides sufficient space for the tendons, while a downwardly curving or hooked acromion compresses the tendons excessively. In one study, 41 per cent of the people had a hooked acromion and, of that 41 per cent, 80 per cent had a positive arthrogram *(Andrews, Wilk, 1994)*.

✦ There are three progressive stages of impingement.

- In **Stage 1**, there is edema and hemorrhage of the subacromial bursa.

- In **Stage 2**, tendinitis and fibrosis are present. Both stages are reversible with conservative care such as rest, stretching and progressive strengthening.

- In **Stage 3**, incomplete tears or complete tendinous rupture occurs. There may be associated bony changes in the acromion and the acromioclavicular joint. Surgery is usually indicated.

Rotator Cuff Tears

Overuse, impingement and normal aging can lead to painful tearing of the rotator cuff tendons. Rotator cuff tears may be partial or full thickness, with supraspinatus the most frequently injured. While the articular and bursal sides can both be affected, most partial tears occur on the articular side, probably due to poorer vascularity here *(Souza, 1997)*.

Medically, tears are treated by open rotator cuff repair surgery in which the rotator cuff is exposed. Acromioplasty is performed — removal of portions of the acromion — and the rotator cuff tendons are reattached to the humerus. The undersurface of the subacromial bursa contains regenerative cells, so this portion may be left to help repair the site post-operatively. Rehabilitation begins with early range of motion and strengthening exercises *(Andrews, Wilk, 1994)*.

Calcific Tendinitis

Calcific tendinitis was once thought to be a degenerative process. Recent studies have shown that it occurs in people aged 30 to 60 years, so this cannot be the case.

Calcific tendinitis is a late-occurring stage of rotator cuff tendinitis, usually developing in the supraspinatus tendon.

Supraspinatus functions to hold the head of the humerus in place. The constant pressure of the head of the humerus seems to "wring out" the blood supply to the poorly supplied tendon even when the arm is in the neutral position. Extreme pressure is put on the rotator cuff in internal rotation at 90 degrees of abduction.

On a cellular level, the tendon's fibrocytes change to chondrocytes, collagen disintegrates and calcific deposits accumulate in the cells. Over time, these deposits are set free into the intercellular spaces. The deposits can be a soft, toothpaste-like material, or hard and chalky. Impingement may occur as the tendon increases in size.

At some point, the deposits are resorbed. There is an increase in vascularity, with painful swelling and inflammation. It is thought that the inflammation and pain are due to the resorption process and not the initial calcification (*Souza, 1994*). Calcific tendinitis may be a mechanism of self-healing.

Complications include tendon rupture secondary to the calcium deposits and bursitis after rupture of the calcific deposit into the bursa. Medically, treatment includes range of motion and strengthening exercises and ultrasound. Steroids have not been found to be useful. NSAIDs may be prescribed (*Andrews, Wilk, 1994*).

Trigger Finger

Through overuse, flexor tendons of any finger may develop a thickened, nodular swelling. This swelling is unable to move through the tendon sheath and gets caught. The finger is stuck in flexion until it is passively extended by an external force (*Travell, Simons, 1983*). Rest, NSAIDs and stretching are the usual treatments.

Repetitive Strain Injury (RSI)

In the workplace, repetitive movements and poor posture lead to muscle fatigue and damage to the muscles, tendons and nerves of the shoulders, neck and arms. Pain, numbness and weakness are experienced. The pain can migrate from one place to another as the person attempts to compensate for the initial discomfort. Inadequate rest breaks and psychological stress can worsen the condition, eventually leading to chronic tissue fatigue and even impaired motor control. The person may be unable to continue working or performing any sports activities.

Japanese researchers used the term "occupational cervicobrachial disorders" (OCD) in the 1960s and 70s to describe musculoskeletal disorders related to work. The term "cumulative trauma disorder" (CTD) was used in the 1980s in North America, while "repetitive strain injury" (RSI) gained popularity in Australia, Great Britain and, later, North America. Tendinitis, tenosynovitis, trigger points, myalgia and nerve entrapment — including thoracic outlet and carpal tunnel syndromes — are some of the diagnosed conditions.

Risk Factors

The development and prognosis of RSI are influenced by several factors both inside and outside the work place. **Intrinsic factors** include joint hypermobility, lack of exercise, increased muscle tension, poor posture and poor nutrition. **Extrinsic factors** include work environment, task repetition, forced speed or rapid movement and lack of movement of the neck and shoulders. **Psychosocial factors** consist of lack of job satisfaction, inadequate co-worker or supervisor support, computer monitoring of task completion, company organizational factors, personal drive to excel and a strong work ethic. Many of these risk factors overlap for a single individual.

The occupations most at risk for developing RSI include computer operation — which implicates those working with keyboards, video display terminals and checkout counters. Telephone operators, emergency vehicle dispatchers, sign language interpreters and technicians working with microscopes are also at risk. Any job where work is continuously performed with raised arms compromises the supraspinatus tendon, adding further complications. This is more of a concern with middle-aged and older workers who already have some tendon degeneration or tearing.

A German study on women showed that neck problems are more frequent and tend to worsen the longer the person works at video display terminals, compared to the expected, age-related neck problems. Those doing repetitive tasks where the head and neck were held relatively motionless, increasing muscular tension, were most at risk *(Fehr, Kreuger, 1992)*. Keyboard operators who pounded the keys or held their wrists in extension while working were also at risk.

Other office work place studies found the following factors associated with RSI symptoms: *neck* injuries were associated with routine work with no decision-making capabilities and fear of being replaced by computers; *shoulder* injuries with greater job pressure; *elbow* injuries with surges in workload and uncertainty about job future; and *hand and wrist* injuries with increased keyboard workloads and lack of supervisor support *(Moon, Sauter, 1996)*.

Medical handling of these conditions also influences the development and outcome of RSI. A physician who does not know the symptoms of RSI or who is skeptical of its existence is unlikely to steer the patient in the direction of help soon enough *(Pascarelli, Quilter, 1994)*.

RSI Treatment

Medically, conservative management — rest and stretching and strengthening exercises with a gradual return to work — is suggested. Massage therapy, physiotherapy and occupational therapy are recommended *(Pascarelli, Quilter, 1994)*. NSAIDs are more useful than steroids. Work place ergonomics should be assessed to prevent recurrence. Splints which limit movement and support the wrist are recommended on an individual basis and surgery is the last approach.

A long-term study on women with RSI showed that those assigned varied tasks, which included different work postures, experienced improvement in their condition, while those with an unchanged job got worse. Therefore, if changes are introduced at an early stage in RSI development, recovery is possible. Data entry operators who were taught to adjust their individual work stations and to intersperse shorter work phases with break activities reduced their neck pain and stiffness from 54 per cent to 16 per cent over a six month period *(Fehr, Kreuger, 1992)*.

Risk factors for deterioration in those who have RSI include poor posture (elevated shoulders and head-forward posture) and high productivity. Those who answered "yes" to questions such as, "Do you get impatient in a line-up?" were more likely to risk worsening over the next few years. Low muscle strength is not a risk factor in the progression of RSI.

Symptom Picture

✦ By nature, tendinitis is a chronic condition with an initial acute inflammatory stage.

Acute

✦ There is a *gradual onset,* with tenderness local to the tendon, one or two days after activity. Initially, pain diminishes with renewed activity. This progresses to pain during activity as the severity increases. Microtearing occurs with adhesion formation as the tendon attempts to heal. Repetitive use tears these new adhesions, causing more inflammation and a cycle of reinjury.

✦ Inflammation, heat and swelling develop along the tendon or tendon sheath.

✦ Crepitus may develop with tenosynovitis and paratendinitis.

✦ There is decreased range of motion of the affected muscle.

Chronic

✦ Pain occurs during and after activity.

✦ Chronic inflammation, fibrosis and adhesions are present.

✦ Chronic swelling or thickening may be observed if the tendon is superficial enough, as with the Achilles tendon.

✦ Crepitus may be present.

✦ There is decreased range of motion and decreased strength.

✦ Flare-ups to the acute stage may occur with repeated overuse.

✦ The tendon may degenerate to such a degree that tendon rupture occurs.

Subjective Information

HEALTH HISTORY QUESTIONS

✦ What activities or movements cause pain?

✦ Where is the pain located?

✦ What are the present symptoms? How long have these symptoms been present?

✦ What is the client's recreational or occupational posture?

✦ Has the client begun a new activity or increased the duration or speed of a previous activity?

✦ Was there a previous injury to the affected limb?

- ✦ Has the condition been diagnosed by a physician?

- ✦ What parallel therapies is the client taking, such as physiotherapy or chiropractic?

- ✦ Are supports or braces used during activities?

- ✦ Is the client taking any medication, such as NSAIDs or steroid injections?

- ✦ Does the client have a stretching and strengthening program and is it being followed?

Objective Information

Observations

Acute

- ✍ Antalgic posture or antalgic gait may be present.
- ✍ Swelling and redness may be noticeable if the tendon is superficial.

Chronic

- ✍ A postural assessment may be performed to determine sources of muscle imbalance.
- ✍ Thickening of the tendon may be observed.
- ✍ Muscle wasting and disuse atrophy occur with complete tendon tears *(Bunker, Wallace, 1991)*.

Palpation

Acute

- ✍ Point tenderness occurs over the tendon.
- ✍ Heat and swelling may be palpated at the tendon.
- ✍ Hypertonicity and trigger points are present in the affected muscle and its antagonists.

Chronic

✍ Pain occurs over or near the tendon.

✍ Swelling and adhesions are present. The tendon may feel granular or hard at the adhesion site.

✍ Hypertonicity and trigger points occur as in the acute stage.

✍ Crepitus may be palpated on movement of the tendon in its sheath.

✍ A snapping sensation may be felt due to tight tendons that snap over bony prominences or bursae *(Souza, 1997)*.

Testing

Acute and Chronic

✍ **AF ROM** of the affected limb is usually painless.

✍ **PR ROM** may reveal pain on actions that fully stretch the affected tendon.

✍ **AR Isometric testing** is painful on contraction of the muscle of the affected tendon, especially if the muscle is contracted in a stretched position. The pain is local to the tendon and increases with the force of the contraction. It is more severe in the acute stage. The therapist may have to move the muscle through its range, testing isometrically in different positions to provoke a positive test. If this fails, the client puts the limb in the position that causes pain and isometric resistance is applied in this position. Weakness may also be present. This is often called the **tendinitis differentiation test.**

Special Tests

✍ Shoulder tendinitis is revealed by a positive **supraspinatus, infraspinatus** or **subscapularis test.**

✍ **Speed's** and **Yergason's tests** are positive with biceps tendinitis.

✍ **Extensor tendinosis test** and **Mill's test** are positive with extensor tendinosis. **Flexor tendinosis test** and **reverse Mill's test** are positive with flexor tendinosis.

✍ **Finkelstein's test** is positive with deQuervain's tenosynovitis.

✍ *Complete rupture* of any tendon has painless **active free** and **passive relaxed** ranges of motion. **Active resisted isometric strength testing** reveals weakness but is painless *(Souza, 1997)*. The **drop arm test** reveals supraspinatus tendon rupture. **Thompson's test** is positive for Achilles tendon rupture.

✍ *Shoulder impingement* is revealed by **painful arc** and **Neer impingement tests,** although these tests do not differentiate which specific structure is compressed *(Andrews, Wilk, 1994)*.

Differential Assessment

✍ **Bursitis** is positive with the **bursitis differentiation test**.

Contraindications

✦ Frictions are avoided if the client is on anti-inflammatory medication.

✍ **Cubital tunnel syndrome** is a peripheral nerve compression. The ulnar nerve is entrapped in a fibro-osseous tunnel behind the medial epicondyle or at the flexor carpi ulnaris aponeurosis. **Tinel's sign** may be positive over the ulnar nerve. Paresthesia and pain are present at the medial epicondyle and the ulnar side of the hand *(Hopkins, 1994; Souza, 1997)*.

Treatment Goals

Treatment Plan

Acute

Reduce inflammation.

🖐 **Positioning** depends on the location of the tendinitis and the client's comfort. The limb is elevated and pillowed securely.

🖐 **Hydrotherapy** is cold, such as an ice pack or a gel pack, applied to the affected tendon.

General Treatment

🖐 If the initial treatment goal is to decrease the edema, lymphatic drainage on the affected limb is performed before any compensatory work is begun.

Reduce pain. Decrease sympathetic nervous system firing.

🖐 If the initial goal is to accustom the client to the therapist's touch and to decrease sympathetic nervous system firing in the context of a relaxation massage, the client is directed to do **diaphragmatic breathing** throughout the treatment.

Treat any compensating structures.

🖐 The trunk and unaffected limbs are treated using effleurage and slow petrissage, such as palmar kneading, fingertip kneading and C-scooping. The focus of the work depends on the muscles that are compensating.

Specific Treatment

Reduce edema.

🖐 Lymphatic drainage techniques are used on the affected limb, beginning with nodal pumping at the proximal lymph nodes. Unidirectional effleurage, stationary circles and the local technique are used proximal to the tendinitis to reduce edema.

Reduce hypertonicity and trigger points.

🖐 The proximal limb is treated to reduce hypertonicity. Trigger points referring into the lesion site are also addressed. Techniques include effleurage and muscle stripping.

🖐 Hypertonicity is decreased in the antagonists of the affected muscle using segmental petrissage instead of techniques that flush circulation through the area.

🖐 Hypertonicity in the affected muscle is treated using Golgi tendon organ release on the *unaffected* tendon of the affected muscle.

444

Treatment Goals   Treatment Plan

Vibrations can be performed on site.

🖐 Muscle squeezing and stroking are used on the distal limb, again avoiding techniques that increase circulation through the lesion site.

Maintain range of motion.

🖐 Pain-free **passive relaxed range of motion** is used on the proximal and affected joints to maintain the succussive action and to help increase lymphatic drainage.

Mobilize hypomobile joints.

🖐 Gentle joint play is applied to hypomobile joints in the affected limb.

Chronic

🖐 All chronic tendon injuries, including impingement syndromes and partial rotator cuff tears *(Souza, 1997; Hertling, Kessler, 1996)*, can be treated with the following protocol.

🖐 **Positioning** is chosen for comfort and for accessibility of the structures that are treated. The limb is only elevated if chronic edema remains. Otherwise, it is positioned comfortably.

🖐 **Hydrotherapy** applications proximal to the tendinitis and on the lesion site itself include deep moist heat to soften adhesions and to increase local circulation. However, the application should not be prolonged.

General Treatment

Decrease sympathetic nervous system firing. Treat compensatory structures.

🖐 Diaphragmatic breathing is encouraged with deeper, potentially painful techniques. The client's trunk and compensating structures are massaged as before. Rhythmic techniques to the trunk and unaffected limb are indicated.

Specific Treatment

Reduce fascial restrictions. Reduce any chronic edema.

🖐 Chronic edema remaining around the tendon may be trapped by proximal and local connective tissue restrictions. Fascial glide is used to assess, then fascial techniques are used to treat the restrictions. These include crossed-hands and ulnar border spreading. Proximal lymphatic drainage is also indicated. A **contrast hydrotherapy** application of alternating hot and cold towels is useful to flush out the edema.

Reduce hypertonicity and trigger points. Improve tissue health.

🖐 The proximal limb is treated to reduce hypertonicity and trigger points and to increase local circulation. Rhythmic techniques, effleurage, repetitive petrissage and ischemic compressions are indicated.

🖐 Antagonists to the affected muscle are treated as in the acute stage. Skin rolling, long effleurage and petrissage techniques are used to increase local circulation.

Treatment Goals

Reduce adhesions.

Mobilize hypomobile joints.
Restore range of motion.
Stretch shortened muscles.

Treatment Plan

🖐 The affected muscle is treated in a similar fashion, working towards the lesion site.

🖐 Adhesions may form in the tendon and between a tendon and a paratendon. They may also form at the musculotendinous junction. To treat, the tendon is first located using bony landmarks. The client is then instructed to isometrically contract the affected muscle, helping to accurately locate the tender lesion site in the tendon.

🖐 Skin rolling, fascial spreading and repetitive muscle stripping are used over the lesion site to break down as many adhesions as possible before frictions are used. Myofascial release through passive lengthening of the muscle by the therapist while applying fascial spreading is also used *(Brukner, Khan, 1993)*.

🖐 Frictions are applied across the tendon over the tender adhesions. If the tendon is adhered to the sheath, a stretch may be placed on the tendon while the technique is performed to allow the sheath to be mobilized over the tendon *(Souza, 1997)*. Afterwards, a passive stretch is placed on the tendon to realign the fibres. An application of **ice** must follow this work *(Brukner, Khan, 1993)*.

🖐 If the client is taking anti-inflammatory medication, the therapist uses fascial techniques and muscle stripping to treat the tendinitis until the medication usage ends.

🖐 The distal limb is treated with effleurage and petrissage to increase local venous return.

🖐 Joint play is used on hypomobile joints in the affected limb.

🖐 **Passive relaxed range of motion** is used on the affected joints.

🖐 A passive stretch is applied to the affected muscle and its antagonists.

Self-care Goals

Educate the client regarding activities.

Stretch shortened muscles.

Self-care Plan

Acute

✍ Relative rest from the activity that causes the tendinitis is important to allow the tissues to heal. Relative rest is continued until the pain and inflammation decrease. This may be difficult to achieve with occupational or sports-related injuries. Rest requires motivation on the client's part to adapt specific activities or temporarily stop them.

✍ **Hydrotherapy** consists of ice applied immediately after activity. Ice should be applied for five to 20 minutes at a time.

✍ A slow, pain-free stretch of the affected muscle and its antagonists is indicated to regain flexibility.

446

Self-care Goals

Self-care Plan

Strengthen weak muscles.

✎ It is crucial to regain full strength in the affected muscle to prevent reinjury. A progressive strengthening program is started when local tenderness on palpation is absent, when there is no pain on activity and when a full, pain-free stretch is obtained *(Brukner, Khan, 1993)*. The client begins with pain-free submaximal isometric exercises for the affected muscle and its antagonists.

Chronic

Educate the client regarding activities.

✎ **Hydrotherapy** contrast bath applications are used to increase tissue health. If a flare-up of acute symptoms is experienced, ice is reapplied after activity.

✎ **Self-massage**, including muscle stripping and skin rolling, may be used on the antagonists and on the affected muscle.

Stretch shortened muscles.
Strengthen weak muscles.

✎ The stretching is continued from the acute stage to maintain flexibility. The client gradually progresses from isometric to isotonic exercise.

✎ To progress to isotonic exercise, the client should be able to perform isometrics throughout the muscle's range without pain for one week. Full passive range of motion must be pain free.

✎ *Eccentric* exercise (the muscle contracts as it lengthens) appears to have a specific strengthening effect on the tendon *(Souza, 1997; Brukner, Khan, 1993)*.

✎ Isotonic exercises are initially slow, gradually increasing in speed over a week. The client should work up to performing three sets of 15 repetitions. The exercises should be pain free for several days in a row. This program continues for three to six weeks. **Ice** is applied after exercise.

✎ The long-term goal is to reach a symptom-free stage, where the client is able to perform functional exercise without pain *(Souza, 1997)*.

Educate the client regarding activities.

✎ The client should modify sport or occupational activities, either by changing the activity if possible or by reducing the repetitions or speed.

✎ The client should change or modify equipment. For example, with racquet sports, reducing string tension and using a smaller racquet will reduce muscle strain.

✎ A routine exercise program, including stretching, should be maintained.

✎ An overzealous progression through the exercise program should be avoided to prevent reinjury.

Refer the client.

✎ Movement therapy, such as the Mitzvah, Feldenkrais or Alexander technique, may be helpful for retraining the client's posture.

Treatment Frequency and Expected Outcome

The optimal treatment frequency to resolve most problems is three times a week for two to three weeks *(Souza, 1997)*, followed by twice a week for one week, then once a week.

Client education is essential, since the client often does not rest for long enough and returns to activity quickly, without gradually strengthening the muscles. This leads to reinjury and, for athletes, a chronic, difficult and often career-limiting disorder.

See also scar tissue, trigger points, bursitis, periostitis and compartment syndromes, dislocations, frozen shoulder, pes planus, understanding compression syndromes, spinal cord injury and hemiplegia.

The outcome also depends on how long the tendinitis has been present before treatment begins. For example, with rest and intense treatment, Achilles tendinitis may respond within four to eight weeks, especially if the symptoms have not been present for more than one or two months. Longer standing tendinitis may require treatment for up to six months *(Brukner, Khan, 1993)*.

BURSITIS

Fiona Rattray

> **Bursitis is inflammation of a bursa.**

A bursa is a small, flat sac lined with synovium. The word bursa means purse *(Buschbacher, 1994)*. Both membranous surfaces of the bursa are normally in contact, separated by only a thin film of lubricating fluid. A bursa reduces friction, usually between tendons and bones. Since it is flat, a bursa is not palpable unless it is inflamed.

A bursa can regrow in six to 24 months if surgically removed *(Souza, 1997)*. Adventitious bursae may form between the scapula and the rib angles *(Zohn, Mennell, 1976)*.

➤ **The cause of bursitis is the overuse** of structures surrounding the bursa, leading to excessive friction and inflammation of the bursal walls. Bursitis is usually secondary to other conditions such as tendinitis.

➤ **Contributing factors** are muscle imbalances, poor biomechanics, postural dysfunctions such as scoliosis or hyperkyphosis and a lack of flexibility.

Less commonly, **acute trauma, infection** and **pathologies** such as osteoarthritis, gout and rheumatoid arthritis can cause bursitis. Acute traumatic bursitis usually occurs to the olecranon, trochanteric, ischial, prepatellar or calcaneal bursae *(Zohn, Mennell, 1976)*. A bursa can become infected, especially if a needle is introduced into it for some therapeutic purpose.

Common Bursitis Locations and Causes

Shoulder Bursae

There are several bursa at the shoulder *(Figure 33.1)*. The *subacromial* (or subdeltoid) bursa lies between the acromion and the supraspinatus tendon, with a portion of the bursa

449

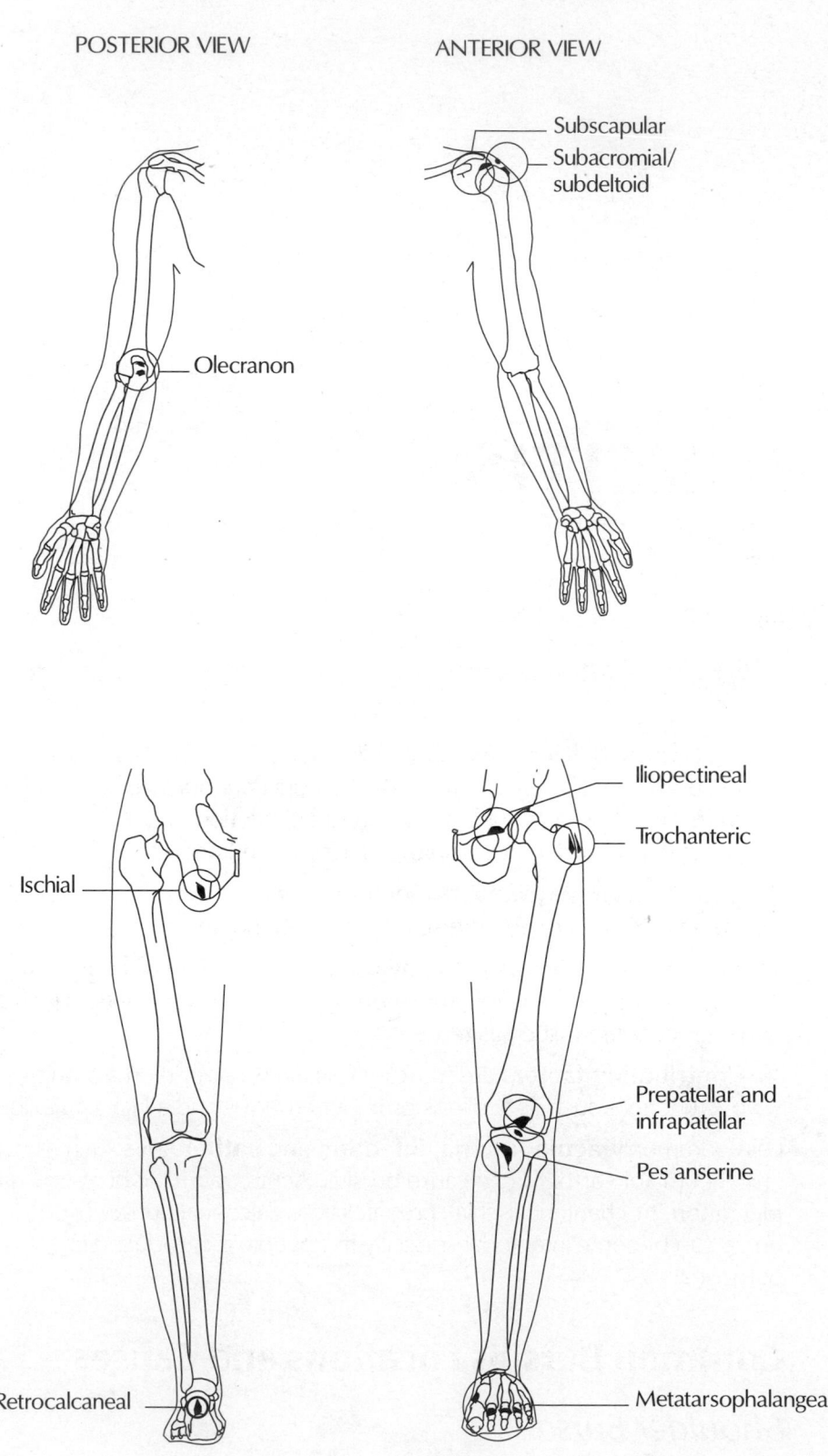

POSTERIOR VIEW

ANTERIOR VIEW

Subscapular

Subacromial/
subdeltoid

Olecranon

Iliopectineal

Trochanteric

Ischial

Prepatellar and
infrapatellar

Pes anserine

Retrocalcaneal

Metatarsophalangeal

Figure 33.1
Locations of various bursa, including shoulder bursa.

450

between the deltoid muscle and the humerus. The subcoracoid portion is not always present *(Bunker, Wallace, 1991)*. The bursa is palpated through the anterior deltoid muscle near the acromion. The *subscapular* bursa lies between the scapula and subscapularis muscle. It is not easily palpable.

Although bursitis does exist at the shoulder, the trend today is to list subacromial bursitis as part of shoulder impingement syndrome. The bursa is painfully irritated as it is compressed between the rotator cuff tendons, the coracoacromial ligament and the acromion *(Pappas, 1995)* or by the biceps tendon *(Andrews, Wilk, 1994)*. Overuse of the shoulder, especially with the arm in an overhead position, is the most common cause.

With acute calcific tendinitis leading to bursitis, there is severe shoulder pain that increases with movement. In the past, it was thought that insidious-onset acute bursitis was due to a degenerative calcific process within the tendon which ruptured the bursa *(Cailliet, 1981)*. However, many people with radiographic evidence of calcific tendinitis are asymptomatic. Furthermore, calcific tendinitis does not occur in persons under 30 or over 60 years of age, so the process cannot be degenerative. Currently, it is thought that the pain occurs in the inflammatory phase when the calcium is resorbed, coinciding with the acute bursitis *(Souza, 1997)*. There is either an insidious onset or history of trauma, such as a fall onto the outstretched arm.

Olecranon Bursa

The olecranon bursa lies between the olecranon and the subcutaneous fascia and is quite swollen and obvious when inflamed. It is irritated by repetitive weight bearing or trauma such as dragging the elbow on the ground when wrestling.

Trochanteric Bursa

There are two main bursae at the greater trochanter. One lies between the gluteus maximus tendon and the trochanter, the other between the gluteus medius tendon and the trochanter. The bursae are palpated through the overlying gluteus maximus tendons. Pain is local to the lateral hip and the client will not be able to sleep on the involved side. Pain is worse on climbing stairs and getting out of a car. Causes include altered hip biomechanics due to a leg length discrepancy, low back pain causing antalgic gait, osteoarthritis and surgery. Repetitive actions and iliotibial band contracture can also cause friction of the bursa.

Iliopectineal Bursa

The iliopectineal bursa lies between the iliopsoas muscle and the iliofemoral ligament. To palpate the bursa, the supine client's hip is flexed to 90 degrees. The bursa is located one or two centimetres inferior to the middle third of the inguinal ligament.

Pain is at the anterior hip and may radiate down the anterior leg due to pressure on the femoral nerve. Antalgic posture is usually hip flexion and external rotation. This bursitis is caused by hip flexor tightness and repetitive activity.

Ischial Bursa

The ischial bursa lies between gluteus maximus and the ischial tuberosity. It is palpated through gluteus maximus. With inflammation, there is well-localized pain over the ischial tuberosity. There may be referral down the posterior leg that mimics sciatic pain. When the client is driving, he may find that pressing down on the brake or gas pedal relieves the pain. This is due to increased tone in muscles that cross the knee which rotates the ischial tuberosity away from the car seat. There is antalgic gait, with the client leaning towards the affected side and shortening his stride. Standing on the toes may be painful *(Souza, 1997)*. This bursitis is caused by sitting for a long time on a hard surface, such as when horseback riding. Today termed "bench warmer's bursitis", in the past it was called "weaver's bottom". Excessive sprinting may also cause this bursitis due to hamstring contraction.

Knee Bursae

There are numerous bursae around the knee. The *pes anserine* bursa lies between the tendons of sartorius, gracilis and semitendinosus muscles and the medial tibia. The *infrapatellar* bursa lies between the patellar ligament and the tibia. Other unnamed bursae lie between the iliotibial band, the lateral collateral ligament and the tibia. All these bursae are palpated through the overlying tendons. Pain is worse on use. Overuse such as occurs in running or cycling is a cause of inflammation. The *prepatellar* bursa lies between the lower half of the patella, the patellar ligament and the skin. It is easily palpated when inflamed and is locally painful. Occupations that involve frequent kneeling cause this bursitis, such as carpet installation.

Retrocalcaneal Bursa

The retrocalcaneal bursa lies between the Achilles tendon and the calcaneus. The bursa is palpated on either side of the tendon. It is locally painful when inflamed. Overuse and a tight gastrocnemius-soleus complex are causes of inflammation.

Medically, acute bursitis is treated with rest, NSAIDs, ultrasound and ice. Superficial bursae such as the olecranon bursa may be protected with a padded donut or pillow. A superficial bursa may also be aspirated, especially if it is infected, then infiltrated with a corticosteroid. Surgical excision is another option. A program of stretching and a gradual return to strengthening for the structures that cross the bursa are recommended.

Other Bursal Injuries

✦ A **Baker's cyst** is a synovial cyst that usually appears at the lateral side of the popliteal space. It is thought to be an enlargement of the extracapsular bursa between the gastrocnemius and semimembranosus muscles, or a herniation of the synovium through the posterior joint capsule wall *(Magee, 1992)*. Baker's cysts can appear in children and adults. One study noted that, when left untreated, 51 of 70 cysts disappeared spontaneously in less than two years, while when they were surgically removed they tended to recur within seven months. One-quarter of the recurrent cysts also spontaneously resolved after five years. Current medical opinion is to leave them alone *(Larson, Grana, 1993)*.

✦ A **bunion** occurs at the first metatarsophalangeal joint capsule. A bunion is formed by excessive bone growth (exostosis), a callus and an inflamed, thickened bursa developing over the joint *(Sammarco, 1995)*. This is in response to joint hypermobility as poor biomechanics allow the first metatarsal bone to deviate medially. The phalanges deviate laterally, forming a hallux valgus. NSAIDs and corrective footwear are used to treat a bunion. Surgery to straighten the toe and reduce the exostosis is an option.

Symptom Picture

Bursitis secondary to overuse is a chronic condition with an initial, acute inflammatory stage.

Acute

✦ The bursa is compressed and irritated by surrounding structures.

✦ Inflammation, heat and swelling are present.

✦ Pain is deep and burning, at rest or on activity. It may refer some distance from the bursa. Pain may disturb sleep, especially if the bursa is compressed.

✦ Range of motion of the affected joint is restricted. Joints distal or proximal may have reduced range if crossed by a muscle or fascia that also crosses the affected bursa.

✦ Other conditions, such as tendinitis, may be present.

Contraindications

✦ With acute bursitis, the therapist should avoid compressing the bursa or applying techniques that place a drag on the surrounding tissues.

✦ On-site techniques are contraindicated with acute bursitis.

✦ If infective bursitis is suspected, the client is referred for medical attention.

Chronic

✦ Pain or achiness is felt with activity or upon direct compression. Pain is more localized to the bursa.

✦ Chronic inflammation, fibrosis and adhesions are present.

✦ Range of motion of the affected joint is less restricted than in the acute stage.

Treatment Considerations

Assessment

✍ **Observation and Palpation in Acute:**

• Swelling and redness are noted over bursae that are more superficial, such as prepatellar, retrocalcaneal or olecranon bursae. These symptoms may not be noticed with deeper bursae, such as the iliopectineal bursa.

- Antalgic posture or gait is present.

- Heat is palpated locally. The bursa is exquisitely painful on direct compression and feels fluctuant.

- Spasm, hypertonicity and trigger points are present in muscles crossing the bursa.

✍ **Observation and Palpation in Chronic:**

- A postural assessment may be performed to determine sources of muscle imbalance.

- Adhesions are palpated. Bogginess may be noted.

- Hypertonicity and trigger points are also present.

✍ **Testing in Acute and Chronic:**

- **AF ROM** of the affected joint is reduced in most directions due to pain, more so in the acute stage. Pain is experienced in a single position in the chronic stage.

- **PR ROM** in the acute stage reveals an empty end feel due to pain, with a markedly reduced range similar to AF ROM. This is not as pronounced in the chronic stage.

- **AR isometric testing** is painful for bursae that are completely surrounded by other structures, such as subacromial, trochanteric and retrocalcaneal bursae. The pain stays constant while the bursa is compressed. This is also called the **bursitis differentiation** test.

- Any specific tests that cause the muscle overlying the bursa to contract are positive, such as **Ober's test** with trochanteric bursitis. Tests that passively compress the bursa are positive, such as the **Faber test** with trochanteric bursitis.

- The **painful arc** and **Neer impingement tests** are positive with shoulder bursitis. Clinically, it may be difficult to differentiate between bursitis and tendinitis with impingement tests. Positional pain relief is less common with bursitis than with tendon or muscle injury *(Souza 1997)*. In the chronic stage, a painful active free arc plus a pain-free passive relaxed arc indicate a muscular or tendinous lesion, not bursitis.

✍ **Differential assessment** for tendinitis utilizes the **tendinitis differentiation test**.

Massage

🖐 The treatment, whether acute or chronic, is in the context of a relaxation massage including unforced **diaphragmatic breathing.**

Acute

🖐 The **hydrotherapy** application is cold to the affected bursa, such as a frozen towel. The application should not be heavy, which would compress the bursa.

🖐 **Positioning** is for comfort, again so the bursa is not compressed. The limb should be comfortably elevated.

🖐 Lymphatic drainage techniques are applied to the affected limb, starting with nodal pumping. The distal limb is treated. Lymphatic drainage is applied to a point just proximal to the edema.

🖐 Swedish techniques such as effleurage and petrissage are applied to the trunk and proximal limb to treat the compensating structures and to decrease sympathetic nervous system firing and pain. Trigger points in the proximal muscles that refer into the affected bursa are treated with muscle stripping and gentle ischemic compressions.

🖐 The attachments of the surrounding muscles are treated using Golgi tendon organ release and the origin and insertion technique. These should only by applied to the attachments that are not local to the bursa. Segmental petrissage techniques are used, working *towards* the bursa, not away from it. The techniques used should not drag on the bursa. There is no on-site work.

🖐 Gentle Grade 1 or 2 joint play is used to decrease the spasm in muscles surrounding the bursa *(Kisner, Colby, 1996)*.

🖐 Stroking and gentle muscle squeezing are applied distal to the affected area.

🖐 Pain-free passive relaxed and active assisted range of motion is interspersed throughout the massage *(Hertling, Kessler, 1996)*.

Chronic

🖐 **Positioning** is the same as for the acute stage.

🖐 The **hydrotherapy** application is deep moist heat before stretching the surrounding fascia. A contrast application is used after treatment to increase local circulation.

🖐 Fascial techniques to treat the muscles crossing the bursa include skin rolling, crossed-hands spreading and fingertip spreading. Connective tissue cutting and longitudinal fingertip spreading are incorporated *(Souza, 1997)*.

🖐 Compensating structures in the trunk and proximal limb are treated with Swedish techniques as in the acute stage.

🖐 Effleurage and petrissage are used, such as wringing and fingertip and palmar kneading, on the agonists and antagonists. Trigger points and taut bands in these muscles are treated with muscle stripping.

🖐 The attachments of the surrounding muscles are treated as before. C-scooping is used, with the bursa in the centre of the scooping motions, and fingertip kneading is applied towards the bursa.

🖐 Pain-free passive relaxed range of motion of the affected joints is interspersed with the massage.

🖐 Frictions to adhered structures surrounding the bursa may be used.

🖐 There is disagreement as to whether the bursa itself should be frictioned. While opinion holds that function should be regained without irritating the bursa *(Kisner, Colby, 1996)*, another view is that, due to the minimal inflammation of a chronic bursitis and the associated fibrosis, frictions may be successful, especially in treating pre-existing tendinitis adhesions *(Hertling, Kessler, 1996; Thomson et al., 1991)*. There may be some irritation in the first three visits and the normal anesthesia effect of frictioning may be difficult to obtain *(Souza, 1994)*. Frictions are followed with a stretch and ice.

- Even if frictions are not used, muscles crossing the affected bursa are stretched to regain flexibility *(Souza, 1997)*.

- Repetitive effleurage and petrissage are used on the distal limb to increase local circulation and remove metabolites.

- Joint play is indicated for any hypomobile joints affecting the bursa *(Hertling, Kessler, 1996)*.

- The treatment is finished with effleurage to the entire limb.

- Secondary conditions such as tendinitis or underlying postural dysfunction are also treated over several appointments.

Self-care

Acute

- The client is instructed to rest, ice and comfortably elevate the affected limb as much as possible.

- Pain-free active free and submaximal isometric exercises are begun as soon as the client can tolerate them.

Chronic

- The client should rest from aggravating activities. Return to activity is gradual. If a flare-up of acute symptoms is experienced, ice is reapplied after activity.

- Self-massage is performed to the muscles surrounding the bursa. Stretching is encouraged.

See also tendinitis, frozen shoulder, osteoarthritis, inflammatory arthritides, pes planus, iliotibial band contracture and scoliosis for related conditions.

- The client gradually progresses from pain-free isometrics to isotonic exercises. The long-term goal is to restore painless, full range of motion and strength *(Pauls, Reed, 1996)*. Altered biomechanics are corrected, such as a leg length discrepancy that may contribute to the bursitis. The client is referred for orthotics if needed. Referrals may also be made to a physiotherapist for ultrasound treatments.

34

FROZEN SHOULDER

Fiona Rattray

> *Frozen shoulder is painful, significant restriction of active and passive range of motion at the shoulder, most frequently in abduction and external rotation.*

With frozen shoulder, the joint capsule becomes tightened and inflexible. Two to three per cent of the population may experience this condition, which affects more women than men. Frozen shoulder rarely occurs in those under 40 or over 70 years of age *(Copeland, 1997)*.

A frozen shoulder progresses through three stages. In the acute stage, the joint capsule becomes painfully contracted, with a loss of the axillary recess. In the subacute stage, capsular fibrosis occurs. In the chronic stage, the range gradually returns.

In 1934, Dr. E. Codman used the term "frozen shoulder" in his original report on the condition, calling it "difficult to define, difficult to treat and difficult to explain from the point of view of pathology". In the past, frozen shoulder was believed to be a progressive, degenerative process, but because it is rarely found in those older than 70 years, this theory is unlikely *(Souza, 1994)*. Today the pathophysiology of the frozen shoulder remains unclear, perhaps because of confusion in terminology and a lack of agreement on the definition and etiology of the condition.

Dr. J. S. Nevasier observed that adhesions developed within the joint capsule, especially in the axillary recess, preventing motion of the humerus. In 1945, he coined the phrase "adhesive capsulitis". Several other terms are used synonymously to describe painful, limited range of motion at the shoulder, such as "capsulitis", "periarticular adhesions", "rotator cuff tendinitis" and "periarthritis" *(Donatelli, 1991)*. One source feels that periarthritis is not an acceptable term to describe frozen shoulder because it also describes bursitis, calcifying tendinitis and rotator cuff tears *(Souza, 1994)*.

Frozen Shoulder Theories

A number of causes have been suggested for frozen shoulder. These include subacromial bursitis, biceps tendon pathology, disuse, supracapsular nerve entrapment leading to muscle dysfunction and small rotator cuff tears. These suggested causes are probably from surgical observations made at different stages of the condition. It has been argued that disuse alone is unlikely to cause frozen shoulder, because the condition does not develop following paralysis and the subsequent loss of function *(Travell, Simons, 1983)*. The concept that a psychiatric personality type is associated with frozen shoulder has been rejected as studies could not agree on the specific personality type *(Souza, 1994)*.

Current thinking is that the joint capsule is primarily involved, with secondary involvement of the surrounding structures. There is a close association among frozen shoulder, referred neck pain, rotator cuff tears and impingement syndrome.

Normally, the superior joint capsule attaches proximal to the greater tuberosity of the humerus and runs medially to the bony rim of the glenoid fossa of the scapula. The inferior joint capsule hangs in a fold or pleat called the "axillary recess". This fold is stretched out when the humerus is abducted. The normal shoulder has a joint volume of up to 35 ml., whereas the frozen shoulder has a volume of 10 ml. or less *(Warner et al., 1997)*. On an arthrogram, the axillary recess is obliterated. Frequently, the bicipital sheath and the subscapularis bursa are also adhered.

Arthroscopic investigation of the glenohumeral joint has revealed inflammatory repair in the subsynovial tissue rather than the synovial layer itself *(Souza, 1994)*. In such a case, the thickened, inelastic synovial membrane tears easily when the humerus abducts or externally rotates, leading to further inflammation. One study found that a triangular section of synovial tissue between the subscapularis and biceps tendons is the area of initial adhesion development *(Figure 34.1)*. Fibrosing then bonds the surrounding rotator

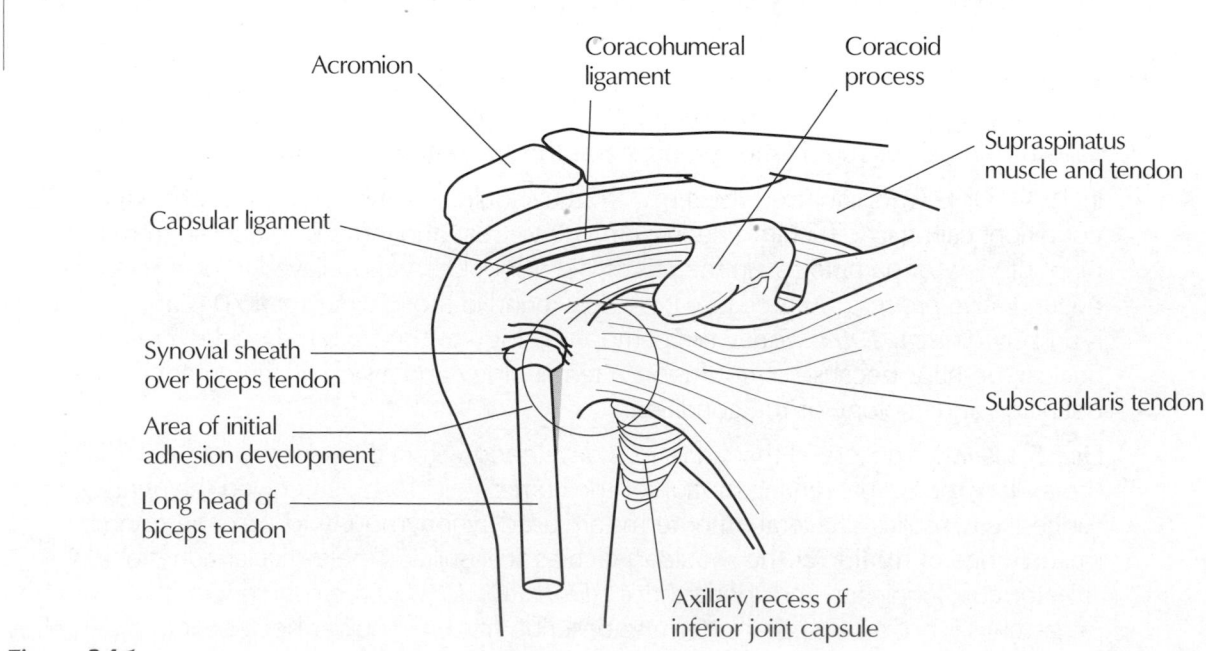

Figure 34.1
Glenohumeral joint anatomy showing the space between the biceps tendon and the subscapularis tendon.

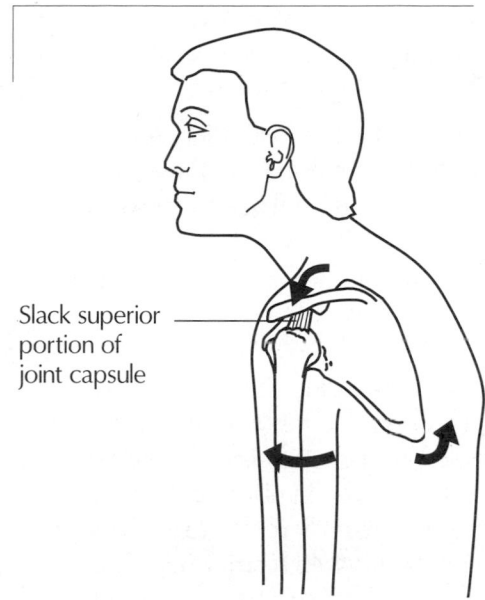

Slack superior portion of joint capsule

Figure 34.2
In hyperkyphosis, the protracted scapula inferiorly rotates, allowing the humerus to hang in a slightly abducted position.

cuff muscles and the glenoid rim. Contractures have been noted in the coracohumeral ligament, which may limit external rotation. These contractures are thought to be analogous to the contractures found in Dupuytren's contracture *(Copeland, 1997)*.

Idiopathic frozen shoulder may also be due to hyperkyphosis causing an alteration of the scapulohumeral alignment, with consequent stress on the joint capsule. In support of this theory, women are more affected by frozen shoulder than men and more women than men have hyperkyphosis. In hyperkyphosis, the scapula assumes an inferiorly rotated position as it protracts over the thorax. The glenoid fossa now faces downward and the head of the humerus takes on a position of slight abduction in the freely hanging arm *(Figure 34.2)*. In this position, the superior portion of the joint capsule loses tension. The rotator cuff muscles must increase their tone in order to maintain the head of the humerus in the glenoid fossa and prevent an inferior subluxation. This increase in tone may increase stress on the joint capsule, leading to increased collagen formation and eventual capsular fibrosis *(Hertling, Kessler, 1996)*.

In another theory, trigger points in the subscapularis muscle restrict external rotation at the shoulder. Referred pain and reduced range of motion activate trigger points in the other muscles of the shoulder, causing further pain and reduced range. Trigger points in the subscapularis, infraspinatus and trapezius muscles also cause vasoconstriction through reflex sympathetic vasomotor control. This vasoconstriction leads to fibrosing in the nearby joint capsule *(Travell, Simons, 1983)*.

Frozen shoulder is described as being **primary** or **secondary**. Primary frozen shoulder is idiopathic, while secondary frozen shoulder results after another pathology such as rotator cuff tears or impingement syndrome. With the increased use of shoulder arthoscopy, primary (idiopathic) frozen shoulder is diagnosed less frequently, because less obvious lesions causing reduced range of motion — such as partial rotator cuff tears — can be observed. In one study of people with shoulder pain, only 50 out of 935 were diagnosed with primary frozen shoulder after arthroscopy *(Copeland, 1997)*.

The causes of frozen shoulder are:

➤ **idiopathic factors**;

➤ **intrinsic musculoskeletal trauma** or **disorder** such as impingement syndrome, subacromial bursitis, rotator cuff tendinitis or tears, dislocations, osteoarthritis, gout and inflammatory synovitis;

➤ **trigger points** in subscapularis muscle;

➤ **postural dysfunctions** such as hyperkyphosis, protracted scapulae and head-forward posture;

➤ **disuse** following shoulder injury or immobilization;

➤ **extrinsic disorders** such as myocardial infarction, hemiplegia, pulmonary disorders such as chronic bronchitis or emphysema, previous breast surgery including mastectomy, lymph node biopsy, coronary bypass surgery and fractures of the humerus *(Warner et al., 1997)*;

➤ **systemic diseases** such as diabetes and hyperthyroidism. People with diabetes have a 10 to 20 per cent incidence. Those who are insulin dependent and who have had diabetes for longer than 10 years are particularly likely to develop frozen shoulder *(Souza, 1994)*.

Motion at the Shoulder

The shoulder joint complex is composed of the sternoclavicular joint, the acromioclavicular joint, the scapulothoracic articulation and the glenohumeral joint. Full abduction of the arm requires rotation of the scapula, elevation of the clavicle, extension and sidebending of the thoracic vertebrae and exaggeration of the lumbar lordosis, as well as elevation of the humerus. In addition, the humerus must externally rotate to prevent the greater tuberosity from impinging on the acromial arch, which would restrict full abduction. The bodies of the first and second ribs must be able to descend to allow full vertebral motion *(Hertling, Kessler, 1996)*. Restriction of any of these joints prevents full abduction of the humerus.

The humerus moves through 180 degrees of abduction, 160 degrees of which occur through combined glenohumeral and scapular movements and 20 degrees of which occur through thoracic and cervical spine sidebending movements. When both arms are raised simultaneously, the spine moves into extension.

In the first 30 degrees of abduction, most of the motion occurs at the glenohumeral joint. After this point, the scapula begins to elevate and rotate on the thorax. The clavicle also elevates, rotates and protracts. The scapula contributes 60 degrees of abduction, with half of that occurring at the sternoclavicular joint.

The ratio of motion between the scapulothoracic articulation and the glenohumeral joint as the arm is abducted through full range is called the "scapulothoracic rhythm". There is an initial setting phase during the first 30 to 60 degrees of abduction, where the relationship of motion between the scapula and humerus is variable depending on the person observed. After 60 degrees the ratio is 2 to 1 glenohumeral to scapulothoracic motion *(Copeland, 1997)*. For every 10 degrees of humeral motion, the scapula moves five degrees. In the frozen shoulder, this scapulothoracic rhythm is altered to a 1:1 ratio.

Medical Treatment of Frozen Shoulder

✦ Analgesics, anti-inflammatories and oral steroids have helped reduce pain symptoms, but have not been shown to change the progression of the condition *(Copeland, 1997)*.

✦ Steroids with local anesthetic have been injected into the subacromial space and the joint capsule. However, studies have not shown this method to have any significant advantage over other forms of treatment *(Souza, 1994)*.

✦ Distention arthrography, where the joint capsule is distended over a series of saline injections has been shown to rupture adhesions. People with mild or moderate restrictions in range of motion have the most success with this method, with pain relief occurring suddenly or over several hours. Relief may be temporary or permanent. There is a risk that the joint capsule may tear at the biceps tendon or the subscapularis bursa. Range of motion does not always increase *(Souza, 1994)*. Arthroscopic surgical release is also used *(Warner et al., 1997)*.

+ Manipulation under anesthesia is performed in cases that do not progress. The arm of the supine person is taken through forced flexion, adduction, external rotation and internal rotation *(Warner et al., 1997)*. After manipulation, anti-inflammatory and analgesic medications are injected into the capsule to prevent post-manipulation adhesions and swelling. Physiotherapy to maintain mobility begins immediately, since the full range gained under anesthesia is rarely maintained after recovery. Results of manipulation under anesthesia are variable, with good range to less than optimal range being recovered *(Copeland, 1997)*. Complications of this technique include: post-manipulation pain; tearing of the capsule, the long head of biceps and the subscapularis tendons; hematoma; shoulder dislocation; and spiral fracture of the humerus *(Souza, 1994)*.

+ In the past, treatment that was too aggressive in the acute stage, such as manipulation under anesthesia and the higher grades of joint play technique, made the condition worse and led to a longer recovery time. Today, the early stages of frozen shoulder are treated with analgesics and passive range of motion *(Souza, 1994)*.

Symptom Picture

Acute

+ The acute stage is also called the **"freezing phase"**, **"first stage"** or **"painful phase"**.

+ There is a gradual onset of pain, perhaps after a minor trauma such as twisting the shoulder while reaching into the back seat of a car. If there was a trauma, the person may immobilize the limb to protect it. Occasionally, there is a major trauma such as a fracture, surgery or myocardial infarction. However, frequently the person may not remember any precipitating factor at all.

+ The pain is severe at night and the person is unable to lie on the affected side. The pain is on the outer aspect of the shoulder and the deltoid insertion *(Copeland, 1997)*, referring to the elbow.

+ Muscle spasm may be present in the rotator cuff muscles *(Hertling, Kessler, 1996)*.

+ Inflammation is present in the capsule.

+ Stiffness is progressive, setting in at two or three weeks after the initial pain begins *(Kisner, Colby, 1996)*.

+ This stage lasts for two to nine months *(Cuillo, 1996)* and longer if aggressive therapy is used *(Warner et al., 1997)*.

+ The condition may be unilateral or bilateral and the non-dominant limb may be more commonly affected. The second shoulder is involved within five years in 10 to 20 per cent of those affected *(Copeland, 1997)*.

+ The acute and subacute stages blend into each other.

Subacute

+ The subacute stage is also called **"frozen phase"**, **"second stage"** or **"stiffening phase"**.

+ The severe pain begins to diminish.

+ Stiffness becomes the primary complaint, interfering with activities of daily living. The primary restriction is in the capsular pattern of external rotation, abduction and internal rotation. There is pain at end ranges of motion.

+ Disuse atrophy of the deltoid and rotator cuff muscles may occur.

+ This stage lasts four to 12 months *(Kisner, Colby, 1996)*.

Chronic

+ The chronic stage is also called the **"thawing phase"**, **"third stage"**, or **"resolution phase"**.

+ Pain is localized to the lateral arm and continues to diminish. The person is not awakened at night by pain, as in the acute stage.

+ Motion and function gradually return. However, full range of motion is not always regained. While many people feel the shoulder is less restricted, objective measurement frequently shows only minor improvements.

+ Although frozen shoulder is often said to resolve spontaneously in two years, several studies have shown that people can remain symptomatic for as long as five to 10 years. The length of the painful phase corresponds to the length of the recovery time *(Souza, 1994)*.

Subjective Information

HEALTH HISTORY QUESTIONS

+ Has there been a history of injury to the shoulder, including surgery to the shoulder or thorax?

+ Does the client have any underlying conditions such as diabetes?

+ Where is the pain located?

+ Does the pain interrupt sleep? Is the client unable to sleep on the affected side? In the acute stage, the client will answer "yes".

+ What actions are limited? Is there an impairment of activities of daily living, such as brushing or washing the hair, putting on a coat, fastening a bra or reaching into a back pocket? The client likely wears shirts that button down the front instead of sweaters that are removed over the head.

+ Has the frozen shoulder been medically diagnosed?

+ Is the client taking any parallel therapies such as physiotherapy?

+ Is the client taking any medication such as anti-inflammatories or analgesics?

Objective Information

Observations

✍ During the gait cycle, the affected arm is held stiffly and its normal swing is absent.

✍ A postural assessment likely reveals a hyperkyphosis and head-forward posture.

✍ The affected shoulder is elevated and protracted.

Palpation

✍ Hypertonicity and trigger points are palpated in the affected muscles, especially upper trapezius, levator scapula and shoulder girdle muscles.

✍ The shoulder girdle muscles and lateral arm are point tender.

✍ In the subacute stage, disuse atrophy and fibrosing are likely present in the muscles of the rotator cuff.

Testing

✍ All testing results are for the glenohumeral joint unless otherwise noted.

Acute

✍ **AF ROM** is restricted by pain in external rotation, abduction and internal rotation. External and internal rotation are measured first with the humerus resting at the client's side, then with the humerus abducted to 90 degrees *(Souza, 1994)* or as much as possible. These two positions of the humerus are used in active and passive movements tested in all stages of presentation. A terminal painful arc is present in the available abduction after 70 degrees *(Bunker, Wallace, 1991)*.

- **Substitute movement patterns**: The client may initiate abduction by hiking the shoulder through upper trapezius contraction or by leaning the trunk *(Souza, 1994)*.

✍ **PR ROM** reveals restrictions in external rotation, abduction and internal rotation due to pain. A muscle-guarding end feel may be noticed.

✍ **AR testing** for rotator cuff muscles reveals full strength. There may be no pain with resisted movement *(Hertling, Kessler, 1996)* or pain if there is an associated tendinitis. In one study, up to 40 per cent of people reported pain on resisted shoulder movement *(Souza, 1994)*.

Subacute

✍ **AF ROM** is most restricted in external rotation, abduction and internal rotation. A pattern of 90 degrees of abduction, 120 degrees of flexion, 60 degrees of external rotation and 45 degrees of internal rotation has been noted *(Hertling, Kessler, 1996)*. A terminal painful arc is noted in the available abduction after 70 degrees *(Bunker, Wallace, 1991)*.

✍ **PR ROM** restrictions are in a capsular pattern of external rotation, abduction and internal rotation, with a painful, leathery end feel.

✍ **AR testing** reveals little pain on any resisted movement at the shoulder if this is kept in the unrestricted range. Strength may be reduced.

Chronic

✍ **AF** and **PR ROM** begin to return to normal.

✍ **AR testing** may reveal reduced strength of the shoulder girdle muscles.

Special Tests

✍ **Apley's scratch test** is positive for restricted motion in abduction and external and internal rotation. AF ROM of the cervical and thoracic spine may show reduced ranges.

✍ **The frozen shoulder passive relaxed abduction test** is positive. In the thoracic and cervical spine, **anterior** and **lateral spinous challenge tests** reveal areas of vertebral hypomobility. The **first rib mobility test** and sternoclavicular joint play may also show hypomobility.

Differentiating Sources of Shoulder Pain and Restricted Abduction and External Rotation

✦ **Posterior dislocation** has a history of trauma, usually a fall forward on the outstretched arm.

✦ **Acromioclavicular joint sprain** is painful very local to the joint and an acromioclavicular shear test is positive.

✦ **Tendinitis** at the shoulder has increasing pain with increasing force of contraction of the affected muscle. Depending on the affected tendon, a Speed's, Yergason's, supraspinatus, infraspinatus or subscapularis active resisted test is positive. A drop arm test is positive with rotator cuff tears. The Neer impingement test is positive with impingement of the supraspinatus tendon.

✦ **Glenohumeral osteoarthritis** has a gradual onset, past history of trauma and X-ray diagnosis.

✦ **Cervical nerve root pathology** has the pain restricted to the specific dermatome affected. Spurling's, cervical distraction and upper limb tension tests are positive.

✦ **Cervical facet joint irritation** has pain distributed over the shoulder and neck; Spurling's and cervical distraction tests are positive.

✦ **Reflex sympathetic dystrophy** has a history of myocardial infarction or trauma such as a Colle's fracture. There is restriction in abduction and external rotation, throbbing pain in the shoulder, as well as sympathetic symptoms. These include swelling of the arm and hand due to venous and lymphatic stasis, sweating of the limb,

Contraindications

✦ Aggressive stretches and joint play mobilizations greater than Grades 1 to 3 are contraindicated in the acute stage *(Souza, 1994).*

✦ Frictions are contraindicated with anti-inflammatory medication.

trophic changes and exaggerated erythema alternating with pallor in response to temperature changes. The wrist and metacarpophalangeal joints are flexed.

✦ **Referred shoulder pain** may also arise from the pleura, the diaphragm *(Copeland, 1997)* and cardiac or gall bladder pathologies.

Treatment Goals

Assess range of motion pre- and post-treatment. Maintain range of motion.

Reduce pain. Reduce sympathetic nervous system firing. Treat any compensating structures.

Treatment Plan

🖐 No single method of treatment seems consistently effective with frozen shoulder. The client may try massage therapy after being treated by a physician, physiotherapist or chiropractor.

🖐 Because progress in this condition occurs in spurts and plateaus, it is necessary for the therapist to keep accurate records of the pre- and post-treatment ranges of motion. Otherwise both the client and therapist can lose track of overall gains in the range.

🖐 The therapist may choose some or all of the following techniques, which may be spread over several treatments rather than all being performed at once.

Acute

🖐 **Positioning** begins in the **prone position**, with pillows under the client's abdomen and ankles. If hyperkyphosis is present, two towel rolls are placed under the shoulders, retracting them. Care is taken in positioning, as the client may be apprehensive and may guard the affected limb. The client is later turned supine.

🖐 **The hydrotherapy** application is ice to the affected shoulder *(Hertling, Kessler, 1996)*. Heat can also be used on the compensating structures.

General Treatment

🖐 The treatment begins on the unaffected shoulder in the context of a relaxation massage, which includes **diaphragmatic breathing** to help reduce any pain the client may experience. The trunk and unaffected shoulder are treated using slow gentle rhythmic techniques, effleurage and petrissage, such as palmar kneading, fingertip kneading and C-scooping. Trigger points are treated using muscle stripping and ischemic compressions according to the client's pain tolerance, followed by effleurage.

Treatment Goals

**Reduce hypertonicity
and trigger points.
Maintain local circulation.**

Treatment Plan

Specific Treatment

✋ The periscapular muscles are treated to reduce pain and hypertonicity. Rhythmic techniques and Swedish techniques are used on trapezius, levator scapulae, rhomboids, latissimus dorsi, serratus anterior, erector spinae, deltoid and rotator cuff muscles. Ulnar border stripping, palmar kneading and muscle stripping are used. See the chapter on hyperkyphosis for more details.

✋ The trigger points in the subscapularis muscle refer to the scapula, posterior shoulder, down the posterior arm to the elbow and around the wrist like a watch strap *(Travell, Simons, 1983)*. Subscapularis is located by placing the client's humerus in 90 degrees of abduction (or as much pain-free abduction as possible with the frozen shoulder) and the elbow in 90 degrees of flexion. If possible, the forearm hangs over the edge of the table. With the therapist's fingers resting against the scapula, the thumbs slide *under* the lateral border of latissimus dorsi and rest against the lateral chest wall. To be sure that the therapist is not palpating through latissimus dorsi, the client is asked to submaximally adduct the shoulder, making the muscle palpably contract. The therapist's thumbs are then angled up between the chest wall and the anterior aspect of the scapula. The client is asked to gently internally rotate the humerus, palpably contracting subscapularis.

✋ Once the muscle is located, muscle stripping, intermittent ischemic compressions and the origin and insertion technique are used on the tissue. Subscapularis may also be treated in the supine position.

✋ Pain-free PIR for subscapularis is performed with the client submaximally resisting external rotation.

✋ Petrissage is used on the periscapular muscles to increase drainage and venous return.

Mobilize hypomobile joints.

✋ Joint play, including spinous process oscillations, is used on hypomobile thoracic vertebrae, ribs and the scapulothoracic articulation.

Maintain range of motion.

✋ The client moves to the side of the table so the glenohumeral joint is over the edge of the table and the affected arm can hang in forward flexion. A pain-free passive pendulum exercise is performed. Gravity acting on the arm distracts the joint surfaces, allowing motion to occur. The therapist slowly moves the humerus back and forth on the forward flexion plane.

Treat other conditions.

✋ For details of hyperkyphosis or other conditions, see the appropriate chapter.

✋ The client is turned supine, with pillows under the knees. If hyperkyphosis is present, a small towel roll is placed along the client's spine to reduce the curve.

Treatment Goals   Treatment Plan

Reduce inflammation.

✋ Lymphatic drainage techniques may be used on the affected shoulder, beginning with pumping at the terminus. Unidirectional effleurage and stationary circles are used over the pectoral and deltoid muscles.

Reduce fascial restrictions.

✋ Fascial techniques are applied to the affected shoulder within the client's pain tolerance. These include slow skin rolling, crossed-hands and fingertip fascial spreading and the connective tissue cutting technique over the pectoral fascia. If hyperkyphosis is present, the unaffected shoulder is treated in a similar manner.

Treat any compensating structures.

✋ The unaffected shoulder, arm and neck muscles, including the scalenes, are treated with Swedish techniques. Golgi tendon organ release is used on the suboccipitals. Intercostal and diaphragm work may be indicated if these structures are tight. See the chapter on asthma for details.

Reduce hypertonicity and trigger points.
Maintain local circulation.

✋ Pectoralis major and deltoid are treated with effleurage and repetitive petrissage. Golgi tendon organ release is used on pectoralis major. The therapist sits at the head of the table and hooks the middle and index fingers of each hand under each tendinous attachment of the pectoralis major at the humerus. This should not feel uncomfortable for the client. The therapist then slowly leans back, stretching pectoralis major and applying a Golgi tendon organ release.

✋ Pectoralis minor and subclavius are also massaged with muscle stripping and intermittent ischemic compressions. Biceps and triceps are worked in a similar manner.

Mobilize hypomobile joints. Reduce spasm. Maintain range of motion.

✋ Mild joint play applied early in the acute stage can possibly prevent the full-blown cycle of freezing and thawing *(Ciullo, 1996)*. Joint play techniques are also effective for reducing pain and spasm *(Hertling, Kessler, 1996)*. Grade 1 oscillation techniques — small amplitude oscillations at the beginning of range — and Grade 2 oscillation techniques — large amplitude oscillations not reaching the end of range — are used in the acute stage to reduce pain and spasm. In addition, Grade 1 mobilization (sustained translation) techniques — small amplitude distraction with no stress on the capsule — and Grade 2 mobilization techniques — enough distraction to tighten the capsule — are used to reduce pain and to normalize joint mechanics. Inferior glenohumeral glide is used first, progressing to lateral glide. See the chapter on non-Swedish techniques for details.

✋ Inferior glide is started with the client's arm at the side. In this example, the client's right shoulder is treated. The therapist's right hand is placed at the client's axilla to stabilize the scapula against the thorax. The thumb is resting on the pectoralis major tendon and the fingers are extended. The web between thumb and fingers stabilizes the inferior aspect of the neck of the glenoid. The client's elbow is flexed

Treatment Goals

Treatment Plan

Mobilize hypomobile joints. Reduce spasm. Maintain range of motion.

to 90 degrees. The therapist's left hand grasps the forearm just distal to the elbow. The scapula is stabilized by superior pressure applied by the right hand. The left hand then draws the humerus inferiorly. This technique increases abduction. Over several repetitions of the technique (either in one treatment or over a series of treatments), the humerus is progressively moved into increasing abduction or flexion.

Lateral glide is performed with the client's arm at the side. Again, this example is for the client's right shoulder. The therapist's right hand grasps the medial portion of the client's humerus, as close to the axilla as possible. The client's elbow is flexed to 90 degrees and the client's hand rests on her abdomen. The therapist's left hand stabilizes at the lateral aspect of the elbow. The therapist's right hand moves the proximal humerus laterally. The left hand allows the distal humerus to move laterally also, so the entire joint capsule is mobilized. This technique increases abduction and external rotation. If the elbow is stabilized against the thorax, the humerus is allowed to tilt. Only the superior portion of the joint capsule is treated with this motion (Hertling, Kessler, 1996).

Any hypomobility in the cervical spine and the sternoclavicular joint is treated with joint play.

Pain-free PIR or a passive stretch is applied to the upper trapezius and levator scapula.

Subacute

Assess range of motion pre- and post-treatment. Increase range of motion.

Positioning is the same as for the acute stage, starting in the **prone** positon. Towel rolls are used if hyperkyphosis is present. **Diaphragmatic breathing** is performed. As pain diminishes, the treatment can be more vigorous, although it is essentially the same as in the acute stage.

Hydrotherapy is a hot application to the posterior shoulder then to the anterior shoulder.

General Treatment

Reduce pain. Reduce sympathetic nervous system firing. Treat any compensating structures.

The work to the client's trunk and unaffected shoulder is the same as in the acute stage.

Specific Treatment

Reduce hypertonicity and trigger points. Maintain local circulation.

Swedish techniques are used on the affected shoulder as in the acute stage. Trigger points, especially in subscapularis, are treated using muscle stripping and ischemic compressions. PIR for

Treatment Goals   Treatment Plan

subscapularis progresses through increasing amounts of abduction and external rotation while the client submaximally resists this action.

Mobilize hypomobile joints.

✋ Hypomobile joints in the thoracic spine, ribs and scapulothoracic articulation are treated with joint play.

Increase range of motion.

✋ With the client moved over to the side of the table and the affected arm hanging over the side, an active pendulum exercise is performed. The client moves the humerus through forward flexion, then adduction and abduction.

✋ A passive stretch with the scapula stabilized can also be used. The client returns to the middle of the table. The arm is at the client's side. The therapist stabilizes the scapula against the thorax with one hand. The other hand grasps the humerus and slowly abducts it.

Treat other conditions.

✋ For details of hyperkyphosis or other conditions, see the appropriate chapter.

✋ The client is turned **supine**, with pillows under the knees. A small towel roll is placed along the spine if hyperkyphosis is present.

Reduce fascial restrictions.

✋ Fascial work to the pectorals is performed as before.

Treat any compensating structures.

✋ The unaffected shoulder, neck and diaphragm are treated with Swedish techniques.

Reduce hypertonicity and trigger points. Maintain local circulation.

✋ Pectoralis major, pectoralis minor, subclavius, deltoid and the arm muscles are treated as in the acute stage.

Reduce adhesions.

✋ Adhesions within the shoulder girdle muscles and tendons are treated with cross-fibre frictions, followed by ice and stretch. For example, the biceps tendon, infraspinatus and subscapularis may be affected (*Thomson et al., 1991*).

Mobilize hypomobile joints.
Increase range of motion.

✋ Grade 4 oscillation techniques — small amplitude oscillations at the limit of range — are used in the subacute stage to stretch the joint capsule. Grade 3 mobilization (sustained translation) techniques — enough distraction to stretch the capsule — are used to increase range of motion (*Souza, 1994*). Inferior and lateral glide joint play are used, gradually increasing the range of abduction.

✋ Active inhibition techniques are also useful in increasing range of motion at the glenohumeral joint. A type of PIR called "rhythmic stabilization" (*Cailliet, 1981*) requires the client to isometrically and reciprocally contract the agonists then antagonists against the therapist's resistance. The therapist grasps the client's forearm, taking up the available range into abduction and external rotation and applying constant long-axis traction to the glenohumeral joint (*Figure 34.3*). The therapist attempts to smoothly move the arm into further abduction and external rotation while the client isometrically, submaximally resists (adduction and internal rotation) for up to 10 seconds.

469

Treatment Goals   Treatment Plan

Increase range of motion.

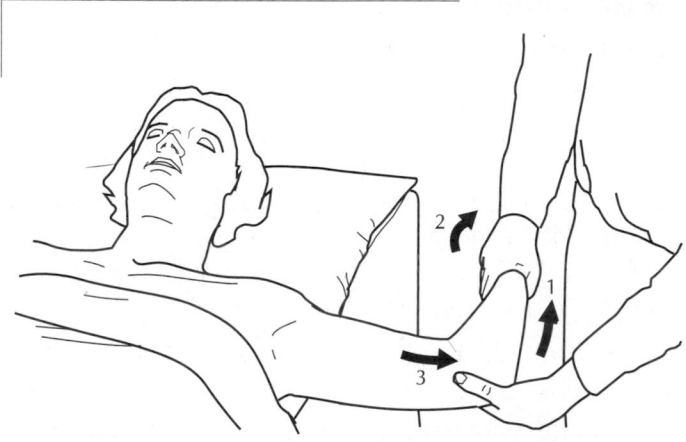

Figure 34.3
First part of "rhythmic stabilization" of the glenohumeral joint. The therapist (1) abducts, (2) externally rotates and (3) applies traction to the arm while the client isometrically resists this action. See text for details.

The therapist's resistance gradually increases, then decreases, as the client meets this resistance. There is no actual motion at the joint. The therapist then reverses the direction of pressure to adduction and internal rotation, while the client isometrically, submaximally resists (abduction and external rotation) for up to 10 seconds. There is no rest period between each reciprocal activation. Once this cycle is completed in the available range of abduction, the therapist moves the arm into more abduction and external rotation and a new cycle begins. Gains in the range are noticed within several minutes. The process is repeated three to four times per week *(Souza, 1994).*

PIR or passive stretch is used on upper trapezius and levator scapula.

Chronic

Assess range of motion pre- and post treatment. Restore range of motion.

The **positioning, hydrotherapy** and techniques are the same as the subacute stage.

Joint play techniques are used to increase the range of the joint capsule, with a focus on the anterior capsule. Inferior and lateral joint play techniques (as described in the subacute stage) in Grade 4 oscillation and Grade 3 mobilization are employed. In addition, the anterior capsule is stretched with a posterior glide.

Posterior glide is begun with the client's humerus as close to 90 degrees of abduction as possible. The elbow is flexed to 90 degrees. In this example, the client's right shoulder is treated. The therapist's left hand grasps the client's wrist and externally rotates the humerus as far as is comfortable, supporting it in this position.

The heel of the therapist's right hand is placed on the proximal portion of the humerus. The humerus is moved posteriorly. The humerus is gradually moved through increasing amounts of external rotation over successive mobilizations *(Hertling, Kessler, 1996).*

Self-care Goals

Self-care Plan

Acute

Educate the client regarding activities.

✍ The client should sleep in a sidelying position with the involved arm uppermost. Several pillows are placed under the involved elbow and forearm to prevent internal rotation and contracture *(Souza, 1994)*.

✍ If the client is sitting or driving for long periods of time, the subscapularis muscle should be stretched frequently in a pain-free manner.

✍ The client should avoid hyperkyphotic and head-forward postures.

✍ Self-massage to the affected muscles is indicated.

✍ Hydrotherapy applications of cold to the affected shoulder and heat to compensating structures are recommended.

Maintain range of motion.

✍ Remedial exercise is limited to passive pendulum (Codman) exercise in pain-free ranges. The client is standing with the unaffected side next to a table and bends forward from the waist, leaning the unaffected hand on the table to support the thorax. The affected arm hangs down, as relaxed as possible. The weight of the arm provides enough traction to separate the glenohumeral joint surfaces. By swaying the body back and forth, the client can passively move the affected arm on the plane of forward flexion and extension without using the muscles surrounding the shoulder. By swaying the body from side to side, abduction and adduction can be achieved passively. Circumduction can be added *(Cailliet, 1981)*.

✍ Wand exercises are also used to maintain range of motion. The client grasps a dowel (or "wand") with both hands shoulder width apart, elbows extended. The wand is held in front of the client and is moved through forward flexion as far as possible. In this position, the wand can then be moved from side to side.

✍ The range of motion of the thoracic and cervical spine must also be maintained through general range of motion exercises and stretches.

Maintain strength.

✍ The client should perform isometric exercises for the muscles of the shoulder girdle.

Refer the client.

✍ The client may be referred to a physiotherapist for transcutaneous electrical nerve stimulation (TENS) treatment or for acupuncture to relieve the pain *(Souza, 1994)*.

✍ Movement therapy, such as the Mitzvah, Feldenkrais and Alexander techniques, may be helpful for retraining the client's posture.

Subacute

Educate the client regarding activities.

✍ Sleeping, driving and posture considerations mentioned in the acute stage are a concern here.

✍ The **hydrotherapy** application is heat to the affected shoulder.

Self-care Goals

Increase range of motion.

Self-care Plan

✍ Active pendulum movements, where the client uses the muscles surrounding the shoulder to move it through its range, are used with clients who are not experiencing acute pain and who have performed passive exercises pain free. Flexion and extension are followed by abduction and adduction and, finally, circumduction. The client can use a small weight to further distract the joint *(Souza, 1994).*

✍ Self-stretches for upper trapezius and levator scapula are indicated, both of which are compensating for the loss of glenohumeral motion. The client should increase the range of motion of the thoracic and cervical spine also through range of motion exercises and stretching.

✍ In the supine position, gravity can be used to **passively stretch** the joint capsule. The client places a thermophore or hot pack on the affected shoulder for 10 to 15 minutes. The arm is placed in as much abduction and external rotation as possible. Discomfort is allowable but pain is not. The position is maintained for 45 minutes to one hour. If the client does not have a thermaphore, the hot packs will need to be changed every 15 minutes. This is repeated daily for one week.

✍ If the client can perform this passive stretch pain free, a small weight can be placed in the hand to increase the pain-free stretch *(Souza, 1994).*

✍ A **gravity-induced PIR** for subscapularis is helpful. The client lies supine with the affected arm over the edge of the bed in as much pain-free abduction and external rotation as possible. The elbow is flexed to 90 degrees. The client slightly internally rotates the humerus, moving it about two centimetres, and holds this position for 20 seconds. The client then relaxes, allowing the arm to move further into external rotation. The cycle is repeated three to five times *(Lewit, 1993).*

✍ Self-mobilization of the glenohumeral joint — with emphasis on inferior glide — can be performed. The client is seated, with the affected arm resting on a table *(Figure 34.4).* To increase *flexion*, the client keeps the elbow in extension and turns the palm down. She presses submaximally against the table for eight to 10 seconds. She relaxes and then carefully attempts to increase the range in a pain-free manner, by pulling the body down and away from the table. To increase *abduction*, the elbow and back of the hand rest on the table with the arm in as much abduction as possible. The client presses the elbow submaximally against the table, relaxes and carefully attempts to increase the range as before. To increase *external rotation*, the client flexes the elbow to 90 degrees and the hand rests palm-down on the table. The palm is pressed submaximally against the table. The client relaxes, then attempts to carefully increase the range by bending forward from the waist *(Souza, 1994).* To increase *internal*

472

Self-care Goals

Self-care Plan

rotation, the client stands with her back to the table and rests her hands behind her on the edge of the table. The hands are pressed submaximally against the table, the client relaxes, then carefully attempts to increase range by bending the knees and slowly lowering the body. The elbows are allowed to flex, internally rotating the humerus *(Hertling, Kessler, 1990).*

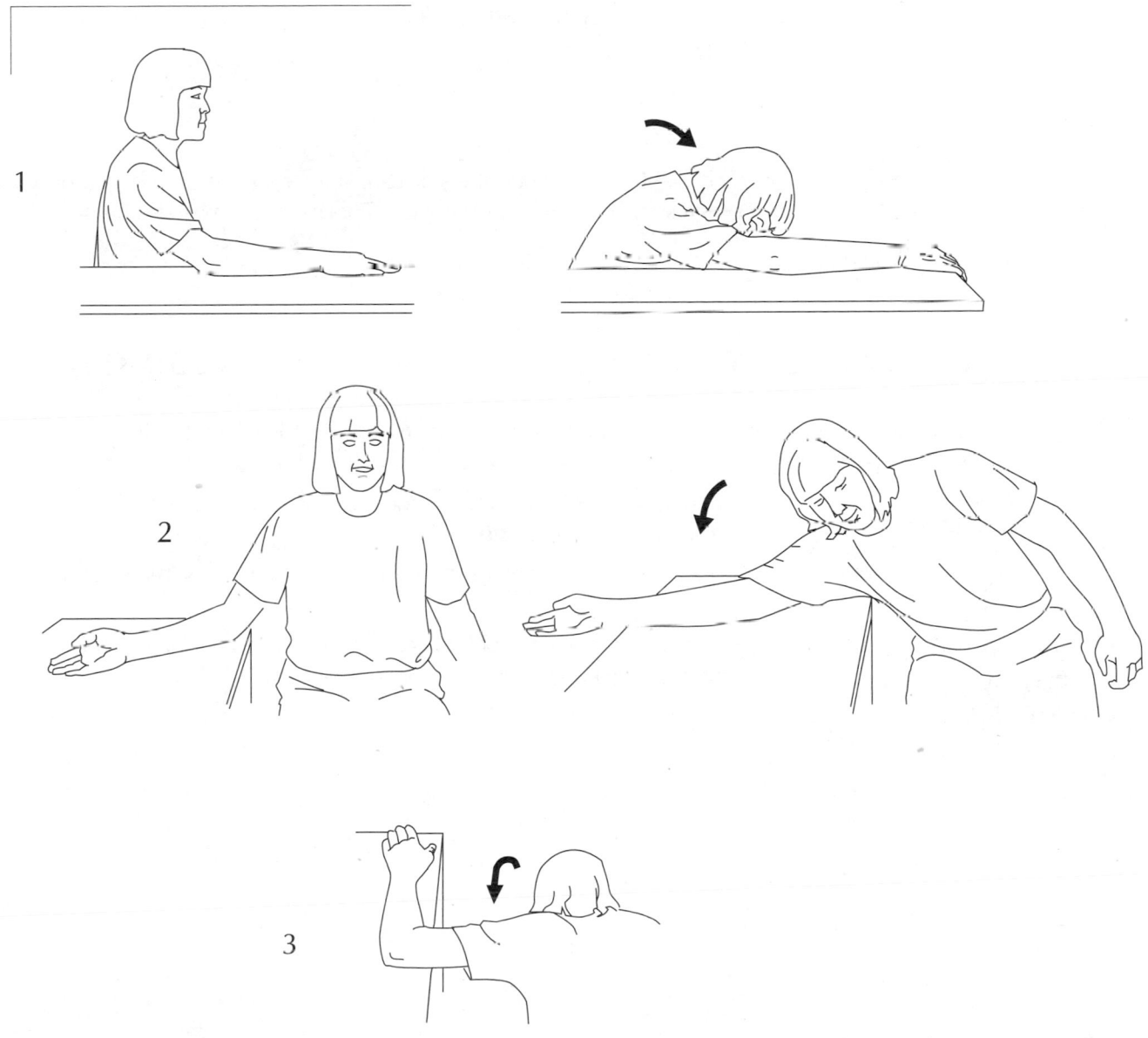

Figure 34.4
Self-mobilization of the glenohumeral joint. (1) Increasing flexion; (2) increasing abduction; (3) increasing external rotation. See text.

Self-care Goals

Self-care Plan

✍ **Wall-walking exercises** have the client standing beside a wall and "walking" the fingers upward to increase range. The client should start with flexion, progressing to abduction. The client can slowly increase abduction by using progressive yet slight changes in angle in relationship to the wall. At home, the client can make a mark on a paper taped to the wall to record the progress that is made.

Increase strength.

✍ Isometric exercises for the shoulder girdle muscles involve interlocking the fingers of both hands and first pushing the hands together, then pulling them apart.

Chronic

✍ The client can continue the self-care suggestions as above, gradually progressing the ranges and strength. Pool exercises may also be helpful.

Treatment Frequency and Expected Outcome

Treatments should be once a week for six weeks. At that point, the client and the remedial exercise self-care plan should be totally reassessed.

See also hyperkyphosis, dislocation, tendinitis, bursitis, Dupuytren's contracture, hemiplegia, chronic bronchitis and emphysema for related conditions.

Progress frequently occurs in spurts and plateaus. Regaining full range of motion may not be possible.

Once the symptoms resolve, they rarely recur in the same shoulder *(Ciullo, 1996)*.

Prevention of frozen shoulder is the best route following shoulder or thoracic surgery. The client should be encouraged to get the humerus moving as soon as possible.

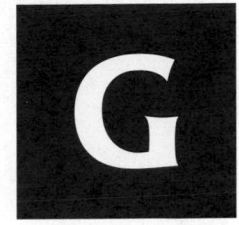

OTHER CONDITIONS AFFECTING THE HEAD AND NECK

35

TORTICOLLIS

Fiona Rattray

> **Torticollis is an abnormal positioning of the head and neck relative to the body.**

The word torticollis is derived from the Latin "tortus", or twisted, and "collum", or neck. A common term is "wry neck". The typical presentation of torticollis has the head and neck sidebent *towards* the affected side, the face turned *away from* the affected side and the shoulder on the affected side *raised (Figure 35.1).* Depending on the specific structures involved, the neck may be in extension, if levator scapula is involved *(Arat, 1973),* or in flexion if sternocleidomastoid is most affected *(Souza, 1997).*

There are several types of torticollis. Since these arise from different causes and have different treatment approaches, it is important for the therapist to determine which type of dysfunction the client has. The affected muscles are the ipsilateral sternocleidomastoid, upper trapezius, levator scapula and scalene muscles and the contralateral splenius cervicis, splenius capitis, multifidi, rotatores and suboccipitals.

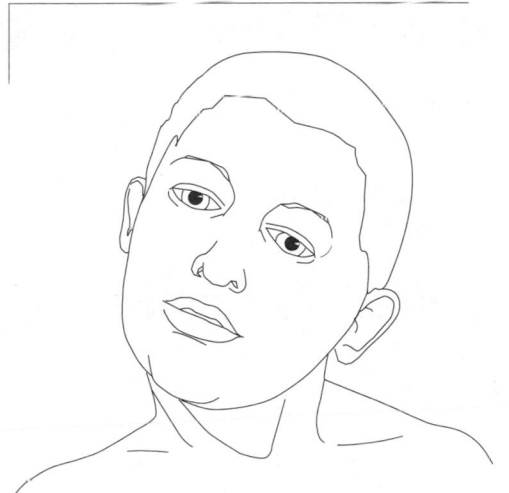

Figure 35.1
Left-sided torticollis with head and neck bent to the left, face turned to the right and left shoulder raised. Note broad, shortened left sternocleidomastoid.

Acute Acquired Torticollis

Acute acquired torticollis is a painful unilateral shortening or spasm of neck muscles resulting in an abnormal head position.

477

The shortening or spasm may result from latent trigger points that have become active by being left in a shortened position (shortening activation). For example, shortened positions arise from holding a telephone to one ear with the shoulder or falling asleep in an awkward position. Sleeping where a cold breeze or air conditioning is blowing on the neck may chill a muscle and activate a trigger point in sternocleidomastoid. Pain is felt if a muscle containing an active trigger point is actively or passively stretched. As the muscle is lengthened to the point of pain, a protective muscle spasm sets in that painfully prevents further lengthening *(Travell, Simons, 1983)*.

"Pseudotorticollis" is described as painful limitation of all neck movement due to idiopathic global muscle spasm *(Souza, 1997)*. While the person cannot move the head in any direction without pain, the head is held in neutral, not in the typical torticollis position of sidebending and rotation. There is no obvious trauma or cause leading to pseudotorticollis.

Causes of acute acquired torticollis are:

➤ **activation of latent trigger points** in cervical muscles, including ipsilateral sternocleidomastoid, scalenes and levator scapula *(Arat, 1973)*, and contralateral splenius capitis and suboccipital muscles;

➤ **subluxation of C1 on C2** due to trauma such as whiplash or sudden turning of the head *(Arat, 1973)* which may be the cause or effect of muscle spasm in the neck. *Reflex muscle guarding* is muscle spasm in response to pain following acute local tissue injury. Muscle guarding may result from referred pain *(Kisner, Colby, 1990; Janda, 1991)*. An *intrinsic muscle spasm* results from the pain of trauma or as a reflex contraction in response to infection, emotional stress or cold. Lack of movement retains painfully irritating metabolites. The muscle responds to the pain by staying in spasm *(Kisner, Colby, 1990; Cailliet, 1993; Rachlin, 1994)*;

➤ **facet joint irritation** with meniscoid entrapment elsewhere in the cervical spine following trauma, jarring of the spine or abrupt movement which may cause cervical spasm *(Brukner, Khan, 1993)*;

➤ **infection** following tonsillectomy, or inflammation of the throat or cervical lymphatic nodes;

➤ **disc-related pain** with cervical degenerative disc disease *(Boyling, Palastanga, 1994)*.

Symptom Picture of Acute Acquired Torticollis

✦ This condition can affect children and adults. The onset is usually sudden; the client may "just wake up with it".

✦ The neck and head are in the typical torticollis position. Some amount of neck extension or flexion may also be present.

✦ The affected muscles are shortened and in spasm.

✦ Pain is pronounced, especially on movement. The person may not move the head, neck or shoulder at all for fear of increasing the pain.

✦ Breathing is often apical and rapid. There is a pained facial expression.

478

✦ If trigger points in sternocleidomastoid are affected, tinnitus, nausea or tearing of the eye on the shortened, affected side may be present. Referred pain is present in the specific pattern of each affected muscle.

✦ If facet joint irritation with meniscoid entrapment is present, the pain came on suddenly following an abrupt neck movement. Pain may also be felt between the scapulae. Forward flexion and sidebending are away from the side with the affected facet joint (*Brukner, Khan, 1993*). The person is usually under the age of 30 years.

✦ If cervical degenerative disc disease is the cause, the pain has a gradual onset; the person wakes up with the torticollis after sleeping in an awkward posture. The sleeping position may allow the nuclear material of the disc to shift slightly (*Edwardson, 1995*). Pain is usually in the lower cervical spine and into the upper thoracic spine, occasionally into the arm (*Boyling, Palastanga, 1994*). The person is usually over 30 years of age.

Medically, acute acquired torticollis is treated with analgesics and muscle relaxants. With pseudotorticollis, chiropractic manipulation or physiotherapy may be used; it may also resolve on its own (*Souza, 1997*).

Congenital Torticollis

Congenital torticollis is a contracturing of one sternocleidomastoid muscle resulting in an abnormal head position.

This type of torticollis is present from infancy. Unless corrected by stretching or surgically dividing the contractured structures, the condition continues through childhood and into adulthood.

There have been several theories as to the cause of congenital torticollis. These include: trauma in the birth process causing inflammation and, later, fibrosing of the affected sternocleidomastoid; malposition of the fetus *in utero*; and torsion of the fetus's cranial bones.

Trauma in the birth process, perhaps due to forceps delivery, cesarean section or breech birth, may lead to intramuscular hemmorrhage in sternocleidomastoid. In the healing process, scar tissue creates fibrosing of the muscle and surrounding connective tissue. Inflammation affecting the cervical lymphatic nodes is also thought to cause fibrosing of sternocleidomastoid.

Tissue ischemia may also be a contributing factor. Interestingly, this ischemia may occur in other muscles, such as vastus lateralis, which are affected by contractures similar to the fibrosis seen in sternocleidomastoid. This ischemia may be caused by intra-uterine pressures and fetal malposition (*Jones, 1968*).

In terms of cranial bones, torsion of the occiput on the sphenoid bone and changes in the angulation of the occiput to the maxillofacial bones are documented as producing torticollis in infants (*Jones, 1968*). Subluxation of C1 on C2 can produce similar results. Over time, fascia surrounding the affected cranial bones and shortened muscles in the neck contracts. Hemihypoplasia (facial bone asymmetry) can occur. The maxilla, zygoma, temporal bone and eye on the affected side are more posterior (*Jones, 1968; Magee, 1992*). A scoliosis then develops secondary to congenital torticollis.

Imbalances in the cranial membranes may also cause congenital torticollis. "The falx [cerebri] and tentorium...could conceivably affect the distribution of gravitational forces" thought to create plagiocephaly *(Jones, 1968)*. Plagiocephaly, a cranial asymmetry where one frontal region and the diagonal occipital area are flattened while the opposite frontal and occipital regions are prominent, is also associated with congenital torticollis and scoliosis.

➤ **Causes of congenital torticollis are idiopathic**, not clearly understood.

Predisposing factors may be trauma, tissue ischemia, cranial bone torsion or cranial membrane dysfunction.

Symptom Picture of Congenital Torticollis

✦ This condition is present from infancy. It may develop over days *(Souza, 1997)* or two to three weeks after birth *(Jones, 1968)*.

✦ The client presents in the typical torticollis position.

✦ There is contracture, thickening and shortening of one sternocleidomastoid and the scalenes and associated fascia; there may or may not be a palpable mass in the muscle.

✦ The person is unable to move the neck normally due to the contracture. The condition is not described as painful.

✦ Other postural dysfunctions such as scoliosis and hemihypoplasia are likely present. Over time, there may be compression on cranial nerves and vasculature, temporomandibular joint dysfunction on the affected side, degeneration of the cervical discs and osteoarthritis of the cervical spine.

Medically, congenital torticollis is initially treated conservatively with muscle stretching. Physical therapy may lengthen sternocleidomastoid if therapy is persistently applied. This may take up to one year *(Souza, 1997)*. If there is no progress, the affected muscle is surgically divided. Areas of fibrosis are removed. The muscle may be left severed, as there have been cases where torticollis returns with reunion of the muscle. Taut bands present in the omohyoid muscle, fascia colli and the carotid fascial sheath are removed. After surgery, the person is immobilized for three days. This is followed by active free and passive relaxed range of motion for the neck. Posture is retrained so the dysfunction does not recur. Surgery has been noted to relieve the facial asymmetry *(Jones, 1968)*.

Spasmodic Torticollis

Spasmodic torticollis is a localized dystonia resulting in an involuntary spasm of cervical muscles and an abnormal head position.

This uncontrollable rhythmic spasm of the neck muscles, often worse when the person is under stress, is embarrassing socially. Spasmodic torticollis is now recognized as being organic in nature. It was once called "hysterical torticollis" and was thought to have a psychogenic origin *(Cyriax, 1991)*.

Causes of spasmodic torticollis are:

➤ **idiopathic** in four out of five cases. It appears linked to depression, severe stress, social or personal upheavals and occupational positioning of the head;

➤ **central nervous system lesions** such as encephalitis and basal ganglion diseases;

➤ **malformation** of the atlanto-occipital articulation;

➤ **postural dysfunction** such as scoliosis;

➤ **trauma** to the head and neck;

➤ **iatrogenic** with treatment of Parkinsons by the drug levodopa.

Symptom Picture of Spasmodic Torticollis

✦ This condition has an adult onset.

✦ The client presents in the typical torticollis position.

✦ The affected muscles in the neck jerk and twitch, and the affected shoulder shrugs uncontrollably. The twitching may spread to both the facial and arm muscles (*Chusid, 1985*).

Contraindications

✦ For any torticollis, avoid full stretches to the sternocleidomastoid muscle if the vertebral artery test is positive or if the client experiences dizziness with the stretch (*Travell, Simons, 1983*). Avoid working over the pulse of the carotid triangle immediately anterior to the sternocleidomastoid muscle and inferior to the angle of the mandible.

✦ For **acute acquired torticollis**, do not passively stretch the spasmodic muscles.

✦ For **congenital torticollis,** if working with infants, use reduced pressure when treating the contractures.

✦ For **spasmodic torticollis**, painful techniques, joint play and local direct massage are contraindicated as they may make the spasm more pronounced (*Bleton, 1994*).

✦ Spasmodic torticollis may be intermittent or permanent. The intensity of the spasm varies according to the position of the person's head. The condition may sometimes spontaneously remit.

✦ Sixty-three per cent of cases resolve while 37 per cent persist or worsen (*Bleton, 1994*).

✦ Factors that *exacerbate* the condition are changes of position, being in public or in stressful situations and wearing a cervical collar.

✦ Factors that *improve* the condition are lying down with the arms raised, applying slight pressure to the chin with one finger, sleeping and carrying something such as a shoulder bag.

Medically, spasmodic torticollis is treated with antispasmodic medication and injections of botulism toxin, which temporarily paralyse the muscles (*Hopkins, 1994*). At one time surgical intervention was used — sectioning the spinal accessory nerve (*Chusid, 1985*). Manipulation and mechanical traction of the cervical spine appear to make the condition worse (*Bleton, 1994*).

Recently, more success has been achieved with biofeedback (*Basmajian, Wolf, 1990*), agonist contraction, relaxation and postural retraining (*Bleton, 1994*).

Treatment Considerations

Assessment

✦ **Health History Questions** (for all types of torticollis): When was the onset and what is the frequency of the condition? Is there any history of neck or spine trauma, or birth trauma (if known)? What is the client's daily posture and sleeping posture? What relieves and aggravates the condition? Is the client taking any specific medication or parallel therapies? Is the condition painful? What is the type and location of the pain? Are there any associated conditions such as temporomandibular joint dysfunction?

✍ **Observations** include a full **postural assessment**, checking for any other postural dysfunctions such as scoliosis. With a typical torticollis posture, there is a cervical scoliosis convex to the unaffected side; that is, with a left torticollis, the neck sidebends to the left, the face rotates to the right, the left shoulder is elevated and there is a right cervical scoliosis *(Kendall et al., 1993)*. The apex is usually at C4 *(Arat, 1973)*. The neck may also be in extension or flexion with acute acquired torticollis. There are often facial bone asymmetries with congenital torticollis. For example, the maxilla, zygoma and temporal bones on the affected side are more posterior, making the eye on the affected side appear more recessed. The mandible may deviate to the affected side *(Magee, 1992)*.

✍ **Palpation** of an acutely spasmodic muscle may reveal heat, point tenderness, firmness and increased tone. A contractured muscle may be tender and feel cool due to ischemia, and be hard and fibrous.

✍ **Testing:**

- **AF** and **PR ROM** on the neck, thorax and shoulder are performed for all types of torticollis. With **acute acquired torticollis** and **spasmodic torticollis**, active free movement is painful and very restricted when attempting to take the neck and head out of the torticollis position. Passive relaxed movement away from the affected side is restricted with a muscle-spasm end feel. With **congenital torticollis**, active free movement away from the affected side is very restricted. Passive relaxed movement away from the affected side is very restricted with a leathery end feel.

- **AR strength testing** with acquired torticollis, performed *once the spasm has reduced*, or with congenital torticollis may reveal weakness of the contralateral **anterior** and **anterolateral** neck muscles, as well as the ipsilateral **posterolateral** neck extensors *(Kendall et al., 1993)*.

- **Compression** and **cervical distraction tests** are used to differentiate a cervical nerve root compression that may underlie an acute acquired torticollis. The **vertebral artery test** rules out cerebral vascular insufficiencies once the spasm has reduced. **Spurling's test** performed after the spasm has reduced may also indicate facet joint irritation.

Massage for Acute Acquired Torticollis

✋ **Positioning** of the client is in supine. Sidelying on the unaffected side with supporting pillows under the head may be possible depending on the client's comfort. The prone position is not tolerated. **Diaphragmatic breathing** is an important part of this treatment, decreasing sympathetic nervous system firing and spasm. **Hydrotherapy** applications depend on the type of spasm or shortening that is present. Local **cold** applications such as an ice pack are used for an analgesic effect, while **heat** is used with trigger points to increase local circulation and flush out metabolites.

- The treatment goals are to decrease pain, spasm and abnormal positioning while working within the client's pain tolerance. Due to the painful nature of this condition, it is important that the therapist gain the client's trust. The client must be reassured that the treatment itself will not be painful. The client's head must be well stabilized during the massage so he is not worried about uncontrolled movement causing more pain.

- Treatment begins on the side that is not in spasm, to accustom the client to the therapist's touch. While supporting the client's head on the affected side with one hand, the therapist uses slow, gentle effleurage and petrissage to the anterior and posterolateral muscles on the unaffected side.

- The therapist then moves to the side in spasm. Techniques that use direct pressure may be too painful for a muscle that is acutely spasmodic. Instead, indirect techniques that employ spinal reflexes, such as agonist contraction *by the client (Lewit, 1993; Chaitow, 1988)*, Golgi tendon organ release and the origin and insertion technique by the therapist, are used. All techniques should be pain free.

- Agonist contraction for the sternocleidomastoid muscle involves contraction in two different directions: sidebending one way and rotation in the opposite direction. It is simpler to break these down into the cardinal planes of motion and perform them one at a time. For example, with a left-sided torticollis, the client isometrically and submaximally resists sidebending to the right. As the spasm diminishes, the therapist passively moves the head a bit out of left sidebending, stopping if there is pain or restriction. This is repeated a few times, until the head is closer to midline. Then the rotation component is addressed as the client isometrically and submaximally resists rotation to the left. The head is again gradually moved out of right rotation.

- Golgi tendon organ release and the origin and insertion technique are performed on the sternal, clavicular and mastoid attachments of the sternocleidomastoid muscle.

- Several applications of the same technique or combinations of different techniques may be necessary to reduce a spasm. The therapist should not focus only on the spasm. After some treatment to the affected sternocleidomastoid muscle, the surrounding tissue and synergists are massaged. This is followed by a return to treatment of the spasm. Work to the side not in spasm, including splenius cervicis, splenius capitis, multifidi, rotatores and suboccipital muscles, is also interspersed with work to the affected side.

- As the spasm of sternocleidomastoid diminishes and disappears, scalenes, upper trapezius and levator scapula on the affected side are treated in a similar manner.

- Initially it may be difficult to reach the scalene muscles directly to perform Golgi tendon organ release until the torticollis is significantly reduced. In this case, agonist contraction is indicated. Continuing with the example of a left-sided torticollis, the client isometrically and submaximally resists: neck sidebending to the right to inhibit left middle scalene *(Figure 35.2)*; neck sidebending to the right followed by head rotation to the left to inhibit left anterior scalene; and sidebending to the right followed by rotation to the right to inhibit left posterior scalene *(Travell, Simons, 1983)*.

- **Once the spasm has decreased** or is less painful for on-site work, gentle direct

483

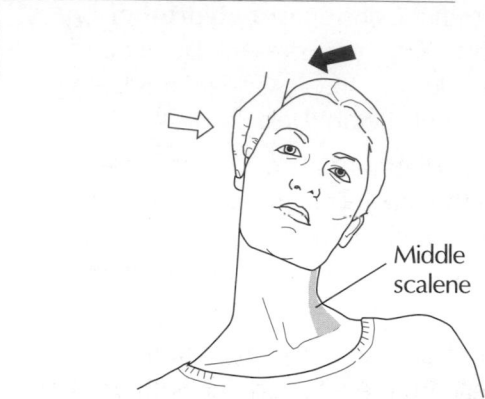

(A) To inhibit spasm of left middle scalene, client isometrically resists sidebending to right (black arrow).

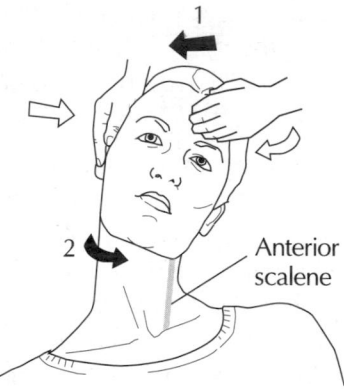

(B) To inhibit spasm of left anterior scalene, client (1) isometrically resists right sidebending (black arrow) then (2) isometrically resists left rotation.

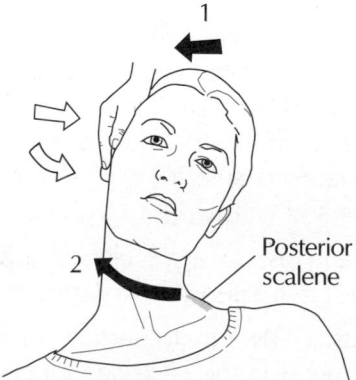

(C) To inhibit spasm of left posterior scalene, client (1) isometrically resists right sidebending (black arrow) then (2) isometrically resists right rotation.

Figure 35.2
Agonist contraction for left scalenes when the neck is in spasm.

techniques such as vibrations, stroking, fingertip kneading and light muscle stripping are used on the affected muscles. Trigger points in sternocleidomastoid can be treated with a light pincer-grasp technique. All other muscles in the neck are assessed for trigger points and hypertonicity and treated within the comfort levels of the client. Strokes that increase local circulation to flush out metabolites are important to include. Pain-free passive relaxed range of motion of the neck is also indicated.

Once the head and neck are in a neutral position, Golgi tendon organ release for the suboccipitals and long-axis traction on the occiput are employed. Joint play to any hypomobile cervical vertebrae is applied in a pain-free manner.

The therapist must significantly decrease the tone in the acutely spasmodic muscles before applying a slow passive stretch to any affected muscles following trigger point treatment. To fully stretch sternocleidomastoid, the client's neck must go into extension. The client may be apprehensive or unwilling to have the neck placed in this position in the current treatment. In this case the therapist may use PIR, which is a less aggressive technique, perform partial stretches that do not go into extension, perform stretches in subsequent treatments or give them for self-care. In all of the following stretches, the shoulder on the affected side is stabilized.

To stretch the clavicular head of the sternocleidomastoid muscle, the client's head is rotated *away* from the side to be stretched and the clavicle is stabilized *(Figure 35.3)*. To stretch the sternal head of sternocleidomastoid, the head is rotated *towards* the affected side and the chin is *tucked into the shoulder*, elevating the mastoid process. The stretch is held for only a few seconds. If the client feels dizzy, the head is returned to neutral immediately. To stretch **middle scalene**, the neck is sidebent to the unaffected side with the client's head in the neutral position. To stretch **anterior scalene**, the neck is sidebent to the unaffected side and the head is rotated to the *affected* side. To stretch **posterior scalene**, the neck is sidebent

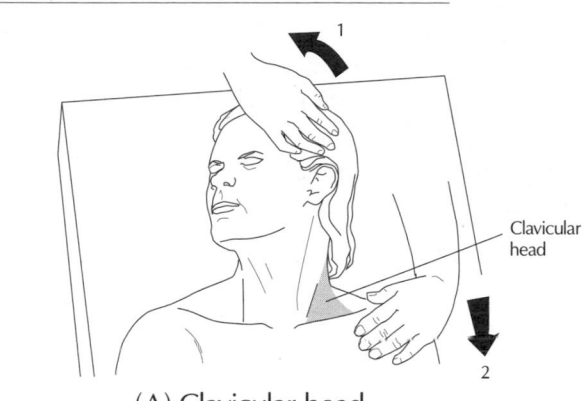

(A) Clavicular head

(1) rotate the head to the right side and (2) stabilize the clavicle.

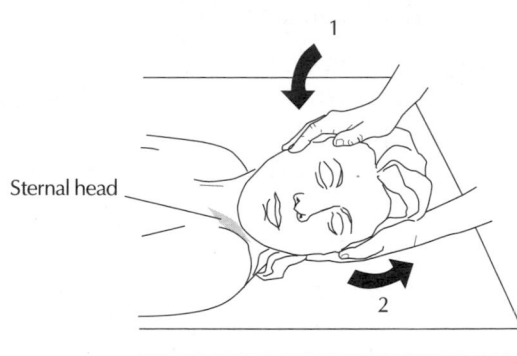

(B) Sternal head

(1) rotate the head to the left side and (2) with therapist's hand on the occiput, elevate the left mastoid process, tucking the chin into the left shoulder.

Figure 35.3
Stretches for left sternocleidomastoid.

to the unaffected side and the head is rotated to the *unaffected* side (*Travell, Simons, 1983*). Upper trapezius and levator scapulae are also stretched.

🖐 The treatment is finished with soothing stroking and petrissage to the muscles of mastication, the forehead and the scalp. In subsequent treatments, once the abnormal head position has gone, postural dysfunctions or hypertonic muscles in the thorax may be treated in the prone position.

🖐 If the torticollis results from facet joint irritation or cervical degenerative disc disease, once the spasm has gone using the above treatment, long-axis traction and pain-free passive relaxed range of motion and joint play are used (*Brukner, Khan, 1993; Edwardson, 1995*). See the chapter on degenerative disc disease for more details.

Self-care for Acute Acquired Torticollis

✍ Diaphragmatic breathing, hydrotherapy, self-massage and the stretches listed above are used by the client. Before stretching, complete active free range of motion is used to prepare the tissues.

✍ Postural imbalances and other contributing factors are addressed to prevent recurrence. For example, if the client reads in bed, the book is held in front instead of to one side, which unequally loads one sternocleidomastoid. If the client sleeps on one side, the pillow is placed between the head and shoulder, keeping the head in midline with the spine. This prevents sternocleidomastoid and scalenes from remaining in a shortened position (*Travell, Simons, 1983*). A travelling neck support pillow is used on long airplane flights to support the head and neck in a neutral position while the client sleeps.

✍ Any weak muscles are strengthened.

✍ The client is referred to a chiropractor if cervical vertebral subluxations are present.

Massage for Congenital Torticollis

✋ If the client is an infant or child, consent to treat is required from the parent(s) or guardian. The parent may wish to be present in the treatment room to learn how to perform the techniques or just to observe the treatment. The treatment may last for five or 10 minutes initially, gradually working up to longer periods of time as the client can tolerate them. It may take months to fully lengthen the tissues.

✋ **Positioning** of the client is in supine. **Hydrotherapy** is heat to the affected structures, applied unilaterally. If the client is old enough to understand instructions for **diaphragmatic breathing**, these are explained. If not, the therapist works with the client's breathing.

✋ The goals of treatment are to lengthen the contractured structures, reduce the abnormal positioning, restore range of motion of the head and neck, strengthen any weak structures and, if necessary, educate the parents regarding self-care.

✋ Initially, gentle fascial stretching is applied to the affected sternocleidomastoid in a segmental fashion. Lighter pressure is used with infants; slightly more pressure may be tolerated by children.

✋ The therapist stabilizes the fascia over the clavicle with the fingers of one hand. The fingers of the other hand grasp the sternocleidomastoid muscle in a pincer grasp one centimetre away from the clavicle. A fascial spread is applied to the tissue. This is repeated segmentally along sternocleidomastoid. Fascial spreading is also used on the scalenes, pectoral fascia, upper trapezius and levator scapulae.

✋ Gentle stretching *(Kisner, Colby, 1990)* is used on the affected muscles, with the long-term goal being to reposition the head in the opposite torticollis position just for the purpose of the stretch *(Thomson et al., 1991; Cyriax, Coldham, 1984)*. See the stretching information in acute acquired torticollis for specifics. Less pressure is used with clients who are very young.

✋ Non-Swedish techniques such as neuromuscular therapy and the craniosacral technique are indicated for cranial bone and cranial membrane distortions.

Self-care for Congenital Torticollis

✍ With an infant, the parents are shown how to perform passive stretching and repositioning of the head *(Thomson et al., 1991)*.

✍ A range of motion retraining exercise is used from about three months of age when the infant is able to focus his eyes. The infant is supine. A brightly coloured object (for example, a rattle) is placed in the infant's line of vision about 40 centimetres away from the head. The baby is allowed to focus on it. The parent stabilizes the infant's torso with one hand to prevent it from moving; the other hand moves the rattle slowly away from the affected side. The motion is restarted each time the infant loses focus on the rattle, until maximum active free range of motion is achieved.

✍ Referrals may be made to practitioners who are trained in neuromuscular therapy and craniosacral techniques if the therapist is not trained in these methods.

Massage for Spasmodic Torticollis

✋ **Positioning** of the client is in supine. Sidelying on the unaffected side with supporting pillows under the head may also be possible. **Diaphragmatic breathing** is an important part of this treatment, decreasing sympathetic nervous system firing and spasm. **Hydrotherapy** is heat to reduce hypertonicity.

✋ Treatment goals are to reduce sympathetic nervous system firing and spasm, to normalize head position, to restore range of motion and to educate the client on preventive techniques and spasm control.

✋ The main focus of the treatment is a full-body relaxation massage. Techniques used are soothing and gentle. Any compensatory structures are treated; the diaphragm, intercostals and pectoral muscles are also worked.

✋ Direct massage on the neck is contraindicated as this may make the acutely spasmodic muscle worse. Instead, submaximal isometric agonist contraction is used *(Bleton, 1994)*. See the acute acquired torticollis section for specific details.

✋ In subsequent treatments, gentle cervical traction and work to correct scoliotic curves may be helpful. Positive results may occur within six months to one year *(Bleton, 1994)*.

Self-care for Spasmodic Torticollis

✍ The client is helped to control the spasm with: diaphragmatic breathing; pain-free active free range of motion of the neck; agonist contraction — for example, using gentle pressure against the mandible on the side to which the head is turned *(Travell, Simons, 1983)*; and slow passive stretches *(Bleton, 1994)*.

✍ The client is referred for biofeedback sessions and relaxation courses to help control the spasm *(Kisner, Colby, 1990)*.

See also stress reduction, trigger points, relevant postural concerns, whiplash, tension headache, degenerative disc disease, osteoarthritis, Parkinsons and temporomandibular joint dysfunction for related treatments.

36

TENSION HEADACHE

Fiona Rattray

Tension headache is a muscle-contraction-type headache.

Tension headaches are headaches with muscular origins and are associated with trigger points and other myofascial pain syndromes *(Travell, Simons, 1983)*.

There are numerous terms used to describe types of headaches. The International Headache Society (IHS) has standardized the terminology and description of headache symptoms; there are 12 categories of headache types according to the IHS. These standard terms are used in this text *(Silberstein et al., 1998)*.

✦ Headaches are divided into primary and secondary conditions.

- **Primary headaches** are those in which the headache *is* the condition, such as tension headache or migraine.
- **Secondary headaches** are a *result* of an underlying pathology, such as hypertension or head trauma. It is important to note that a person may suffer from more than one category of headache at a time.

The cause of a headache can range from a life-threatening disease to a minor complaint. It is, therefore, important for the therapist to be alert for signs that the client's headache is a red flag for an underlying pathology. If this is suspected, the client is referred for medical diagnosis. However, only 0.004 per cent of all headaches are due to a serious pathology *(Cady, Fox, 1995)*.

Other Headaches with Muscular Origins

✦ **Cervicogenic headache** describes a headache that is unilateral and frontal, arising from structures in the neck *(Davidoff, 1995)*.

✦ **Spinally mediated headache** describes a headache with origins in trigger points (in muscles of the neck and thorax as low as the 10th thoracic vertebra), as well as in cervical facet joints, cervical interspinous ligaments and the cervical intervertebral discs *(Cady, Fox, 1995)*. Spinal dysfunction can affect the sympathetic nervous system and lead to headaches. Under certain circumstances, stress (including pain) in the muscles, tendons and ligaments at any level of the spine leads to afferent hyperactivity (increased nerve firing) of the sympathetic nervous system at that vertebral level. This hyperactivity allows stimuli, that are normally ineffectual, to produce efferent firing from the specific segment of the spine. Consequently, the skeletal muscles (such as erector spinae) and visceral organs innervated by that segment of the spine are kept in a state of overactivity *(Chaitow, 1988)*. This is termed "spinal facilitation". In one study, spinal facilitation occurred with a 3/8-inch heel lift. Areas affected by facilitation may have a skin temperature up to 10 degrees cooler than surrounding skin *(Cady, Fox, 1995)*.

- The process of facilitation is not completely understood, and why some postural dysfunctions and traumas cause facilitation and others do not is not known. It is thought that emotional excitation such as stress may also increase facilitation, as the spinal cord may amplify intense input.

- Facilitation is also possible in the cranial nerves, such as the trigeminal nerve (CNV) supplying the muscles of the face *(Vander et al., 1994)*. Facilitation of this nerve could occur by teeth-clenching. The accessory nerve (CNXI) innervates the trapezius muscle; facilitation could occur through faulty head posture. People with chronic headaches have increased tension in trapezius, temporalis and masseter muscles.

- Spinal facilitation is also reported with migraine and cluster headaches. Perhaps facilitation of the vagus nerve (CNX) which synapses with the smooth muscle of the stomach and small and large intestines is involved in the nausea people with migraines experience.

✦ **Chronic daily headache** (CDH) is a term used to describe chronic daily or near-daily headaches that are constant but with fluctuations in pain levels. There are often disturbances of deep, restorative sleep. Chronic daily headaches may consist of several types of head pain: tension headaches, post-traumatic headaches, migraines, drug-associated headaches, fibromyalgia headaches, spinally mediated headaches and temporomandibular headaches. Chronic pain lowers the quality of life of the sufferer; there is increased stress and a lower irritability threshold.

➤ **Causes of tension headache are trigger points** that refer pain into the head and neck.

Predisposing factors are:

➤ **trigger point stimuli** and **perpetuating factors** including trauma (to head, neck or spine), acute muscle overload, infection (such as sinusitis), fatigue, chilling of the muscle, referred pain and emotional stress;

➤ **sleep disturbance** of deep restorative sleep. This is present with myofascial pain syndromes;

➤ **postural imbalances** such as hyperkyphosis, head-forward posture and scoliosis;

➤ **temporomandibular joint** dysfunction.

Medically, tension headache is treated with analgesics such as Aspirin and Tylenol. Some physicians may inject trigger points with a 0.5 per cent procaine solution, followed by a stretch to the muscle *(Travell, Simons, 1983)*.

490

Referrals may be made by the physician for stress management with chronic daily headaches. Persons suffering chronic daily headaches are first slowly detoxified from medication use to prevent rebound headaches. A combination of physical therapy, appropriate medication, psychotherapy, sleep management and stress reduction (including biofeedback for muscle relaxation) is currently used in some headache clinics (*Silberstein et al., 1998*).

In a recent study, dissatisfaction with their medical encounter was reported by almost three-quarters of headache patients. Perhaps this is due to medical training which often focuses on headache as a symptom, rather than a primary condition. When diagnostic tests fail to reveal an underlying pathology, physicians may feel their responsibility to the patient has ended (*Cady, Fox, 1995*).

Symptom Picture

- Estimates of the prevalence of tension headaches vary; figures suggest that up to 63 per cent of men and up to 86 per cent of women experience them; chronic tension headaches occur in 3 per cent of people (*Silberstein et al., 1998*).

- There is a family history in 40 to 50 per cent of these headache sufferers (*Silberstein et al., 1998*).

- The pain is bilateral, diffuse and constant with tension headaches. It may be dull or vise-like. The location of the pain is often in the referral pattern of trigger points in specific muscles (*Travell, Simons, 1983*). Cervicogenic and spinally mediated headaches may have associated neck and shoulder pain. Chronic daily headache tends to have accompanying shoulder and periscapular pain.

- These headaches begin in early adulthood.

- The frequency is variable; tension headaches may be episodic, and may or may not have easily identifiable times of onset or end. Episodic headaches have clearly identifiable endpoints and occur one after another; chronic daily headaches are constant, with fluctuations in pain levels. Chronic headaches may also be associated with a history of childhood abuse (*Cady, Fox, 1995*).

- The duration of the symptoms is from 30 minutes to weeks. A chronic tension headache is one that lasts more than 15 days (*Cady, Fox, 1995*).

- The onset of tension headaches is usually later in the afternoon after latent trigger points have been activated.

- Associated symptoms are muscle tenderness and stiffness, hypertonicity in the affected muscles and loss of appetite. If sternocleidomastoid is affected with trigger points, the client may experience nausea, vertigo and tinnitus (*Travell, Simons, 1983*).

- Aggravating factors include stress, fatigue, cold, hypoglycemia and poor posture or decrease in range of motion of the head and neck. Infections such as herpes simplex or sinusitis can perpetuate trigger points.

- During the headache, the person wishes to rest; there is mild disability, but the person can usually function in activities of daily living. Stretching or heat applied to the shoulder muscles may help.

Contraindications

✦ Do not work deeply during a tension headache. Avoid vigorous techniques or deep pressure when treating hyperirritable trigger points, since "kick-back" pain may result. Kick-back pain is a recurrence of the client's symptoms hours or days after treatment. This is especially true if ischemic compressions are applied too quickly and deeply, released too quickly and not followed by either a passive stretch and heat or slow, full active free range of motion and heat.

✦ There may be associated postural dysfunctions. Temporomandibular joint dysfunction may be present.

Differentiating Other Headaches

✦ With new headaches that begin later in adult life, especially after age 50, the client should be referred to a physician. New primary headache is rare in the elderly; the headache may be secondary to an underlying pathology (Davidoff, 1995).

✦ See the migraine chapter for differentiating other types of headaches.

Treatment Considerations

HEALTH HISTORY QUESTIONS

✦ Does the client have a headache now?

✦ When was the onset of the present headache? If the client has a history of headaches, at what age did they begin? Many primary headache symptoms begin in adolescence or early adulthood.

✦ Was there a trauma to the head, neck or spine that may indicate a post-whiplash or post-concussion headache?

✦ Does the client have a temperature, transient rash or stiff neck, indicating possible meningitis?

✦ Does the client experience sleep disturbances?

✦ What is the location and quality of the pain? Does it refer anywhere?

✦ What are other symptoms? How frequent are they?

✦ What is the duration of the headache?

✦ What was the time of onset? Is this the same for recurring headaches?

✦ What relieves the headache?

✦ What aggravates the headache?

✦ Does the client take medication for this condition, including prescription drugs, over-the-counter medication, herbal preparations or supplements?

✦ Are there any underlying pathologies such as fibromyalgia, degenerative disc disease, osteoarthritis of the cervical spine or dental abnormalities such as temporomandibular joint dysfunction?

✦ Has the client suffered a recent cold or influenza attack that could precipitate a tension headache?

✦ Is the client using parallel therapies such as chiropractic or osteopathic manipulation, biofeedback or acupuncture?

Further Assessment

✍ **Observations** include a full postural assessment, looking for head-forward posture, hyperkyphosis, hyperlordosis, scoliosis or pes planus.

✍ **Palpation:**

- The neck, shoulder and thoracic muscles and muscles of mastication may be hypertonic and tender. The muscles of respiration are also likely to be hypertonic, including the diaphragm, intercostals, scalenes and sternocleidomastoids.

- Ischemia produces areas of coolness in the skin of the neck or thorax with trigger points and with spinally mediated headaches.

✍ **Testing:**

- **AF** and **PR ROM** are performed on the neck, thorax, shoulder and mandible. There is reduced cervical and thoracic mobility in AF and PR ranges of motion in muscles affected by trigger points. There may also be reduced ranges in mandibular motion.

- **AR strength testing** may reveal the affected neck, head and shoulder girdle muscles to be weaker.

- **Special tests,** including both **motion** and **static palpation**, are performed in the cervical and thoracic spine and may reveal areas of hyper- and hypomobility. **Passive relaxed atlanto-occipital** and **atlanto-axial articulation** may have restrictions. **Passive relaxed anterior** and **lateral spinous challenges**, as well as **first rib mobility** and **rib motion tests** may show areas of hypo- or hypermobility.

- **Spurling's, cervical compression** and **cervical distraction tests** are used to differentiate a facet joint irritation that may underlie the headache.

Massage

Sources recommend massage therapy for the treatment of tension headaches (*Travell, Simons, 1983 and 1992; Silberstein et al., 1998; Cady, Fox, 1995*).

During Headache

🖐 The treatment is in the context of a relaxation massage including unforced **diaphragmatic breathing.**

🖐 The **pre-treatment hydrotherapy** is heat to the *affected muscles.* Cold may be placed on the *referral pattern* for an analgesic effect.

🖐 **Positioning** may be in supine or sidelying. Prone may be poorly tolerated, as the face cradle may compress painful areas on the face. A towel may be used to cover the client's eyes in the supine position if the light is too bright.

🖐 Treatment goals are to reduce sympathetic nervous system firing, pain, hypertonicity, trigger points and joint dysfunctions and to increase range of motion and tissue health. All work is performed within the client's pain tolerance. An enriched lotion using pure essential oils such as lavender, peppermint or blue chamomile can be used. Twenty-five drops of essential oil are added to 50 ml. of vegetable oil *(Lawless, 1995).*

🖐 Treatment in the **supine** or **sidelying** position uses soothing Swedish techniques, such as effleurage, stroking and fingertip kneading on the pectorals and posterior neck muscles such as upper trapezius and levator scapulae to reduce hypertonicity. Petrissage is used on the muscles of mastication, facial muscles and scalp. Pain-free joint play is also used on hypomobile cervical vertebrae.

🖐 Trigger points are treated with muscle stripping and gentle ischemic compressions. Some common patterns:

- Upper trapezius referral is above the eye, around the ear and down the lateral neck in the shape of a question mark.

- Splenius capitis referrals are to the top of the head.

- Splenius cervicis referrals are to the temporal region and back of the neck.

- Occipitalis trigger points send pain to the posterior head; frontalis trigger points refer locally above the eye.

- The suboccipitals refer pain around the ear.

- Sternocleidomastoid trigger points refer to the occiput, around the eye, into the ear and across the forehead. Sternocleidomastoid can activate secondary trigger points in the anterior scalene muscle. Trigger points in temporalis refer to the temporal region and the teeth.

- The occipitofrontalis muscle refers above the eye and the back of the head. Masseter trigger points refer above the eye and into the ear, jaw and teeth *(Travell, Simons, 1983).*

🖐 PIR is used to gently increase range of motion at the neck following trigger point work.

🖐 As the treatment progresses, the therapist asks if the headache has substantially reduced or disappeared. If this is the case, all the affected muscles have been treated. If not, the therapist should include synergist and antagonist muscles that also refer to the headache area. However, in one massage appointment the therapist should maintain a balance between the desire to thoroughly inactivate all trigger points causing the headache and overtreatment.

🖐 The head, neck and shoulder massage is finished with passive range of motion, gentle long-axis traction or Golgi tendon organ release to the occiput.

If tolerated, work in the prone position includes general, soothing Swedish work to the shoulders and upper thoracic area. Areas of hypomobility in the thoracic spine and ribs are treated with joint play *(Edeling, 1994)*.

✋ Any underlying postural or joint dysfunctions are treated in subsequent visits. See the appropriate chapters for details.

Between Headaches

✋ Treatment goals are to reduce sympathetic nervous system firing, hypertonicity, trigger points and joint dysfunctions as well as to increase range of motion and tissue health.

✋ The treatment is similar to that which is performed during a headache, except that the therapist can be more vigorous; areas of restricted range of motion are addressed using joint play and fascial techniques.

Self-care

✍ The client should rest from activity following the treatment of trigger points.

✍ A hot bath or other hot hydrotherapy application is indicated for the affected muscles after trigger point therapy. Self-care hydrotherapy that may relieve a tension headache is contrast towels applied to the neck and head *(Moor et al.,1964)*.

✍ Diaphragmatic breathing is recommended to reduce stress levels and pain

✍ Self-massage, consisting of muscle stripping and alternating ischemic compressions and stretch, is recommended.

✍ The client should frequently repeat either slow, full, pain-free stretches or active free range of motion to the affected muscles. Slow stretching should also be performed before and after any activity.

✍ Strengthening exercises are given for any weak muscles. Isometric resistance can be performed for various neck muscles with the client using her hands to provide the resistance.

✍ Perpetuating factors should be reduced or eliminated; any postural imbalances should be corrected. Postural re-education such as Mitzvah or Feldenkrais movement therapy may be helpful.

See also stress reduction, trigger points, the postural dysfunction section, whiplash, torticollis, migraine, degenerative disc disease, temporomandibular joint dysfunction, sinusitis, constipation and osteoarthritis for related treatments.

✍ Sleeping in the prone position is avoided, as this stresses the neck muscles and facet joints.

✍ In terms of trigger point perpetuating factors, the client can be referred to a physician if metabolic imbalances may be present, to a naturopath or nutritionist if nutritional inadequacies are suspected or for orthotics if structural imbalances are present.

MIGRAINE

Fiona Rattray

> **Migraine headache is a paroxysmal neurological disorder with many signs and symptoms (Davidoff, 1995).**

While many studies have been published on migraine, there is not yet a satisfactory definition for the disorder. This may be because the symptoms of migraine differ from person to person, and even in a single individual or during a single episode.

The term "migraine" derives from the Greek word "hemicrania", or half the head, the common distribution of pain for this headache. While most people consider tension headache, migraine and cluster headaches to be distinct entities with head pain as the common symptom, some researchers believe they represent points on a continuum *(Cady, Fox, 1995)*.

✦ Headaches in general are divided into primary and secondary conditions.

- **Primary headaches** are those in which the headache *is* the condition, such as tension, migraine, mixed, transformational and cluster headaches. Episodic headaches have clearly identifiable endpoints.
- **Secondary headaches** are a *result* of an underlying pathology.

Since the cause of a headache can range from a life-threatening disease to a minor complaint, it is essential to accurately assess the client and refer out for medical diagnosis if necessary. However, only 0.004 per cent of all headaches are due to a serious pathology *(Cady, Fox, 1995)*.

Migraine Theories

Migraine headache is a poorly understood condition that affects the lives of millions. The concept that migraines may have a vascular origin was first put forward by the physician

Thomas Willis in 1672. By the 1930s this theory had become the **vascular model** of migraine, in which some unknown mechanism triggers vasoconstriction of the intercranial arteries. At this point the person may experience a migraine aura, or visual distortions. After the headache onset, vasodilation occurs in the arteries, producing pain.

However, the vascular model does not explain the migraine sufferers who do not respond to vasoconstricting drugs in the vasodilation stage and those who do not experience auras. The **neurogenic theory** (or trigeminovascular system theory) proposes that migraine is a primary disorder of the central nervous system. Pain-sensing neurons surrounding the blood vessels and dura mater of the brain arise from the trigeminal ganglion and the upper cervical dorsal roots of C1 and C2 *(Silberstein et al., 1998; Davidoff, 1995)*.

When a *migraine attack* begins, the trigeminovascular system may have been activated by triggers such as trauma, chemicals, acute hypertension or ischemia. A reduction in cerebral blood flow (oligemia) occurs, usually starting at the occiput. It moves in a wave across the cortex at two to three millimetres per minute. Studies indicate that aura is associated with this wave and that the same reduction in blood flow appears to be true for migraine without aura *(Sandler et al., 1996)*.

When the *headache* occurs, the pain-sensing neurons of the trigeminal system may be reacting to plasma proteins. These proteins are released by antidromic stimulation of the trigeminal nerve (nerve impulses travelling in the opposite direction of usual flow). The proteins cause cerebral blood vessel dilation, or a neurogenic inflammatory process. Over time, this may sensitize the nerve fibres to previously innocuous stimuli such as blood vessel pulsations or cervical muscle pain *(Silberstein et al., 1998; Olesen, Schmidt, 1993)*.

Migraine is, therefore, likely an instability in the control system that modulates incoming pain and cortical blood flow. This seems analogous to the "facilitation" process mentioned in the tension headache chapter *(Olesen, Schmidt, 1993)*. Serotonin, a neurochemical that helps regulate cerebral vasodilation and vasoconstriction, may also be involved in the whole process.

Other aggravating factors may play a part in migraine, especially those that influence the nerve roots of C1 and C2. One study found that 26 out of 27 people suffering headaches, including migraine, had postural dysfunctions such as hyperlordosis and head-forward posture *(Cady, Fox, 1995)*. Neck pain, including pain from whiplash, has precipitated migraines *(Davidoff, 1995)* as have trigger points in the neck.

History of Migraine

The agony of migraine has been described by people around the world for centuries. Many early cultures thought that headaches were a curse from the gods and goddesses, and appealed to them for help. A Sumerian inscription (from about 4000 BC) recommends that a "wise woman spin [the hair of a kid]...bind the head of the sick man [with the string]...cast the water of incantation...over him, that the headache may ascend to heaven" *(Cady, Fox, 1995)*. Ancient Egyptian physicians (about 1200 BC) tied a clay crocodile effigy to the head of the migraine sufferer with a strip of linen inscribed with the names of the gods. The pressure from either of these remedies may have alleviated the pain *(The College of Family Physicians of Canada, 1995a; Silberstein et al., 1998)*.

Other cultures used more pharmacological remedies. The ancient Incas used coca juice, containing cocaine, dripped on an incision in the scalp to relieve pain. In North America,

Native Americans used willow bark extract, a natural analgesic, for head pain. The ancient Chinese recognized several types of headaches, listed in **The Yellow Emperor's Classics of Internal Medicine** (about 1000 BC). These were treated with combinations of acupuncture, herbs, diet and lifestyle changes — techniques that work to this day (*Cady, Fox, 1995*).

While most people experience migraine as excruciating pain, some have found that the visual disturbances associated with vascular headache unlock creativity. In the twelfth century, Hildegaard von Bingen, a German abbess, scientist, artist and musician, painted and wrote descriptions of "visions" experienced during the aura of migraine. She described "a great star, most splendid and beautiful, with [an] exceeding multitude of falling stars" and images of zig-zag lines; the former is recognized today as scintillating scotoma, the latter as fortification spectra (*Silberstein et al., 1998*). Lewis Carroll, the author of Alice in Wonderland, used the perceptual disturbances he experienced during migraine in his stories. Alice grows tall or becomes short "like a telescope"; today these accurate descriptions are called Alice-in-Wonderland syndrome (*Davidoff, 1995*).

Causes of migraine headache are:

➤ **unknown**, perhaps a central nervous system disorder that produces secondary intracranial vasodilation followed by vasoconstriction;

➤ **genetics** may play a part; familial hemiplegic migraine is associated with chromosome 19 (*Sandler et al., 1996*).

✦ Triggering factors:

- **stress**, either emotional or physical;

- **foodstuffs and food additives** such as chocolate, cheese, citrus fruits, pickles, sour cream, onions, sausages, pork, alcoholic beverages (especially red wine), chocolate, monosodium glutamate and aspartame;

- **hunger** from skipping meals, dieting or eating inadequately;

- **medication** such as oral contraceptives and nitroglycerine used to treat angina;

- **weather change** where there is an alteration in barometric pressure;

- **visual stimuli** such as reflected sunlight, bright lights or computer screens;

- **auditory stimuli** such as loud music;

- **olfactory stimuli** such as perfumes, colognes, aftershave lotions, tobacco smoke, paint, diesel fuel and gasoline;

- **sleeping** too long, too little or at unusual times;

- **hormonal shifts** around ovulation, menstruation, pregnancy or breast-feeding;

- **allergies** to foods such as eggs, wheat, meat and milk.

✦ Aggravating factors:

- **movement** or change in position;

- **trigger points** in muscles that refer to the head and neck (*Davidoff, 1995; Travell, Simons, 1983*);

- **postural dysfunction** such as hyperkyphosis or hyperlordosis (*Edeling, 1994*).

Medically, migraine headache is often treated with prescription medication; however, the inappropriate use of medication can cause adverse reactions and even perpetuate the headache. Many migraine sufferers have found medical therapy ineffective, partially due to the undesirable side-effects of some of the prescribed medication *(Cady, Fox, 1995)*.

Medications can be symptomatic or preventative. In the 1880s the use of bromide combined with cannabis was recommended for acute migraines. Ergotamine tartrate, a vasoconstrictor, was first isolated in 1928 and used for migraine. Today, numerous drugs are used to treat migraine; the following are only some examples: isometheptene (Midrin) is a vasoconstrictor; Aspirin, naproxen and Anacin are analgesics; Fiorinal and Fioricet combine analgesics with barbiturates and sometimes codeine; Compazine and Thorazine are tranquillizers; and Sumatriptan (Imitrex) mimics serotonin.

The herb feverfew, fish oils with omega-3 fatty acids and magnesium supplements *(Cady, Fox, 1995; Theisler, 1990)* are used to reduce migraines.

At one time the migraine sufferer was believed to have a certain psychological profile of repressed feelings, perfectionism and anxiety, called the "migraine personality". However, studies have failed to support this concept *(Cady, Fox, 1995)*.

Symptom Picture

+ Twenty-five per cent of women and eight per cent of males are affected by migraines *(Sandler et al., 1996)*.

+ There is a family history in 70 per cent of people with migraines.

+ Before an attack, 50 per cent of migraine sufferers report fluid retention; moreover, an increase in stress and fatigue in the 24-hour period before the migraine seems to be a trigger *(Hogenhuis, Steiner, 1994)*.

+ The pain is pulsating and of moderate to severe intensity; it is unilateral in 60 per cent of migraine sufferers. It often begins as a dull ache or sensation of pressure which gradually localizes to one area and becomes more intense and pounding over several minutes or hours. It may also begin abruptly, spreading into a more global, throbbing migraine. Physical exertion may exacerbate symptoms. In some cases a migraine may be persistent and severe enough to require hospitalization (status migrainosus). However, some migraine sufferers experience bilateral, non-throbbing headaches *(Cady, Fox, 1995)*.

+ These headaches can begin in childhood, adolescence or early adulthood *(Cady, Fox, 1995)*.

+ The frequency is rarely greater than one per week.

+ The symptoms last for four to 72 hours.

+ The onset is variable, with an early morning onset common.

+ Associated symptoms include: muscle soreness; hypersensitivity to light (photophobia) and sound (phonophobia); and autonomic nervous system dysfunctions such as gastrointestinal problems (nausea, vomiting and diarrhea) and cutaneous vasoconstriction producing cold extremities and sweating.

+ There are multiple triggering and aggravating factors. In general, sensitivity to a particular trigger may take years or decades to evolve. Triggers may be multifactorial, requiring more than one factor to precipitate an attack. The number of triggers increases with age *(Davidoff, 1995)*.

✦ During the headache, the person withdraws from activity, often to a quiet, darkened room if possible, suffering pain and disability.

✦ Usually, the headache resolves over several hours, during sleep or rest; however, there may be vomiting or an intense emotional release abruptly ending the migraine.

✦ There is a period of 24 to 48 hours following migraine resolution termed the "postdrome", when the person may feel fatigued and drained. Depression, muscle achiness and emotional volatility may also be felt.

✦ Other types of headaches, such as tension headaches, may be experienced at other times *(Travell, Simons, 1983)*.

✦ Chronic pain lowers the quality of life of the migraine sufferer.

✦ Migraine is divided into two main categories: with and without aura.

Migraine without Aura

✦ Formerly called "common migraine", this condition affects 85 per cent of people with migraines.

✦ In the 24- to 48-hour period before the migraine, the person experiences premonitory symptoms, or alteration of central nervous system activity. This may include mood changes, food cravings, altered sensory perception, excessive yawning and memory dysfunction. These symptoms may originate in the hypothalamus.

Migraine with Aura

✦ Formerly called "classic migraine", this affects 15 per cent of people with migraines.

✦ The aura is associated with a reduction in cerebral blood flow. It develops gradually over five to 20 minutes, lasting for less than one hour and resolving with the headache. Auras are usually visual, often perceived as flashing lights, zig-zag lines or visual distortion *(Figure 37.1)*. They may also be sensory, such as a sensation of pins and needles around the lips and hands. Auditory disturbances include hissing or rumbling noises, while olfactory hallucinations include strong smells such as of burning rubber.

Migraine in Children

✦ Migraine may affect 5 per cent of all children.

✦ In early childhood, boys are more affected than girls; in the teen years, migraine is more prevalent in girls.

✦ Headache is less prominent; instead, abdominal pain, cramping, vomiting, episodic vertigo and autonomic symptoms are more common.

✦ While migraines have been reported in infants, they usually first occur after five years of age, with a peak occurrence between 10 and 13 years of age *(Davidoff, 1995)*.

✦ Usually one or both parents have a history of migraine *(Today's Health, 1991)*.

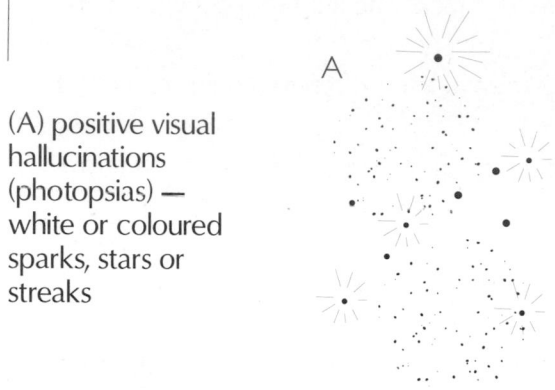

(A) positive visual hallucinations (photopsias) — white or coloured sparks, stars or streaks

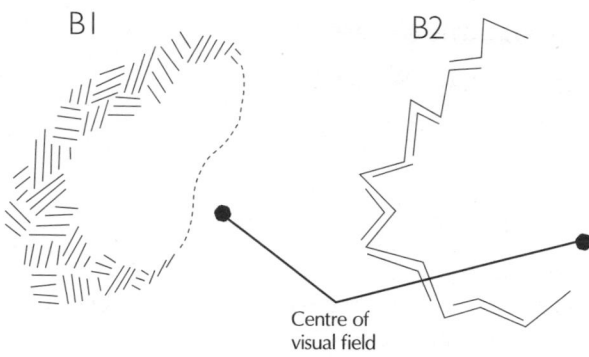

Centre of visual field

(B) negative visual phenomena (scotomas) with partial or complete obliteration of the field of vision.
(B1) and (B2) fortification spectra with central scotoma — a glittering zig-zag border to the scotoma is termed a scintillating scotoma.

The Path Travelled
The radial nerve is a continuation of the posterio
62.1) From the posterior axillary wall between t
continues in the spiral groove of the humerus, de
the humerus to the lateral side which then trav
superficial at this point before it travels between
extensor carpi radialis longus and extensor carpi
It crosses the elbow   tor. At this poin
branches. The positi   enters the s
aspect of the radius, innerva   sor digito
longus and brevis, abductor   ongus, extenso
branch terminates at the wr
    The superficial branch   contiues down the
pronator teres and the raidal attachments of the f

Centre of visual field

(B3) progressive central scotoma, spreading slowly from the centre over 10 to 30 minutes then fading (*Davidoff, 1995*).

Figure 37.1
Visual symptoms of migraine auras.

Differentiating Other Types of Headaches

With new headaches that begin later in adult life, especially after age 50, the client should be referred to a physician. New primary headache is rare in the elderly; the headache may be secondary to an underlying pathology (*Cady, Fox, 1995*).

High-Risk Headaches: Report to Physician

- There is onset of a new headache after age 50.

- There is onset of a new or different headache.

- The client reports the "worst" headache ever experienced.

- There is a recent history of acute head trauma.

- There is onset of a headache that steadily worsens over time or worsens with exertion, coughing or straining.

- The headache is associated with changes in neurological status, such as drowsiness, confusion, weakness, ataxia and loss of coordination and deep tendon reflexes or Babinski response.

- There is a new headache in a person with cancer or HIV.

- The headache is associated with fever and neck rigidity.

- The headache is associated with hypertension (*Silberstein et al., 1998; Davidoff, 1995*).

WARNING SYMPTOMS — CONSIDERED SERIOUS AND WARRANTING IMMEDIATE REPORTING TO PHYSICIAN:

- **Meningitis** signs include severe headache, nuchal rigidity, fever, nausea, vomiting, pain behind the eyes which worsens with eye movement, photophobia and transient rash.

- **New headache with a pregnancy** usually affects clients in the second trimester. Continuous, severe frontal or occipital headache, accompanied by visual disturbances, which is not relieved by usual remedies may indicate pregnancy-induced hypertension, also referred to as pre-eclampsia. These symptoms are more serious if also accompanied by swelling in the face and hands (*Bourne 1995*).

- A **cerebral aneurism** (stroke) producing a subarachnoid hemorrhage has abrupt, explosive pain; there may be a transient loss of consciousness at the headache onset. Nausea, stiff neck and photophobia may be present. Half the people with cerebral aneurisms die if not medically treated (*Alexander, 1994*). A sentinel headache, also with abrupt pain onset, can occur if the blood vessel does not rupture. This headache usually subsides over two days but can continue until a major hemorrhage occurs within days or even weeks (*Silberstein et al., 1998; Davidoff, 1995*).

- **Brain tumour** pain is generally not severe; however, there are associated neurological signs such as loss of coordination, weakness, dizziness, double vision, nausea, vomiting, lethargy, personality changes and sleep interruption (*Alexander, 1994*).

THESE SYMPTOMS WARRANT EARLY REPORTING TO THE PHYSICIAN (WITHIN 24 HOURS):

- **Diabetes mellitus hypoglycemia** headache is one of a number of symptoms indicating insulin reaction. Other symptoms include sweating, blurred vision, slurred speech, impaired motor function and tachycardia. People with diabetes mellitus usually recognize their symptom profile and will ingest a concentrated carbohydrate source such as sugar which is rapidly absorbed. If a concentrated carbohydrate source is not taken, it is a medical emergency as the person may progress to convulsions and coma.

- **Temporal arteritis pain** is persistent and non-throbbing, over the affected artery and inside the eye, and associated with diminished pulse in the temporal arteries. It is usually seen in the elderly client.

- **Lyme disease** headache pain is bilateral and gradual in onset; there is an associated skin rash. It is caused by an infection by spirochete acquired from a tick bite.

- **Trigeminal neuralgia pain** is over the distribution of the trigeminal nerve. Pain occurs several times a day and there are associated facial tics.

- **Acute sinusitis pain** is often severe and is located over the affected sinus. There is a low-grade fever and a feeling of fullness and pressure in the affected sinus, with nasal discharge.

- **Low pressure headache syndrome pain** is aggravated by upright posture and head shaking. It is relieved in less than 30 minutes by lying down. Nausea, vomiting and dizziness may also occur. Some of the causes are lumbar punctures for spinal anesthesia or myelograms which decrease cerebrospinal fluid pressure.

Mixed and Transformational Headaches

Headaches that share tension- and migraine-type symptoms are termed "mixed headaches". Often there is an underlying tension headache with periods of migraine symptoms. Episodic migraine may evolve into chronic near-daily headaches which have been termed a "transformational headache" *(Cady, Fox, 1995)*. In this case, there is a family history of migraine, precipitating factors such as menstruation and migraine-related gastrointestinal symptoms. Overuse of medication is commonly associated with these headaches.

Symptom Picture

+ The pain is bilateral with mixed headaches.
+ The headaches begin when the client is between 20 and 40 years of age.
+ The frequency is often daily.
+ Episodic headaches have clearly identifiable endpoints, whereas chronic daily and near-daily headaches are constant, with fluctuations in pain levels.
+ The headaches may come on at any time of the day.
+ Associated symptoms are nausea, vomiting, irritable bowel syndrome, sleep disturbances and depression.
+ Aggravating factors are mental or physical activity.
+ During the headache, the person presents differently depending on the associated symptoms.

Cluster Headache

Cluster headaches affect an estimated 0.1 per cent of the population, men five times more frequently than women. They may be caused by abnormal hypothalamic function. Cluster indicates a grouping of headaches, often once a day for several weeks. The headaches may then disappear for months or years. There is rarely a family history with cluster headaches; however, tobacco use is more prevalent than with any other type of headache.

Symptom Picture

+ The pain of a cluster headache is always unilateral, often periorbital. It may refer into the nose, jaw or teeth. It is devastating in intensity, described as sharp, boring and burning.
+ These headaches begin when the person is between 20 and 40 years of age.
+ During an active cluster period, there may be one to six headaches per day.
+ The symptoms last for 30 minutes to three hours. Chronic cluster headache occurs when the cluster period exceeds 12 months.
+ The onset is one to three hours after the person goes to sleep.

+ There are ipsilateral autonomic dysfunctions such as nasal congestion, lacrimation, facial swelling and partial Horner's syndrome of ptosis (drooping of the eyelid) and miosis (pupil constriction).

+ Aggravating factors include vasodilators, such as alcohol, and reduced oxygen levels experienced at altitudes above 5,000 feet.

+ During the headache, the person is agitated and hyperactive and may pace the room. It is difficult for the person to find a comfortable position.

+ Medically, 70 per cent of cluster headache sufferers respond favourably to oxygen therapy. Medication such as ergotamine, verapamil and lithium may also help.

Drug-Associated Headaches

Some headaches are related to medication or drug use. Certain substances may be effective against headaches, such as over-the-counter headache medication, prescription analgesics, ergotamines and caffeine, but when taken indiscriminately may cause "rebound headaches". Drug-associated headaches often begin in the early morning when blood levels of the drug are lower. The specific drug that causes the headache is required for relief. Slow reduction of drug levels over a period of several weeks is required for detoxification.

Symptom Picture

+ The pain of a drug induced headache is bilateral, constant, dull and fluctuating in intensity. Periods of migraine-like intensity may occur, although nausea and photophobia are not frequent symptoms.

+ The frequency is often daily.

+ The duration of the symptoms is related to drug use.

+ The onset is related to abstinence from drug use.

+ Associated symptoms are memory impairment and medication-related symptoms.

+ Aggravating factors are withdrawal of the offending drug.

+ The person has severe pain during drug withdrawal.

Chronic Paroxysmal Hemicrania

This rare, excruciating headache disorder shares some features with the cluster headache. However, it occurs more frequently in women.

Symptom Picture

+ The pain of a paroxysmal headache is always unilateral.

+ These headaches begin in early adulthood.

✦ The frequency is daily, with an average of 14 attacks and up to 75 attacks a day.

✦ The symptoms last for one to two minutes or up to 30 minutes.

✦ The onset is during the daytime.

✦ There are ipsilateral autonomic dysfunctions similar to cluster headaches, such as unilateral eyelid drooping and eye tearing.

Contraindications

✦ During a migraine, massage may be contraindicated depending on the client's symptoms.

✦ Avoid the use of heat on the neck or head during migraine as heat causes painful vasodilation.

✦ Do not work deeply during a migraine.

✦ Avoid music or bright lights if the client is sensitive to them during the headache.

✦ Either during or between attacks, avoid the use of fragrances with those whose migraine triggers are perfumes; these may include essential oils.

✦ Aggravating factors are head movements.

✦ During the headache, the person is agitated and hyperactive and may pace the room.

✦ Medically, there is good response to indomethacin.

Trauma-Related Headaches

Trauma to the head, neck or spine may result in headaches. Falls that create a shear at the sacroiliac joint may cause headaches *(Kuchera, Kuchera, 1993)*. Falls on the coccyx may result in headaches due to tension placed on the dural tube and membranes surrounding the spinal cord and brain *(Upledger, Vredevoogd, 1983)*.

✦ See also tension headaches for other types of headaches.

Treatment Considerations

HEALTH HISTORY QUESTIONS

✦ Does the client have a migraine now?

✦ When was the onset of the present migraine? If the client has a history of migraines, at what age did they begin?

✦ Was there a trauma to the head, neck or spine, which may indicate a post-whiplash or post-concussion headache?

✦ Has the client experienced a lumbar puncture procedure for spinal anesthesia or a myelogram indicating that the headache is likely due to low cerebrospinal fluid pressure?

✦ Does the client have a temperature, transient rash or stiff neck, indicating possible meningitis?

✦ Does the client experience sleep disturbances, indicating chronic daily headaches?

✦ What are the location and quality of the pain? Does it refer anywhere?

✦ What are the symptoms? How frequent are they? Do they include systemic manifestations such as anorexia, nausea, vomiting, aura and irritability to sensory input?

✦ What is the duration of the migraine?

✦ What was the time of onset? Is this the same for recurring headaches? Did the headache waken the person early in the morning before the usual time of awakening?

✦ What relieves the migraine?

✦ Does the client take medication for this condition, including prescription drugs, over-the-counter medication, herbal preparations or supplements?

✦ Are there any underlying pathologies such as fibromyalgia, degenerative disc disease or osteoarthritis of the cervical spine, dental abnormalities such as temporomandibular joint dysfunction or dental abscess?

✦ Has the client suffered a recent cold or influenza attack which could precipitate a migraine?

✦ Is the client using parallel therapies such as chiropractic or osteopathic manipulation, biofeedback, acupuncture or naturopathy?

Further Assessment

✐ **Observations** include a full postural assessment, looking for head-forward posture, hyperkyphosis, hyperlordosis, scoliosis or pes planus.

✐ **Palpation:**

• The neck, shoulder and thoracic muscles and muscles of mastication may be hypertonic and tender. The muscles of respiration are also likely to be hypertonic, including the diaphragm, intercostals, scalenes and sternocleidomastoids.

• Ischemia produces coolness in the skin of the neck or thorax.

✐ **Testing:**

• **AF** and **PR ROM** are performed on the neck, thorax, shoulder and mandible. There is reduced cervical and thoracic mobility in **AF** and **PR** ranges of motion. There may be reduced ranges in mandibular motion.

• **AR strength testing** may reveal the neck and shoulder girdle muscles to be weaker and overused.

• **Special tests** include the **vertebral artery test**, which is used to rule out any vertebral artery insufficiency before performing any test that extends, sidebends and rotates the cervical spine, such as **Spurling's test**.

• Both **motion** and **static palpation** are performed in the cervical and thoracic spine and may reveal areas of hyper- and hypomobility. **Passive relaxed atlanto-occipital** and **atlanto-axial articulation** may have restrictions. **Passive relaxed anterior** and **lateral spinous challenges**, as well as **first rib mobility** and **rib**

507

motion tests may show areas of hypo- or hypermobility.

- **Blood pressure** is taken if the client is pregnant or an adult over 50 years of age who is experiencing a new headache.
- **Kernig's/Brudzinski test** is positive with meningitis.
- **Spurling's, cervical compression** and **cervical distraction tests** are used to differentiate a cervical nerve root compression that may underlie the headache. Spurling's may also indicate facet joint irritation.

Massage

☝ Massage therapy has been described as "promoting a headache-protective environment for the migraine sufferer" *(Cady, Fox, 1995)*, and as "bring[ing] about a degree of relief" to abort an attack in progress *(Theisler, 1990).*

During an Attack

☝ The treatment is limited to 30 to 45 minutes in length to avoid exhausting the client. The treatment is in the context of a relaxation massage including unforced **diaphragmatic breathing.**

☝ **Positioning** may be supine or sidelying, as is comfortable for the client. The prone position may be poorly tolerated, since there may be a sensation of too much blood rushing to the head. A towel may be used to cover the client's eyes in the supine position if the light is too bright. **Hydrotherapy** is cold or ice to the head and neck.

☝ The treatment goals are to decrease pain and hypertonicity and to work within the client's pain tolerance. If the client is unable to tolerate any direct work on the head, scalp and neck, hand and foot massage may be tolerated while cold cloths are applied to the head and neck.

☝ If the client can tolerate direct work, in the supine position, lymphatic drainage for the head and neck is indicated. General soothing Swedish work to the shoulder girdle, neck muscles and scalp includes stroking, vibrations and fingertip kneading. Gentle pressure point work to the frontal, temporal, maxillary and occipital areas may be tolerated by some *(Theisler, 1990)*. Golgi tendon organ release for the suboccipitals, long-axis traction on the occiput and Swedish techniques for the temporalis and masseter may also help. Trigger points that refer into the head and neck are treated with muscle stripping and intermittent ischemic compressions. For example, trigger points in upper trapezius refer into the temporal region *(Travell, Simons, 1983)*. PIR with associated eye movements may be used to gently increase range of motion at the neck.

Between Attacks

☝ Treatment goals are to reduce sympathetic nervous system firing, hypertonicity, trigger points and joint dysfunctions and to increase range of motion and tissue health.

☝ The treatment is similar to that which is performed during an attack, except that the therapist can be more vigorous; areas of restricted range of motion are addressed. In addition, the prone position is used to treat the thoracic and lumbar areas, reducing hypertonicity and trigger points. Hot hydrotherapy applications are now appropriate if needed. Migraine may be relieved using pure essential oils; however, it is important to assess if the client has triggers to smell before using them. Lavender or peppermint can be used. Twenty-five drops of essential oil are added to 50 ml. of vegetable oil *(Sellar, 1992)*. Joint mobilizations for cervical and thoracic hypomobile segments are indicated. Grade 1 mobilizations repeated five to 10 times are appropriate *(Edeling, 1994)*. Any postural or temporomandibular joint dysfunctions that are present are also addressed. See the appropriate chapters for details.

Self-care

✍ Self-massage of the neck, face and scalp can abort a migraine in progress; it is also useful between attacks.

✍ **Hydrotherapy applications before a migraine:** hot, full-immersion baths when the client feels cold can help to abort the headache *(Today's Health, 1991; Moor et al., 1964)*. **Hydrotherapy applications during a migraine:** ice packs applied to the arteries of the scalp and neck reduce pain.

✍ Aerobic exercise between attacks may help to decrease the frequency of migraines *(Davidoff, 1995)*.

✍ Stretching the neck and shoulder muscles is indicated.

✍ Behavioural modifications such as regulating sleep, taking regular meals and exercise, avoiding food-related triggers and managing stress may help decrease the symptoms. Migraines in children can be significantly reduced by eliminating food triggers.

See also stress reduction, trigger points, tension headaches, the postural dysfunction section, whiplash, torticollis, understanding peripheral nerve lesions (for trigeminal neuralgia), degenerative disc disease, osteoarthritis, diabetes mellitus, fibromyalgia and chronic fatigue syndrome, HIV, sinusitis and inflammatory arthritides for related treatments.

✍ The client is referred to a physician if the headache worsens; a chiropractor, osteopath, craniosacral practitioner, dentist or acupuncturist may also be appropriate. In one study chiropractic manipulation had a success rate of 72 per cent in treating migraines, especially if neck problems are associated with low back or sacroiliac joint dysfunction *(Theisler, 1990)*. Biofeedback has been found helpful in controlling headaches. A naturopath can help with nutrition counselling, herbal remedies or other supplements. Self-help organizations such as the Migraine Foundation also offer information and support.

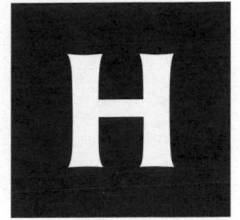

POSTURAL DYSFUNCTION

STRATEGIES:
Fascial and Muscle Imbalances

Fiona Rattray

Normal Postural Curves

At birth, the spine is in flexion. This curve is considered a primary curve. At three months of age, as the infant holds the head up, the secondary cervical lordotic curve begins to develop, while the lumbar lordotic curve appears between six and eight months when the child sits up and walks. The knees have a varus orientation until about 18 months of age. After this point, a valgus orientation is seen until the child reaches three years of age. The knees are usually straight by the time the child is six years old. For a child, it is normal to have an increase in the lumbar lordotic curve or hyperlordosis *(Magee, 1992; Kendall, McCreary, 1983)*.

Theories about Postural Dysfunctions

Bones may be seen as building blocks piled on top of each other, connected by ligaments and fascia. Muscles move and stabilize the bones. Relative symmetry in length and strength of the muscles, fascial tension and mobility of the joints are necessary for full and proper functioning of the musculoskeletal system, including proper posture.

It is important to note that postural dysfunctions may be **functional** or **structural**. A functional postural change means that the soft tissues, such as muscles, fascia and ligaments, have adapted by either shortening or lengthening. Because the changes are in soft tissue, the posture can be altered. The therapist is able to stretch the shortened tissues during treatment, while the client can voluntarily alter the posture by changing position. A structural postural change means that the bones have an altered shape due to a pathological process or malformation. For example, vertebrae may be wedge shaped or only half formed. The bony changes that are present cannot be altered by the client or the therapist. However, the soft tissues have also adapted and may be treated to maintain tissue health.

In the past, a functional curve in the spine was called Arvedson's first degree curve. Minor bony changes were second degree curves, while severe bony changes were third degree curves *(Wale, 1980)*.

Muscles can be categorized into two groups according to their reaction to dysfunction: **postural** and **phasic**. Skeletal muscles are composed of two main types of fibres, slow twitch (or type 1) fibres and fast twitch (or type 2) fibres. So-called postural muscles have a higher proportion of slow twitch fibres. These muscles fatigue slowly (after several hundred contractions) and respond to disuse or stress by *shortening*. Those described as phasic muscles have a higher proportion of fast twitch fibres. These muscles fatigue rapidly (sometimes after a few contractions) and respond to disuse or stress by *weakening* *(Dvorak, Dvorak, 1990; Neumann, 1989)*.

Postural muscles primarily maintain upright posture, for which they require endurance. Phasic muscles are responsible for movement, for which they require speed. While most muscles have both functions, one function predominates. Some studies show that specific use of a muscle can change the proportion of each fibre type. For example, slow twitch fibres are more numerous in the quadriceps of marathon runners than in non-athletes, giving the runners' endurance *(Dvorak, Dvorak, 1990)*.

With postural dysfunctions, patterns of tightness and weakness emerge once the muscle type is known. For example, the pectoral muscles are postural, shortening in response to disuse. The rhomboids are phasic, weakening under stress. The combined action of these two muscle groups at the shoulder girdle leads to an increase in shoulder protraction and thoracic curve, known as hyperkyphosis.

Muscles that are primarily postural are (Figure 38.1):

✦ gastrocnemius, soleus, rectus femoris, biceps femoris, semimembranosus, semitendinosus, pectineus, the adductors, tensor fascia lata, piriformis, iliopsoas, quadratus lumborum, erector spinae, multifidi, rotatores, diaphragm, intercostals *(Zadai, 1992)*, pectoralis major (sternal and clavicular heads), upper trapezius, levator scapulae, sternocleidomastoid and wrist and elbow flexors *(Neumann, 1989; Janda, 1984; Lewit 1993)*.

Muscles that are primarily phasic are (Figure 38.1):

✦ the peroneals, tibialis anterior, vastus lateralis, vastus medialis, gluteus maximus, gluteus medius, gluteus minimus, rectus abdominus, rhomboids, lower trapezius, middle trapezius, serratus anterior and wrist and elbow extensors *(Neumann, 1989; Dvorak, Dvorak, 1990)*.

There is disagreement over the category of some key muscles. The scalenes may be postural *(Neumann, 1989; Lewit, 1993; Dvorak, Dvorak, 1990)* or phasic *(Janda, 1984)*; this book considers them to be postural. The internal and external abdominal obliques are considered phasic *(Janda, 1984; Neumann, 1989)* or postural *(Lewit, 1993)*; this book considers them phasic.

The **tight-loose** concept, which suggests that tightness creates asymmetry and looseness permits it to continue, is another component of postural dysfunction *(Greenman, 1989)*. Tightness and looseness are due to reflexive and biomechanical causes. For example,

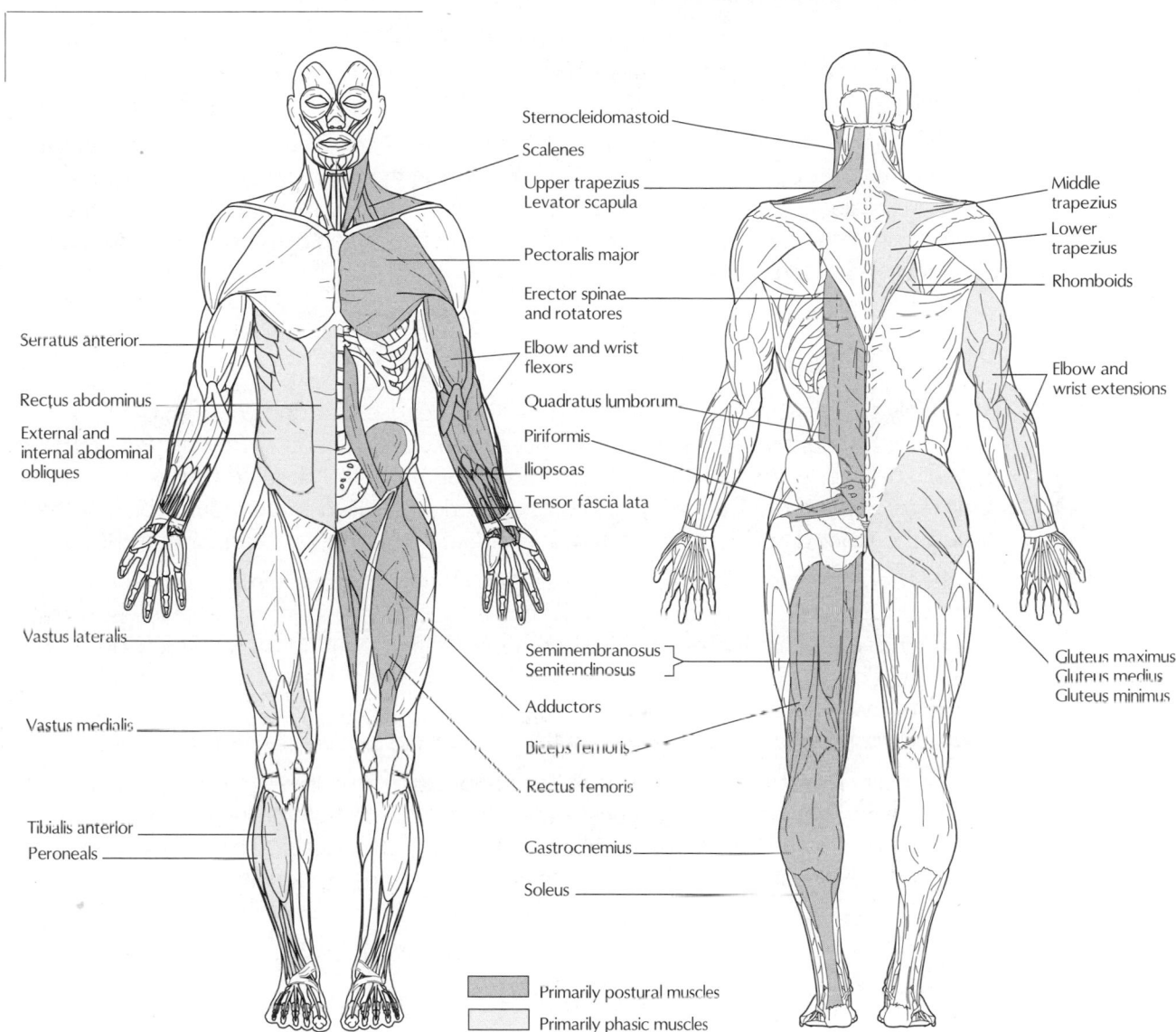

Sternocleidomastoid
Scalenes
Upper trapezius
Levator scapula
Pectoralis major
Erector spinae and rotatores
Elbow and wrist flexors
Quadratus lumborum
Piriformis
Iliopsoas
Tensor fascia lata

Middle trapezius
Lower trapezius
Rhomboids
Elbow and wrist extensions

Serratus anterior
Rectus abdominus
External and internal abdominal obliques

Vastus lateralis
Vastus medialis

Tibialis anterior
Peroneals

Semimembranosus
Semitendinosus
Adductors
Biceps femoris
Rectus femoris
Gastrocnemius
Soleus

Gluteus maximus
Gluteus medius
Gluteus minimus

Primarily postural muscles
Primarily phasic muscles

Figure 38.1
Primarily postural muscles respond to dysfunction by shortening.
Primarily phasic muscles respond by weakening.

tightening of an agonist muscle reciprocally inhibits its antagonist. Because a muscle and its covering fascia are closely bonded, the fascia over the hypertonic agonist muscle shortens. The fascia over the antagonist must correspondingly loosen. Biomechanically, trauma to muscles and fascia may also cause shortening due to scar tissue and adhesions. Occupational postures may allow some fascia and muscles to shorten and others to loosen.

These altered myofascial relationships have both local and distant effects on the body — not just on muscle and fascia but also on nerves and vasculature *(Basmajian, Nyberg, 1993)*.

The looseness of the tight-loose concept is a relative one, however, as palpation of phasic muscles will often reveal that they feel tight. Muscles can be weak and stretched, yet still be

515

tight, because they are trying to prevent further postural distortion. An example of this is the increase in erector spinae activity and tightness on the convex, or outside, portion of a scoliotic curve as these muscles try to prevent the curve from increasing *(Robin, 1990)*.

Another theory describes the tight muscles in a postural condition as either in **concentric** (shortening) or **eccentric** (lengthening) contraction. In the example of hyperkyphosis, pectoralis major and minor are acting concentrically — that is, they are shortening and contracting. Rhomboids and middle trapezius are acting eccentrically or lengthening and contracting *(St. John, 1994)*.

Pain of Postural Origin

Pain solely of a postural origin is seen in people 30 years of age and younger, often in people with sedentary occupations and those who do not exercise *(Boyling, Palastanga, 1994)*. The pain is often intermittent. The more frequently the affected tissues are put under stress, the more frequently the pain is experienced. Pain is, therefore, worse at the end of the work day. When the posture is changed, the pain disappears or diminishes.

For the therapist, it is difficult to tell by palpation alone whether a tender and tight muscle is short and tight or weak, stretched and tight. Is the muscle tender because it is ischemic or is it tender because it is constantly stretched? It is important not to rely solely on symptomatic areas of tenderness when creating a treatment plan. In the hyperkyphosis example, giving the client stretches for the painful and already stretched rhomboids will only make matters worse and will allow the postural dysfunction to remain.

This difficulty illustrates the necessity of both performing a postural assessment, using a plumb line and goniometer for accuracy, and checking the length of the muscles involved in the postural dysfunction using muscle length tests. In this way, the therapist will be certain of appropriately treating the shortened muscles. See Appendix B for details of a postural assessment.

General Treatment Principles

The basic principle for treating postural dysfunctions, after assessment, is first to **stretch** the short muscles, then to **strengthen** the weak muscles. If strengthening of the weak, inhibited phasic muscles is attempted first, the shortened postural muscles and fascia will prevent the phasic muscles from regaining their full strength.

The majority of the stretching and mobilizing work is performed by the therapist during treatment, using fascial techniques, joint play, post-isometric relaxation and trigger point techniques. The majority of the strengthening is done by the client as self-care active resistance exercises.

It is worth remembering that people are not completely symmetrical. A person may have one shoulder slightly higher than the other or an increase in pelvic tilt and be asymptomatic for pain, because the body has been able to successfully adapt to the imbalances. Pain may only arise when an activity or event places extra stress on the tissues, overwhelming the body's ability to adapt. An asymmetry that is not painful does not necessarily need to be corrected. In other words, if it's not broken, don't fix it.

PES PLANUS

Fiona Rattray

Pes planus is a decreased medial longitudinal arch and a pronated hindfoot.

The terms **pes planus, pronated foot** and **flat foot** are often used interchangeably *(Kisner, Colby, 1990)*.

Pronation is a combined movement of the foot and ankle that includes eversion of the calcaneus, abduction of the forefoot and some dorsiflexion at the subtalar joint *(Hertling, Kessler, 1990; Magee, 1992)*. **Hindfoot valgus** is another term for eversion of the calcaneus, which leads to foot pronation.

The converse movement is **supination,** which involves inversion, adduction and some plantarflexion at the subtalar joint.

There are two types of pes planus: functional and structural. **Functional pes planus** indicates ligamentous laxity or muscle weakness as a contributor to the condition. It can be corrected. **Structural** or **rigid** pes planus results from bony malformation or change. It cannot be altered by positional changes or voluntary effort.

At one point, it was believed that the arches in the normal, static foot, especially the medial longitudinal arch, were primarily supported by muscles *(Wale, 1980)*. This has been disproved by electromyographic tests *(Basmajian, DeLuca, 1985)*. A combination of bones, ligaments and muscles support the arches of the normal foot *(Basmajian, DeLuca, 1985; Hertling, Kessler, 1990)*.

There are three main arches: the medial longitudinal, lateral longitudinal and anterior transverse arches. The bones that form the **medial longitudinal arch** are the calcaneus, talus, navicular, three cuneiforms and three medial metatarsals *(Pansky, 1979)*. The medial longitudinal arch is not a true arch in an architectural sense, since its configuration is not formed by the shape of the bones alone. In the static or weight bearing foot, the medial

517

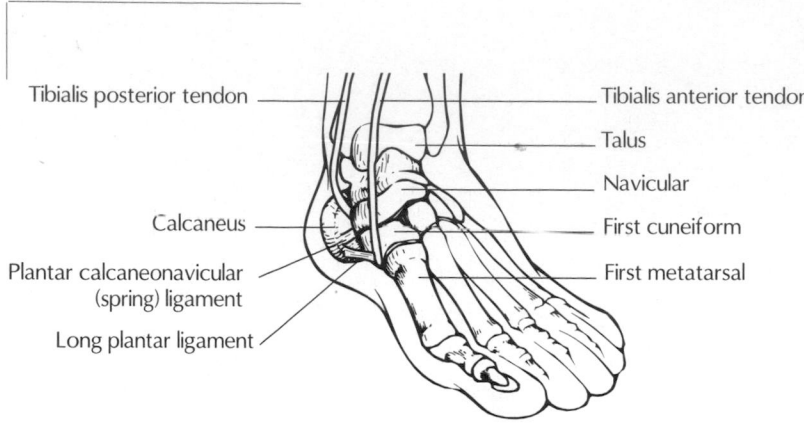

Figure 39.1
The medial longitudinal arch.

Tibialis posterior tendon

Calcaneus

Plantar calcaneonavicular (spring) ligament

Long plantar ligament

Tibialis anterior tendon

Talus

Navicular

First cuneiform

First metatarsal

arch is maintained by the long and short plantar ligaments, the plantar calcaneonavicular (spring) ligament and the plantar aponeurosis. In the active or dynamic foot, tibialis posterior, tibialis anterior and, to a lesser extent, peroneus longus provide a muscular sling to support the arch, which prevents it from flattening into a pronated position (*Figure 39.1*). Other muscles that provide support for the medial longitudinal arch are flexor hallucis longus, flexor digitorum longus and the intrinsic muscles of the foot. The shape of the **anterior transverse arch,** composed of the metatarsal heads, also depends on muscular support from the lumbricals and interossei. The **lateral longitudinal arch,** however, is a true architectural arch, with the cuboid bone forming the keystone between the calcaneus and the fourth and fifth metatarsals. Newborn babies lack all these arches. The medial longitudinal arch begins to develop after about two years of age, so it is normal for infants to have pes planus (*Magee, 1992*).

To illustrate the configuration of the arches, the foot may be represented as a twisted osteoligamentous plate (*Hertling, Kessler, 1990*). In the standing foot, the metatarsal heads, representing one end of the plate, are positioned horizontally; the calcaneus, representing the other end, is positioned vertically. The medial arch relies on this twisted configuration of the foot (*Figure 39.2*). Pronation of the foot occurs primarily at the subtalar joint and secondarily at the midtarsal joint. When the foot pronates, the twisted plate flattens along the medial arch. When the foot supinates, the twist on the plate increases, raising the medial arch.

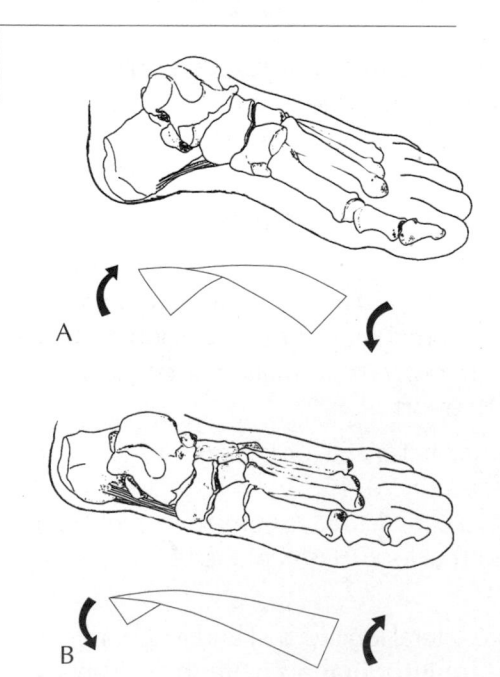

Figure 39.2
The medial longitudinal arch: A) twisting into supination; B) untwisting into pronation.

In a normal gait cycle, some pronation is important during the contact phase following heel strike. This allows the foot to adapt to uneven terrain and enables the lower leg to internally rotate (*Buschbacher, 1994*). Toe off causes the plantar aponeurosis to tighten, supinating or raising the medial arch and adding stability to the foot. See Appendix B for information on the gait cycle.

In pes planus, the talar head is displaced medially and inferiorly from the navicular bone. The ligaments, joint capsules and fascia which support and form the medial longitudinal arch become overstretched. The lack of ligamentous stability in the flatfooted person forces the muscles to provide most of the arches' stability both in standing and walking, because the foot is in a pronated, untwisted position. For example, it has been shown that in the normal, static foot, tibialis anterior, tibialis posterior, peroneus longus, the long toe flexors and the intrinsic

518

muscles of the foot do not support the medial longitudinal arch. However, they do show activity in the static foot of a person with pes planus *(Basmajian, DeLuca, 1985; Travell, Simons, 1992).*

The muscles supporting the arch in the dynamic foot — tibialis anterior and the peroneal muscles — are primarily phasic; that is, they respond to stress by fatiguing. Gastrocnemius and soleus are primarily postural muscles and respond to stress by adaptively shortening *(Dvorak, Dvorak, 1990).* These characteristics of the muscles help to perpetuate pes planus.

Muscles that evert the foot are peroneus longus, brevis and tertius. Although the three peroneals are all evertors of the foot, the tendon of peroneus longus wraps around the lateral surface of the cuboid and inserts onto the medial plantar surface of the first cuboid and first metatarsal. It indirectly everts the foot. In weight bearing, it supports the medial arch by causing the head of the first metatarsal to press into the floor. In contrast, peroneus brevis and tertius insert laterally onto the base of the fifth metatarsal, directly everting the foot. In the pronated foot, these muscles are prone to developing trigger points and taut bands *(Travell, Simons, 1992).* Shortening of these muscles reinforces eversion, maintaining pes planus *(Kendall, McCreary, 1983).* The same is true of gastrocnemius and soleus *(Hertling, Kessler, 1990).*

Functional pes planus can worsen if the arches are not adequately supported. In one study, 44 persons completed a 100 kilometre hike. Those with pes planus before the walk had a further drop in the arches at the end, while those with normal feet had no change *(Basmajian, DeLuca, 1985).*

Other foot problems the therapist may see:

✦ **Forefoot varus** involves inversion of the forefoot on the hindfoot at the midtarsal joint; clinically, it looks like pes planus and can contribute to tibialis posterior tendinitis and Morton's neuroma *(Magee, 1992).*

✦ **Heel spurs** may result from continuous pulling on the attachments of the plantar aponeurosis. As the medial longitudinal arch flattens, increased stress is placed on the aponeurosis.

✦ A **spreading of the anterior transverse arch,** especially between the first and second metatarsal heads, allows **hallux valgus** to form *(Magee, 1992).* **Hallux valgus** is a valgus orientation of the big toe or hallux, with an accompanying medial deviation of the first metatarsal bone. It may be caused by, or contribute to, pes planus. The first metatarsophalangeal joint capsule becomes hypermobile; a callus and an inflamed, thickened bursa develop over the joint, which form a bunion. This is often due to poor footwear *(Buschbacher, 1994).*

✦ **Pes cavus** is the opposite foot configuration of pes planus. It presents as a high medial arch due to increased twisting or supination of the foot. The calcaneus is inverted. Tibialis anterior, tibialis posterior and the toe flexors are shortened.

✦ **Hindfoot varus** is an inversion of the calcaneus, seen with supination. **Forefoot valgus** is an eversion of the forefoot on the hindfoot at the midtarsal joint; clinically, it looks like pes cavus *(Magee, 1992).*

✦ **Metatarsalgia** is a general term for foot pain experienced at the metatarsal heads. It may occur with either pes planus or pes cavus *(Hertling, Kessler, 1990; Buschbacher, 1994).*

✦ A **Morton's foot structure**, where the second metatarsal is longer than the first, allows the first metatarsal to become hypermobile. The body's weight is abnormally distributed through the head of the second metatarsal on the toe off phase of the gait cycle. This often results in callus formation and tenderness under the second metatarsal head. A Morton foot structure places stress on tibialis posterior and may occur with pes planus *(Travell, Simons, 1992)*.

✦ **Morton's neuroma** is a swelling of the distal interdigital nerves of the foot, usually between the third and fourth metatarsals. It may be caused by hypermobility of the metatarsals. Pain results on compression or weight bearing, as the nerve is compressed between the bones. Morton's neuroma may be exacerbated by shoes that are too tight *(Magee, 1992)*.

Pes planus can contribute to other postural dysfunctions because medial displacement of the talus leads to an internal rotation of the tibia when the client is standing. This can result in altered knee and hip biomechanics, such as knee valgus, patellar tracking disorders, iliotibial band contracture *(Brukner, Khan, 1993)*, piriformis syndrome, hyperlordosis, scoliosis and osteoarthritis of the hip. Conversely, these dysfunctions can cause pes planus. Overuse injuries, such as Achilles tendinitis, shin splints and stress fractures of the metatarsals and navicular, may also result from pes planus *(Brukner, Khan, 1993)*. The client may not view a foot condition as the source of the problem. The therapist must be aware that pes planus may be a contributing factor to the client's presenting complaint.

The causes of pes planus are:

➤ **hypermobilty** in the foot due to joint capsule and ligamentous laxity. This may be inherited or due to a pathology such as rheumatoid arthritis;

➤ **poor biomechanics** of the subtalar joint and midtarsal joint *(Brukner, Khan, 1993)*;

➤ **shortened muscles,** such as gastrocnemius, soleus and Achilles tendon, which reduce the ability of the ankle to dorsiflex. This leads to compensation by the midtarsal joint; the foot must untwist into pronation to allow the midtarsal joint to unlock *(Hertling, Kessler, 1990)*. Peroneus longus, brevis and tertius are shortened by pronation. In addition, a shortened iliotibial band and internal tibial rotation can cause, or result from, pes planus;

➤ **weakness** of the muscles that support the arch in the dynamic foot, especially tibialis posterior *(Travell, Simons, 1992; Kendall, McCreary, 1983)*;

➤ **congenital abnormalities in the bones of the foot**, usually a fixation of the talus and calcaneus by ligamentous or osseous union *(Hertling, Kessler, 1990)*. A longer second metatarsal also allows weight bearing to occur through the head of this bone, leading to pain and possible transverse arch spread. Hallux valgus may cause, or result from, pes planus;

➤ **congenital abnormalities in the bones of the leg and thigh**, such as femoral anteversion or an increase in torsion of the femur. When viewed from above, the distal end of the femur is internally rotated. A person with femoral anteversion has increased internal rotation of the leg in the stance phase, which internally rotates the subtalar joint, pronating the foot *(Hertling, Kessler, 1990)*. This can lead to, or result from, pes planus. Internal tibial torsion can also contribute to pes planus;

➤ **habitual poor posture** such as standing with the feet wide apart, which pronates the hindfoot *(Hertling, Kessler, 1990)*;

➤ **nerve lesions** to the common peroneal or posterior tibial nerve resulting in paralysis or muscle weakness;

➤ **trauma** to the foot or ankle. Landing heavily on the feet after jumping or falling may result in fractures to the calcaneus or in a third degree sprain of the spring ligament *(Magee, 1992).* In elderly persons, acquired pes planus is associated with tibialis posterior tendon rupture *(Buschbacher, 1994);*

➤ **footwear** that does not provide medial arch support can allow pes planus to worsen, especially with activities such as running or hiking.

Hypermobility and ligamentous laxity that occur during **pregnancy** can be contributing factors to pes planus *(Kisner, Colby, 1990).*

Symptom Picture

✦ Hypermobility of the medial arch is present and the foot is pronated.

✦ Pes planus can be functional or structural, unilateral or bilateral.

✦ With existing pes planus, overuse of the feet without adequate arch supports may worsen the condition.

✦ Pain may or may not be present. Pain is usually due to fatigue of the affected muscles and ligaments. It is most frequently noticed on the plantar surface, although it may also occur in the fatigued tibialis anterior and posterior *(Hertling, Kessler, 1990).* Pain may occur with regular activities or with increased stress during activities such as running. It may also be located in the knee, hip or low back due to compensation.

✦ With pronation, peroneus longus, peroneus brevis, peroneus tertius, gastrocnemius and soleus are likely short and hypertonic. Trigger points may be present in these muscles *(Travell, Simons, 1992).* Adhesions may be present around the peroneal and Achilles tendons. The ankle joint and superior tibiofibular joints may be hypomobile.

✦ Tibialis posterior, tibialis anterior, the long toe flexors and the intrinsic muscles of the foot are lengthened and possibly weak.

✦ Other conditions, such as plantar fasciitis, shin splints and iliotibial band contracture, may be present.

✦ Occupational or recreational factors may perpetuate or worsen pes planus.

Subjective Information

HEALTH HISTORY QUESTIONS

✦ How long has pes planus been present? Was the client born with it or has it been acquired?

✦ What areas are painful, if any? Is there any pain in the client's foot, ankle, leg, knee, hip or low back? Does this occur when the client is standing for prolonged periods or when the client is walking or running? For example, at midstance in the gait cycle, pain may be noted in the plantar surface. Are there any relieving factors?

✦ Do the client's feet tire easily or only with activity?

✦ What are the client's postural habits, including occupational or recreational sources of postural stress?

✦ Is there any inflammation present at the first metatarsophalangeal joint, indicating a bunion, or at the plantar surface, indicating plantar fasciitis?

✦ What type of footwear does the client wear? Are orthotics or other supportive footwear used?

✦ Is the client having any other parallel therapy, such as chiropractic, physiotherapy or chiropody, for this condition?

Objective Information

Observations

Gait Assessment

✐ In a normal gait cycle, pronation occurs 15 to 20 per cent into the contact phase. With pes planus, pronation occurs throughout the stance phase (*Hertling, Kessler, 1990*).

Postural Assessment

✐ A **mild** pes planus has four to six degrees of hindfoot valgus when measured in a standing posterior view (*Hertling, Kessler, 1990*). A **moderate** pes planus has six to 10 degrees of hindfoot valgus (*Figure 39.3*). A **severe** pes planus has 10 to 15 degrees of hindfoot valgus (*Magee, 1992*).

✐ The Achilles tendon has a valgus orientation.

✐ Internal tibial torsion is possible.

✐ Valgus may occur at the knees.

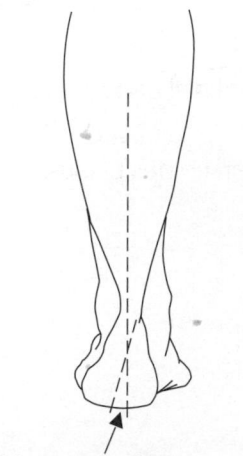

Moderate pes planus: 6 to 10º

Figure 39.3
Left hindfoot valgus.

522

- Internal rotation may occur at the hip.

- The medial arch is flattened and the foot is pronated.

- The talar head bulges medially. There is redness or a callus formation where the client's shoe rubs against the talar head.

- A valgus orientation of the first metatarsal joint may be present. A bunion may also be noticeable.

- The forefoot may be abducted.

- With a Morton foot, the head of the second metatarsal is longer than the first. Callus formation over the heads of the first and second metatarsals may be present.

- If the client is wearing older shoes that have no arch or calcaneal supports, the therapist checks for wear patterns and overhanging uppers. Excessive medial displacement or bulging of the heel counter over the sole of the shoe indicates pes planus (Hertling, Kessler, 1990).

Palpation

- Tenderness, if present, may be at the spring ligament, the navicular, the calcaneal attachment of the long plantar ligament and plantar fascia, the first and second metatarsal heads and the first metatarsophalangeal joint. Tenderness may also be present in the muscles and tendons of the leg.

- There may be areas of local heat on the first metatarsophalageal joint with associated bunions and on the plantar surface with associated plantar fasciitis.

- The texture of the skin over the talar head and the first and second metatarsal heads may be thick and rough.

- The intrinsic foot muscles, tibialis anterior, tibialis posterior and the long toe flexors are hypertonic and lengthened. Gastrocnemius, soleus, peroneus longus, peroneus brevis and peroneus tertius are hypertonic and shortened. Trigger points are likely in peroneus longus and brevis.

Testing

- **AF ROM** of the foot, ankle, knee and hip is performed. With pes planus, eversion in the non-weight-bearing calcaneus is greater than 10 degrees (Hertling, Kessler, 1990). Dorsiflexion of the ankle may be limited with severe pes planus (Magee, 1992). Increased internal rotation may be present with femoral anteversion.

- **PR ROM** is assessed in the foot, ankle, superior tibiofibular joint and hip. The tarsal joints and the other joints of the medial longitudinal arch are hypermobile.

- With a restricted ankle joint capsule, plantarflexion and dorsiflexion are both reduced, with dorsiflexion at less than 10 degrees (Hertling, Kessler, 1990).

- With low-grade inflammation of the ligaments or plantar fascia, passive eversion of the calcaneus, supination of the foot and extension of the toes provoke pain.

- With pronation, the superior tibiofibular joint may be hypomobile.

- With femoral anteversion, internal rotation of the hip is increased while external rotation

Contraindications

✦ Do not mobilize the hypermobile joints on the medial longitudinal arch.

✦ Do not passively stretch tibialis anterior and posterior, since this will allow increased pronation of the foot.

✦ Avoid using heat on the plantar surface of the foot in the presence of an inflammatory process such as plantar fasciitis.

✦ Friction techniques are contraindicated if the client is using anti-inflammatory medication.

is decreased (*Hertling, Kessler, 1990*).

✍ **AR testing** of tibialis anterior, tibialis posterior and extensor hallucis longus may reveal reduced strength.

✍ **Length testing** of gastrocnemius, soleus and the peroneals may reveal shortening of these muscles.

Special Tests

✍ A **functional** or **structural pes planus test** is positive.

✍ **Morton's neuroma test** may also be positive.

Treatment Goals

Assess the client to determine if the pes planus is functional or structural.

Decrease sympathetic nervous system firing.

Treat compensating structures.

Treat other conditions.

Treatment Plan

🖑 With functional pes planus, the therapist lengthens the shortened structures and the client strengthens the fatigued muscles. With structural pes planus, the therapist maintains tissue health and treats the compensatory structures.

🖑 **Positioning** is started prone, with pillows under the abdomen and ankles, to reach the compensating structures and to allow the heat of hydrotherapy to take effect.

🖑 **Hydrotherapy** applications are pre-treatment contrast foot baths to stimulate local circulation. Deep moist heat can be used before stretching the fascia of gastrocnemius and the peroneals.

General Treatment

🖑 The massage is performed in the context of a relaxation treatment, which includes **diaphragmatic breathing.**

🖑 In the **prone** position, the low back, gluteals and thighs are treated, with the focus on increasing circulation, reducing hypertonicity and treating trigger points. Techniques include effleurage, petrissage and muscle stripping.

🖑 Other conditions, such as iliotibial band contracture, may be treated at this time or left for subsequent treatments.

Treatment Goals

Treatment Plan

Specific Treatment

Reduce fascial restrictions.

☝ Fascial techniques to treat the shortened gastrocnemius include skin rolling, crossed-hands spreading and fingertip spreading. Connective tissue cutting and longitudinal fingertip spreading are used along the peroneals. Fascial techniques may also be used on the lateral border of the plantar surface but not on the medial border since these tissues are stretched.

Reduce hypertonicity.

☝ Effleurage and petrissage, including wringing, muscle stripping and palmar kneading, are used on the shortened, hypertonic gastrocnemius, soleus and peroneus longus, brevis and tertius. Deep muscle stripping is avoided along the distal posterior medial border of the tibia where tibialis posterior is situated, since this muscle is lengthened.

Reduce pain if present.
Reduce trigger points.

☝ Trigger points in peroneus longus and brevis refer pain into the lateral leg and around the lateral malleolus *(Travell, Simons, 1992)*. These are treated with ischemic compressions.

Reduce any adhesions.

☝ Frictions may be appropriate on the Achilles and peroneal tendons and on the lateral border of the foot. These are followed by ice and a stretch.

☝ Passive relaxed dorsiflexion and inversion of the ankle may be interspersed through the treatment. Eversion is avoided.

Stretch shortened muscles.

☝ PIR may be used to lengthen peroneus longus, brevis and tertius. In a passive stretch for gastrocnemius or soleus, the forefoot is not used as a lever, since this places a stress on the overstretched midtarsal joints. Instead, the calcaneus is used *(Hertling, Kessler, 1990)*. The client is asked to slide down the table a few centimetres, until the feet are handing over the edge so the ankle can be dorsiflexed.

Increase local circulation to remove metabolites.

☝ Repetitive effleurage is used on the posterior leg and foot muscles.

☝ The client is turned **supine** and pillowed appropriately. Further work to the gastrocnemius may be performed, if necessary, with the client's knee and hip flexed. The therapist covers the client's foot with the sheet and sits on the foot to stabilize it. To treat gastrocnemius, the therapist reaches behind the tibia and grasps the border of the muscle. A connective tissue stroke is used, working obliquely from one side of the muscle to the other. The therapist changes hands, this time working in the opposite oblique direction. The overall effect is to wring the muscle away from the tibia and reduce fascial contractures.

Encourage circulation in weak, taut structures.

☝ The knee and hip are returned to the table and stimulating Swedish techniques are used for the overstretched muscles supporting the medial longitudinal arch. Tibialis anterior, tibialis posterior, toe flexors and intrinsic foot muscles are treated using brisk repetitive petrissage, tapotement and point kneading. The inferior aspects of tibialis posterior and flexor digitorum longus may be treated at the inferior

525

Treatment Goals

Mobilize hypomobile joints.

Treatment Plan

medial aspect of the tibia. It is important to avoid long stretching techniques on these muscles.

✋ Joint play techniques are used on the hypomobile superior tibiofibular joint and ankle, excluding the hypermobile medial arch.

✋ The gastrocnemius and soleus may be stretched again in the supine position.

✋ The treatment is finished with local circulation techniques, such as effleurage, on the entire limb.

Self-care Goals

Reduce stresses placed on the overstretched structures. Educate the client regarding activities.

Stretch shortened muscles.

Strengthen weak muscles.

Refer the client.

Self-care Plan

✍ The client should avoid activities that stress the medial longitudinal arch if there is no footwear support for the arches. Moreover, the client should wear support sandals instead of walking in bare feet.

✍ Contrast foot baths are indicated after prolonged standing or activities that stress the feet.

✍ The client should apply ice locally if there is any inflammation, as may happen with plantar fasciitis.

✍ Self-massage to the leg, foot and ankle is performed, following the principles of lengthening work to the shortened muscles and stimulating work to the fatigued muscles.

✍ The client should stretch gastrocnemius, soleus and peroneus longus, brevis and tertius.

✍ Active resisted strengthening of tibialis anterior and posterior and the intrinsic foot muscles is important. To strengthen tibialis anterior, inversion, dorsiflexion and adduction are performed, using a theraband or rubber tubing to provide resistance. Tibialis posterior is strengthened by the client resisting inversion and plantarflexion. To strengthen the intrinsic foot muscles, the client is instructed to grip pencils or pebbles, or to scrunch up towels, with the toes.

✍ The client with postural pes planus may be referred for partial shoe inserts, supportive shoes or orthotics. These devices provide arch support and control calcaneal movement. An adjustment period to orthotic use may be necessary to prevent the client from experiencing foot, calf, knee and low back pain. At first, the client may wear the orthotics for one or two hours and gradually increase the time spent wearing them. The client should consult with the health care professional who fitted the orthotics, for specific advice.

Treatment Frequency and Expected Outcome

Treatment should be given once a week for six weeks. The client is then reassessed at which time the remedial exercise self-care plan is also reassessed.

See also sprains, tendinitis, plantar fasciitis, periostitis and compartment syndromes, patellofemoral syndrome, iliotibial band contracture, piriformis syndrome, hyperlordosis, scoliosis, pregnancy, osteoarthritis and fractures for related conditions.

The outcome for a client with functional pes planus who is compliant with the self-care program is favourable. Once the ligaments have stretched, they cannot return to their original length. However, strengthening exercises and arch supports for activities that stress the foot will allow the client to function for longer periods without fatigue and pain. This is especially important for a high-activity client, such as a runner or hiker, to prevent further dropping of the medial longitudinal arch and injuries such as tendinitis.

40

ILIOTIBIAL BAND CONTRACTURE

Fiona Rattray

Iliotibial band contracture is a contracture or thickening of the iliotibial band (Thomson et al., 1991).

Iliotibial band friction syndrome is inflammation and pain where the iliotibial band crosses the lateral femoral condyle (Booher, Thibodeau, 1989).

Iliotibial band contracture and iliotibial band friction syndrome may present unilaterally or bilaterally.

The iliotibial band (ITB) is a reinforced tract of fascia connecting proximally to the tensor fascia lata and gluteus maximus muscles, and distally to the lateral tibia. It provides lateral support at the knee, especially when the knee is in extension.

When this fascia becomes contractured, the biomechanics of the knee and hip are restricted. Other structures, such as the ankle or sacroiliac joint, may compensate. The trochanteric bursa located between the greater trochanter and the iliotibial band can also become inflamed.

While the iliotibial band itself may be contractured, the presence of trigger points or an increase in tone in tensor fascia lata and gluteus maximus may also contribute to iliotibial band tightness *(Travell, Simons, 1992).*

Some knee surgery procedures use a portion of the iliotibial band to provide lateral support following a rotational instability injury to the knee. Lateral scarring along the distal portion of the iliotibial band results from this surgery.

Causes of iliotibial band contracture are:

➤ **activities or occupations that place the knee and hip in flexion,** allowing the iliotibial band and tensor fascia lata to shorten. Examples of this are cycling, horseback riding or prolonged sitting. Other causes include activities that shorten tensor fascia lata, such as running in only one direction on a track that is sloped or banked. A runner with pronated feet who wears shoes with inadequate arch supports may develop iliotibial band contracture;

➤ **postural imbalances,** such as anterior pelvic tilt or hyperlordosis, which can shorten the iliotibial band. Examples of this are a weak gluteus medius which will allow tensor fascia lata to tighten and pull the pelvis into an anterior pelvic tilt, a shortened rectus femoris which will also increase an anterior pelvic tilt and habitual weight bearing on one leg which shortens the opposite iliotibial band;

➤ **prolonged wheelchair use or bedrest,** which can lead to a slow, progressive contracture.

Causes of iliotibial band friction syndrome are:

➤ **prolonged, repetitive activities** where the knee and hip are flexed, such as running or cycling.

Contributing factors are poor tensor fascia lata stretching procedures and an anterior pelvic tilt.

Symptom Picture

✦ Pain is frequently gradual at onset and worse with activity *(Thompson et al., 1991)*. The pain is felt along the lateral thigh and into the lateral aspect of the knee.

✦ Shortening of the iliotibial band occurs.

✦ Thickening, adhesions and possible fibrositic nodules can be found along the affected iliotibial band.

✦ Inflammation is possible due to the tight iliotibial band rubbing over the lateral femoral condyle.

✦ Hypertonicity and trigger points in tensor fascia lata, hip flexors and rectus femoris lead to reduced circulation and shortening of these muscles.

✦ With an anterior pelvic tilt, lumbar pain and sacroiliac joint hypermobility may occur.

✦ A valgus or a hyperextension orientation of the affected knee may be present.

✦ Secondary trochanteric bursitis can develop.

Subjective Information

HEALTH HISTORY QUESTIONS

✦ How is the client's general health?

✦ What are the client's recreational activities?

✦ Has there been a change in the client's activity levels? For example, has the distance cycled or run been increased?

✦ What is the client's occupation? Does the work involve a lot of sitting — for example, driving a vehicle or a desk job?

✦ Has there been a change in the client's posture, such as an anterior pelvic tilt with advanced pregnancy?

✦ Does the client have a stretching program that includes the hip flexors, iliotibial band and tensor fascia lata?

✦ Is there any pain present? Where is it? What is the quality of the pain? With an iliotibial band contracture, the pain may be described as an achiness on the lateral aspect of the thigh, with a gradual onset. The pain of iliotibial band friction syndrome is directly over the lateral femoral condyle and is worse on activity.

✦ With iliotibial band friction syndrome, is the client taking medication such as anti-inflammatories or analgesics?

Objective Information

Observations

✍ A well-defined iliotibial band may create an indentation in the lateral aspect of the affected thigh.

✍ With a unilateral iliotibial band contracture, viewed anteriorly, there is a lateral pelvic tilt that is low on the affected or contractured side *(Figure 40.1)*.

✍ The knee on the affected side may present with a valgus orientation.

✍ Pes planus may be present on the affected side.

✍ With a bilateral presentation, viewed laterally, an anterior pelvic tilt is due to the shortened iliotibial band and tensor fascia lata *(Figure 40.2)*.

✍ Hyperlordosis results from an anterior pelvic tilt caused by shortened hip flexors and rectus femoris.

✍ Bilateral valgus orientation of the knees may be observed from the anterior or posterior view.

✍ Pes planus may be present bilaterally.

✍ In the case of iliotibial band friction syndrome, redness or local edema may be observed at the affected lateral femoral condyle.

531

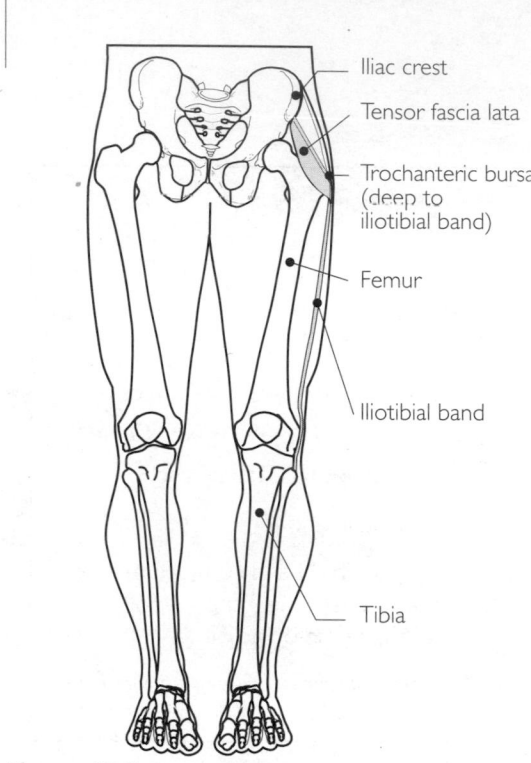

Figure 40.1
Unilateral presentation of iliotibial band contracture showing lateral pelvic tilt and possible
valgus knee and pes planus.

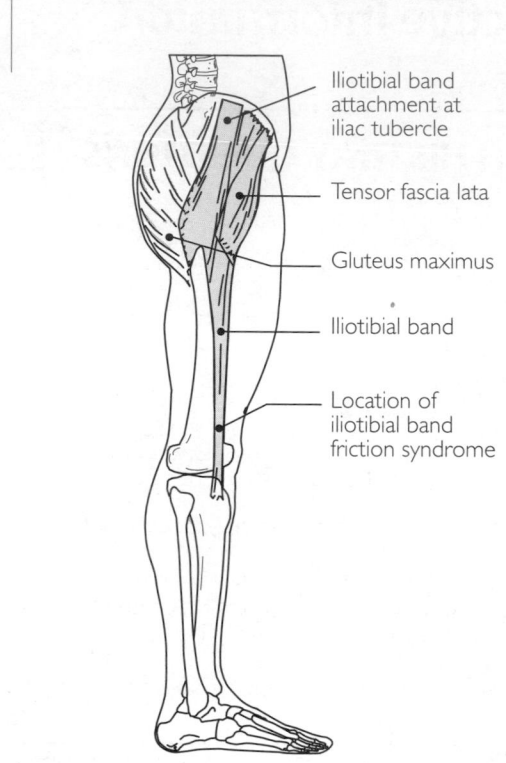

Figure 40.2
Bilateral presentation of iliotibial band showing anterior pelvic tilt and hyperlordosis and possible knee
hyperextension.

Palpation

✍ Tenderness may be present along the iliotibial band, especially the distal third section
and at the greater trochanter.

✍ The affected iliotibial band is thickened and reinforced. Adhesions may be present.

✍ If the presentation is unilateral, on the contractured side increased tone and trigger
points are likely palpated in tensor fascia lata and gluteus maximus. On the non-
contractured leg, increased tone may be present in iliopsoas and, possibly, the
adductors *(St. John, 1994).*

✍ If the presentation is bilateral, there is likely increased tone and possible trigger points in
tensor fascia lata, gluteus maximus, rectus femoris, iliopsoas, adductors and quadratus
lumborum.

✍ With **iliotibial band friction syndrome,** inflammation consisting of heat, swelling and
point tenderness is present local to the affected lateral femoral condyle.

Testing

✍ **AF ROM** of the affected knee, hip, sacroiliac joint and lumbar spine is performed. There
is reduced extension and adduction of the hip. Painful extension of the knee may be
present (knee extension is always painful with iliotibial band friction syndrome). These

findings are bilateral or unilateral depending on the presentation.

✎ **PR ROM** of the affected knee, hip and sacroiliac joint may reveal painful extension at the lateral aspect of the knee, especially with iliotibial band friction syndrome.

✎ **AR testing** of tensor fascia lata, rectus femoris, gluteus maximus, gluteus medius, iliopsoas and quadratus lumborum may indicate stronger tensor fascia lata, hip flexors and gluteus maximus, with a weaker gluteus medius (*Travell, Simons, 1992*).

Contraindications

✦ Do not randomly stretch fascia. Assess the fascia and only treat areas of restriction.

✦ Frictions are contraindicated if the client is on anti-inflammatory medication.

Special Tests

✎ **Length testing** of rectus femoris and iliopsoas (Thomas and Ely's tests) reveals a shortness of these muscles. A positive **Ober's test** or a positive **modified Ober's test** indicates a shortened tensor fascia lata or iliotibial band. A positive **Noble's test** indicates the presence of iliotibial band friction syndrome.

Treatment Goals

Reduce the contractured fascia.

Treatment Plan

✋ The results of palpation and testing determine whether the treatment focus is on reducing the contractures and fascial adhesions or on the muscular origins and the tibial insertion of the band or both. The assessment also indicates whether the treatment is performed unilaterally or bilaterally.

✋ The focus of this treatment is on reducing the contractured fascia. Therefore, this tissue is usually treated first. However, in a unilateral presentation, this is contrary to the treatment principle of treating the unaffected or non-contractured side first.

✋ **Positioning** is determined by the specific structures to be treated. For example, a sidelying position, with supporting pillows under the client's knee to flex and abduct the hip, shortens the iliotibial band and tensor fascia lata. These structures are, therefore, less taut and treatment is more comfortable for the client. Sidelying or prone position can be used to treat the low back and gluteals.

✋ **Hydrotherapy** is a pre-treatment application of deep moist heat, such as a hydrocollator. Strips of cheesecloth dipped in wax are applied to the iliotibial band. Following the fascial work, cool or contrast is used to increase local circulation. Cold is applied to any inflammation.

General Treatment

Decrease sympathetic nervous system firing.

✋ This treatment is performed in the context of a relaxation massage. However, there is some degree of discomfort or pain possible with

Treatment Goals   Treatment Plan

the treatment of this condition. This is clearly stated by the therapist in the consent to treatment statement, so the client may alter or stop the treatment at any point if she wishes. The therapist must ensure that the discomfort or pain is tolerable for the client at all times, working with the client rather than pushing her past her pain limits. To facilitate this, the client is directed to do **diaphragmatic breathing** during any deep and painful techniques. The therapist also intersperses the deeper fascial techniques with effleurage and lighter techniques.

Reduce the hypertonicity and trigger points.

A general low back massage is performed while the hydrotherapy application is taking effect. Rocking, shaking, effleurage and petrissage are used to reduce any hypertonicity or trigger points that are present. Trigger points in quadratus lumborum refer into the gluteus maximus muscle and sacroiliac joint on the same side (*Travell, Simons, 1992*).

Treat other conditions.

If hyperlordosis or trochanteric bursitis is present, refer to those chapters for more specific techniques. These conditions are addressed over a series of appointments.

Specific Treatment

Depending on the results of the assessment, the therapist may choose to start the specific massage with either fascial techniques or work to the muscular origins of the iliotibial band.

Reduce fascial restrictions.

Fascial techniques to treat the iliotibial band itself include skin rolling, crossed-hands spreading and deep longitudinal spreading. Specific transverse work includes C-bow and S-bow techniques. The J-stroke is effective on the most adhered tissues, always within the client's pain tolerance. Fascial techniques are applied in varying directions to thoroughly reduce all restrictions in the fascia. This includes the insertion of the iliotibial band on the tibia, working proximally along the band to the most adhered areas. These fascial techniques are alternated with repetitive light effleurage to increase local circulation.

Reduce any adhesions.

Adhesions are treated with frictions. This technique is always followed by a stretch and ice.

Reduce any inflammation.

If **iliotibial band friction syndrome** is present, the inflammation local to the lateral femoral condyle may make direct, on-site fascial work impossible. **Cold hydrotherapy** or ice is applied to the tissue to reduce the inflammation. Lymphatic drainage techniques are used on the proximal leg. Tightness of the fascia over the lateral condyle should be sufficiently reduced by treatment of the proximal iliotibial band as previously described. In subsequent treatments, when inflammation has subsided, specific frictions are performed to the adhesions in the distal iliotibial band.

Treatment Goals

Treatment Plan

👋 The tensor fascia lata is treated specifically for any hypertonicity, adhering or trigger points. Trigger points in tensor fascia lata may refer tenderness to the greater trochanter (*Travell, Simons, 1992*). Techniques include skin rolling, repetitive petrissage and cross-fibre stripping to the muscle attachments at the iliac crest and around the trochanter. Golgi tendon organ release is used at the greater trochanter. Muscle stripping and ischemic compressions are applied to any trigger points.

👋 Gluteus maximus is specifically treated for hypertonicity and trigger points using the above techniques.

Encourage local circulation to remove metabolites.

👋 This specific work is finished with repetitive effleurage to the lateral leg and gluteals to increase local circulation.

👋 Local **contrast hydrotherapy** applications are used post-treatment to increase local circulation.

👋 The rest of the affected leg is treated, including iliopsoas, quadriceps, hamstrings, adductors and muscles of the lower leg and foot to reduce hypertonicity and trigger points. Vastus lateralis trigger points specifically refer pain into the lateral thigh and knee (*Travell, Simons, 1992*).

👋 If the ankle, superior and inferior tibiofibular joints, knee, hip or sacroiliac joints are hypomobile, joint play techniques are used. Passive relaxed range of motion of the hip and knee are interspersed throughout the treatment.

Stretch the shortened muscles.

👋 Post-isometric relaxation will lengthen the tensor fascia lata and stretch any muscles treated for trigger points.

Treat compensatory structures.

👋 If the contracture is unilateral, the client can remain in the sidelying position with the affected hip and knee uppermost and in flexion. The non-contractured leg is in slight extension. This allows the hypertonic adductors on the non-contractured leg to be treated with repetitive petrissage and muscle stripping. The client can then be turned prone or supine for a general massage to increase local circulation and decrease the hypertonicity of the non-contractured thigh and leg.

👋 If the contracture is bilateral, the therapist has the client turn over so the other leg is treated in a similar manner.

Self-care Goals

Self-care Plan

✍ Deep moist heat and contrast applications to the thigh are used. Local ice or cold will reduce the inflammation and pain of an iliotibial band friction syndrome.

535

Self-care Goals

Self-care Plan

✍ Self-massage, such as skin rolling, can be done on the iliotibial band and tensor fascia lata.

Stretch short muscles.

✍ To stretch tensor fascia lata, the client places the hand on the affected side against a wall, crosses the affected leg into adduction behind the unaffected leg and leans the body towards the wall.

✍ Alternatively, the client can stretch tensor fascia lata by lying on the unaffected side, extending and externally rotating the affected leg and then relaxing the leg to allow for adduction and stretch.

✍ If the client is seated for extended periods of time, frequent stretching of the tensor fascia lata and iliotibial band is also important.

✍ To stretch gluteus maximus, the client brings the knee to the shoulder on the same side.

✍ Refer to the chapter on hyperlordosis for specific remedial exercises if an anterior pelvic tilt is present.

Educate the client regarding activities.

✍ The client should try to avoid or minimize activities that shorten the iliotibial band and tensor fascia lata. For example, the client should avoid running uphill, but should run on level ground as much as possible; instead of running in one direction only on a sloping track, the client should run in both directions.

✍ Sleeping on the unaffected side with a pillow under the affected knee will reduce the compression of the tight iliotibial band (*Travell, Simons, 1992*).

Treatment Frequency and Expected Outcome

Treatment should be once a week for six weeks. At that point, the therapist should totally reassess both the client and the remedial exercise self-care plan.

See also bursitis, pes planus, hyperlordosis, scoliosis and pregnancy for related conditions.

Outcome of treatment depends on the length of time the contracture has existed and the perpetuating factors. For example, if a client has recently increased the mileage cycled and has no postural contributing factors, there may be a noticeable improvement after the initial treatment. However, if long-term postural imbalances are contributing to the condition, the progress will depend on correcting these imbalances and ongoing client compliance.

41

PATELLOFEMORAL SYNDROME

Fiona Rattray

Patellofemoral syndrome, also called patellofemoral tracking disorder, describes various painful degenerative changes to the articular cartilage on the underside of the patella.

Sixty-five per cent of patellofemoral pain is due to tracking or instability problems *(Larson, Grana, 1993)*.

The patella is a sesamoid bone that covers the anterior portion of the knee joint. It attaches superiorly to the quadriceps tendon and inferiorly to the patellar tendon. The patella is stabilized medially and laterally by the patellar retinacula.

The patella and its articulating surfaces, the femoral condyles, the patellar tendon and its attachment to the tibia, the retinaculum, the synovium and the quadriceps muscle, make up the extensor mechanism of the knee. When the knee is extended, the patella glides superior to the femoral condyles. When the knee is flexed, the patella glides inferior to the condyles. This gliding occurs along the longitudinal axis of the femur in response to the contraction of the quadriceps muscle. The pull of the patellar tendon is along the longitudinal axis of the tibia. Due to the slight valgus angulation that most knee joints assume when the knee is in extension, the long axis of the femur and the long axis of the tibia are at a slight angle to each other *(Figure 41.1)*. This angle is called the Q (quadriceps) angle *(Hertling, Kessler, 1990)*.

The Q angle results in a slight lateral pull on the patella. The lateral femoral condyle and the patellar groove on the femur help to prevent this lateral movement. When the knee is in flexion, the quadriceps muscle pulls the patella tightly into the femoral groove. However, as the knee approaches full extension, the patella glides in a superior direction into the shallower portion of the femoral groove. Both the vastus medialis obliquus and the medial retinaculum must function to prevent the patella from tracking laterally. This is especially important when the knee is bearing a load.

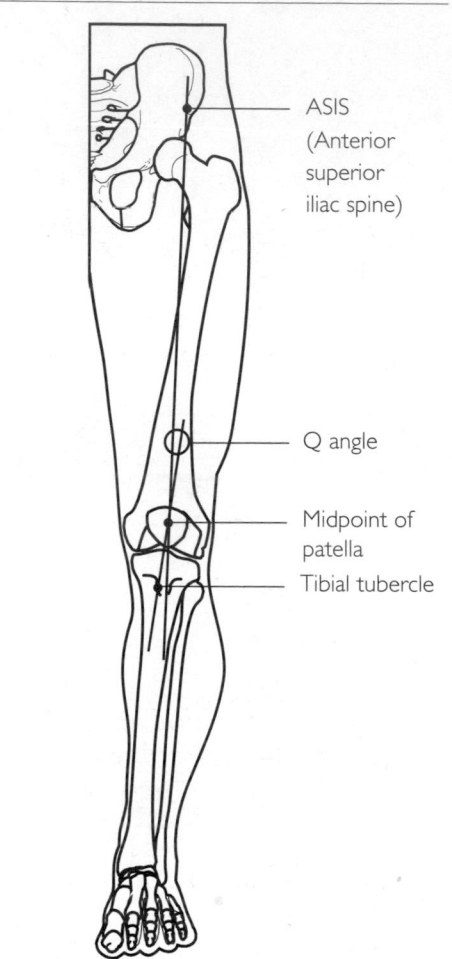

Figure 41.1
Landmarks for measuring the Q angle.

Labels in figure:
ASIS (Anterior superior iliac spine)
Q angle
Midpoint of patella
Tibial tubercle

In order to withstand loads, the patellar cartilage, at five millimetres, is the thickest cartilage in the human body. Cartilage is a unique structure designed to produce almost frictionless motion between the joint surfaces. It has a friction equivalent to one-eighth that of ice gliding on ice. The patellar cartilage is hyaline cartilage, named after the Greek word for mirror, because it is smooth and mirror-like. Cartilage is self-renewing and self-lubricating. In children, cartilage is a blue-white colour; as people age, it becomes increasingly yellow. The reason for this is not known and there is no evidence that this colour change affects the function of the cartilage *(Fox, Del Pizzo, 1993)*.

The posterior articulating surface of the patella consists of a lateral and medial facet. A small, odd medial facet is present in 30 per cent of the population *(Larson, Grana, 1993)*. The areas of contact between the articulating surfaces of the patella and the femoral condyles vary with the position of the knee from extension through full flexion. With normal knee biomechanics, compressive forces apply to both the lateral and medial articulating facets.

The mechanism of **patellofemoral syndrome** is not completely understood. There are several predisposing factors to this condition, including abnormal biomechanics, soft tissue dysfunction and previous injury.

Contributing factors include:

➤ **abnormal biomechanics,** such as increased foot pronation, internal tibial rotation and internal femoral rotation (femoral anteversion), any of which can lead to an increased Q angle;

➤ **a small, high-riding patella** (patella alta), which is less stable because it lies in the shallower superior portions of the femoral groove. A less prominent lateral femoral condyle will allow the patella to track laterally;

➤ **tight lateral structures**, such as the vastus lateralis, lateral retinaculum, iliotibial band and tensor fascia lata. These increase the lateral pull on the patella;

➤ **tight posterior and anterior structures**, such as hamstrings, gastrocnemius and rectus femoris; any of these can restrict normal movement at the ankle and knee;

➤ **weakness** of muscles, such as vastus medialis obliquus, which allows the lateral motion of the patella, and weakness in gluteus medius, which permits medial rotation of the femur;

➤ **knee injury**, including patellar subluxation, as well as knee surgery. These can injure the articular surfaces and result in weakness of vastus medialis obliquus;

➤ **arthroscopic procedures**, which can cause iatrogenic lesions of the cartilage *(Glinz, 1987)*;

➤ **repeated knee stress** and overuse *(Brukner, Khan, 1993)*.

All these predisposing factors may have an effect on the patellofemoral contact, on the tracking of the patella in the femoral groove or on both these mechanisms. With repeated knee flexion there is an increased stress on the articular cartilage. This can produce degenerative changes, synovial irritation, inflammation and pain. The problem with this theory of the development of patellofemoral syndrome is that many persons with patellofemoral pain have intact articular surfaces and no evidence of synovial irritation (Larson, Grana, 1993).

Another theory holds that the subchondral bone of the odd medial facet is less dense than the rest of the patella. This facet only articulates in extreme knee flexion and, therefore, does not receive enough compressive stresses to increase its density and strength. If the patella tracks too far laterally during loaded knee extension, the patella will rotate slightly, causing the odd medial facet to become a contact point. The less dense subchondral bone is less able to bear loads and breaks down more rapidly than the rest of the articulating surface (Hertling, Kessler, 1990). However, the odd medial facet is only present in 30 per cent of the population, so this may not be the whole picture.

Finally, one study has shown that fibrillation of collagen in the intermediate and deep portions of the articular cartilage can occur without being initially observable on the surface. This has been called "basal degeneration". A failure of the cartilage to absorb stresses in the knee joint could place more load on the subchondral bone. An increase in subchondral interosseous pressure has been proven to cause pain. Because bone is innervated for pain and cartilage is not, this is a more feasible explanation for the syndrome (Larson, Grana, 1993).

The Medical Treatment of Patellofemoral Syndrome

In the past, the medical approach to a patellar tracking problem included a lateral release of the retinaculum from the inferior pole of the patella to one or two centimetres above the superior pole. Following surgery, occasional signs of over-release were the knee giving way, knee weakness and pain, a palpable defect in vastus lateralis, excessive patellar tilt of 80 to 130 degrees and possible medial subluxation of the patella. Because of these possible complications, a lateral release is currently not considered if there is patella alta or an excessive lateral tilt of the patella or an insufficient medial restraint on the patella (for example, with weakness in vastus medialis obliquus).

In more recent studies performed on cadavers with chondromalacia, the lateral release did not unload the lateral patellar facet as had been empirically assumed. Instead, there were inconsistent and unpredictable effects on the pressure at the patellofemoral contact. In some cases, the contact pressure was redistributed to different areas of the patella (Fox, Del Pizzo, 1993).

The conservative medical approach now is to use non-steroidal anti-inflammatories (NSAIDs) for one month in combination with remedial exercises, such as straight leg raises and knee extensions. The exercises are continued for eight to 12 weeks. The patella is also taped for this period of time to correct its abnormal position and relieve the pressures on the articulating surfaces. Surgery is used in only a minority of cases. The importance of remedial exercise in reducing the symptoms of patellofemoral syndrome is illustrated by one study where the majority of persons failed to follow the rehabilitation program and their symptoms remained (Larson, Grana, 1993).

The use of knee supports or braces to relieve patellofemoral syndrome is not completely agreed upon. Few studies have been done on the effects of knee braces and those that have been performed do not conclusively show which types of braces are useful. Braces may work by altering proprioception at the knee or by altering the actual tracking of the patella. One source stresses the need for a comprehensive remedial exercise program to rehabilitate the knee, instead of relying only on knee supports *(Fox, Del Pizzo, 1993)*.

Associated Conditions

Chondromalacia patella is literally a softening of the cartilage of the patella. In the past, this was thought to be the cause of patellofemoral pain. However, arthroscopic observations have revealed that true chondromalacia is often asymptomatic and is a part of the normal aging process *(Larson, Grana, 1993)*. It may develop secondary to patellar tracking disorders. Development of chondromalacia occurs in the deeper layers of the cartilage. This is in contrast to the development of osteoarthritis where a superficial fraying of the cartilage is noted. The literature on chondromalacia patella is often contradictory, because the terminology used is not consistent *(Fox, Del Pizzo, 1993)*.

Plica syndrome may be a cause of knee pain. Synovial folds at the knee, also called "plica", are frequently observed during arthroscopic examination. The medial plica runs from the superiomedial portion of the knee obliquely and laterally to the infrapatellar fat pad at the tibia. This thickened band is present in up to 55 per cent of the knees studied. These folds are usually asymptomatic unless repeated overuse or injury to the knee results in fibrosing of the plica. The band can then compress the patella and the medial femoral condyle, causing changes in the articular surfaces. The knee is painful and may mimic patellofemoral pain. Clicking or swelling is variable with plica syndrome. A taut, palpable tender band is noted just medial to the patella *(Fox, Del Pizzo, 1993)*.

Symptom Picture

✦ The symptom picture of patellofemoral syndrome includes peripatellar and subpatellar pain. The client experiences difficulty in sitting for long periods of time due to pain, the so-called movie theatre sign. Activities such as walking down stairs, squatting and running downhill are painful and the knee may give way. There is pain on patellar compression.

✦ Crepitus is present in the joint. Swelling may be present, especially if arthritic change is also present. This is associated with disuse atrophy of the quadriceps muscles.

Treatment Considerations

Assessment

🖾 **Observations:**

• A **postural assessment** is performed. In a posterior view, pronation of the foot and a valgus orientation of the knee may be contributing factors. In an anterior view, with the client's feet parallel, a medial orientation of the patella (squinting patella) may be caused by internal femoral and tibial rotation. If the client is allowed to stand in his normal posture, the feet appear externally rotated while the patella seems to have a medial position. Some hypotrophy of vastus medialis may be noticed. In a lateral view, hyperextension of the knees may be present, as may patella alta.

- In terms of **gait assessment**, in an anterior view, the thigh internally rotates and adducts to midline, so the weight bearing foot is placed under the centre of the pelvis. With gluteus medius weakness, a Trendelenburg gait may be present *(Larson, Grana, 1993)*.

- When the client is seated, hypotrophy of the vastus medialis may be noticed.

✍ **Palpation** of the medial and lateral borders of the patella reveals tenderness and possible swelling. The tissue just medial to the patella is palpated for a vertical taut band that may indicate a plica cord.

✍ **Testing:**

- **AF ROM** of the knee may reveal excessive lateral motion of the patella in the first 45 degrees of flexion. The patella is then lightly palpated for snapping of soft tissue over medial or lateral retinaculum while the client flexes and extends the knee *(Fox, Del Pizzo, 1993)*.

- In **PR ROM** the patella is palpated for crepitus and to check if the patella tracks in the same lateral manner as in the AF ROM testing. Tightness of the lateral retinaculum is present when the patella is mobilized medially. The ankle, hip, sacroiliac joints and lumbar spine are also assessed for any contributing hypomobility.

- **AR strength** of gluteus medius may be reduced. A functional test for hip abductors is a single leg squat, with a weakness revealed by the pelvis dropping on the untested side.

- **Length tests** of hamstrings reveal reduced knee extension when the hip is first flexed to 90 degrees *(Fox, Del Pizzo, 1993)*. Gastrocnemius may also be short, placing the knee in slight flexion.

- The **Q angle** is greater than 18 degrees when the client is standing *(Fox, Del Pizzo, 1993)*.

- **Waldron's, McConnell's** and **Clarke's patellofemoral grind tests** are positive. A **patellar apprehension test** may be positive. This test may be performed with the knee in full extension and at a functional position of 30 to 45 degrees of flexion *(Fox, Del Pizzo, 1993)*. An **Ober's test** is positive with a tight iliotibial band.

✍ **Differential assessment** for patellar tendinitis is pain with compression at the tendinous insertion at the inferior patella and pain at the inferior patella with knee squats *(Fox, Del Pizzo, 1993)*.

Contraindications

✦ If any inflammation is present, avoid using hot local hydrotherapy or local techniques, such as frictions, at the lesion site.

✦ Full flexion passive relaxed range of motion with overpressure is contraindicated if this produces pain.

Massage

- In terms of massage, the primary focus is on the compensating structures that have contributed to the condition — for example, iliotibial band friction syndrome.

- **Positioning** is prone, supine or sidelying.

- **Hydrotherapy** can include deep moist heat to the iliotibial band and lateral retinaculum or contrast applications to encourage local circulation.

- General Swedish techniques are used on the low back and gluteals in the prone position. Hypomobile joints in the lumbar spine and sacroiliac joints are mobilized using joint play.

- Fascial techniques are used on the iliotibial band and the hamstrings. For details see the iliotibial band contracture chapter. Transverse fascial spreading and skin rolling are indicated for the lateral knee and retinaculum. The patella is mobilized in a medial direction. Specific petrissage is used on the tensor fascia lata, gluteus medius, hamstrings and gastrocnemius to reduce their tone.

- In the supine position, adductors and quadriceps muscles are treated with petrissage. Trigger points in the quadriceps muscles can refer pain to the knee joint; trigger points in vastus medialis can cause weakness and buckling of the knee while walking (*Travell, Simons, 1992*). Muscle stripping and ischemic compressions are indicated. Pain-free passive relaxed range of motion of the knee will help with succussive action. Passive stretches and post-isometric relaxation techniques for the shortened hamstrings and gastrocnemius are interspersed throughout the massage.

- Hypomobile joints, such as the hip and ankle, are treated using joint play. Massage to the distal leg and foot is performed. See the chapter on pes planus for details. Repetitive effleurage to the entire leg and thigh is used to increase local venous return and flush metabolites from the tissues.

Self-care

- The self-care program for patellofemoral syndrome should include the entire limb, not just the knee. The vastus medialis obliquus is often dysfunctional and weak, allowing the patella to track laterally. Regaining the strength of this muscle is important. However, the vastus medialis obliquus is difficult to strengthen in isolation from the vastus lateralis.

- The client can begin with quadriceps setting, straight leg raises with the knees held in extension or knee extension over a towel roll to strengthen the vastus medialis obliquus. The forces on the articular surfaces of the patella are lowest at 0 to 30 degrees of extension (*Fox, Del Pizzo, 1993*).

- To isometrically strengthen the adductors and vastus medialis obliquus, the client sits on the floor with the knees extended. The client pushes the first metatarsophalangeal joints of both great toes together. This is progressed to AR isometric exercises where the client is sitting, squeezing a ball or towel roll between the knees.

- The client can progress to short arc and long arc extensions of the knee as tolerated. Some sources feel that short arc extensions for tracking should be done from 90 to 40 degrees of knee flexion only, because, even though contraction of the vastus medialis obliquus is maximal at terminal extension, so is the contraction of vastus lateralis (*Fox, Del Pizzo, 1993*). This maximal contraction of vastus lateralis would overpower the medialis.

✍ If these exercises exacerbate symptoms, the client can try rapid full range of motion exercises that have a low impact, such as swimming. The frog kick is avoided *(Larson, Grana, 1993)*.

✍ To strengthen the hip abductors, the client is sidelying on the unaffected leg and abducts the affected leg against gravity.

✍ To strengthen the adductors, the client is sidelying on the affected leg. The hip and knee of the unaffected leg are flexed so the foot can be placed flat on the table. The affected leg is adducted against gravity.

✍ For exercises to strengthen the supinators of the foot, see the chapter on pes planus.

✍ The client can also perform self-mobilization of the patella in a medial direction. This can be combined with self-massage of the lateral retinaculum. If the iliotibial band is involved, self-massage is indicated here also.

✍ Flexibility exercises are started early, because a combination of a tight lateral retinaculum and a lack of adequate vastus medialis obliquus strength contributes to this condition.

✍ The hamstrings and gastrocnemius muscles should be stretched because, when tight, they have been shown to increase stress on the patellofemoral joint. One source notes that knee pain is often relieved by one or two months of hamstring stretches *(Fox, Del Pizzo, 1993)*. For exercises to stretch the iliotibial band, refer to the iliotibial band contracture chapter.

✍ In later stages of healing, closed kinetic chain exercises are better for rehabilitation because forces are distributed more evenly over the joint. Examples of closed kinetic chain exercises include: step-downs with the leg to be strengthened remaining on the top step while the other leg steps back up; and partial squats where the client leans back against a wall, isometrically squeezing a ball or towel roll between the knees. To retrain the extensor mechanism, the client is given partial lunges with the affected knee flexed to 30 degrees. The vastus medialis obliquus is isometrically contracted for 10 seconds while the client supinates the foot then returns it slowly to the neutral position. The exercise is repeated, then the knee is extended and the entire cycle is performed again *(Hertling, Kessler, 1990)*. The client progresses to a stationary bike with the resistance set to low. The stress placed on the knee by step machines can be reduced by the client using short steps that do not emphasize knee flexion.

See also iliotibial band contracture, pes planus, hyperlordosis, pregnancy and osteoarthritis for related conditions.

✍ If the knee continues to be symptomatic, the client can be referred to a physiotherapist for patellar taping that includes correction of lateral glide, lateral tilt and rotational components. This system was developed by Jenny McConnell, an Australian physical therapist *(Brukner, Khan, 1993)*.

✍ The client should be referred for orthotics if foot pronation is a contributing factor.

42

HYPERLORDOSIS

Fiona Rattray

Hyperlordosis is an increase in the normal lumbar lordotic curve with increased anterior pelvic tilt and hip flexion.

It has been noted that muscles respond to stress by either shortening or fatiguing and that there are patterns to these reactions. One of these patterns, which is present in hyperlordosis, is described as pelvic-crossed syndrome *(Janda in Twomey, Taylor, 1987)*. In this syndrome, the shortened hip flexors and lumbar muscles inhibit the muscles that are antagonists across from them *(Figure 42.1)*.

Contraction of iliopsoas in the standing person increases the normal lumbar lordotic curve *(Travell, Simons, 1992)*. This muscle runs from the anterolateral portions of the lumbar vertebrae and the iliac fossa of the pelvis, across the anterolateral portion of the pubic ramus to attach to the femur. It also tilts the pelvis anteriorly when it shortens, reinforcing the postural dysfunction.

With hyperlordosis *(Figure 42.1)*, muscles that are short and tight bilaterally are iliopsoas, rectus femoris, tensor fascia lata, quadratus lumborum and lumbar erector spinae; these are postural muscles, responding to stress by adaptively shortening. The adductors are postural muscles and are likely to adaptively shorten. Piriformis is also a postural muscle and shortens with foot pronation.

Muscles that are stretched, weak and taut in hyperlordosis are rectus abdominius, external and internal abdominal obliques and gluteus maximus; these are phasic muscles, responding to stress by fatiguing. Although hamstrings are postural muscles, the anterior pelvic tilt of hyperlordosis increases the distance between the attachments on the ischial tuberosity and the tibia, making the hamstrings adaptively stretched and tight *(Kendall, McCreary, 1983; Janda in Twomey, Taylor, 1987)*.

Hyperlordosis can contribute to other postural dysfunctions. There may be a

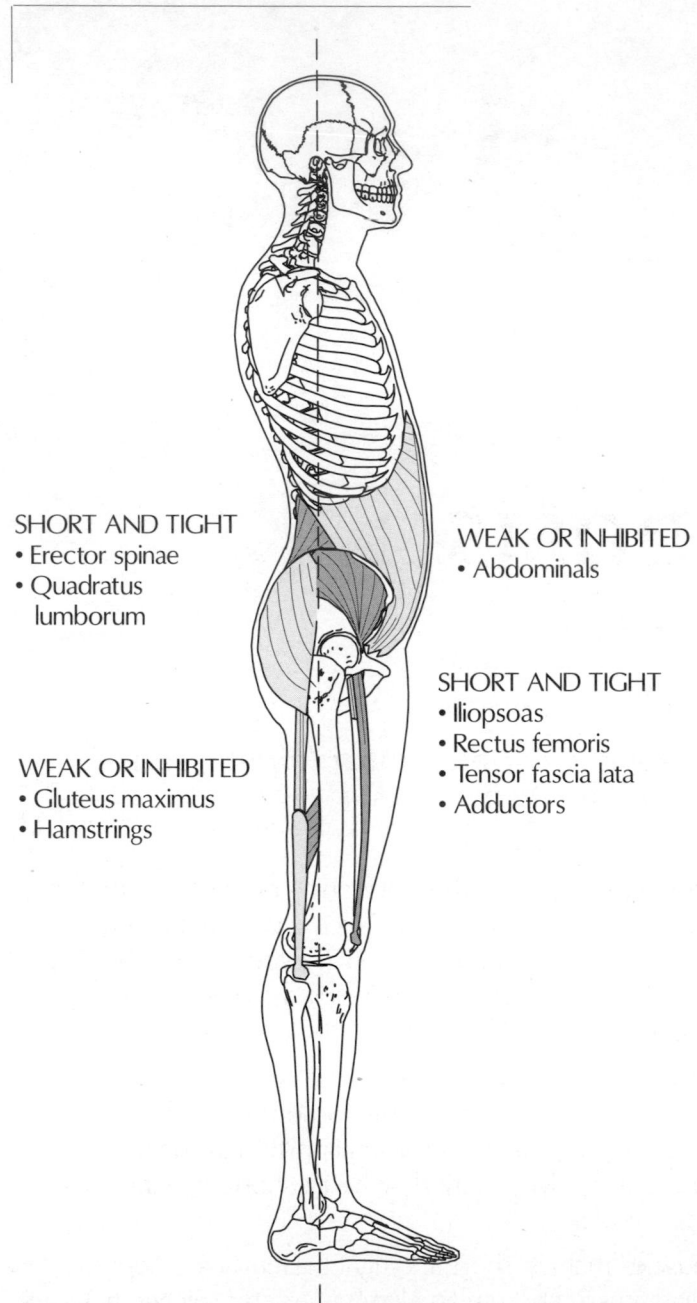

SHORT AND TIGHT
• Erector spinae
• Quadratus
  lumborum

WEAK OR INHIBITED
• Abdominals

SHORT AND TIGHT
• Iliopsoas
• Rectus femoris
• Tensor fascia lata
• Adductors

WEAK OR INHIBITED
• Gluteus maximus
• Hamstrings

Figure 42.1
Tight and weak muscles in hyperlordosis
illustrating pelvic-crossed syndrome.

compensatory hyperkyphosis and head-forward posture. Conversely, other postural dysfunctions such as pes planus, iliotibial band contracture or hyperkyphosis may cause hyperlordosis.

A pathology that may be present with hyperlordosis :

✦ **Spondylolisthesis**, a defect of the neural arch, consists of anterior slippage of the lumbar vertebrae following a bilateral fracture of the pars interarticularis. It can be caused by hyperlordosis, congenital deformity or stress fracture *(Kuchera, Kuchera, 1993)*. Spondylolisthesis is most common between L5 and S1. It may be asymptomatic or painful *(Buschbacher, 1994)*. Spondylolysis is a unilateral fracture of the pars *(Hertling, Kessler, 1990)*.

Causes of hyperlordosis are:

➤ **sustained poor posture.** A person may feel comfortable in a slouched posture and habitually adopt this position;

➤ **prolonged standing.** This may be occupationally related *(Boyling, Palastanga, 1994)*;

➤ **other postural conditions**: bilateral iliotibial band contracture *(Kendall et al., 1993)* and pes planus;

➤ **weak abdominal muscles**, from either disuse or abdominal surgery;

➤ **pregnancy**;

➤ **obesity** *(Kisner, Colby, 1990)*.

Swayback Posture

There is no agreement in literature as to the specific definition and attributes of swayback or slouched posture. It is generally noted that, in the lateral view, the pelvis is projected anteriorly from the gravity line and associated thoracic hyperkyphosis and head-forward posture are present. The anterior shifting of the pelvis may cause the thoracic curve as a compensatory mechanism or vise versa *(Kendall, McCreary, 1983; Thomson et al., 1991; Kisner, Colby, 1990)*. Swayback posture may arise from an increase in the lumbosacral angle, causing the person to lean the thoracic cage posteriorly to compensate *(Cailliet, 1995; Magee, 1992)*.

There is marked disagreement on the direction of pelvic tilt. It is noted as being a posterior tilt with shortened hamstrings and with the compensatory posterior bending of the thorax to counter the anterior shifting of the pelvis. This makes it appear as if the person has a hyperlordosis *(Kendall, McCreary, 1983)*. On the other hand, the pelvic tilt is also shown as being anterior *(Thomson et al., 1991)*; and both an anterior and a posterior pelvic tilt are shown as contributing to swayback posture *(Magee, 1992)*. The hip joints are either described as being in extension *(Kendall, McCreary, 1983; Kisner, Colby, 1990)* or shown in flexion *(Thomson et al., 1991)*.

Given these disagreements, it is therefore important for the therapist to perform his own assessment of posture and muscle length when the client is described as being swaybacked. See also the chapter on hyperkyphosis for related assessments.

Symptom Picture

✦ There is an increased lumbar lordotic curve with associated bilateral anterior pelvic tilt and hip flexion. Other possible altered biomechanics are bilateral pes planus, knee hyperextension or bilateral iliotibial band contracture.

✦ Muscle imbalances are present. The hip flexors and lumbar extensors are short and tight, while the abdominals are weak and stretched. The hamstrings and gluteus maximus are stretched and taut to compensate for the anterior pelvic tilt. The adductors may be short and tight also to compensate for the anterior tilt.

✦ Pain may arise from tight ischemic tissue, overstretched tissue or trigger points.

✦ Range of motion at the hip is reduced in extension.

✦ Pain may arise from a stretched anterior longitudinal ligament or from facet joint approximation which may lead to the facets weight bearing and becoming irritated. It may also be caused by posterior disk and intervertebral foramen narrowing with possible nerve root irritation *(Kisner, Colby, 1990)*.

✦ Poor postural habits are present.

✦ Other postural imbalances such as hyperkyphosis may be noted.

Subjective Information

HEALTH HISTORY QUESTIONS

✦ How long has the hyperlordosis been present? Did it occur or worsen during pregnancy?

✦ What areas are painful, if any? What aggravates or relieves the pain? For example, do positions such as standing at work or at home aggravate the back pain? Is the pain relieved by placing a footrest under one foot or by changing position?

✦ How is the client's general health? Are there any underlying pathologies or injuries that may cause back pain?

✦ What are the client's postural habits, including occupational or recreational sources of postural stress?

✦ Has the client had abdominal or lumbar surgery? This may cause muscular and fascial weakness *(Gracovetsky, 1988).*

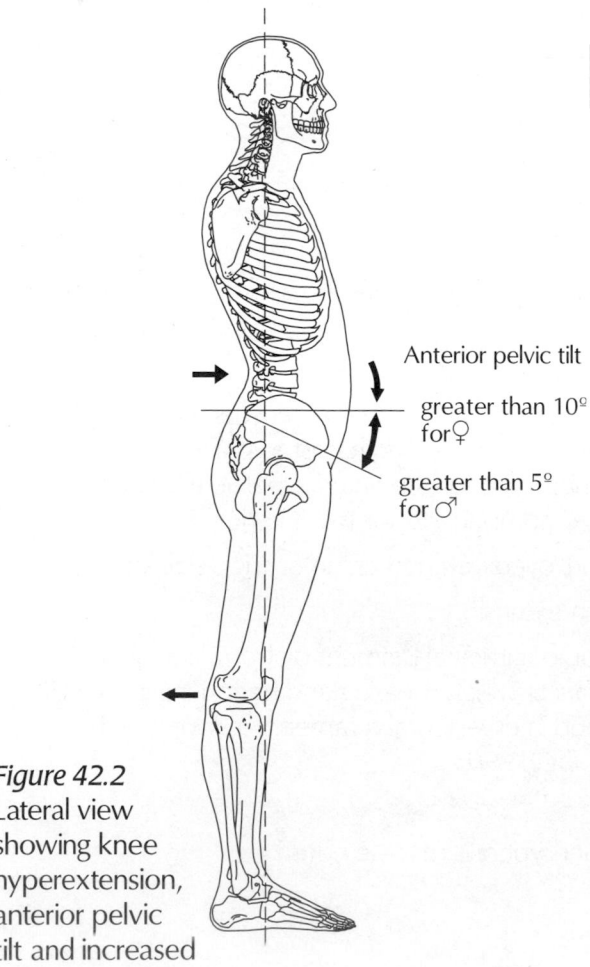

Anterior pelvic tilt

greater than 10° for ♀

greater than 5° for ♂

Figure 42.2 Lateral view showing knee hyperextension, anterior pelvic tilt and increased lordotic curve.

Objective Information

Observations

Postural Assessment – Lateral View

✍ Slight ankle plantarflexion is possible.

✍ Slight knee hyperextension is possible.

✍ The hip joints are flexed.

✍ Bilateral anterior pelvic tilt in hyperlordosis is greater than 10 degrees in female clients and greater than five degrees in male clients. Normal values for pelvic tilt are five to 10 degrees of anterior tilt for females and zero to five degrees of anterior tilt for males *(Figure 42.2).*

✍ The lumbar lordotic curve is increased.

✍ Often there is a compensatory hyperkyphosis and head-forward posture.

✍ Bilateral pes planus may be noted in a posterior view.

✍ Abdominal or lumbar scarring may be present from surgery.

Palpation

✍ Tenderness, hypertonicity and trigger points may be present in the lumbar erector spinae, quadratus lumborum, iliopsoas, tensor fascia lata and rectus femoris.

✍ The texture of the lumbar and iliotibial tract fascia is thickened and reinforced.

Testing

✍ **AF ROM** to test trunk and hip flexion reveals shortened lumbar extensors and lengthened hamstrings. AF extension of the lumbar spine in the standing position may aggravate low back pain associated with hyperlordosis *(Cailliet, 1995)*.

✍ **PR ROM** of the hip is reduced in extension.

✍ **AR strength testing** reveals that both iliopsoas are strong while the abdominals are weak.

Special Tests

✍ A **Thomas test** is positive bilaterally, indicating that both iliopsoas and rectus femoris are short. **Ely's test** is positive bilaterally, indicating rectus femoris shortness. **Ober's test** is positive bilaterally, indicating tensor fascia lata shortness. The **hip adductor length test** is positive, indicating adductor muscle shortness. **Piriformis length test** is also likely positive. **Straight leg raise test** shows an increase in hamstring length.

✍ In the lumbar spine and thoracolumbar junction, **anterior** and **lateral spinous challenge tests** may reveal areas of vertebral hypo- or hypermobility.

Differentiating Sources of Low Back Pain

✦ **Space-occupying lesions** such as a disc herniation give positive results with Valsalva's, Kemp's, Kernig's, straight leg raise, deep tendon reflexes and gastrocnemius strength tests.

✦ **Facet joint irritation** is revealed with a positive Kemp's test.

✦ **Sacroiliac joint mobility** is assessed with motion palpation.

✦ **Sacroiliac joint dysfunction** results in positive sacroiliac joint mobility, sacroiliac joint gapping, sacroiliac joint squish, Gaenslen's and Faber tests.

✦ **Hip pathologies** referring pain are revealed by positive hip quadrant and Faber tests.

✦ **Spondylolisthesis** is sometimes palpated as an anterior displacement of L5 on S1, but is most clearly identified through referral to a physician for X-rays.

✦ **Visceral pathologies** may also refer to the back — for example, renal and urological pathologies. Bone cancer may also cause bilateral back pain that is unrelieved by positional changes and worse at night. Prostate cancer, most commonly presenting in males over 50 years of age, has back and lateral leg pain as a symptom. See Appendix D for more details. The client should be referred to a physician if orthopedic testing results are negative or inconclusive for a neuromuscular source of the pain.

Contraindications

+ If low back pain is present, rule out potential pathological sources before treatment. Refer the client to a physician if necessary.
+ Avoid mobilizing hypermobile vertebral segments.
+ Do not randomly stretch fascia. Assess the fascia and only treat areas of restriction.
+ Do not compress over palpable vasculature, including the aorta, when massaging the abdomen or the femoral artery when massaging the upper medial thigh.
+ Avoid lengthening techniques on weak, overstretched tissues.

Treatment Goals

Treatment Plan

🖐 The therapist may choose several or all of the following techniques to treat the hyperlordotic client. Techniques may be spread out over a series of treatments rather than being done all at once. The techniques chosen should, however, be performed bilaterally within the same treatment.

🖐 **Positioning** is started supine with pillows under the knees to reduce the hyperlordosis. This allows the tight hip flexors to be released first. The client is then turned prone, with pillows under the abdomen and ankles.

🖐 **Hydrotherapy** is pre-treatment heat to the fascia over one rectus femoris. The heat is then moved to the other thigh. When the client is turned prone, heat is applied to the lumbar fascia. Cool applications are used to stimulate the gluteals and hamstrings.

General Treatment

Decrease sympathetic nervous system firing.

🖐 The session is performed in the context of a relaxation treatment, which includes **diaphragmatic breathing** to help reduce any pain experienced with the direct fascial work.

Specific Treatment

Reduce fascial restrictions.

🖐 Fascial techniques are used on the pre-heated anterior hip, including slow skin rolling and connective tissue cutting along the rectus femoris and tensor fascia lata. Ulnar border stripping from the patella to the anterior superior iliac spine along rectus femoris is also indicated. The other limb is treated in a similar manner.

🖐 Myofascial release may also be used on the hip flexors. The client is draped so the abdomen and affected thigh are uncovered. A towel is

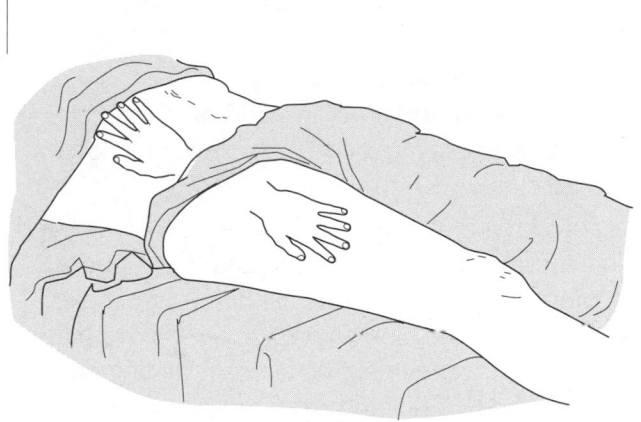

Figure 42.3
Draping and hand position for fascial work to anterior hip.

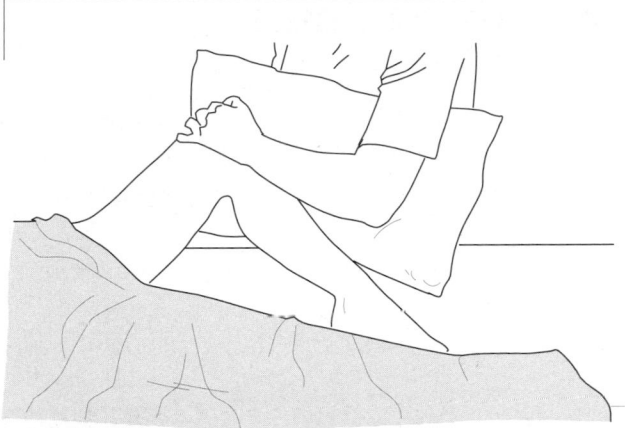

Figure 42.4
Position for work to adductors with limb position and pillow between client's knee and therapist's torso.

Treatment Goals   Treatment Plan

used to cover the client's chest (*Figure 42.3*). The therapist's forearms are crossed and the proximal hand is placed gently on the client's abdomen over the iliopsoas muscle. The distal hand is placed on the upper thigh and the slack is taken up. The pressure used by the proximal hand is just sufficient to stabilize the abdominal fascia, while the distal hand applies the majority of the pressure in a distal direction. This technique can be facilitated by allowing the client's leg to hang off the table, while the other leg is flexed at the hip and knee.

If the adductors are also affected, first the client's abdomen is redraped. The client's lower limb is positioned so the plantar surface of the foot is on the medial side of the untreated knee, with the affected knee flexed and the hip flexed, medially rotated and abducted. A pillow is placed between the client's affected knee and the therapist's torso, allowing the affected knee to rest against the torso (*Figure 42.4*). Slow ulnar border stripping is applied to the adductors, working in a distal to proximal direction.

Reduce hypertonicity and trigger points. Reduce pain if present.

Swedish techniques for rectus femoris, tensor fascia lata and the adductors include effleurage, palmar kneading, wringing and muscle stripping. The trigger point in rectus femoris is located inferior to the anterior superior iliac spine. It refers pain into the knee (*Travell, Simons, 1992*).

Increase local circulation to remove metabolites.

Work to the thigh is finished with repetitive effleurage. The limb is placed back on the table with the hip and knee in flexion to relax the abdominal muscles. The abdomen is undraped again in preparation for

551

Treatment Goals   Treatment Plan

treating iliopsoas. It may be necessary to do an abdominal massage prior to working on the iliopsoas, or it may be possible to start on the iliacus if the client is comfortable with this.

✋ In rhythm with the client's breath, increasing pressure is slowly applied through the abdominal muscles just medial to the anterior superior iliac spine. The fingers apply tolerable pressure as the client exhales and are held in place as the client inhales. To help locate the muscle, if necessary, the client is asked to gently flex the hip, contracting iliacus, and then relaxing. Once iliacus is contacted, slow muscle stripping and the origin and insertion technique are used to treat the muscle belly. The fingers are smoothly and softly withdrawn when the work to iliacus is completed.

✋ The same careful approach is used for psoas major. The lateral border of rectus abdominis is landmarked at the level of the umbilicus. Slowly increasing pressure is applied at this location, allowing the viscera to slide away from the palpating fingers. Pressure is applied at an oblique angle towards the spine. If a pulse is palpated, the pressure is redirected. If necessary, the muscle is located again with active resisted contraction. Slow muscle stripping and ischemic compression are used on the muscle belly.

✋ There are three trigger points in iliopsoas. One is located in iliacus, in the iliac fossa on the inside surface of the pelvis, just superior to the anterior superior iliac spine and deep to the abdominal muscles. The second is located in psoas at the level of L3. Both of these trigger points refer pain into the low back, in an ipsilateral horizontal pattern. The third trigger point is located at the insertion of the tendon onto the lesser trochanter of the femur. This trigger point refers to the anterior thigh and the low back (Travell, Simons, 1992). Abdominal work is finished with effleurage and stroking.

Stretch the shortened muscles.

✋ PIR is used to lengthen iliopsoas. The client slides to the side of the table so the limb to be treated can hang freely over the side of the table. The hip and knee of the untreated limb are flexed with the foot flat on the table. This stabilizes the low back against the table. Further stabilization is applied at the anterior superior iliac spine of the untreated side with the proximal hand. The thigh of the treated side is moved into extension with the distal hand, until the iliopsoas is beginning to be stretched. The client submaximally flexes the hip against the therapist's resistance for 10 seconds and relaxes, allowing the limb to fall into extension. The cycle is repeated at least three times.

Mobilize hypomobile joints.

✋ If a sacroiliac joint is hypomobile, joint play is used. One hand is placed palm upwards between the client's lumbar spine and the table. The thumb points towards the client's head and the fingertips stabilize the sacrum at S2. The posterior superior iliac spine rests on the proximal

Treatment Goals   Treatment Plan

phalanges. The other hand cups the client's anterior superior iliac spine, with the heel of the hand resting on the bone. The forearm is pronated so the thumb points towards the client's feet and the fingertips are on the lateral hip. The pelvis is mobilized posteriorly by the hand on the anterior superior iliac spine. The motion between the sacrum and posterior superior iliac spine is monitored. The pelvis is then mobilized anteriorly by the proximal phalanges under the posterior superior iliac spine. The technique is repeated several times until the joint is mobilized.

🖐 In another joint play technique, medially directed pressure is applied bilaterally to the outsides of both anterior superior iliac spines, flaring the posterior superior iliac spines.

Restore range of motion.

🖐 A combination of full **passive hip flexion** and submaximal isometric contraction of the hamstrings is used to decrease the anterior pelvic tilt *(Hertling, Kessler, 1996; St. John, 1991)*. The client's hip and knee are fully flexed so the thigh is against the client's abdomen. The therapist leans against the client's anterior leg to maintain this full flexion, first placing a pillow between his torso and the client. The ischial tuberosity is carefully grasped and used as a lever to rotate the pelvis posteriorly at the sacroiliac joint *(Kapandji, 1974)*. When the slack is taken up in the hip and sacroiliac joint, the client's untreated thigh will come slightly off the table. When this happens, the client is instructed to submaximally, isometrically contract the hamstrings by pushing into the therapist's torso. This helps to pull the pelvis into a posterior tilt. The contraction is maintained for 10 seconds while the therapist continues to carefully, passively rotate the pelvis posteriorly.

🖐 In the **prone** position, hot **hydrotherapy** is applied to the lumbar fascia. Rhythmic techniques can be used to mobilize the low back.

Reduce fascial restrictions.

🖐 Fascial techniques are used on the lumbar fascia. These include skin rolling, crossed-hands spreading, fingertip spreading and the connective tissue cutting technique around the superior attachments at the iliac crest, the inferior attachments at the twelfth rib and the lateral attachments at the lumbar vertebrae.

Mobilize hypomobile joints.

🖐 Any hypomobility of the lumbar spine or thoracolumbar junction is treated with spinous process oscillations, anterior challenge or lateral challenge joint play.

Reduce hypertonicity and trigger points.

🖐 Swedish techniques are used on the lumbar erector spinae and quadratus lumborum, including effleurage and ulnar border stripping. Trigger points in quadratus lumborum refer into the lateral hip, sacroiliac joint and inferior portion of the gluteals *(Travell, Simons, 1992)*.

Stretch the shortened muscles.

🖐 PIR may be used to lengthen rectus femoris. The client's knee is flexed, bringing the heel towards the gluteals until the client feels a stretch on rectus femoris. The client submaximally extends the knee

Treatment Goals   Treatment Plan

against the therapist's resistance for 10 seconds and relaxes, allowing the knee to be moved into more flexion by the therapist. The cycle is repeated at least three times.

✋ For quadratus lumborum PIR, see the chapter on scoliosis.

✋ If piriformis is short, Golgi tendon organ release is used on the insertion at the greater trochanter, followed by PIR with the client's knee flexed.

Encourage local circulation in weak, taut structures.

✋ The gluteals and hamstrings are treated with brisk, stimulating Swedish techniques such as alternating palmar kneading and tapotement. Cool **hydrotherapy** can be used to stimulate the gluteals and hamstrings.

✋ The treatment is ended with effleurage to encourage local circulation.

Treat other conditions.

✋ Other conditions, such as iliotibial band contracture, can be treated during subsequent appointments.

Self-care Goals   Self-care Plan

Re-educate the client regarding activities.

✎ The client should avoid postures that encourage hyperlordosis and must avoid maintaining one position for prolonged periods. If possible, short, frequent breaks for stretching are taken during the day. Chairs and seats should have adequate lumbar support and, when sitting, the client's femurs should be horizontal to the ground to maintain a normal lordosis. A footrest may be needed to achieve this.

✎ The client is encouraged to be aware of her standing posture, and make an effort to maintain an increased posterior pelvic tilt.

✎ The client is instructed to avoid sleeping with the hips in flexion to prevent iliopsoas trigger points from being activated.

✎ Self-massage for hip flexors is indicated.

Stretch shortened muscles.

✎ For gravity-induced PIR for the left **iliopsoas,** the client lies supine on a table with the gluteals at the edge. The right limb is flexed at the hip and knee and the client holds this knee to the chest. The left limb is allowed to hang over the edge of the table. The client contracts the left iliopsis for 20 seconds, very slightly raising the hanging limb, then exhales and lets the leg relax and drop into extension. This cycle is repeated at least three times and is then performed on the right limb.

✎ To treat the left **rectus femoris,** the client is supine with the right knee and hip flexed, this time with the hamstrings at the edge of the table, allowing the left leg to hang from the knee. The client pulls the right knee to the chest. The client contracts the left rectus femoris, extending the knee, and holds this for 20 seconds. The client exhales and allows the hanging leg to relax and drop into flexion at the knee.

✍ A similar approach is used to stretch the **adductors** in the supine position, only here the hip and knee are flexed so the foot rests on the table. The client allows the hip to drop into abduction *(Lewit, 1993)*.

✍ Seated flexion-extension exercises are also useful for retraining the lumbar and abdominal muscles. The client kneels on the floor with the legs tucked under the gluteals. Starting with the head, the client slowly exhales and curls into flexion, one vertebrae at a time until full relaxed flexion of the torso is reached. This stretches the lumbar muscles. The client then lifts the head to look to the ceiling, moving the spine into extension one vertebrae at a time while inhaling. The flexion-extension cycle is repeated.

Strengthen weak muscles.

✍ To **strengthen** the inhibited abdominal muscles, the client can begin with supine pelvic tilt exercises. The hips and knees are flexed to 90 degrees and the feet are flat on the floor. The client flattens the low back into the floor while concentrating on contracting the abdominal muscles to roll the pelvis into a posterior pelvic tilt. The tilt is held isometrically for 15 seconds. The client relaxes and then repeats the exercise. Pelvic tilts can also be performed in a seated or standing position.

✍ These exercises can progress to where the client lies supine, maintaining a posterior pelvic tilt. The hips and knees are flexed to greater than 90 degrees bringing the feet off the floor. The client slowly flexes and extends the lower limbs in a small range. Over time, as the abdominals strengthen, the client can progress to reducing the amount of knee and hip flexion, moving towards straight leg raises *(Kisner, Colby, 1990)*. As strength returns, the client can move on to torso curl-ups and flexed-knee sit ups.

✍ Gluteus maximus should also be strengthened. To do this, the prone client extends the hip with the knee flexed and holds this isometrically for 15 seconds.

Refer the client.

✍ If pes planus is a contributing factor, the client should consider wearing arch supports.

✍ Movement therapy, such as Mitzvah and Alexander techniques, may be helpful for retraining the client's posture.

Treatment Frequency and Expected Outcome

See also pes planus, iliotibial band contracture, hyperkyphosis, scoliosis, pregnancy, piriformis syndrome and degenerative disc disease for related conditions.

Treatment should be given once a week for six weeks. The client should then be reassessed. The remedial exercise self-care plan should also be reassessed at six weeks.

The outcome for reducing hyperlordosis is favourable, especially with client compliance in postural retraining and strengthening of weak muscles.

43

HYPERKYPHOSIS

Fiona Rattray

> **Hyperkyphosis is an increase in the normal thoracic kyphotic curve, with protracted scapulae and head-forward posture.**

Functional or postural curves may be voluntarily altered or reversed by positional changes. They can be corrected with passive soft tissue stretching, joint mobilization and strengthening exercises *(Porth, 1990)*. **Structural** curves are fixed, due to bony changes, and cannot be corrected by positional changes or voluntary effort.

With hyperkyphosis, a pattern of muscles responding to stress by shortening or adaptively weakening appears in the shoulder and neck region *(Janda in Twomey, Taylor, 1987; Lewit, 1993)*. In this shoulder-crossed syndrome, the shortened shoulder protractors and neck extensors inhibit the posterior thoracic muscles, anterior neck flexors, suprahyoids and infrahyoids, producing an increase in the thoracic curve and a compensatory increase in the cervical lordotic curve *(Figure 43.1)*.

An increase in the thoracic curve has several implications for the upper body. Inefficient breathing patterns found with restricted thoracic mobility and rib motion can lead to respiratory conditions such as bronchitis. Thoracic outlet syndromes occur with tight anterior chest muscles. Protraction of the scapula alters the position of the glenohumeral joint, turning it inferiorly. This forces the rotator cuff muscles to contract to maintain the humeral head in its proper position. An increase in stress on the joint capsule may precipitate frozen shoulder *(Hertling, Kessler, 1990)*.

An increase in the cervical curve as seen with a head-forward posture also has implications for the head and neck. There is increased pressure on the facet joints of the upper cervical spine leading also to increased wear on the discs *(Kisner, Colby, 1990)*. The mandible is moved posteriorly by the stretched anterior throat muscles, leading to stress on the temporomandibular joint *(Hertling, Kessler, 1990)*.

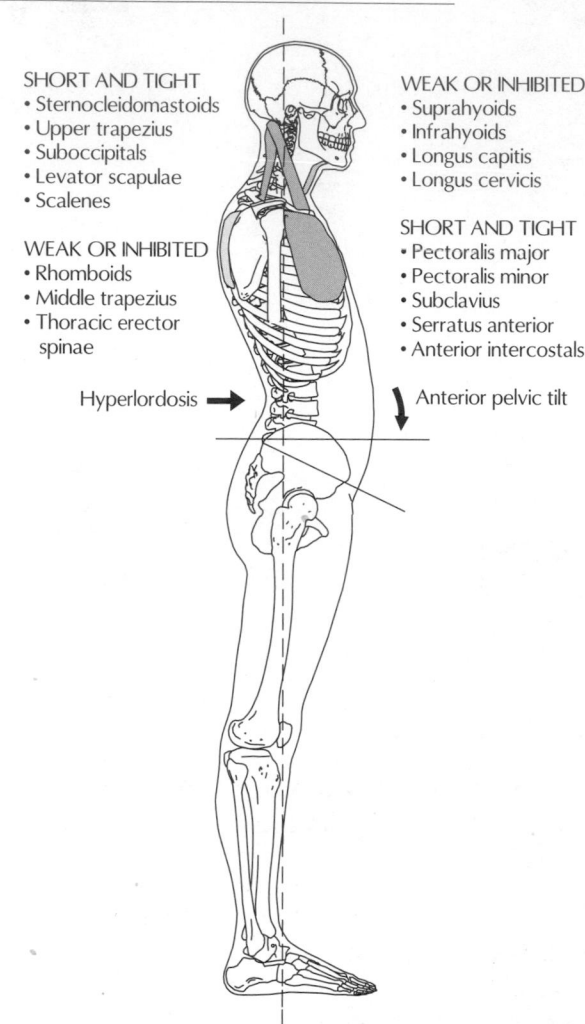

SHORT AND TIGHT
• Sternocleidomastoids
• Upper trapezius
• Suboccipitals
• Levator scapulae
• Scalenes

WEAK OR INHIBITED
• Rhomboids
• Middle trapezius
• Thoracic erector spinae

Hyperlordosis ➔

WEAK OR INHIBITED
• Suprahyoids
• Infrahyoids
• Longus capitis
• Longus cervicis

SHORT AND TIGHT
• Pectoralis major
• Pectoralis minor
• Subclavius
• Serratus anterior
• Anterior intercostals

↘ Anterior pelvic tilt

Figure 43.1
Tight and weak muscles in hyperkyphosis, illustrating shoulder-crossed syndrome and head-forward posture; there is an accompanying hyperlordosis and anterior pelvic tilt.

With hyperkyphosis and shoulder protraction, muscles that are short and tight are pectoralis major, pectoralis minor, subclavius, serratus anterior and anterior intercostals. With internal rotation of the humerus, subscapularis is tight. Latissimus dorsi is tight with depressed shoulders.

With head-forward posture, levator scapulae, upper trapezius, sternocleidomastoids, scalenes and the suboccipitals are short and tight. Serratus posterior superior is tight with elevated upper ribs and apical breathing patterns. Pectoralis major, levator scapulae, sternocleidomastoids, upper trapezius and scalenes have a clearly postural role, responding to stress by adaptively shortening.

Muscles that are stretched, weak and taut are rhomboids and middle trapezii; these are phasic muscles, responding to stress by fatiguing. With head-forward posture, longus cervicis, longus capitis, the suprahyoids and infrahyoids are stretched and weak. The thoracic erector spinae and lower cervical extensors, despite being postural muscles, are adaptively stretched (*Kisner, Colby, 1990; Kendall, McCreary, 1983*).

If hyperkyphosis is combined with hyperlodosis, the abdominals are stretched, weak and taut, and the hip flexors and lumbar erectors are short and tight. An increase in the thoracic curve and head-forward posture also accompany swayback posture, which is variously described as having either an anterior or posterior pelvic tilt. See the hyperlordosis chapter for a discussion of these conditions.

Pathologies that may lead to hyperkyphosis:

✦ **Osteoporosis** of the thoracic and cervical spine can lead to vertebral wedging and hyperkyphosis. See the chapter on osteoporosis for details.

✦ **Ankylosing spondylitis** results in fusion of the spine in a hyperkyphotic position. It is described in the inflammatory arthritides chapter.

✦ **Pott's disease,** or osteitis of the thoracic vertebrae, is usually due to tuberculosis. Wedging of the vertebrae results in a gibbus deformity or severe structural hyperkyphosis. Compression of the nerve roots causes symmetrical epigastric or intercostal pain. If the disease is also in the cervical spine, there is paresthesia in the hands, a tickling cough and pain on swallowing. This disease affects children and adults up to age 40.

✦ **Scheuermann's disease,** or idiopathic juvenile osteochondrosis of the thoracic vertebrae, is a condition where the growth ossification centres stop functioning or

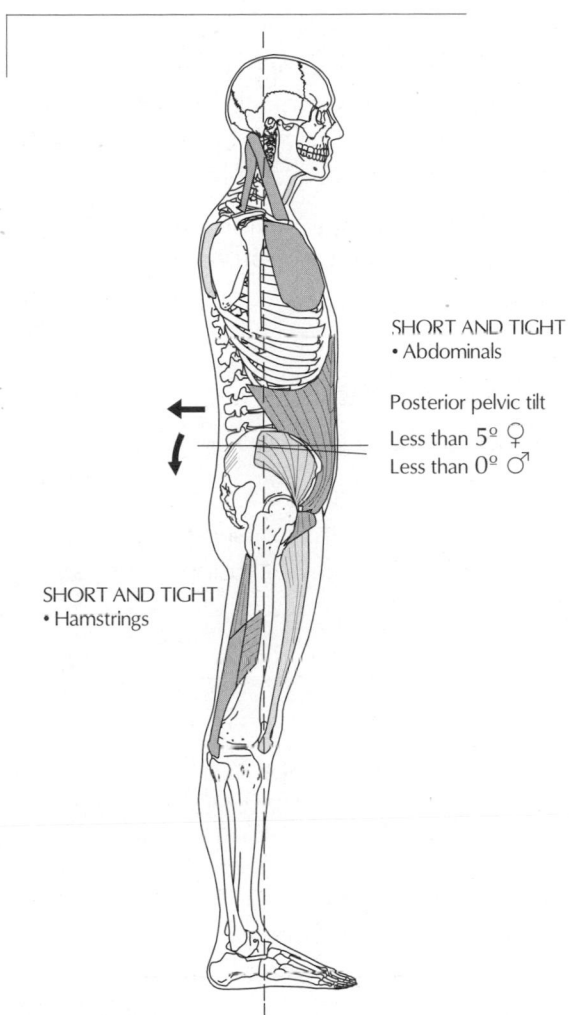

SHORT AND TIGHT
• Abdominals

Posterior pelvic tilt

Less than 5º ♀
Less than 0º ♂

SHORT AND TIGHT
• Hamstrings

Figure 43.2
Flatback posture showing posterior pelvic tilt due to tight hamstrings and abdominal muscles, with accompanying hyperkyphosis.

degenerate, resulting in wedging of the vertebrae. There is an increase in the normal thoracic curve which may be asymptomatic or mildly painful. It occurs mainly in males *(Schumacher, 1993)*.

Causes of hyperkyphosis are:

➤ **sustained poor posture,** either habitual (slouching or sleeping in a curled-up position) or emotional (the person protracts the shoulders and depresses the sternum protectively or rounds the shoulders and slouches to appear shorter);

➤ **occupational sources,** such as sitting at a computer or being on the phone;

➤ overemphasis on **flexion or pectoralis strengthening exercises;**

➤ **pathology** such as osteoporosis or ankylosing spondylitis.

Flatback

Hyperkyphosis may also accompany flatback or a *decrease* in the lumbar lordosis *(Figure 43.2)*. This presents with a flattened appearance to the low back, posterior pelvic tilt and hip extension. The hamstrings and abdominals are tight and short, while the lumbar extensors and the hip flexors are somewhat weak and inhibited. Flatback may result from habitual slouched posture. Pain may result from overstretched posterior longitudinal ligaments and a lack of shock-absorbing capabilities of the normal lordotic curve.

Symptom Picture

✦ There is an increased thoracic curve with associated protraction of the scapulae and a head-forward posture.

✦ Hyperkyphosis can be functional or structural.

✦ **In a functional hyperkyphosis:**

• Pain may arise from a stretched posterior longitudinal ligament in the thoracic spine and from facet joint approximation and intervertebral foramen narrowing in the upper cervical spine *(Kisner, Colby, 1990)*. Pain may also be caused by tight ischemic tissue, overstretched tissue or trigger points.

Breathing is often apical and the ribs may be hypomobile.

- Muscle imbalances are present. The shoulder protractors and upper cervical extensors are short and tight, while the shoulder retractors, thoracic extensors and anterior neck muscles are weak and stretched. Protraction of the scapulae rotates the glenoid fossa inferiorly so there is increased tone in the rotator cuff muscles.

- Entrapment of lymphatic vessels, which travel through a tight pectoralis major, may lead to same-side breast tissue congestion and edema *(Travell, Simons, 1992)*.

- Range of motion of the thoracic spine, cervical spine and ribs is reduced.

- Poor postural habits, such as slouching, are present.

- Other postural conditions, such as hyperlordosis or flatback, may be present.

- Secondary conditions may develop. These include thoracic outlet syndrome or temporomandibular joint dysfunction.

✦ **In a structural hyperkyphosis:**

- In addition to the above, there is associated vertebral wedging or fusion. There is posterior displacement of the nucleus pulposus.

Subjective Information

HEALTH HISTORY QUESTIONS

✦ How long has the hyperkyphosis been present?

✦ What areas are painful, if any? What aggravates or relieves the pain?

✦ Does the client have any other conditions or underlying pathologies, such as asthma, frozen shoulder, thoracic outlet syndrome, osteoporosis or jaw, head or neck pain?

✦ What are the client's postural habits, including occupational or recreational sources of postural stress?

✦ Does the client have uncorrected vision or hearing problems? Either of these conditions can contribute to a head-forward posture.

✦ Has the client had any parallel therapies for the hyperkyphosis, such as chiropractic, physiotherapy or bracing?

Objective Information

Observations

Postural Assessment – Lateral View

✍ Slight ankle plantarflexion is possible with knee hyperextension.

✍ With an accompanying hyperlordosis, the hip joints are flexed, the lumbar lordotic curve is increased and the bilateral anterior pelvic tilt is greater than 10 degrees in female clients and greater than five degrees in male clients.

✍ With flatback, the hip joints are extended, the lumbar lordotic curve is decreased and the bilateral pelvic tilt is less than five degrees in female clients and less than zero degrees in male clients.

✍ The thoracic curve is increased.

✍ The acromioclavicular joints may be anterior.

✍ The cervical lordotic curve is increased.

✍ The external auditory meatus is anterior to the plumb line with a head-forward posture.

✍ In a posterior view, the scapulae are protracted and often winged. The shoulders may be bilaterally elevated, neutral or depressed.

Palpation

✍ The pectoral muscles, sternocleidomastoids and anterior and upper cervical extensors are tender and hypertonic and contain trigger points.

✍ The pectoral fascia may be thickened and tender.

Testing

✍ **AF ROM** of the thoracic spine reveals a decrease in extension.

✍ **PR ROM** of the cervical spine is reduced in forward flexion and lateral flexion. With shoulder protraction, there is reduced external rotation of the glenohumeral joint.

✍ **AR strength testing** reveals weakness in the middle trapezius and rhomboids.

Special Tests

✍ **Pectoralis major, pectoralis minor** and, likely, **shoulder adductor length tests** are positive bilaterally. **The straight leg raise test** reveals an increase in hamstring length with an anterior pelvic tilt and a decrease in hamstring length with a posterior pelvic tilt.

✍ In the thoracic and cervical spine, **anterior** and **lateral spinous challenge tests** reveal areas of vertebral hypo- or hypermobility. **Rib motion** and **levatores costarum fixation tests** are positive with rib fixation. **Spurling's test** is positive with facet joint irritation. **Adson's, Wright's hyperabduction** or **costoclavicular syndrome test** is positive with thoracic outlet syndrome.

Contraindications

✦ If a pathology is suspected but undiagnosed, such as osteoporosis, refer the client to a physician.

✦ Avoid mobilizing hypermobile vertebral segments. Joint play techniques for the ribs and rib springing are contraindicated with rib hypermobility and a history of rib subluxation.

✦ Do not randomly stretch fascia. Assess the fascia and only treat areas of restriction.

✦ Avoid lengthening techniques on weak, overstretched tissues.

Differentiating Types of Thoracic Pain

✦ **Nerve root compression** is characterized by a decrease in reflexes and a positive Valsalva's or Spurling's test.

✦ **Pott's disease** is characterized by an increase in pain on active free extension and rotation of the thoracic spine. Pain on jumping and landing on the feet is also significant. Medical diagnosis is made by X-ray (*Taber's Cyclopedic Medical Dictionary, 1981*).

✦ **Scheuermann's disease** is diagnosed medically with X-rays (*Schumacher, 1993*).

Treatment Goals   Treatment Plan

Assess to determine if the hyperkyphosis is functional or structural.

🖐 Due to the possibility of either anterior or posterior pelvic tilt that accompanies hyperkyphosis, an assessment is necessary to determine the treatment plan for the muscles that cross the pelvis. With anterior pelvic tilt, the hip flexors are shortened, while with posterior pelvic tilt, the hamstrings are shortened.

🖐 With a functional hyperkyphosis, the curves can be altered. If the hyperkyphosis is structural, the treatment plan involves maintaining tissue health, reducing pain and treating secondary conditions, such as frozen shoulder. There is no possibility of changing the curve. With more severe structural curves, a towel roll or thin pillow may be needed under the client's head for support and comfort in the supine position.

🖐 The therapist may choose several or all of the following techniques, which may be spread over several treatments rather than all being performed at once. Whatever techniques are used, they should be applied bilaterally.

🖐 Positioning begins in the **supine position,** with pillows under the client's knees. A small towel roll is placed longitudinally along the client's spine to flatten the curve. The client is later turned prone.

🖐 **Hydrotherapy** applications are pre-treatment heat applied over one pectoralis major muscle before treating the fascia, then moved to the other side. Cool applications are used on the stretched rhomboids.

Treatment Goals

Treatment Plan

General Treatment

🖐 This treatment addresses a functional curve without including work to the pelvis.

Decrease sympathetic nervous system firing.

🖐 The treatment is performed in the context of a relaxation treatment, which includes **diaphragmatic breathing** to help reduce any pain the client may experience with direct fascial work.

Specific Treatment

Reduce fascial restrictions.

🖐 The hydrotherapy is moved to the other pectoralis major muscle. Fascial techniques are applied to the pre-heated side, which include slow skin rolling, crossed-hands and fingertip fascial spreading as well as connective tissue cutting over the pectoral muscles. The other side is treated in a similar manner after removing the heat.

🖐 To treat the fascia over the lower anterior intercostals and pectoralis major attachments, the client is draped so the abdomen is uncovered. A towel is used to cover the client's chest. Slow skin rolling and fascial spreading are used on the affected tissue.

Reduce hypertonicity and trigger points. Reduce pain if present.

🖐 Swedish techniques for pectoralis major, pectoralis minor, subclavius, deltoids and anterior intercostals include effleurage, fingertip kneading, muscle stripping and the origin and insertion technique. The diaphragm is treated with costal border scooping and specific muscle stripping under the costal border, using the client's breathing. After redraping the abdomen, the therapist applies muscle stripping and ischemic compressions to trigger points in the shoulder protractors.

🖐 The sternal attachments of pectoralis major are treated with fingertip kneading and fascial spreading. With a female client, a V-shaped draping method can be used (*Figure 43.3*). If this is not comfortable for the client, fingertip kneading is used through the sheets.

🖐 Pectoralis major trigger points refer into the shoulder, chest and breast.

🖐 Pectoralis minor is located by placing the client's hand on the abdomen, with the humerus in slight abduction. The therapist's thumbs are placed under the lateral border of pectoralis major to palpate the smaller muscle. The client is asked to depress the shoulder, making pectoralis minor palpably contract. Once the muscle is located, muscle stripping and the origin and insertion technique are used on the tissue. Trigger points in pectoralis minor refer to the anterior shoulder. Subclavius is palpated immediately inferior to the clavicle. The trigger point in this muscle refers pain down the arm into the lateral hand. See the thoracic outlet syndrome chapter for more technique details.

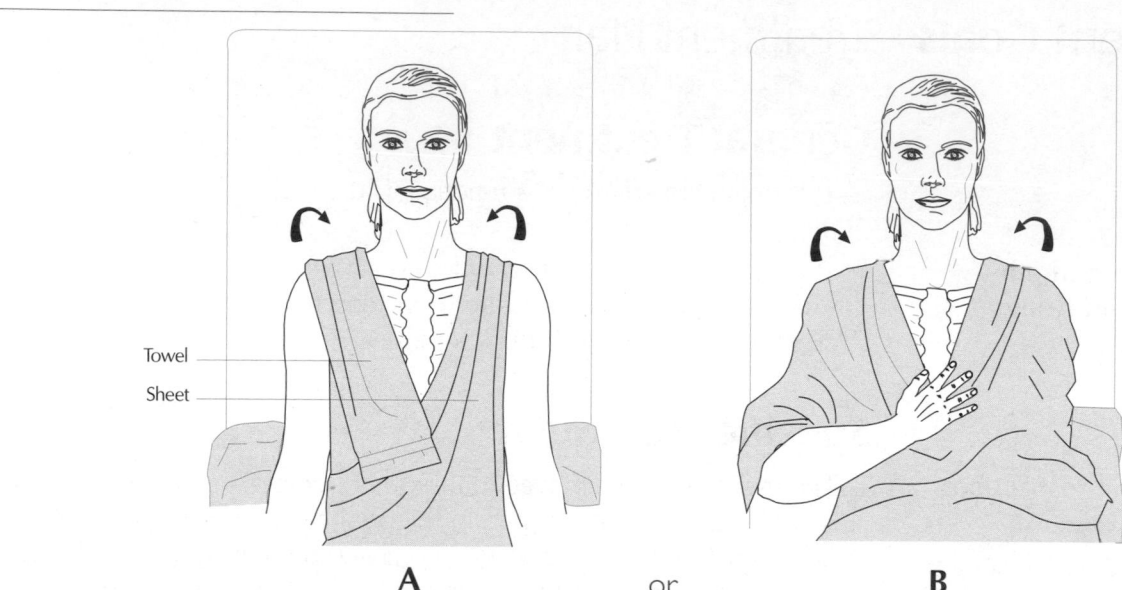

A   or   B

Figure 43.3
V-drape method for working directly on sternal attachments of pectoralis major with the client supine.

In (A), the therapist has first tucked the sheet behind the left shoulder, leaving the right shoulder uncovered. A towel is placed lengthwise over the right shoulder and sheet covering the thorax. The towel is tucked behind the right shoulder. The sheet under the towel is slid down, uncovering the sternum only.

or

In (B), the therapist has asked the client to anchor the sheet over the inferior aspect of the sternum after tucking the ends behind the shoulders.

Treatment Goals

Increase local circulation to remove metabolites.

Mobilize hypomobile joints.
Increase thoracic capacity.

Stretch shortened muscles.

Treatment Plan

- Repetitive effleurage and petrissage are used on the shoulder protractors.

- Joint play to the sternoclavicular and acromioclavicular joints is indicated. Rib springing is also used to mobilize the ribs and stretch the anterior intercostals, allowing for fuller respiration.

- PIR for the clavicular portion of pectoralis major has the humerus at 90 degrees of abduction and the upper limb hanging off the table. The sternum is stabilized with one of the therapist's hands while the other hand is placed on the distal humerus. The client submaximally horizontally flexes the humerus against the therapist's resistance for 10 seconds and then relaxes, allowing the limb to fall into extension. The cycle is repeated at least three times. To treat the sternal portion, the client's humerus is positioned in more than 120 degrees of abduction and the stretch is repeated. Latissimus dorsi is treated by repeating the stretch with the arm in 180 degrees of abduction of the glenohumeral joint, which is also full forward flexion. To stabilize the pelvis, the client's hips and knees are flexed so the feet are flat on the table and the lumbar spine is pressed into the table.

564

Treatment Goals   Treatment Plan

⚕ To treat pectoralis minor, the arm is at the client's side with the hand on the abdomen. The client slides to the side of the table so the scapula is free to hang over the side of the table. The heel of the therapist's hand is placed on the coracoid process and the client submaximally protracts and depresses the scapula against the therapist's resistance.

Reduce hypertonicity and trigger points.

⚕ The tight upper cervical muscles, including the suboccipitals, are treated with fascial fingertip stroking, effleurage, fingertip kneading and Golgi tendon organ release. The tight sternocleidomastoids, upper trapezius, scalenes and levator scapulae are treated with muscle stripping. Passive range of motion in all ranges is used on the cervical spine.

⚕ The client is turned **prone,** with pillows under the abdomen and ankles. Two towel rolls are placed under the shoulders, retracting them.

Reduce hypertonicity and trigger points.

⚕ Rhythmic techniques and Swedish techniques are used on latissimus dorsi, serratus posterior superior, subscapularis and the rotator cuff muscles.

⚕ To specifically treat a short latissimus dorsi, the client's upper limb on the side to be treated is placed in full forward flexion, placing a stretch on the muscle. Ulnar border stripping is used in an inferior to superior direction along the muscle.

⚕ Trigger points in latissimus dorsi refer inferior to the scapula and, sometimes, down the extensor surface of the arm. The trigger point in serratus posterior superior is covered by the medial superior angle of the scapula. To locate it, the therapist allows the client's arm to hang off the side of the table, abducting the scapula and uncovering the trigger point.

⚕ Rhomboid trigger points are activated by shortening of pectoralis major. They refer locally and are treated with ischemic compressions only, to avoid lengthening the tissues.

⚕ Subscapularis is treated with muscle stripping and ischemic compressions. See the frozen shoulder chapter for more details.

Mobilize hypomobile joints.

⚕ Joint play including spinous process oscillations is used on hypomobile vertebrae and ribs. The recoil technique is used for posterior rib fixation due to levator costarum tightness. See the asthma chapter for details.

Encourage local circulation in weak, taut structures.

⚕ The middle trapezius, rhomboids and thoracic erector spinae are treated with brisk, stimulating Swedish techniques such as alternating palmar kneading and tapotement. Cool **hydrotherapy** can be used to stimulate these muscles.

⚕ The treatment is ended with effleurage to encourage local circulation.

Treatment Goals

Treat other conditions.

Treatment Plan

✋ The **sidelying** position may be more comfortable for the client with extremely tender shoulder protractor muscles. The uppermost elbow is flexed and the limb is allowed to adduct with gravity's help across the torso, shortening the pectoralis muscles and making them less tender.

✋ The serratus anterior muscle is located by the therapist extending the client's humerus and letting the arm hang behind the torso. Muscle stripping is used from the lateral attachments posteriorly around the rib cage, as far under the scapula as possible. Serratus anterior trigger points refer locally to the lateral thorax. The client may report that he is unable to take a deep breath when this trigger point is activated *(Travell, Simons, 1983)*. PIR for this muscle is achieved by the therapist stabilizing the client's pelvis while extending and adducting the humerus against the client's resistance. The client is asked to inhale, which further stretches the muscle *(Travell, Simons, 1983)*.

✋ Other conditions, such as temporomandibular joint dysfunction are treated during subsequent treatments.

Self-care Goals

Educate the client regarding activities.

Stretch shortened muscles.

Self-care Plan

✍ The client should avoid postures that encourage hyperkyphosis. He is instructed to avoid maintaining one posture for prolonged periods. If possible, short, frequent breaks for stretching are taken during the day.

✍ A lumbar support or roll for the client's chair will help to maintain the normal lumbar lordosis. This helps move the head posteriorly, retracting the scapula.

✍ If the standing posture is slouched with rounded shoulders, the client is instructed to lift the sternum up without contracting the rhomboids. This moves the head out of a forward posture.

✍ The client should avoid sleeping in a curled-up, sidelying posture.

✍ If the client's breathing is apical, diaphragmatic breathing is useful.

✍ Self-massage to the shoulder protractors is indicated.

✍ **Self-stretching** for pectoralis major is performed in an open doorway. The client stands with both hands and forearms resting on the doorframe. One foot is in front of the other with the knee of the forward foot in flexion. The client keeps the head upright, not allowing it to move forward. To stretch the clavicular fibres of pectoralis major, the hands are held just above shoulder height and the client leans through the doorway. To stretch the sternal fibres, the hands are held above the head so both shoulders are abducted to 90

Self-care Goals

Self-care Plan

degrees. To stretch the costal and abdominal fibres as well as pectoralis minor, the client moves the arms above 120 degrees of abduction. Each stretch is held for at least 30 seconds *(Travell, Simons, 1992).*

Strengthen weak structures.

✍ Active resisted strengthening for rhomboids is performed in the prone position. The client holds both arms at 90 degrees of abduction, with both humeri in *internal* rotation, and squeezes the scapulae together. The resistance is progressed — at first it is only against gravity and eventually the client uses weights. To strengthen the middle trapezii, the exercise is repeated but with the humeri *externally* rotated *(Kisner, Colby, 1990; Kendall, McCreary, 1983).*

Refer the client.

✍ Movement therapy, such as the Mitzvah, Feldenkrais or Alexander technique, may be helpful for retraining the client's posture.

Treatment Frequency and Expected Outcome

Treatments should be once a week for six weeks. At that point the client and the remedial exercise self-care plan should be totally reassessed.

See also frozen shoulder, hyperlordosis, scoliosis, pregnancy, thoracic outlet syndrome, temporomandibular joint dysfunction, degenerative disc disease, osteoarthritis, osteoporitis, inflammatory arthritides, chronic bronchitis and asthma for related treatments.

The outcome for treatment of functional hyperkyphosis is favourable with a client who is compliant with a remedial exercise program.

44

SCOLIOSIS

Fiona Rattray

> **Scoliosis is a lateral rotatory deviation of the spine.**

Scoliosis curves are described according to the side that the **convexity** is on — for example, a right thoracolumbar curve *(Figure 44.1)*. While curves are also traditionally labelled as **C-curves** (one curve) or **S-curves** (two curves), these terms describe only the appearance of the thoracic and lumbar spine. There is usually also a compensatory curve in the cervical spine. A person can have an S-curve scoliosis and still have the occiput centred over the sacrum because the intervening curves cancel each other out *(Cailliet, 1975)*.

Functional curves, also known as postural or non-structural curves, may be voluntarily altered or reversed by positional changes or muscular action. They can be corrected with passive soft tissue stretching, joint mobilization and active strengthening *(Porth, 1990)*.

Structural curves are fixed due to bony changes and cannot be corrected by positional changes or voluntary effort. They usually have a childhood onset and correction requires bracing or surgery.

The **span** is the distance on the spine that the curve covers — for example, a thoracolumbar curve spanning T8 to L3 or a cervical curve between C1 and C7.

+ The **apex** vertebra is the one in any curve that is farthest from the midline.

+ The **major** curve in an S-curve scoliosis is the largest curve with the greatest angulation.

+ The **minor** curve is a smaller, compensatory curve.

+ A **transitional** vertebra is the one that marks the end of one curve and the beginning of the next.

The **severity** of a scoliosis is measured in degrees. It may also be described as mild (up to 20 degrees), moderate (20 to 50 degrees) or severe (greater than 50 degrees). Mild scoliosis of less than 10 degrees is considered within normal limits. A mild curve, especially if it is detected early, may be corrected with stretching and strengthening. Moderate scoliosis is associated with the beginnings of bony change and is usually treated with bracing. Severe scoliosis is associated with decreased life expectancy in children, due to reduced pulmonary function, and osteoarthritis in adults. Severe scoliosis is treated by surgery (Kisner, Colby, 1990).

To completely understand the presentation of a scoliosis, it is necessary for the therapist to think of the pelvis, spine and rib cage as a three dimensional structure. In scoliosis, not just the spine but also the ribs and pelvis are laterally bent, rotated and distorted. The pelvis may be torqued — that is, one innominate bone may be more anterior than the other. This may also occur at the shoulder girdle.

To understand the compensation that occurs with scoliosis, it is important to recognize the actions of the righting reflex. This reflex is likely responsible for the development of secondary compensatory curves (Hoppenfeld, 1967; St. John, 1994). The righting reflex is the body's attempt to establish a centre of gravity, keep the eyes on a horizontal plane and permit normal function (Travell, Simons, 1992). With a single curve, this is not possible, because the head would always be tilted.

The effects of the righting reflex can be easily demonstrated by the reader tilting the head to one side for several minutes while trying to perform activities of daily living. This creates a primary cervical curve. It is extremely difficult for a person to maintain the tilt without raising the shoulder on the same side to compensate, creating a secondary thoracic curve. Another way to demonstrate the righting reflex is for the reader to wear one shoe that has a moderate heel. To compensate for this leg length inequality and tilted pelvis, the spine must curve to keep the eyes on the horizontal plane.

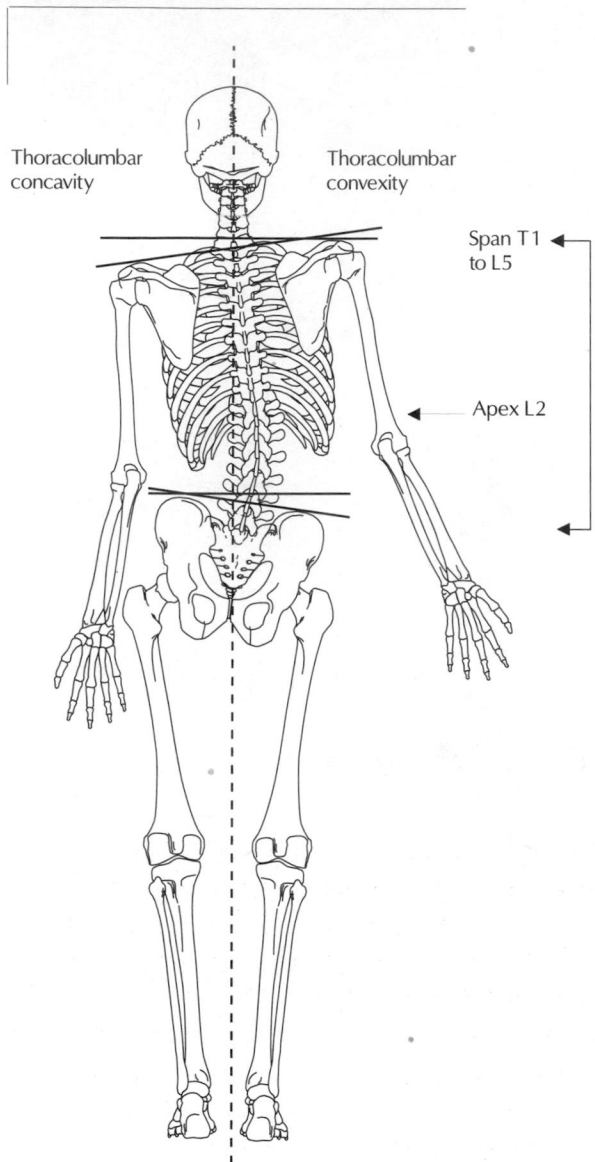

Thoracolumbar concavity

Thoracolumbar convexity

Span T1 to L5

Apex L2

Figure 44.1
A functional right thoracolumbar C-curve scoliosis, span T1 to L5, apex at L2.

The entire body, from feet to cranium, can be involved in a scoliosis. This is an example of Wolff's principle. The principle states that, over time, bones remodel themselves along the lines of force that are placed on them. This concept is also be extended to connective tissue, muscles and viscera (Hoppenfeld, 1967; Caillet, 1975).

Some degree of mild scoliosis is found in children and adolescents of both sexes around the world. The exact numbers depend on the degree of curve that is deemed significant. For example, taking 16 years as a sample age, 10 degree curves are found in 3 per cent of the population, 20 degree curves are found in 0.3 per cent of the same age group, while 30 degree curves appear in 0.15 per cent (Robin, 1990).

Causes of scoliosis are idiopathic, functional, neuromuscular, congenital and introgenic.

One authority notes that many of the studies performed on spinal curves have lumped together the data on the many varieties of scoliotic curves and differing age groups in which these curves appear. This makes determining the cause of idiopathic scoliosis difficult, since not all curves are the same *(Nachemson, 1984)*.

The Scoliosis Research Society has developed a classification system for spinal curves which lists over 70 causes of scoliosis *(Bunch, Patwardhan, 1989)*. The most common, which are listed above, have many different characteristics.

➤ **Idiopathic** scoliosis comprises approximately 85 per cent of all reported scoliosis cases and occurs in approximately eight per cent of the population *(Porth, 1990)*. It appears in three age groups. Infantile scoliosis is more common in boys from birth to three years, adolescent scoliosis in girls from 10 to 16 years and juvenile scoliosis affecting both males and females equally between the ages of four and nine years. It is possible that idiopathic scoliosis is a symptom rather than a single disease *(Nachemson, 1984)*. Scoliosis may develop in adults also. It is estimated that lumbar scoliosis with associated rib humping develops in almost six per cent of persons over 50 years of age *(Bunch, Patwardhan, 1989)*.

✦ *Central nervous system input through altered proprioceptive and vestibular sources:* Abnormal muscle spindle response to proprioception in the paraspinal muscles may cause idiopathic scoliosis. Asymmetry in the labyrinth of the inner ear may be a factor influencing spinal posture. There may also be a breakdown in the mechanisms of postural control. One study found an increase in labyrinth sensitivity on the convex side of the curve and that right eye dominance may be associated with left-sided curves *(Jacobs, 1982)*.

✦ *Biomechanical factors:* These could cause imbalances. On average, the right halves of the vertebral bodies, the right ribs and the right humerus are larger than the left. The femur, fibula, clavicle and bones of the skull are slightly larger on the left side *(Robin, 1990)*. In one study, adolescents with idiopathic scoliosis were 17 per cent more flexible than a comparable non-scoliotic age group *(Miller, 1984)*. Another study suggested that torsion of the spine in a mechanical model was due to the actions of paraspinal muscles. There does not seem to be a connection between hand dominance and the direction of the curve. However, few electromyographic studies have been performed on the numerous muscles involved in scoliosis other than the paraspinals *(Robin, 1990)*.

✦ *Muscle imbalances:* While there is fibrosing and associated fatty deposits in muscles on the *concave* side of the curve, numerous studies have shown an increase in muscle activity on the *convex* side. This is believed to counter the pull from the concave side *(Robin, 1990)*. Although the significance is unclear, biochemical changes, such as collagen abnormalities, were reported with scoliosis. These may be the result of the curve, not the cause.

✦ *Hereditary factors:* Heredity has been proposed as a cause of spinal curves, yet it is more likely that *environmental factors* play a role. For example, infantile idiopathic scoliosis is much less common today in Europe than it was in the 1930s and 1940s when there was widespread malnutrition *(Robin, 1990)*.

✦ *Growth and sex hormones:* These may play a role in the development of scoliosis. Several studies have shown that within all racial groups, both female and male adolescents with idiopathic scoliosis were taller and thinner than non-scoliotic adolescents in the same age groups *(Bunch, Patwardhan, 1989)*. With minor curves, there is little difference in distribution between the sexes. However, the risk of progression of the curve is higher in females than in males. This leads to a female-male ratio of 1.5 to 1 for 10 degree curves, 5 to 1 for 20 degree curves and 10 to 1 for 30 degree curves *(DeSmet, 1985)*. It has been suggested that the difference in these ratios reflects the different ages at which the "normal" kyphotic curve develops in the two sexes *(Robin, 1990)*.

➤ **Functional** causes are musculoskeletal in nature. They relate to functional scoliosis. This term is perhaps confusing because a spinal curve caused by a short tibia or small hemipelvis (left or right half of a pelvis) seems to be a result of a structural asymmetry. However, a functional scoliosis is one that can be changed by altering position. This is certainly true of a leg length inequality because a shoe lift will correct the imbalance in the pelvis, reducing the scoliosis *(Cailliet, 1975)*.

✦ *Bony asymmetries below the pelvis:* A leg length inequality due to unilateral pes planus, a short tibia, short femur or small hemipelvis places the sacral base on an oblique angle in a standing person. A fracture of the tibia or femur may shorten the limb length. In a seated person, a small hemipelvis can cause pelvic obliquity. The spine must curve to compensate.

✦ *Bony asymmetries above the pelvis:* A short humerus causes the seated person to lean to the affected side, creating compensation in the lumbar, thoracic and cervical spine *(Travell, Simons, 1992)*. Plagiocephaly, or cranial asymmetry where one frontal region and the diagonal occipital area are flattened while the opposite frontal and occipital regions are prominent, is also associated with scoliosis. Torsion of the occiput on the sphenoid bone is documented as producing a cervical curve in children *(Jones, 1968)*.

✦ *Trigger points:* Trigger points in quadratus lumborum cause shortening of this muscle, raising the pelvis on the affected side and giving the appearance of a short leg *(Travell, Simons, 1992)*.

✦ *Habitual asymmetric postures:* This is where the person stands or sits with the weight shifted to one side. These postures result in asymmetric soft tissue shortening. Some causes are an occupational posture or sitting for long periods of time with a wallet in one pocket.

✦ *Soft tissue restrictions or contractures:* These occuring above or below the pelvis can lead to scoliosis. Unilateral tensor fascia lata and iliotibial band contracture can produce lateral pelvic tilt *(Kendall et al., 1993)*. Unilaterally shortened abdominal obliques or latissimus dorsi muscles can also lead to curving of the thoracic spine and lateral pelvic tilt *(Kendall, McCreary, 1983)*. Several studies on infants and children with pelvic distortions and scoliosis revealed an accompanying atlanto-occipital joint hypomobility *(Lewit, 1993)*.

✦ *Antalgic scoliosis:* This is a temporary curve caused by muscle spasm accompanying disc herniation or sciatic nerve irritation. The convexity may be towards, or away from, the affected side *(Magee, 1992)*.

➤ **Neuromuscular** conditions, such as cerebral palsy, Friedreich's ataxia, muscular dystrophy or spinal cord lesions, lead to muscular weakness and imbalance. Paralysis following polio can result in a long C-curve scoliosis on the side of muscular impairment.

➤ **Congenital** bony abnormalities can cause spinal curves. A *hemivertebra* is the incomplete formation of one side of the vertebra. With *vertebral wedging*, increased pressure on a bone's epiphyseal plate slows its rate of growth. Slowed growth occurs on the concave side of a scoliotic curve, resulting in asymmetric wedge-shaped vertebrae. This process can cause progression of a scoliosis in a child or adolescent (*Hoppenfeld, 1967*). In *vertebral bridging*, there is a failure of vertebral segmentation, and bony bars exist between vertebrae. These tether the growing bones together on one side, causing a curve. Malformed or congenitally absent ribs also cause scoliosis.

➤ **Iatrogenic** causes, such as pneumonectomy or open heart surgery, where the ribs are resected, may allow lateral curves to develop later. Incisions through the intercostals alone are recorded as provoking scoliosis in children (*Barral, Mercier, 1988; Hoppenfeld, 1967*).

Progression of Curves

A scoliosis can progress, stay the same or even regress. It is not clearly understood why some curves progress and some do not. Two factors prevent a curve from increasing. One is the normal passive resistance of the spine, ribs and ligaments that will limit excessive movement; the other is the contraction of the muscles on the convex side (*Miller, 1984*). Infantile idiopathic scoliosis often regresses spontaneously, while regression of adolescent scoliosis is much less common. Single curves tend to increase more than double curves (*Robin, 1990*).

The damaging effects of scoliosis on pulmonary function seem to occur in children where the curves have progressed past 60 degrees, while adolescents with a similar degree of curve rarely show signs of significantly reduced pulmonary function (*Robin, 1990*).

Bony and Soft Tissue Imbalances in Scoliosis

True leg length inequality is measured precisely to the millimetre only with an X-ray technique that includes both the legs and the pelvis. Other methods, such as measuring from the medial malleolus to the anterior superior iliac spine in the supine client, are useful only in a general way, because of variations in the pelvis. A clearer idea of which bones are short is achieved by assessing each component of the limb: the malleolar height and the length of the tibia and the femur (*Travell, Simons, 1992*).

On the transverse plane, each vertebra rotates around the axis of the spinal foramen so the spinal cord is not compressed. In a lateral curve, the vertebral bodies rotate around this axis *towards the convexity* of a curve (*Figure 44.2*). The vertebral bodies have greater mass and the convex side of the curve has more space for them to rotate into. The spinous processes, having less mass, rotate to the concave side where there is less space (*Hoppenfeld, 1967*). As the curve increases, the vertebral rotation increases. The greatest vertebral rotation occurs at the apex of the curve.

The degree of curve that is present with a scoliosis may be much greater than that which is indicated by the apparent position of the spinous processes pushing against the skin. The true position of the vertebral bodies is observable only on X-rays.

The ribs, articulating with the vertebral bodies and transverse processes, also become distorted. From a posterior view, the transverse processes are more posterior on the convex

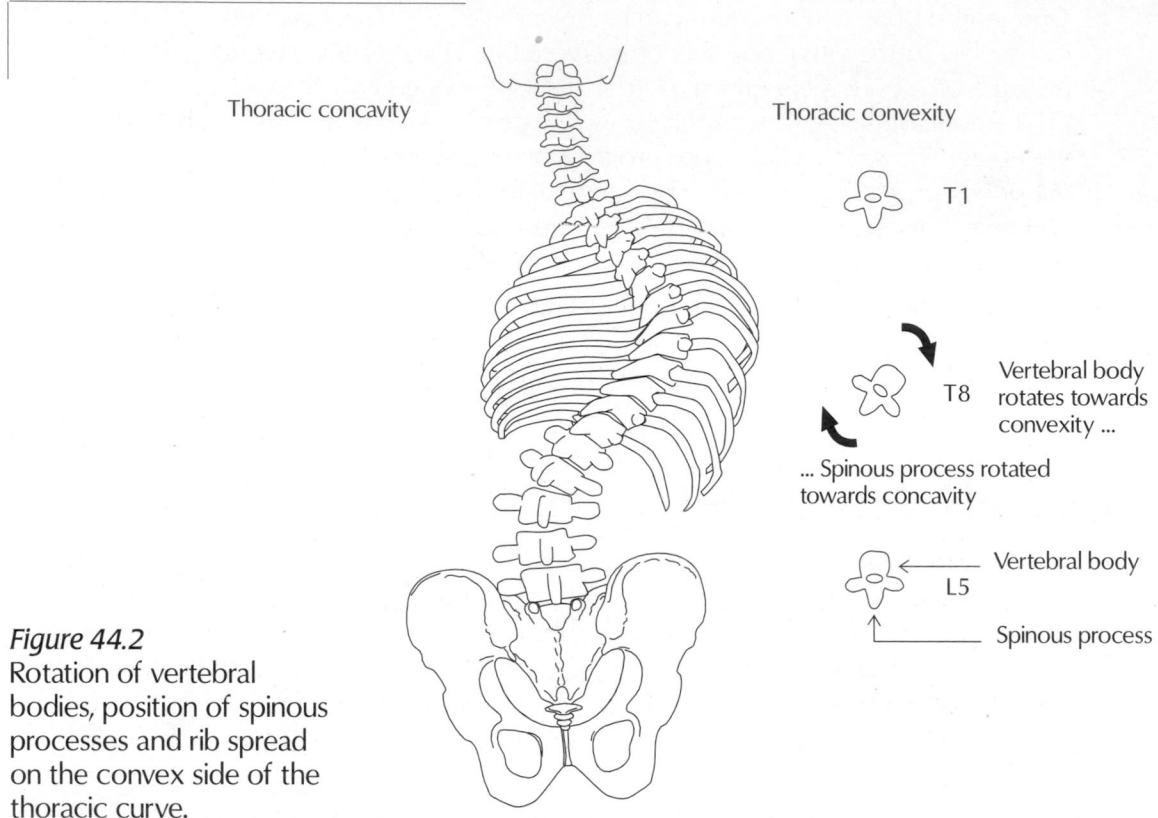

Thoracic concavity

Thoracic convexity

T1

T8 — Vertebral body rotates towards convexity ...

... Spinous process rotated towards concavity

L5 — Vertebral body

Spinous process

Figure 44.2
Rotation of vertebral bodies, position of spinous processes and rib spread on the convex side of the thoracic curve.

side. Therefore, the attached ribs on the convex side are also more posterior and prominent. This is called "rib humping". On the concave side, the transverse processes and ribs are more anterior and the ribs, therefore, appear flattened. On the convex side the ribs are also farther apart, whereas on the concave side, they are closer together. From an anterior view, the ribs are prominent on the concave side and flattened on the convex side *(Hoppenfeld, 1967)*.

The true muscle bulk of the paraspinal muscles is misleading. The muscles appear bigger on the convex side because they are pushed posteriorly by the ribs and transverse processes, and smaller on the concave side because they are pulled anteriorly by the bones *(Figure 44.3)*.

As previously mentioned, most studies on the muscles involved in scoliosis have focused on the paraspinal muscles. It appears that the deeper transverse muscles, including the multifidi, seem to play a larger part in scoliosis than do the more lateral and superficial erector spinae group. The multifidi, erector spinae and intercostal muscles on the *concave side* of the curve become shorter, tighter and fibrosed, further facilitating the curve. This is similar to how a bowstring pulls a bow into a curve.

In the paravertebral and intercostal muscles on the *convex side*, there is increased activity in an attempt to keep the spine upright. The attachments of these muscles are pulled farther apart by the tethering effect of the fibrosed muscles on the concave side. The convex activity has been shown to disappear following spinal fusion in idiopathic scoliosis *(Robin, 1990)*.

The actions of the abdominal obliques, iliopsoas, latissimus dorsi, intercostals and erector

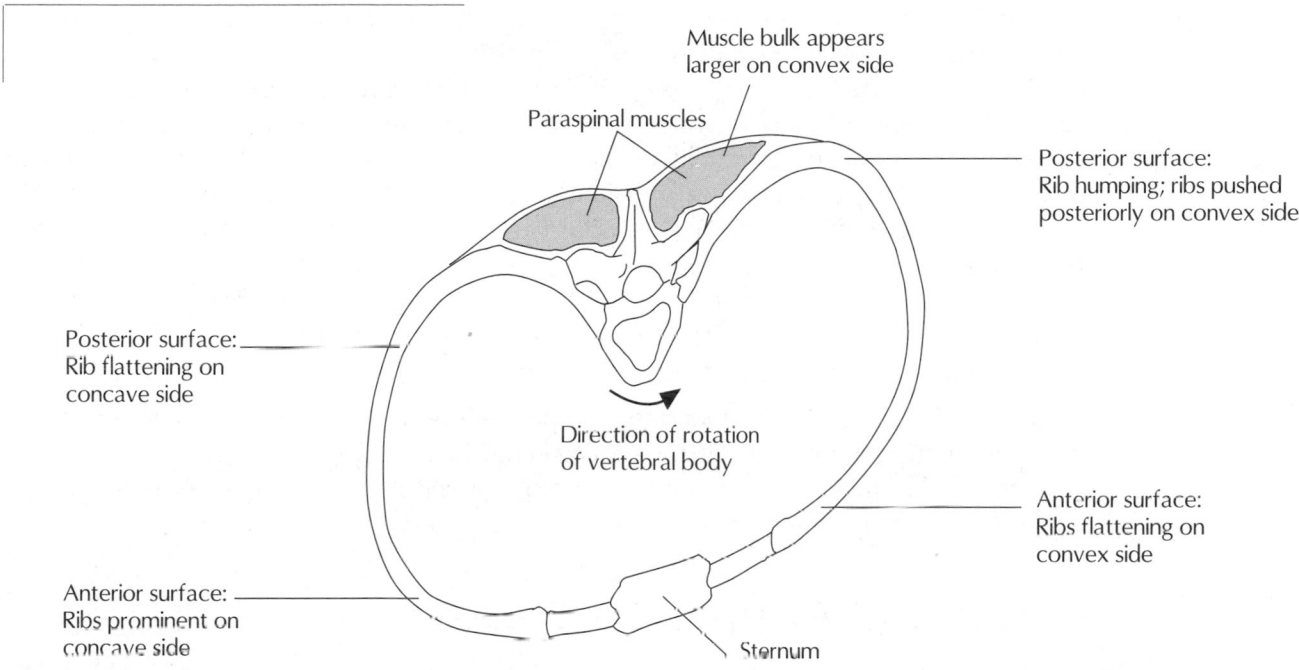

Muscle bulk appears
larger on convex side

Paraspinal muscles

Posterior surface:
Rib humping; ribs pushed
posteriorly on convex side

Posterior surface:
Rib flattening on
concave side

Direction of rotation
of vertebral body

Anterior surface:
Ribs flattening on
convex side

Anterior surface:
Ribs prominent on
concave side

Sternum

Figure 44.3
True bulk of paraspinal muscles is misleading.

spinae muscles acting unilaterally were shown to increase the severity of a curve *(Robin, 1990; Kendall, McCreary, 1983)*. Tight quadratus lumborum, iliopsoas and adductors on one side, plus tensor fascia lata and gluteus medius on the other side of the body, can maintain a pelvic obliquity *(Kendall, McCreary, 1983)*. The shoulder on the convex side of the thoracic curve is elevated by the actions of upper trapezius and levator scapula. The scapula is more prominent on this side.

A Historical Perspective of Scoliosis

References to "crook-backed" persons can be found in ancient Greek, Chinese and Indian medical literature. Biblical sources thought that no cure for this condition was possible. Hippocrates believed that a deformed spine could be straightened using traction after the patient was strapped to a frame. The next advance in the treatment of scoliosis came in the 1500s, when corsets, braces and suspension were used. The concept of exercise therapy for spinal deformities was introduced in the first "back school" in the early nineteenth century. At this time, plaster casting was also used to straighten the spine.

Spinal fusion was successfully used in 1911 to stabilize the spine in tuberculosis. By 1963, Paul Harrington, MD, had developed an internal fixation system to stabilize scoliosis resulting from polio. Electrical muscle stimulation, initially popular in the 1980s as a promising approach to reducing spinal curves, is now used in only very few cases *(Robin, 1990)*.

In the early 1970s, school screening programs to detect early signs of scoliosis were implemented, first in North America and later in many places worldwide. The screening programs were used to refer children for treatment if necessary and also to collect data on scoliosis. At this time, it was thought that curves of greater than 10 per cent in adolescents aged 10 to 16 years warranted observation, including full spinal X-rays. It was believed that because the curves were occurring in growing spines, these curves would increase with growth. However, follow-up studies showed that 80 per cent of the curves did not, in fact, progress. Some curves even regressed. Of those that did progress, the majority did not deteriorate beyond 20 to 30 degrees of curve *(Nachemson, 1984)*. Most of these progressed curves were treated conservatively with braces and only a minority required surgery. In one study of 26,000 children in Canada who were screened for scoliosis, 150 had curves of more than 10 degrees. More than half of these children had stable curves after diagnosis, one-third had curves that progressed and 15 children had curves that regressed. Only 31 children (0.12 per cent of the total study group of 26,000) were referred for any kind of treatment. Recently, the cost effectiveness of these school screening programs has been questioned *(Robin, 1990)*.

Another study of adolescents found that 40 per cent of the curves were due to minor leg length inequalities, not deformities originating in the spine. Fifty per cent of the curves originating in the spine were considered to be of no clinical significance, while only 10 per cent were truly progressive, increasing five degrees or more each year *(Robin, 1990)*.

The Medical Treatment of Scoliosis

In cases where curves are thought to be progressive, a scoliosis may be treated with a brace. If this does not reduce or halt the curve, surgery is usually performed, especially in cases where a severe scoliosis is deemed life threatening.

Braces, such as the plastic Milwaukee brace, generate force on the thorax to reduce the curve. This force is at the apex of a curve. Pressure is also applied on the opposite side of the body at the axilla and the pelvis *(DeSmet, 1985)*. Braces are used for curves of less than 40 to 60 degrees in children and adolescents, where the spine has not stopped growing. It is most common to recommend that these braces to be worn 23 hours a day for several years, although a few studies indicate part-time use of a brace is just as effective *(Bunch, Patwardhan, 1989; Robin, 1990)*.

Surgically, there are several methods of correcting a scoliosis. Surgery is the usual choice for curves over 40 or 50 degrees *(Kisner, Colby, 1990)*. Spinal fusion and Harrington and Luque rod instrumentation are common techniques. The massage therapist should understand where fusion and immobilization have taken place in order to perform a safe and effective massage treatment.

Spinal fusion involves a posterior midline longitudinal incision along the spinous processes. The paraspinal muscles are not cut but are reflected back to the transverse processes. Ligaments and facet joints are removed and the spaces left by the excision of the joint capsules are packed with bone grafts. Further bone grafts are placed over the fusion site *(DeSmet, 1985)*. Types of grafts include: autografts, where bone is taken from the individual with the scoliosis, usually from the posterior surface of the ilium; allografts, where bone is harvested from other persons and frozen for later use; and xenografts from animals — for example, cow bone *(Bunch, Patwardhan, 1989)*.

If **Harrington rod** instrumentation is the method chosen to reduce the scoliosis, the rods are inserted during a fusion procedure just before the facet joints are fused. Each rod has two hooks that are inserted onto the vertebral lamina at each end of the curve. Two kinds of rods may be used. Harrington distraction rods generate force to straighten the curve from the concavity, while Harrington compression rods pull the convex side straight.

Depending on the type of curve, wiring may be used to stabilize the rods to the vertebrae. Additional bone grafts are placed over the rods. The paraspinal muscles and skin are repositioned over the fusion site.

There are **complications** arising from Harrington rod placement. These include rod breakage or migration, hook dislocation, peripheral nerve damage and, in children and adolescents, the halt of spinal growth in the fused section *(DeSmet, 1985)*. In addition, the vertebrae, facet joints and discs immediately superior and inferior to the fused section have to compensate for the immobility in the spine. They are subject to increased wear and tear, as are the peripheral nerves that exit at these hypermobile vertebrae sections.

With **Luque instrumentation**, two L-shaped rods generate force from the sides of the vertebrae to straighten the curve *(DeSmet, 1985; Bunch, Patwardhan, 1989)*. The L-rods are placed on each side of the spinous processes and are secured together by wires passing under each lamina inside the neural canal. This method eliminates the need for post-operative immobilization. The initial belief that a formal spinal fusion could be avoided using the L-rods was later disproved. **Complications** from Luque instrumentation are a high level of neurological complications, such as motor weakness and sensory disturbances associated with nerve damage from passing wires under the lamina.

A combined method was developed to avoid the complications associated with the Luque method. The Wisconsin Drummond system uses both Harrington rods and Luque rods; wires for the L-rods are passed through the base of the spinous processes, avoiding the neural canal *(Bunch, Patwardhan, 1989)*.

Symptom Picture

+ There is one or more lateral and rotational curves to the lumbar, thoracic and cervical spine, with associated rib humping on the convex side of the thoracic curve. There is a lateral pelvic tilt.

+ The scoliosis may be a C-curve or an S-curve. It may also be functional or structural. A scoliosis can be mild, moderate or severe.

+ **In a functional scoliosis:**
  • Muscle imbalances and shortening are present. The specific muscles that are affected depend on the type of curve. See Observations. Hypertonicity and trigger points are present in the shortened muscles.
  • Range of motion is reduced away from the concave side. Rib mobility is restricted.
  • Pain may arise from tight ischemic tissue or from overstretched tissue.
  • Poor postural habits are present.
  • Other postural imbalances, such as pes planus, may be present.
  • Secondary conditions may develop, such as thoracic outlet syndrome or intercostal neuralgia.

+ **In a structural scoliosis:**
  • In addition to the above, there are also associated lateral displacement of the nucleus pulposus, vertebral body wedging and possible osteoarthritis. Facet joint

approximation and irritation may occur. Concave-side compression of the posterior disc and intervertebral foramen narrowing with possible nerve root irritation are likely.

- Idiopathic scoliosis in children is rarely painful. Pathologically caused scoliosis, however, often causes constant pain, which is worse at night and alleviated by anti-inflammatories *(Robin, 1990)*.

- Severe curves have associated pulmonary and visceral dysfunction from compression *(Porth, 1990)*.

Subjective Information

HEALTH HISTORY QUESTIONS

✦ How is the client's general health?

✦ At what age did the scoliosis became noticeable?

✦ In the past, did the client fracture any bones in the lower limb, creating a leg length inequality?

✦ What areas are painful, if any? What aggravates or relieves the pain?

✦ What are the client's postural habits, including occupational or recreational sources of postural stress?

✦ Is there a medical or chiropractic diagnosis for the degree of curvature?

✦ What other parallel therapies, if any, has the client had, such as braces, chiropractic or traction?

✦ Has the curve been surgically corrected? Does the client know the extent of the fusion? Were rods used? Does the client have any complications from the surgery, such as peripheral nerve damage?

✦ Are there any complications from the scoliosis? These are most likely with severe curves and may include impaired respiratory capacity, nerve impingement, osteoarthritis or visceral dysfunction.

Objective Information

Observations

✍ When recording a scoliosis, the therapist should list:

- whether it is an S- or C-curve and the direction of the convexity;
- the span of the scoliosis;
- the apex of the curve;
- the transitional vertebra with an S-curve;
- whether it is a functional or structural curve.

✍ The therapist observes the client standing in a relaxed, habitual posture. In an attempt to make the pelvis level and straighten the spine, a person with a short leg weight bears on this leg. By slightly flexing the hip and knee of the longer leg, or placing the longer leg to one side or in front, the pelvis on the high side drops down *(Travell, Simons, 1992)*. This is also true when there is no inequality in leg length and the person has a habit of standing with one knee slightly flexed *(Kapandji, 1974)*.

✍ If the client extends both knees, locking them in place, a different picture emerges. The pelvis is now laterally tilted, lower on the side of the short leg, regardless of whether there is a C-curve or an S-curve above it *(Travell, Simons, 1992)*. The client weight bears more on the convex side of a C-curve *(Hoppenfeld, 1967; Robin, 1990)*.

✍ With pelvic torsion, anterior rotation of the innominate bone *raises* the PSIS and sacrum on the same side, while posterior rotation *lowers* the PSIS and the sacrum on the same side *(Figure 44.4)*. Compensatory anterior rotation of the innominate bone is associated with a short lower limb on that side, while compensatory posterior rotation of the innominate is associated with a long lower limb *(Hertling, Kessler, 1990; Travell, Simons, 1992)*.

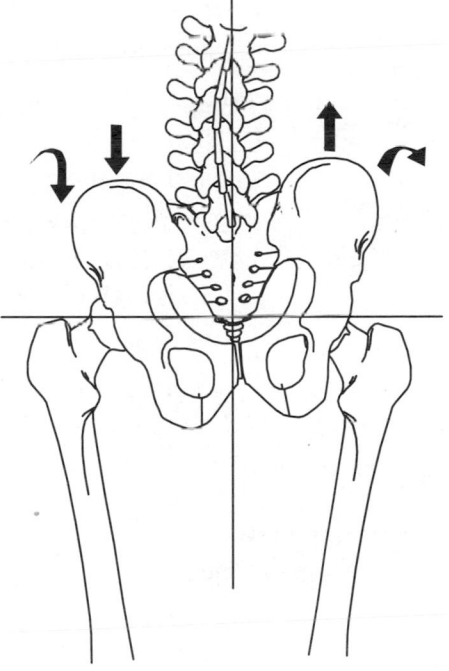

Posterior rotation of innominate bone on long leg side lowers the PSIS

Anterior rotation of innominate bone on short lleg side raises the PSIS

Figure 44.4
Pelvic torsion.

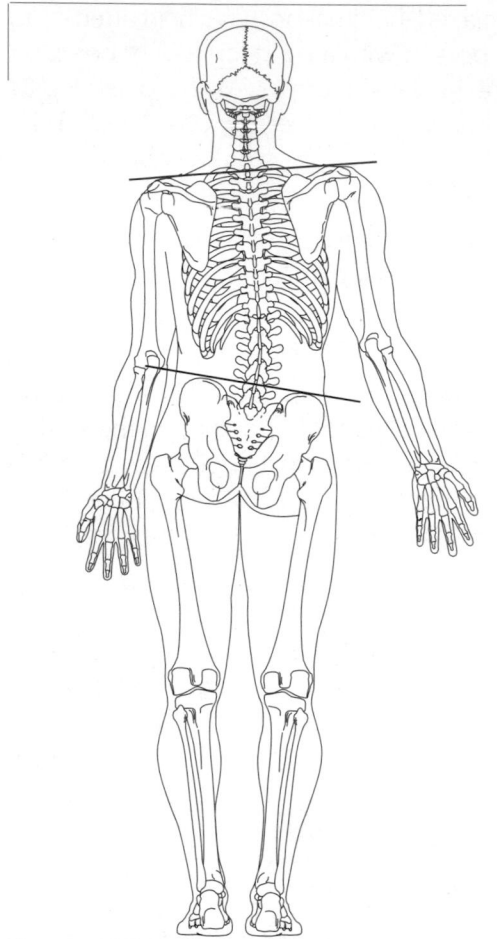

Figure 44.5
C-curve scoliosis: Right thoracolumbar
functional curve, span T2 to L4, apex at L2.

Postural Assessment

C-curve Scoliosis: Right Thoracolumbar Functional Curve

✎ This curve is also described and shown as a wedge (*St. John, 1994; Travell, Simons 1992*).

Posterior View (see *Figure 44.5*)

✎ With the plumb line as reference, the occiput is checked to see if it is centred above a point midway between the calcanei.

✎ The level of the occiput is assessed.

✎ There may be a left cervical compensatory curve.

✎ The right acromioclavicular joint is higher.

✎ Humeral lengths are assessed bilaterally.

✎ The right scapula is higher and possibly winged.

✎ The distance between the medial borders of both scapulae and the spine is checked.

✎ Right rib humping is present.

✎ There may be asymmetrical skin folds on the torso, with more folds on the concave side.

✎ Iliac crest levels are higher on the left.

✎ There is an asymmetrical negative space between the torso and the arms.

✎ PSIS levels are checked — with lateral pelvic tilt only, the PSIS is **low** on the dropped side; with pelvic torsion, the PSIS is **high** on the anteriorly rotated, short-leg side.

✎ Knee valgus is possible.

✎ Heights of the malleoli, fibular heads and greater trochanters are checked — any of these on the right may be lower with a short right leg as the scoliosis source (*Magee, 1992*).

✎ Right foot pronation is possible.

Lateral View

✎ Knee hyperextension is possible.

✎ Increased anterior pelvic tilt is seen on the short limb side (females five to 10 degrees, males zero to five degrees are normal limits — the pelvis should be compared bilaterally for torsion).

Anterior View

✎ The right ASIS is lower than the left with a short right limb or pelvic torsion (*Hertling, Kessler, 1990*).

✎ The left ribs are prominent (*Hoppenfeld, 1967*).

✎ Facial bones are frequently smaller on the same side as a small hemipelvis (*Travell, Simons, 1992*).

Superior View

✎ It is possible that the ASIS and acromioclavicular joint on one side are anterior, giving a unilateral torsion, or that one ASIS and the other acromioclavicular joint are anterior, giving an opposing torsion (*St. John, 1994*).

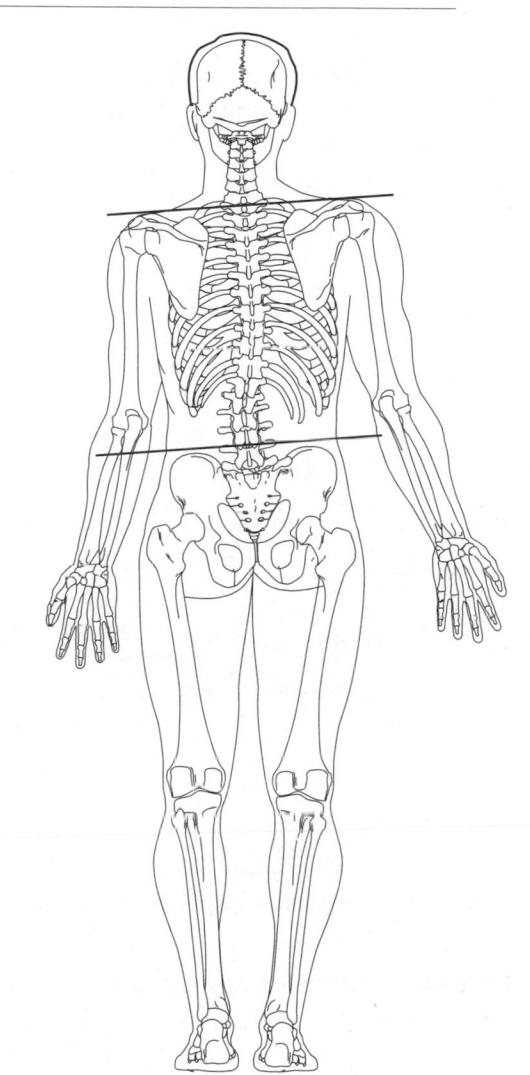

Figure 44.6
S-curve scoliosis: Right thoracic, left lumbar functional curve; left lumbar curve spans L2 to L4, apex at L3; transitional vertebra L1; right thoracic curves span T3 to T12, apex at T8.

S-curve Scoliosis: Right Thoracic, Left Lumbar Functional Curve

✍ This curve is also described and shown as a parallelogram *(St. John, 1994; Travell, Simons, 1992)*.

Posterior View (see *Figure 44.6*)

✍ With the plumb line as a reference, the occiput is checked to see if it is centred above a point midway between the calcanei.

✍ The level of the occiput is assessed.

✍ There may be a left cervical compensatory curve.

✍ The right acromioclavicular joint is higher.

✍ Humeral lengths are bilaterally assessed.

✍ The right scapula is higher and possibly winged.

✍ The distance between the medial borders of both scapulae and the spine is checked.

✍ Right rib humping is present.

✍ There may be asymmetrical skin folds on the torso, with more folds on the concave side.

✍ Iliac crest levels are higher on the right.

✍ There is an symmetrical negative space between the torso and the arms.

✍ PSIS levels are checked — with lateral pelvic tilt only, the PSIS is **low** on the dropped side; with pelvic torsion, the PSIS is **high** on the anteriorly rotated, short leg side.

✍ Knee valgus is possible.

✍ Heights of the malleoli, fibular heads and greater trochanters are checked — any of these on the left may be lower with a short left leg as the scoliosis source *(Magee, 1992)*.

✍ Left foot pronation is possible.

Lateral View

✍ Knee hyperextension is possible.

✍ Increased anterior pelvic tilt is seen on the short limb side (females five to 10 degrees, males zero to five degrees are normal limits — the pelvis should be compared bilaterally for torsion).

Anterior View

✍ The left ASIS is lower than the right with a short left limb or pelvic torsion *(Hertling, Kessler, 1990)*.

✍ The left ribs are prominent.

Superior View

✍ It is possible that the ASIS and acromioclavicular joint on one side are anterior, giving a unilateral torsion, or that one ASIS and the other acromioclavicular joint are anterior, giving an opposing torsion *(St. John, 1994)*.

Structural Scoliosis

✍ The most common pattern for idiopathic scoliosis is a right thoracic curve spanning T5 to T11, with the apex at T8 and with a compensatory left lumbar curve from T12 to L4 *(Bunch, Patwardhan, 1989)*.

✍ Non-idiopathic scoliosis resulting from congenital bony changes frequently has a left thoracic pattern. There may be café au lait spots, a patch of hair over the vertebrae, a short leg, trunk and neck, or a small foot.

✍ Scoliosis resulting from neurological conditions usually appears as a lumbar or thoracolumbar curve extending to the pelvis. There is pelvic obliquity with a very prominent hip and adduction of the femur *(Bunch, Patwardhan, 1989)*.

Palpation

✍ Depending on the shape of the curve, the therapist palpates the erector spinae, quadratus lumborum, intercostals, trapezius and gluteus medius for hypertonicity and trigger points.

✍ The therapist palpates for fibrosing in the concave side of the curve.

Testing

✍ **AF ROM** of the spine in lateral bending and flexion reveals decreased range towards the convex side.

✍ **PR ROM** of the hip reveals decreased range in extension with an anterior pelvic tilt. PR ROM of the protracted shoulder is decreased in external rotation. PR ROM of the cervical spine may also be decreased.

✍ **AR strength testing** reveals weakness in the abdominals and in the muscles on the concave side of the curve. With an anterior pelvic tilt, gluteus maximus is weak on the side with the anterior tilt. With a lateral pelvic tilt, gluteus medius is weak on the high side.

Special Tests

✍ A **functional** or **structural scoliosis test** is positive, as are **scoliosis small hemipelvis** (*Figure 44.7*) and **scoliosis short leg tests** (*Figure 44.8*) with these conditions.

✍ Functional leg length is assessed with the **supine to sit test**, while **true tibia and femur length** are assessed with the client supine.

✍ Sacroiliac joint motion is assessed with the **sacroiliac joint motion test** and **Gillet's test.**

✍ **Anterior spinous challenge, lateral spinous challenge, motion palpation** and **static**

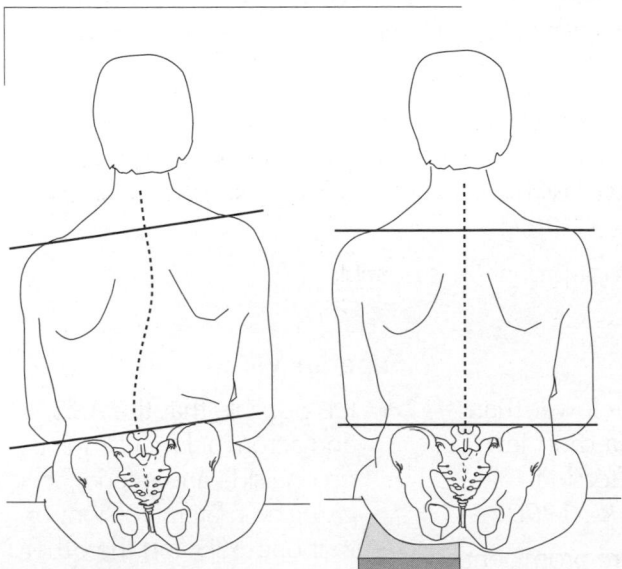

Figure 44.7
A small left hemipelvis causing a functional S-curve is assessed with a lift placed under the ischium. If the curve neutralizes the scoliosis is functional.

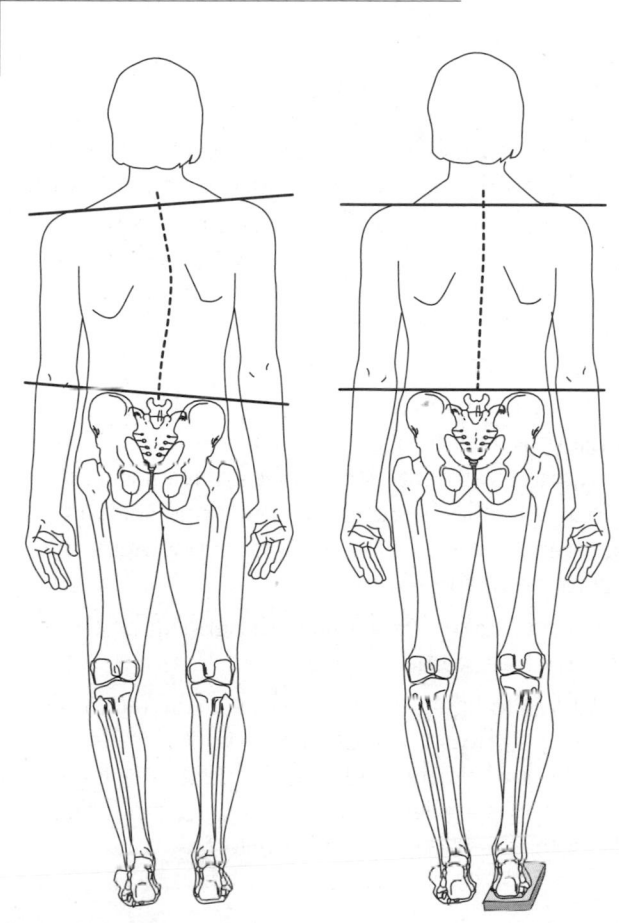

Figure 44.8
A short right leg causing a functional C-curve is assessed with a lift placed under the heel. The lift placed under the short leg balances the curves in a functional scoliosis.

palpation of the spine may reveal areas of hypo- and hypermobility in functional and structural curves. In addition, **rib motion** is asymmetrical and hypomobile.

✍ Length tests for muscles attaching to the pelvis and shoulder girdle should be performed. This includes **Thomas, Ely's, adductor length, piriformis length, Ober's, quadratus lumborum, shoulder adductors, pectoralis major and pectoralis minor.** The results will vary depending on the type of curve and amount of torsion present in the pelvis and shoulders.

✍ There is disagreement on the length of some muscles in scoliosis. For example, one source lists iliopsoas as being short on the convex side of a C-curve *(Kendall, McCreary, 1983)*; another source shows iliopsoas short on the concave side *(St. John, 1994)*. Pectoralis minor may be short because it is depressing one shoulder, or short because it is protracting the shoulder *(St. John, 1994)*. The therapist is advised to bilaterally compare and record the lengths of the involved muscles and *lengthen the ones that are short.*

✍ **Valsalva's, Kernig's** and **straight leg raise tests** are positive with space-occupying lesions. **Kemp's** is also positive with space-occupying lesions or facet joint irritation.

Contraindications

✦ If a pathology is suspected but undiagnosed, such as a spinal lesion, osseous change or degeneration, or decreased pulmonary function, refer the client to a physician.

✦ If the client has a fusion or immobilization from rods, do not attempt to mobilize these vertebrae.

✦ Avoid mobilizing hypermobile vertebrae, especially if they are adjacent to fused vertebrae. Joint play techniques for the ribs and rib springing are contraindicated with rib hypermobility and a history of rib subluxation.

✦ Do not use longitudinal work or stretching techniques on the muscles on the convex side of a curve because these muscles are already overstretched.

✦ Avoid applications of heat over metal rods as these may painfully retain heat for some time.

✦ Do not randomly stretch fascia. Assess the fascia and only treat areas of restriction.

Treatment Goals   Treatment Plan

Assess the client to determine if the scoliosis is functional or structural.

Due to the complexity of scoliosis, it is recommended that, after thoroughly assessing the client, the therapist chooses one area of the body to work on at a time. For example, with a pelvic obliquity or pelvic torsion, muscles that attach to the pelvis are treated over several appointments. As the pelvis levels out, fewer imbalances affect the structures above it. Over several more treatments, the thorax, shoulders and neck are treated.

If the curves are functional or even mildly idiopathic, the curves can be altered. If the scoliosis is structural or the spine has been straightened surgically, the treatment plan involves maintaining tissue health, reducing pain and treating secondary conditions, such as thoracic outlet syndrome. In these cases, there is no possibility of changing the configuration of the spine.

Positioning may be prone, supine or sidelying depending on the location of the tight structures to be treated.

Hydrotherapy is heat to the tight structures. Heat is applied in one area, then another. This patchwork effect allows work on the pre-heated area while the hydrotherapy is heating the next area to be treated. Cool hydrotherapy is applied in the same patchwork manner to the weak muscles after these muscles are treated.

General Treatment

The treatment described below addresses a right thoracic, left lumbar functional S-curve (see *Figure 44.9*).

Decrease sympathetic nervous system firing.

Treatment is performed in a relaxation context. This includes **diaphragmatic breathing** to help reduce any pain experienced with the direct fascial work.

Specific Treatment

In this example, the treatment is begun with the client in the **prone** position. The client is pillowed under the abdomen and ankles. A small towel folded or rolled up can be placed under the ASIS of the anteriorly rotated left pelvis to encourage a posterior rotation.

Reduce fascial restrictions.

Following the pre-heated areas, the fascial work to the *short and tight muscles on the concave sides* zigzags across the client's body, inferior to superior. **Heat** is applied to the left lateral hip while petrissage is used on the short right adductors. The heat is then moved to the right quadratus lumborum while fascial spreading and connective tissue cutting techniques are used on the left gluteus medius. The heat is next moved to the left thoracic erector spinae and intercostals while the muscles in the concavity of the lumbar curve are treated. Skin rolling and crossed-hands spreading are used

584

Treatment Goals Treatment Plan

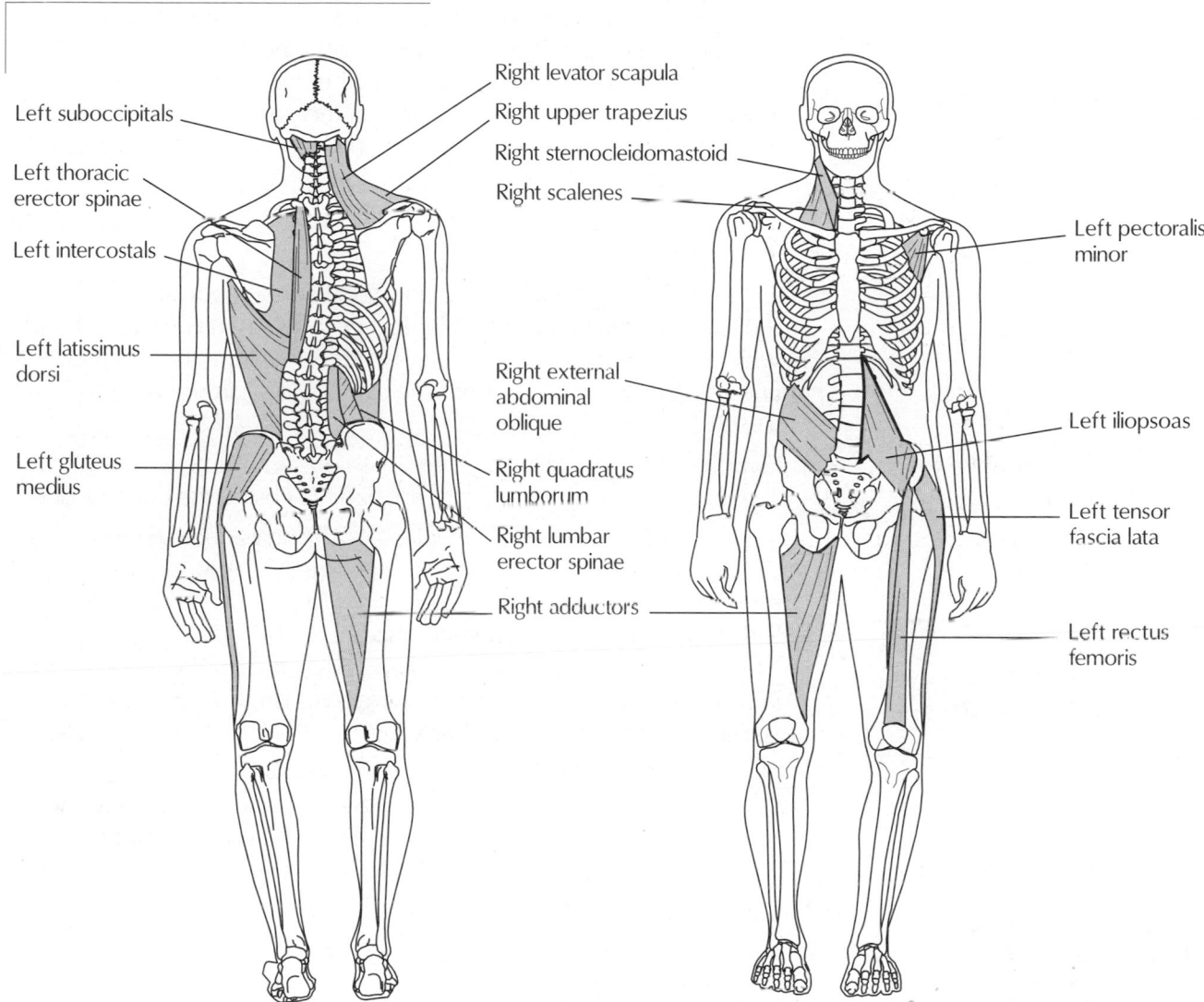

Left suboccipitals

Left thoracic
erector spinae

Left intercostals

Left latissimus
dorsi

Left gluteus
medius

Right levator scapula

Right upper trapezius

Right sternocleidomastoid

Right scalenes

Right external
abdominal
oblique

Right quadratus
lumborum

Right lumbar
erector spinae

Right adductors

Left pectoralis
minor

Left iliopsoas

Left tensor
fascia lata

Left rectus
femoris

Figure 44.9
Right thoracic, left lumbar S-curve, showing short muscles. As well as a lateral tilt, there is an anterior pelvic tilt on the left, and a protracted right shoulder in the described treatment.

over the entire lower right quadrant.

🖑 The right lumbar erector spinae are treated with longitudinal and transverse spreading. The attachments of quadratus lumborum at the iliac crest, lumbar vertebrae and twelfth rib are outlined using connective tissue cutting and fascial spreading.

🖑 The heat is moved to the right upper trapezius while fascial techniques are used on the left latissimus dorsi, left erector spinae and left intercostals. One group of intercostals is systematically treated with fingertip fascial stoking laterally to medially. This is

Treatment Goals   Treatment Plan

repeated three or four times, with the pressure tolerably increased each time. The technique is repeated on the next intercostals. A group of three or four intercostals may be the maximum treated in a single appointment. If necessary, fascial techniques are used on the right upper trapezius and levator scapula.

**Reduce hypertonicity.
Increase local circulation
to remove metabolites.**

A variety of Swedish techniques is used on the tight structures, working inferiorly to superiorly, including effleurage, ulnar border stripping and muscle stripping.

**Reduce trigger points.
Reduce pain if present.**

Trigger points in gluteus medius and quadratus lumborum refer into the sacroiliac joint and lateral hip. Trigger points in multifidi refer locally, while those in iliocostalis and longissimus refer along these muscle groups, occasionally down into the gluteals (*Travell, Simons 1983, 1992*).

Mobilize hypomobile joints.

Hypomobile vertebrae are treated with posterior-anterior and lateral joint play. Rib springing is used to mobilize the ribs on the concave side.

**Encourage local circulation
in weak, taut structures.**

The stretched, weak and tight intercostals and paraspinal muscles on the *convex* sides of the curves are now treated. Any stimulating petrissage technique may be used, providing the work is transverse to the muscle fibres. Tapotement is also used. The left adductors, right gluteus medius, left upper trapezius and levator scapula are included in this work. Trigger points in the rhomboids on the convex side, which are activated by scapular winging, are treated with ischemic compression (*Travell, Simons, 1983*).

Strengthen weak muscles.

Active resisted exercise is used to strengthen the intercostals on the convex side. The therapist compresses the ribs with both hands while the client inhales against this resistance.

Cool washes are applied to the stretched muscles.

Stretch shortened muscles.

PIR may be used to lengthen the left rectus femoris. See hyperlordosis treatment for details.

With the client **sidelying** on the left side, a small towel roll is placed under the left waist, between the ribs and pelvis. The client is asked to position the right lower limb on the table so the right hip is extended, while the left hip and knee are flexed. The right arm is placed in full flexion in front of the head. This allows the pelvis to be pulled away from the rib cage, stretching the tight right quadratus lumborum.

Skin rolling and fascial stroking are used on the tight right external abdominal obliques, following the attachments at the iliac crest and costal margins. This is followed by petrissage to these muscles.

PIR for quadratus lumborum proceeds from the sidelying position described above. The client allows the lower limb to drop off the table. Both the therapist's arms are crossed, stabilizing the inferior ribs with one hand and the iliac crest with the other. The client minimally

Treatment Goals   Treatment Plan

contracts the quadratus lumborum against the therapist's resistance for 10 seconds and then relaxes, allowing the lower limb to drop farther off the table. The cycle is repeated at least three times.

- In the **supine** position, for the pelvis, both fascial and Swedish techniques and PIR are used for the tight and short left iliopsoas, rectus femoris and right adductors. A hypomobile sacroiliac joint is mobilized with joint play. The left anterior pelvic tilt may also be treated with passive range of motion and active resisted techniques. For details see the hyperlordosis chapter.

Reduce hypertonicity.
Stretch shortened muscles.

- In terms of the shoulder girdle, the tight left latissimus dorsi and right pectoralis minor are also treated with fascial and Swedish work and PIR. For details see the hyperkyphosis chapter.

- The flattened right anterior ribs are treated with fascial and Swedish techniques and rib springing as outlined in the prone section above. The prominent left anterior ribs are strengthened with active resisted exercise.

- The diaphragm, if tight, is treated using ischemic thumb pressure inferior to the costal margins. Working with the client's breathing, the therapist applies pressure with exhalation and the thumbs are held in place with inhalation. Cross-fibre thumb kneading is used on the diaphragm attachments. The thumbs are drawn out slowly on completion of the technique.

- The tight right scalenes, right sternocleidomastoid (*Travell, Simons, 1983*) and left suboccipitals are treated with muscle stripping.

Treat other conditions.

- Other conditions, such as pes planus and iliotibial band contracture, are treated on subsequent appointments.

Self-care Goals   Self-care Plan

Educate the client regarding activities.

- The client should avoid postures that encourage the scoliosis. For example, clients with one humerus shorter than the other should raise the arm of a workstation chair either with padding or by using adjustable-height arm rests.

Stretch shortened muscles.

- **Self-stretching** for the shortened muscles is important. Although exercise alone cannot halt the progression of a moderate scoliosis, it is useful for functional and mild idiopathic curves (*Kisner, Colby, 1990*).

- **PIR** for many of the shortened muscles is listed in the hyperlordosis and hyperkyphosis treatments. In addition, the client is given **heel-sitting exercises** for spinal flexibility. The client is seated on the floor with the heels under the gluteals. The client bends forward from the

587

Self-care Goals

Self-care Plan

hips so the abdomen rests on the anterior thighs and the arms are stretched out above the head, hands resting on the floor. The client laterally bends the trunk away from the concavity by walking the hands to the convex side. When a full stretch has been reached, the client inhales and then exhales completely. The stretch is increased towards the convexity. The cycle of inhalation, exhalation and stretch is repeated several times. The action of the ribs while breathing may possibly decrease rotation of the vertebrae (*Kisner, Colby, 1990*).

Strengthen weak muscles.

✍ Strengthening for the weaker convex muscles, such as in the lumbar spine, is achieved by the client sidelying on the concave side with the lower limbs stabilized. The client raises the shoulders off the floor and holds this position. The uppermost arm may rest on the client's side with this exercise. Other strengthening exercises for weaker muscles are found in the hyperlordosis, hyperkyphosis and asthma chapters.

✍ If the client is in the care of another health care practitioner, such as a physiotherapist, with the client's permission the therapist should contact the other practitioner to coordinate the overall treatment plan.

Refer the client.

✍ The client can be referred for medical or chiropractic assessment of the severity of the curve if this is not known or for orthotics if leg length discrepancy is a contributing factor. Clients with asymmetries of cranial and facial bones can be referred to practitioners of St. John Neuromuscular Technique. See Non-Swedish Techniques for details.

✍ Movement therapy, such as the Mitzvah, Feldenkrais or Alexander technique, may be helpful for retraining the client's posture.

Treatment Frequency and Expected Outcome

With functional scoliosis or mild idiopathic scoliosis, treatments may be once a week for six weeks. The therapist should then totally reassess both the client and the client's exercise plan.

See also myofascial trigger points, pes planus, iliotibial band contracture, hyperlordosis, hyperkyphosis, torticollis, thoracic outlet syndrome, temporomandibular joint dysfunction, cerebral palsy, poliomyelitis, spinal cord injury, understanding peripheral nerve lesions, degenerative disc disease and osteoarthritis for related treatments.

The outcome for a functional scoliosis is favourable with a client who is compliant with a remedial exercise program. Correcting a leg length inequality with shoe supports is also important.

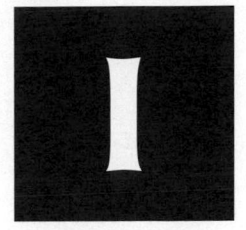

JOINT DYSFUNCTIONS

45

HYPERMOBILITY AND HYPOMOBILITY

Fiona Rattray

Hypermobility

Hypermobility is an increased degree of motion at a joint.

Hypermobility can occur at one joint (often trauma-related) or several joints, or can be generalized throughout the body. It can range from mild joint laxity to extreme mobility or even joint instability. In general, women and children tend to be more flexible than men and the elderly *(Lewit, 1993)*. Racial origin can have an influence on range of motion. Asians have a greater range of motion than Blacks, and Blacks have greater range than Caucasians *(Travell, Simons, 1992)*.

Hypermobility and compensatory weakness can be created in the body by soft tissue tightness and hypomobility in another place *(Greenman, 1989)*. This is most obvious in postural dysfunctions. In the spine, a hypermobile joint may be found next to a hypomobile joint *(Neumann, 1989)*.

Physiological hypermobility occurs in some body types and occupations and during pregnancy. The ectomorphic body type, where there is a greater proportion of tissues, such as nerves and skin, which are derived from the embryonic ectoderm layer, is linear, delicate, slightly developed and has hypermobile joints *(Greenman, 1989)*. In addition, gymnasts and dancers tend to be more flexible or strive to develop more flexibility than average people. The hormone relaxin, secreted during pregnancy, allows joint capsules and ligaments to become hypermobile to facilitate labour and delivery of the baby. Joints, especially noticeable in the pelvis, ankle and feet, remain hypermobile for up to six months postpartum *(Brayshaw, Wright, 1994)*.

While hypermobility itself does not necessarily mean pain and dysfunction *(Neumann, 1989)*, people with joint laxity may be at risk for musculoskeletal symptoms and injuries, including sprain, tendinitis, osteoarthritis and entrapment neuropathies such as carpal tunnel syndrome *(Greenman, 1989)*. There is an interplay between articular dysfunction and myofascial pain syndromes *(Travell, Simons, 1992)*. **Hypermobility syndrome** occurs in up to five per cent of those with hypermobility *(Beighton et al., 1989)*; the person experiences symptoms including muscle and joint pain, overuse syndromes such as tendinitis, abdominal muscle weakness, hyperextensible skin and mitral valve prolapse.

Certain pathologies and conditions predispose people to hypermobility. **Rheumatoid arthritis**, a systemic autoimmune disorder characterized by inflammation and destruction of connective tissue, results in hypermobility of the affected joints. The **Ehlers-Danlos syndromes** are a group of inherited disorders characterized by joint hypermobility, sometimes dislocation, skin hyperextensibility, increased bruising and tissue fragility. **Marfan's syndrome** is an inherited disorder with fragmentation of elastin, leading to joint hypermobility (dislocation is not common), elongated bones, aortal widening, mitral valve prolapse and changes in the eye, specifically in the lens *(Schumacher, 1993)*. In either of these syndromes, hypermobility increases substantially following joint injury.

Medically, if damage to a joint is sufficient, a hypermobile joint may be treated one of several ways: with injections to sclerose the joint capsule or vertebral disc; with surgical shortening of ligaments or muscles crossing the joint; or with fixation externally with splints or internally with pins, plates or other appliances.

Causes of hypermobility are:

➤ **compensation** due to hypomobility or postural dysfunction elsewhere in the body;

➤ **increased flexibility** due to body type, occupation or activity;

➤ **hormonal influences** during pregnancy;

➤ **joint trauma** such as sprain or dislocation;

➤ **pathologies and conditions** causing joint laxity, such as rheumatoid arthritis, Ehlers-Danlos syndromes and Marfan's syndrome; and peripheral nerve lesions and central nervous system lesions, such as hemiplegia, which lead to flaccidity and in turn, unsupported joints.

Symptom Picture of Hypermobility

✦ The affected joint has a greater-than-normal range of motion.

✦ When symptomatic, hypermobility may be *painful* if the ligaments crossing the joint are intact but overstretched or if intra-articular adhesions are stretched; or *painless* if the ligaments are ruptured *(Magee, 1992; Beighton et al., 1989)*.

✦ The joint capsule is lax. Greater stress is placed on the joint capsule, articular surfaces of the joint, intervertebral discs and menisci.

✦ Muscles crossing the affected joint may be hypertonic in an attempt to support the joint.

Contraindications

✦ Do not mobilize a hypermobile joint.

✦ Do not stretch muscles that cross a hypermobile joint past the accepted range for that joint *(Travell, Simons, 1983)*.

Treatment Considerations

Assessment

✍ **Observations** including a full postural assessment may reveal areas of imbalance.

✍ **Palpation** may reveal tenderness in the muscles crossing the hypermobile joint *(Beighton et al., 1989)*.

✍ **Testing:**

- **AF ROM** and **PR ROM** are greater than normal at a hypermobile joint.

- End feel is encountered at a point later than normally expected for the specific joint. It may be painfully or painlessly hypermobile.

- A **nine-point scoring system** has been developed to measure hypermobility for the spine and the paired fingers, thumbs, elbows and knees *(Beighton et al.,1989; Greenman, 1989)*. Higher scores indicates greater joint laxity, with between four and six points indicating hypermobility syndrome *(Travell, Simons, 1992)*:

  — passive dorsiflexion of the little fingers past 90 degrees — one point for each finger;

  — passive apposition of the thumbs to the flexor surface of the forearms — one point for each thumb;

  — hyperextension of the elbows beyond 10 degrees — one point for each elbow;

  — forward flexion of the trunk with the knees extended, with the palms of the hands flat on the floor — one point;

  — hyperextension of the knees beyond 10 degrees — one point for each knee.

- In the spine and rib cage, **anterior spinous challenge, lateral spinous challenge, motion palpation, static palpation of the spine, rib motion** and **rib palpation** reveal areas of hypermobility.

- A **ligamentous stress test** for joints of the limbs will reveal hypermobility. See the chapter on sprains for more details of individual tests. Other stress tests include **acromioclavicular shear test** for the acromioclavicular joint and **sacroiliac joint gapping, sacroiliac joint "squish"** and **Gaenslen's tests** for the sacroiliac joint.

Massage

🖐 No techniques are used specifically on the hypermobile joint. Instead, if hypermobility is combined with compensatory *hypomobility* at another joint proximal or distal to the hypermobile joint, joint play is used on the *hypomobile* joint *(Neumann, 1989)*.

🖐 For example, a person with hyperkyphosis has reduced thoracic mobility and protracted shoulders. With protraction, the glenohumeral joint turns inferiorly, allowing the humeral head to slip inferiorly. If the rotator cuff muscles do not work harder to keep the humeral head in place, the joint capsule stretches and the glenohumeral joint becomes hypermobile. Joint play is used on the hypomobile thoracic spine to normalize the biomechanics and reduce the stress on the glenohumeral joint.

🖐 Trigger points may be present in muscles that cross a hypermobile joint. These are treated with muscle stripping or ischemic compression followed by heat only, no stretch *(Travell, Simons, 1992)*.

Self-care

✍ An important factor in treating a hypermobile joint is to strengthen all the muscles crossing the joint, since hypermobility requires stabilization. The client should begin with isometric exercises, progressing to isotonic exercises when the muscles are able to support the joint in a physiologically normal position.

✍ The client is referred to a physician or chiropractor if an undiagnosed pathology is suspected as the underlying cause of the hypermobility.

Hypomobility

Hypomobility is loss of motion at a joint, including the loss of normal joint play movements.

Hypomobility can occur at one joint (often due to soft tissue contractures) or several joints, or can be generalized throughout the body. Joints on the dominant side of the body tend to be more hypomobile than those on the non-dominant side *(Magee, 1992)*. The mesomorphic body type, where there is a relative preponderance of muscle, bone and connective tissue, and the body is rectangular in shape, is often less flexible. Hypomobility often requires nearby joints to become hypermobile to compensate.

A **minor intervertebral derangement** in the spine is an isolated, painful, hypomobile vertebra. It has a mechanical, postural or traumatic cause *(Basmajian, 1985)*. Static and mobility X-rays of the affected vertebra reveal nothing abnormal. Palpation and vertebral mobility tests reveal the painful, hypomobile segment.

In general, hypomobile joints can lead to strained muscles, peripheral nerve compression, tendinitis *(Magee, 1992)* and decreased ability to perform activities of daily life.

Causes of hypomobility are:

➤ **compensation** due to hypermobility or postural dysfunction elsewhere in the body;

➤ **decreased flexibility** due to body type or occupation;

➤ **intra-articular and extra-articular adhesions** following joint trauma, surgery and immobilization including prolonged bedrest and wheelchair use;

➤ **surgical fixation** by pins, screws, plates or rods, or by surgical shortening of ligaments or muscles that cross the affected joint;

➤ **pathologies and conditions** causing contractures, such as Dupuytren's contracture, frozen shoulder, ankylosing spondylitis, peripheral nerve lesions and central nervous system lesions.

594

Symptom Picture of Hypomobility

+ The affected joint has a reduced range of motion and reduced joint play movements.
+ Stiffness and pain are present *(Hertling, Kessler, 1996)*.

+ The joint capsule may be fibrosed. Intra-articular adhesions may be present. Shortened fascia, scar tissue or contractures may be present in muscles that cross the joint.
+ Structures such as nerve roots, intervertebral discs, peripheral nerves, blood vessels and menisci may be entrapped or compressed by the hypomobile joint.
+ Proper nutrition is reduced to the articular surfaces of the joint.
+ There are frequently associated myofascial pain syndromes, including trigger points, in the muscles that cross a hypomobile joint.

Contraindications

+ Do not attempt to mobilize a hypomobile joint that has been surgically repaired with metal appliances.
+ Where the ligaments have been surgically shortened, do not restore full range of motion of the affected joint in the direction that will stretch the repaired ligament.

Treatment Considerations

Assessment

✍ **Observations** including a full postural assessment may reveal areas of imbalance.

✍ **Testing:**

- **AF ROM** and **PR ROM** are reduced from normal ranges with hypomobility. An end feel is encountered before it is usually expected for a specific joint. In addition, depending on the cause of the hypomobility, the end feel may be capsular or bony.

- In the spine and rib cage, **anterior spinous challenge, lateral spinous challenge, motion palpation, static palpation of the spine, rib motion** and **rib palpation** reveal areas of hypomobility and minor intervertebral derangement.

- The **sacroiliac joint gapping, sacroiliac joint "squish"** and **Gaenslen's tests** may indicate hypomobility of the sacroiliac joint.

- The **upper limb tension tests, slump test** and **straight leg raise test** are used to assess restrictions to the peripheral nerves *(Hertling, Kessler, 1996)*.

Massage

✋ Heat is used to make the soft tissue crossing the hypomobile joint more flexible.

✋ Joint play techniques are used on the hypomobile joint, with increasing grades of oscillations over subsequent treatments. Mobilization is only performed to the point of pain, never beyond it *(Hertling, Kessler, 1996)*.

Fascial techniques, passive stretching and treatment of trigger points that reduce range of motion, followed by PIR techniques, are also indicated. Frictions, followed by a stretch and ice, may be used to reduce any adhesions.

To mobilize neural tissue that has been restricted by hypomobility, the upper limb tension, slump and straight leg raise tests are repeated as mobilizing techniques *(Hertling, Kessler, 1996)*. The specific test that is positive (for example, upper limb tension test) is then used for mobilizing the peripheral nerve.

See also trigger points, osteoarthritis, inflammatory arthritides, degenerative disc disease, temporomandibular joint dysfunction, all postural dysfunctions, pregnancy, compression syndromes, peripheral nerve lesions, central nervous system conditions, tendinitis, Dupuytren's contracture, frozen shoulder, dislocation, fractures and sprains for related treatments.

Self-care

Heat is applied to the soft tissues surrounding the hypomobile joint.

Passive self-stretches and gravity-induced PIR are used to maintain flexibility. If the client has someone to help out, regular PIR is also useful.

The client is referred to a physician or chiropractor if an undiagnosed pathology is suspected as the underlying cause of the hypomobility.

46

TEMPOROMANDIBULAR JOINT DYSFUNCTION

Fiona Rattray

Temporomandibular joint (TMJ) dysfunction is a disorder of the muscles of mastication, the temporomandibular joints and associated structures.

There are several synonyms for this condition, including temporomandibular disorder, temporomandibular joint pain dysfunction syndrome and temporomandibular joint syndrome. There has been confusion in the terminology surrounding the naming of face and jaw pain. Some authors have argued that the term "TMJ disorder" is misleading, since the masticatory muscles are involved and it is not strictly a *joint* disorder at all *(Hertling, Kessler, 1996)*. Other authors have attempted to differentiate among temporomandibular muscle pain, calling it myalgia and fibromyalgia and joint pain, naming this temporomandibular arthralgia *(Jacobson, Donlon, 1990)*.

Further complicating matters, the terminology used by dentists and physicians to describe the jaw positions used in evaluating proper mandibular motion is not clear. All terminology has not been universally adopted by those investigating TMJ dysfunction *(Hertling, Kessler, 1996)*.

While TMJ disorders may be thought of as a recent phenomenon, a combination of jaw, head and ear pain has been described clinically for centuries. Patients "whose teeth were disposed irregularly, crowding one on another [who experience] headaches" were noted by Hippocrates *(Gelb, 1985)*.

In 1934, Dr. J. Costen described headaches and ear pain in 11 people who were missing molars. His theory was that the height of the posterior teeth helped to maintain proper space at the TMJ; pain resulted from the mandible mechanically compressing the auriculotemporal nerve once the molars were lost. This theory was later disproved and replaced by the concept that a predisposition to TMJ problems, plus dysfunction of the masticatory muscles and articular disc, plus psychosocial factors such as stress, lead to TMJ dysfunction. Tooth loss and malocclusion, or tooth misalignment, likely play a secondary role instead of a primary one *(Cady, Fox, 1995)*.

In the past, TMJ dysfunction was often misdiagnosed and improperly treated, perhaps due to the varying pain locations and other seemingly psychological symptoms such as increased stress and tinnitus. The pendulum seems to have swung in the opposite direction, and TMJ dysfunction may now be overdiagnosed, as it is often diagnosed only on the basis of clicking sounds *(Foreman, Croft, 1995)*. For example, as 35 to 40 per cent of normal adults have clicking sounds in the temporomandibular joint, joint noise can only be used as an indicator of dysfunction if other symptoms such as limited jaw opening and tenderness are present *(Davidoff, 1995)*.

TMJ Anatomy and Function

The two temporomandibular joints are the most superior synovial joints in the body. Motion occurring at the temporomandibular joints has two components, rotation and glide. The inferior portion of the joint — the condyle — allows for rotation, which occurs mostly in the first third of mandibular depression, or opening of the jaw. The superior portion of the joint — the temporal bone — allows for the gliding motion. The articular eminence, a widening of the temporal bone, marks the normal limit of anterior translation of the condyle.

Between the two bones is a meniscus or articular disc, a biconcave structure composed of connective tissue. This biconcave shape allows the disc to centre itself above the condyle. The disc is hypovascular and not pain sensitive *(Figure 46.1)*. Posteriorly, it is attached to retrodiscal connective tissue, which is highly vascularized, well innervated and covered with a synovial membrane. Anteriorly, the disc is attached to the superior portion of the lateral pterygoid muscle. Coordination of movement between the disc and the condyle is maintained by the lateral collateral and capsular ligaments.

When the jaw opens, the muscles that close the jaw — temporalis, masseter and medial pterygoid — must relax to allow the supra- and infrahyoids to depress the mandible. The inferior portion of the lateral pterygoid pulls the condyles forward while the superior portion of the lateral pterygoid pulls the disc anteriorly. Lateral movement is caused by ipsilateral contraction of the temporalis and masseter muscles and by contralateral contraction of the lateral and medial pterygoids and temporalis muscles *(Souza, 1997)*.

One concept that is important to maintaining the health of the muscles of mastication is the rest position of the mandible when the head is upright. The muscles that elevate the jaw must work continuously to overcome the effects of gravity, as

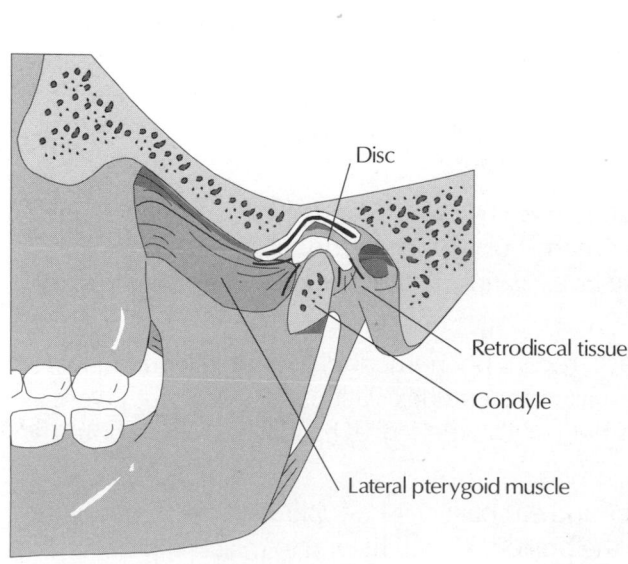

Figure 46.1
The temporomandibular joint.

Disc

Retrodiscal tissue

Condyle

Lateral pterygoid muscle

well as working when a person is chewing, swallowing and talking. In the rest position, the jaw is almost closed and there is a balance in tone between the muscles that open and the muscles that close the mandible. The tongue rests against the roof of the mouth. This creates a slight space between the tooth surfaces, allowing the tone of the jaw elevator muscles to normalize.

The TMJ is part of a musculoskeletal mechanism that not only has to do with jaw movement, but also influences head position. The head is balanced on the spine at C1 by posterior cervical muscles including the suboccipitals. It is counterbalanced by the mandible and the anterior cervical muscles including the supra- and infrahyoids and the other muscles of mastication.

Conversely, the mandible hangs in a ligamentous and muscular sling that is influenced by the position of the head, neck *(Hertling, Kessler, 1996)* and rest of the body. To demonstrate how head position affects these joints, the reader is asked to sit upright, head aligned in the anatomical position. The teeth are gently rubbed together, noting their occlusion, or how they fit together. If the head is tipped even slightly to one side, the occlusion is altered laterally as the mandible moves at the TMJs. If the head is moved into a head-forward position, the mandible is retracted by the pull of the infra- and suprahyoid muscles. If either of these postures is habitual, over time the TMJs will be affected.

Factors Contributing to TMJ Dysfunction

Three components must be present for TMJ dysfunction to occur: **predisposition, tissue alteration** and **stress** *(Gelb, 1985)*. Predisposition can be *intrinsic* — the genetic development of muscles, ligaments and bones — or *extrinsic* — trauma to the neck, face or jaw. Tissue alteration can occur to the skeletal, dental and neuromuscular structures. Malocclusion, tooth loss, cranial bone misalignment, hypermobility, postural dysfunction, spasm, ischemia and trigger points are examples of tissue alteration. Stress results in increased tone of the muscles of mastication due to jaw clenching, bruxism (tooth grinding during sleep) or habits such as gum chewing. Joint noises, such as popping or clicking, may be present with tissue alteration and stress.

However, a person can have one or two of these components without developing TMJ dysfunction. For example, popping or clicking noises are possible in normal joints, perhaps due to separation of the articular surfaces or ligament movements *(Magee, 1992)*. Joint sounds, range of motion changes and malocclusion without pain do not indicate the need for treatment *(Jacobson, Donlon, 1990)*.

A typical pattern of tissue alteration in terms of the position of the disc occurs when the resting position of the mandible is altered by forward-head posture. As the posterior cervical muscles, especially the suboccipitals, contract to hold the head upright in a head-forward posture, the infra- and suprahyoids and omohyoids are stretched. The mandible moves posteriorly, changing the pattern of occlusion and stretching the joint capsule and lateral pterygoid. This can lead to hypertonicity and trigger points in the superior fibres of lateral pterygoid, causing an anterior displacement of the articular disc *(Travell, Simons, 1983; Hertling, Kessler, 1996)*.

Another mechanism of disc displacement is hypertonicity or trigger points in the posterior portion of temporalis, which may pull the condyle posteriorly in relationship to the disc.

With anterior disc displacement, the condyle rests on the thicker posterior portion of the

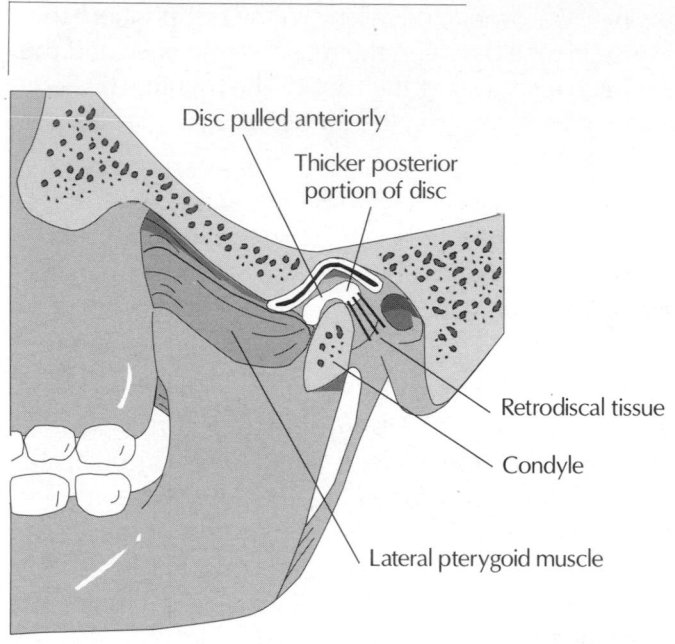

Figure 46.2
Anterior disc displacement.

disc, instead of in its normal position in the thinner middle portion *(Figure 46.2)*. When the condyle moves forward, it must first ride over the posterior disc, causing an initial opening click or pop, before it reaches the middle portion. The disc and condyle then glide forward to allow jaw opening.

Clicking during mid-range of mandibular opening may indicate incoordination of the lateral pterygoid which controls disc motion. The closer to full opening that the pop occurs, the more anterior the displacement of the disc *(Jacobson, Donlon, 1990)*. Clicking near full opening may indicate that the condyle is moving over the anterior portion of the disc *(Hertling, Kessler, 1996)*. If a pop is heard when closing the jaw, the condyle is pulled back into position behind the disc *(Souza, 1997)*. Reciprocal clicking refers to clicking which occurs on both opening and closing the mandible.

An **opening lock** or subluxation occurs when the condyle is anterior to the articular eminence; the condyle is unable to return posteriorly and the jaw cannot close. A **closing lock** occurs when the disc is displaced anteriorly and the condyle cannot reduce over the posterior portion of the disc into the disc depression; the jaw cannot open more than 10 millimetres and often there is premature dental contact on the same side as the disc displacement.

Stretching of the joint capsule can lead to joint hypermobility and **capsulitis**, or inflammation of the joint capsule. This stretching can occur either with direct trauma, such as whiplash, or indirect trauma, such as a prolonged dental procedure.

Over time, with disc displacement, when the jaw is closed the condyle may rest posterior to the disc on the retrodiscal tissue, which is not designed for load bearing. **Synovitis** and joint effusion can occur if the retrodiscal tissue is irritated. Both compression of the retrodiscal tissue and the swelling that follows increase the pressure in the joint and may cause pain. If the disc has degenerated, there is limitation of movement and clicking or popping at the joint *(Souza, 1997)*.

Other factors in TMJ dysfunction are incorrect swallowing patterns, mouth breathing and incorrect respiration. An example of incorrect swallowing patterns is protruding the tongue when drinking from a glass. Mouth breathing prevents the tongue from sitting against the hard palate. This also occurs with prolonged thumb or finger sucking. In a child, pressure from the tongue creates the internal shape of the mouth; loss of this pressure can lead to developmental abnormalities. Mouth breathing facilitates a head-forward posture in both children and adults. Apical breathing alters the relationship of the thorax and cervical spine.

Interestingly, the opening width of the mouth is also restricted by trigger points in muscles that are distant from the joint itself: sternocleidomastoid, trapezius, the scalenes and the pectoral muscles; and by trigger points in leg muscles resulting from a Morton foot structure, where the second metatarsal is longer than the first *(Travell, Simons, 1983)*. The therapist should, therefore, assess the client's entire body when treating TMJ dysfunction, not just the joint itself.

The causes of temporomandibular joint dysfunction are:

➤ **imbalances in the muscles of mastication** resulting from hypertonicity, spasm, trigger points and abnormal joint mechanics;

➤ **muscle overuse** due to habits such as chewing gum, chewing on one side of the mouth only, repetitive, prolonged yawning, and pipe or cigar smoking; or in an occupation or activity where a mouthpiece or mouthguard is required, such as clarinet playing, scuba diving or hockey;

➤ **malocclusion**, including loss of the vertical dimension of the bite (due to tooth loss — for example, molar extraction — or to tooth-surface grinding) which increases the compression on the disc;

➤ **cranial bone misalignment**, especially temporal bone misalignment, which can lead to altered joint mechanics (*Gelb, 1985*);

➤ **postural dysfunction** such as hyperkyphosis and scoliosis which lead to neck and shoulder muscle imbalances and, therefore, increased activity in the jaw muscles to counterbalance the head position (*Gelb, 1985*). Lateral pelvic tilt due to leg length discrepancy or a small hemipelvis (*Travell, Simons, 1983*), and foot and ankle problems which alter gait, such as pes planus and ankle sprain, also affect head position (*Milne et al., 1997*). A difference of one centimetre in leg length has been documented as producing altered occlusion, thereby altering the resting position of the mandible (*Gelb, 1985*);

➤ **increased stress** leading to jaw clenching ("holding back" words by gritting the teeth) and bruxism (tooth grinding during sleep). This can include apical breathing which also leads to neck and shoulder muscle imbalances;

➤ **trauma**, either direct or indirect; direct trauma includes a blow to the jaw, the hyperextension phase of whiplash when the mandible opens forcefully, mandibular fracture and surgery; indirect trauma can result from prolonged dental work when the mouth is held open for long periods of time, from intubation during general anesthesia, from prolonged cervical traction or from supporting the head under the chin by the cupped hand when sitting;

➤ **sinus blockage or infection** can lead to mouth breathing, forward-head posture to open the airway and abnormal jaw position (*Gelb, 1985*);

➤ **joint pathology,** such as hypermobility (*Beighton et al., 1989*), capsulitis or synovitis which leads to joint contractures, osteoarthritis and rheumatoid arthritis.

Locating the Muscles of Mastication

The muscles of mastication can be palpated both externally and intra-orally. Palpation inside the mouth requires the use of vinyl or latex gloves. Because the therapist cannot see the structures being palpated, it is suggested that she practise landmarking and palpation first on a model skull, then with a gloved hand inside her own mouth, in order to make intra-oral palpation accurate. Active resisted isometric contraction of the specific muscle is extremely important in aiding correct muscle location, especially with lateral and medial pterygoids. Once the therapist is confident with intra-oral landmarking, she can progress to actual treatment.

Temporalis

Temporalis runs from the temporal fossa to the coronoid process of the mandible *(Figure 46.3)*. It **elevates** the mandible (closes the jaw). The posterior fibres acting bilaterally retract the jaw and, acting unilaterally, they move the mandible to the same side. To palpate this muscle, the therapist asks the client to gently clench the jaw.

Masseter

This muscle has a superficial and a deep layer, running from the zygomatic arch to the angle of the mandible. It acts to **elevate** the mandible; the deep fibres also retract the mandible. To palpate this muscle *externally,* the therapist asks the client to gently clench the jaw to isolate the muscle while the therapist palpates inferior to the zygomatic arch. To palpate the muscle *intra-orally,* the therapist places her gloved finger into the client's open mouth between the cheek and the molars; the client slowly elevates the mandible so the teeth meet — not on the therapist's finger (!) — and gently clenches the jaw; the muscle is clearly palpated between the finger inside and the thumb outside the cheek.

Medial Pterygoid

Medial pterygoid runs from the lateral pterygoid plate of the sphenoid bone to the inner aspect of the angle of the mandible *(Figure 46.4)*. Bilaterally, both medial pterygoids **elevate** the mandible; unilaterally, one muscle moves the mandible to the opposite side.

To palpate this muscle *externally,* the therapist first slightly sidebends the client's head to the side being palpated, creating slack in the skin covering the angle of the mandible. The therapist palpates along the inner surface of the mandible at the angle while the client is asked to gently clench the jaw to isolate the muscle.

Intra-orally, the therapist's gloved finger is first placed on the last lower molar, then slid around to the medial surface of the molar and inferiorly past the gum towards the floor of the mouth.

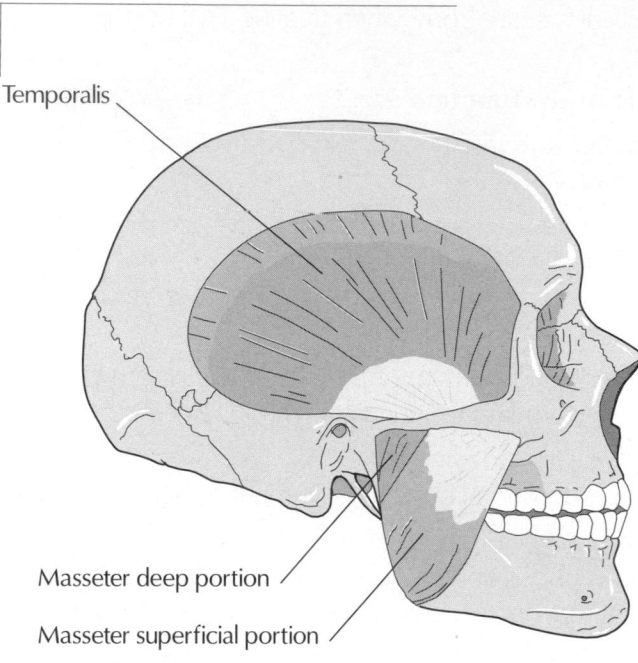

Figure 46.3
Temporalis and masseter muscles.

Temporalis

Masseter deep portion

Masseter superficial portion

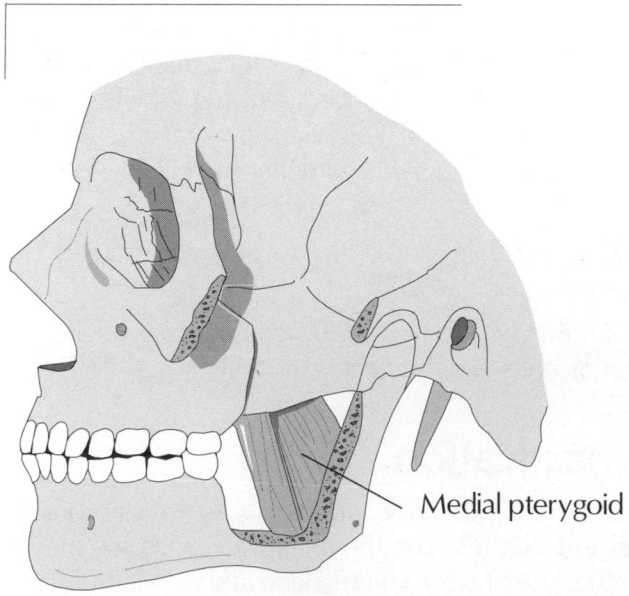

Figure 46.4
The medial pterygoid (zygomatic arch and portion of mandible removed to show the location of the muscle).

Medial pterygoid

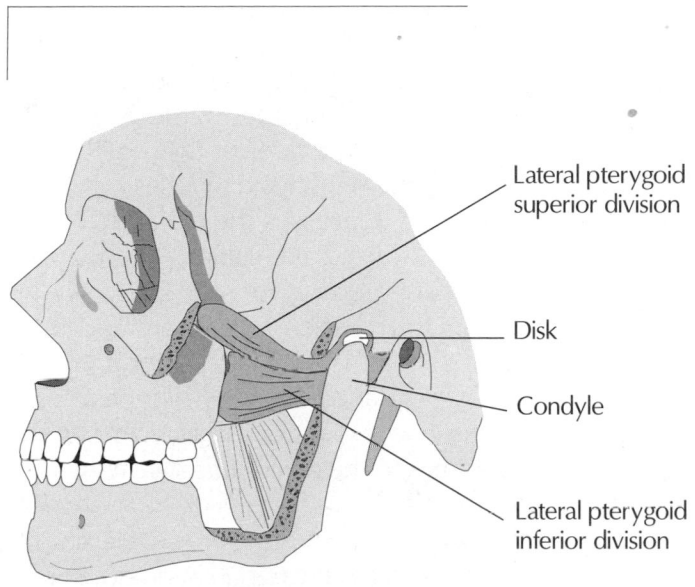

Figure 46.5
The lateral pterygoid (zygomatic arch and portion of mandible removed to show the location of the muscle).

Keeping the pad of the finger against the inner surface of the mandible, the finger is then slid posteriorly to medial pterygoid. To have this muscle isometrically contract, the therapist first hooks two fingers of the non-palpating hand over the lower front teeth. This prevents the client from biting down on the palpating finger. The client is then asked to *gently* attempt to close the jaw.

Lateral Pterygoid

Lateral pterygoid has superior and inferior portions *(Figure 46.5)*. The superior portion runs from the sphenoid bone posteriorly to the temporomandibular joint capsule and articular disc. It acts to pull the disc anteriorly when the mandible opens and to check-rein the disc as the mandible closes. The inferior portion runs from the lateral pterygoid plate to the neck of the mandible, acting to **depress** (or open the jaw) and protrude the mandible bilaterally and to pull the jaw to the opposite side when acting unilaterally.

To palpate this muscle *externally,* the therapist asks the client first to open the jaw two centimetres to move the ramus of the mandible out of the way. Lateral pterygoid is palpated about two centimeters anterior to the external auditory meatus, inferior to the zygomatic arch and through the mandibular notch. The muscle is palpated through masseter muscle. To isolate lateral pterygoid, the therapist asks the client to gently resist depression of the mandible.

Intra-orally, the therapist's gloved finger is placed between the cheek and the teeth, with the fingernail against the last upper molars. The client may need to open the jaw and move it to the side being palpated to allow the next movement. The finger is slid superiorly and posteriorly between the maxilla and the coronoid process of the mandible, into the hollow at the roof of the cheek pouch. Lateral pterygoid is isolated once again by resisting mandibular depression.

Digastric

The digastric muscle has two bellies. The posterior belly of digastric attaches to the mastoid notch and to a common tendon that threads through a loop attaching to the hyoid bone *(Figure 46.6)*. It then continues as the anterior belly, which attaches to the inside of the mandible at the symphysis. Bilaterally, digastric **depresses** and retracts the mandible; unilaterally, it moves the mandible to the same side *(Travell, Simons, 1983)*.

To palpate this muscle, the therapist asks the client to open the jaw gently against resistance. The posterior belly is located between the angle of the mandible and the mastoid process, while the anterior belly is close to midline between the hyoid and the mandible.

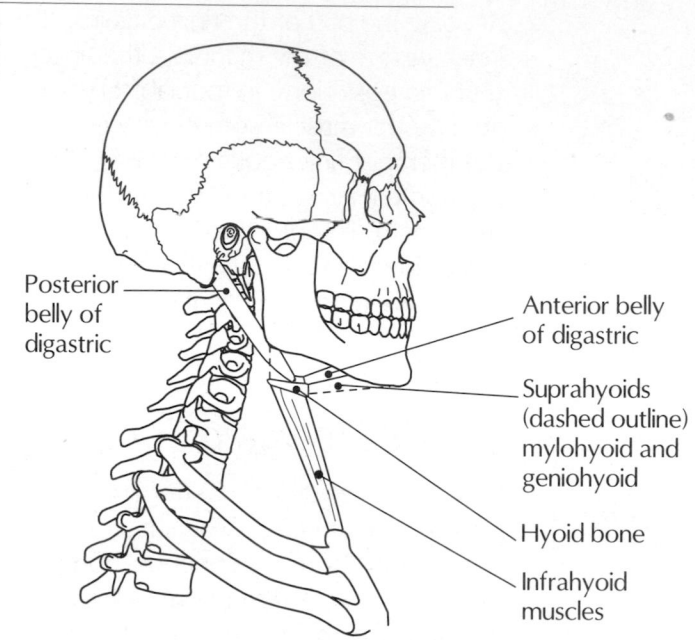

Figure 46.6
Digastric, supra- and infrahyoid muscles with the hyoid bone.

Posterior belly of digastric

Anterior belly of digastric

Suprahyoids (dashed outline) mylohyoid and geniohyoid

Hyoid bone

Infrahyoid muscles

Mylohyoid

Mylohyoid attaches to the inside of the entire mandible and runs to the hyoid bone. It forms the floor of the mouth and is one of the suprahyoid muscles. Mylohyoid **depresses** the mandible when the hyoid is fixed and tightens the floor of the mouth (*Hertling, Kessler, 1996*). To palpate this muscle, the therapist asks the client to depress the mandible gently against resistance. *Externally,* it is palpated on the inner aspect of the mandible, from the ramus to the angle. *Intra-orally,* the therapist's gloved finger is placed between the lower teeth and the tongue. Starting at the incisors, the finger pad is slid down the inner surface of the mandible to the floor of the mouth. Palpation continues posteriorly as far as the last molar, where mylohyoid ends.

Geniohyoid

This muscle runs from the inferior mental spine of the mandible to the hyoid bone. Geniohyoid is one of the suprahyoid muscles and **depresses** the mandible. It lies on top of mylohyoid and supports the root of the tongue. The anterior portion of geniohyoid is palpated in conjunction with mylohyoid.

Infrahyoids

Infrahyoid muscles also **depress** the mandible. To locate these muscles accurately, the therapist uses the hyoid bone as an initial reference. The infrahyoid muscles run inferior from the hyoid to the sternum, just anterior to the trachea, while the suprahyoids run superior from the hyoid to the mandible. Gentle resisted depression of the mandible makes these muscles palpable. See Whiplash for more details.

The Medical Treatment of TMJ Dysfunction

In the past, the surgical approach to TMJ problems has included disc repositioning via arthroscopy, discectomy (both with and without disc replacement by teflon implant) and total joint replacement. Disc replacement has been a controversial procedure and osteoarthritis development is common with discectomy (*Souza, 1997*).

Today, the medical strategy to TMJ dysfunction has shifted to a more conservative chronic pain management approach including medication, dental splints, physical therapy and behavioural therapy such as stress management. Surgery is considered if these other methods have not succeeded (*Cady, Fox, 1995*).

Medication may include NSAIDs to reduce pain and inflammation, and muscle relaxants to reduce the spasm.

A bite plate or interocclusal splint may be recommended to reduce pain and muscle hypertonicity and to reposition the disc. A soft splint is used for protection if bruxism is present, reducing the stress placed on the TMJ. A hard splint repositions or stabilizes the mandible. The splint is worn for six weeks to three months; if the symptoms subside, the splint may be used at night only. In one study, stabilization had a success rate of 55 per cent while of those who opted for no splint use, 42 per cent had a resolution of disc displacement *(Souza, 1997)*.

It had been thought that a "TMJ personality" existed; however, no such psychosocial personality type has been proven *(Cady, Fox, 1995)*.

Symptom Picture

+ TMJ dysfunction may be unilateral or bilateral.

+ Symptoms of TMJ dysfunction are most common in people between 15 and 45 years of age, and more common in women by a ratio of 5:1 *(Cady, Fox, 1995)*.

+ The triad of **predisposition, tissue alteration** (neuromuscular, skeletal and dental) and **stress** sufficient to cause jaw clenching or bruxism is necessary to provoke TMJ dysfunction.

+ Postural dysfunctions such as head-forward posture may be present.

+ Other pathologies such as fibromyalgia, osteoarthritis and rheumatoid arthritis may also be present.

+ In the **early stage**, there is muscular incoordination and subluxation.

  • Temporomandibular joint sounds (clicking, popping) occur with jaw movement.

  • Jaw pain is precipitated by movement or jaw clenching. Pain is often worse in the morning. Tenderness is noted in the muscles of mastication and the joint capsule.

  • A headache may be present, often frontal or temporal.

  • Spasm occurs in the muscles of mastication.

  • Hypertonicity and trigger points are present in the muscles of mastication and the muscles of the shoulders and neck.

  • There is decreased range of motion, especially opening of the jaw; the mandible has irregular opening or closing motions; the mandible may catch or lock on opening or closing.

  • Ear stuffiness, blockage and hearing loss may result from trigger points and hypertonicity in medial pterygoid; taut bands in this muscle may restrict opening of the eustachian tube by the tensor velli palatini muscle *(Travell, Simons, 1983)*.

  • Trauma, either direct or indirect, may produce inflammation, edema, adhesions, capsulitis or synovitis. Capsulitis pain and tenderness are located at the joint. They are worse with lateral movement or on opening widely. Synovitis pain is worse on the ipsilateral side with full closure.

- Occasional symptoms include tinnitus, nausea, lacrimation, sensitive teeth and paresthesia which may be due to trigger points.
  ✦ In the **later stage**, if not corrected, the muscles of mastication may develop contractures, limiting range of motion.
  - Degeneration of the disc, condylar head and articular eminence may occur *(Jacobson, Donlon, 1990)*.

Subjective Information

HEALTH HISTORY QUESTIONS

✦ What is the client's overall health history? Are there any contributing or underlying pathologies such as osteoarthritis or rheumatoid arthritis? For example, women with TMJ dysfunction may be more disposed to hypothyroidism, since this condition can contribute to the trigger points present with TMJ *(Gelb, 1985)*.

✦ Is there a history of direct head or face trauma, such as whiplash or impact to the jaw?

✦ When was the onset of the current symptoms?

✦ What is the location and type of pain, such as jaw, face, neck or shoulder pain?

✦ Does the client have any pain on jaw opening or closing or chewing? Pain experienced on full opening may indicate an extra-articular problem such as capsulitis or trigger points in lateral pterygoid. Pain experienced on biting or clenching may be intra-articular or due to trigger points in masseter, medial pterygoid or temporalis.

✦ Is pain worse with jaw protrusion or lateral deviation of the jaw? This may indicate lateral pterygoid involvement.

✦ Are there any noises on jaw opening or closing, such as clicking, popping, grinding or grating?

✦ Is there reduced range of motion with jaw opening or closing?

✦ Has the jaw ever locked? Locking in an open position indicates anterior subluxation of the condyle, while locking in a closed position is likely due to the disc being displaced anteriorly *(Foreman, Croft, 1995)*.

✦ Does the client have a history of headaches? What are their type, location and frequency?

✦ Is the client under increasing or high levels of stress at home or work?

✦ Is the client a mouth breather?

✦ Does the client smoke, chew gum, yawn repeatedly, grind or clench the teeth, chew the nails or have any habits that overuse the TMJ and muscles of mastication? Does the client have fatigue with chewing?

✦ Does the client habitually compress the TMJ — for example, when sitting, by resting the chin on one hand?

✦ Are there any other symptoms such as ringing in the ears, changes in hearing, dizziness or swelling around the TMJ?

- ✦ Are there signs of inflammation? This may indicate an ear or throat infection or mumps.
- ✦ What is the client's dental history? Has the client had any prolonged dental work or tooth extractions, or worn braces? Painful, sensitive or missing teeth can lead to improper chewing patterns.
- ✦ Is there sensitivity to hot, cold or sweet foods which may indicate dental caries or abscess?
- ✦ What relieves the pain or other symptoms?
- ✦ Has the client seen any other health care practitioner for this condition, such as a dentist, physiotherapist or chiropractor? What treatment was given? Is the client still receiving this treatment?
- ✦ Is the client using a bite plate or dental splint?
- ✦ Is the client taking any medication for the condition, such as analgesics, muscle relaxants or anti-inflammatories? This includes self-medication such as Aspirin or other over-the-counter products.

Objective Information

Observations

Postural Assessment

- ✍ A full postural assessment is performed. Scoliosis, hyperkyphosis, hyperlordosis or pes planus may be present; see the appropriate chapter for details. The following upper body observations may be present.
- ✍ In an **anterior view,** the shoulders may be elevated or one may be higher than the other. The symmetry of the face is assessed, observing levels of both external auditory meatus, frontal ridges, zygomatic arches, angles of the mandible and alignment of the jaw and teeth.
- ✍ In a **lateral view**, a habituated antalgic head-forward posture may be observed, with an accompanying increase in the cervical lordotic curve. Assessment for mandibular protraction or retraction is performed.
- ✍ With a head-forward posture, the sternocleidomastoid muscle assumes a more vertical orientation. In a normal posture, this muscle angles posteriorly from the inferior to superior attachments.
- ✍ The scapula may be protracted.
- ✍ In a **posterior view**, the level of the occiput is observed for lateral tilting.
- ✍ The person may have a pained or medicated facial expression.
- ✍ The masseter or temporalis muscles may be obviously clenched. There may be ridging on the inside of the cheek (buccal mucosa) and lateral tongue scalloping due to jaw clenching.

Palpation

✍ Tenderness is present in the muscles of mastication. Tenderness is also present either anterior to the TMJ itself or inside the external auditory meatus on the anterior aspect.

✍ With inflammation, there is an increase in temperature over the affected TMJ. Edema may be palpable.

✍ The affected muscles may be fibrosed. There is popping, clicking or crepitus palpable in the affected joint with movement. A click on initial opening may indicate an anterior disc displacement, with the condyle moving over the posterior portion of the disc. Clicking during mid-range of mandibular opening may indicate incoordination of lateral pterygoid, while clicking near the end of opening may indicate that the condyle is moving over the anterior portion of the disc *(Hertling, Kessler, 1996)*.

✍ There are hypertonicity and trigger points in the muscles of mastication and also in the muscles of the neck and thorax, including upper trapezius, suboccipitals, scalenes, erector spinae and intercostals.

Testing

✍ Since mandibular motion and restriction of motion is complex, some detail is given below.

✍ **AF ROM** of the mandible on the cardinal planes is reduced due to pain. Depression, elevation, lateral deviation, protraction and retraction are all assessed. Range of motion of the mandible *(Figure 46.7)* is recorded on a special section of the client's health history chart *(Foreman, Croft, 1995)*.

• Assessment is made to see if condylar movement is symmetrical; one condyle may move before the other.

• A ruler may be used to record mandibular depression: normal range measured from maxillary to mandibular incisor edge is between 35 to 50 millimetres *(Magee, 1992)*.

• Normal lateral motion to each side is eight to 10 millimetres using the midline of the maxillary and mandibular incisors. Restriction of 50 per cent or more may be due to capsular restriction on the contralateral side. For example, only four millimetres of movement to the left may indicate right capsular restriction *(Hertling, Kessler, 1996)*.

• Mandibular protrusion is five millimetres, measured from the position where both maxillary and mandibular incisors are opposed; normal retrusion is three to four millimetres, measured from the same position of opposed incisors *(Hertling, Kessler, 1996)*.

✍ The **temporomandibular joint AF ROM test** is performed. A **positive** test reveals either a C-wobble, indicating a capsular source on the side the jaw deviates towards, or an S-wobble, indicating a muscular source such as trigger points.

• Reduced mandibular depression may be due to bilateral trigger points in masseter.

• Lateral mandibular deviation may be due to trigger points in masseter, temporalis and posterior digastric on the side the mandible deviates *towards*. Masseter trigger points pull with full opening; temporalis trigger points pull on opening or closing; posterior digastric trigger points pull the mandible over on initial jaw opening only.

• Lateral deviation may also result from trigger points in lateral pterygoid on the side it moves *away from*. This is confirmed by having the client place the tip of the tongue

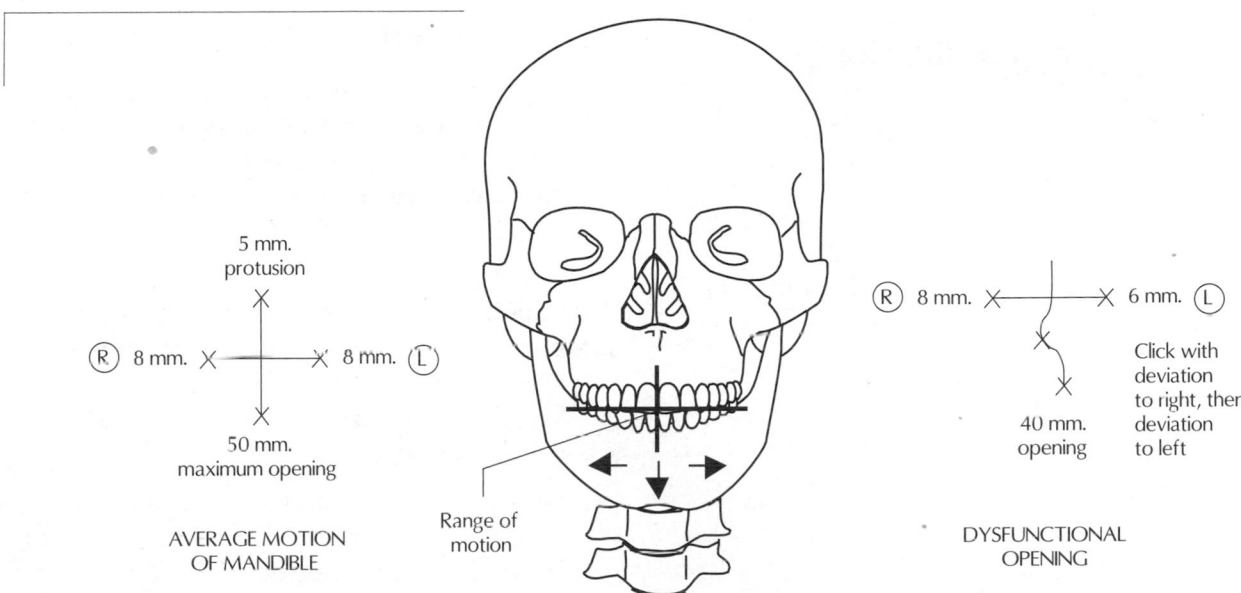

5 mm.
protusion

(R) 8 mm. ——— 8 mm. (L)

50 mm.
maximum opening

AVERAGE MOTION
OF MANDIBLE

Range of
motion

(R) 8 mm. ——— 6 mm. (L)

40 mm.
opening

Click with
deviation
to right, then
deviation
to left

DYSFUNCTIONAL
OPENING

Figure 46.7
Range of motion measured from the starting position with the jaw closed, noting alignment of the teeth; then the jaw is moved into maximum depression, left and right lateral motion and protrusion.

on the hard palate as far back as possible while opening the mouth. If lateral motion stops, trigger points are responsible *(Travell, Simons, 1983)*.

✍ **AF ROM** of the cervical spine on the cardinal planes may also be reduced.

✍ **PR ROM** of the mandible is performed on the cardinal planes of motion, with the range that stretches the affected muscles tested **last**. A painful, muscle-spasm end feel is present with muscular involvement; clicking and springy block end feel are present with disc derangement; a capsular restriction is present with joint hypomobility or capsulitis; and, on initial opening, a large anterior glide (instead of initial rotation) is present with hypermobility *(Hertling, Kessler, 1996)*. Closed lock end feel is soft.

✍ **PR ROM** of the cervical spine may also be reduced.

✍ **AR isometric testing** of the mandible is performed. With resisted depression, weakness or pain may be due to lateral pterygoid or supra- or infrahyoid muscles; with resisted lateral motion, weakness is due to lateral or medial pterygoid on the opposite side; with resisted protrusion, weakness is due to lateral or medial pterygoids.

Special Tests

✍ A **three-knuckle test** is positive with trigger points in the muscles that elevate the jaw *(Travell, Simons, 1983)*.

✍ **Passive relaxed atlanto-occipital** and **atlanto-axial articulation tests** may be restricted with a capsular pattern. **Passive relaxed anterior** and **lateral spinous challenges** may be hyper- or hypomobile in the cervical spine.

Contraindications

+ Do not compress over the carotid artery or carotid sinuses when treating the anterior neck muscles.

+ Do not use massage techniques on both sternocleidomastoid muscles at the same time, as the carotid arteries may be compressed. Also, the client may feel choked. Similarly, avoid bilateral treatment of infra- and suprahyoid muscles.

+ Avoid deep work over the styloid process of the temporal bone, as it is a potentially fragile structure.

+ Frictions are contraindicated if the client is taking anti-inflammatories or blood thinners.

+ Do not use techniques that compress the mandible superiorly against the TMJ.

+ Do not use latex gloves for intra-oral work if the client has a latex allergy.

+ Avoid using heavy or deep pressures when working intra-orally, as the muscles are delicate and often tender.

+ TMJ dysfunction may be a result of a history of abuse, which the client may or may not disclose. The therapist should be mindful of this possibility, especially if working intra-orally, and respect any limits the client may have.

Differential Assessment

✍ **Tension headache** pain may be bilateral and vise-like, often worse in the afternoon. The pain is located in the referral pattern of affected shoulder and neck muscles. These muscles are stiff and achy.

✍ **Migraine** pain is usually unilateral and throbbing. There are associated symptoms such as nausea, vomiting, cold extremities and achiness of the shoulder and neck muscles. Visual disturbances such as flashes of light may be reported.

✍ **Sinusitis** pain is located over the affected sinus: frontal or maxillary. There is a feeling of congestion in the affected sinus. The person may have a low-grade fever and feel generally debilitated.

✍ **Trigeminal neuralgia** pain is sudden, paroxysmal, "lightening like" and often throbbing. It is located along the distribution of the affected nerve. A "trigger zone" in the skin supplied by the nerve causes an attack when stimulated. Movement of the affected area also increases pain.

✍ **Toothache** pain is local to the affected tooth and its root; the tooth is often sensitive to hot, cold or sweet foods.

✍ **Fibromyalgia** pain is diffuse and achy. There are characteristic tender points in muscles throughout the body. Other symptoms include sleep disturbances, headaches and debilitating fatigue.

Treatment Goals

Treatment Plan

☝ Massage therapy, especially relaxation, trigger point therapy and focused work on the muscles of mastication, is effective for treating TMJ disorders *(Cady, Fox, 1995; Kisner, Colby, 1996)*.

☝ **Positioning** is chosen for comfort and for access to the structures that are treated. Prone, sidelying or supine are all indicated. In the prone position, a face cradle may be used for comfort and to prevent compression on the TMJ.

☝ **Hydrotherapy** is heat to the affected muscles in the shoulder girdle, neck and jaw. If inflammation is present, cold such as a gel pack is applied to the affected joint instead.

General Treatment

Reduce pain. Decrease sympathetic nervous system firing.

☝ If the initial goal is to accustom the client to the therapist's touch and to decrease the sympathetic nervous system firing in the context of a relaxation massage, the treatment begins, in the prone position, on the trunk and shoulder girdle. The client is directed to do **diaphragmatic breathing** throughout the treatment. Relaxation is a key component of the treatment *(Gelb, 1985)*.

Treat any compensating structures. Maintain local circulation.

☝ The trunk and shoulder girdle are treated to reduce hypertonicity as well as to increase drainage and venous return to the affected tissues. Rhythmic techniques, effleurage and slow petrissage such as palmar kneading, fingertip kneading and C-scooping are used.

Specific Treatment

☝ Specific work is performed in the supine position. Initially the therapist is seated.

Reduce inflammation and edema if present.

☝ Assuming that the initial treatment goal is to reduce the edema, lymphatic drainage techniques are used, beginning with nodal pumping at the terminus (just superior to the clavicle, immediately lateral to the sternocleidomastoid muscle), then at the proximal lymph nodes in the neck and axilla. Nodes are found in chains anterior and posterior to sternocleidomastoid, below the angle of the mandible and at the occiput. Unidirectional effleurage, stationary circles and the local technique are used proximal to the affected joint to reduce edema and prevent adhesion formation. For specific lymphatic drainage patterns of the neck and trunk, see the chapter on edema.

Reduce fascial restrictions if present. Stretch short muscles.

☝ Fascial glide is used to assess, then fascial techniques are used to treat, the restrictions around the neck and jaw. Techniques include skin rolling, crossed-hands and fingertip spreading and the connective tissue cutting technique over the pectoral muscles.

Treatment Goals

Treatment Plan

Reduce hypertonicity and trigger points.

🖐 Passive stretches are used on the tight postural muscles such as pectoralis major.

🖐 Effleurage and petrissage are used on the muscles of the shoulder girdle and neck to reduce hypertonicity.

🖐 Posteriorly, these muscles include upper trapezius, levator scapulae, splenius cervicis and capitis, semispinalis capitis, the suboccipitals, cervical multifidi and rotatores.

🖐 Anteriolaterally, the scalenes are also treated. See the chapter on thoracic outlet syndrome for details of scalene palpation and treatment.

🖐 Anteriorly, pectoralis major, pectoralis minor and subclavius are treated, especially with clients who have a head-forward posture. There is an additional focus on muscles of respiration, including intercostals, in clients who are apical breathers.

🖐 Sternocleidomastoid muscles are treated unilaterally to avoid giving the client a feeling of being choked and reducing circulation to the head. Direct compression over the deep carotid artery, located in the carotid triangle, is avoided *(Pansky, 1979)*. The area is bordered posteriorly by the upper half of sternocleidomastoid, superiorly by the posterior digastric muscle and anteriorly by the omohyoid muscle. The therapist should also work around the external jugular vein which runs over sternocleidomastoid *(Travell, Simons, 1983)*. Pincer grasp and origin and insertion techniques can be used. See the chapter on whiplash for details of palpation, trigger point referral and treatment of sternocleidomastoid.

Mobilize hypomobile joints.

🖐 Joint play techniques are indicated for hypomobile cervical vertebrae and other joints in the thorax and shoulder.

Reduce hypertonicity and trigger points. Reduce spasm if present.

🖐 The muscles of mastication are now treated from outside the mouth. Palpation and specific location of these muscles using active resisted contraction are listed earlier in this chapter. Temporalis, masseter, lateral pterygoid and medial pterygoid are treated with fingertip kneading, muscle stripping and ischemic compressions according to the client's pain tolerance. Gentle fascial spreading can also be used on temporalis and masseter.

🖐 When temporalis and masseter are massaged, the direction of strokes is from superior to inferior to avoid compressing the mandible. The origin and insertion technique is used on temporalis attachments to the frontal and parietal bones, and also on the zygomatic and mandibular attachments of masseter.

🖐 Trigger points in temporalis refer to the upper teeth and temporal regions. The client is asked to partially depress the mandible to make taut bands in this muscle more palpable.

Treatment Goals

**Reduce hypertonicity.
Treat trigger points.**

Treatment Plan

- Masseter trigger points refer into the TMJ, the mandible, and the molars and above the eye. They also produce tinnitus in the affected ear. Lateral pterygoid refers to the TMJ and the zygoma; tinnitus is also produced. Medial pterygoid refers to the TMJ and into the back of the mouth and pharynx (*Travell, Simons, 1983*).

- Next, the infra- and suprahyoids including omohyoid are treated. Specific client consent is recommended to treat these muscles which run over the front of the throat. The therapist stands at the client's shoulder, facing the client so the client's comfort levels are constantly monitored during palpation and treatment. After the hyoid bone is located as a reference, cross-fibre strokes are used on the infrahyoid muscles, moving from *lateral to medial,* systematically along the muscles. The therapist's thumb (or finger) gently stabilizes the lateral trachea on the side not being treated. The therapist avoids the carotid triangle. Gentle ischemic compression is used to treat trigger points. Infrahyoid muscles are treated unilaterally to prevent the client from feeling choked. Clinically, infrahyoid muscles seem to refer into the throat. See the chapter on whiplash for more details on palpation and treatment.

- The suprahyoids, including mylohyoid and anterior and posterior digastric muscles, are treated next. They are also treated using a stabilizing thumb (or finger) on one side, while short cross-fibre strokes are used to locate trigger points in the other side of the muscle. Specific palpation of these muscles is described earlier in this chapter. Clinically, mylohyoid trigger points seem to refer into the tongue and throat. Anterior digastric refers to the lower incisors, while posterior digastric refers below the ear (*Travell, Simons, 1983*). Care should be taken when treating the posterior digastric muscle, as the styloid process of the temporal bone lies superior to the muscle belly.

- Masseter, lateral pterygoid, mylohyoid and medial pterygoid can also be treated intra-orally. Specific consent is required to work inside the mouth. A signal should be arranged so treatment can be stopped if necessary, as the client will be unable to clearly communicate when the therapist is working intra-orally. For example, the client raising one hand is an indication for the therapist to stop and remove the treating hand from the client's mouth.

- Vinyl or latex gloves must be worn by the therapist for intra-oral work. After putting the gloves on, the therapist should wash the powder from the outside of the gloves and rinse the gloves thoroughly to remove any soap before treating. Due to the increase of allergies to latex, it is suggested that vinyl gloves be used instead; if latex gloves are used, the therapist must check beforehand that the client is not allergic.

Treatment Goals

Treatment Plan

🖐 Palpation and isometric active resisted contractions to accurately locate muscles inside the mouth are listed earlier in this chapter. It is suggested that the order of treatment be masseter and lateral pterygoid, then mylohyoid and medial pterygoid; usually, work to masseter is most easily tolerated and work to medial pterygoid is least easily tolerated by the client. Pressures used need not be heavy as these muscles are not generally worked on and they respond well to treatment. Often they are quite tender. The origin and insertion technique, gentle muscle stripping, cross-fibre work and ischemic compressions to the client's pain tolerance are indicated. If a barrier to massage pressure is noted, the therapist should allow the tissue to release, not push past the barrier. One finger is used to treat; the index finger is perhaps best, although therapists with larger hands may find the little finger is more appropriate.

Reduce any adhesions.

🖐 Muscle stripping in short strokes is used to reduce adhesions intra- and extra-orally.

Restore proprioception to affected muscles.
Maintain range of motion.

🖐 Pain-free **active free range of motion** is used to normalize proprioception. Between treatment of each muscle, the therapist takes the treating finger out of the client's mouth and allows the client to gently open and close the mandible a few times, normalizing proprioception at the TMJ.

Mobilize hypomobile joints.

🖐 Joint play techniques may be used for hypomobile temporomandibular joints.

Reduce hypertonicity and trigger points.

🖐 Once the work inside the mouth is completed, the therapist removes the gloves and sits down again. Suboccipital hypertonicity is reduced with Golgi tendon organ release. Specific passive stretching for short suboccipitals in the prone position is achieved by the therapist first stabilizing the spinous process of C2 with the index and middle finger of one hand (Kisner, Colby, 1990). The fingertips of the other hand grasp the occiput and slowly traction the occiput into flexion.

🖐 Long-axis traction of the cervical spine is also indicated.

🖐 Inferior traction of the mandible is perfomed by the therapist contacting the angle of the mandible with the fingertips. A light, steady traction is applied in an inferior direction. This is not rotation of the mandible, as in the initial opening motions the mandible usually makes; rather it is a motion towards the client's feet. The client should feel that the TMJ is "opening up". The traction is released gently.

Restore range of motion.

🖐 **Passive relaxed range of motion** is used on the cervical spine.

Stretch shortened structures.

🖐 PIR for a tight digastric muscle is performed by the therapist placing one hand under the mandible; the thumb of the other hand is on the lateral aspect of the client's hyoid bone on the tight side. The client submaximally isometrically resists jaw depression for up to 10 seconds, then exhales and relaxes completely; the therapist moves

Treatment Goals	Treatment Plan

the hyoid medially *(Hertling, Kessler, 1996).*

✋ The treatment is finished with effleurage to the neck and shoulders and a scalp massage.

Treat other conditions.

✋ Any other conditions, including hyperkyphosis or scoliosis, are also treated.

Self-care Goals	Self-care Plan

✍ **Self-massage**, both extra- and intra-oral, to the affected muscles, is very effective. Muscle stripping and gentle ischemic compressions are indicated. The therapist must educate the client regarding the muscle locations and gentleness of the pressure used.

✍ **Hydrotherapy** is applied as appropriate. Heat is used to reduce hypertonicity and cold is applied with inflammation.

Stretch short structures.

✍ Masseter is most effectively stretched when the client is supine. The client hooks two fingers behind the lower incisors and pulls the mandible anteriorly and inferiorly *(Travell, Simons, 1983).*

✍ The client can also perform PIR for tight digastric muscles, described in the treatment section.

✍ Mandibular self-distraction is performed by the client placing the heel of each hand on each side of the jaw, at the angle of the mandible. Gentle traction is applied in an inferior direction, taking care that *distraction,* not rotation, occurs.

✍ Gentle hinge-like motions, where the client opens the mouth only slightly, are indicated. The client places the fingers of both hands over the condyles while doing this, to be sure that only rotation and not glide is occurring at the TMJ. As pain diminishes, this can be progressed to yawning, which is helpful as both a stretch and as an inhibitor of the muscles that elevate the mandible.

✍ The suboccipitals are stretched with the client in a seated position. This stretch also distracts the occiput, C1 and C2 from each other. The client places the hands behind the neck, with the fingers interlaced. The palms rest against the neck, stabilizing the cervical spine from C3 to C7. The client then *flexes the head* 15 degrees on the cervical spine five or six times. It is important that the client understand that this is a movement of the head only, not the cervical spine *(Gelb, 1985).*

✍ Any postural imbalances, such as hyperkyphosis or head-forward posture, should be corrected. See the appropriate postural chapters for details.

Self-care Goals

Self-care Plan

Educate the client regarding activities.

✍ Relaxation exercises are important for the client, such as practising diaphragmatic breathing. Diaphragmatic breathing also helps to restore proper biomechanics of the cervical spine.

✍ The client avoids activities that stress the TMJ, including compressing the mandible superiorly while leaning the chin on the cupped hand and oral habits such as chewing gum.

✍ The client should understand and practise the resting position of the mandible to reduce muscular strain. The client's lips are closed and the teeth are slightly apart. The tongue rests on the hard palate just behind the front incisors and the client breathes through the nose, not the mouth (*Kisner, Colby, 1996*).

✍ To restore correct motion at the TMJ, the client retracts the mandible, then places the tongue on the roof of the mouth as far back as possible while opening the mouth; this prevents gliding from occurring first. The client can also palpate the condyles bilaterally to be sure that rotation occurs before glide.

✍ If the jaw deviates to one side when opening, the client can look in a mirror while opening and closing the jaw, and practise moving the jaw to the opposite side.

✍ A routine exercise program is important to reduce overall stress and to stretch the affected postural muscles.

✍ During dental procedures, the client should take breaks to open and close the mouth.

Strengthen weak muscles.

✍ Isometric active resisted exercises are used for specific muscles; for example, resisting jaw depression to strengthen lateral pterygoid.

Refer the client.

✍ The client may need to be referred to a dentist, osteopath, chiropractor, physician (ear, nose and throat specialist) or craniosacral therapist.

✍ Relaxation therapy such as biofeedback may also be indicated.

✍ Movement therapy, such as the Mitzvah, Feldenkrais or Alexander technique, may be helpful for retraining the client's posture.

Treatment Frequency and Expected Outcome

See also stress reduction, edema, trigger points, whiplash, tension headache, migraine, torticollis, fibromyalgia, understanding peripheral nerve lesions and all postural dysfunctions for related treatments.

Treatment frequency is two times a week for two weeks, followed by reassessment, then once a week for several months (*Souza, 1997*).

The prognosis is good if the client has had the condition for a short period of time (*Foreman, Croft, 1995*). Client education is essential, because often the client aggravates the condition by clenching the jaw in response to stress.

47

DEGENERATIVE DISC DISEASE

Fiona Rattray

> **Degenerative disc disease is degeneration of the annular fibres of the intervertebral disc.**

Intervertebral discs function as shock absorbers between the vertebrae when these bones are load bearing. The discs also allow for movement to occur between the vertebrae; therefore, they are flexible yet strong.

Discs have two distinct components, the annulus fibrosus and the nucleus pulposus *(Figure 47.1).* The annulus fibrosus, also called annular fibres, are concentric layers of collagen forming a laminated band which holds two vertebrae together; each layer is on a diagonal at right angles to its neighbour. The annular fibres are thicker anteriorly and laterally and are firmly attached to the end plates of the vertebrae above and below. The posterior portion is thinner and less firmly attached.

The nucleus pulposus is a transparent jelly in the central part of the disc, surrounded by the annular fibres. The nucleus has a high water content and behaves as a viscous fluid. The water content is 88 per cent at birth, decreasing over time to 65 to 70 per cent in old age *(Souza, 1997).*

The disc has a capacity to swell when compressive forces are reduced. For example, a person is taller in the morning than at night. Water is forced out of the disc to the vertebral bodies during the day because of gravity, movement and compression. It returns to the disc at night.

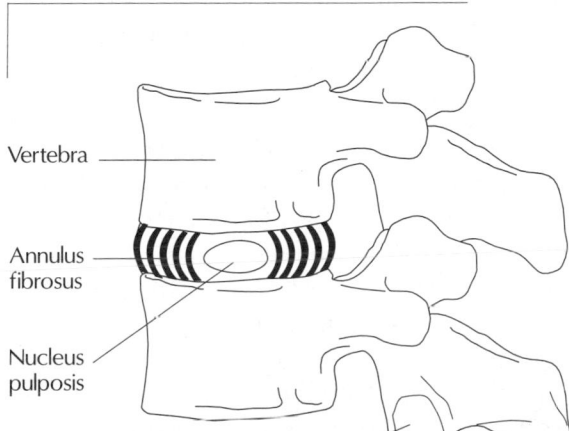

Vertebra

Annulus fibrosus

Nucleus pulposis

Facet joint

Figure 47.1
Disc and vertebrae.

There is more movement possible in the lumbar and cervical spine than in the thoracic spine, with motion restricted in the thorax primarily by the ribs. Rotation in the lumbar spine is restricted more than rotation in the cervical spine due to the orientation of the lumbar facet joints.

The disc and facet joints are a three-joint structure between each pair of vertebrae. Force is directed through the discs and facet joints when the spine is weight bearing. A disc maintains the separation of the two adjacent vertebrae through its inherent internal pressure; the fluid of the nucleus exerts a pressure that keeps the vertebrae apart and the annular fibres taut. The nucleus moves slightly posteriorly when the spine is in flexion and slightly anteriorly when the spine is in extension. The annular fibres bulge slightly, then recover when the spine straightens.

Facet joints between the vertebrae direct and control the degree of vertebral movement, whether flexion, extension, sidebending or rotation. They are surrounded by joint capsules that are looser in the cervical region than in the thoracic and lumbar spine. The capsule is lined with synovium. Meniscoids, fat-filled synovial folds that extend between the facet joints, probably act as shock absorbers.

Vertebral discs are not very pain sensitive, with only the posterior peripheral aspect of the annulus fibrosus being innervated. The anterior and posterior longitudinal ligament, nerve roots and vertebral bodies are pain sensitive, as well as the highly innervated facet joints.

Discs are hypovascular, making repair a slower process. Only the periphery is vascularized. Nutrition diffuses into the disc primarily through the cartilaginous vertebral end-plates.

Lumbar Intra-Discal Pressure in the Seated Position

The design of the modern work chair with its horizontal seat and vertical back was developed in 1884 by the German orthopedic surgeon F. Staffel. At that time, work surfaces were usually in an inclined position. Staffel thought that a straight back, hips and knees in 90 degrees of flexion and a horizontal gaze were the ideal posture for the seated worker. Today, this position is still considered optimal.

However, present-day office work — especially work at a computer — often requires the worker to lean forward for convenience of vision. Lumbar flexion may increase depending on the height of the work surface. This often results in 60 degrees of hip flexion and 30 degrees of lumbar spine flexion, which varies greatly from the degree of hip flexion envisioned by Staffel.

A study on intra-discal loading revealed that 140 per cent of body weight was recorded between L3 and L4 in Staffel's seated position with the eyes horizontal. When seated subjects leaned forward, the pressure at L3 and L4 increased to 185 to 250 per cent of body weight, depending on the task performed. Over time, these pressures can result in microtrauma, intra-discal fissures and low back pain. When the seat surface was inclined forward, so that hip flexion was up to 120 degrees, and the desk top was sloped to prevent lumbar flexion *(Figure 47.2)*, the intra-discal loading on the three lower discs was reduced by 33 per cent compared to Staffel's position, and 55 per cent compared to the forward-leaning posture. In the study, the most comfortable seat surface position was 10 degrees of forward inclination. While improving the ergonomics of the office chair will help to reduce stresses on the lumbar discs, the entire work station must be modified, from work-surface height to layout of the work area *(Fehr, Krueger, 1992)*.

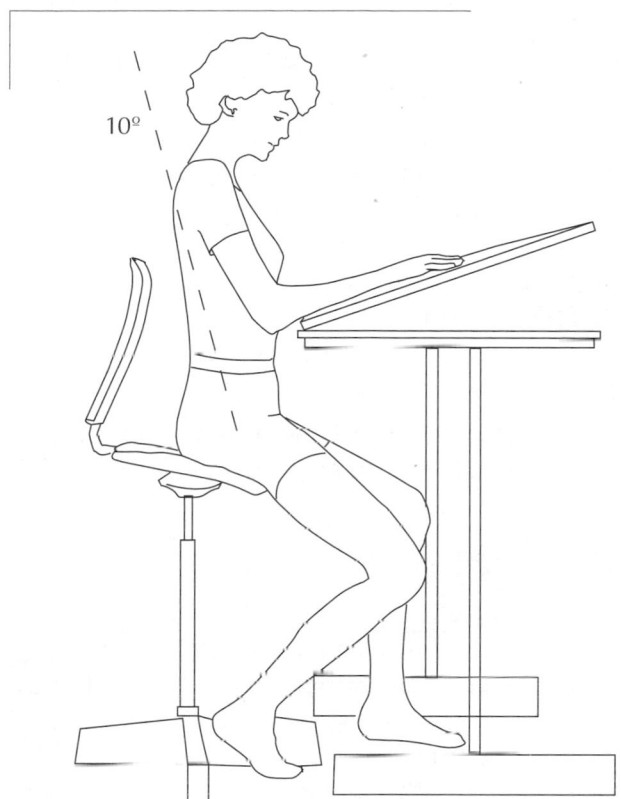

Figure 47.2
Optimal seat position for comfort in lumbar spine.

Degeneration of the Disc

Degeneration of the disc is a normal process. As a person ages, the vertebral discs undergo slow wear and tear. This typically consists of fibrous changes in the nucleus and in the organization of the annulus fibrosus rings, and disappearance of the cartilaginous end-plates. The discs of the lumbar and cervical spine are most affected. As early as 20 years of age, changes in the lumbar discs can be noticed as the vascular supply to the disc becomes occluded, affecting its nutrition. The posterior portions of the annulus become compressed and bulge as a result of the lumbar lordosis. These posterior annular fibres appear to be thinner and shorter than the anterior ones. The discs become somewhat wedge-shaped, narrower posteriorly than anteriorly. The nucleus gradually changes from a gel to a fibrous structure; its water-binding capacity decreases while its collagen content increases. The overall height of the disc decreases and the disc space narrows.

By the third decade of a person's life, the facet joints become involved in the degenerative process. They experience abnormal stress due to the altered disc mechanics; synovitis and joint effusion may occur *(Hertling, Kessler, 1990)*.

The posterolateral portion of the disc fibres weaken first. One contributing factor is the functional movements of the spine. These are often diagonal combinations of flexion and rotation, placing more stress on the posterolateral portion of the annular fibres by the nucleus. Another factor that leads to weakness is that the posterior longitudinal ligament is thicker and stronger than the thinner, more lateral portions of the annulus. Over time, as the posterolateral annular fibres compress and bulge, clefts appear between the layers of the annulus. The individual layers of the annulus may separate, allowing nuclear material to infiltrate between them. The clefts may meet and form gaps. Eventually these clefts and gaps become radial and horizontal tears; the nucleus is allowed to protrude into the annular space.

The annular fibres, over time, become weaker and less elastic, creating tension on the outer fibres. This, combined with altered disc mechanics and weight bearing in the spine, encourages bone reinforcement at the outer edges of the vertebrae. Osteophytes form anteriorly and posteriorly.

While between the ages of 40 and 50, discs in the lumbar spine are still capable of imbibing water, it is during this decade that the nucleus gradually changes to a fibrous material almost indistinguishable from the annular fibres. Then the disc space narrows considerably and range of motion is reduced. This narrowing occurs in 70 per cent of men and 55 per cent of women between ages 55 and 64 years *(Hertling, Kessler, 1996)*. The intervertebral foramen space is also reduced, leaving less room for the nerve roots. This process occurs earlier in the cervical spine. By age 40 the nucleus pulposus in the cervical spine is essentially non-existant, having also changed to fibrous material *(Souza, 1997)*.

Disc breakdown is not surprising when the forces the discs usually endure are measured. Pressure within the healthy lumbar disc varies with different postures and activities. Intradiscal pressure increases with flexion and decreases with extension. This is true in both sitting and lifting. When the spine is rotated, pressures are increased 20 per cent from those measured when the person is standing straight. When the person is laughing, pressures increase up to 50 per cent. With flexion, pressures increase 150 per cent. When a 20 kilogram weight is lifted with the knees straight and the back flexed, pressures increase up to 169 per cent *(Magee, 1992)*.

Although this degenerative process is a normal one, pathological disc degeneration occurs when changes happen either at an accelerated rate or prematurely. Pain and disability result when the surrounding tissues cannot adapt to the changes.

Acute Injuries to the Disc

At any point in this continuum of degeneration, an acute rupture can occur. Between ages 30 and 45, it is most common for a traumatic rupture in the lumbar spine to occur, as the annular fibres are weaker and less able to withstand higher stress. However, it is possible for an acute rupture to occur before 20 years of age in discs that show no signs of degeneration *(Boyling, Palastanga, 1994)*. In people over the age of 50 years, rupture is less likely as the nucleus of the disc has fibrosed.

Herniation is a commonly used term to describe a disc injury that results from rupture of the annular fibres. In terms of lumbar injuries, men are affected more than women in a ratio of 3:2. Herniation at L4 to L5 or L5 to S1 accounts for 98 per cent of all low back disc injuries *(Hertling, Kessler, 1996)*.

The suggested mechanism of disc herniation is a combination of flexion and torsional (twisting) forces. In laboratory studies, this torsion produced a lateral shear as well as peripheral separations of the annular layers in degenerated lumbar discs *(Foreman, Croft, 1995)*.

The damage to the annular fibres may extend through many or all layers at one time. As a result, the disc bulges; if it bulges far enough posteriorly or posterolaterally, pain-sensitive structures such as nerve roots and ligaments are compressed. This gives rise to symptoms of paresthesia, pain and possibly motor weakness. With a severe tear, escaped nuclear material can also compress or irritate pain-sensitive structures.

Despite the above information, the exact cause and mechanism by which disc degeneration and injury occur are not completely understood. There is also no universal agreement on the terminology used to describe the types of annular fibre breakdown and the position of the nucleus.

According to one source, before the injury occurs, the disc may bulge, usually posterolaterally, with the annular fibres intact *(Figure 47.3)*. This is referred to as *protrusion*. Herniation may then follow as the annular fibres tear. Herniation has the following subcategories: in a *prolapse*, only the outermost annular fibres hold the nucleus; with *extrusion*, the annulus fibrosus is pierced, allowing the nucleus to enter the epidural space; and with *sequestration*, fragments of the nucleus and annulus are found outside the disc *(Magee, 1992)*.

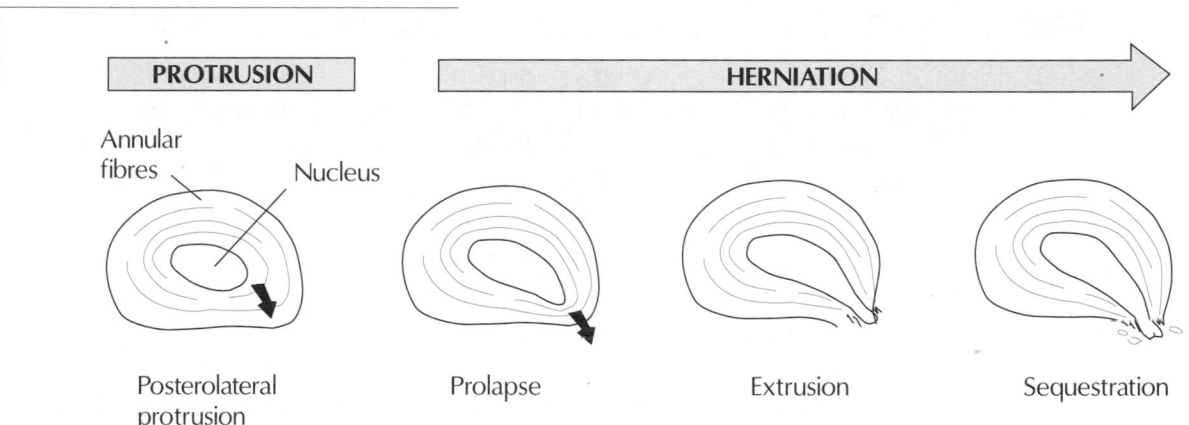

PROTRUSION   HERNIATION

Annular fibres   Nucleus

Posterolateral protrusion   Prolapse   Extrusion   Sequestration

Figure 47.3
Stages of acute disc herniation.

Another source describes herniation as the nucleus being partially expelled into the epidural space, while prolapse is a complete rupture of the nucleus into the vertebral canal (*Kisner, Colby, 1996*). A third description of the process begins with radial fissures of annulus fibres, followed by an annular bulge, then protrusion of the nucleus into the epidural space (*McKenzie, 1989*).

Other terms that are used with degenerative disc disease:

- **Spondylosis** is degenerative changes in the facet joints and eventual ankylosing of the joint capsules.

- **Slipped disc** is a lay term for disc herniation.

- **Lumbago** is a general, non-specific term for low back pain.

- **Sciatica**, when used as a lay term, means pain in the back of the leg; it does not identify the origin of the pain. True sciatica is compression or inflammation of the sciatic nerve. This could occur for several reasons such as disc herniation, vertebral osteophytes or a piriformis syndrome. However, pain that refers down the posterior leg could also arise from lumbar facet joint irritation, sacroiliac joint dysfunction or trigger points.

➤ **The cause of degenerative disc disease is chronic overloading of the disc** leading to annular fibre microtearing and migration of the nucleus.

➤ **Contributing factors** include trauma, muscle imbalances leading to asymmetric loading of the spine, postural dysfunction such as head-forward posture, chronic degenerative changes in the disc, poor blood supply to the disc, lack of flexibility, improper back support and poor posture.

➤ Other factors are biomechanical changes such as asymmetrically shaped facet joints or facet joints that are hypermobile or hypomobile; either of these situations leads to increased wear on the annulus. Annular breakdown can occur at the affected level with hypermobility and with the unequal stresses that arise from unequal motion. It can also occur at discs above or below a hypomobile segment.

The Medical Treatment of Disc Injury

Medically, the disc is the most researched structure in the back as a source of low back and referred back pain. The disc is considered by many to be the primary cause of back pain (*Hertling, Kessler, 1996*). However, many structures outside the disc also refer pain and may mimic symptoms of disc disease. Therefore, differential assessment is important. Diagnosis is made through subjective information, and orthopedic and laboratory testing.

A study on the reliability of orthopedic testing with cervical disc disease shows that while cervical compression and distraction tests reliably indicated the specific disc lesion, not all persons with cervical disc disease were positive for the tests (*Souza, 1997*). In addition, degenerative changes visible on X-rays are not necessarily indicative of a person's symptoms. A person with severe degenerative change may have few or no symptoms, while another person with little obvious change may have severe, ongoing pain. With acute injuries, myelograms have clinically proven to be unreliable for assessing disc lesions. Flexion and extension X-rays may be used to differentiate annulus rupture from nuclear protrusion (*McKenzie, 1989*).

Degenerative disc disease is usually treated conservatively at first. This includes analgesics and muscle relaxants, a few days of bedrest and functional positioning so the person finds and maintains a position of symptom reduction and optimal comfort. Simple movements and exercises are interspersed with maintainance of the functional position. As symptoms resolve, strengthening exercises are used.

In the past, prolonged bedrest and immobilization were routinely prescribed for disc herniations. As most back pain was thought to be of discal origin, this led to a legacy of bedrest prescribed for any back pain and a reluctance to assign any form of active exercise (*Buschbacher, 1994*). Today it is becoming recognized that bedrest is only useful with extremely painful conditions that are worsened by standing; bedrest ultimately adds to muscle weakness and facet joint dysfunction at the level of the lesion (*McKenzie, 1989*).

If reduction of symptoms does not occur after three months of conservative treatment, surgery such as laminectomy or discectomy may be performed as a last resort. Intervertebral foramina are enlarged and the unstable segments may be fused. Alternatively, sclerosing or hardening agents may be injected into the disc to reduce movement and to stabilize a particular level. However, hypomobility of one segment or several segments means hypermobility of surrounding segments due to compensation. This may lead to more biomechanical problems at a later date.

One study divided patients with low back and sciatic pain into two groups. One group was given conservative care; 90 per cent of these people were better one year later. The other group received surgery; 100 per cent were better only in the first two months following surgery. One year later, this had dropped to 90 per cent, the same as the group that had not received surgery. Early return of symptoms usually means adhesion and scar formation that surgery cannot repair and prognosis is poor. To reduce adhesion formation following surgery the performance of a straight leg raise once every two hours is suggested (*McKenzie, 1989*).

Other forms of conservative care for degenerative disc disease include chiropractic and physiotherapy, especially the McKenzie exercises mentioned at the end of this chapter. Chiropractors do not usually manipulate the affected level, but manipulate at other levels. There is no evidence that manipulation will draw the nuclear material back into place, as is sometimes claimed (*Edmond, 1993*). Traction and physical therapy may be of benefit. A response is usually evident in a few days; if the patient is unresponsive, she is referred for medical co-management *(Souza, 1997)*. Physiotherapists use modalities such as cold and heat, exercises and traction.

Symptom Picture of Degenerative Disc Disease

Stages of Degeneration

✦ Degenerative disc disease is thought to go through three stages of degeneration: dysfunction, instability and stabilization *(Hertling, Kessler, 1996)*. Pain and other symptoms may occur at any stage. On the other hand, the person may remain asymptomatic if a threshold of tissue damage is not reached; this threshold varies from person to person.

- In the **dysfunction stage**, biomechanical changes over many years result in weakness, bulging and minor tears in the annulus which heal slowly. These disc protrusions may be symptomatic. There may also be painful chronic facet joint irritation, joint effusion and muscle spasm. In the cervical spine, the meniscoids, folds of the inflamed synovium, can become trapped between the joint surfaces, reducing range of motion *(Souza, 1997)*. An acute acquired torticollis can result *(Boyling, Palastanga, 1994)*. The dysfunction stage is considered reversible.

- In the **instability stage**, the posterior annular fibres and joint capsules become lax causing the vertebral segment to become hypermobile. Pain may result from the stress on the ligaments and joint capsules due to this increased mobility. Nerve entrapment may occur. Spondylolisthesis, or an anterior displacement of L5 on S1, may occur with lower lumbar involvement. The disc is secured by peripheral osteophytes as the body attempts to restabilize the vertebral segment with bony reinforcement along spinal ligaments. Tissue change in this stage is considered permanent.

- In the **stabilization stage**, there is loss of disc material and decreased disc height, the intervertebral foramen narrows, the joint capsules and posterior ligaments fibrose. Osteophytes form, causing a decreased range of motion at the affected segment. Stenosis, or narrowing of the spinal canal, may occur. Degeneration may spread to other vertebral levels.

✦ With cervical degenerative disc disease, there is a gradual onset of neck stiffness and pain into the shoulders which is often worse on one side. As the condition progresses, symptoms may get worse, from paresthesia, to loss of reflexes, then muscle weakness. These symptoms may have a slow or rapid onset. There are frequent occipital headaches.

✦ With lumbar degenerative disc disease, pain is noted across the lower back and hip, occasionally into the leg; it is worse with prolonged activity. There is a history of back injuries.

Symptom Picture of Acute Disc Herniation

Acute Herniation

✦ Acute herniation can occur at any stage, but is more common at the end of the dysfunction or beginning of the instability stage, usually between 30 and 45 years of age. A posterolateral protrusion is most common.

✦ A single severe strain, repeated minor strains or sustained flexion may cause an **acute rupture.** The person may have been sitting for a prolonged period with the spine in flexion before the rupture occures. There may or may not be a sensation of something tearing. Edema and protective muscle spasm set in around the affected level. There may be associated ligamentous sprains.

✦ **Pain** arises from compression of pain-sensitive structures by the protrusion. These structures include nerve roots, ligaments, dura mater and blood vessels. With a herniation where the nucleus is still contained by the annulus, pain is usually worse first thing in the morning. At this time of day the disc has imbibed more water and exerts more compression on surrounding structures. Pain also increases when the person is inactive.

• The pain is likely sclerotomic, deep and poorly localized. For example, the pain of a developing lower lumbar disc lesion starts centrally at the level of the affected disc, then over time moves laterally, increasing in intensity *(Figure 47.4).* It eventually spreads across the back, into the gluteal muscles, then down the thigh to the leg and foot. A reversal of this pattern is seen as the lesion is corrected. The acute stage usually lasts up to six days.

✦ An **acute scoliosis** or other spinal distortion may occur in response to the acute herniation. The position of the nucleus pulposus holding the vertebral surfaces apart is responsible for the direction that the traumatic scoliosis takes. Ninety per cent of these scolioses have a lateral shift away from pain, while 10 per cent have a lateral shift towards the pain; the latter is more difficult to treat *(McKenzie, 1989).*

Neurological Signs of Herniation

✦ Neurological signs occur with pressure on the nerve roots or spinal cord. **True neurological** signs are motor weakness specific to the level of the lesion and specific dermatomal sensory changes such

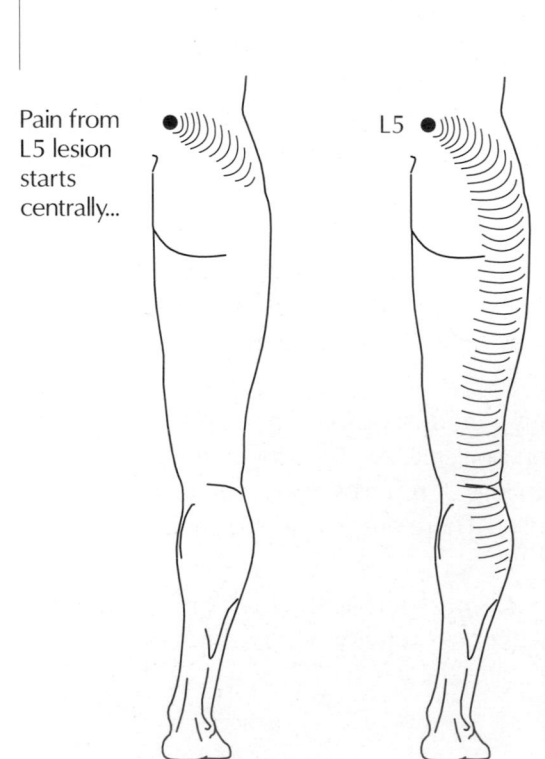

Pain from L5 lesion starts centrally...

L5

...over time, it moves peripherally down the leg.

Figure 47.4
Pain from disc injury.

as numbness. These are more likely to occur with prolapse and sequestration, where the nucleus leaks out of the annular fibres and impinges on the nerves. Neurogenic pain — that is, pain of neurological origin — is present. Irritation of the dura or nerve roots may result from the leaked nuclear material; symptoms persist for some time and are not relieved by movement.

✦ A **nerve root impingement syndrome**, where the symptoms change with ongoing pressure, may also occur. Less frequently, a central prolapse can lead to upper motor neuron lesions in the cervical spine. In the lumbar spine, a central prolapse can lead to compression of the sacral nerve roots with bladder or bowel dysfunction and numbness across the low back, gluteals and around the hips (saddle anesthesia).

How Herniation Position Affects the Symptom Picture

✦ Symptoms of a protrusion vary depending on the vertebral level, direction of protrusion, as well as the amount of protrusion. For example, posterolateral and posterior disc injuries are worse with activities that increase the interdiscal pressure, such as flexion, sitting, coughing and standing from a sitting postion. Symptoms usually decrease with walking.

✦ A **large cervical posterolateral protrusion** may cause nerve root signs in the upper limbs.

✦ A **small lumbar posterolateral protrusion** may produce pain spreading across the back into the gluteals and thighs.

✦ A **large lumbar posterior protrusion** may cause spinal cord compression with loss of bladder control. Less commonly, an anterior protrusion causes back pain and possibly no neurological signs, as the bulge compresses the anterior longitudinal ligament.

✦ Symptoms may shift if the annulus is intact. On the other hand, if the annulus ruptures, this allows material to leak and the hydrostatic mechanism is no longer intact; in this case, the symptoms cannot be relieved by movements of the spine.

✦ Acute posterior neck lesions may refer pain and paresthesia across the shoulder and down the affected arm in a specific dermatomal pattern. Pain may be sharp or deep and aching; it is worse with weight bearing such as carrying a bag or purse. Acute anterior disc bulges may produce difficulty in swallowing.

✦ Acute lumbar lesions start as sudden back pain that progresses to mainly leg pain. The pain may be sharp, deep or aching. Herniation is always painful, with the onset often before noon when the disc is most hydrated and the nucleus is able to move the most *(McKenzie, 1989)*. Calf cramping may be present with herniation. Standing and walking are less painful than sitting with a posterior or posterolateral lesion, while pain on standing or walking suggests an anterior lesion.

✦ Healing is slow due to the hypovascular nature of the disc. As the condition resolves through the subacute to chronic stages, the spinal deformity reduces, range of motion increases and orthopedic tests such as the straight leg raise, slump and upper limb tension tests are negative. Worsening signs in the lumbar spine are a lack of back pain but an escalation of neurological symptoms.

Subjective Information

HEALTH HISTORY QUESTIONS

✦ Standardized forms, such as the Vernon-Mior Neck Pain and Disability Index or the Revised Oswestry Low Back Pain Questionnaire *(Chapman-Smith, 1996)* can be used to measure the client's initial symptoms.

✦ What are the type, onset and location of pain and other symptoms? What are the client's activity levels?

✦ How long has the current episode lasted?

✦ Have there been any previous injuries to the affected area with cervical involvement, such as whiplash?

✦ With the low back, is there a history of episodes of back pain, perhaps a sensation of the back locking? Has there been a history of injuries to the lower limbs that would alter gait or posture, creating biomechanical imbalances? Has the client experienced surgery, such as abdominal surgery, that would create scar tissue, again affecting biomechanics?

✦ What factors aggravate and relieve the symptoms? Does coughing or sneezing aggravate the symptoms? Does walking or lying down relieve symptoms?

✦ Has the condition been medically diagnosed? Has the client had surgery for this condition? Is the client taking any medication or parallel therapies?

Objective Information

Observations

✎ A postural assessment is performed. Underlying postural contributors may be present. With degenerative disc disease of the cervical spine, in the lateral view, a head-forward posture is likely revealed. In the lumbar spine, lateral view, either a hyperlordosis (anterior pelvic tilt) or "flatback" (posterior pelvic tilt) may be present; in the seated position, the client may slouch, placing the lumbar spine in flexion.

✎ Muscle atrophy may be present depending on the stage of degeneration.

✎ With acute herniations in the cervical spine, in the posterior view, the neck may be rotated and sidebent. In the lumbar spine, in the lateral view, a decrease in the normal lordosis may be noted; in a posterior view, a leg length discrepancy or an acute scoliosis may be observed.

Palpation

✎ Palpation with degenerative disc disease may reveal point tenderness, trigger points, fascial restrictions, as well as fibrosed and hypertonic muscles crossing the affected level. There may be distal muscle atrophy.

✍ With acute disc herniation, tenderness, heat, spasm and active trigger points are likely present in muscles that cross the affected areas.

Testing

Degenerative Disc Disease

✍ **AF** and **PR ROM** of either the cervical or lumbar spine may reveal reduced ranges in AF and PR ROM, with PR ROM having more available range. In both, cervical and lumbar spine extension is most restricted. Stiffness is likely. Pain may or may not be present, depending on numerous factors including stage of degeneration. The end feel is likely capsular in the affected areas.

✍ **AR isometric testing** may reveal weakness in affected muscles, depending on the stage of degeneration.

Acute Herniation

✍ **AF** and **PR ROM** in either the cervical or lumbar spine reveal ranges limited by pain and muscle spasm, passive range less so than active.

✍ In the lumbar spine, **active free flexion** may have a deviation to one side. If the movement is away from the painful side, vertebral joint derangement may be present; if the movement is towards the painful side, an entrapped or adhered nerve root may be present (*McKenzie, 1989*). Another source states that if sidebending away from the painful side increases the symptoms, the problem may be a disc herniation medial to the nerve root, or it may be muscular or articular in origin. If sidebending towards the painful side increases the symptoms, disc herniation is lateral to the nerve root, or the lesion is inside the vertebral joints (*Magee, 1992*).

✍ **With posterior or posterolateral herniations that are contained by the annular fibres:** movements can reduce the symptoms; flexion is limited and symptoms peripheralize with movement; extension is also limited and symptoms centralize with movement.

✍ **With a complete annular rupture and sequestered nucleus:** movement cannot relieve the symptoms as the hydrostatic disc mechanism is no longer intact.

Special Tests

✍ Key findings for **nerve root impingement** are motor weakness and dermatomal sensory changes such as paresthesia or sensation loss in the distribution for the specific affected vertebral level. Decreased ability to perform straight leg raising, dermatomal radiating pain and depressed deep tendon reflexes may be associated with referred pain from facet joints, interspinous ligaments and spinal muscles as well as the disc; therefore, they are not considered true signs of lumbar nerve root compression (*Kisner, Colby, 1996*).

✍ A cervical disc herniation may give positive results with **upper limb tension tests, Spurling's, Valsalva's** and **deep tendon reflex tests.** Specific **active resisted** and

sensory tests are performed to isolate the lesion.

- For C5 lesions, shoulder abduction is weak; sensory changes are over the lateral forearm.
- For C6 lesions, elbow flexion or wrist extension is weak; sensory changes are over the thumb or index finger.
- For C7 lesions, elbow extension or wrist flexion is weak; sensory changes are over the middle, index and ring fingers.
- For C8 lesions, thumb abduction is weak; sensory changes are over the little and ring fingers.
- For T1 lesions, finger adduction is weak; sensory changes are over the medial forearm *(Hertling, Kessler, 1996)*.

✍ A lumbar disc herniation may give positive results with **slump, Valsalva's, Kemp's, Kernig's, straight leg raise and deep tendon reflex tests.** Again, specific **active resisted** and **sensory tests** are performed to isolate the lesion; however, nerve root compression must occur before these tests are positive.

- For L4 lesions, ankle dorsiflexion or heel walking is weak; sensory changes are over the medial aspect of the ankle.
- For L5 lesions, big toe extension is weak; sensory changes are over the dorsum of the foot.
- For S1 lesions, plantarflexion or toe walking is weak; sensory changes are on the lateral aspect of the ankle.

Differentiating Sources of Neck and Arm Pain

✍ **Facet joint irritation** is revealed with a positive Kemp's test.

✍ The various **thoracic outlet syndromes** are indicated using Adson's, Travell's variation, costoclavicular, Eden's and Wright's hyperabduction tests.

✍ **Scalene trigger points** will yield positive scalene cramp and scalene relief tests.

✍ **Carpal tunnel syndrome** will yield a positive Phalen's test.

✍ **Tendinitis** of the rotator cuff muscles will result in a positive active resisted test.

✍ **Osteoarthritis** in the glenohumeral joint is diagnosed medically by X-ray and other diagnostic tests.

✍ **Visceral pathologies** may also refer to the shoulder and arm. Liver and gall bladder pathologies refer pain to the right shoulder, while pancreatic pathologies and angina refer pain to the left shoulder. See Appendix D for more details. The client should be referred to a physician if orthopedic testing results are negative or inconclusive for a neuromuscular source of the pain.

Differentiating Sources of Low Back and Leg Pain

✍ **Facet joint irritation** is revealed with a positive Kemp's test.

✍ **Sacroiliac joint mobility** is assessed with motion palpation.

✍ **Sacroiliac joint dysfunction** results in sacroiliac joint gapping, sacroiliac joint squish,

Contraindications

✦ Treatment is contraindicated with saddle anesthesia and bladder weakness; this indicates herniation and compression of the fourth sacral nerve root. The client is referred for immediate medical attention.

✦ If no position can be found that relieves the pain, treatment is contraindicated until the client is referred to a physician for assessment.

✦ Positions that aggravate symptoms are avoided.

✦ Do not mobilize hypermobile joints.

✦ Do not remove all protective spasming with acute disc lesions; spasm stabilizes the hypermobile segments.

✦ Pressure and direction of techniques are modified and deep or longitudinal techniques are not used on areas of muscle atrophy.

Gaenslen's and Faber tests being positive. Sacroiliac joint motion may be either hyper- or hypomobile.

✍ **Hip pathologies** referring pain are revealed by positive hip quadrant and Faber tests.

✦ **Spondylolisthesis** is sometimes palpated as an anterior displacement of L5 on S1; pain may be relieved by placing one hand on the client's sacrum, the other hand on the abdomen and gently compressing the sacrum and abdomen *(McKenzie, 1989)*. It is most clearly identified through referral to a physician for X-rays.

✦ **Visceral pathologies** may also refer to the back, such as renal and urological pathologies. Bone cancer may also cause bilateral back pain that is unrelieved by positional changes and is worse at night. See Appendix D for more details.

Treatment Goals

Assess the client to determine the stage of degeneration.

Decrease sympathetic nervous system firing. Reduce pain. Reduce spasm.

Treatment Plan

General Treatment for Degenerative Disc Disease

✋ Treatment goals for degenerative disc disease depend on the presenting symptoms and stage of degeneration. Massage is recommended to reduce spasm and pain *(Buschbacher, 1994)*. In the later stages, focus is on maintenance of tissue health and symptomatic relief.

✋ The treatment is in the context of a relaxation massage including unforced **diaphragmatic breathing.**

Specific Treatment

✋ The **pre-treatment hydrotherapy** is heat to affected areas and areas of fascial restriction.

✋ **Positioning** may be prone, sidelying or supine, depending on the structures to be treated and the areas affected. Pillowing should support the client in a pain-free position of ease and relaxation.

Treatment Goals   Treatment Plan

Reduce compressive forces on the disc and nerves. Reduce fascial restrictions, hypertonicity and trigger points. Maintain tissue health.

✋ **For DDD of the cervical spine**, if the client has a postural dysfunction such as a head-forward posture, treatment begins on the anterior thorax. Fascial techniques such as skin rolling and fascial spreading are used over the pectorals, intercostals and scalene muscles. Swedish techniques such as effleurage and kneading are used on these muscles, as well as the sternocleidomastoid. Trigger points that refer into the painful areas are treated. PIR is used to stretch short, tight scalenes.

Mobilize hypomobile joints.

✋ Joint play for adjacent hypomobile vertebrae will relieve stresses on the affected level (*Thomson et al., 1991; Hertling, Kessler, 1996*).

Stretch shortened muscles.

✋ On the shortened suboccipitals and posterior cervical muscles, Golgi tendon organ release, petrissage, gentle long-axis traction, passive stretching and fascial techniques are used. These are followed by soothing massage to the muscles of the face.

Encourage circulation in overstretched muscles.

✋ The client is turned prone and petrissage is used on the shoulder girdle and thoracic erector spinae. Brisk, stimulating work is performed on the scapular retractors. See hyperkyphosis treatment for more details.

Reduce compressive forces on the disc and nerves. Reduce fascial restrictions, hypertonicity and trigger points. Maintain tissue health.

✋ **For DDD of the lumbar spine, if the client has a postural dysfunction such as hyperlordosis,** the massage begins with treatment of the hip flexors. Skin rolling and crossed-hands fascial spread are applied over rectus femoris and the iliotibial band. Swedish techniques are indicated for the short hip flexors. Trigger points in iliopsoas and tensor fascia lata are addressed. Joint play for hypomobile sacroiliac joints is used.

✋ The client is turned prone and fascial techniques are employed over the lumbar erector spinae. General Swedish work is used on erector spinae, quadratus lumborum and gluteal muscles; any trigger points in these muscles are treated.

Mobilize hypomobile joints.

✋ Joint play is again used on hypomobile vertebrae. Long-axis traction to the lumbar vertebrae is achieved by placing one hand on the sacrum, the other on the lumbothoracic junction and applying traction inferiorly on the sacrum and superiorly on the thorax. See the chapter on hyperlordosis for more details.

Stretch shortened muscles.

✋ Stretch the shortened hip flexors using passive strength or PIR. See chapter on hyperlordosis for more details.

Reduce fascial restrictions, hypertonicity and trigger points.

✋ **For DDD of the lumbar spine if the client has flatback, or posterior pelvic tilt,** the focus is on lengthening the shortened hamstrings. The therapist uses fascial and Swedish techniques, as well as PIR. Stimulating Swedish techniques are used on the lengthened hip flexors and lumbar extensors. See hyperkyphosis treatment for details.

Mobilize pelvis to restore optimal orientation.

✋ To decrease the posterior pelvic tilt, a combination of **passive hip extension** and submaximal isometric contraction of the quadriceps is

Treatment Goals

Treatment Plan

used *(Boyling, Palastanga, 1994).* The supine client lies close to the edge of the table so the leg can move off the table into extension. (If the client experiences back pain with this position, the unaffected leg is flexed at the hip and knee so the foot rests on the table; this may relieve the back pain.) The therapist stabilizes the unaffected anterior superior iliac spine with one hand and places the other hand on the affected thigh proximal to the knee, extending the leg until the slack is taken up. The client is instructed to submaximally, isometrically perform a straight leg raise by pushing into the therapist's hand. This helps to pull the pelvis into an anterior tilt. The contraction is maintained for 10 seconds while the therapist continues to resist.

✋ Alternatively, the prone client lies on the table without a pillow under the abdomen. The therapist places his own leg on the table, with his hip and knee flexed, tibia flat on the table and a towel across his thigh. The client's affected thigh rests on top of the therapist's thigh which acts as a wedge to move the client's leg into extension. The client's anterior superior iliac spine is carefully grasped and used as a lever to rotate the pelvis anteriorly at the sacroiliac joint. When the slack is taken up in the hip and sacroiliac joint, the client is instructed to submaximally, isometrically contract the quadriceps by pushing into the therapist's thigh. This helps to pull the pelvis into a anterior tilt. The contraction is maintained for 10 seconds while the therapist continues to carefully, passively rotate the pelvis anteriorly.

Self-care Goals

Self-care Plan

For Degenerative Disc Disease

Educate the client.

✍ Heat is used on shortened tissues. Self-massage is helpful for hypertonic areas. Diaphragmatic breathing is encouraged for pain management.

Maintain range of motion.

✍ Pain-free range of motion is maintained. Over time, stretching of specific shortened muscles is followed by isometric strengthening of weaker muscles. Spine extension exercises are important.

Relieve compressive forces on the disc and nerves.

✍ For the cervical spine, a passive positional traction of the cervical spine is used to relieve pain. This is also termed unloading the spine. The supine client rests the head on a small towel roll, positioning the neck in flexion and sidebending away from the painful side *(Hertling, Kessler, 1996).*

✍ For the lumbar spine, positional traction is achieved by lying prone on a kitchen or dining room table so the pelvis and legs hang over the end of the table. The hips and knees are in flexion, the feet do not

Self-care Goals	## Self-care Plan

touch the ground. Unloading of the spine is also achieved with swimming.

Refer the client.

✍ If pes planus or leg length inequality is a contributing factor to pain, the client may consider orthotics. Postural re-education and movement therapy, such as Mitzvah and Alexander techniques, may be helpful for retraining the client's posture.

Educate the client about posture.

✍ A slumped sitting posture exacerbates and perpetuates low back pain and is to be avoided (*McKenzie, 1989*).

Treatment Goals	## Treatment Plan

General Treatment for Acute Herniation

🖐 Massage is recommended in acute disc injuries to relieve pain and to promote relaxation (*Kisner, Colby, 1996*).

Decrease sympathetic nervous system firing.

🖐 The treatment is in the context of a relaxation massage including unforced **diaphragmatic breathing.** The treatment is a half-hour to avoid overtaxing the client.

🖐 The **pre-treatment hydrotherapy** is ice to reduce spasm and pain.

🖐 **Positioning** may be prone, sidelying or supine, depending on the structures to be treated and the position of the herniation.

Specific Treatment

Reduce compressive forces on the disc through positioning and pillowing.

🖐 Passive positioning and the location of the pillows is crucial to the acute treatment. The client should assume a position that reduces the symptoms and is most comfortable (*Kisner, Colby, 1996*). For example, with a *lumbar posterior or posterolateral protrusion*, in the **supine** position lumbar extension is most comfortable; the legs are extended with no pillow under the knees. With a *cervical posterolateral protrusion*, a small towel roll under the neck while the client is supine maintains a cervical lordosis.

🖐 In the **prone** position, the *lumbar spine* is extended with no pillow under the abdomen. The neck is kept in alignment using a face cradle. In the **sidelying** position, pillows are placed under the head so the *cervical spine* is in alignment. A towel roll is placed at the curve of the waist to stabilize the pelvis and a pillow is placed between the knees. If the client needs to change position — for example, from prone to supine — the pelvis and shoulder girdle are kept in alignment. The client will be most comfortable if she turns over without twisting the spine.

Treatment Goals

Treatment Plan

✋ With the less common *anterior protrusions,* the symptoms are relieved by flexion of the lumbar or *cervical spine,* depending on the location. In the **supine** position, the *lumbar spine* is flexed with pillows under the knees; the cervical spine is flexed with a pillow under the head. In the **prone** position, the lumbar spine is maintained in flexion with an abdominal pillow; pillowing under the thorax maintains cervical flexion.

✋ Whether the affected area is the lumbar or cervical spine, gentle long-axis traction should reduce symptoms, using either the sacrum or the occiput as the traction area. The therapist always works within the client's pain tolerance.

Reduce spasm. Reduce pain. Reduce edema.

✋ Massage is performed to reduce edema, spasm and pain in muscles that cross the affected area. Techniques include lymphatic drainage, effleurage, kneading and stroking. Isometric agonist contraction may also reduce spasm.

Reduce some fascial restrictions. Reduce trigger points.

✋ Gentle fascial techniques may be used on shortened fascia (*Kisner, Colby, 1996; Thomson et al., 1991*). Trigger points that refer into the affected areas are treated with muscle stripping and gentle ischemic compressions.

✋ As the condition resolves into subacute and chronic stages, the treatment can become more vigorous. For example, hypomobile joints distant from the lesion can be mobilized. Fascial restrictions and hypertonicty are treated with fascial and Swedish techniques.

Self-care Goals

Self-care Plan

For Acute Herniation

Maintain pain-free range of motion.

✍ Periods of rest in a pain-reduced position interspersed with slow, controlled pain-reduced movement are indicated.

Reduce the herniation.

✍ The client is taught to find a pain-reduced position, whether standing, sitting or lying. With *posterolateral protrusions,* maintaining the lumbar lordosis is important. Lying prone is gradually progressed to passive lumbar extension where the client props herself up on her elbows. With the cervical spine, extension and sidebending to the unaffected side are likely to relieve symptoms. The less common *anterior protrusions* are usually relieved by flexion.

Educate the client.

✍ Hydrotherapy application is cold to reduce pain and spasm. Stress reduction, diaphragmatic breathing and self-massage are also helpful.

✍ Self-traction mentioned in the degenerative disc section is implemented as long as symptoms are reduced by the activity.

Self-care Goals

Self-care Plan

Strengthen weakened muscles.

- Gentle pain-free strengthening exercises are introduced.

- Posterior pelvic tilts performed in the acute stage worsen a posterolateral protrusion as they flex the spine; anterior pelvic tilts are preferred as they maintain the lordosis *(Kisner, Colby, 1996)*.

- As the condition progresses to the subacute and chronic stages, strengthening exercises that maintain the lordosis either in the neck or low back are used with posterolateral protrusions. Back extension while lying prone is used; the client lifts the arm on one side and the leg on the other side into extension. Strengthening the cervical multifidi is performed by the client placing the fingertips of both hands on the back of the neck at the level to be strengthened and isometrically resisting anterior fingertip pressure.

- Range of motion is gradually increased into previously painful ranges; strenghtening of all muscles that cross the affected level is also introduced.

Educate the client on correct posture.

- Correct lifting procedures and correct posture during activities of daily living are taught. If symptoms begin to return, the client should immediately resume the corrective postures and exercises.

- The client is taught correct posture. For example, in the seated position, a lumbar support such as a towel roll or Obus form is used with lumbar posterolateral protrusions. When moving from one position to another, the client maintains a protective posture.

- Pain-free range of motion is introduced while keeping the appropriate protective posture. Gradually movements of the limbs are introduced as long as these are pain-reduced and the protective posture is maintained.

Refer the client.

- The client is referred to a physician for assessment if the condition worsens or does not resolve. A chiropractor, physiotherapist or osteopath can also help with managing the symptoms.

- Orthotics may also be useful. If there is no history of increased pain with standing or walking, then leg length discrepancy is not likely to be relevant. If leg length is a contributing factor, a correction using an orthotic on the short leg should diminish the pain within a few days *(McKenzie, 1989)*.

- The client can also be referred for postural training such as the Mitzvah or Alexander technique.

Treatment Frequency and Expected Outcome

Treatment frequency for degenerative disc disease and acute disc lesions is two times a week for three weeks, followed by reassessment, then once a week for a month. Daily postural awarenes and self-care strengthening exercises are needed for both degenerative

See also stress reduction, spasm, trigger points, strain, sprain, postural dysfunctions, temporomandibular joint dysfunction, tension headaches, torticollis, conditions of the peripheral nervous system, thoracic outlet syndrome, piriformis syndrome and osteoarthritis for related treatments.

disc disease and disc herniation.

The prognosis for cervical degenerative disc disease is better if the symptoms are of recent and sudden onset; a gradual onset with muscle weakness and atrophy has a poorer prognosis. There may be a few weeks of symptoms, then an asymptomatic period, followed by occasional bouts brought on by overuse or poor posture.

In the lumbar spine a similar pattern occurs.

The prognosis for acute disc herniation symptoms in the cervical spine is good. The most severe symptoms may diminish in a few days (Hertling, Kessler, 1996) with full healing taking up to six months (Buschbacher, 1994). In the lumbar spine, acute disc herniation can take up to eight weeks to heal in most cases (Buschbacher, 1994). Asymptomatic periods may be interspersed with acute episodes of disc bulging that occur for no apparent reason in either the cervical or lumbar spine.

McKenzie Exercises

Physiotherapists may recommend McKenzie exercises for the client. These are often thought of as extension exercises only. However, New Zealand physiotherapist Robin McKenzie developed a successful system of assessment and treatment of low back and cervical pain whether of muscular, connective tissue, facet joint or disc-related origin (McKenzie, 1989; Grant, 1988). He noted that, in the seated position, people tend to slump and flex their lumbar spine, stretching the posterior vertebral ligaments and placing stress on the discs. His theory is that most back pain results from the abnormal biomechanics that arise as the nucleus pulposus migrates posteriorly inside the disc, rather than actual disc herniation.

McKenzie divided low back pain into three categories: postural syndrome, dysfunction syndrome and derangement syndrome. With McKenzie's postural syndrome, there is muscle shortness due to postural stress; intermittent pain occurs with certain postures (in this text, functional hyperlordosis and "swayback" affecting muscle). With his dysfunction syndrome there is connective tissue shortness due to adaptive shortening; there is intermittent pain and partial loss of movement (in this text, functional hyperlordosis and "swayback" affecting fascia). With his derangement syndrome there is deformation of the soft tissues due to movement of the nucleus pulposus and annulus, causing a disturbance of the normal resting position of the vertebrae; there is constant pain and partial loss of movement (in this text, acute disc lesion).

McKenzie's system to assess patients uses range of motion and repetitive movement. While initially developed for the low back, the same principles are applied to the cervical spine. Test movements described in the next section of active free flexion, extension and lateral pelvic shift to right and left are assessed by repeating each range 10 times. Symptoms are termed centralized when they diminish or become more central to the spine; peripheralized symptoms are those experienced farther along the affected limb.

Testing

With a derangement syndrome (acute disc lesions) the pain should either diminish or centralize to the spine during one of the test movements if the condition is appropriate for treatment with McKenzie's exercise therapy. If no position or movement decreases the symptoms, the condition is not suitable for exercise therapy, eliminating people with "true, constant severe sciatic pain with neurological deficit" *(McKenzie, 1989)*. McKenzie notes that these people require traction and bedrest, then reassessment in one or two weeks to see if exercise therapy is appropriate.

With a lumbar *posterior nuclear derangement*, extension of the lumbar spine, while initially limited, centralizes symptoms; flexion peripheralizes symptoms. If extension increases symptoms, the protrusion is either posterolateral or it cannot be mechanically reduced.

With a lumbar *posterolateral nuclear derangement*, extension initially increases the symptoms due to a lateral vertebral shift. The shift is corrected by the therapist first standing on the side to which the thorax is shifted. The therapist's shoulder is placed against the client's arm which is held against the client's ribs. The therapist's hands are placed on the client's opposite hip, fingers interlaced. The therapist simultaneously glides the thorax away while gliding the pelvis towards him. Once the shift is corrected, extension centralizes the symptoms.

With the less common lumbar *anterior nuclear derangement*, flexion of the lumbar spine centralizes symptoms; extension peripheralizes symptoms.

Remedial Exercises

While not all of McKenzie's exercise variations are described here, the following gives the massage therapist a brief understanding of the protocol.

McKenzie's exercises are progressive. Ten to 15 repetitions of an exercise are adequate; repetitions should be fluid and have a relaxation phase between them.

To treat **acute lumbar posterior nuclear derangement,** the person first lies prone for 10 minutes to let the nucleus return to the normal position, then lies prone with arms above the head. The client progresses to passive extension lying prone, with the torso propped up on the elbows. At this point, the pain should be localized more centrally. Later in the day, the person progresses to a few gentle flexion exercises in the supine position (knees to chest) followed by extension lying prone. The client finally, carefully, performs flexion in standing. The client is educated about proper lordosis in sitting and lifting.

To treat an **acute posterolateral nuclear derangement,** with the example of a lateral pelvic shift to the right, torso to left, the person is taught to correct the lateral shift first. This is achieved by the therapist standing behind the client with one hand on the client's left shoulder and the other hand on the client's right iliac crest. Slight pressure is applied with both hands. The hand on the left shoulder pushes to the right, while the hand on the right iliac crest pushes to the left. In effect, this squeezes the client's torso between the therapist's hands into a postion of overcorrection in the opposite direction: now the pelvis is shifted to the left and the torso to right. The person is held in this position for a minute or two.

The client is then taught to perform this exercise standing. The client's left hand is placed on the left lower ribs and guides the torso to the right; at the same time, the client's right hand is placed on the iliac crest and guides the pelvis to the left. This is followed by extension of the lumbar spine while in a standing position. As long as a lordosis is maintained, the person is not likely to go back into scoliosis.

To treat an **anterior nuclear derangement,** any lateral shift is corrected first by having the standing person flex the hip and knee on the side opposite to which the lateral deviation occurs; the foot is placed on the seat of a chair. The leg on the side of the lateral shift stays straight. The person flexes the torso onto the raised thigh. This is repeated several times. After correcting the lateral shift, or if no shift was present, the person progresses into lying supine, bringing both knees to the chest and holding them there. Over several days, the person can progress to careful flexion in standing *(McKenzie, 1989)*.

OSTEOARTHRITIS

Fiona Rattray

Osteoarthritis (OA) is a group of chronic, degenerative conditions that affect joints, specifically the articular cartilage and subchondral bone.

Degenerative joint disease and osteoarthrosis are other terms used to describe this disease process. The term *spondylitis* is used for arthritis affecting the vertebral column. The prevalence of osteoarthritis increases with age, although it is not caused by aging. Osteoarthritis is the most common form of arthritis, or inflammation of a joint.

Primary osteoarthritis is idiopathic and either local (involving one or two joint groups) or generalized (involving three or more joint groups). **Secondary osteoarthritis** is the result of a known cause, such as joint trauma or an underlying pathology *(Brandt et al., 1998)*. It is possible that primary osteoarthritis may be the result of biomechanical stress and that there is little difference between primary and secondary osteoarthritis in terms of pathological process *(Hertling, Kessler, 1996)*.

Arthritis is one of the most ancient pathological conditions affecting animals, including humans. Some fossilized dinosaur bones exhibit arthritic changes, although it is not always possible to distinguish between osteoarthritis and mild rheumatoid arthritis in fossil records. Arthritic change is also visible in Neanderthal fossils and Egyptian mummies, with the spine, hips and knee joints being affected.

Massage therapy and exercise have traditionally been used to treat arthritis in cultures around the globe. The ancient Chinese in 3000 BC and Hippocrates around 400 BC mention rubbing and "frictions" to ease joint pain from arthritis. In more recent times, deep massage and careful passive movements were recommended for pain relief with arthritis and rheumatism by medical authors in the first half of the twentieth century *(Walker, Helewa, 1996)*. Massage is recommended today for pain management *(Lorig, Fries, 1995)*.

The social and economic costs of osteoarthritis are enormous. Pain and the reduced ability to move affected joints diminish the quality of life for those with the disease. In Canada, 2.7 million people have osteoarthritis *(The Arthritis Society, 1998a)*. For many people it is possible to continue working, with an average of 2.5 days per month lost due to the disease *(Schumacher, 1993)*. For many in the later stages of osteoarthritis, the disease becomes physically and emotionally debilitating. Physician and hospital visits, medication and devices to help activities of daily living are factors in economic costs.

Pathological Process of Osteoarthritis

A synovial joint is composed of hyaline-cartilage-covered bone ends connected by a fibrous joint capsule and reinforced by extra-capsular ligaments. Muscles and tendons cross the joint and control its movement. The joint capsule is lined with synovial tissue, which produces synovial fluid to nourish and lubricate the cartilage.

Healthy cartilage of synovial joints is resilient and able to yield under compression. Once the load on the cartilage is removed, the cartilage recovers its original shape. The resiliency is due to the high water content — up to 80 per cent — of the ground substance that makes up cartilage. Within the ground substance, proteoglycans, molecules that give elasticity to cartilage, are interwoven with collagen fibres.

When slightly stretched during joint motion, muscles that cross a joint function as active shock absorbers as well as movement controllers. This mechanism is important for protecting articular cartilage. For example, up to four times the body weight is transmitted through the knee when walking. Without the energy absorption of gastrocnemius, quadriceps and hamstrings, the energy of normal walking would tear the knee ligaments, severely affecting the cartilage *(Schumacher, 1993)*. Proper coordination of muscle activity is, therefore, important for healthy, moving joints.

With osteoarthritis, the load-bearing portions of articular cartilage are affected first. Repeated stress causes the collagen fibres to break. The cartilage initially responds by increasing both its water content and the number of proteoglycans present in an attempt to repair itself. However, cartilage is avascular and not able to repair itself using the normal inflammatory response. Osteoarthritis in its **early stage** is, therefore, considered non-inflammatory. In the early stage, which may last for years, the cartilage is actually thicker than normal *(Schumacher, 1993)*.

Over time, as the collagen fibres continue to break, proteoglycans are depleted and the cartilage softens and becomes thinner *(Figure 48.1)*. Vertical clefts develop in the cartilage surface. These clefts deepen and small portions of the cartilage fragment off into the synovial fluid. With joint motion, the clefts eventually extend to the subchondral bone which underlies the cartilage. When seen on an X-ray, this loss of cartilage narrows the space between the joint surfaces. The subchondral bone eventually becomes exposed. While cartilage is aneural and does not register pain, subchondral bone is pain sensitive.

In the **later stage**, other changes occur besides the degeneration of cartilage. The subchondral bone remodels and thickens; its exposed surface becomes polished, or eburnated, from the contact of bone on bone. Microfractures and cysts appear below the surface of the bone and weaken it. To support the affected joint, new bone and cartilage grow at the margins of the joint. These bone spurs, or osteophytes, alter the shape of the joint; they may also restrict movement. Vertebral osteophytes can painfully compress nerve roots.

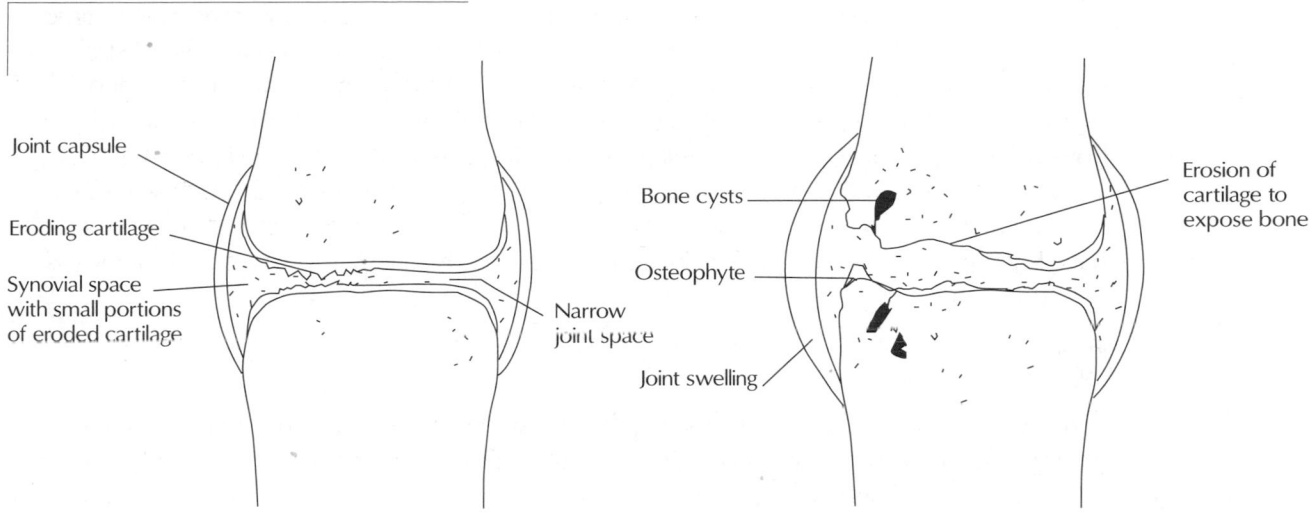

Figure 48.1   Early stage of osteoarthritis.   Later stages of osteoarthritis.

A mild chronic synovitis can occur in the later stage when cartilage fragments and enzymes released by inflammation irritate the synovial lining. The synovium and joint capsule thicken in response to the irritation, reducing range of motion at the joint. Muscle wasting occurs in muscles that cross the affected joint.

Causes of osteoarthritis are:

➤ **idiopathic**, not clearly understood;

➤ **altered biomechanics**, such as leg length discrepancy, congenital hip dislocation, valgus or varus knee orientation, joint hypermobility *(Beighton et al., 1989)* and muscular incoordination;

➤ **immobilization**, which reduces circulation of synovial fluid to the cartilage;

➤ **trauma**, either acute, such as a fracture, or chronic, such as occupational overuse or minor repetitive stress;

➤ **pathology** such as diabetes mellitus and rheumatoid arthritis *(Brandt et al., 1998)*.

Contributing factors include genetic predisposition with Heberden's nodes (distal interphalangeal joint osteoarthritis) and obesity with knee osteoarthritis *(Schumacher, 1993)*.

Gender and racial differences exist for the prevalence of the disease and the joint affected. For example, Black women are twice as likely as Caucasian women to get knee osteoarthritis, and women in general are twice as likely to have this joint affected than men. Osteoarthritis of the hip is less common in Chinese and East Indian populations than in those of Caucasian ancestry.

Medically, diagnosis may be made by health history questioning, physical examination and laboratory tests that differentiate other pathologies. While used in diagnosis, X-rays do not always indicate the degree of cartilage degeneration in the early stages of osteoarthritis. In addition, fewer than one-half of those whose X-rays show degeneration have symptoms of osteoarthritis *(Schumacher, 1993)*.

Osteoarthritis is treated with medication, physical therapy and surgery. Treatment is aimed at controlling pain and maintaining range of motion. Medication is used to manage pain and in later stages to control inflammation. Analgesics include Aspirin and acetaminophen. NSAIDs include ibuprofen and naproxen. Steroid injections are not commonly used. Physical therapy involves strengthening the muscles crossing the affected joints without stressing the joint. In the later stage, protection of the joint is achieved through splint or appliance use. Balanced eating habits are recommended for clients who are obese and have knee joints affected. Client education about the disease is important and therapy is tailored to the individual.

In some cases, synthetic synovial fluid (Synvisc) injected into the joint may bring temporary relief in later stages of the disease.

Surgery in advanced cases includes angulation osteotomy, where joint misalignment — for example, a valgus deformity — is corrected, and joint replacement by prosthetics, especially of the knee and hip.

Symptom Picture

+ While osteoarthritis can occur in people 25 to 34 years of age, it is more common in later decades of life. More than 85 per cent of those over 70 years of age have some degree of osteoarthritis (*The Arthritis Society, 1998a*).

+ Joints can be affected unilaterally or bilaterally.

+ In the **early stage**, cartilage degeneration is initially painless.

+ Later, pain follows extensive joint use and is relieved by rest. The pain is local to the affected joint; it is achy and difficult to pinpoint initially. Reduced range of motion and joint stiffness are noticed in the morning or with periods of immobility and last until the person "works it out" — less than 30 minutes.

+ In the **later stage**, as cartilage erodes, pain-sensitive subchondral bone is exposed. Pain follows moderate joint use; this progresses to pain with minimal active motion, passive motion and even rest. Pain may also occur at night. The joint is locally tender. Crepitus is present with movement. Stiffness and reduced range of motion are present. Contractures form in the joint capsule and in the muscles surrounding the joint; there may be reduced strength in these muscles. There is further reduction in range of motion as a result of osteophyte formation and synovitis. Joint misalignment may result, such as valgus deviation at the first metatarsophalangeal joint. Instability may develop with cartilage erosion at some joints, such as the knee. Periods of acute inflammation may occur, accompanied by muscle spasm and edema. With reduced mobility and activity, the cardiopulmonary system is eventually affected.

Common Osteoarthritis Locations

+ In the **hand**, Heberden's nodes are osteophyte formations at the distal interphalangeal joints, accompanied by lateral joint deviation (*Figure 48.2*). These nodes may develop over years or have a sudden onset following acute inflammation. Bouchard's nodes are

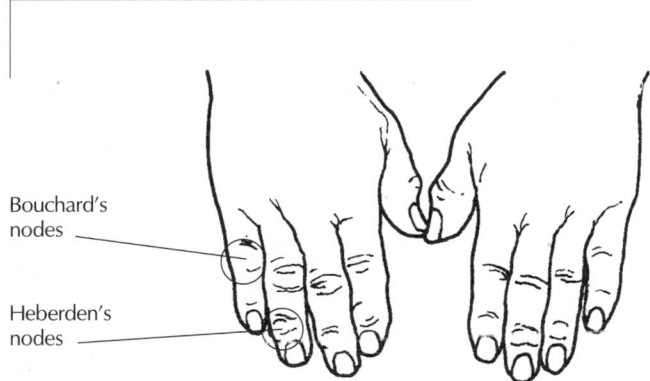

Figure 48.2
Osteoarthritis in the hand.

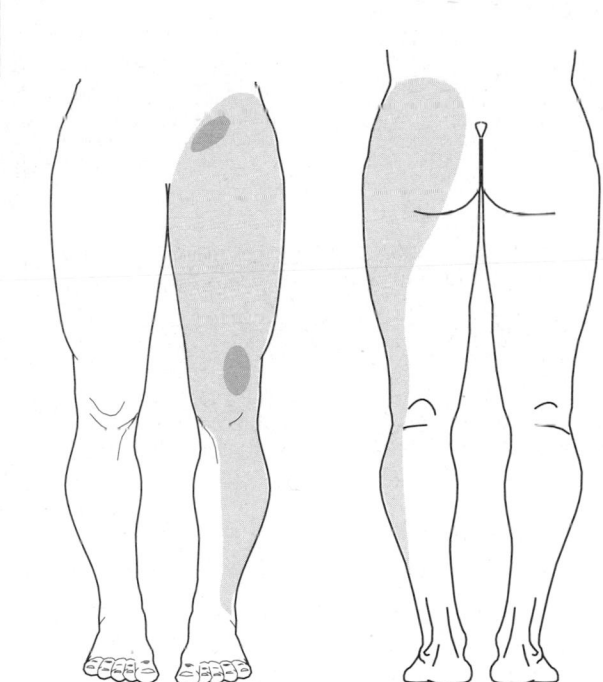

Figure 48.3
Pain locations with OA of the hip: darker areas are most common locations.

found at the proximal interphalangeal joints. The trapezioscaphoid joint is also commonly affected.

✦ In the **spine,** the intervertebral discs, vertebrae and facet joints of L4 to L5, C4 to C7 and the upper thoracic vertebrae are commonly affected. While degeneration of the spine can be asymptomatic, pain and stiffness can occur. Degeneration occurs where the spine experiences the most angular motion; as the intervertebral discs degenerate and become thinner, the facet joints become malaligned, allowing bone to contact bone *(Walker, Helewa, 1996).* Osteophyte formation can lead to narrowing of the intervertebral foramen and spinal stenosis, or narrowing of the spinal canal. Both of these situations can compress the nerve roots, leading to constant or intermittent radicular pain.

✦ In the **hip,** pain has an insidious onset. Internal rotation and extension are reduced. The person walks with a limp. Pain occurs over the groin and adductors, although gluteal and knee pain may occur *(Figure 48.3).* In some cases, there may be compensatory low back pain.

✦ In the **knee,** pain is local to the joint and worse on climbing or standing. Synovitis may occur in the early stage. Crepitus is present on active or passive motion. Cartilage degeneration leads to valgus or varus knee orientation. Muscle atrophy occurs in quadriceps and hamstrings, with the possibility of shortening of the hip flexors on the affected side.

Contraindications

✦ Avoid using heat with acute inflammation.

✦ Exercise caution when applying overpressure with osteophyte formation.

Treatment Considerations

HEALTH HISTORY QUESTIONS

✦ What is the client's general health?

✦ Do any other conditions, such as hypertension, exist?

✦ What joint or joints are affected?

✦ Is there a history of previous injury to the joint?

✦ When was the onset of symptoms?

✦ Is there pain? Stiffness? In the morning? After a period of immobility?

✦ Does stiffness disappear with use?

✦ Has the condition been diagnosed by a physician?

✦ What medications, if any, is the client taking, including self-medication and over-the-counter drugs?

✦ Is the client seeing a chiropractor, physiotherapist or other practitioner for treatment?

Further Assessment

✎ **Observation and Palpation:**

- With a **chronic** presentation, joint enlargement and swelling may be observed. Antalgic posture or gait is present.

- A postural assessment may be performed to determine sources of muscle imbalance.

- Hypertonicity, adhesions and trigger points are palpated in muscles that cross the joint and in compensatory muscles. In later presentations of osteoarthritis, osteophytes, crepitus, fibrosing and disuse atrophy may be present.

- In an **acute** episode, heat, swelling, edema and redness are noted over a superficial joint. This may not be noticed with deeper joints such as the hip.

- Spasm, hypertonicity and trigger points are palpated in muscles crossing the affected joint.

✎ **Testing:**

- **AF ROM** of the affected joint is reduced in most directions due to pain. Pain is experienced throughout the range in an acute episode.

- **PR ROM** reveals a painful, leathery end feel in the capsular pattern for the affected joint; bony end feel may also be present with osteophyte formation. Muscle spasm and empty end feel are present with an acute episode.

- **AR isometric testing** reveals weakness and possibly pain in the muscles crossing the affected joint. A modified blood pressure cuff is used to accurately record strength. See Appendix C for details.

✍ **Differentiating Sources of Joint Pain:**

- Other conditions can mimic the joint pain of osteoarthritis, such as trigger points (*Travell, Simons, 1983*) and tendinitis. It is also important to differentiate osteoarthritis from rheumatoid arthritis, as the treatments are different; see inflammatory arthritides for more information.

- **Trigger point** pain is in the referral pattern for the muscle that contains the taut band and trigger point.

- **Tendinitis** pain is positive with the tendinitis differentiation test.

- **Bursitis** pain is positive with the bursitis differentiation test.

- **Space-occupying lesions** such as a disc herniation or osteophytes which compress peripheral nerves give positive results in radicular patterns with the slump, Spurling's, Kemp's, Kernig's, straight leg raise and upper limb tension tests. Weakness is present in affected muscles.

- **Facet joint irritation** is revealed with a positive Kemp's test.

- The client should be referred to a physician if orthopedic testing results are negative or inconclusive for a neuromuscular source of the pain.

Massage

✋ Treatment goals include reducing stiffness, pain, edema and spasm, increasing range of motion and reducing inflammation if present. In the early stage, the focus is on relieving the compressive forces on the joint if possible. In the later stage, maintenance of tissue health and symptomatic relief are important.

✋ The treatment is a half-hour to one hour in duration, depending on the number of joints affected and the client's overall health. The treatment is in the context of a relaxation massage including **diaphragmatic breathing**. Techniques are used within the client's pain tolerance, especially since this is a chronic, painful condition.

✋ **Positioning** may be prone, sidelying or supine, again depending on client comfort and affected joints.

✋ **Pre-treatment** deep moist heat, such as a wax bath or hydrocollator, is applied before mobilizing or stretching soft tissue contractures, provided no inflammation is present.

✋ Essential oils added to the massage oil or lotion may help with the treatment of osteoarthritis. Lavender can help reduce pain and roman chamomile has anti-inflammatory properties. A 2.5 per cent solution, or 25 drops total of pure essential oil in 50 ml. of carrier oil, is suggested (*Lawless, 1992*).

Early Stage

✋ Pain-free rhythmic techniques, rocking and shaking may be used to begin the treatment. Contralateral and compensatory structures are treated to reduce hypertonicity and trigger points, especially in muscles that cross the affected joint. Working proximal to distal on the affected limb, the therapist should apply soothing Swedish techniques, such as effleurage, stroking and various petrissage techniques, to reduce hypertonicity. Trigger points are treated with muscle stripping and gentle ischemic compressions. Gentle long-axis traction *(Walker, Helewa, 1996)* and Golgi tendon organ release are also indicated.

🖐 Fascial techniques are employed if soft tissue contractures are present *(Souza, 1997)*. Gentle passive stretching, PIR and passive relaxed range of motion are interspersed with Swedish techniques.

🖐 Joint play techniques are used to mobilize the affected joint capsule and encourage the movement of nutrition to the cartilage *(Kisner, Colby, 1996)*. Other conditions, such as postural dysfunctions, are addressed.

Later Stage

🖐 The treatment proceeds as above. When muscle spasm is present, joint play is used to reduce spasm, with caution used with osteophyte formation.

🖐 Cold hydrotherapy to the client's tolerance is used with **acute inflammation**; proximal lymphatic drainage is indicated for both acute and chronic presentations *(Kurz, 1990)*.

🖐 Treatments are of an ongoing nature as this is a chronic, degenerative condition.

Self-care

✍ Appropriate hydrotherapy, such as deep moist heat for chronic presentations or cold for acute episodes, is indicated. Self-massage to the muscles surrounding the affected joint can help to control pain *(Lorig, Fries, 1995)*. Relaxation techniques such as diaphragmatic breathing are also helpful.

✍ Rest from activities which aggravate the joint and relaxation exercises are suggested.

✍ Gentle pain-free stretching and pain-free range of motion are important, as are gravity-reduced activities such as swimming. Especially in the early stage, careful strengthening of muscles that cross the affected joint may relieve the pain. Isometric exercise for muscles crossing the affected joint are progressed to isotonic exercises. It is important to maintain cardiovascular activities; permission may be needed from the client's physician for these exercises. The client should avoid working in ranges of motion that aggravate the joint when exercising; there should be no pain during or after exercise.

✍ Activities of daily living can be made less painful. It is recommended that the client plan the day so that activities or tasks are combined so as to minimize stair climbing or excessive running around. The client should rest when the joint feels irritated *(Lorig, Fries, 1995)*. If a client has one hip joint affected and is using a cane for walking, the cane is used on the opposite side to the affected hip; loads are carried on the affected side *(Walker, Helewa, 1996)*. Special devices to aid in daily activities are available. Door handles can be changed from knobs to lever-type fittings; kitchen implements are now made with large, soft handles for easier gripping.

✍ The client is referred to a physician, physiotherapist, naturopath, nutritionist or the Arthritis Society for assessment, treatment and more self-help information.

✍ Increasingly, people are using complimentary therapies and supplements to control osteoarthritis. These therapies are not always endorsed by the medical establishment, perhaps due to lack of accepted research *(Walker, Helewa, 1996)*. However, acupuncture, used for thousands of years in China, is gaining acceptance for managing arthritis symptoms *(Rodrigues, n.d.)*.

✍ Dietary supplements and modifications are also popular. Glucosamine sulphate is favourably referenced in European medical journals, but is only now being studied in Canada *(Arthritis News, n.d.)*; anecdotal reports find this supplement beneficial.

✍ One study suggests that inflammation may be alleviated by omega-3 fatty acids found in cold-water fish oils *(The Arthritis Society, 1998c)*. Vitamin C supplements and foods containing sulphur such as asparagus and eggs are said to reduce inflammation and repair cartilage and bone. On the other hand, plants in the nightshade family (tomatoes, bell peppers, eggplant and white potatoes) contain solanine, a compound that may cause muscle pain and discomfort *(Balch, Balch, 1997)*.

See also stress reduction, edema, trigger points, spasm, tendinitis, bursitis, inflammatory arthritides, postural dysfunctions and degenerative disc disease for related treatments.

✍ Some people use folk remedies such copper bracelets and vinegar applications around the affected joint; these remedies have not been approved by Western medical authorities.

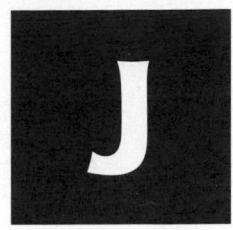

CONDITIONS OF THE CENTRAL NERVOUS SYSTEM

STRATEGIES:
Central Nervous System Conditions

Linda Ludwig

> *The central nervous system (CNS) is comprised of the brain and spinal cord (Figure 49.1). Lesions in this system can result in sensory, motor and autonomic dysfunction.*

Necrosis of the tissue in the CNS results in the formation of scar tissue, which is referred to as a lesion. Specific dysfunctions and their severity are dependent on the cause, location and size of the lesion.

The CNS conditions presented in this section are hemiplegia, multiple sclerosis (MS), Parkinsons (Parkinson's disease or PD), cerebral palsy (CP) and spinal cord injuries (SCI). This chapter examines global signs and symptoms, and treatment goals. A general treatment strategy is provided as well as specific treatment approaches for spasticity and emotional support.

Progressive and Non-progressive Conditions

The dysfunctions that result from a CNS lesion can be progressive or non-progressive. Parkinsons and multiple sclerosis are progressive conditions in the majority of cases. The symptoms and degree of disability increase over time as a result of the disease process.

Hemiplegia, spinal cord injuries and cerebral palsy are non-progressive conditions that result from a trauma, a cerebrovascular accident, a vertebral fracture that injures the spinal cord or a birth trauma. The specific symptoms caused by the lesion do not get worse.

Symptom Severity

The person with any of the above conditions may fully recover or may have permanent disabilities. The disability can range from relatively asymptomatic to severe. It is possible,

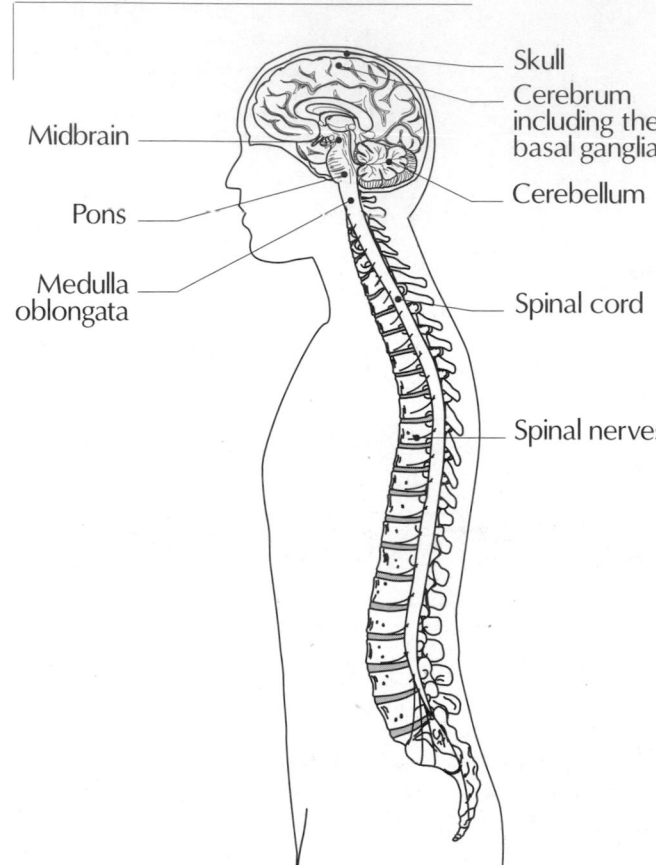

Figure 49.1
The central nervous system.

Labels on figure:
Midbrain
Pons
Medulla oblongata
Skull
Cerebrum including the basal ganglia
Cerebellum
Spinal cord
Spinal nerves

with hemiplegia, that a person may fully recover with no disability. In some cases of benign multiple sclerosis, the person has only a few attacks but fully recovers and remains symptom-free for life. Some people have been found to be asymptomatic for multiple sclerosis all their lives, although lesions are found on autopsy (*Porth, 1990*).

The severity of symptoms varies widely depending on the extent of the lesions. Some people with cerebral palsy, multiple sclerosis and hemiplegia can have relatively mild disabilities, whereas others with the same conditions may need to use a wheelchair and may require constant care.

Secondary symptoms often develop over time, generally causing an increase in dysfunction. For example, altered posture as a result of being in a wheelchair can result in contracture formation in the weak, short or spastic muscles. These contractures can dramatically affect the range of motion of the joints crossed by the contractured muscle. Severe disability can occur in the affected limb as a result. Each client is seen as an individual and the condition is treated according to how that particular client presents.

Symptom Picture

✦ **Motor dysfunctions include:**
- spasticity, rigidity;
- weakness, flaccidity;
- resting tremors, intention tremors.

✦ If the client is ambulatory, **altered gait** may be present. Circumducted gait is often present with hemiplegia or MS. Bradykinesic or festinating gait is a common symptom of Parkinsons. A cane is frequently used on the unaffected side. The person may use a wheelchair.

✦ Decreased **tissue health** and **edema** may be present. These, in turn, can lead to **decubitus ulcers** and other skin ulcers if tissue damage occurs.

✦ **Contractures** develop in short or weak muscles leading to a decrease in the range of motion and limiting function in the affected joints. For example, contractures in the flexors of the hand will cause it to form a fist. But some contractures are encouraged to take a functional form. An example of a functional contracture of the hand is finger flexors which have been splinted to encourage a hook-like shape. This allows for access to the electric wheelchair control stick as well as hooking onto objects. In this case, the therapist would not decrease the contracture since it is actually enhancing the client's function.

✦ Decreased **joint health** results from a lack of successive action in the joint. This is secondary to motor dysfunctions and contractures.

✦ Eventually, **postural imbalances** occur, such as hyperlordosis, hyperkyphosis, head-forward posture and scoliosis. These can lead to altered biomechanics of the joints. Combined soft tissue and joint problems result in numerous secondary conditions in the affected limbs, such as tendinitis, subluxation or dislocation, adhesive capsulitis in the shoulder, peripheral nerve compressions, degenerative disc disease and osteoarthritis.

✦ **Pain** can be a primary symptom of a CNS lesion or a result of secondary conditions.

✦ **Sensory and autonomic dysfunction** can also result from the lesion. There may be areas of paresthesia or dysesthesia. In more severe cases, such as complete spinal cord lesions, total sensory impairment can occur in parts of the body. There may be increased sweating or secretions, primarily with Parkinsons, or general abnormalities in temperature regulation with MS, Parkinsons or SCI.

✦ The sympathetic nervous system may respond excessively to a specific stimulus. This is known as **autonomic dysreflexia** and is usually associated with spinal cord injuries. It is a potentially serious condition.

✦ **Compensatory changes** in unaffected limbs result in muscle hypertonicity and fascial restrictions as well as tendinitis and other overuse syndromes.

✦ **Behaviour and emotional changes** can result, possibly due to neurological damage and possibly due to the significant life changes that have occurred because of the lesion.

✦ **Seizures** are possible whenever a brain lesion is present.

✦ **Speech dysfunction** can be present with most CNS lesions and can cause difficulty with communication. Dysphasia is impaired speech. Aphasia is an inability to speak. Dysphasia may be due to an inability to coordinate the muscles to produce words; the person knows what she wants to say but cannot. On the other hand, aphasia can be a lack of comprehension of the meaning of words.

✦ **Bowel and bladder function** may be affected.

Motor Dysfunctions: Spasticity

Spasticity can exist with hemiplegia, multiple sclerosis, spinal cord injuries and cerebral palsy. Spasticity occurs when there is a loss of inhibition of alpha motor neuron firing. Usually, smooth movement involves a finely tuned adjustment of firing and inhibition of the motor neurons. If a lesion occurs in an area of the CNS which controls movement, inhibition is lost and movement becomes uncontrolled.

Spasticity is often defined as the resistance of a limb to passive movement, if the limb is moved against the patterns of the client's spasticity. It also follows that the client will have excessive involuntary assisted movement when the limb is moved **into** the patterns of spasticity. In both cases, the client is unable to control the movement. The amount of spasticity is variable.

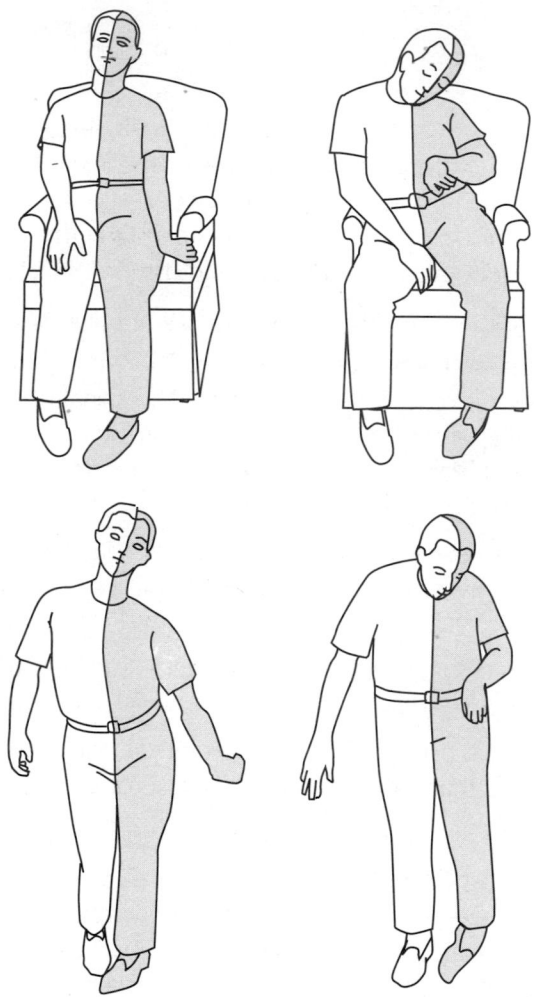

Extensor pattern, sitting   Flexor pattern, sitting

Extensor pattern, standing   Flexor pattern, standing

Figure 49.2
Patterns of spasticity.

Spasticity will appear in particular patterns in the upper and lower body. These are flexor patterns or extensor patterns (*Figure 49.2*). Any combination of patterns is possible (*Lynch, Grisogono, 1991*).

The flexor pattern of the upper body consists of flexion of the client's head and trunk towards the affected side, depression of the shoulder, retraction of the scapula, internal rotation and adduction of the glenohumeral joint, flexion of the elbow, pronation of the forearm and flexion of the wrist and fingers with thumb adduction.

The extensor pattern of the upper body consists of slight extension of the client's neck and head, with the trunk bent away from the affected side. However, the scapula is retracted as with the flexor pattern. There is internal rotation of the glenohumeral joint. The elbow is rigidly extended with pronation of the forearm. The hand is either in flexion forming a tight fist or in flexion at the proximal interphalangeal joints (PIPs) and distal interphalangeal joints (DIPs). The palm faces backwards.

The flexor pattern of the lower body consists of abduction, external rotation and flexion of the hip, flexion of the knee, dorsiflexion and inversion of the ankle and flexion of the toes.

The extensor pattern of the lower body consists of adduction, internal rotation and extension of the hip, extension of the knee and plantarflexion and inversion of the ankle.

In addition to these patterns, the therapist may sometimes observe different movements associated with spasticity, known as **associated reactions:**

✦ The **extensor thrust pattern** causes the person to vigorously extend the limbs while arching the back. It can be triggered by stimulation or pressure to the back of the head or trunk.

✦ The **bite reflex** can accompany the extensor thrust pattern. The teeth are clenched together with extreme force. This is most common with head injuries.

✦ The **positive supporting reaction** is stiffening of the legs in extension or tight flexion. This can occur in response to pressure on the ball of the foot or stretching of the plantar surface of the foot by dorsiflexing the toes.

✦ Stimulus to the palmar surface of the hand can elicit the **grasp reflex** which results in withdrawal of the entire arm into a tightly flexed position.

These reactions are not necessarily present in each client. While taking the health history, the therapist asks the client if she is aware of having any of these associated reactions. This is asked in lay terms, such as, "Do you experience any reactions when the bottoms of your feet or palms of your hands are touched?"

Factors Influencing Spasticity

An individual's spasticity will change according to the position of the limbs, emotional state, physical exertion, autonomic activity and pain, and when certain areas are touched *(Thomson et al., 1991)*. The positioning of the head and torso can increase spasticity. For example, rotation of the head away from the affected side can reinforce flexor patterns in the upper limb whereas turning the head towards the affected side can increase the extensor patterns of the upper limb *(Bobath, 1990)*.

Emotional upsets, such as frustration or fear, difficulties in communication or even meeting a new person, can increase spasticity. With this awareness, the therapist may find that initial testing results will yield spasticity levels higher than usual for the client.

Increased autonomic activity and pain will influence the excitability of the nervous system. Since the person with hemiplegia is unable to moderate and inhibit this excitation, spasticity will increase *(Bobath, 1990)*.

As the client continues the rehabilitation process, spasticity will often diminish or be relatively more controlled. Generally, reducing spasticity will increase functional ability; however in some cases, the spasticity is useful to the client. Spasticity in the legs can assist standing up or with transferring from a wheelchair to a bed. The therapist must not assume that reducing spasticity is an aim of treatment; consent must be given by the client.

Techniques to Reduce Spasticity

A variety of techniques reduce spasticity temporarily:

✦ **Each client will have an individual reaction to each technique. The therapist must discover which methods are the most effective for a particular client.** For example, one client will respond well to gentle, repetitive stroking whereas another will find Golgi tendon organ inhibiting techniques helpful. Yet another client may find that rhythmical rocking actually increases spasticity. It is useful to ask the client if she is aware of a technique that works particularly well.

✦ Each technique should be performed slowly and gently, with soft, broad hand contact. The transition between techniques should be smooth and rhythmical. Movements are **never** forced. Along with the following techniques, hydrotherapy can be used. The response to the particular hot or cold application is individual.

Positioning

Positioning the client in alignment and moving the limbs out of the pattern of spasticity as much as possible can reduce the spasticity. For example, if the client is supine and has a flexor pattern in the upper body, the following positioning can be attempted:

• the head is kept in neutral alignment with the spine, shoulders and pelvis;

• the head and torso are placed in midline;

• the shoulder is pillowed into protraction and slight elevation;

- the glenohumeral joint is brought into slight external rotation and abduction;

- the elbow is brought out of flexion as much as possible. If the client is supine on a massage table, it may be possible to place the arm comfortably and securely in full extension even if this were impossible for the client to do herself;

- the wrist is extended as much as possible;

- the fingers are extended as much as possible. A towel roll is placed in the palm to encourage the hand to stay open.

For the lower limbs, with an extensor pattern, the following position can be attempted:

- the hip is brought forward into flexion. A towel can be used under the back and hip for support;

- the knee is brought into flexion and supported with a pillow;

- the femur is placed into a slightly externally rotated position using a towel or pillow under the lateral thigh.

Massage Techniques

✋ A variety of Swedish techniques applied repeatedly in a slow rhythmical manner can reduce spasticity. For example, stroking, palmar kneading and even vibrations can be applied along the affected limb until the spasticity is reduced.

✋ Slow rhythmical shaking of the limb may be performed. For some clients it is most effective to begin with a rhythmical shaking of the distal limb and slowly bring the shaking to each joint while moving in a proximal direction. For example, shaking is started at the fingers. Then, as they release, the shaking moves to the wrist, the elbow and, finally, the shoulder.

✋ Golgi tendon organ release can reduce a spastic response. This technique works best on easily accessible tendons, especially the Achilles tendon at the ankle, the biceps femoris tendon just above the patella and the hamstring tendons at the knee.

✋ For some clients, stimulation of the antagonist muscle will cause a reflexive release of the spastic muscle. For example, in the arm, firm tapping of the triceps can release spasticity of the biceps muscle.

✋ Passive range of motion of affected joints can be applied. This movement must be performed carefully. If performed too quickly, the stretch reflex will cause the affected muscles to go into their spastic pattern. If the wrist flexors are drawn into a spastic contraction, they will be held in tight flexion. The therapist gently tries to move the wrist into extension as the spasticity releases. The wrist is slowly moved into extension as far as possible without force. The therapist can add a gentle stretch at the end of the pain-free available range to encourage non-spastic movement patterns. This is generally based on the concepts of proprioceptive neuromuscular facilitation therapy (PNF). To enhance its effectiveness, passive range of motion can be combined with the slow application of Swedish techniques. The limb is moved passively until resistance is encountered. Swedish techniques are applied. As the resistance reduces, the limb is moved further.

✋ If the spine is accessible during treatment, stroking down the spine and over the sacrum will decrease sympathetic firing and, in turn, reduce spasticity.

Rigidity

Rigidity is described as resistance to movement in flexion, extension and rotation. It is commonly present in clients with Parkinsons. Rigidity can result in painful cramps as well as pain, numbness and achiness. Unfortunately, Aspirin and other analgesics do not seem to ease the discomfort *(Lieberman, Williams, 1993)*.

Lead pipe rigidity is palpated as a uniform resistance throughout the range of motion of an affected joint.

Cog wheel rigidity is the term used to describe a ratchet-like movement of an affected limb. The limb can be moved a short distance through the range of motion but the movement is interrupted by a tremor. The movement stops for a moment and then can be resumed again. This cycle is repeated throughout the range of motion.

Techniques to Reduce Rigidity

Massage Techniques

- Decreasing sympathetic nervous system firing will help reduce rigidity.
- Swedish techniques such as effleurage and palmar and fingertip kneading are applied to the rigid muscles. These can be followed by an application of heat.
- Slow passive stretches have a positive effect on these muscles.

Subjective Information

HEALTH HISTORY QUESTIONS

- What is the client's general health? Are there other conditions such as hypertension, diabetes and kidney pathologies, all of which require specific treatment modifications? Is there a family history of any of these conditions?

- What is the date of diagnosis? What is the progression of the condition? What are the present symptoms — sensory, motor and autonomic? What is the prognosis of the condition?

- Is the client taking any medications? What are their side effects? Are there any restrictions imposed by the physician? Is the client receiving any treatment currently?

- Is the client experiencing any pain? Where is it? How would the client describe the pain (hot, burning, sharp, achy)? What aggravates the pain and what alleviates the pain?

- What is the client's functional ability? What are the fine and gross motor skills? Is the client independent or relatively dependent in lifestyle? Are aids such as a cane, walker or wheelchair required occasionally or regularly? Is a leg bag used?

- Specific questions for each condition are included in that chapter.

Objective Information

Symptoms and manifestations will vary greatly from one client to another, depending on the condition, its severity and its progression.

Observations

✍ Altered gait, such as circumducted or festinating gait, may be present.

✍ Posture is observed for spasticity or rigidity, noting which limbs are affected and what pattern is present. For example, if spasticity is present the therapist notes if there is a flexor or extensor pattern in the upper body and in the lower body. See Spasticity in this chapter for more details.

✍ Muscle bulk differences may be apparent. These may be noted from one side of the body to another, as with hemiplegia and hemiplegic CP, or from the upper body to the lower body, as with clients using wheelchairs.

✍ Functional ability is easily observed as the client performs actions while at the clinic — removing a coat, holding a pen and writing, standing up and sitting down. The ease of movement is also noted. Ambulation aids that are used also indicate functional abilities — for example, using a cane versus a wheelchair.

✍ Trophic changes of the skin may occur. Edema may be present. The skin may be pale, dry or oily.

✍ Decubitus ulcers may be present, especially in people using wheelchairs or requiring prolonged bedrest. Any red areas, especially over bony prominences, are recorded, as well as reported to the client.

Palpation

✍ Muscle tone is palpated, assessing for the hypertonicity of spasticity or rigidity as well as the hypotonicity of flaccid muscles.

✍ Contractures are likely. These would be present in the agonist in the case of spasticity, in both agonist and antagonist with rigidity and in the unopposed antagonist with flaccidity.

✍ Edematous tissue may be present, especially in the distal extremities due to the lack of movement. Fragility in the overlying tissue may be present if the edema is long-standing. The edematous tissue may be cool due to ischemia. Pitted edema is possible with longstanding edema.

✍ Some areas palpated may feel tender or painful to the client as a result of altered sensation.

✍ Muscle imbalances and altered posture may result in secondary changes. Tenderness, adhesions or signs of inflammation may be palpated as the result of soft tissue or joint pathology or trauma.

Testing

✍ The usual range of motion and strength testing protocol is attempted.

✍ **AF** and **PR ROM** will reveal a decrease in range of motion, if spasticity or rigidity is present. The more severe the spasticity or rigidity, the more severely compromised the range of motion will be. In the most severe cases, no movement is possible.

✍ **AR strength testing** will not yield useful results if spasticity or rigidity is present.

Special Tests

✍ **Pitted edema test** is done.

✍ **Sensory testing** for light touch, deep pressure, pain and temperature perception, two-point discrimination and proprioception is performed. Results will vary depending on the severity of the condition.

✍ Active free and passive relaxed **muscle spasticity grading** will determine the degree of spasticity present.

✍ **Specific orthopedic tests** are performed for secondary conditions such as tendinitis. If spasticity or rigidity is present, the test may not yield viable results.

Treatment Considerations

Positioning

✋ Positioning varies according to the client's presentation and the presence of complications such as hypertension. Prone, supine, sidelying, seated and in wheelchair positions are considered.

Lifting and Transferring

✋ Lifting and transferring the client onto a massage table may be necessary if the client is in a wheelchair. This requires careful consideration by the therapist. First, the therapist establishes how much the client can assist the transfer. Can the client stand temporarily if supported? Does the client have an intention tremor that may affect the transfer? How heavy is the client compared with the therapist? Is someone available to assist the therapist with the transfer if the client is unable to support some of her own weight? If there is any concern that the therapist will have difficulty transferring the client, the treatment is done as an "in chair" massage. The therapist should never risk injury in transferring a client. In fact, whenever possible, the transfers should be performed by two people, even if the client is light in weight. A back injury can happen in a split second.

✋ If the transfer seems possible and reasonable without compromising the client or the therapist, clear communication is of primary importance. The desired outcome of the transfer is explained to the client. For example, the client will be "on the table, on your back with your head at the far end of the table". The client is asked how she usually gets out of her chair and onto a bed. This allows the therapist to use a method that is familiar to the client and to get a sense of how much she can help. The therapist then explains what is to be done. "I'll support you under the arms while you get up on to your feet.

Then you can turn slightly to the right side (pointing out the direction) so that your buttocks are on the table. I will then lift your legs onto the table and help you lay back with your head here (indicate the place)." The therapist also explains that this will be done at the count of three and then counts off, "1, 2, 3"; in this way the actions are coordinated.

When a transfer is performed with the help of another person, the movements are coordinated among all three people. Even if the client is not directly assisting in the transfer, her inclusion in the planning is an affirmation of her importance as a person — she is not simply "something to be moved". Stress levels are reduced when people feel a measure of control. Inclusion in transfer planning and implementation gives this control.

Once on the table, the client is pillowed securely and safely. If edema is present, the affected limb is elevated.

Hydrotherapy

Hydrotherapy applications vary according to the client's presentation. **Extremes of temperature** are avoided if:

- the client's tissue is in poor health;
- edema is present;
- there are skin lesions or ulcers;
- sensory perception is compromised or lost;
- the client has hypertension;
- the client has multiple sclerosis.

The **weight and the location** of the application are also considered and modified as necessary. For example, a hot application on the torso of a person with hypertension is contraindicated because of the stress this places on the heart. Broad hot applications used on a client with MS cause fatigue and, in turn, exacerbate symptoms. In both of these cases, local warm treatments might be used as a modification. Heavy application such as a hydrocollator or thermophore is inappropriate on fragile tissue. If fragile tissue is present, washes might be safe to use.

Treatment Goal	Treatment Plan
	## General Treatment
Decrease sympathetic nervous system firing.	Treatment is in the context of a relaxation massage. Slow, deep breathing is encouraged throughout. Decreasing sympathetic nervous system firing leads to a decrease in many of the symptoms experienced by a person with a CNS lesion, including spasticity, rigidity, both resting tremors (Parkinsons) and intention tremors (multiple sclerosis) and pain (*Thomson et al., 1991*).

Treatment Goal	Treatment Plan

Specific Treatment

Maintain tissue health.

🖐 Tissue health is affected by the decreased functional ability of the client. This affects circulation including venous and lymphatic return. A variety of general Swedish techniques is used to improve circulation and venous return. Pressure, direction and length of the strokes are modified according to sensory loss, dystrophic tissue, spasticity or secondary conditions such as hypertension.

🖐 Edema is commonly found in the distal part of affected limbs. If the client is using a wheelchair, the feet and ankles can be edematous. Elevation of the affected limbs combined with lymphatic drainage techniques and passive range of motion of the joints are indicated. If hypertension or a joint pathology is present, range of motion is performed in mid-range. The therapist is vigilant in identifying decubitus ulcers or any other skin lesion that could easily become infected.

Decrease spasticity and rigidity, temporarily.

🖐 With a clear understanding of the factors that affect spasticity (the position of the person and the limb; the emotional state of the person), a variety of techniques that reduce spasticity is used. Each client will react differently to the techniques and the therapist needs to find the specific techniques that work for each individual client.

🖐 Spasticity is positively influenced by a stress reduction treatment.

🖐 Rigidity is affected by the client's emotional state. With this in mind, the therapist increases the person's overall relaxation. Specific Swedish techniques, such as kneading strokes, followed by heat are applied to the achy, rigid muscles to help the client feel more comfortable (*Lieberman, Williams, 1993*).

Maintain joint health and range of motion.

🖐 Movement dysfunctions can drastically affect the full range of motion. Subsequently, through a lack of successive action, joint health is compromised.

🖐 Contractures eventually form in the shortened, weak muscles. This leads to a further decrease in range of motion. The more compromised the range of motion, the more compromised the functional ability of the joint and, ultimately, the limb. The therapist uses passive range of motion to maintain and, if possible, increase the range of motion of affected joints. This exercise will also maintain joint health. Passive stretches are applied to specific shortened muscles in an attempt to prevent contracture formation.

Address secondary postural changes.

🖐 Movement disorders result in muscle imbalances and alterations in biomechanics. These lead to a variety of secondary conditions, which are often painful. Tendinitis, adhesive capsulitis, dislocations, peripheral nerve compression syndromes, headaches, hyperkyphosis, hyperlordosis, scoliosis and pain in the shoulder, hip and knees are only some of the possibilities. The use of aids such as canes, walkers

659

Treatment Goal

Treatment Plan

and wheelchairs (see the Ambulation Aids chapter) contributes to secondary changes.

✋ For the most part, these conditions are treated as usual with modifications to pressure and length of treatment. For example, trigger points are treated in the least invasive way using repetitive petrissage or gently, gradually applied ischemic compressions. Frictioning of adhesions in a tendinitis is progressive over several treatments. The pressure used is moderate or light in some areas and increased gradually. Strokes are applied segmentally versus long and dragging.

Provide emotional support.

✋ When a person who was able becomes less able or disabled, there is a major emotional impact as she redefines her concept of self. This process will be different for each individual and some people will be more successful than others. Some people will not be able to come to terms with the new self. Eventually, however, most people do develop a new self-image leading to dynamic and satisfying lives.

✋ A person goes through a period of adjustment after a life-altering incident. Many people experience a period of self-blame. Self-esteem and self-worth can diminish as the person feels helpless and dependent. Apathy can arise and confusion can result due to the impairment of memory, movement or sensory perception.

✋ During this process and beyond, the therapist can focus on providing emotional support to the client. Giving emotional support means actively listening to the client and offering encouragement of, and support for, the client's belief in overcoming her disability *(Heart and Stroke Foundation of Ontario, N.d.e.)*. Emotional support can also be conveyed through the therapist's hands. Rather than a specific technique, it is developed as a quality of touch and the intent to be supportive.

Encourage whole body integration.

✋ It is important for the client's optimal recovery that she be actively aware of the affected areas of her body. This awareness can be promoted during the massage process.

✋ When one side is weaker than the other (with hemiplegia, MS and possibly Parkinsons, SCI and cerebral palsy), the therapist stands on the affected side of the client so the client must look towards that side.

✋ The therapist can reinforce sensory stimulation through massage techniques by asking the client questions such as, "How is this pressure?" or "Is this tender?", while working on the affected side.

✋ When the therapist performs passive movement, the client is encouraged to visualize and feel the movement. If possible, she is asked to do the same movement on the unaffected side while the

Treatment Goal	Treatment Plan

therapist continues on the affected side. Actions can be verbally reinforced by explaining clearly and simply what is being done.

🖐 Slow bilateral stroking or muscle squeezing from the head along both sides of the body to the feet is incorporated at any point in the massage. The therapist may wish to begin and end the massage in this way.

Self-care Goal	Self-care Plan

✍ **Self-care, treatment frequency** and **prognosis** are specific to each condition. See the individual chapters.

COMMUNICATION SKILLS

Linda Ludwig

It is essential that the therapist remember that the degree of a person's physical disability does not indicate the person's level of intelligence. Negative stereotypes and images in our culture are damaging to persons with disabilities; respect and caring should be shown at all times. The client is an individual; a therapist needs to see the person first rather than the disability.

Using Appropriate Terminology

Medical terms such as hemiplegic or spastic are used to describe the condition and symptoms of a client with a CNS lesion. It is important not to label the person with these terms.

Identifying a client by the disability diminishes him as a person. Therefore, therapists should avoid saying "my hemiplegic client" or, even worse, "my hemiplegic". Instead, by saying "my client who has hemiplegia", the client is identified as a person first. Terms such as "inflicted with", "victim of", "crippled" or "invalid" also reinforce the sense that these clients should be pitied. It is more appropriate to say the client "has a particular condition" which was "caused by" a particular accident or pathology.

If the client uses a wheelchair, referring to this as "wheelchair bound" focuses on limitations. Saying the person "uses a wheelchair" states the fact with no judgement.

If the therapist feels uncertain about how to refer to an aspect of the client's condition, the client can be told this directly and then asked what terms should be used. Often he will offer the preferred terminology.

Communication Strategies

A client's eyesight, hearing and speech may be affected as a result of a CNS lesion. The therapist needs to be creative and flexible in order to communicate effectively with these clients.

Visual impairments can include diplopia (double vision), nystagmus (a constant, involuntary, cyclical motion of the eyeball) and even blindness (*Taber's Cyclopedic Medical Dictionary, 1981*). If a visual impairment is present, in addition to the consent to treatment, the therapist clearly explains the treatment as it is proceeding so the client experiences no surprises.

In the case of a **hearing impairment** or loss, writing is often a necessary form of communication. If the client is unable to write, a symbol board may be used.

A variety of **speech dysfunctions** can occur, such as dysphasia (slurred speech or an inability to pronounce certain words), aphasia (a pronounced loss of the ability to speak, grasp simple concepts or follow simple instructions) and dysarthria (an incoordination of the muscles affecting speech), among others. If the person is unable to verbalize, specialized systems of communication may be used, such as symbol boards and electronic voice synthesizers.

If the client has a speech or **comprehension difficulty**, the following communication skills are useful (*Heart and Stroke Foundation of Ontario, N.d.c*). Each client has different needs, so the therapist is encouraged to experiment to determine the techniques that are most effective for the individual.

✦ The therapist should speak slowly and clearly rather than loudly. Aphasic people need more time to follow and process what they are hearing.

✦ Short, clear sentences are more easily understood. Therefore, complex ideas or instructions should be avoided.

✦ Repetition can be helpful when trying to describe a particular task.

✦ The therapist should not be condescending. It is possible the person with aphasia or dysphasia understands more than it appears. Difficulty in communicating and the severity of physical disability do not necessarily reflect the person's ability to comprehend.

✦ The therapist needs to take time to think out what will be said to the client. Understanding is improved if the task to be done, such as the positioning for a massage, is described in a clear and logical sequence.

✦ Using gestures and looking at the client when speaking are helpful. Writing, pictures or photographs can also be used to convey messages.

✦ Background noise should be kept to a minimum. If music is usually playing, it should be turned off while asking questions or explaining things to the client.

✦ The client can be helped to use hand signals or gestures to show that he understands. If necessary, the client can be guided through the process of doing the gesture, first by watching the therapist demonstrate it, then by trying to imitate the gesture.

✦ A client who mimics or passively repeats what has been said may have echolalia — a possible symptom of hemiplegia. This should not be mistaken for actual understanding.

AMBULATION AIDS

Linda Ludwig

Information regarding functional ability may be gathered by observing the ambulation aids used by a client. These include canes, walkers, wheelchairs and scooters.

Canes and Walkers

If ambulation is possible, canes and walkers are used to support the lower limbs or to assist balance. Upper body strength and coordination are necessary for using a cane. Generally, the cane is held on the unaffected or stronger side. When taking a stride, the person shifts the weight of the body to this side to create stability. The affected leg is then swung forward. Ideally, the cane reaches up to the level of the greater trochanter, allowing for about 20 degrees of elbow flexion in the supporting arm *(Braddon, 1996)*.

Less upper body strength and coordination are required for using a walker. It offers maximum support for ambulation but results in slower movement.

Wheelchairs

Wheelchairs are used when ambulation is difficult or impossible. Manual wheelchairs require upper body strength and coordination. They offer a form of exercise for the person but are not suitable if fatigue is a concern.

A motorized wheelchair is used if a manual wheelchair cannot be propelled due to inadequate strength and coordination of the upper body. Movement of the chair is controlled with a joystick located on the arm rest. A chin or mouth control mechanism can be used if there is limited upper body control.

Scooters are electronic chairs with three or four wheels. Movement and direction are controlled by a T-shaped handlebar situated in front of the seat. Generally, the person using

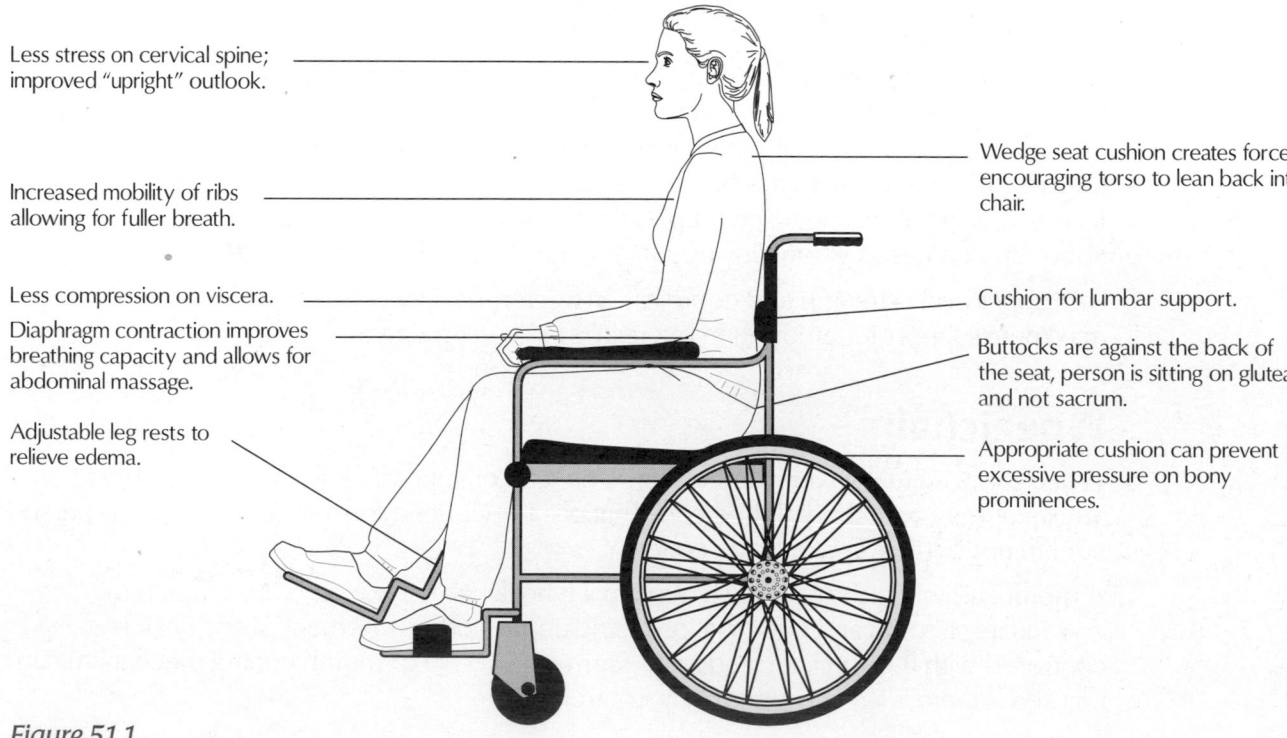

A. Compromised Positioning

"Depressed" posture with shoulders collapsed in.

Breathing is compromised from hyperkyphosis and compressed diaphragm. Susceptibility to respiratory conditions.

Constant pressure on viscera increase constipation and incontinence.

Compressed diaphragm also contributes to constipation and edema in legs through lack of abdominal movement.

Dependent edema with prolonged sitting.

Tension in neck and shoulders caused by cervical lordosis and head-forward posture.

Back is convex and rigid.

Pain in lumbar and gluteal areas caused by prolonged sitting and poor positioning.

Potential for decubitus ulcers over bony prominences.

B. Optimal Positioning

Less stress on cervical spine; improved "upright" outlook.

Increased mobility of ribs allowing for fuller breath.

Less compression on viscera.

Diaphragm contraction improves breathing capacity and allows for abdominal massage.

Adjustable leg rests to relieve edema.

Wedge seat cushion creates force encouraging torso to lean back into chair.

Cushion for lumbar support.

Buttocks are against the back of the seat, person is sitting on gluteals and not sacrum.

Appropriate cushion can prevent excessive pressure on bony prominences.

Figure 51.1
(A) Compromised and (B) optimal positioning.

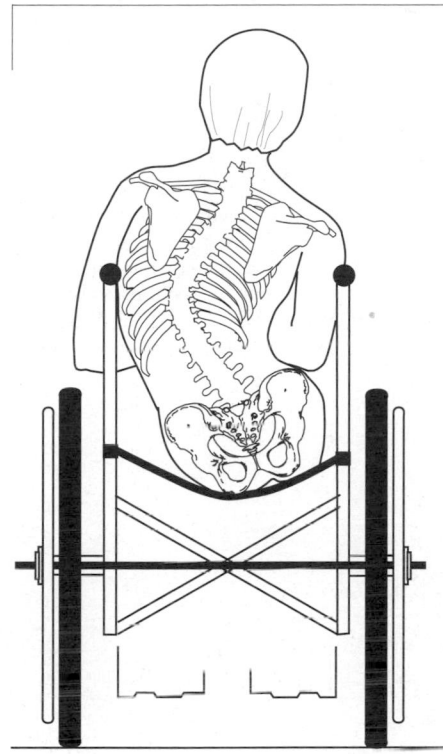

Figure 51.2

Sling seat of a standard chair, as well as improper support of sitting posture, can lead to scoliosis.

a scooter is capable of transferring herself in and out of the chair. She has some ability to walk but lacks the endurance to go long distances or use a manual wheelchair.

Treatment Considerations

With cane, walker and wheelchair use, compression and overuse syndromes, pain, trigger points and muscle hypertonicity develop in the shoulder, arm and hand controlling the device. Clients using a wheelchair can also experience neck pain in the sternocleidomastoid, scalene, upper trapezius and suboccipital muscles due to hypertonicity and trigger points. Pain is caused by overuse of these muscles for balance when in the chair *(Figure 51.1)*. All overuse syndromes are treated in the usual manner with modifications made for the client's specific condition.

Dependent edema occurs in the lower limbs and feet for those using wheelchairs. Elevation is encouraged throughout the day. Some chairs have adjustable leg rests. Supportive socks can be worn to prevent the edema. Lymphatic techniques are performed.

Decubitus ulcers can result with prolonged sitting, which places excessive pressure on tissue. This is especially likely over bony prominences such as the lower lumbar spine, the sacrum and the ischial tuberosities. Frequent changes of position are encouraged. Air cell or gel cushions can relieve some of the pressure on high risk areas.

Postural imbalances such as scoliosis and hyperkyphosis develop from poor positioning in the wheelchair. Scoliosis can appear when there is a tendency to collapse on the weaker side *(Figure 51.2)* or if the chair has a "sling" or soft seat *(Braddon, 1996)*. A structural support is added to the chair or a pillow is placed on the convex side of the scoliosis. A solid seat cushion encourages a midline position of the torso.

Hyperkyphosis results with "sacral seating" and the tendency to slump forward from weak truck extensors.

A solid seat cushion or a wedge-shaped cushion can be used with the thick edge placed under the knees.

Treating a Client in a Wheelchair

The therapist checks that the castor wheels (the small wheels on the front) are aligned with the large wheels and facing forward. With a manual chair, the brakes must be on; with a motorized chair the power may be turned off or care is taken not to hit the joystick. The arm rests and neck support are removed. The therapist carefully notes how to replace these parts after the massage.

Pillows are placed in any area that requires support. If the back is being treated, the client leans forward on pillows placed on a table. When the anterior chest is treated, a pillow is

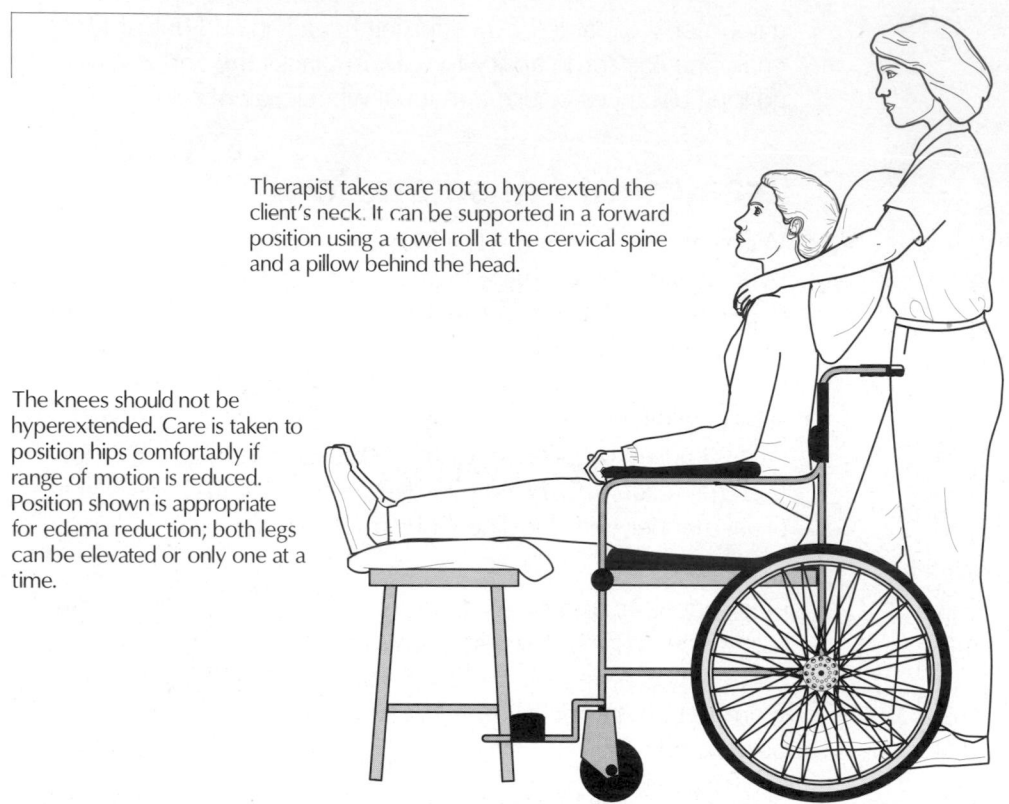

Therapist takes care not to hyperextend the client's neck. It can be supported in a forward position using a towel roll at the cervical spine and a pillow behind the head.

The therapist must take care not to stress her posture by hunching over or arching the low back while massaging. Frequent changes of position are optimal.

The knees should not be hyperextended. Care is taken to position hips comfortably if range of motion is reduced. Position shown is appropriate for edema reduction; both legs can be elevated or only one at a time.

Figure 51.3
In-chair massage.

placed between the therapist and the client. The client is assisted to lean back onto the pillow. The therapist reaches over the shoulders of the client to treat the pectoral muscles, shoulder and upper arm *(Figure 51.3)*.

If edema is present in the legs, the therapist raises the leg supports if possible. Elevation can also be achieved using a stool and pillows, or the therapist can be seated with pillows on her lap and the client's legs placed in her lap. There may be restrictions in hip movement. The leg is moved into an elevated position slowly, with consideration shown for the end of range of hip flexion. The leg is not forced beyond this point. Care is taken not to place the knee in hyperextension. The usual hydrotherapy, passive range of motion and lymphatic drainage techniques are employed. Some therapists may be skeptical about the effectiveness of treating edema in a seated position. In clinical practice, pre- and post-treatment measurements have demonstrated successful temporary reduction of edema.

DECUBITUS ULCERS

Linda Ludwig

Decubitus ulcers, also called "pressure sores", are skin lesions caused by an external pressure, shearing or friction force that is sufficient to locally impair circulation and lymphatic flow in susceptible individuals. The lesions may result in ulcerations.

Throughout history, decubitus ulcers have plagued those with disabilities and chronic illnesses. The duration and intensity of pressure are two factors that affect the severity of a pressure sore. Pressure as little as 33 mm Hg can effectively block venous return and removal of metabolic waste, leading to edema and local tissue injury *(Ozer, 1988)*. Low pressure can cause damage if it is applied over several hours. Higher pressure can cause tissue damage in only a few minutes. In either case, this leads to ischemia and irreversible tissue damage due to a deficiency of oxygen to the cells (known as hypoxia) and a retention of toxic metabolic waste. Pressure sores are serious if left untreated, leading to septicemia and even death *(Porth, 1990)*. Most pressure sores are preventable (up to 95 per cent) if susceptible people are identified and a specific prevention program is undertaken *(Simpson et al., 1996)*.

Causes of decubitus ulcers are:

➤ **pressure** from prolonged immobilization or use of a wheelchair;

➤ **friction** damage, which usually strips away the epidermis, such as if the skin over the elbow or heel is rubbed against sheets when someone is moved in bed. Usually a shallow dermal ulcer results. Though this type of sore is less serious initially, the area becomes more susceptible to pressure;

➤ **shear forces** that torque tissue in opposite directions, such as when a person lying in a semi-supine position slips down the bed. The epidermis is often stationary while the underlying tissue moves forward. This force damages the capillaries; tissue damage follows. Full-thickness ulcers can occur, particularly over the sacral area and heel.

Factors Contributing to the Development of Decubitus Ulcers

Sensory perception and motor losses, which are present with people who have neurological disorders, such as spinal cord injuries, place these people at risk. Due to the loss of sensation, these clients may not notice the development of pressure sores and, in turn, may not take action to reduce excessive pressure. With motor losses, the person may be unable to change position without assistance. Those restricted to bed or to a sitting position are at greater risk for developing pressure sores *(Simpson et al., 1996)*.

Persons with **severely compromised tissue health** through illness, such as elderly persons who are bedridden and those who have long-term, severe diabetes mellitus, are also prone to decubitus ulcers. Those who smoke seem to be four times more susceptible to pressure sores than non-smokers *(Simpson et al., 1996)*. In addition, conditions that result in edema compromise metabolic exchange and contribute to toxin retention.

Incontinence can be a contributing factor, because enzymes in urine and fecal matter can compromise local tissue health. This area is then more vulnerable to developing a decubitus ulcer. Generally, any amount of moisture on exposed skin could put a susceptible person at risk.

Poor nutrition, such as inadequate protein intake, and vitamin deficiencies, such as in vitamin C, vitamin B12, iron and zinc, can lead to poor tissue health *(Simpson et al., 1996; Webster, 1991)*.

Medication including tranquillizers, sedatives and opiates reduce a person's sensory perception and mobility, increasing the risk of pressure sores. The anti-inflammatory property of steroids causes a disruption in the normal healing process of damaged tissue, reducing tissue health.

Symptom Picture

✦ Pressure sores commonly occur over bony prominences, especially the sacrum and ischial tuberosity, as well as the greater trochanter, spinous processes, calcaneus and elbow *(Figure 52.1)*.

✦ As with other types of wounds, decubitus ulcers can be classified as partial- or full-thickness wounds.

• **Stage 1:** The earliest stage of a pressure sore is evident with local erythema, accompanied by palpable warmth and a hardened swelling over the fragile but intact tissue. Usually, the redness associated with areas where pressure is applied will diminish upon release of the pressure, often within a few minutes. A sign that a pressure sore may be developing is if the erythema does not resolve after 30 minutes of pressure release *(Krasner, 1990)*. Discolouration is often red, but may be reddish-brown, even purple-blue. At this stage, the edema and erythema are reversible but require intervention.

• **Stage 2:** More tissue damage occurs, with the epidermis and often the dermis being affected. This is classified as partial-thickness damage. A blister, abrasion or shallow

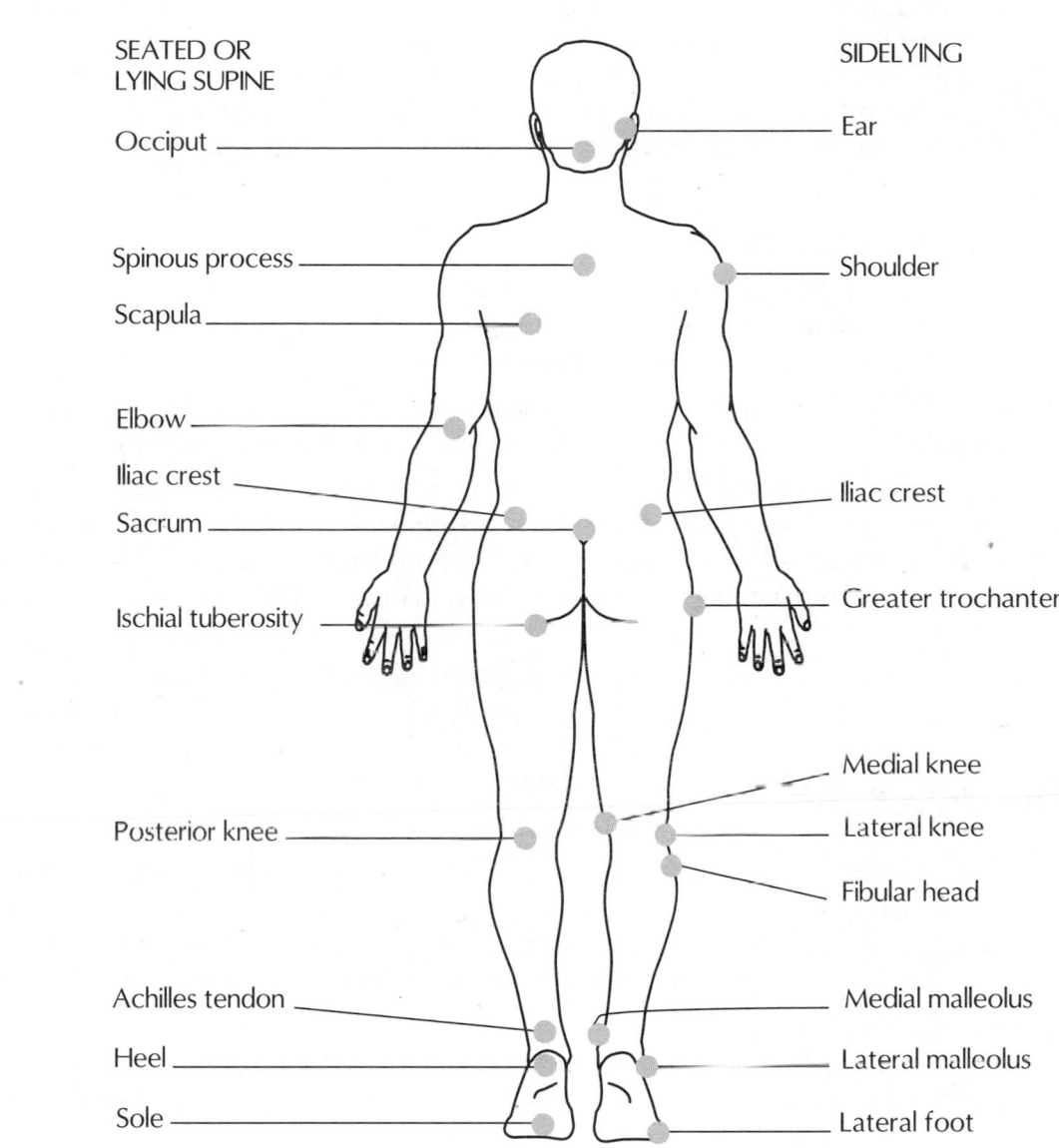

SEATED OR
LYING SUPINE

SIDELYING

Occiput — Ear

Spinous process — Shoulder

Scapula —

Elbow —

Iliac crest — Iliac crest

Sacrum —

Ischial tuberosity — Greater trochanter

Medial knee

Posterior knee — Lateral knee

Fibular head

Achilles tendon — Medial malleolus

Heel — Lateral malleolus

Sole — Lateral foot

Figure 52.1
Areas at risk of developing pressure sores.

ulcer may be present. The area is moist, pink and painful.

- **Stage 3:** Full-thickness damage involves skin loss down to the subcutaneous layers. A cavity is created. There may be exudate and a crust over the cavity. The crust, referred to as eschar, is thick and leathery necrotic tissue.

- **Stage 4:** The most severe lesion includes not only full-thickness tissue damage but also necrosis to underlying muscle and bone. A deep cavity may be covered with a crust and lead to sepsis *(Fernandez, 1987)*.

✦ Infection is a risk whenever the epidermis is interrupted.

✦ Healing of the ulcerated area is through the inflammatory response. In stages 3 and 4, debridement of the tissue — removal of the necrotic tissue — is necessary to promote better healing. Occasionally, surgery is used to remove the ulcer if it is full thickness and larger than two centimetres in diameter *(Webster, 1991)*. In such cases, a full-thickness skin graft may be used to replace the tissue lost from ulceration. Treatment usually occurs over several weeks or often months and is carefully monitored. To prevent a repeat occurrence, the cause is determined and eliminated, if possible.

Prevention Is the Key

Prevention of decubiti is extremely important, since treatment is difficult and time-consuming. There is often an extended absence from work, even hospitalization if the ulcer is severe. Healing may require months.

Changing position regularly, or having someone do this for the person, is essential. The frequency of position changes depends on how susceptible the person is.

The initial positioning of a person should be done properly and then maintained to avoid shear forces and excessive pressure over bony prominences. Extra padding or sheepskin is used if one is in bed for a prolonged time; a gel cushion is useful in dispersing pressure with prolonged sitting. Friction to the skin is avoided through careful movement and lifting of the person.

Proper nutrition and adequate hydration will promote better tissue health and healing, especially a diet high in calories and protein *(Krasner, 1990)*. Vitamin deficiencies must be corrected, especially that of vitamin C, zinc, iron or vitamin B12 *(Simpson, et al., 1996)*.

The skin is kept dry and clean.

The person and any care givers must be vigilant for the early signs of a pressure sore. Mild pressure sores are reversible, but even with these, by the time the sore is noticed a large amount of damage to the intervening tissue has occurred.

Care is taken so clothing, shoes, orthoses and wheelchairs are properly fitted with no areas of excessive friction or pressure.

Contraindications

◆ Local massage is contraindicated once a decubitus ulcer begins to develop, with heat, redness and swelling apparent. If a sore is detected during massage, the client and any care givers are informed immediately so medical attention is received as soon as possible.

Treatment Considerations

Before Decubitus Ulcer Development

🖑 The therapist should monitor the skin and tissue health of those clients at risk for pressure sores.

🖑 To prevent pressure sores from developing, local circulation is promoted. Circulatory techniques such as effleurage and petrissage are performed, taking into account tissue fragility. Modifications are made to the pressure used and techniques are applied segmentally to avoid drag on the tissue. A study was conducted to assess the effectiveness of massage (with soap and water) performed by nurses on the pressure areas in elderly patients. The control group was not treated with massage. A 38 per cent reduction of pressure sores resulted in the control group *(Fernandez, 1987)*. The contradictory results reflect the potential danger of applying overly vigorous massage on fragile tissue and they reinforce the importance of appropriate technique applications. Moreover, the medium of the massage in this study — soap and water — can dry out and crack the skin. This increases susceptibility to the development of pressure sores *(Krasner, 1990)*.

- Lymphatic drainage massage is important to reduce edema and beneficial in preventing pressure sores *(Bader, 1990)*. Lymphatic drainage techniques include appropriate nodal pumping followed by stationary circles and unidirectional effleurage.

After Decubitus Ulcer Development

- In the early stages, the client and care giver are told immediately.

- Hydrotherapy applications of cold for five-minute intervals, through the day, can be used to decrease swelling. In the case of only epidermis and dermis damage, treatment primarily involves the relief of the pressure. Preventative measures are used to stop further tissue damage.

- Local massage is contraindicated.

- **Medical attention is required immediately.**

See also edema, spinal cord injury, cerebral palsy, hemiplegia, multiple sclerosis, Parkinsons, diabetes mellitus and fractures.

SEIZURES

Linda Ludwig

A seizure is characterized by the spontaneous, uncontrolled, abnormal discharge of neurons in the brain.

A seizure is not a disease but a symptom of an existing disorder that affects the brain. It is important to note that seizures and epilepsy are not necessarily the same thing. Seizures can be caused by trauma to the brain or a variety of other conditions, such as head trauma, drug and alcohol abuse, infections and cerebrovascular lesions. In some cases, the cause is metabolic abnormalities, as with toxemia in pregnancy, hypoxia and the rapid withdrawal of drugs. In children, a fever of over 104 degrees Fahrenheit can result in seizures. In fact, anyone is capable of having a seizure.

Epileptic seizures are spontaneous and have an irreversible cause.

Causes of epilepsy can be:

➤ primary (idiopathic);

➤ secondary to cerebral scarring from a head injury, birth trauma, infection or CVA (cerebrovascular accident). Epilepsy often coexists with cerebral palsy. There are many types of epilepsy, depending on the specific part of the brain that is involved.

Various types of epilepsy exist in about 0.5 per cent of the total population *(Hueston, Tubiana, 1985)*.

In susceptible individuals, certain stimuli may be triggers for epileptic seizures. These stimuli may be flashing lights, patterns on material or walls, touch, noise, perfumes or essential oils, a lack of sleep, pain or an altered body chemistry due to food allergies. It is generally agreed that emotional stress can precipitate a seizure *(Hopkins, 1994)*.

Types of Seizures

There are various types of seizures:

✦ With **partial seizures**, there is no impairment of consciousness; an aura or prodromal symptoms are the only manifestation. It is possible that a partial seizure could lead to a generalized seizure.

✦ **Generalized seizures** include what are often referred to as petit mal and grand mal seizures:

- **Petit mal** is also known as an absence seizure. The symptoms include a blank stare, a transient loss of consciousness and an increase or decrease in postural muscle tone. They may last for a few seconds to almost a minute.

- **Grand mal** is also referred to as a tonic-clonic seizure. In this case, there are tonic contractions of muscles, loss of consciousness and bladder and bowel incontinence, followed by bilateral, rhythmic contraction and relaxation of the limbs.

After the seizure there is a slow return to consciousness *(Porth, 1990)*. The person recovering from the episode may experience confusion, and fatigue may last a few days.

Medical treatment involves addressing the underlying cause of the seizures, if possible. Anticonvulsant medication such as Tegretol and Dilantin, can be taken for the condition, with 60 to 80 per cent of people experiencing good seizure control *(Porth, 1990)*. Initially though, finding the proper dose can be a long and frustrating process.

Symptom Picture

Seizures may include the following:

✦ There may be altered motor activity.

✦ An aura or prodromal symptoms may include sensory, visual and auditory disturbances.

✦ Autonomic symptoms may manifest such as flushing, pupillary change and tachycardia.

✦ Following the seizure the person is often disoriented and fatigued for a few days.

✦ **Status epilepticus** is a seizure that does not stop spontaneously or seizures that occur in a rapid succession without recovery of full consciousness. It is considered a medical emergency if this occurs with the tonic-clonic type of seizure because cardiorespiratory failure can result due to hypoxia. A primary cause of this serious condition in a person who is already diagnosed with epilepsy is non-compliance with medication use *(Porth, 1990)*.

Contraindications

✦ Deep, vigorous or painful techniques that increase sympathetic nervous system firing are contraindicated. New treatment techniques and hydrotherapy should be introduced gradually, to avoid triggering a seizure.

Treatment Considerations

HEALTH HISTORY QUESTIONS

- ✦ What is the seizure type experienced?

- ✦ When was the last seizure?

- ✦ What are the frequency and severity of the seizures?

- ✦ Is medication used? If so, are the seizures controlled?

- ✦ Has the client ever experienced status epilepticus? What were the circumstances surrounding the episode?

- ✦ What are the triggers of the client's seizures? If possible, they are removed from the treatment environment.

- ✦ A verbal contract is suggested to establish a protocol should the client have a seizure during treatment. The protocol may involve the client signalling the seizure onset. It may entail an agreement to send the client to a hospital if the seizure is prolonged (longer than 10 minutes), if an injury occurs, or if the client stops breathing.

Massage

🖐 If the client's seizures usually involve large, uncontrolled movements, the therapist may offer to perform the massage on a mat on the floor. As much as possible, the treatment environment should be made safe by the removal of any sharp or dangerous objects that could injure the client. Pillows are kept nearby to place between the client and anything that could harm her, in case a seizure occurs.

🖐 The massage treatment will not be specifically for the seizures. The focus of treatment will reflect the client's request but is performed in the context of a stress reduction massage modified for the possibility of seizures. Slow, gentle techniques are indicated, avoiding abrupt actions.

🖐 If a seizure occurs during treatment:

- The therapist should not leave the room but should stay with the client. The primary concern is the client's safety. The therapist does not try to control the movements but simply prevents the client from hitting anything. If possible, the client is placed in the recovery position.

- Nothing is placed between the client's teeth or administered to her. The seizure is timed and heart rate and breathing are monitored. After the seizure stops, the client is given time to recover.

See also hemiplegia, cerebral palsy and stress reduction for related treatments.

54

HEMIPLEGIA

Linda Ludwig

Hemiplegia is a non-progressive condition of paralysis on one side of the body as a result of a brain lesion.

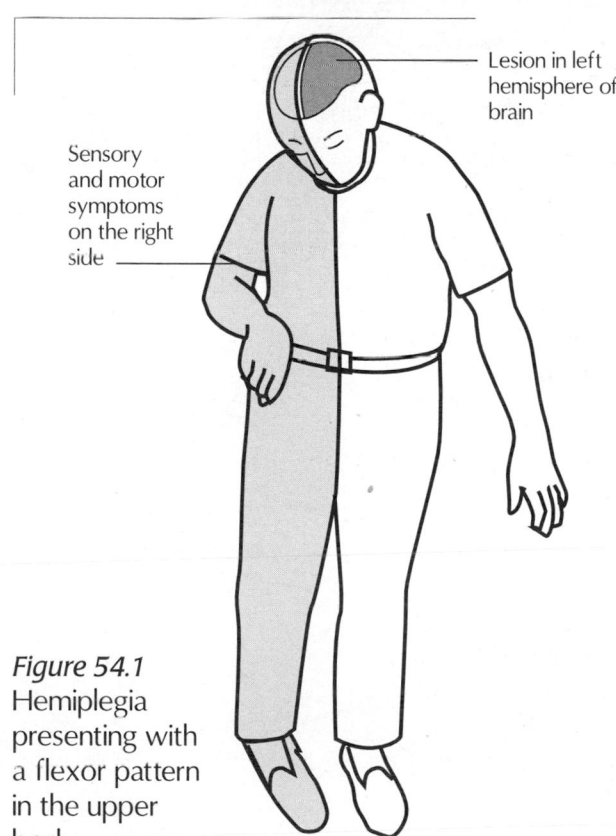

Lesion in left hemisphere of brain

Sensory and motor symptoms on the right side

Figure 54.1 Hemiplegia presenting with a flexor pattern in the upper body.

Hemiplegia occurs on the side of the body **opposite** to the side on which the brain lesion has occurred. Therefore, a left-sided cerebrovascular accident will result in right-sided hemiplegia and vice versa *(Figure 54.1)*. Hemiplegia that results from a cerebrovascular accident is also referred to as a stroke; a stroke that lasts for less than 24 hours is called a transient ischemic attack (TIA). After this type of an attack, there are no residual symptoms *(Thomson et al., 1991)*.

Depending on the location and extent of damage to the brain, the effects on the person with hemiplegia may be temporary or permanent. They also range from almost imperceptible to severely disabling with profound spasticity and extreme sensory or perceptual loss. The body will attempt some repair to those areas of the brain whose functions have been disturbed by the interruption of blood flow. Neighbouring arteries will grow larger and take over the damaged artery's work. In turn, this allows recovery of some of the affected nerve cells. Recovery from embolism or thrombosis in a small artery is usually better than recovery from a ruptured artery (*Heart and Stroke Foundation of Canada, 1993*).

Causes of hemiplegia are:

➤ **cerebrovascular pathology** such as cerebral thrombus, cerebral hemorrhage due to aneurysm and cerebral embolism. These are the most common causes of strokes which result in hemiplegia. Thrombic strokes account for up to 66 per cent of cases, whereas embolisms account for 5 to 14 per cent and hemorrhage for 14 to 20 per cent (*Porth, 1990*);

➤ **head trauma**, as a result of a fall or motor vehicle accident (MVA), which can result in a cerebral hemorrhage, leading to hemiplegia;

➤ **a brain tumour**, which can result in an erosion of blood vessels, causing cerebral hemorrhage and, in turn, hemiplegia.

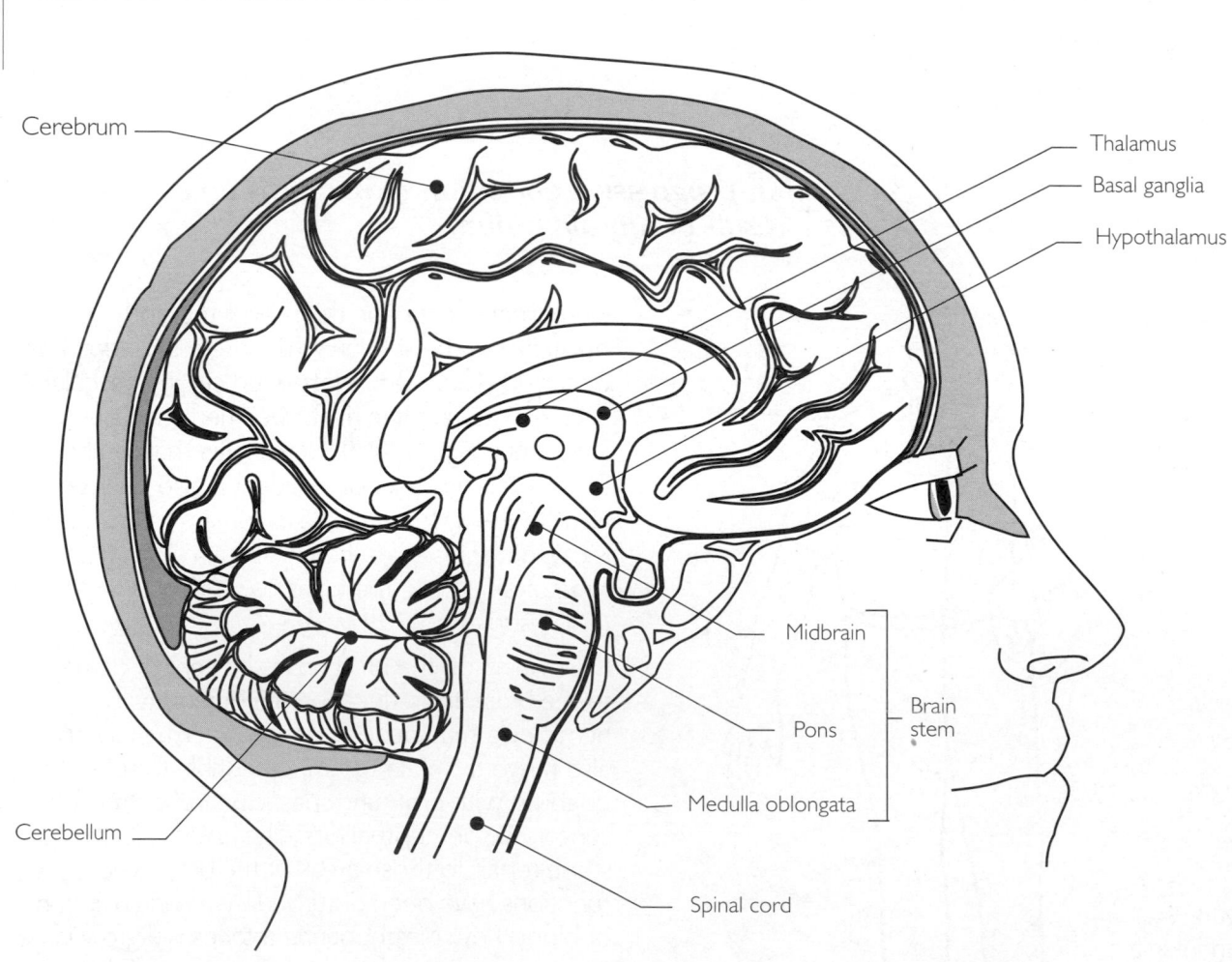

Figure 54.2
Areas commonly affected by stroke.

An area in the central nervous system commonly affected by strokes is the internal capsule. The internal capsule contains fibres that connect the cerebral cortex with the basal ganglia, thalamus, brain stem and spinal cord *(Figure 54.2)*. Lesions in this structure result in motor disabilities. The vestibular system may also be affected by stroke. The resulting lesions can cause excessive tone in the muscles which hold the body upright, also known as anti-gravity muscles.

Immediately after a stroke or head trauma, muscles on the affected side will be weak or flaccid. This is considered the acute phase.

Gradually, over a period of weeks, the flaccid paralysis will yield to spastic paralysis, though some flaccidity may remain. Spasticity occurs because lesions have interfered with the brain's control over spinal cord activity. The result is uninhibited alpha motor neuron firing. This type of paralysis will take on particular flexor and extensor patterns reflecting the uninhibited dominant reflexes *(Kaplan, Cerullo, 1986)*. These patterns are evident in the orientation of the head, the torso and the upper and lower limbs. Inferior subluxation of the shoulder may occur during the flaccid stage, since the glenohumeral joint is not supported. Known as "hemiplegic shoulder", it may continue as spasticity sets in. The person may experience loss of speech and sensation, decreased awareness of the affected side and impaired perceptual abilities, among others, depending on which centres of the brain have been affected. Initially, rehabilitation efforts will focus on reducing the reflex patterns, bringing spasticity under control and providing speech therapy and any other training necessary to increase the client's abilities to function daily.

Massage therapy can temporarily decrease spasticity, increase the client's awareness of the hemiplegic side and improve tissue and joint health. It can also offer emotional support. In the chronic stage, the focus is on treating secondary tissue and joint changes that result from ongoing postural imbalances and poor biomechanics.

Symptom Picture

✦ In the acute phase after the stroke, the muscles on the affected side are **flaccid**. This will last for a few days to several weeks and possibly longer. At this stage, the muscles lack tone and feel heavy to lift. No spasticity or reflex patterns are evident.

✦ Gradually, **spasticity and reflex patterns** will develop. Some flaccidity may remain. Certain people will have a spontaneous recovery, experiencing no residual symptoms. In many cases, people will have a good recovery because the lesions did not cause significant CNS damage while others will have improvement due to therapy. At this stage, the person may resume many activities, including work, since the spasticity is often mild and will not significantly interfere with movement. However, the spasticity can increase with effort, physical exertion and emotional stress. In the most serious cases, the person's physical abilities will be severely restricted, creating the need for ongoing care.

✦ Spasticity contributes to functional disability and potentially disabling postures. The amount of spasticity of each individual client is variable.

✦ The client will have an **altered posture** due to the spasticity patterns on the affected side. The most common pattern is a flexor pattern in the upper limbs combined with an

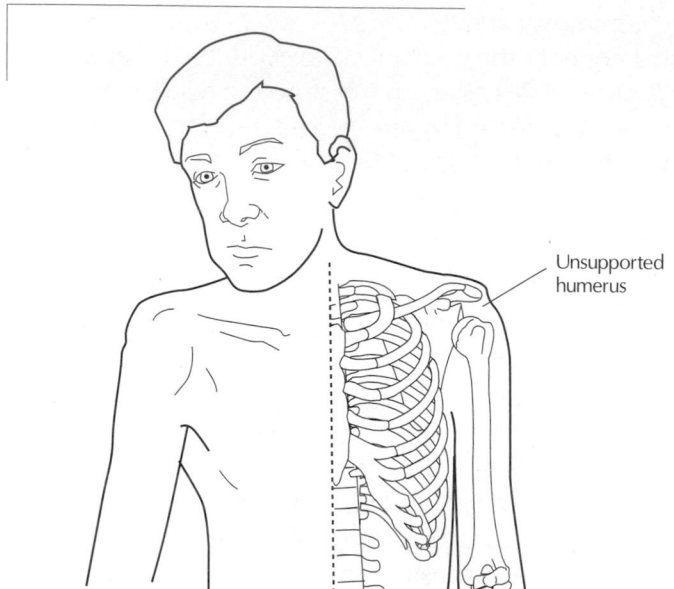

Unsupported
humerus

Figure 54.3
Subluxation of hemiplegic shoulder.

extensor pattern in the lower limbs. Other pattern combinations are possible.

✦ **Altered gait** can be the result of spasticity in the lower limb, as well as balance, proprioception and perception problems. Spasticity will require the person to support his weight on the unaffected leg and then swing the affected leg forward in circumduction, because of the lack of knee flexion. Poor balance and difficulty shifting weight will affect the speed, smoothness and accuracy of the movement.

✦ A **hemiplegic shoulder** may be present *(Figure 54.3).* This is a painful condition. It refers to the adduction and internal rotation of the glenohumeral joint combined with the retraction of the scapula which is due to the reflex patterns and spasticity. The condition may begin in the early stages post-stroke.

Flaccidity in the shoulder girdle muscles and poor positioning of the person's body often result in an inferior subluxation of the humerus. In later stages, as spasticity develops, impaired movement is compounded by contracture formation and other secondary conditions, such as tendinitis, bursitis, rotator cuff tear and adhesive capsulitis. Splints may be used to encourage functional contractures.

✦ **Seizures** may result from the brain lesion.

✦ The presence of **edema** is common. If edema is not addressed and becomes long-standing, tissue fragility will result. In this case, any injury could develop into an ulcer and, potentially, gangrene.

✦ **Pain** may be present and is often related to reduced range of motion of the joint, an altered plane of joint movement, muscle weakness, trigger points or tissue dystrophy, such as edema in the extremities. The shoulder is often affected.

✦ **Shoulder-hand syndrome** can develop in at least 12.5 per cent of clients with hemiplegia. This condition presents with a decrease in range of motion of the shoulder and hand, followed by throbbing pain and edema. The elbow remains symptom-free. The syndrome usually occurs with a lesion of the premotor cortex, in the first to third month and up to the sixth month post-stroke *(Cailliet, 1980).*

✦ **Compensatory changes** will occur on the unaffected side and a variety of overuse syndromes could develop depending on the amount of functional loss on the hemiplegic side.

✦ **Sensory deficit** may be present including light touch, temperature and pain perception, two-point discrimination and proprioception. The more severe the sensory impairment, the less chance there is of functional recovery.

✦ There may be **neglect of the affected side**. This may manifest as the person's inability to recognize the hemiplegic side as part of himself or extreme cases where the person completely denies ownership of the affected limbs *(Ingram, 1995).*

✦ **Behavioural and emotional changes** may be present. At least 25 per cent of people with hemiplegia experience depression, though it is not clear how much of this is due to brain damage versus an emotional response to the condition *(Lynch, Grisogono, 1991)*. It has been found that in a right-handed person, a lesion in the left hemisphere can result in personality changes, such as increased passivity and caution, whereas traits such as overestimation of ability and a tendency to quick action are noted with a lesion in the right hemisphere *(American Heart Association, 1994)*.

✦ A variety of **visual impairments** is possible. The client may have difficulty distinguishing between vertical and horizontal or difficulty in assessing an object's spatial relationship to his body. There may be an inability to perceive anything in the field of vision on the hemiplegic side. In such a case, the client may eat only food on one side of the plate or comb only one-half of the hair on his head *(Johnstone, 1991)*.

✦ **Speech difficulties** may occur, particularly aphasia or dysphasia. These conditions arise from damage to the dominant hemisphere. For right-handed people, aphasia would result from a lesion in the left hemisphere. Due to the diffuse organization of the speech centre in left-handed people, there is less chance of aphasia occurring in this group. Likewise, the recovery rate from aphasia is better for left-handed people *(Kaplan, Cerullo, 1986)*.

✦ **Cognitive impairment**, such as with language comprehension and memory, can occur. Apraxia is the inability to properly organize attempts at movement. This results in difficulty with movement despite having the physical ability to move.

Subjective Information

HEALTH HISTORY QUESTIONS

✦ Are there any conditions that can affect cardiovascular health, such as diabetes, kidney disease, atherosclerosis, heart disease, hypertension or emphysema? Is there a family history of stroke or any other condition?

✦ When did the stroke occur? Is there a previous history of stroke or transient ischemic attack?

✦ What was the cause? What treatment has been received? Was surgical repair done?

✦ What medications have been prescribed? Does the client take them as directed?

✦ Is the client's blood pressure stable? When was it last checked?

✦ Has the client had seizures since the stroke? If so, how often do they occur? Can the client describe what happens? Is medication being taken to control them?

✦ Does the client's physician know he is seeking massage therapy?

✦ Does the client experience any pain? Can the client describe the type of pain as well as where, when and how long it is experienced?

✦ What therapy was done — physiotherapy, occupational therapy, speech therapy, massage therapy? How long was it received? What was the purpose of the therapy?

✦ Has the physician restricted any activities, such as prolonged or vigorous walks or hot baths?

✦ What activities of daily living is the client able to do — walk, shop, cook, dress? How long can the person do these activities before feeling fatigued or short of breath? Are these activities done with or without assistance? Are supports used, such as splints, orthotics or a cane?

✦ What is the client's general lifestyle, including activities that can improve cardiovascular health, such as stopping smoking, reducing or eliminating caffeine and alcohol consumption, exercising and modifying diet, particularly limiting fat and sugar intake? Is the client compliant with these changes to improve his cardio-vascular health?

Objective Information

Observation

✍ The therapist should observe for the spasticity pattern on the affected side. If the client is able to walk, he may have a circumducted gait. The ability to balance and shift weight may be impaired. A cane or walker may be used.

✍ The client is checked for edema on the affected side, specifically in the distal limbs.

✍ Muscle bulk differences may be noticed when comparing the affected side of the body with the unaffected side.

✍ Functional abilities of the hemiplegic side will vary for each client depending on the severity of the stroke and the resulting spasticity or residual flaccidity.

✍ A postural assessment can be performed, noting asymmetries and altered biomechanics on the affected side or by compensation by the unaffected side.

✍ The therapist should observe the client's treatment of the affected side to determine if the client attempts to use it or ignores it (called "neglect") (Ingram, 1995).

Palpation

✍ Hypertonicity is palpated in the muscles affected by spasticity. Flaccidity or muscle hypotonicity may be present in muscles on the affected side.

✍ Over time, contractures are likely to develop in the muscles experiencing spasticity. For example, a flexor pattern in the arm could result in contractures in the wrist flexors.

✍ Edema may be present in the distal part of the affected limbs. The edematous tissue may be cool due to ischemia.

✍ Numerous shoulder pathologies of the affected limb may be present. Additional care should be taken when palpating this area. There is the possibility of shoulder-hand syndrome in the acute stages after the stroke. In chronic cases, pain may be experienced due to soft tissue dysfunction (tendinitis or bursitis), joint pathologies (osteoarthritis) and reduced tissue health (ongoing edema). The therapist may also detect tenderness, adhesions or signs of inflammation. While not common, heterotopic calcification is a possible complication of hemiplegia, which would be accompanied by heat and swelling.

Testing

✍ **AF and PR ROM testing** will show a decrease in range of motion if spasticity is present. The more severe the spasticity, the more severely compromised the range of motion. In the most extreme cases, no movement is possible. Flaccidity will also result in a decreased range of motion in the joints crossed by those muscles.

✍ **AR strength testing** will not yield useful results if spasticity is present.

Special Tests

✍ **Sensory testing**: Light touch, temperature and pain perception, two-point discrimination and proprioception may all be affected. There are wide varieties and degrees of sensory loss from slight and patchy to profound.

- Sensory discrimination is often less accurate in the arm and hand than in the leg and foot. This is thought to be due to the added sensory stimulation that occurs with standing and walking. These activities are encouraged early in the rehabilitation process. More accurate light touch perception and two-point discrimination are likely in the distal limb compared to the proximal limb *(Bobath, 1990).*

✍ Specific orthopedic tests are performed for secondary conditions. If spasticity is present, the test may not yield viable results. In particular, tests should be conducted for shoulder conditions on the affected side. Tendinitis, bursitis, adhesive capsulitis and rotator cuff tear may be present. The therapist should exercise additional care if glenohumeral subluxation is present. This is usually present in the acute stage post-stroke but may linger if spasticity is significant.

Contraindications

✦ If hemiplegia was the result of a cerebrovascular accident and assessment indicates a concern for cardiovascular health, modifications should be made to treatment and hydrotherapy applications. See Hypertension Treatment for details.

✦ Special care should be taken when treating the sternocleidomastoid muscle. Light pressure or Golgi tendon organ techniques on the attachments should be used. Techniques that apply pressure on the muscle belly are avoided because the carotid artery travels beneath this muscle. If atherosclerosis is present in the carotid arteries, deep pressure may dislodge sclerotic material into the bloodstream, which then becomes an embolus. This could precipitate a stroke.

♦ With the exception of light stroking, massage techniques should be performed on one side of the neck at a time. It is contraindicated to place the client's head in a position of neck extension and head rotation. This may dangerously occlude the vertebral artery.

♦ Modifications of temperature and weight of hydrotherapy applications will be necessary if sensory deficit or tissue fragility is present. Heat applications on the torso should be specific and not diffuse in the case of a client with a cardiovascular pathology.

Treatment Goals Treatment Plan

Make treatment safe.

🖐 Before the massage can begin, the therapist needs to clearly think through the modifications necessary to make the treatment safe. Considerations will include treatment duration, positioning of the client and hydrotherapy modalities to be used.

🖐 **Duration** of each treatment will depend on the client's cardiovascular health. Since hemiplegia is often the result of a cerebrovascular accident, a full-body treatment may be too taxing for the client.

• A treatment of 30 to 45 minutes is often more appropriate than one hour. The focus of each treatment could alternate between the upper and the lower body, with the client's entire body being treated over a number of sessions.

• For a partial treatment, the therapist can apply gentle muscle squeezing and stroking to those areas of the body that are not the primary focus for that treatment. In this way the client feels some integration of the body. If the client responds well to these treatments, the duration could be extended to one hour, provided appropriate modifications are made (see the chapter on hypertension).

Modify position for cardiovascular concerns.

🖐 **Positioning** possibilities will again be limited by the cardiovascular health of the client as well as by his degree of spasticity. The more spasticity that is present, the fewer the changes of position. Effort the client exerts to change position will generally increase spasticity; this must be weighed against possible gains from treating the client in a different position. Mild spasticity does not pose as great a concern.

• The client will often collapse on the hemiplegic side or sit improperly so it is important to position his body in proper alignment. This neutral position is attempted regardless of whether the client is seated, supine or sidelying. If prone is deemed to be a safe position, a face cradle should be used. If possible, the limbs are moved slowly and gently out of their reflex pattern and pillowed

Treatment Goals

Modify hydrotherapy for cardiovascular concerns.

Decrease sympathetic nervous system firing. Provide emotional support.

Maintain tissue health. Decrease edema, if present.

Limit contractures, if possible.

Decrease pain. Address secondary postural changes and muscle imbalances.

Treatment Plan

comfortably and securely. See Spasticity in CNS Strategies for more details.

🖐 **Hydrotherapy** applications to reduce spasticity can be hot or cold. Heat will reduce muscle tone and cold will depress afferent and efferent firing.

- Wet cold applications, such as wraps, can be used to cover all or part of an affected limb. Cold packs can be used for more local applications (*Pederson, 1969; Cailliet, 1980*).

- When addressing contractures, applications of heat can be used as a pre-treatment hydrotherapy. Reduced temperature whirlpools may be appropriate for the lower leg before treating ankle contractures if no edema is present.

General Treatment

🖐 The treatment is performed in the context of a relaxation massage. Slow, easy breathing is encouraged. Supportive, soothing and rhythmical techniques are used.

Specific Treatment

🖐 Techniques will be modified if cardiovascular health is a concern. See Hypertension Treatment for specific details.

🖐 Lymphatic drainage techniques are interspersed with **mid-range passive range of motion.** Cool hydrotherapy also assists in reducing edema. If the client has a cardiovascular condition, care should be taken not to elevate the limb above the heart.

🖐 Swedish massage techniques can be used to improve circulation and overall tissue health. These must be modified for depth and speed if sensory impairment is present.

- Massage techniques are applied segmentally when cardiovascular pathologies and tissue fragility are present, since long massage strokes can create drag on the tissue.

🖐 Contractures are treated with a local application of heat followed by a slow **prolonged passive stretch with overpressure.**

🖐 If hemiplegic shoulder is present, the scapula is pillowed in a protracted position. The humerus is supported in a slightly superior orientation. The therapist should avoid placing an inferior pressure on the glenohumeral joint.

- Swedish techniques focus on increasing local circulation, reducing pain (through decreasing sympathetic nervous system firing) and reducing spasticity in the scapular retractors, such as rhomboids,

Treatment Goals   Treatment Plan

and in the internal rotators, such as pectoralis major and minor.

- If tendinitis, adhesive capsulitis, osteoarthritis or other such conditions are present, standard treatment approaches apply, with appropriate modifications for hemiplegia. For example, frictions would not be performed if the client is on anti-inflammatories. If it is safe to do this usually painful technique (pain can increase sympathetic nervous system firing), application would be less aggressive and interspersed with soothing techniques. If necessary, the painful work can be performed over a series of treatments.

- In the case of tendinitis and adhesive capsulitis, shoulder joint motion relies on free scapular movement. Treatment of the rhomboids, subscapularis, supraspinatus and rotator cuff muscles is essential in order to maintain good shoulder mobility. Segmental effleurage and petrissage are used.

- Trigger points are treated with the least invasive techniques, such as gentle repetitive muscle stripping and skin rolling or gradually applied ischemic compressions.

Decrease spasticity, temporarily.

- Reducing spasticity will contribute to joint health as it allows improved limb movement. In addition to the positioning considerations already discussed, there are a variety of techniques used to reduce spasticity. See the CNS Strategies chapter for details about each technique.

- **Techniques to reduce spasticity:**

  - slow rhythmical Swedish techniques such as stroking and palmar kneading;

  - slow rhythmical shaking of the limb;

  - Golgi tendon organ pressure, if the tendon is accessible;

  - stimulation of the antagonist muscle;

  - slow steady performance of passive range of motion to an affected limb;

  - slow rhythmical stroking along the spine.

- Each client will have an individual reaction to each technique. The therapist will need to determine which techniques are most effective for a particular client. For example, one client may respond well to gentle repetitive stroking, whereas another may find rhythmical techniques more beneficial.

- A key point the therapist must remember is that stressful emotional responses on the part of the client will increase spasticity. This reaction can be controlled if the therapist maintains a relaxation focus throughout the treatment, using appropriate speed and application.

Maintain joint health and range of motion.

- **Passive movement** is used to improve joint health and mobility. This should be performed slowly and gently on each joint of the affected

Treatment Goals

Treatment Plan

limb, so as not to elicit a stretch reflex.

✋ **Passive range of motion** of the affected joints is interspersed throughout the massage. Care should be taken not to perform a repetitive full-limb movement with a client who has a cardiovascular pathology.

✋ Hemiplegia is distinct because of its clear left-right, affected-unaffected separation of the body. Every opportunity is used to bring the client's awareness to the affected side. See the CNS Strategies chapter for more details.

✋ **Techniques to integrate the body:**

Encourage whole body integration. Maintain awareness of the affected side.

- the therapist stands on the affected side when talking to the client;

- feedback is elicited when performing massage on the affected side;

- passive or active assisted movements are performed with an affected limb and the client is asked to follow this action with the unaffected limb;

- techniques or movements performed on the affected side are verbally reinforced;

- techniques are applied simultaneously to both sides of the body.

Self-care Goals

Self-care Plan

Increase functional ability through improvement of strength, range of motion and balance.

✍ The client is encouraged to do activities of daily living at the level of his ability.

✍ A modified exercise program is encouraged. A referral to a physiotherapist is appropriate.

✍ Self-massage and self-movement of the client's affected side by the unaffected side will maintain range of motion of some joints, give sensory stimulation to the area and improve awareness and proprioception of that limb. Specific stretches are given, as appropriate. For example, rhomboids and pectoralis major stretches will affect scapular retraction and internal rotation of the humerus.

Educate about maintenance of tissue health.

✍ To treat distal edema, the client is taught basic lymphatic drainage techniques and cool hydrotherapy applications, such as towel wraps. The client is also educated about signs of gangrene, which is tissue necrosis due to an interference of blood supply (Porth, 1990). Medical help should be sought if black or brown discolouration develops in distal digits. This may be accompanied by inflammation or by coolness and swelling in the affected tissue.

Encourage relaxation.

✍ Relaxation techniques such as diaphragmatic breathing, which is contraindicated if diabetes or kidney disease is present *(Fried, 1990)*, visualization and meditation are encouraged. Relaxation decreases spasticity as well as pain perception.

✍ The client is encouraged to participate in movement rehabilitation programs if difficulty develops with balancing and shifting weight. Yoga and Tai Chi will improve flexibility, balance and coordination. A regular aerobic program, such as swimming or walking, could be undertaken. If cardiovascular health is compromised, permission from the physician is obtained first.

Refer the client.

✍ Biofeedback techniques have been found to reduce spasticity. Therefore, a referral may be appropriate. A local support or social group, such as a Stroke Club, can benefit the client.

Treatment Frequency and Expected Outcome

The brain lesion in hemiplegia is non-progressive. While some people will recover fully, others will have varying degrees of ongoing symptoms. Therefore, the treatments are ongoing.

A good prognosis for recovery is dependent on several factors:

✦ the person's general health;

✦ acceptance of the disability;

✦ the presence of a supportive person at home to assist in care giving;

✦ good visual and motor coordination;

✦ an early return of muscle tone from the flaccid stage;

✦ the presence of deep tendon reflexes;

✦ voluntary motor activity;

See also Strategies: Central Nervous System Conditions, hypertension, stress reduction, hyperkyphosis, scoliosis, adhesive capsulitis, tendinitis, bursitis, osteoarthritis, dislocation, edema, peripheral nerve compression syndromes and seizures for related treatments.

✦ good strength in the hand and trunk muscles;

✦ skill in feeding and bladder control.

A potentially poor prognosis is likely in the case of:

✦ a long time lapse between hemiplegia onset and rehabilitation efforts;

✦ persistent muscle hypotonicity or extreme flaccidity;

✦ contractures;

✦ severe cognitive dysfunction;

✦ severe sensory or perceptual impairment;

✦ visual field defects.

Despite a potentially poor prognosis, it was found that rehabilitation efforts led to significant gains of functional ability for the person with hemiplegia *(Kaplan, Cerullo, 1986)*.

55

MULTIPLE SCLEROSIS

Linda Ludwig

Multiple sclerosis (MS) is a condition in which demyelination of the nerves occurs.

Demyelination results in scar tissue formation that affects nerve transmissions in widely scattered areas of the brain and spinal cord. "The diversity of the symptoms, signs and course of MS continues to astonish even the most experienced physician" *(DeSouza, 1990)*.

MS begins with an inflammatory process, followed by the loss of myelin that surrounds the nerve axons. This process is referred to as demyelination. Myelin functions to provide insulation to the axon in order to speed transmissions along the nerve. Scar tissue, known as sclerotic plaques, develops at the sites of demyelination. These plaques cause a slowing, disruption or blockage of nerve transmissions. As the plaques increase, symptoms become more severe.

It is suggested that, in the early stages of MS, myelin is able to regenerate through the work of the oligodendrocytes. This results in the improvement in the person's symptoms. Over time, these cells fatigue and less recovery occurs *(Porth, 1990)*.

The specific symptoms that each person experiences with MS will vary according to the location of the lesion in the central nervous system (CNS) and the extent of that lesion. In particular, the white matter of the CNS is affected. Lesions are most commonly found in the brain stem, cerebellum and spinal cord.

Some cranial nerves can also be involved, namely the optic nerve and the trigeminal nerve. Lesions of the optic nerve can result in the loss of visual acuity and in colour blindness, visual field defects and diplopia (double vision). Total blindness is uncommon. Lesions of the trigeminal nerve result in trigeminal neuralgia.

There are several different **types of MS** based on the progression of the condition:

✦ **Benign MS** is a mild form of this disease. A few exacerbations are followed by complete recovery and the client remains asymptomatic.

✦ **Attack-remitting MS** has repeated cycles of exacerbation and remission. Symptoms such as double vision, slurred speech, numbness and tingling anywhere in the body can occur during the attacks.

  • **Benign or mild attack-remitting MS** causes only mild disability when the attack subsides.

  • **Chronic progressive attack-remitting MS** results in increased symptoms following attacks. In some cases, the remission periods become less and less frequent, and disability increases continuously.

✦ **Acute progressive MS** results in a rapid progression of symptoms and disability. It can be fatal within a few years *(DeSouza, 1990; Schapiro, 1994)*.

Fortunately, the more severe forms of MS are also the least common. In fact, two-thirds of those diagnosed with MS remain functional and ambulatory after 20 years *(Schapiro, 1994)*.

Multiple sclerosis is difficult for physicians to diagnose, particularly if the person has the attack-remission type of MS. Because the earliest symptoms are often slight, the person does not seek medical attention. As the condition progresses, the signs and symptoms resemble many other nervous system disorders.

Clinical diagnosis of MS by a physician usually follows: two attacks with signs of nervous system damage, such as unexplained weakness and numbness or tingling in the hands and feet; an erratic pattern of symptoms that appears and disappears suddenly; and involvement of two or more parts of the CNS. Recently, magnetic resonance imaging (MRI) has been useful in detecting the sclerotic plaques in the central nervous system that indicate MS.

The diagnosis of multiple sclerosis can have a substantial emotional impact on a person. The disease's progression is unpredictable over the course of a lifetime as well as from day to day. This disease strikes people during a very active time in life. The average age of onset is between 20 and 40 years, although it can occur as early as 15 and as late as 45 *(Schapiro, 1994)*. Women are affected slightly more than men.

The causes of MS are unclear, although it is thought that many factors interact in a specific way to result in the disease process *(Schapiro, 1994)*. The following four factors are all considered to be in some way involved in the cause of multiple sclerosis:

➤ **Genetic Factor:** Some genetic link is present. Recent studies in Canada have shown that, likely, more than one gene is responsible for a predisposition to MS. This condition has been found in 25 per cent to 30 per cent of monozygotic twins. There also seems to be an increased risk to relatives of affected individuals *(Mohr, Gautier, 1995)*.

➤ **Environmental Factor:** This condition is most prevalent in temperate climates, such as North America and Northern Europe, between 40 degrees and 60 degrees north and south latitudes. Therefore, the closer one is to the equator the less likely one is to get MS. To further suggest an environmental link, if a person immigrates to a temperate climate before the age of 15 years, she has the same risk as the local population of contracting the disease *(Porth, 1990)*.

➤ **Viral Factor:** Some researchers believe that a virus is responsible for stimulating overactivity of the immune response. This overactivity results in the demyelination of the axons.

➤ **Immunological Factor:** The overactivity of certain types of white blood cells leads to attacks on the myelin as if it were a foreign substance. Susceptibility to this autoimmune disorder is thought to be, in part, genetically predisposed *(Schapiro, 1994)*.

While not actual causes, some factors seem to **exacerbate symptoms:**

✦ Deficiencies in zinc, vitamins B6 or B12 or essential fatty acids are possible links. Essential fatty acids are components of myelin. Their lack or mishandling by the body is thought to result in weak or susceptible myelin *(Graham, 1989)*.

✦ Amalgam dental fillings seem to affect some people with MS. One theory is that mercury and lead pass through the blood-brain barrier and allow toxins into the CNS *(Graham, 1989)*.

✦ Food allergies to dairy products and increased intake of polyunsaturated fats can exacerbate symptoms in some people with MS *(Graham, 1989)*.

✦ Stressful events, overexertion, heat, fever, injury and emotional upset can exacerbate symptoms.

Currently, there is no cure. Despite this, many strategies enable people with MS to lead full lives. These strategies involve diet, nutrition, exercise, support groups, stress reduction and a realistic organization of activities around whatever limitations, such as fatigue, spasticity or muscle weakness, this condition has created. Medications include Betaseron, which seems to reduce the number and severity of attacks as well as actually reducing the number of lesions in the CNS. It is useful for people who have the attack-remitting form of MS. Massage therapy improves physical awareness, temporarily decreases spasticity, improves soft tissue and joint health, decreases contractures, reduces stress and can give feelings of emotional support and well being to people with multiple sclerosis.

Symptom Picture

✦ No client will have all of the symptoms listed. In fact, no two clients will have the same presentation because symptoms will vary according to the location and extent of the lesions in the CNS. Because the client's symptoms can change from one treatment to the next, the therapist needs to get a clear picture of the client's current picture. The short-term aims reflect these changes. During an acute attack, the client is unlikely to come for massage. During remission, new symptoms or exacerbation of previous ones are possible. The percentages listed below reflect the likelihood of that symptom being present *(Rowland, 1995)*.

✦ **Fatigue** is common. A feeling of overwhelming tiredness can also increase other symptoms such as tingling and numbness, blurred vision or slurred speech. Fatigue (59 to 85 per cent) is normally experienced after vigorous activity but, in the case of MS, fatigue can set in after only a short time into the activity. A few factors contribute to this fatigue: inefficient neuronal transmissions resulting from demyelination and the presence of scar tissue on the axons; and inefficient movement caused by spasticity, weakness, reduced range of motion and tremors. The stress response, as well as the presence of infections, can worsen the feeling of exhaustion. Fatigue results in a decrease in functional ability. Rest is required to restore nerve and muscle function. "MS fatigue" is a term used to describe the lassitude or feeling of sudden sleepiness after almost no activity. This type of fatigue often is treated with drug therapy *(Schapiro, 1994)*.

✦ **Spasticity** (73 to 100 per cent) is often present. Spasticity results in inefficient movement, muscle imbalances and altered posture. **Weakness** (65 to 100 per cent) can come from lesions in the spinal cord. The lesions cause a partial or complete block of nerve transmissions along the axon. Weakness will often be experienced on one side more than the other. **Proprioception** (48 to 72 per cent) may be impaired. **Tremors** (36 to 81 per cent), usually intention tremors, are frequently present. These tremors occur when the person is actively attempting a movement. They may vary from small amplitude, rhythmical movements of a limb or hand to powerful, large amplitude rhythmical movements of the limbs and trunk.

✦ All these symptoms contribute to **inefficient movement patterns.** Altered gait, primarily circumducted gait, and dragging of the foot can result from weakness and spasticity in one leg. Increasing the efficiency of movement will benefit the client's energy levels and maintain better tissue and joint health.

✦ **Altered posture** is caused by muscle imbalances, weakness and spasticity. These factors can alter biomechanics and contribute to secondary conditions. If the client is using a wheelchair, scoliosis or hyperkyphosis can develop. Contracture formation is also possible. When muscles are weak, contractures can develop in the unopposed antagonist muscles. For example, contractures would develop in the forearm extensors if the forearm flexors were weak. With spasticity, the contractures are likely to form in the spastic muscles. For example, spastic forearm flexors would develop the contractures.

✦ **Compensatory changes** occur in the unaffected or overused limbs; this is most notable on the strong side if the client presents with a stronger and a weaker side. Depending on the severity of symptoms, the client might use a cane, a walker or a wheelchair occasionally or regularly. It is not unusual that a client will arrive for a treatment using a cane one week but require a wheelchair a few weeks later, then require only a cane again later.

✦ **Paresthesia** (16 to 72 per cent), such as numbness, tingling or burning, may be experienced. Pain can be a primary symptom of conditions such as trigeminal neuralgia. Pain can also be a symptom secondary to muscular imbalances and dysfunction. For example, knee or hip pain may be due to altered gait; increased stress to the muscles and joints occurs from the abrupt actions involved in circumducting a weak leg. Often a cane is used to assist with walking. Shoulder pain and overuse syndromes result from holding the cane.

✦ **Cold extremities or sweating abnormalities** may result from autonomic dysfunction (38 to 43 per cent). **Edema** may be present. This is likely if the client is in a wheelchair or if weak muscles affect the efficiency of venous and lymphatic return. If edema is not addressed and becomes longstanding, tissue fragility and pitted edema will result. In such a case, any injury could develop into an ulcer and, potentially, gangrene.

✦ **Mood swings**, depression (8 to 55 per cent), euphoria (4 to 18 per cent), as well as cognitive problems, such as forgetfulness and inattentiveness, may be present.

• Depression may be physiological due to the presence of MS lesions or psychological due to the strain of having a progressive degenerative condition. MS is unpredictable.

From day to day, the client does not know how her symptoms will present and how much fatigue will be experienced. This creates ongoing stress and uncertainty. Medications prescribed for depression can alter muscle tone.

- Euphoria may, at first, seem to be a positive symptom but it does have its drawbacks. The client may take unnecessary risks without clearly considering the consequences. The client may not understand that a thermophore or a brisk, vigorous massage will likely cause extreme fatigue and could increase the MS symptoms. This client would encourage the therapist to "go ahead and try it".

✦ **Other symptoms:**

- vertigo (7 to 27 per cent), loss of balance and lack of coordination;
- diplopia (18 to 39 per cent), nystagmus (54 to 73 per cent), decreased visual acuity, reduced visual field and colour blindness;
- speech disturbances such as dysarthria (29 to 62 per cent) and slurring;
- bladder dysfunction (49 to 93 per cent) and, secondary to this, frequent urinary tract infections. The presence of infection can increase fatigue levels and exacerbate symptoms;
- bowel dysfunction (39 to 64 per cent) and constipation.

Subjective Information

HEALTH HISTORY QUESTIONS

✦ Are other conditions present, such as a cold, flu or infection? These conditions can increase the client's susceptibility to fatigue.

✦ When was the diagnosis of MS made? When were the first symptoms experienced? What were the symptoms?

✦ How has the MS progressed for the client?

✦ What are the symptoms currently being experienced by the client?

✦ Does the client have attacks and remissions?

✦ When was the last attack? How long did it last? Have any of the symptoms remained?

✦ Is the client taking any medication?

✦ Is pain present? Can the client describe the type of pain as well as where, when and how long it is experienced?

✦ Is there diminished or lost sensory perception or limb proprioception?

✦ Does the client experience fatigue? When does it occur? How does this feels for her? How long does it take her to recover?

✦ Is the client seeking any other treatment, such as physiotherapy, naturopathy or chiropractic?

✦ How functional is the client with activities of daily living? Is she independent, working? What are the client's gross and fine motor skills?

✦ Are supports used? Are they used occasionally or daily?

✦ What are the client's current stress levels?

✦ How is the client affected by heat? By exercise, hot weather, showers or baths? Stress and heat affect fatigue levels as well as exacerbating symptoms.

✦ Is the client participating in any rehabilitation, exercise or other program?

✦ Has the client had previous massage experience?

✦ What is the client's treatment focus for that day?

Objective Information

Observations

✍ There is no typical MS client. See the CNS Strategies chapter for general observations for a CNS lesion.

Contraindications

✦ **Techniques or modalities that will fatigue the client are contraindicated.**

• Painful techniques, such as frictions, and vigorous work increase sympathetic nervous system firing and, in turn, induce fatigue.

• Heat applied over a large area will affect nerve conduction and exacerbate fatigue in the vast majority of people.

✦ Deep techniques are contraindicated in areas with altered sensation.

✦ If decubitus ulcers are present local massage is contraindicated.

• If the therapist notices red, inflamed areas over bony prominences the client should be immediately referred to a physician.

Palpation

✍ There is no typical MS client. See the CNS Strategies chapter for general palpation for a CNS lesion.

Testing

The usual range of motion and strength testing protocol is attempted.

✍ **AF** and **PR ROM** will reveal a decrease in range of motion, if spasticity or weakness is present. The more severe the motor dysfunctions, the more severely compromised the range of motion.

✍ **AR strength** testing will not yield useful results with the limbs affected by spasticity.

• Some people with MS have a weak side. In such cases, AR testing will reveal diminished strength of the muscles on that side of the body.

Special Tests

✋ **Sensory testing** for light touch, deep pressure, pain and temperature perception, two-point discrimination and proprioception are performed. Results will vary depending on the client; there may be a variety of sensory changes from anesthesia to paresthesia.

✋ **Specific orthopedic tests** are performed for secondary conditions. If spasticity is present, the tests may not yield viable results.

Treatment Goals

Treatment Plan

✋ The symptoms of multiple sclerosis can change from treatment to treatment. Therefore, the massage treatment will change to reflect short-term goals, as determined by the current symptoms. The therapist must be adaptable to this changing picture. Some considerations never change:

The therapist will always aim to decrease sympathetic nervous system firing, avoid inducing fatigue and provide caring touch and a supportive environment for the client.

✋ Before massage can begin, the therapist needs to clearly think through the modifications necessary to make the treatment safe.

Avoid exacerbating spasticity.

✋ **Positioning** possibilities may be limited by the degree of spasticity or the size of the client, if transferring from a wheelchair is considered. The more spasticity is present, the fewer the changes of position. The effort exerted by the client to change position will generally increase spasticity and must be weighed against what might be gained by treating the client in a different position. Mild spasticity does not pose a concern.

Maintain proper body alignment.

• The client is positioned in proper alignment, whether she is on a massage table, in a wheelchair or seated. To reinforce good posture, the head is kept in line with the spine; the shoulders and pelvis are placed in a midline position. For some clients, head position can increase spasticity in the upper limbs, in which case the head should be in a neutral position regardless of whether the client is seated, supine or sidelying. If prone is deemed to be a safe position, a face cradle is used.

• Just as some positioning can increase spasticity, there are other positions that act to inhibit spasticity. Generally, this is achieved by taking the limbs out of their reflex pattern, if possible. The limbs are moved slowly and gently, and pillowed comfortably and securely.

✋ **Hydrotherapy** for clients who have an intolerance to heat is generally limited to cool and cold applications, which are usually well tolerated. These are appropriate for edema or inflammation. Cold can sometimes reduce spasticity, as it depresses afferent and efferent

Treatment Goals

Treatment Plan

firing. Wet cold applications, such as wraps, are used to cover all or part of an affected limb. Cold packs are used for more local applications *(Pedersen, 1969; Cailliet, 1980)*. Although heat may feel good to the client, large applications (such as a thermaphore on the back) for a prolonged time can exacerbate fatigue and, potentially, the symptoms of the client's MS.

- **Local** warm and hot applications can be appropriate, such as after the treatment of trigger points. If a specific local application of heat is indicated, a mild temperature is used and the client is monitored for any negative effects post-treatment.

General Treatment

Decrease sympathetic nervous system firing. Prevent fatigue. Provide emotional support.

The treatment is performed in the context of a relaxation massage, using smooth rhythmical techniques. A supportive touch is used. Diaphragmatic breathing is encouraged throughout the massage.

Specific Treatment

The client's current specific requests help to focus the treatment — for example, to address tendinitis, bursitis or stress. Due to the variability of symptoms from week to week or from day to day, the treatment requests will likely vary.

Improve and maintain tissue health. Decrease edema, if present. Be vigilant for decubitis ulcers.

Techniques are modified to prevent fatigue. If edema is present, inguinal or axillary pumping is followed by drainage techniques. These are interspersed with **passive range of motion.** Elevation of the limb and cool hydrotherapy also assist to reduce edema. Swedish massage techniques are used to improve circulation and overall tissue health. These must be modified for depth (lighter) and speed (slower) if sensory impairment is present. The strokes are applied segmentally if the tissue is fragile, as long strokes can create drag on the tissue.

Limit contractures, if possible.

Contractures, which reduce range of motion in a joint, are treated with a slow **prolonged passive stretch with overpressure.**

Address postural changes and muscle imbalances. Decrease pain.

Secondary conditions are addressed. To promote functional and efficient movement, postural changes such as scoliosis, hyperlordosis, hyperkyphosis and head-forward posture are addressed as usual using Swedish techniques and movement. Modifications of pressure are made as required.

Address secondary conditions.

If tendinitis, osteoarthritis (often in the hip and knee because of circumducted gait) or other such conditions are present, the standard treatment approaches apply; appropriate modifications are made.

Frictions are not performed if the client is on anti-inflammatories. If it is

Treatment Goals   Treatment Plan

safe to do this usually painful technique (pain can increase sympathetic nervous system firing), application would be modified and interspersed with soothing techniques. This work would also be performed over a series of treatments. Trigger points are treated with the least invasive techniques, such as gentle repetitive muscle stripping and skin rolling or gradually applied ischemic compressions.

🖐 When performing painful techniques, communication with the client is essential. If the client becomes fatigued the specific work is stopped. The client is consulted to determine if the massage should continue.

Decrease spasticity, temporarily.

🖐 Reduction of spasticity contributes to joint health as it allows improved limb movement. This, in turn, reduces fatigue levels. In addition to the positioning considerations already discussed, there are a variety of strategies to reduce spasticity. See the CNS Strategies chapter for added details about each technique.

🖐 **Techniques to reduce spasticity:**

- slow rhythmical Swedish techniques such as stroking and palmar kneading;

- slow rhythmical shaking of the limb;

- Golgi tendon organ pressure, if the tendon is accessible;

- stimulation of the antagonist muscle;

- slow steady performance of passive range of motion to an affected limb;

- slow rhythmical stroking along the spine.

🖐 Each client will have an individual reaction to each technique. The therapist will need to determine which techniques are most effective for a particular client. For example, one client may respond well to gentle repetitive stroking, whereas another may find rhythmical techniques more beneficial.

🖐 A key point the therapist must remember is that stressful emotional responses on the part of the client will increase spasticity. This reaction can be controlled if the therapist maintains a relaxation focus throughout the treatment, using appropriate techniques with modified speed and application.

Maintain joint health and range of motion.

🖐 **Passive movement** is used to improve joint health and mobility. It should be performed slowly and gently on each joint. If spasticity is present, extra care is taken so as not to elicit a stretch reflex. Passive range of motion of the affected joints is interspersed throughout the massage.

Provide emotional support. Encourage whole body integration.

🖐 With MS, one side of the client's body is usually weaker than the other side. Therefore, the therapist uses every opportunity to bring the client's awareness to this weaker side. See the CNS Strategies chapter for more details.

Treatment Goals

Treatment Plan

✋ **Techniques to integrate the body:**

- the therapist stands on the weaker side when talking to the client;
- feedback is elicited when performing massage on areas that have sensory dysfunction or increased spasticity. If the client is totally focused on the symptomatic areas, the therapist redirects the awareness to the unaffected areas;
- techniques are applied simultaneously to both sides of the body.

Self-care Goals

Self-care Plan

Increase functional ability through improving strength, range of motion and balance.

✍ The client is encouraged to do activities of daily living at the level of her ability, but to pace the activities to avoid fatigue. The client is encouraged to participate in movement rehabilitation programs if difficulty develops with balancing and shifting weight. Yoga and Tai Chi will improve flexibility, balance and coordination. A regular aerobic program, such as swimming or walking, could be undertaken. Modifications are necessary to prevent fatigue.

✍ A modified strengthening program is encouraged. The weakness experienced by a client with MS is due to problems with nerve transmissions from the CNS to the muscle. Traditional weight training has poor results with people who have MS and often increases fatigue and leads to further weakness.

- The strengthening program is done in a cool environment because an increase in body temperature will increase fatigue. Rest periods of up to five minutes are built in throughout the exercise program.

- Resistance is submaximal; the client does not use her full strength. Initially, gravity may be the only resistance; rubber tubing or Therabands can be gradually introduced. The proximal muscles are worked first, followed by the distal muscles.

- The client begins with eight to 10 repetitions of a movement, with an increase of one to two repetitions every few weeks. This continues until 20 repetitions are achieved. At this time, more resistance is added in the form of a one pound weight or rubber tubing. The cycle is repeated. The client monitors her own progress. Modifications in progression, resistance and rest periods are made as needed.

Educate about the maintenance of tissue health.

✍ To treat distal edema, the client is taught basic lymphatic drainage techniques and cool hydrotherapy applications, such as towel wraps. The client is also educated about signs of gangrene, which is tissue necrosis due to an interference of blood supply *(Porth, 1990)*.

Medical help should be sought if black or brown discolouration develops in distal digits. This may be accompanied by inflammation or by coolness and swelling in the affected tissue.

Encourage relaxation.

✍ Relaxation techniques such as diaphragmatic breathing, which is contraindicated if diabetes or kidney disease is present *(Fried, 1990)*, visualization and meditation are encouraged.

Refer the client.

✍ Biofeedback techniques have been found to reduce spasticity. Therefore, a referral may be appropriate. In addition, referral to a local support or social group, such as an MS Society, can be made.

Treatment Frequency and Expected Outcome

One-hour treatments on a weekly basis have been found to be beneficial for stress reduction, increased functional ability and a greater sense of well being. If the client has specific needs, such as tendinitis or bursitis, two half-hour treatments may be appropriate, with painful work distributed over several treatments.

Multiple sclerosis is a progressive degenerative condition. Progression of the condition will vary depending on the individual. The average life expectancy is 25 to 30 years from onset.

See also Strategies:
Central Nervous System
Conditions, stress
reduction, hyperlordosis,
hyperkyphosis, scoliosis,
tendinitis, bursitis,
osteoarthritis, edema and
decubitus ulcers for
related treatments.

Factors that affect the client's prognosis:

✦ women fare better than men;

✦ a person with sensory symptoms at onset fares better than one with motor symptoms at onset;

✦ incoordination at or near onset is the least favourable onset;

✦ long remission between the first and second attacks is favourable;

✦ the state of the disability five years after onset correlates with the progression that can be expected in the following five to 10 years.

56

PARKINSONS

Linda Ludwig

Parkinsons is a progressive disorder involving diminishing basal ganglia function. The disorder results in slow, increasingly difficult movement, accompanied by resting tremors and muscular rigidity.

Parkinsons was first clinically documented by Dr. James Parkinson in 1817. With only a few exceptions, his observations of Parkinsons prove thorough and accurate even today. Named after Dr. Parkinson, this condition is known by several terms. Through common usage, Parkinson's disease, Parkinsonism, Parkinson's syndrome and Parkinsons are often used interchangeably. "Parkinson's disease" can imply a known cause; "idiopathic Parkinson's disease" suggests an unknown cause. In deference to those with the condition, who object to the term "disease" and the implication of debility and illness, this text uses the term "Parkinsons" (PD).

With usual brain function, the substantia nigra, located in the basal ganglia, communicates to other areas of the brain to control movement. Neurons use the neurotransmitter dopamine. Concentrations of this substance will gradually decrease over the course of the normal aging process. In Parkinsons, the supply of dopamine is diminished due to necrosis of the dopamine-producing cells in the substantia nigra, which results in a deterioration of the body's proper movement and balance. The symptoms occur when the concentration of dopamine diminishes to 60 to 80 per cent in the neurons and 80 per cent in the basal ganglia *(Hopkins, 1992)*.

Parkinsons strikes people later in life, usually in the mid- to late sixties with an increasing likelihood as the person gets older. It affects one out of 1000 under the age of 60, with only one of seven diagnoses made of people under the age of 50. Five out of 1000 are affected at age 70 and as many as 20 out of 1000 at age 85 *(Caird, 1991)*. Young-onset Parkinsons can occur between the ages of 21 and 39, accounting for about five per cent of those with the condition. The symptoms are the same as with older onset with the

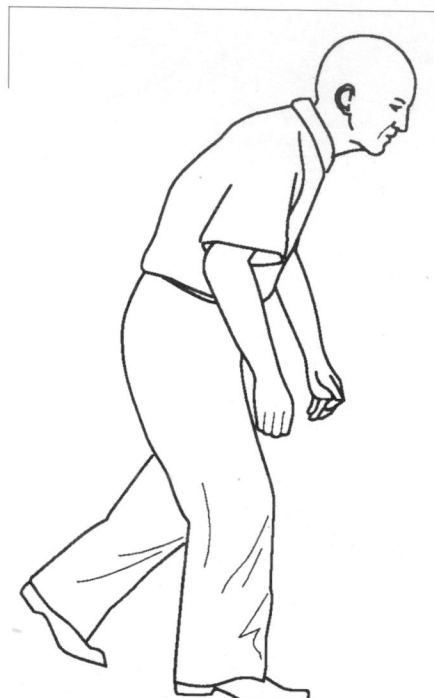

Figure 56.1
Over time, postural changes include head-forward posture, hyperkyphosis and increased flexion of the elbow, hips and knees.

addition of dystonia (twisting movements). The progression of symptoms with early onset is more gradual and has a good response to drug therapy *(Grimes et al., 1994)*.

The initial onset of Parkinsons is insidious. It may begin with a slight stoop in the shoulders, a lack of swing in one arm when walking, obscure muscular aches and cramps or a tremor in one finger. Seventy per cent of those with this condition experience a tremor as the initial symptom. A person in the early stages of the condition can easily ignore these symptoms, although the signs are often noticed by those around him. Usually the person does not seek medical attention for years.

The symptoms begin unilaterally and eventually become bilateral. After a few years, early postural changes will appear. What began as a slight stoop to the shoulders will also include a head-forward posture and hyperkyphosis of the torso. Over time, increased flexion of the elbows, hips and knees will occur *(Figure 56.1)*.

Tremors in the hands often progress to the point where the person is unable to perform controlled fine motor movements, such as writing. The person may now notice difficulty in changing positions in bed or in standing up. These are the first signs of bradykinesia, a difficulty in initiating movement.

When the person finally does seek medical help, the physician assesses the presence of bradykinesia, resting tremor and rigidity, as well as fixed posture, loss of postural reflexes and freezing phenomenon, a sudden, involuntary cessation of movement. A diagnosis of Parkinsons is made if two of the six symptoms listed above are present, with one of these symptoms being bradykinesia, resting tremor or rigidity.

The cause of Parkinsons is unknown.

➤ Genetics do not appear to play a role; studies of monozygotic twins show that if one twin gets Parkinsons, the risk of the other twin getting the condition is no greater than in the average population *(Hopkins, 1992)*.

So-called "Parkinsons-plus" syndromes (Parkinsons as a symptom of some other brain condition) **has several causes:**

➤ **repeated head trauma** as occurs with boxing *(Stern, 1990)* or, possibly, a **cerebrovascular accident** *(Porth, 1990)* can lead to injury of the central nervous system (CNS) including the basal ganglia;

➤ **toxins** have been indicated, such as severe carbon monoxide poisoning *(Porth, 1990)*. Recently, the condition has been linked to exposure to epoxy resins in paint and glue *(Lipovenko, 1995)*;

➤ **iatrogenic drug-induced** Parkinsons can occur as a result of antipsychotic medications that block dopamine receptors. A synthetically produced street drug, MTPT, also produces Parkinsons' symptoms. This drug's effect on dopamine cells is currently being studied in order to better understand the mechanisms of PD and to develop a cure for the condition *(Lieberman, Williams, 1993)*;

➤ **pathologies** such as a brain tumour, Huntington's disease, Creutzfeld-Jacob disease, Alzheimer's disease and hydrocephalus can cause Parkinsons. Encephalitis was a common cause in the first half of this century but is not common now *(Stern, 1990)*.

Progression

Parkinsons progresses slowly or rapidly, with mild or severe symptoms. The Hoehn-Yahr Scale is used to evaluate the disability of PD *(Grimes et al., 1994; Lieberman, Williams, 1993)*:

✦ **Stage 1:** One side of the body is involved. Usually rigidity or tremors are present. If the symptoms are mild, no treatment is given; if they are moderate, physiotherapy and massage are helpful.

✦ **Stage 2:** Both sides of the body are involved. Moderate tremors, rigidity and bradykinesia are present. Balance is not affected. Levodopa drug therapy may begin.

✦ **Stage 3:** Significant tremors, rigidity and bradykinesia are present. Balance and walking are now impaired. Other symptoms include unsteadiness, dystonia and freezing.

✦ **Stage 4:** Increasingly severe disability results because of severe bradykinesia. While walking is still possible, there is marked impairment. Some assistance is required with activities of daily living.

✦ **Stage 5:** There is a loss of ability to function independently. The person is immobile.

The Medical Treatment for Parkinsons

At present, there is no cure for Parkinsons. The condition is treated symptomatically with drug therapy. Levodopa (L-dopa) is commonly used, often in combination with other drugs. There are some side effects with levodopa, such as nausea, anorexia and dizziness. Generally, levodopa is combined with either carbidopa (Sinemet) or benserazide (Prolopa) because these drugs facilitate the medication reaching the brain. In addition, the combination of these drugs reduces nausea, low blood pressure and heart problems that can arise when levodopa is taken on its own *(Grimes et al., 1994)*. Unfortunately, the beneficial effects of levodopa are limited to the first three to five years of use. About 50 per cent of those on the drug find that the effects diminish and the PD symptoms worsen. After this time, increased doses are needed to achieve improvement. After 10 years, up to 80 per cent of people feel the drugs are less effective as their function and mobility decrease.

During this three- to 10-year period, the effects of the drugs can be unpredictable and may include involuntary choreiform-like movements (dystonia), altered behaviour (hallucinations and confusion) and "on-off" phenomenon. When "on-off" phenomenon occurs, the drug ceases to be effective and turns "off", with no forewarning. The "off" period can last for a few minutes to hours. It is obviously frustrating for the person; others may misinterpret the person's slower responses or inability to respond as not trying or inattention. It is during this "off" stage that choreiform movements also occur. These same movements occur when the dose is wearing off, when the dose is too high or at the peak of the dose. Dystonia is sustained during the "off" stage or when the medication is wearing off. Dystonia that occurs at the peak dose is intermittent *(Grimes et al., 1994)*.

A variety of other drugs is used and, occasionally, brain surgery is performed. Physical, occupational and massage therapy are also incorporated in the treatment of this condition. Massage therapy increases body and postural awareness, encourages movement of the limbs, maintains tissue and joint health, reduces stress and offers a supportive and accepting environment to the person with Parkinsons.

Symptom Picture

✦ **Bradykinesia** is the slow initiation and performance of movements. The symptom of bradykinesia has a wide range of effects on the body.

  • Compromised basal ganglia function causes increasing impairment of automatic sequential actions and complex repetitive actions such as walking or writing. Ordinary actions take additional time and effort, which increases as the condition progresses.

  • Changes of position, going from sitting to standing and turning over in bed pose problems. There is a loss of spontaneous movement including facial expressions, blinking and gesturing.

✦ **Rigidity** is the resistance to movement in all ranges, including rotation. It increases with voluntary movement and standing *(Stern, 1990)*. Rigidity can affect all muscles and generally feels like a stiffness or achiness that never goes away, as if the client "has not stretched for 100 years" *(Lieberman, Williams, 1993)*.

  • The rigidity of *facial muscles* and the loss of spontaneous facial expression cause a frozen expression, sometimes referred to as a "mask of Parkinsons". This can affect the person's functional ability and has a profound social effect. Some may mistakenly interpret this rigid facial expression as a reflection of the person's personality or emotional state. Dysarthria, or impairment of the tongue and muscles affecting speech, can cause a slow, soft monotone form of speech, with difficulty in articulating words. Excessive production of saliva and difficulty swallowing result in drooling. These factors, combined with the embarrassment many people with PD feel about tremors, can lead to social isolation and depression.

  • In the *upper limbs*, increased muscle tone of the suboccipital and posterior cervical muscles can cause headaches. Increased tone of the pectoralis and latissimus dorsi muscles can cause chest pain; backache can result from increased tone in the quadratus lumborum muscle. Walking, eating, speaking, breathing and making facial expressions may be compromised.

  • Rigidity of the *trunk muscles* can decrease thoracic mobility which could lead to compromised respiratory function. Respiratory complications frequently occur; pneumonia is one of the leading causes of death in people with PD *(Turnbull, 1992)*.

  • Rigidity in *leg muscles* can lead to swelling *(Lieberman, Williams, 1993)*.

✦ **Resting tremors** occur most often in the hand, at a rate of four to five, and up to eight, cycles per second. They often start in one hand, then appear in the foot on the same side. After some time, often two years or more, a tremor will then begin in the limbs of the other side. Trembling in the hands may be accompanied by a "pill rolling" tremor.

Pill rolling is the action of the thumb moving across the index and middle fingers. Resting tremors occur when the person is at rest, but they slow or stop when an action is initiated, as well as with relaxation and during sleep. In the early stages of the condition, these tremors can often be consciously controlled. This changes as the disorder progresses.

- The person often finds tremors to be the most debilitating aspect of the condition (*Elble, Koller, 1990*), although, as the PD progresses, bradykinesia becomes an even greater disability than tremors or rigidity (*Grimes et al., 1994*).

- The resting tremors of Parkinsons should not be confused with *benign essential tremor*. Benign essential tremor has a familial tendency. It can begin at any age, usually appearing as a trembling in both hands and often spreading to the head and voice. Benign essential tremor is slowly progressive, with long periods of remission. Generally, the tremor occurs when the hand is held in a particular position, such as holding a cup, or when doing an action. It does not occur at rest and will cease when the limb is supported.

✦ **Breathing** is affected. Rigidity of respiratory muscles contributes to shallow breathing and an increased risk of pneumonia and other respiratory conditions. In addition, dysfunction of the central respiratory control centres, as a result of the disease process, also contributes to intermittent dyspnea (difficulty breathing), tachypnea (rapid breathing), chest discomfort and involuntary gasping (*Cohen, Weiner, 1994*).

✦ **Fatigue** is experienced. Compromised function requires a greater expenditure of energy to complete actions.

✦ **Postural changes** result. The forward flexion and lateral tilt of the trunk and forward flexion of the head can initially be lessened through the client's effort to stand straighter. Eventually, the posture will become more fixed, leading to postural imbalances and joint dysfunction. The lateral tilt of the trunk can lead to a scoliosis. Hyperkyphosis is increasingly pronounced. Contractures can occur.

✦ **Gait** is affected. There is less arm swinging while walking and a loss of spontaneous gestures. Postural changes, combined with the effects of bradykinesia, alter the gait. Flexed posture will force the person to walk with quick, shuffling steps to keep from falling forward. Due to the difficulty of initiating movements, the commencement of a stride is a problem. It is challenging when the person wants to change direction or stop, since each of these actions requires initiation of a new motion. Over time, as gait alterations continue, the person is almost running with short, shuffling steps. This is called **"festinating gait"**.

✦ **Balance** is affected. The righting reflexes enable a person to stay upright and balanced. With Parkinsons, "retropulsion" may occur, making the person unable to stop from falling backward. "Propulsion" results in the inability to stop from falling forward. This leads to falls which can result in injury; even while seated, the loss of the righting reflexes can cause the person to fall over.

✦ **Freezing phenomenon** is the sudden inability of the person to move. This occurs if the person becomes distracted or interrupted while doing an action. For example, when walking, the freezing phenomenon can occur if the person sees a real or imagined obstacle, such as a line on the pavement. He is suddenly unable to lift his feet, as if the feet were glued to the ground. To start moving, he must relax and think about unsticking his feet and then step over the perceived obstacle (*Calne et al., 1995*).

✦ **Pain syndromes** can result from altered biomechanics, postural imbalances and muscle disuse with the resultant ischemia. Pain can also result from the cramping and spasm in muscles of the affected limb. It can be severe, especially in people with a younger onset. Pain is more likely during "off" drug periods, usually in the morning, when medication levels are low.

✦ **Sensory changes** can occur in glove and sock patterns, which result in hyperesthesia and pain when the area is touched. The reason is not known but may be a side effect of medication use.

✦ **Autonomic dysfunction** is relatively common. Salivation and sweating increase. Salivation, combined with difficulty swallowing, can lead to drooling and difficulty holding food in the mouth. Episodes of profuse sweating may occur. An increase in sebaceous secretions results in a greasy skin texture around the face and neck. The skin may be dry over the rest of the body.

✦ **Constipation** can result, often as a side effect of some medications as well as from hyperkyphosis.

✦ **Hypotension** is experienced in greater numbers of people with Parkinsons than in the general population. Low blood pressure can occur while resting, as well as when standing (referred to as orthostatic hypotension). It is thought to be related to autonomic dysfunction as well as to the effects of levodopa therapy. Hypotension is indicated if systolic pressure falls by 20 to 30 mm Hg or diastolic pressure falls by 10 to 20 mm Hg with a postural change from the supine position to standing.

✦ **Speech** is affected by swallowing difficulties as well as incoordination or decreased muscle movements.

✦ **Writing ability** is affected. Written letters become increasingly small and cramped. This is known as micrographia.

✦ **Depression** can result from chemical imbalances in the brain, as part of the disorder. It can be exacerbated by stress from social isolation and physical limitations. It may also be a side effects of drugs, particularly anticholinergic medications such as Artane or Cogentin (*Lieberman, Williams, 1993*).

✦ **Dementia** may occur. Prevalent statistics suggest that dementia occurs in 40 per cent of people with PD, though many suggest this is exaggerated. If factors such as depression, pseudodementia and Alzheimer's disease are considered, some physicians suggest the incidence of true Parkinsons dementia is likely 10 to 15 per cent (*Hopkins, 1992*).

Subjective Information

HEALTH HISTORY QUESTIONS

✦ What is the client's general health? Are there any cardiovascular problems, diabetes or kidney disease?

✦ When was the client diagnosed?

✦ What were the first symptoms experienced? How have they progressed? What are the current symptoms?

✦ What medications are currently being taken? Are any side effects being experienced?

✦ Does the client experience "on-off" phenomenon? The client should be encouraged to book massage appointments for when the medication is working to get the most benefit and allow the therapist to do the most effective work.

✦ What other treatment is the client receiving, such as physiotherapy or chiropractic?

✦ Is the client experiencing any pain? Can the client describe the type of pain as well as where, when and how long it is experienced?

✦ What is the functional ability of the client's fine and gross motor skills? How able is the client to do activities of daily living? Is the client independent? Is he working? Is he retired? Does he have any hobbies or perform regular exercise?

✦ Are any difficulties experienced with changing positions, such as turning over in bed or getting up from a supine position? This helps the therapist know how much assistance the client will need during the massage.

✦ Does the client use any aids, such as a cane or walker?

Objective Information

Observations

✐ The typical Parkinsons posture includes forward flexion and bowing down of the head, forward flexion and lateral tilt of the trunk, flexion of the elbows, hips and knees and inversion of the feet with the big toes dorsiflexed.

✐ A postural assessment will allow measurement of the degree of the hyperkyphosis and head-forward posture, as well as revealing the presence of a scoliosis and a posterior or anterior pelvic tilt.

✐ Gait abnormalities are observed.

✐ Resting tremors may be apparent in the hand and foot, unilaterally or bilaterally.

✐ Difficulty in maintaining an upright posture, due to the loss of righting reflexes, is observed.

✐ Movements generally appear stiff and rigid.

✍ A frozen facial expression may be accompanied by a lack of eye blinking and an increase in drooling.

✍ See also the CNS Strategies chapter, observation section.

Palpation

✍ Rigidity is palpated in muscles throughout the body, due to increased tone in the agonist and antagonist muscles.

✍ Skin may be oily on the face, but dry on the rest of the body.

✍ See also the CNS Strategies chapter, palpation section.

Testing

✍ The usual range of motion and strength testing protocol is attempted.

✍ **AF ROM testing** will reveal a decrease in range of motion if rigidity is present. The more severe the rigidity, the more severely compromised the range of motion.

✍ **PR ROM testing** will reveal uniform resistance in the flexor and extensor groups acting on an affected joint, which will decrease the range of motion. This type of rigidity is referred to as lead pipe rigidity. Muscle resistance that is interrupted intermittently by a tremor, creating a ratchet-like movement, is referred to as cog wheel rigidity. This type usually occurs in the wrist and elbow.

✍ **AR strength testing** will not yield useful results with the limbs affected by rigidity.

Special Tests

✍ **Bradykinesia testing:** A positive test results if the movement becomes slower and increasingly difficult.

✍ **Sensory testing** for light touch, deep pressure, pain and temperature perception, two-point discrimination and proprioception is performed. Results will vary depending on the client; there may be sensory impairment or facilitation.

✍ **Specific orthopedic tests** are performed for secondary conditions. If rigidity is present, the tests may not yield viable results.

Contraindications

✦ Sympathetic nervous system firing should not be stimulated as this will increase the symptoms. Prolonged vigorous or painful techniques should be avoided.

✦ Areas sensitive to touch are avoided.

✦ Pressure and hydrotherapy applications are modified on areas of altered sensation.

✦ Positioning, techniques and hydrotherapy are modified if **hypertension** is present. Due to the usually advanced age of persons with Parkinsons, increased blood pressure and heart disease are concerns.

✦ **Hypotension** is a threat as a result of autonomic dysfunction or as a drug side effect. Added care should be taken when the client changes position. The therapist may need to give support to the client when he is getting on and off the table.

Treatment Goals — Treatment Plan

- **Positioning** possibilities may be limited by the degree of rigidity and the severity of forward flexion of the thorax.

- The more rigidity and the more difficulty the client has with positional changes, the fewer the changes of position. The effort exerted to change position can increase sympathetic nervous system firing and, in turn, increase tremors and rigidity. This must be weighed against the potential benefits of treating the client in another position. If turning is a problem, the supine position is the most effective.

Maintain proper alignment.

- The client is positioned in proper alignment, whether on the massage table or seated. To reinforce good posture, the head is kept in line with the spine. The shoulders and pelvis are midline.

- Positioning should encourage a less flexed posture. In the **prone** position, one or two pillows are placed lengthwise under the trunk; towels are used to support the shoulders. An adjustable face cradle enables the client to keep the neck in alignment without overly encouraging a head-forward posture. If a face cradle is not available, pillowing is used to support the head as it is turned to one side.

- The **supine** position requires pillowing to comfortably support the forward flexion of the trunk and the forward position of the head. The therapist takes care not to increase or exaggerate the already flexed posture.

- **Sidelying** can be used but this position can promote flexion of the trunk. The therapist must ensure that the trunk is as straight as possible. The client is encouraged to avoid curling forward. A few pillows placed anteriorly may help. A towel roll under the waist helps to decrease a lateral lumbar curve and creates less compression of the ribs and intercostal muscles on the side away from the table. A pillow is also placed between the knees.

- If the client produces excess saliva, a cloth is kept beside the client during the treatment. If the therapist needs to assist the client in cleaning off the saliva, the therapist wears vinyl gloves.

- **Hydrotherapy** modifications are necessary with decreased tissue health and lost sensory perception or the presence of hypertension. If no problems exist, deep moist heat is used to increase relaxation and decrease muscle tone. If edema is present, cool applications are used in conjunction with elevation.

General Treatment

Decrease sympathetic nervous system firing. Provide emotional support. Decrease tremors, temporarily.

- The treatment is performed in the context of a relaxation massage. Slow relaxed breathing is encouraged. A supportive touch is used throughout the massage, while performing smooth rhythmical techniques.

Treatment Goals Treatment Plan

Specific Treatment

Decrease edema, if present.

🖐 If edema is present, drainage techniques are interspersed with **passive range of motion.** Elevation of the limb and cool hydrotherapy also assist to reduce edema.

Maintain tissue health.

🖐 Swedish massage techniques are used to improve circulation and overall tissue health. These must be modified for depth and speed if sensory impairment is present. Strokes are applied segmentally if the tissue is fragile as long strokes can create drag on the tissue.

Decrease pain.

🖐 Pain is decreased through promoting relaxation and addressing secondary postural changes and compensation. Areas that may be touch-sensitive are avoided. Pain can also be caused by too much or too little treatment. The therapist needs good client feedback from treatment to treatment.

Address postural changes and muscle imbalances.

🖐 To minimize the effects of postural changes, a variety of Swedish techniques are used to massage the affected soft tissue. Range of motion of joints is maintained and the client is made aware of his postural restrictions.

🖐 A primary treatment focus is on decreasing the forward flexion of the trunk and cervical spine, as well as addressing any scoliosis. With the client in a supine position, the areas addressed are the upper trunk, including the anterior chest and shoulder girdle, and the cervical spine.

🖐 The anterior chest and neck are treated as in a hyperkyphosis treatment. Fascial release, through skin rolling or spreading techniques, is applied to the anterior chest and neck.

🖐 The pectoral muscles, major and minor, are thoroughly treated with Swedish techniques. A passive stretch of the muscles is included by abducting and extending the arm (see the thoracic outlet syndrome chapter).

🖐 **Passive range of motion** and joint play are applied to the glenohumeral and sternoclavicular joints. Work to the shoulder girdle increases the client's mobility and awareness, encouraging conscious arm swinging movements while walking.

🖐 Sternocleidomastoid, scalenes, hyoid and suboccipital muscles are treated with Swedish techniques to decrease muscle tone. Pincer grasp techniques, Golgi tendon organ release, muscle stripping and ischemic compressions are used. **Passive stretches** are performed on all these muscles.

🖐 If an anterior pelvic tilt is found during the postural assessment, the iliopsoas, rectus femoris and quadratus lumborum muscles are the focus of treatment to reduce hypertonicity and trigger points.

🖐 If a posterior pelvic tilt is observed during the postural assessment, the

712

Treatment Goals   Treatment Plan

gluteal, hamstring and abdominal muscles are treated to reduce hypertonicity and trigger points.

Limit contractures, if possible.

☙ Contractures are treated using pre-treatment heat followed with a slow **prolonged passive stretch with overpressure.**

Reduce constipation, if appropriate.

☙ A general abdominal massage is performed using Swedish techniques, such as over-handed palmar kneading and wringing. Specifically, fingertip kneading is applied to the colon.

Address the diaphragm muscle.

☙ Fascial techniques, such as spreading and skin rolling, are gradually applied over the abdomen and lower intercostal area. These are followed by specific muscle stripping to the accessible intercostal muscles, done gently and slowly so as not to increase sympathetic nervous system firing. As this work is time-consuming, only a few muscles are treated each appointment.

☙ To treat the diaphragm, specific compressions and kneading techniques are applied along, and just under, the costal border. Point pressure can be applied at several points along the diaphragm. The thumb pressure is directed under up and under the costal border with exhalation — this is when the diaphragm is relaxed and most accessible.

Maintain thoracic mobility.

☙ General full-body rhythmical rocking is appropriate. Rib springing is performed in the supine and the prone positions to mobilize the thorax. With the client in a supine position, following the abdominal massage, the therapist stands opposite the side to be mobilized. The lower hand is placed under the ribs and positioned as if to do unilateral wringing. The heel of the other hand is placed along the medial costal border. The lower hand lifts the ribs upward and medially while the upper hand applies a pressure on the ribs downward and laterally. As the pressure from the upper hand increases, the lower hand releases the ribs. The mobilization is done in a rhythmical manner, similar to kneading bread. It is performed several times on each side.

☙ Further **active resisted mobilizations** are performed by compressing the ribs medially with exhalation. The therapist's hands are placed on either side of the ribs, the fingers oriented towards the head but following along the ribs at an oblique angle. The technique works well if the therapist directs the client's inhalation and exhalation. Mobilizations are performed for two to three breaths.

☙ The client is directed to take full breaths encouraging diaphragm, rib and sternal movement.

☙ **Rotational movements of the trunk** are encouraged. The client bends the knees while lying supine and rotates them to one side. The head is turned to the opposite side within the available range.

  • The therapist holds the knees and supports them as they rotate

713

Treatment Goals | Treatment Plan

towards the table. This exercise does not require that end of range is achieved; the client should not feel a large stretch but rather relaxation in the muscles. This is held for up to 10 seconds.

- The therapist then walks to the other side of the table and brings the knees to that side for about 10 seconds. The client's head is rotated to the other side. This is repeated several times.

- The hip-knee movements assist in relaxing the muscles of the pelvis and lumbar and thoracic spine. The cervical movements assist in relaxing the cervical and upper thoracic spine.

- Lateral and anterior challenge are used to mobilize the spine.

- The following techniques decrease rigidity:

  - overall reduction of sympathetic nervous system firing;

  - Swedish techniques such as effleurage, palmar kneading and fingertip kneading;

  - slow passive stretches.

- Specifically, the rigid facial muscles can be massaged with passive movements performed to the temporomandibular joint.

Decrease rigidity, temporarily.

Encourage integration of the body.

- Feedback is elicited from the client when performing massage on the areas that have sensory dysfunction or increased rigidity. In the case of a client who is totally focused on the symptomatic areas, the therapist redirects awareness to unaffected areas.

- When finishing the treatment, the therapist may use techniques such as stroking or gentle muscle squeezing, applied simultaneously along both sides of the body. Techniques are started at the shoulder, then continued along the length of the body finishing at the feet.

- See the CNS strategies chapter for more details.

Self-care Goals | Self-care Plan

Encourage relaxation.

- Relaxation techniques, such as diaphragmatic breathing, are encouraged, though contraindicated if advanced diabetes or kidney disease is present (*Fried, 1990*). Visualization and meditation are useful.

Maintain functional ability through improving flexibility, range of motion and balance.

- The client is encouraged to do activities of daily living at the level of his ability, but to pace the activities to avoid fatigue. The client is also encouraged to participate in movement rehabilitation programs if difficulty develops with balancing and shifting weight. Yoga and Tai Chi will improve flexibility, balance and coordination. Diaphragmatic breathing helps to maintain maximal respiratory capacity and mobility of the thorax. A regular aerobic program, such as walking, could be

Self-care Goals   Self-care Plan

undertaken. The client is encouraged to consciously stand as straight as possible and swing the arms while walking.

✍ Remedial exercises are done at a relaxed and easy pace. If movements become complicated and difficult for the client, the sympathetic nervous response will increase and create more rigidity. Exercises should be performed when the medications are working and not during "off" periods. Exercising to music helps to create more rhythmical movements *(Duvoisin, 1991)*.

✍ **Trunk rotation exercises** done during the treatment are given as self-care *(Figure 56.2)*:

• They can be done on a bed or on the floor — whatever is easier for the client. However, as self-care, each movement is not held for

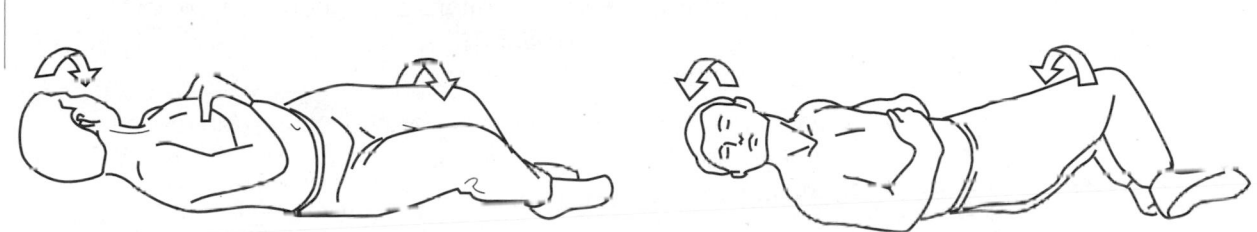

Part 1: The head rotates in one direction while the legs (with the knees flexed) rotate in the opposite direction.

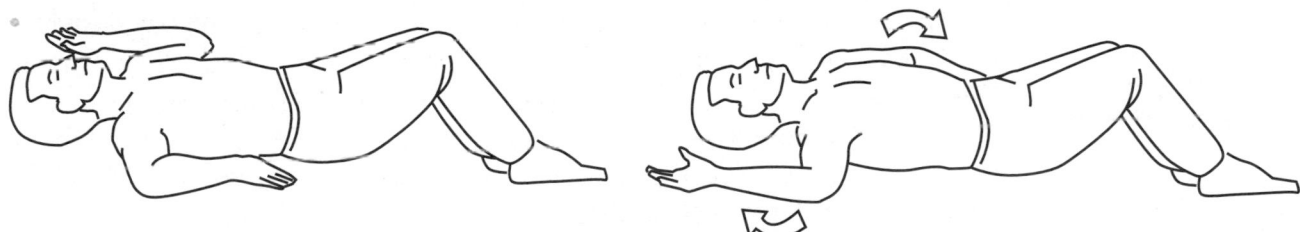

Part 2: Ninety degrees of shoulder abduction, 90 degrees of elbow flexion. One shoulder internally rotates while the other externally rotates. These are performed alternately in a slow rhythmical manner. The legs are not involved.

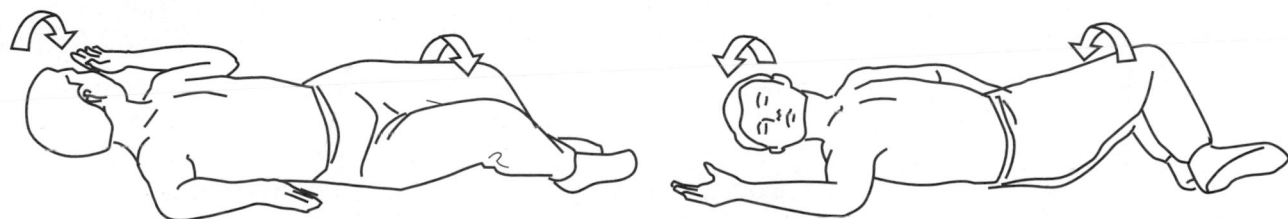

Part 3: The above actions are combined in a smooth relaxed manner.

Figure 56.2
Trunk rotation exercises.

Self-care Goals

Maintain functional ability through improving flexibility, range of motion and balance.

Self-care Plan

10 seconds; instead, a relaxed rhythm is established. Once the client can easily perform the alternating hip-knee and neck rotation *(Figure 56.2: Part 1)*, the exercise is made more complex by adding arm movements. These arm movements help to release the shoulder girdle, including the internal and external rotators of the humerus.

- Initially, the client places the arms at 90 degrees of abduction. With the humerus in external rotation, the elbow of one arm is flexed to 90 degrees with the palm facing up and the fingers parallel to the head.

- The other humerus is in internal rotation, with the elbow similarly flexed but the palm of the hand facing down and the fingers pointing towards the feet.

- The client alternates the position of the shoulder from internal rotation to external rotation in a rhythmical manner *(Figure 56.2: Part 2)*.

- When the arm movement is performed easily, head movement is added. The head is turned towards the side where the palm is **facing upwards.**

- Finally, when this becomes easy, the initial hip-knee movement is added *(Figure 56.2: Part 3)*.

✐ The client may not be able to do this last combined movement and should be encouraged to do only what can be accomplished easily and without stress.

✐ If necessary, each of the movements can be done separately or in combinations of two. For example, the hip-knee exercise is combined with the neck rotation and the arm-shoulder exercise is combined with the neck rotation.

✐ The **spine and shoulder girdle mobilization** can also be performed in a sidelying position:

- The pelvis is stabilized in a midline position.

- The trunk is slowly rotated forward and backward *(Figure 56.3: Part 1)*.

- The scapula is then protracted with forward rotation and retracted with backward rotation *(Figure 56.3: Part 2)*. Protraction of the scapula is achieved with the shoulder flexed to 90 degrees and the elbow extended. The action is one of reaching out with the arm. Retraction of the scapula is achieved by bringing the shoulder back into extension, with the elbow bent to 90 degrees of flexion. This action is one of pulling away from something.

- The movements should be slow and rhythmical

Self-care Goals

Self-care Plan

✍ Initially, the therapist can educate a care giver to place a hand on the pelvis to help stabilize it or to guide the movement of the scapula. This is only necessary until the exercise is easy for the client.

✍ Pelvic rocking exercises are performed in a seated portion:

- The client supports himself in order to gently tilt the pelvis forward (anteriorly) and then backward (posteriorly).

- A rhythm is established and the rocking repeated until the client feels the movements are relaxed and easy. The trunk stays upright with minimal movement forward and backward.

✍ The above exercises were modified from Feldenkrais therapy (*Turnbull, 1992*).

Educate the client.

✍ The client is encouraged to maintain tissue health. To treat distal edema, the client is taught basic lymphatic drainage techniques and cool hydrotherapy applications, such as towel wraps. The client is also educated about signs of gangrene, which is tissue necrosis due to an interference of blood supply *(Porth, 1990)*. Medical help should be sought if black or brown discolouration develops in distal digits. This

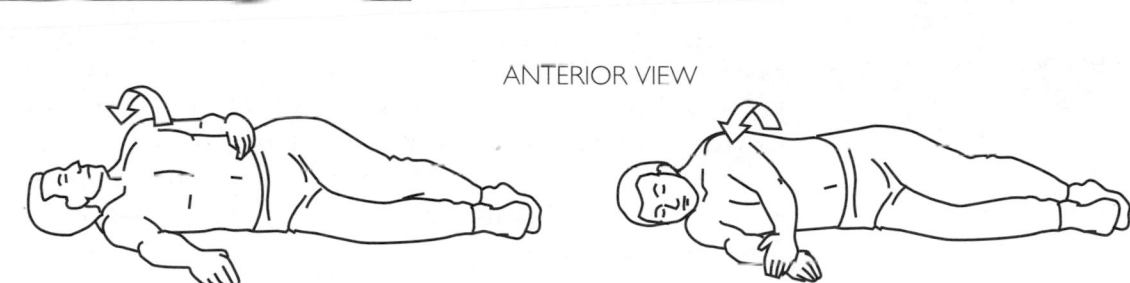

Part 1: In sidelying, the trunk is slowly rotated forward and back with the hips relatively stable.

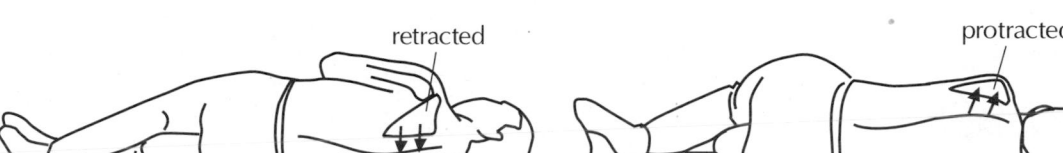

Part 2: The shoulder is retracted when the trunk is rotated back.
The shoulder is protracted when the trunk is rotated forward (the extended arm reaches forward).

Figure 56.3
Spine and shoulder girdle mobilization in sidelying.

Self-care Goals

Self-care Plan

may be accompanied by inflammation or by coolness and swelling in the affected tissue. The client is encouraged to be aware of posture and to maintain the best possible posture for as long as possible. The client should engage arm swinging when walking and should try to stand and sit with the upper body straighter.

Refer the client.

✍ The client can be referred to a local support or social group such as the Parkinsons Society.

Treatment Frequency and Expected Outcome

Because Parkinsons is a permanent condition, the treatments are regular and ongoing. One-hour weekly treatments have been shown to be beneficial.

Parkinsons is a progressive condition. The progress may be slow or rapid. People whose initial symptom is a tremor will tend to have a slower progression *(Grimes et al., 1994)*.

See also Strategies: Central Nervous System Conditions, stress reduction, constipation, hyperkyphosis, hyperlordosis, scoliosis, bronchitis and the other respiratory conditions, hypertension and edema for related treatments.

Before levodopa drug therapy was introduced, 50 per cent of those with the condition were either unable to work or completely disabled within four years of the onset. The average life span was nine years from onset to death. Since levodopa drug therapy has been used, over 50 per cent of people with PD are in better shape six years after starting treatment than before treatment. The average lifespan has improved to 14 years from onset. With onset occurring in one's sixties, this begins to approach normal life expectancy of the general population *(Hopkins, 1992)*.

57

CEREBRAL PALSY

Linda Ludwig

Cerebral palsy (CP) is a term used for motor function disorders that result from damage to the immature brain.

"Cerebral" means brain and "palsy" refers to a lack of movement control. This non-progressive condition is the result of lesions that occur during the perinatal period, from half-way through pregnancy to seven days postpartum, and up to three years of age.

In 1862, Dr. Little, an English physician, first described one type of cerebral palsy known as spastic diplegia *(Hopkins, 1994)*. This type of cerebral palsy accounts for 75 per cent of all cases and involves spasticity of the lower limbs and hips as one of the primary symptoms *(Ontario Federation for Cerebral Palsy, N.d.a.)*.

Fetal brain development begins approximately midway through pregnancy. At this stage and into early infant life, the brain is susceptible to damage which, in turn, can result in cerebral palsy.

There is a variety of possible causes of cerebral palsy:

➤ **Hypoxia** and **ischemia** can occur in utero from a kink in the umbilical cord or the cord wrapping around the fetus's neck, maldevelopment of the placenta or shock in the mother from an accident. Postpartum hypoxia or ischemia can result from suppression of the respiratory centres because of overmedication of the mother just before birthing, or pneumonia, a collapsed lung or drowning of the infant.

➤ **Trauma to, or rupture of, cerebral blood vessels** can occur in utero due to separation of the placenta. Difficult or prolonged delivery, such as with a breech birth or the birth of a very large baby, can result in trauma and injury to the brain. Postpartum head injury from an accident or abuse accounts for 18 per cent of people with cerebral palsy *(Ontario Federation for Cerebral Palsy, N.d.a.)*. The brain of a premature baby is particularly susceptible to hemorrhage. Strokes can occur as a result of dehydration.

➤ **Toxicity** and **infection** can lead to brain damage. In utero, rhesus (Rh factor) incompatibility or an infection in the mother, such as measles, shingles or a virus, can damage brain cells. Postpartum meningitis, viral encephalitis and lead and carbon monoxide poisoning account for 57 per cent of people with cerebral palsy *(Ontario Federation for Cerebral Palsy, N.d.a.).*

It is estimated that one in every 500 babies and up to one in three premature babies are affected to some extent with cerebral palsy *(Ontario Federation for Cerebral Palsy, 1995).* Boys are affected slightly more than girls at a ratio of 1.5 to 1 *(Hopkins, 1994).* The symptoms can be as variable as the causes. The type and severity of symptoms will depend on the location and extent of the brain lesion, from few or no obvious signs to a severe lack of motor control.

Cerebral palsy is named according to the main movement disorder and the limbs that are affected. There are **four main types of movement disorders:** spastic (increased tone); athetoid (uncontrolled movement); ataxic (poor coordination); or mixed (usually spastic and athetoid). The most common is spastic cerebral palsy and the least common is ataxic cerebral palsy. CP can manifest in the limbs in a variety of ways including: monoplegia (one arm or leg); diplegia (usually both legs); triplegia (three limbs); quadriplegia (all four limbs); and hemiplegia (the arm and leg on one side of the body).

Senses such as vision and hearing are commonly affected to varying degrees. These sensory losses result in compromised learning and communication skills. Epilepsy as well as mental developmental delay and emotional disturbances may be present. While the original lesion is non-progressive, the original symptoms change as the child ages and the central nervous system matures *(Hopkins, 1994).*

Since cerebral palsy occurs at such an early age, the long-term effects can result in increased functional losses. These are due to chronic stresses that occur as the person compensates for the effects of the disability. Postural dysfunctions, such as scoliosis and hyperkyphosis, can compromise respiratory and gastrointestinal function. Pain syndromes, acute or chronic, can be musculoskeletal (altered posture), neurological (peripheral nerve compression or entrapment) or arthritic (altered biomechanics of joints). Osteoporosis and, in turn, fractures are common as a result of limited weight bearing and inactivity. The side effect of some medications can compromise bone density. For example, Dilantin, an anticonvulsant used to treat seizures, has been found to contribute to osteoporosis *(Ontario Federation for Cerebral Palsy, N.d.c.).* It is also thought that the original disease process of CP causes certain tissues, organs and organ systems to be weak. Over a lifetime this may speed the aging process in these structures.

The Medical Treatment for Cerebral Palsy

There is no cure for cerebral palsy but for the child much can be done to lessen the disabling effects of the condition. Physical and occupational therapy are commonly used to increase functional ability and encourage as much independence as possible. Usually, as the child reaches adolescence, the preference is for sports activities with therapeutic benefits, such as swimming or horseback riding, rather than organized therapy. Speech therapy is often required.

Surgery may be performed to lengthen tendons that are shortened and, therefore, interfere with functional movement. In the leg, surgery is usually performed on the Achilles tendon to increase ankle dorsiflexion. In the arm, surgery is often done on the flexor tendons in the forearm to increase wrist flexion. Occasionally, specific nerve roots in the spine are surgically severed (referred to as posterior rhizotomy) to reduce spasticity. Medications are prescribed to treat spasticity, rigidity and seizures.

Massage therapy addresses spasticity, temporarily, as well as the many secondary conditions that can result from the motor disorders. The therapist is also able to provide supportive and sensitive touch.

Symptom Picture

✦ A client's symptom picture reflects initial symptoms as well as those associated with aging with CP. A 35-year-old client will have had the condition for over 30 years. Long-term tissue, joint and postural changes, often accompanied by pain, are present.

✦ **Impaired movement** is usually hemiplegic, diplegic or quadriplegic but can be monoplegic or triplegic.

✦ There is a variety of movement disorders.

  • **Spasticity** is the most common. It increases with pain, stress and emotions such as fear or anxiety. Rigidity is possible.

  • **Athetoid** movements are slow and writhing. They increase with voluntary movement and stop with sleep.

  • **Choreiform** movements are quick, uncontrolled and without purpose. They do not stop with sleep.

  • **Ataxia** is a lack of coordination and clumsiness of movements. Ataxia in the face causes grimacing. It is sometimes accompanied by an intention tremor.

  • **Flaccidity** may be present in the first year or two. It will then change to spasticity or athetoid movement.

  • **Reflex movements** may be present. These may be early developmental reflexes that would usually disappear as the child develops. The affected muscles are usually sensitive to stretching.

✦ **Pain** can result from muscular, neurological and bony changes. It can be acute or chronic. Pain can be caused by long-term postural changes and imbalances, which result from impaired movement and compensation.

✦ CP causes many **postural dysfunctions.**

  • Scoliosis can be present. As the person with CP ages this can lead to respiratory difficulties due to decreased rib movement and compression of the lung and diaphragm on the concave side.

  • Hyperlordosis and hyperkyphosis may be present.

✦ **Contracture formation** reduces range of motion and increases functional losses. Surgery is often performed during childhood to lengthen the affected tendons.

  • Equinus deformity is caused by a short Achilles tendon which reduces dorsiflexion.

  • Internal rotation of the hip is common with spastic diplegia.

- Hip flexion contracture is common.

✦ Permanent skeletal changes and **arthritis** develop from poor joint biomechanics. These occur in a younger population, becoming more extensive with age. The lower limbs seem particularly vulnerable. The hip, knee and ankle joints often present with problems such as hip subluxation, dislocation and cartilage degeneration.

✦ **Stenosis** of the cervical spine is a risk, especially with athetoid cerebral palsy.

✦ **Osteoporosis** is likely if the person is non-weight-bearing or inactive for many years.

✦ **Peripheral nerve compressions** are possible, as a result of postural imbalances.

✦ **Epilepsy** may be present as a result of the CNS lesion.

✦ **Tissue health** is often compromised. Disuse atrophy is likely in people over 60 who are not able to carry out traditional forms of exercise. If the person is in a wheelchair, edema in the legs will likely develop and there is a risk of decubitus ulcers.

✦ There can be a variety of **sensory losses.** There is an inability to distinguish objects by touch alone (agnosia). For example, to tell the difference between a block and a ball, the person must look at the objects. Proprioception may be decreased.

✦ **Generally, perception of pain, temperature and pressure is not affected.**

✦ **Bowel and bladder function** are usually compromised. Esophagitis, gastritis and ulcers may be present. Constipation and gastrointestinal problems can be secondary to medication use as well as to decreased activity, postural dysfunction and aging.

✦ **Speech** may be affected by dysarthria, which is an impairment of the muscles involved in producing speech. The person may speak slowly and be difficult to understand. There can be difficulty swallowing and an inability to control saliva. Some people with CP liken their speech to a different language. As the listener becomes attuned to it, words are easier to comprehend.

✦ **Hearing** impairment may be slight or profound.

✦ **Vision** can be normal or limited. The person may be cross-eyed or may squint excessively. Blindness is possible.

✦ Frustration and anger may result if the person is severely physically disabled but of average cognitive awareness. This is due to the difficulty in communication and extreme functional limitations.

✦ Many associate intellectual impairment with CP but, in fact, intellect may or may not be affected. Estimates vary because of the difficulty in assessment when communication skills are affected. It is most important to be aware that the degree of physical disability in a person with cerebral palsy does not indicate her level of intelligence.

Subjective Information

HEALTH HISTORY QUESTIONS

✦ Are any other conditions present, such as hypertension, diabetes or kidney disease?

✦ What type of cerebral palsy does the client have?

✦ What are the client's general symptoms?

✦ What medication is the client taking?

✦ Is the client experiencing any pain? Can the client describe the type of pain as well as where, when and how long it is experienced?

✦ Are there any sensory losses? Hearing? Vision? Speech?

✦ Does the client have seizures? What type is experienced? What are the triggers?

✦ What movement is affected? How are the fine and gross motor skills? Are ambulation aids used?

✦ What activities can the client do? Does the client work? What are the client's hobbies?

Objective Information

Observations

✍ A spasticity pattern or other movement dysfunction may be observed in the affected limbs.

✍ If the client is able to walk she may have a circumducted gait. The ability to balance and shift weight may be impaired. A cane, walker or wheelchair may be used.

✍ Edema is often present in the distal limbs.

✍ Muscle bulk differences may be noticed when comparing the affected limbs with the unaffected limbs.

✍ A postural assessment can be performed, noting asymmetries as a result of motor dysfunction (spasticity or athetoid movements), altered biomechanics of the affected limbs and compensation by the unaffected limbs.

Palpation

✍ Hypertonicity is palpated in the muscles affected by spasticity or athetoid movements.

✍ Contractures are likely in the muscles experiencing spasticity. For example, contractures may be palpated in the wrist flexors, hip flexors and Achilles tendons.

✍ Edema may be palpated in the distal part of the affected limbs. This tissue may be cool due to ischemia.

✍ Numerous shoulder, hip and knee pathologies on the affected limbs may be present. There may be adhesions or signs of inflammation as a result of soft tissue or joint pathology.

✍ Tenderness is often present. In adults with CP, this pain is due to arthritic changes, peripheral nerve compression or secondary postural changes.

Testing

✍ Some clients may be reluctant to take part in testing because of childhood experiences with continual physical examinations. A respectful and clear consent to the testing process will often help the client overcome her reluctance. Testing is performed over a series of treatments.

✍ **AF** and **PR ROM** will reveal a decrease in range of motion if spasticity is present. The more severe the spasticity the more severely compromised the range of motion. In the most extreme cases, no movement is possible.

✍ If athetoid movements are present, range of motion testing may not yield useful or accurate results.

✍ **AR strength testing** will not yield useful results if spasticity or athetoid movements are present.

Contraindications

✦ Avoid joint play and aggressive mobilization techniques such as rib springing if osteoporosis or osteoarthritis is present in an older adult with CP.

✦ Do not increase sympathetic nervous system firing as this will increase the symptoms. Avoid vigorous or painful techniques.

✦ Modify pressure and hydrotherapy applications on areas of altered sensation.

✦ Modify positioning, Swedish techniques and hydrotherapy if **hypertension** is present.

✦ The presence of decubitus ulcers is a contraindication to local massage. If the therapist observes the early signs of an ulcer — redness and, possibly, heat, swelling and pain — the client is referred for medical attention.

✦ Avoid frictions if the client is on anti-inflammatories.

Special Tests

✍ **Sensory testing:** There are wide varieties and degrees of sensory losses, from slight and patchy to profound; pain, temperature and touch perception may not be affected.

✍ **Specific orthopedic tests** are performed for secondary conditions. If spasticity or athetoid movements are present in the limbs to be tested, the test may not yield viable results.

Treatment Goals | Treatment Plan

🖐 This treatment reflects the added concerns for adult clients with CP. If seizures are experienced by the client, appropriate modifications are made. See the seizures chapter.

🖐 **Positioning** prone, supine, sidelying, seated and in a wheelchair are possible. Any position can be used that is comfortable for the client and allows access to the structures to be massaged. Sidelying allows good overall access in treating the neck, anterior and posterior shoulder, low back, gluteals and leg.

🖐 Athetoid movements can make positioning difficult and will require discussion with the client. The client's sleeping position can be used as a guide to a comfortable and familiar choice. Modifications are made to reflect any secondary conditions such as hypertension.

🖐 **Hydrotherapy** reflects the needs of the client and is modified if poor tissue health, hypertension or other secondary tissue concerns are present. Sensory perception of pain, heat and cold is not usually affected with cerebral palsy. The client's temperature preference is individual. For some clients, colder temperatures increase spasticity. Generally, heat applications are used to increase relaxation and decrease excessive muscle tone. Contrast applications are used to improve circulation and tissue health. Cool applications are used with elevation to reduce edema.

General Treatment

Decrease sympathetic nervous system firing. Provide emotional support.

🖐 The treatment is performed in the context of a relaxation massage. Diaphragmatic breathing is encouraged. Supportive touch is used to apply smooth rhythmical Swedish techniques.

Specific Treatment

Decrease edema, if present. Maintain tissue health. Be vigilant for decubitus ulcers.

🖐 The limb is elevated and cool hydrotherapy is applied to reduce edema. Axillary or inguinal pumping is performed followed by drainage techniques. This is interspersed with **passive range of motion** to the joints of the affected limb. If edema is not addressed and becomes long-standing, tissue fragility will result. Then any injury could develop into an ulcer and, potentially, gangrene.

🖐 Swedish massage techniques are used to improve circulation and overall tissue health. The strokes are applied with reduced pressure and segmentally if the tissue is fragile, as long strokes can create drag on the tissue.

Reduce contractures, if possible. Support functional contractures, if present.

🖐 Contractures, which contribute to a reduced range of motion in a joint, are often present in the hip flexors, external rotators and Achilles tendons. Pre-treatment hydrotherapy of a warm or hot application is followed by a slow **prolonged passive stretch.** This

725

Treatment Goals Treatment Plan

should not be forced or abrupt. If no joint pathology is present, overpressure is applied at the end of range.

Address postural changes and muscle imbalances. Decrease pain.

🤚 Muscle imbalances that lead to altered posture affect the efficiency of movement and lead to fatigue. To promote functional and efficient movement, postural changes such as scoliosis, hyperlordosis and hyperkyphosis are addressed as usual, with modifications to speed and depth of techniques as necessary.

🤚 Trigger points are treated with the least invasive techniques such as gentle repetitive muscle stripping and skin rolling or gradually applied ischemic compressions.

🤚 Frictions should not be performed if the client is on anti-inflammatories. If it is safe to do this usually painful technique (pain can increase sympathetic nervous system firing), its application should be modified and interspersed with soothing techniques. This work can also be performed over a series of treatments.

🤚 When painful techniques are performed, communication with the client is essential. If the client becomes agitated, the specific work is stopped. The client is consulted to determine if the massage should be continued.

Encourage diaphragmatic breathing.

🤚 Long-term postural changes can lead to respiratory difficulties. The diaphragm, intercostal, scalene and sternocleidomastoid muscles are treated.

🤚 The client is directed to take full breaths which include diaphragm, rib and sternal movements.

Reduce spasticity, temporarily.

🤚 Reduction of spasticity will contribute to joint health as it allows improved limb movement. This in turn reduces fatigue levels.

Techniques to reduce spasticity:

- slow rhythmical Swedish techniques such as stroking and palmar kneading;
- slow rhythmical shaking of the limb;
- pressure on the Golgi tendon organ if the tendon is accessible;
- stimulation of the antagonist muscle;
- slow steady performance of passive range of motion to an affected limb;
- slow rhythmical stroking along the spine.

🤚 Each client will have an individual reaction to each technique. The therapist will need to determine which techniques are most effective for a particular client. For example, one client may respond well to gentle repetitive stroking, whereas another may find rhythmical techniques more beneficial.

Treatment Goals

Treatment Plan

✋ A key point the therapist must remember is that stressful emotional responses on the part of the client will increase spasticity. This reaction can be controlled if the therapist maintains a relaxation focus throughout the treatment, using appropriate speed and application.

Maintain joint health and range of motion.

✋ Modifications are made for joint pathologies or osteoporosis by decreasing the vigour of joint play and passive movements. **Passive movement** is used to improve joint health and mobility. This should be performed slowly and gently on each joint of the affected limb, so as not to elicit a stretch reflex. If a restriction in movement is felt, the limb is held at that particular place in the range until a release is felt. The movement then continues slowly. The joints with the least restriction are moved first, followed by those that are most restricted. The entire limb is addressed. Passive range of motion of the affected joints is interspersed through the massage.

Encourage whole body integration.

✋ Techniques to integrate the body:

- if the client's CP presents as hemiplegic, monoplegic or triplegic, the client is spoken to while the therapist stands on the affected side;

- when massage is performed on areas that have sensory dysfunction, spasticity or that experience athetoid movements, the client is asked to give feedback. On the other hand, if the client is totally focused on the symptomatic areas, the therapist redirects awareness to the unaffected areas;

- techniques are applied simultaneously to both sides of the body. In the case of diplegia, the focus is to integrate the affected legs with the unaffected arms.

✋ See the chapter Strategies: Central Nervous System Conditions for more details.

Self-care Goals

Self-care Plan

Encourage relaxation.

✍ Relaxation techniques such as diaphragmatic breathing, which is contraindicated if diabetes or kidney disease is present (*Fried, 1990*), visualization and meditation are encouraged.

Improve functional ability through the improvement of strength, flexibility and balance.

✍ The client should perform activities of daily living at the level of her ability.

✍ Yoga and Tai Chi will improve flexibility, balance and coordination.

✍ If possible, a regular aerobic program such as swimming or walking is undertaken.

✍ A stretching program is encouraged overall and for specific muscles that affect an individual client.

Self-care Goals

Self-care Plan

✍ A modified resistance program can build strength. Strength is lost due to the loss of muscle mass from lack of use and aging.

✍ The client is urged to do whatever activity is comfortable.

Educate the client about maintaining tissue health.

✍ To treat distal edema, the client or a care giver is taught basic lymphatic drainage techniques and cool hydrotherapy applications, such as towel wraps. The client is also educated about signs of gangrene, which is tissue necrosis due to an interference of blood supply *(Porth, 1990)*. Medical help should be sought if black or brown discolouration develops in distal digits. This may be accompanied by inflammation or by coolness and swelling in the affected tissue. Decubitus ulcers are also a concern. The client must be vigilant for redness with heat or swelling of the skin over a bony prominence. These lesions are the result of pressure, friction and heat or moisture. They can develop within hours. Therefore, immediate medical attention is urged.

Refer the client.

✍ Referral to a support group or local cerebral palsy organization can offer the client contacts for social interaction, special events and programs.

Treatment Frequency and Expected Outcome

Cerebral palsy is a permanent condition. Therefore, treatments are regular and ongoing. One-hour weekly treatments have been shown to be beneficial.

Cerebral palsy is non-progressive, but over time there are secondary changes as a result of the original disabilities.

Many clients do not participate in rehabilitation programs as adults although these are helpful in increasing tissue and joint health. There also seems to be a tendency to visit physicians less frequently than would be healthy. This is attributed in part to people's negative childhood experiences with the medical profession *(Ontario Federation for Cerebral Palsy, 1993)*.

See also Strategies: Central Nervous System Conditions, stress reduction, constipation, dislocations, scoliosis, hyperkyphosis, hyperlordosis, hypertension, respiratory conditions, seizures, decubitus ulcers and edema for related treatments.

Many of those with CP are able to live with relative independence. Spastic CP, particularly diplegic or hemiplegic, offers a more favourable prognosis for independence than athetosis. Likewise, independent mobility and the presence of fine motor skills offer a good prognosis for independence.

58

SPINAL CORD INJURY

Linda Ludwig

A spinal cord Injury (SCI) is an injury to the vertebral column, spinal cord or both due to a direct or indirect trauma.

SCI is a non-progressive condition that results in a complete or incomplete loss of sensory, motor or autonomic function at the level of the lesion and distal to the lesion.

Up until the Second World War, as many as 80 per cent of those with a spinal cord injury died within two years of the trauma. The development of antibiotics in the 1940s dramatically changed this prognosis. It was Sir Ludwig Guttmann in Britain who introduced rehabilitation programs for patients with an SCI. This has allowed them to go beyond just surviving and move towards leading productive lives *(Hammell, 1995)*.

The spinal cord itself is a column of nerve tissue that begins at the medulla oblongata, just superior to the foramen magnum, and ends at L2 *(Figure 58.1)*. Here it becomes the conus medullaris and then the cauda equina. The cord is surrounded by the pia mater, the cerebrospinal fluid, the arachnoid and the dura mater. The spinal cord is made up of grey matter centrally, which is H-shaped when viewed in cross-section, and of white matter around the periphery. The grey matter has three horns. The anterior (ventral) horn contains lower motor neurons whose axons terminate in skeletal muscle. The lateral horns in the thoracic region contain sympathetic fibres from the autonomic nervous system. The posterior (dorsal) horns contain sensory fibres *(Figure 58.2)*. Also within the spinal cord are motor and sensory pathways that serve as lines of communication between the brain and spinal cord. These are called "tracts". The descending tracts are from the brain to the spinal cord. For example, the corticospinal tract consists of upper motor neurons that arise from the motor cortex and travel down the spinal cord for the purpose of controlling movement of the neck, trunk (the ventral tract) and limbs (the lateral tract).

The ascending tracts are located in the white matter and the posterior horn of the grey matter. These send sensory information to the brain. For example, the spinothalamic tract carries crude touch and pressure (the ventral tract) as well as pain and temperature (the lateral tract). Proprioception, vibration, two-point discrimination and fine touch perception are carried on the posterior tract.

The spinal cord is, finally, surrounded and protected by the bony spinal column. The spinal column consists of 33 vertebrae: seven cervical, 12 thoracic, five lumbar, five fused sacral (forming one bone) and four fused coccygeal (forming one bone). There are 31 pairs of spinal nerves that come off the spinal cord and exit between these vertebrae.

The space between the spinal cord and the vertebrae is known as the spinal canal. The canal is relatively small except in the cervical spine where the spinal cord occupies only 50 per cent of the spinal canal. This allows for more freedom of movement but also creates relative instability and vulnerability to injury. Most spinal cord traumas are sustained not by a direct blow but rather from indirect force created by a violent motion of the neck and trunk. This is most common where comparatively immobile segments meet mobile segments. Therefore, about 53 per cent of spinal cord injuries occur in the cervical spine. The most vulnerable segments are C4 to C6. Another area commonly

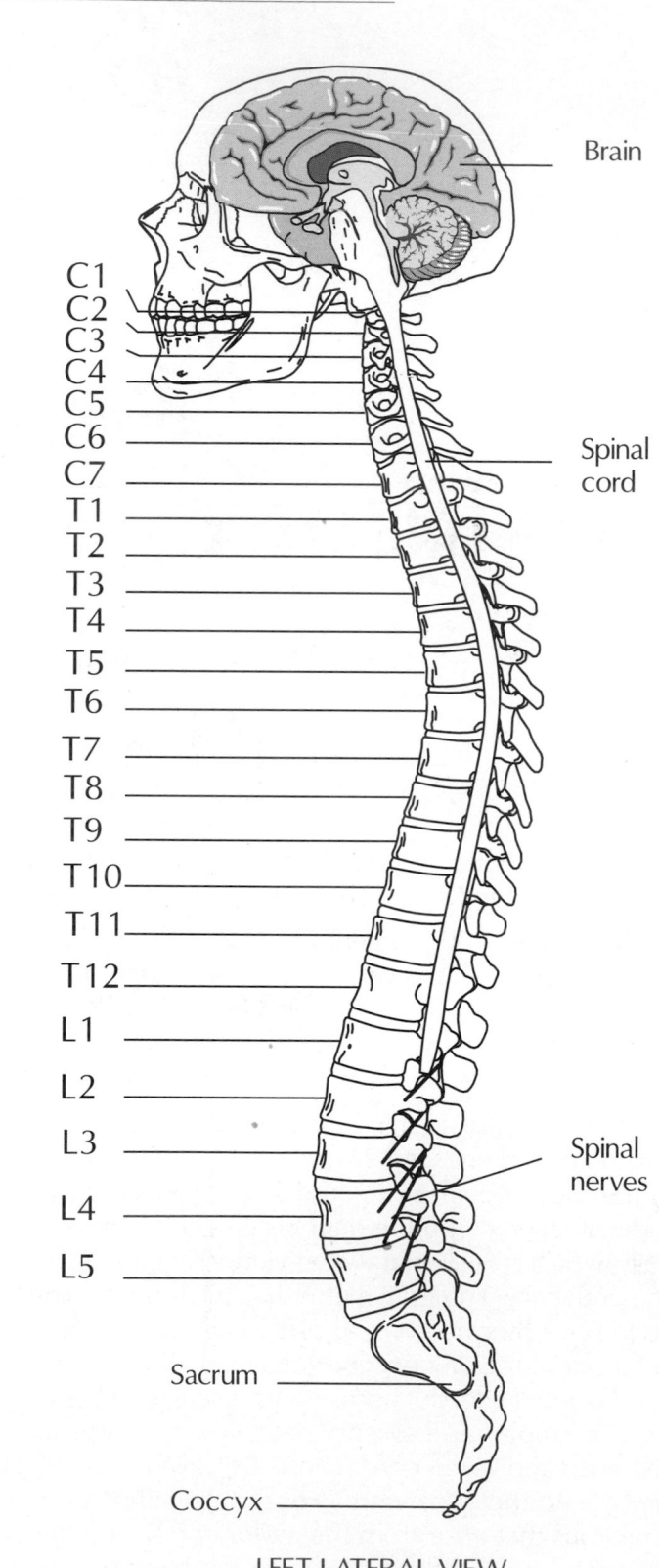

C1
C2
C3
C4
C5
C6
C7
T1
T2
T3
T4
T5
T6
T7
T8
T9
T10
T11
T12
L1
L2
L3
L4
L5

Brain

Spinal cord

Spinal nerves

Sacrum

Coccyx

LEFT LATERAL VIEW

Figure 58.1
The vertebral column and spinal cord.

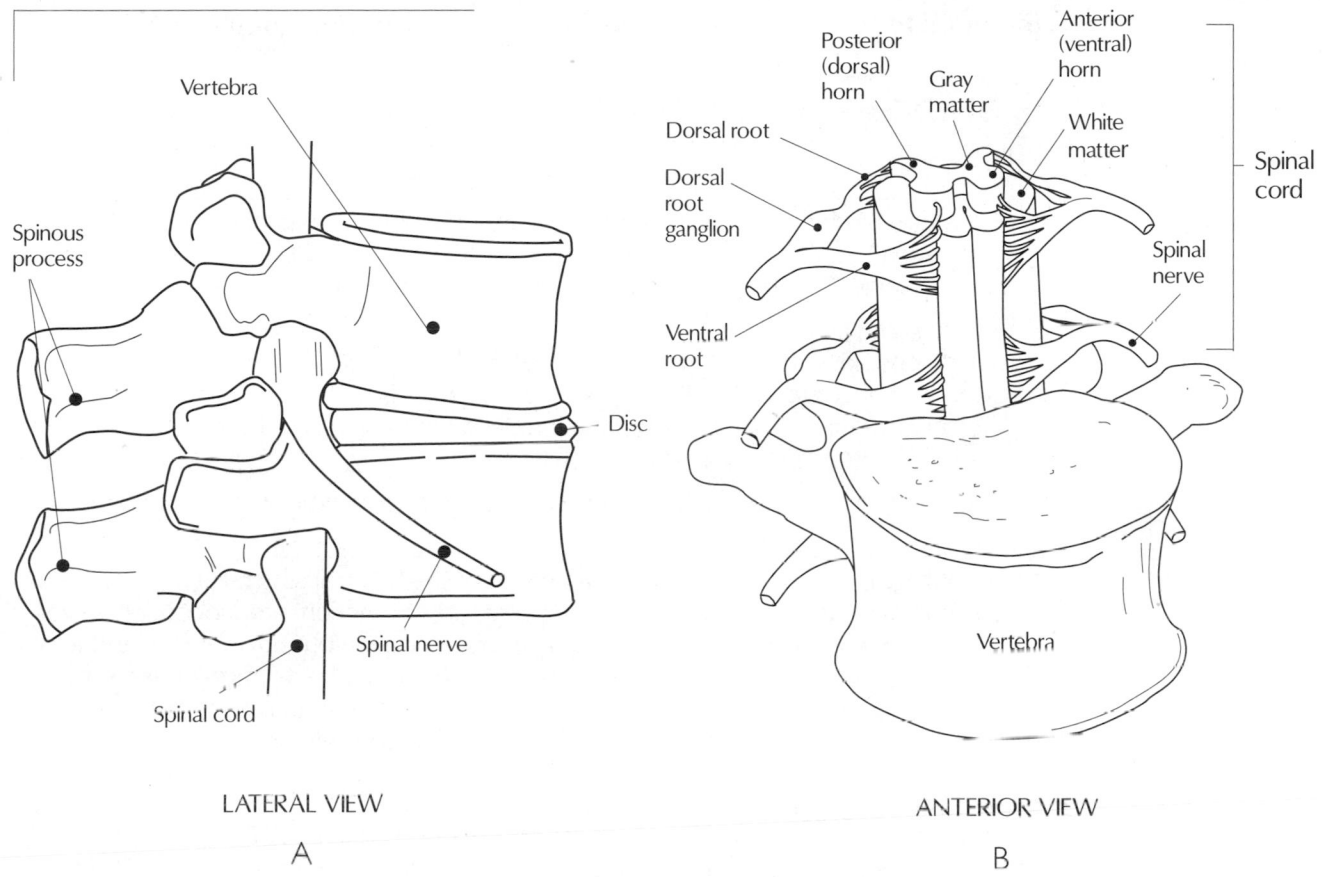

Figure 58.2
(A) The spinal cord within the vertebral column. (B) A cross section of the spinal cord.

affected is T12 to L1.

Spinal cord injuries can result in quadriplegia, which is also referred to as tetraplegia, or paraplegia. Both involve impairment or loss of motor, sensory or autonomic function. The terms **quadriparesis** and **paraparesis** refer to weakness as opposed to total functional loss.

- **Quadriplegia** affects the four limbs and the trunk and pelvic organs. It results when spinal cord damage occurs in the cervical segments — T1 and above.

- **Paraplegia** affects the lower limbs. In this case, the spinal cord lesion occurs in the thoracic, lumbar or sacral segments — T2 and below. Depending on the specific area damaged, trunk or pelvic organs may be involved.

Spinal cord injuries are said to be complete or incomplete. This refers to the amount of motor and sensory impairment rather than the amount of severance of the spinal cord.

- A **complete lesion** results in a total loss of function below the level of the lesion. There may be nerve breakage because the spinal cord is stretched, ischemia because of loss of the vascular supply to the spinal cord or, in rare cases, total transection of the spinal cord (*Somers, 1992*).

• An **incomplete lesion** results in some function below the level of the lesion.

Specific Types of Incompete SCI

NAME	CAUSE	IMPAIRMENT OR DYSFUNCTION
Central Cord Syndrome is damage in the centre of the cord with the periphery of the cord unaffected.	✦ hyperextension injury, usually in the cervical spine ✦ often affects elderly people with arthritic changes to the cervical spine	✦ Motor and sensory abilities of the upper limbs are affected. Muscles are weak or flaccid. The lower limbs are spared or less affected. This occurs because the cortico-spinal tract is organized such that the control of the arms is located centrally and control of the legs located laterally. ✦ If damage is severe, there is greater loss of motor and sensory function below the lesion and the legs are often spastic. ✦ Bowel and bladder function remain intact or are only partially affected.
Brown-Sequard Syndrome is damage to one side of the cord.	✦ stabbing and gunshot wounds	✦ On the same side of the lesion (ipsilaterally), there is decreased or absent motor function, proprioception, vibration and two-point discrimination but **normal** pain and temperature perception. While most tracts travel on the same side that they serve, when the spinothalamic tract enters the spinal cord it crosses to the opposite side of the cord. This tract then travels on the side opposite to the side it serves. Therefore, with an injury that damages the left side of the cord, all other sensory perception is affected, except pain and temperature perception. This is intact for the left side. ✦ On the right side, opposite the lesion, motor function is normal but there is a loss of pain and temperature perception. The spinothalamic tract controlling the right side pain and temperature perception was travelling on the left side, which sustained the injury.
Anterior Cord Syndrome is damage to the anterior spinal artery or anterior aspect of the cord resulting in cortico-spinal and spinothalamic tract injury.	✦ direct trauma, often a hyperflexion injury	✦ There is variable bilateral loss of motor function and pain, temperature and crude touch perception. Proprioception, vibration and two-point discrimination are **normal** because these are carried on the undamaged posterior tract.

Causes of spinal cord injury are:

➤ **direct or indirect trauma** to the spinal cord, sustained in a variety of ways,

• **motor vehicle and motorcycle accidents**, which account for the largest percentage of SCIs: in Canada, 41 per cent; in the UK, 39 per cent; in the USA, 47.7 per cent. The usual type of accident is a high-speed roll-over on a rural road at night. The result is cervical spinal cord injuries. No seat belts are worn in 97 per cent of the accidents that result in spinal cord damage. Of these injuries, 28.4 per cent result in complete paraplegia, 23 per cent result in complete quadriplegia and 30.8 per cent result in incomplete quadriplegia. Better car safety standards, air bags and seat belt regulations have reduced the number and severity of SCIs *(Hammell, 1995)*;

- **diving,** especially into unknown waters, which may result in a SCI that is often fatal. Those who survive are often quadriplegic;

- **sports and recreation** injuries, which vary with the culture. In the USA, football has the highest incidence of SCIs; in the UK, South Africa and Ireland, rugby is the main culprit; and, in Canada, it is ice hockey. People injured are usually not professional athletes. Amateur athletes often have poorer conditioning programs and are less aware of how to sustain an impact. Sports injuries account for 6 per cent of all SCIs in Canada and up to 17 per cent in the UK. Unfortunately, of the spinal cord injuries sustained, 91.8 per cent result in quadriplegia; 44 per cent are complete and 47 per cent are incomplete *(Hammell, 1995)*;

- **penetrating wounds as a result of violent trauma from gunshots or stabbing.** This accounts for a larger percentage of SCIs in war-torn countries. The USA has a higher percentage of SCIs from gun and stab wounds than countries such as Canada and the UK. The numbers have almost tripled in the last 10 years, up to 35 per cent of all SCIs in larger urban centres such as Los Angeles, New York and Washington. Of these, 42.2 per cent result in complete paraplegia and 16 per cent result in complete quadriplegia;

- in other countries, causes vary. For example, in Singapore 24 per cent of the spinal cord injuries from 1973 to 1984 were the result of falls from unsafe construction sites and unsafe bamboo scaffolding. In India, 66 per cent of SCIs resulted from falls from a height or into unprotected wells. In countries with limited health care resources, many people die within two years of the spinal cord injury due to the lack of proper treatment facilities;

- in 10 per cent of SCIs, no vertebral injury is sustained yet spinal cord damage occurs *(Somers, 1992)*. Damage likely occurs because the spinal canal narrows, such as with stenosis or with spondylosis (vertebral immobility and fixation). In these cases, a relatively mild hyperextension accident can result in a SCI. This is increasing likely in elderly people;

➤ **non-traumatic injuries** include: spinal hematoma, infection, radiation, neoplasm and interruption of the cord's vascular supply due to surgery, cardiac arrest or aortic aneurysm.

It is estimated that 8,000 to 10,000 new traumatic SCIs occur each year, based on 1980 statistics from the USA. Generally, males are affected 4 to 1 compared to females. The average age is between 19 and 30 years old *(Somers, 1992)*.

When an injury is sustained to the spinal cord, spinal shock occurs almost immediately. There is a loss of voluntary motor control, sensory and autonomic function and spinal reflexes below the level of the lesion. The specific cause of this is unknown. Within the first 24 hours and over the next several weeks, the spinal shock resolves and those tracts that are undamaged resume functioning. If the reflex function returns by the time the person reaches the hospital there is a good prognosis for a full recovery *(Porth, 1990)*.

The injury can result in direct trauma to the neurons at the level of the injury. But most serious is the secondary damage that results from the body's response to the injury and damage to the spinal cord's blood supply. Gross edema compresses the spinal cord against the meninges. Interruption of the blood supply due to damage to the vasculature results in ischemia or hemorrhage and hematoma. This leads to necrosis of, and, ultimately, scar tissue formation in, the spinal cord. The damage spreads up or down the spinal cord for one to three segments in either direction. The grey matter is affected first and, with severe injuries, damage will spread to the white matter within a few hours.

Virtually all systems in the body are affected by a spinal cord injury: motor, sensory, autonomic, respiratory, cardiovascular, gastrointestinal and integumentary. Better management of these injuries means lesions that were once complete are now often incomplete.

It is obvious that emotional and psychosocial aspects of spinal injuries are profound. It was thought that those who experienced an SCI went through prescribed emotional stages: shock, denial, depression, anger, dependency and, finally, adjustment. It was expected that the person should progress through each stage; if this did not occur, the person was often said to be in denial and not progressing appropriately *(Somers, 1992)*. In some cases, discharge from the hospital was delayed if the person failed to exhibit depression *(Hammell, 1995)*.

Recently, there has been a move to see each person as an individual who will experience a variety of emotions at various times. Generally, it has become more accepted that people will grieve and adapt in their own ways. The level of injury — quadriplegia versus paraplegia — makes no difference in a person's ability to adjust successfully.

Because this condition often affects people in early adulthood, it creates not only physical dependence but financial dependence too. While many people with an SCI have successful careers, about 50 per cent remain unemployed after the injury *(Somers, 1992)*.

Initially, treatment is emergency medical care that may include surgery to stabilize the spine and prevent further damage. Rehabilitation programs include physiotherapy, occupational therapy and nutrition counselling. Massage therapy promotes good tissue and joint health, stress and pain reduction *(Yarkony, 1994)*, as well as providing emotional support.

Studies have demonstrated that health care professionals have had a tendency to interpret the emotions of people with an SCI as depressive far more often that the injured person would consider himself depressed *(Hammell, 1995)*. It is important that the therapist does not expect certain emotions but is supportive of the client's true feelings, which may include hope and optimism.

Symptom Picture

✦ The dysfunction resulting from an SCI is dependent on the level at which the injury occurred and the amount of spinal cord damage. There can be a total loss of sensory and motor function from a complete lesion. Partial losses result from an incomplete lesion. Most people experience some recovery of function one or more levels distal to the level of injury. Commonly, one side of the body will be stronger than the other. This is thought to be due, in part, to the recovery of the spinal nerves *(Somers, 1992)*. Immediately after the trauma, flaccidity and loss of reflexes occur below the level of the injury as part of spinal shock. This can last for up to eight weeks.

✦ With an **upper motor neuron lesion,** at or above T12, spasticity results distal to the lesion as spinal shock subsides. This includes muscles, the bowel and the bladder. Spasticity may be accompanied by hyperreflexia *(Somers, 1992).*

✦ With a **lower motor neuron lesion,** at T12 or below, muscles innervated by the damaged cord segments remain partially or fully flaccid. This affects the lower limbs, bowel, bladder and genitals. Reflexes are disrupted or absent *(Hammell, 1995).*

✦ **Mixed lesions** occur at T12/L1 and lead to mixed responses, such as spastic lower limbs and a flaccid bladder *(Hanak, Scott, 1993).*

✦ **Spasticity** is often a complication of an SCI. All people with cervical lesions will have spasticity. About 75 per cent with thoracic lesions and under 60 per cent with lumbar lesions also experience spasticity *(Hammell, 1995).* There is a higher incidence of spasticity with incomplete lesions *(Somers, 1992).* During the year following the trauma spasticity gradually increases. Spasticity in the flexors (usually in the arms) is often affected first, followed by the extensors (usually in the legs). A plateau is reached after the first year and spasticity is maintained at a particular level. Spasticity can be mild, moderate or severe. If mild or moderate, the person can learn to trigger the spasticity and use the resulting increased muscle tone to assist with activities such as transfers to or from a wheelchair. The spasticity can also result in feelings of tightness in the limb and can interfere with movement. This is especially apparent with severe spasticity. Not only does it interfere with function, but a sudden flexor spasm can throw a person from his wheelchair. In these cases, medication such as Baclofen is used. Sudden increases in spasticity can signal a medical problem such as a bladder or urinary tract infection or the presence of a pressure sore.

✦ **Hypertonicity** is experienced in the unaffected muscles. These muscles are overworked, particularly with **breathing**, because they are recruited to perform actions that are weak or lost.

  • The diaphragm is innervated by C3 to C5, the intercostal and abdominal muscles from T1 to T12, the sternocleidomastoid by CNXI and the scalene muscles from C2 to C7. Muscles of respiration are affected if the SCI is above C5. With a C1 or C2 lesion, the person is dependent on artificial ventilation. A C3 lesion has weak function of the diaphragm and cervical muscles, allowing for some independent respiration along with intermittent ventilator use.

  • A C4 lesion has diaphragm, cervical and some shoulder muscle function. These muscles are used for respiration. The breathing pattern is primarily apical due to the compression of the diaphragm from poor posture in the wheelchair and the loss of intercostal muscle function. In order to maintain adequate oxygen intake, the rate of respiration is increased, resulting in achy, overworked cervical muscles with trigger points. There is difficulty coughing and an increase in fatigue. Respiratory conditions which occur can easily become life threatening.

✦ **Pain** can come from muscular, neurological or psychological sources. At least 33 per cent and up to 95 per cent of those with SCIs experience some amount of pain or discomfort as a complication to their injury *(Yarkony, 1994).* Secondary to the injury, pain is experienced in muscles that retain innervation. This pain is a result of overuse in the neck, shoulder, arm and supportive trunk muscles.

  • The onset of pain can be shortly after the injury, such as the short bursts of burning, stabbing peripheral nerve pain which improve with activity. Weeks to months after the injury there can be constant tingling and numbness associated with central cord pain or dull, achy muscular pain. In both of these cases, rest is a relieving factor. Visceral pain has a diffuse, burning quality and is often associated with bowel and bladder distention. Psychogenic pain is variable in both perception and onset.

✦ A small percentage of people experiences severe, disabling pain. This is associated with incomplete lesions, lesions that affect the central cord and lesions caused by gunshot wounds. Diffuse pain affects the legs, back and abdomen in a person with paraplegia and particularly the arms and hands in a person with quadriplegia. The triggers are variable, including prolonged inactivity, cold, damp weather, spasticity and pressure sores.

✦ **Heterotopic ossification** occurs in 16 per cent to 53 per cent of those with SCIs (*Somers, 1992*). The formation of bone in the muscle or connective tissue happens generally one to four months after the injury. There is swelling, heat, pain and a reduced range of motion.

✦ **Contractures** can develop due to immobilization, spasticity or muscle imbalances. They result in pain and loss of function. Flexion contractures are most common, with the hand, hip, knee and ankle usually affected. Splints and braces are often used to place the limb in a neutral position or to create functional contractures. With cervical SCIs, splinting is done within 48 hours of hospital admission.

✦ **Range of motion** is affected by spasticity, flaccidity and contractures. Limited range of motion, in turn, affects functional ability as well as joint and tissue health.

✦ **Tissue health** is affected by the presence of edema. Clients with paraplegia and flaccidity are especially likely to have edema. Long-standing edema results in tissue fragility. Any injury could develop into an ulcer and, potentially, gangrene.

✦ There is an increased risk of **decubitus ulcers** (also called pressure sores or bed sores) due to the lack of sensation, which would normally signal the person to move and relieve pressure on an area. Immobility, prolonged exposure to moisture and heat as well as shear or frictioning forces on the skin can contribute to ulcer formation. This is a life-long concern for a person with an SCI. Some sources suggest there is an increased risk in those with paraplegia *(Ozer, 1988)* while others suggest an increased risk in those with quadriplegia and complete lesions *(Somers, 1992)*. Diffuse, burning pain over the buttocks or heels after a prolonged period of inactivity or a sudden change in spasticity could signal the beginning of a decubitus ulcer.

✦ **Deep vein thrombosis** is a risk in the early stages post-trauma. It is fatal for 2 per cent to 16 per cent of those with an SCI within two to three months of the injury. Anticoagulants such as Heparin and range of motion exercises beginning shortly after the trauma are helpful in preventing this *(Ozer, 1988; Yarkony, 1994)*.

✦ Partial or complete **sensory** loss occurs below the level of the lesion. If there is partial sensory perception, the awareness that remains depends on the specific tracts that are intact. For example, pain and temperature perception are retained if the spinothalamic tract is undamaged.

✦ **Autonomic dysreflexia** is an acute episode of exaggerated sympathetic response. This response occurs in those with a lesion at or above T6, more commonly if they are quadriplegic. Autonomic dysreflexia is evoked primarily by painful or uncomfortable stimuli in the abdomen or pelvic area, such as the distention of a full bladder, muscle spasms, an extensive stretch placed on the muscle, a kink in the catheter bag or in the presence of infection such as decubitus ulcers. The person will experience severe hypertension, as high as 300/160, bradycardia and a sudden pounding headache. Below the level of the lesion, vasospasms, pilorector response and skin pallor occur. Above the lesion, flushed skin and sweating result and the person experiences anxiety *(Porth, 1990)*. This is considered an emergency because convulsions, loss of consciousness and even death can result. If dysreflexia occurs the client is placed in an upright position with the head raised up to 45 degrees. Supportive hose or tight clothing is removed or loosened. The noxious stimuli is removed. If this is not possible or the episode continues, medical attention is sought.

+ **Thermoregulation,** or the ability to control blood vessel response, is lost. The person loses the ability to dissipate heat through blood vessel dilation and sweating. The person also loses the ability to conserve heat with vasoconstriction and shivering. In turn, the body tends to take on the temperature of the external environment. The higher the level of the lesion, the greater the area of the body that is affected *(Porth, 1990)*. This is generally seen with lesions of T6 and above.

+ **Gastrointestinal problems** can occur. In the early stages, this includes ulcers and gastrointestinal (GI) tract bleeding. In the late stages, paralytic ileus (weak, distended intestines resulting in an obstruction), fecal impaction and bowel obstruction may occur *(Somers, 1992)*.

+ **Cardiac problems** such as bradycardia are present in the acute stage. Orthostatic hypotension occurs with lesions at T4 to T6 and above. Positional changes need to be made slowly or dizziness, pallor, sweating and, possibly, fainting can result.

+ **Bowel and bladder incontinence** are present. Depending on the level of the lesion, these organs may be flaccid or spastic. More than one-third of those with an SCI surveyed felt that this was the most significant loss from the injury *(Yarkony, 1994)*. Until recently, bladder complications were the leading cause of death after an SCI.

+ **Sexual function** is affected in the male in that erection or ejaculation may be impaired, depending on the level of the lesion. Generally, a woman's sexual function and ability to become pregnant are not altered but giving birth requires special precautions.

+ **Clinical depression** occurs in 15 per cent to 30 per cent of people with an SCI. Suicide, which accounts for 4 per cent to 21 per cent of deaths, is the leading cause of death for those with traumatic complete paraplegia. Younger people commit suicide within the first five years *(Yarkony, 1994)*. In some cases, suicide is committed through the conscious neglect of serious conditions such as decubitus ulcers.

Subjective Information

HEALTH HISTORY QUESTIONS

✦ Are any other conditions present, such as hypertension, diabetes or kidney disease?

✦ When did the injury occur? Some clients may be reluctant to talk about how the injury happened in the initial meeting. They may become more willing after a level of trust is established.

✦ What is the type of injury (complete or incomplete) and at what level is the lesion?

✦ Was surgery performed to stabilize the spine? Are pins, wires or rods present?

✦ Does the client experience spasticity? If so, which limbs are affected, how severe is it and are there any specific triggers?

✦ What medication is the client taking? When was it last taken?

✦ Is the client experiencing any pain? Can the client describe the type of pain as well as where, when and how long it is experienced?

✦ Are there any sensory losses? What specifically was lost — pain and temperature or deep touch perception, for example?

✦ Does the client have autonomic dysreflexia? What are the triggers? Who should be contacted if this occurs during the massage?

✦ Does the client experience hypotension?

✦ Does the client experience difficulty in regulating body temperature? For example, is sweating or shivering functioning appropriately?

✦ If it is not obvious, is a leg bag used? This bag is used to hold urine and must be carefully positioned during the massage.

✦ What movement is affected? How are the client's fine and gross motor skills?

✦ What activities can the client do? Does the client work? What are the client's hobbies?

Objective Information

Observations

✐ A postural assessment can be performed, noting asymmetries as a result of the motor dysfunction, altered biomechanics of the affected limbs and compensation by the unaffected limbs. The client's posture in the wheelchair is observed. He may be leaning to one side. A head-forward posture may be observed. Most people with a functional level of C6, or occasionally C5, or lower use a manual wheelchair. If the functional level is C5 or above, an electric wheelchair is used. Frequently, one side of the body will be stronger than the other.

✍ Apical breathing may be observed in a person with an SCI at or above C5.

✍ The therapist observes specifically for edema in the distal limbs.

✍ Muscle bulk differences may be noticed when comparing the affected limbs with the unaffected limbs.

✍ Scars may be present at the lesion site as surgery is often performed to repair or stabilize the affected structures.

✍ Spasticity patterns and contractured areas are noted.

✍ Functional abilities, which will vary for each client, are observed. If there is a lack of fine motor ability, a mouthstick may be used. This aid can be used to turn pages or work on a keyboard.

Palpation

✍ Increased tone is palpated in the muscles affected by spasticity. Hypertonicity is also palpated in the muscles shortened from altered posture and in the functional muscles from overuse (for example, the muscles of mastication may be hypertonic and the jaw may be misaligned if a mouthstick is used; neck and shoulder muscles are hypertonic from balancing in the chair). Trigger points may be present in these muscles.

✍ Contractures are likely in the muscles experiencing spasticity. For example, contractures may be palpated in the wrist flexors as well as the hip, knee and ankle flexors.

✍ Decreased tone is palpated in flaccid muscles.

✍ Edema may be present in the distal part of affected limbs. The edematous tissue may be cool due to ischemia.

✍ Numerous soft tissue and joint pathologies, such as tendinitis or osteoarthritis, may be present in the affected limbs. There may be adhesions or signs of inflammation.

✍ Tenderness and severe pain can be present. These can be from muscular (biomechanical), neurological, visceral and idiopathic sources.

Testing

✍ Due to multiple innervation of most muscles, there will often be intact partial innervation. While the client performs tests, the therapist observes for substitute movements. These are movements where functioning muscles are recruited to perform for the lost or weak muscles. This is useful for improving functional ability but hinders accurate assessment.

✍ **AF and PR ROM testing** will show a decrease in range of motion if spasticity is present. The more severe the spasticity, the more severely compromised the range of motion. In the most severe cases, no movement is possible. Flaccidity will result in a decrease in range of motion.

✍ **AR strength testing** will not yield useful results if spasticity is present.

Special Tests

✍ **Sensory testing** for light touch, temperature and pain perception, two-point discrimination and proprioception may all be affected.

✍ There are wide varieties and degrees of sensory loss from slight and patchy to profound.

✍ **Specific orthopedic tests** are performed to assess for any particular secondary conditions. If spasticity is present in the limbs to be tested, the tests may not yield viable results.

Contraindications

◆ If diaphragm function is severely compromised, prone and supine positioning is not used as it will interfere with the ease of respiration.

◆ The therapist should check with the physician regarding risk of **deep vein thrombosis.** If a thrombosis is present, massage to the specific limb is contraindicated.

◆ Triggers that might cause **autonomic dysreflexia** are avoided if the client is subject to this reaction.

◆ With **heterotopic ossificans**, deep, aggressive techniques such as frictions are contraindicated on the affected tissue.

◆ Sympathetic nervous system firing should not be increased as this will increase the symptoms. Vigorous or painful techniques are avoided.

◆ Pressure and hydrotherapy applications should be modified on areas of altered sensation.

◆ Positioning, techniques and hydrotherapy are modified if **hypertension** is present.

◆ The therapist should be aware of the potential for **hypotension**, as a result of autonomic dysfunction. Added care should be taken when the client changes position. The therapist may need to give support to the client when he is getting on and off the table.

◆ Both temperature and duration of hydrotherapy applications should be modified if dysfunction in thermoregulation is present.

◆ The presence of decubitus ulcers is a contraindication to local massage. If the therapist observes the early signs of an ulcer — redness and, possibly, heat, swelling and pain — the client is referred for medical attention.

◆ Joint play and aggressive mobilization techniques such as rib springing are avoided if osteoporosis is present. This is most likely in a person who has a long-term SCI. Joint play or passive range of motion are not performed locally if the lesion site has not been stabilized.

◆ If a leg bag is used, it should not be elevated above the level of the kidneys.

Treatment Goals

Maintain tissue and joint health. Promote body integration.

Provide a safe position.

Decrease sympathetic nervous system firing. Provide emotional support.

Treatment Plan

✋ While a full-body massage is beneficial, some clients see no purpose in receiving treatment in areas of reduced sensation. The therapist can educate the client as to the benefits of maintaining tissue and joint health as well as integration of the body. Ultimately, the client will choose the focus of the treatment, perhaps reducing edema in the legs, reducing spasticity in the limbs (often the wrists and hands) or relieving pain and hypertonicity in the overused head, neck and shoulder muscles. Some people, often those who are younger or recently injured with an SCI are particularly uncomfortable with their changed bodies. Initially, massage may be performed through the clothing and in a limited area, until the client feels comfortable.

✋ **Positioning** includes prone, supine, sidelying, seated and in a wheelchair. Any position can be used that is safe and comfortable for the client while allowing access to the structures to be massaged. Sidelying allows good overall access in treating the neck, anterior and posterior shoulder, low back, gluteals and leg. The client's sleeping position can be used as a guide to offering a comfortable and familiar choice. Modifications are made to reflect any secondary conditions such as hypertension.

✋ If diaphragm function is compromised, a seated position was found to reduce the work of breathing *(Irwin, Tecklin, 1995)*. Sidelying on the least affected side or semi-supine, with the trunk, arms and head well supported by pillows, may be used.

✋ **Hydrotherapy** reflects the needs and symptoms of the individual client and is modified if poor tissue health, hypertension or other secondary tissue concerns are present. Thermoregulation may be affected to the extent that extremes of temperature are not adequately dissipated. Therefore, they should not be used in hydrotherapy applications. If this is not a problem, check with the client for his temperature preference. For example, for some clients, colder temperatures can reduce spasticity whereas for others they increase spasticity.

✋ Generally, heat applications are used to increase relaxation and decrease excessive muscle tone. Contrast applications are used to improve circulation and tissue health. Cool applications are used with elevation to reduce edema.

General Treatment

✋ The treatment is performed in the context of a relaxation massage. Slow relaxed breathing is encouraged and soothing rhythmical techniques are used. A supportive touch is essential.

Treatment Goals   Treatment Plan

Specific Treatment

Maintain tissue health.
Decrease edema if present.
Be vigilant for decubitus ulcers.

If edema is present, axillary or inguinal pumping is performed followed by drainage techniques interspersed with **passive range of motion.** Elevation of the limb and cool hydrotherapy also assist to reduce edema. If the client has a leg bag, it is removed and laid beside him before the leg is elevated.

Swedish massage techniques are used to improve circulation and overall tissue health. The strokes are applied with reduced pressure and segmentally if the tissue is fragile, as long strokes can create drag on the tissue.

Limit contractures,
if possible.

Contractures, which contribute to a reduced range of motion in a joint, are addressed in the hip flexors, the hamstrings, the low back muscles as well as the wrist and finger flexors. Pre-treatment hydrotherapy of a warm or hot application is followed by a slow **prolonged passive stretch.** Care is taken not to overstretch the muscles since too much length can interfere with some functional movements. One example is a lesion at or above C5 which generally requires maintenance of range of motion of the wrist and fingers as well as some functional contractures. A functional contracture of the fingers in some degree of flexion allows the hand to function as a hook, as well as allowing for tenodesis, which is the tendency of the thumb to move towards the fingers in the action of prehension when the wrist is extremely extended (Hanak, Scott, 1993). All actions of the wrist and fingers are encouraged, especially wrist extension. However, care is taken not to overextend the fingers and, in turn, lose the functional contracture that contributes to functional movements (Hill, 1986).

All stretches should not be forced or applied abruptly. If no joint pathology is present, overpressure may be applied at the end of range to further increase range of motion, if this is desired.

Address postural changes
and muscle imbalances.
Decrease pain.

Scoliosis, hyperlordosis, hyperkyphosis and head-forward posture are addressed as usual. Overworked muscles are treated, such as the shoulder girdle muscles or the muscles that control the jaw if a mouthstick is used. Modifications in pressure and movement are made for joint pathologies, osteoporosis, poor tissue health and sensory losses.

Address abdomen.

Abdominal massage promotes the movement of fecal matter through the colon. The techniques usually used in a constipation treatment are appropriate, such as fingertip kneading along the colon.

Address muscles of
respiration.

Long-term postural changes can lead to respiratory difficulties. To strengthen functional but weak intercostal muscles, the therapist applies resistance with the palms of the hands against the client's ribs. The resistance is held constant with exhalation and then gently but

Treatment Goals   Treatment Plan

firmly increased with each inhalation. This is repeated for a few breaths. Diaphragmatic breathing is introduced. The therapist encourages as much full breathing as possible. Spasticity requires the slow application of any techniques.

✋ If the intercostal muscles are not functional or are weak, or the client has a lesion above C5, the other respiratory muscles such as the diaphragm, scalene and sternocleidomastoid muscles will be hypertonic from overwork. They may also be only partially innervated and, in turn, weak. These muscles are treated with effleurage followed by petrissage such as repetitive muscle stripping, thumb kneading and fingertip kneading.

✋ Fascial techniques are applied to the anterior or lateral cervical region or over the anterior chest or as indicated from palpation assessment.

✋ If congestion is present in the lungs, drainage techniques are performed, modifying the pressure used as necessary. See the bronchitis chapter for details.

✋ Trigger points are treated with the least invasive techniques such as gentle repetitive muscle stripping and skin rolling or gradually applied ischemic compressions so as not to increase sympathetic nervous system firing.

✋ When potentially painful techniques are performed, communication with the client is essential. If the client becomes agitated or spasticity increases, the specific work is stopped. The client is consulted to determine if the massage should be continued.

✋ Slow gentle stretching to the cervical spine is performed **only** if the spine is stable. There may be instability around the lesion site. In the early stages post-trauma, the therapist obtains permission from the physician about which ranges of motion are safe, if any. Eventually, surgery will usually be performed to stabilize the lesion site. If this has not been done, clients will retain some instability in specific ranges of motion. In this case, the therapist gets this information from the client and **avoids** these ranges.

Decrease spasticity, temporarily.

✋ Reducing spasticity will contribute to joint health, as it allows improved limb movement. This in turn reduces fatigue levels.

✋ Techniques to reduce spasticity:
- slow rhythmical Swedish techniques such as stroking and palmar kneading;
- slow rhythmical shaking of the limb;
- Golgi tendon organ pressure, if the tendon is accessible;
- stimulation of the antagonist muscle;
- slow steady performance of passive range of motion to an affected

Treatment Goals

Treatment Plan

limb, ensuring that the joint is stable if the passive movement places a stretch on the lesion site;

- slow rhythmical stroking along the spine.

☝ Each client will have an individual reaction to each technique. The therapist will need to determine which techniques are most effective for a particular client. For example, one client may respond well to gentle repetitive stroking, whereas another may find rhythmical techniques more beneficial.

☝ A key point the therapist must remember is that stressful emotional responses on the part of the client will increase spasticity. This reaction can be controlled if the therapist maintains a relaxation focus throughout the treatment, using appropriate speed and application.

Maintain joint health and range of motion.

☝ **Passive movement** is used to improve joint health and mobility. This should be performed slowly and gently on each joint of the affected limb, so as not to elicit a stretch reflex, and only if the joint is stable in that range. If a restriction in movement is felt, the limb is held at that particular place in the range until a release is felt. The movement then continues slowly.

☝ The joints with the least restriction are moved first, followed by those that are most restricted. The entire limb is addressed. Passive range of motion of affected joints is interspersed through the massage.

Provide whole body integration.

☝ Techniques to integrate the body:

- feedback is requested when performing massage on areas that have partial sensory dysfunction or spasticity;

- if the client is totally focused on the symptomatic areas, the therapist redirects awareness to the unaffected areas;

- techniques are applied simultaneously to both sides of the body. In the case of paraplegia, the focus is to integrate the affected legs with the unaffected arms.

☝ See the CNS Strategies chapter for more details.

Self-care Goals

Self-care Plan

Encourage relaxation.

✍ Relaxation techniques such as diaphragmatic breathing are taught; this is contraindicated if diabetes or kidney disease is present (*Fried, 1990*). Visualization and meditation are encouraged. These, along with biofeedback and acupuncture, have been shown to give pain relief (*Yarkony, 1994*).

Self-care Goals

Increase functional ability through improving strength and range of motion.

Educate about maintenance of tissue health.

Refer the client.

Self-care Plan

✍ The client is encouraged to do activities of daily living at the level of his ability as well as to take part in recreational activities. A stretching program is encouraged overall and for specific muscles. A modified resistance program can build strength. Ongoing strengthening is required for muscles that are functional. Some muscles will be required to take over the weak or lost actions. Others, such as muscles in the leg, may suffer from disuse atrophy. As the person ages, there is a natural loss of muscle mass which can be prevented with resistance training.

✍ To treat distal edema, the client or a care giver is taught basic lymphatic drainage techniques and cool hydrotherapy applications, such as towel wraps. The client is also educated about signs of gangrene, which is tissue necrosis due to an interference of the blood supply *(Porth, 1990)*. Medical help should be sought if black or brown discolouration develops in distal digits. This may be accompanied by inflammation or by coolness and swelling in the affected tissue. Decubitus ulcers are also a concern. The client must be vigilant for redness with heat or swelling of the skin over a bony prominence. These lesions are the result of pressure, friction, heat or moisture. They can develop within hours. Therefore, immediate medical attention is urged.

✍ Referral to a support group can offer the client contacts for social interaction, special events and programs.

Treatment Frequency and Expected Outcome

A spinal cord injury is a permanent condition. Therefore, treatments are regular and ongoing. One-hour weekly treatments have been shown to be beneficial.

An SCI is non-progressive, but over time there are secondary changes as a result of the original disabilities. Some studies suggest that the body experiences stress as a result of functioning with ongoing disabilities and this, in turn, causes slight speeding of the aging process.

There is a functional decline as the person ages, which usually begins about 20 years after the trauma *(Hammell, 1995)*. This includes: decreased muscle mass and strength; the presence of osteoarthritis with pain and decreased range of motion; a general decline in most other body systems such as the gastrointestinal, genitourinary, cardiovascular and respiratory systems; and an increased susceptibility of the skin to decubitus ulcers.

Life expectancy after a spinal cord injury that occurred at age 20 is 60 to 65 years. If the injury occurred at age 40, the life expectancy is 60 to 68 years. The worst prognosis is for an SCI that results in complete quadriplegia. Life expectancy is 50 to 58 years, no matter

See also Strategies: Central Nervous System Conditions, stress reduction, scoliosis, hyperkyphosis, hyperlordosis, hypertension, respiratory conditions, decubitus ulcers, constipation and edema for related treatments.

when the onset *(Hopkins, 1994)*.

Overall, general life satisfaction was found to increase with age and increased time post-trauma. It is important that clients maintain strength and range of motion throughout life and are prepared for early aging changes *(Hammell, 1995)*.

POLIOMYELITIS

Linda Ludwig

> **Poliomyelitis is an acute viral infection specifically affecting the motor neurons in the spinal cord and brain stem.**

Poliomyelitis (or polio) can be asymptomatic but can also result in flaccid paralysis and muscle weakness. Although it had been around a long time, polio was first clearly described in 1840 by Jacob Heine. In the early part of the twentieth century, it was discovered that polio was caused by a virus. During this time, it was, in fact, the most common form of viral infection. Prior to 1956, 25,000 to 50,000 cases were reported annually in the USA. The Salk and Sabin vaccine was developed in 1955. By this time, almost 50,000 Canadians were affected and another 4,000 had died from poliomyelitis. By the mid 1960s, the condition was under control. Now, in countries where inoculation programs and immunization with oral vaccine occur, poliomyelitis has become clinically rare.

Most polio infections end in full recovery. Of those infected, only one in 1,000 children develops paralysis. In adults, the risk increases to one in 100 of those infected developing paralysis *(Aminoff, 1995)*. In 1979, 28 cases of paralytic poliomyelitis were reported in the USA: 13 occurred in an epidemic in an unvaccinated Amish community; 11 occurred in association with vaccination; and four were isolated cases *(Rowland, 1995)*.

Types of Polio

✦ There are several types of polio that can lead to paralysis.

✦ The most common type is **spinal poliomyelitis**, where inflammation and destruction of the anterior horn cells may occur at any level of the spinal cord.

✦ The most serious type is **bulbar poliomyelitis**, which involves cranial nerves and sometimes the cardiorespiratory centre. Bulbar poliomyelitis has a poor prognosis with a very high mortality rate if paralysis of the respiratory muscles and failure of the medulla (the respiratory centre in the brain) occur *(Rowland, 1995)*.

The polio virus enters the system through direct contact. It is thought to enter through the mouth, from where it invades the lymphatic tissue. At this stage, the person is relatively asymptomatic with only a slight temperature and other flu-like symptoms. The virus then gains access to the nervous system, possibly by way of the gastrointestinal tract or the sympathetic pathways. The polio virus has an affinity for motor neurons. Therefore, in the spinal cord, it destroys the anterior horn cells but leaves the sensory cells intact. Necrosis of the motor cells is followed by local inflammation of the meninges. During this process, the person's symptoms progress to severe headaches along with intense muscular pain and stiffness, especially in the neck and back. **Kernig's/Brudzinski's tests** would be positive, indicating meningeal irritation *(Porth, 1990)*.

✦ **Non-paralytic polio** involves flu-like symptoms and meningeal irritation. In **paralytic polio**, the symptoms progress further.

Symptom Picture for Paralytic Polio

✦ Over a three to five day period, there is progressive, asymmetrical flaccid weakness in the muscles, usually involving the proximal muscles of the legs *(Rowland, 1995)*. This results because of necrosis of the motor cells which leads to degeneration of the specific peripheral nerves associated with those cells. Other motor cells cease to function or have compromised function because of compression from the inflammatory process.

✦ These symptoms may improve because undamaged neurons, which have been compressed, recover their function as the inflammatory process resolves. Weakness will be left in those muscles innervated by motor cells that were only partially damaged. In these cases, peripheral nerve regeneration may also occur and further enhance functional ability. By six months after the initial onset, 80 per cent of people make a good or full recovery *(Aminoff, 1995)*. The amount of permanent paralysis of the involved muscles is dependent on whether the anterior horn cells were completely destroyed or only slightly damaged.

✦ Permanent function loss occurs in those muscles innervated by cell that suffered necrosis.

✦ Reflexes are also lost in the paralysed muscles.

✦ If the infection occurred when the client was a child, bone growth may be affected, causing shortening of the limb.

✦ Eventually, the flaccid tissue is replaced by fibrous or fatty tissue *(Wale, 1980)*.

✦ There are muscle imbalances due to muscular flaccidity which lead to soft tissue contractures and postural deformities, such as scoliosis.

✦ Over time, joint pathologies can also develop. For example, osteoarthritis may develop, along with soft tissue conditions such as tendinitis, bursitis and sprains from poor biomechanics.

Post Polio Syndrome

Post polio syndrome (PPS) is considered a late complication of paralytic poliomyelitis. It occurs after the person has been stable for years, often for decades, after the initial infection. Especially at risk are those who had onset when they were older, those who had a severe case of polio and those who were very active after recovery *(Aminoff, 1995)*. Approximately 20 to 25 per cent of those who previously had polio will develop PPS.

➤ **The cause of PPS is unknown** but it is generally thought not to be a reactivation of the polio virus. Some sources suggest it is exhaustion of motor neurons from the excessive demand placed on them. The specific motor cells affected are those that were only partially damaged after the initial infection, years ago. Another thought is that the current damage is the result of an immune-mediated response *(Hopkins, 1994; Aminoff, 1995)*.

Symptom Picture for Post Polio Syndrome

✦ There are varying degrees of PPS severity, from mild to seriously disabling.

✦ The condition presents as a slow, progressive weakness in the muscles previously affected and spreads to the same muscles on the other side of the body as well as muscles that were previously thought to be unaffected.

✦ Often debilitating fatigue is experienced, as are muscle cramps, weakness and joint pain.

✦ Secondary contractures and joint and soft tissue conditions can increase postural deformities and, often, cause loss of functional ability.

Contraindications

✦ Decreased tissue health may contraindicate deep or vigorous techniques to flaccid and atrophied muscles. If arthritis is present, joint play and overpressure are modified or avoided.

✦ Dysarthria (difficulty with speech due to dysfunction of the tongue or other speech muscles), dysphagia (difficulty with speech due to dysfunction in the brain) and respiratory difficulties such as sleep apnea (a cessation of breathing while sleeping likely due to a dysfunction in the respiratory centre in the brain) may be experienced.

✦ Some drugs that combat the extreme fatigue are being tested. Other drugs being tested enhance nerve cell survival and function. Unfortunately, these are years away from being available to those affected with PPS.

Treatment Considerations

Assessment

✎ **Observation** includes a **postural assessment** to better understand the individual's compensation pattern.

✎ **Testing** for **length** and **strength** will reveal the presence of contractures. This testing also shows how the client uses the synergists to do particular movements in order to be more functional.

Massage

It is most likely that the therapist will be treating an adult client whose initial onset was many years previous. Since flaccid paralysis results from the destruction of motor neurons, the condition is permanent and the specific functional loss of affected muscles will not return. This results in progressive muscle atrophy and, eventually, contracture formation in the unopposed antagonist muscles. Total loss of a particular action often does not result if the synergists are intact and strengthened. Ultimately, paralysis depends on the degree of neurological involvement, which will determine whether the muscles involved are in one small group or an entire limb. The muscles frequently involved are tibialis anterior and posterior, the peroneals, quadriceps and gluteus medius.

🖐 Maintaining tissue health, range of motion and strength of the compensating muscles are aims of treatment. An overall stress reduction focus is used if pain is present.

🖐 **Post polio syndrome** requires an additional stress reduction component because of the anxiety that accompanies the return of acute symptoms and, in some cases, a decrease in functional ability.

🖐 In both cases, the therapist is observant for secondary postural changes that result from a long-term disability. Scoliosis, hyperlordosis or hyperkyphosis are treated if present. Techniques are modified to accommodate compromised tissue, joint and bone health. The same approach applies for tendinitis, bursitis or any other secondary condition to that may be present. Compensatory changes may result from the use of lifts, braces and other supports.

See also stress reduction, scoliosis, hyperkyphosis, hyperlordosis, tendinitis, bursitis, sprains, osteoarthritis and peripheral nerve lesions for related treatments.

🖐 Reduction of contractures can facilitate better movement and function. These are addressed using pre-treatment hydrotherapy of deep moist heat followed by fascial techniques, overpressure and stretches.

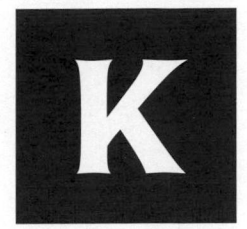

CONDITIONS OF THE PERIPHERAL NERVOUS SYSTEM

UNDERSTANDING PERIPHERAL NERVE LESIONS

Linda Ludwig

A peripheral nerve lesion is an injury to a peripheral nerve which, depending on the severity, results in motor loss (flaccidity) or weakness (paresis), sensory loss (anesthesia), sensory Impairment (paresthesia) or pain (dysesthesia), as well as autonomic dysfunction.

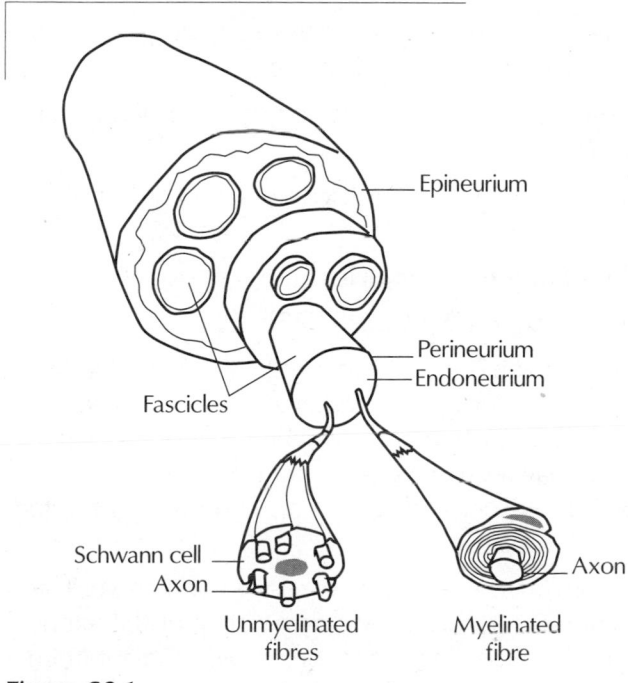

Epineurium

Perineurium
Endoneurium

Fascicles

Schwann cell
Axon

Unmyelinated
fibres

Axon

Myelinated
fibre

Figure 60.1
A peripheral nerve.

The peripheral nervous system (PNS) refers to the portion of the nervous system that lies outside the brain and spinal cord. This system includes spinal nerves and cranial nerves. Nerves *(Figure 60.1)* consist of many nerve fibres (axons). Individual fibres can be myelinated, which means they have an insulating layer that speeds nerve impulse conduction, or unmyelinated. Several connective tissue layers provide protection to the many fibres within a nerve. First, the endoneurium surrounds the individual fibres. A group of fibres, called a fascicle, is contained within a mechanically strong perineurium. The epineurium provides a further protective barrier around the fascicles which make up the nerve. It is within this final layer that the main intraneural blood supply is found.

The fibres that make up each nerve may have different functions. Some conduct information to (via afferent fibres) or from (via efferent fibres) the central nervous system *(Figure 60.2)*. The afferent

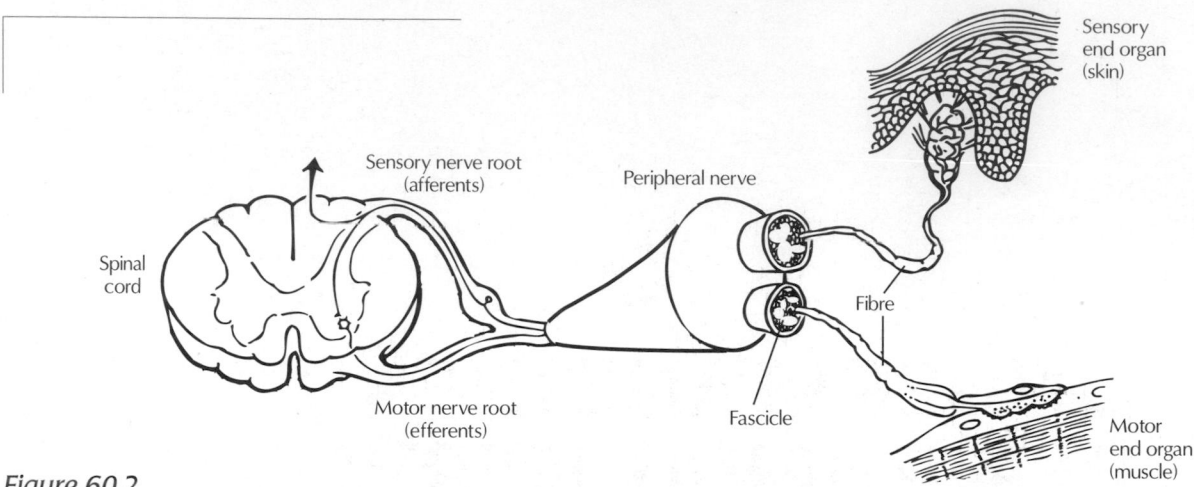

Figure 60.2
The connection between the peripheral and central nervous systems.

fibres, or **sensory neurons**, convey sensory stimuli from the skin and deeper structures (referred to as sensory end organs) to the central nervous system. The somatic efferent fibres are also known as **motor neurons**. Their cell bodies are found in the brain stem and spinal cord, with their axons innervating skeletal muscle cells (referred to as motor end organs). When firing, these motor neurons lead to muscular contractions. A combination of these fibres is known as a **mixed nerve**. Autonomic fibres, which influence vasomotor function, sweating and skin, hair and nail health as well as neuropathic pain *(Stewart, 1993)*, usually travel with these nerves or along the walls of arteries.

Causes of peripheral nerve lesions are:

➤ **compression** either internally (from a bony callus, hypertonic muscles or a tumour) or externally (from crutches or prolonged leaning);

➤ **trauma** such as crushing or severance wounds; this may result from a variety of incidences such as car accidents, industrial accidents or knife injuries;

➤ **systemic disorders** such as leprosy. Leprosy is the most common cause of peripheral nerve lesions worldwide *(Hopkins, 1994)*;

➤ **systemic edematous conditions** such as pregnancy, hypothyroidism and diabetes, kidney and heart conditions.

There are two recognized systems for **classifying nerve injuries.**

✦ The following is the method organized by Seddon *(Seddon, 1972)*:

• **Neuropraxia** (first degree) is the compression of a nerve causing a local conduction block, with no structural damage to the axon or to tissue distal to the lesion. The conduction block is caused by a local demyelination of nerve fibres. Recovery occurs as the damaged area is repaired, which may require weeks or months. This type of injury involves loss of motor function but sensory and autonomic fibres are unaffected. Prognosis is usually good.

• **Axonotmesis** (second degree) is the prolonged, severe compression of a nerve. This causes a lesion at the site of the compression followed by degeneration of the axons distal to the injury. The endoneurial tube remains intact. Sensory, motor and autonomic losses occur. Regeneration of the axons to the peripheral end organs results in functional recovery. Prognosis is good since the endoneurial tube provides an appropriate pathway through which the axons can regenerate to the correct end organs.

- **Neurotmesis** (third degree through fifth degree) is an injury to the nerve as a result of severance of part or all of the nerve trunk, including the endoneurial tube. This category of injury results in degeneration of the nerve. Axons may have difficulty regenerating to distal end organs because of scar tissue at the lesion site from local edema and bleeding. The same losses occur as with axonotmesis. In this case, the prognosis for recovery is poor because there is no clear pathway to orient the regenerating axons. Surgical repair is usually required to ensure some functional recovery.

✦ Sunderland's system *(Sunderland, 1978)* is more detailed than Seddon's, using a first through fifth degree classification. The first two categories correlate to Seddon's first and second degrees. Sunderland divides the more severe injuries into three categories. The third degree is similar to Seddon's except that while the axon and epineurial tube are severed, the perineurium remains intact. The fourth degree lesion is the loss of continuity of the perineurium, with the endoneurium intact; this degree may include the development of a neuroma (see section later in this chapter) within the continuity of the proximal nerve fibres or endoneurial tube. The fifth degree lesion is the total loss of continuity of the nerve including the endoneurium. This is often due to the retraction of proximal and distal nerve stumps. In degrees three to five, scar tissue develops and there is the loss of a clear pathway to guide the regenerating axons to the appropriate end organs. Surgery is required to improve a generally poor prognosis.

✦ Nerve lesions may be **complete** — all fibres within the nerve are affected — or **partial** — only some fibres are affected. In terms of the healing process, the lesion may be **regenerating** — repairing itself — or **permanent** — the nerve is unable to regrow.

Peripheral Nerve Pain

Peripheral nerve pain can be due to neuritis, neuralgia, causalgia, reflex sympathetic dystrophy (RSD) and neuromas.

Neuritis

Neuritis is inflammation of the nerve. However, the term may be incorrectly used to denote non-inflammatory lesions of the peripheral nervous system.

Primarily, the sheath and connective tissue are affected; usually the axon is not affected. The condition is characterized by constant dull pain. Irritative phenomena, such as paresthesia or dysesthesia, may be present. In cases of long duration, there may be motor and sensory deficit.

Causes of neuritis are:

➤ **secondary to a pathology** such as diabetes, leprosy or tuberculosis.

➤ **trauma** to the nerve;

➤ **chronic exposure** to a toxin such as lead, drugs or alcohol.

Treatment is by a physician and neurologist. Massage is ideally contraindicated.

Neuralgia

Neuralgia is defined as nerve pain. It is characterized by recurrent attacks of sudden, paroxysmal (excruciating) pain along the distribution of the affected nerve. It is described as "lightening like" and often throbbing. Unlike neuritis, there is no appreciable pathological change in the nerve. The condition is characterized by a "trigger zone", an area that causes an attack when stimulated. The trigger zone is often the cutaneous region supplied by the nerve. Movement of the affected area also increases pain. Commonly affected are the trigeminal and intercostal nerves. Other common conditions include phrenic, lumbar, brachial and sciatic neuralgia.

Causes of neuralgia are:

➤ **local compression** from a trauma, with inflammation leading to scar tissue, a subluxation of the vertebrae or a bony callus;

➤ **prolonged exposure to cold.**

Treatment of neuralgia is directed by a physician. Massage therapy can, however, play a significant role in alleviating the discomfort of neuralgia and, in particular, managing those cases caused by pressure from soft tissue or local swelling.

Massage is locally contraindicated in the acute stages of neuralgia.

Trigeminal Neuralgia

Trigeminal neuralgia is also known as *tic douloureux* or painful tic. It affects the trigeminal nerve, which is cranial nerve V (CNV). This nerve supplies sensory awareness to the face and motor function to the muscles of mastication and the tensor tympani of the middle ear. The nerve consists of three divisions: the ophthalmic, maxillary and mandibular (*Figure 60.3*).

The primary causes of trigeminal neuralgia are:

➤ **local compression** such as that caused by a neuroma;

➤ **demyelinating conditions** with subsequent scarring, such as multiple sclerosis.

This condition affects women more than men, usually at middle age or older. Sudden painful attacks occur unilaterally, along one or more divisions of the nerve. Facial tics or spasms are observed, often resembling grimaces. If the ophthalmic division is affected, inflammation of the sclera or iris can occur and glaucoma is possible. Loss of hearing is due to paralysis of the tensor tympani. Paralysis of the muscles of mastication leads to locking of the jaw and muscle spasms. A loss of sensation in the face is often experienced (*Figure 60.4*). The **trigger zone** may be the lips, face or tongue. Afferent stimulation of this very sensitive area, which can be light touch, changes in temperature, especially cold, or facial movement such as chewing, shaving or talking, can bring on an attack.

Medical treatment consists of antiseizure medication, such as carbamazepine, sold as Tegretol; the side effects may be drowsiness, headaches and dizziness. In extreme cases, surgery may be performed. Relaxation strategies combined with biofeedback can decrease the intensity of the pain and often reduce attacks. Acupuncture is helpful for some people. Though it seems contradictory, inactivity increases the pain and a regular routine of facial exercises is suggested. The client's physician should be consulted first.

Local massage over the trigger zone is contraindicated.

🖐 A full-body relaxation massage is appropriate between attacks. The trigger zone, as indicated by the client, is avoided. Swedish massage techniques are applied slowly and rhythmically to decrease sympathetic nervous system firing. Diaphragmatic breathing is

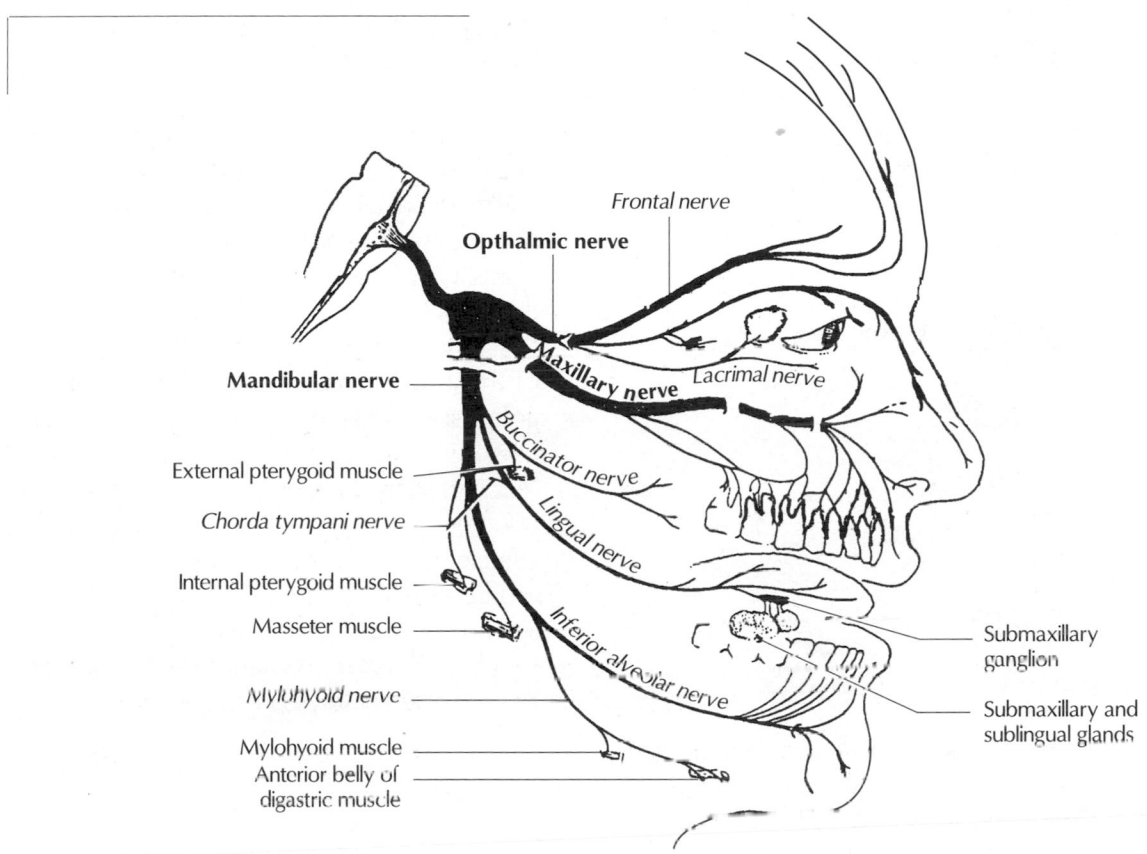

Figure 60.3
Cranial nerve V (CNV) and its three divisions: ophthalmic, maxillary and mandibular.

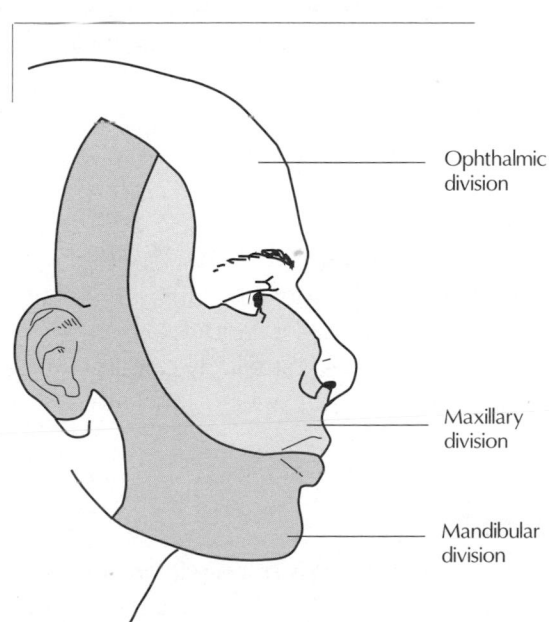

Figure 60.4
Sensory distribution of the trigeminal nerve.

encouraged. Platysma trigger points are treated, if present. These refer into the lower jaw, over the cheek and up to the zygomatic arch.

Intercostal Neuralgia

This condition affects the intercostal nerve that travels between the internal and innermost intercostal muscles *(Figure 60.5)*. The nerve travels as a neurovascular bundle from the spine to the sternum for ribs 1 to 6, and from the spine to the abdomen for ribs 7 to 11. Below the twelfth rib there is no intercostal muscle; therefore, this nerve is called the "subcostal nerve".

Causes of intercostal neuralgia are:

➤ **diabetes**, due in part to metabolic changes. Attacks may recur at different areas of the trunk or they may remain localized. Usual recovery time is one to two years.

➤ **Post-herpes zoster (shingles).** When first contracting this virus, the person gets chicken pox.

757

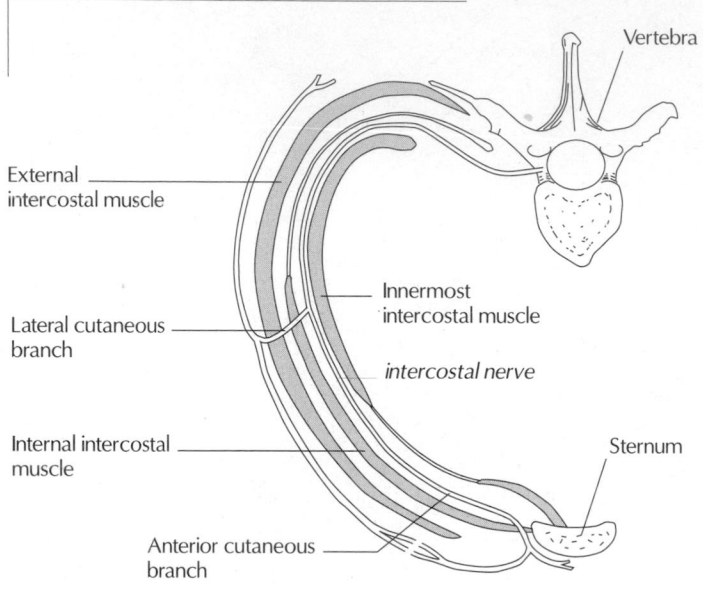

External intercostal muscle

Lateral cutaneous branch

Internal intercostal muscle

Anterior cutaneous branch

Vertebra

Innermost intercostal muscle

intercostal nerve

Sternum

Figure 60.5
Intercostal nerve pathway.

The virus then invades the dorsal root ganglion of the intercostal and, occasionally, the optic nerve. Years later, when the person is immune suppressed, the virus reactivates. Usually only one nerve is affected. Shingles results in pain, followed by skin eruptions which eventually dry into scabs. Usually as the vesicles fade so does the pain. Unfortunately, up to 10 per cent of those with younger onset, and 50 per cent of those with onset at over 60 years of age, get post-herpetic neuralgia. This condition consists of intermittent attacks of deep, burning, sharp pain shooting along the affected intercostal nerve. Pain is especially intense where the cutaneous branches emerge at the spine, at the lateral axillary line and at the sternum. The trigger is often light touch and movement over the affected area. It often resolves in about two years.

Treatment is by a physician and a neurologist. Drugs may be of help to some people, but often the condition will resolve with time. Local massage over the trigger zone is contraindicated.

🖑 Stress reduction massage and referral for biofeedback are helpful to enable the client to better cope with the pain. When the condition is no longer acute, massage, using a variety of Swedish techniques, is performed to increase local circulation and reduce intercostal muscle spasms. Diaphragmatic breathing is encouraged and an abdominal massage is performed, the goal being to decrease hypertonicity of the diaphragm. Thoracic mobility is maintained using rib springing and vertebral mobilization techniques. Rib springing is contraindicated if local muscle spasms are present or with any condition that compromises bone and joint health.

Causalgia

Causalgia is considered a severe pain syndrome. It is characterized by the sudden onset of an intense, persistent, usually burning pain, most often associated with a traumatic injury to a peripheral nerve. The lesion to the nerve is often incomplete and there may be accompanying arterial injuries *(Wilson, 1981)*. This condition was first widely documented during the American Civil War. It was commonly seen with gunshot wounds and other weapons-related injuries *(Mumenthaler, 1992)*.

Causes of causalgia are:

➤ **gunshot wounds** — a major cause of causalgia;

➤ **iatrogenic nerve injuries**, particularly secondary to surgery, less often with injections;

➤ **electrocution**;

➤ **amputations**;

> ➤ **injuries from high velocity sharp objects**, such as with industrial machinery *(Hooshmand, 1993)*.

Accompanying the pain are severe autonomic and trophic disturbances such as poor vasomotor control, swelling and dystrophic skin changes *(Stewart, 1993)*. The most commonly affected nerves are those rich in autonomic fibres, namely the median nerve of the brachial plexus and the tibial division of the sciatic nerve. Some sources note that the pain pattern follows the distribution of the affected nerve, distal to the lesion site *(Hopkins, 1994)*; others suggest a pattern that lies primarily on the dorsum of the hand or foot, eventually expanding to the entire limb *(Hooshmand, 1993)*. Aggravating factors include emotional stress, loud or sudden noises and tactile stimulation *(Hopkins, 1994)*.

Theories about the physiological mechanism of causalgia focus on overactivity of the sympathetic nervous system. This may be due to the failure of "opioid peptides in modulating the system" *(Hopkins, 1994)* or from a "short circuit" which transfers excitation from the sympathetic fibres to the pain fibres in an abnormal fibre contact or synapse formation *(Mumenthaler, 1992)*.

Medical treatment, in the past, consisted of sympathectomies, the surgical severance of the affected sympathetic fibres. Unfortunately, in 50 to 70 per cent of cases, the client would remain pain free for only six months to five years, at which time the causalgia would return *(Mumenthaler, 1992)*. Currently, this type of surgery is generally performed on those with a limited life expectancy. Antidepressants and drugs that are sympathetic nerve blockers have sometimes proven effective.

🖐 Although it may seem that local stimulation should be avoided, including massage therapy, use of the limb is encouraged in an attempt to normalize the nerve pathway *(Hooshmand, 1993)*. This includes active assisted movements, which could be performed during the massage treatment, as well as active free and active assisted movements that could be given as self-care. Both movement exercise regimes are within the client's pain tolerance and include rest periods *(Wilson, 1981)*. A relaxation massage can be given in order to decrease sympathetic nervous system firing and to alleviate the client's pain, as well as to provide emotional support.

Reflex Sympathetic Dystrophy (RSD)

Reflex sympathetic dystrophy is considered a pain syndrome. While this term is often used interchangeably with causalgia, it actually refers to a different pain syndrome. Some authors refer to the condition as minor causalgia.

It is thought that an abnormal sympathetic reflex results in arterial spasm. This causes a spontaneous burning pain in the limb beyond the area of a nerve injury. The onset of pain may be immediately following an injury or within a few weeks of a trauma. Pain is often out of proportion to the injury. Edema is present, accompanied by dystrophic tissue. At this stage of onset of pain, tissue may be warm and hyperemic or cool and pale. Sweating is usually increased but may also be decreased, and muscular wasting often occurs. Pain is aggravated by movement and emotional excitation. The person often immobilizes the area in an attempt to stop the pain but, unfortunately, this leads to increased edema and ischemia in the tissue which then cause more pain. A vicious pain cycle develops. Over time, three to six months after the injury, constant pain affects the limb distal to the injury site. The joints become stiff and the tissue is cool and cyanotic. Osteoporosis may be present *(Kline, Hudson, 1995)*.

Causes of reflex sympathetic dystrophy are:

➤ **trauma**, often from relatively minor injuries, which may be followed by prolonged immobilization;

➤ **surgery** involving the wrist, hand, ankle or foot, which may be followed by prolonged immobilization.

Medical treatment of this condition using sympathetic nerve blocks or sympathectomy is not especially successful *(Kline, Hudson, 1995)*.

As with all pain syndromes, an integral part of massage treatment includes support and encouragement of the client. Edema is controlled using lymphatic drainage techniques and elevation. Active assisted movement and maintenance of the joint's range of motion are performed to the affected area within the client's pain tolerance. Heat applications, such as a thermaphore or parrafin, can be used on the affected area. These allow the client to perform active movement with greater ease. **Tissue dystrophy or lack of vasomotor control would contraindicate the use of heat.** Techniques are done within the context of a relaxation massage to decrease sympathetic nervous system firing. As self-care, active free and active assisted movements are encouraged within client's pain tolerance and incorporating sufficient resting time. Further desensitization is promoted through the application of various textures to the skin; initally, soft smooth materials are used, followed by rough, firm textures, applied over the affected area *(Wilson, 1981)*.

Neuromas

A neuroma is a tumour composed of nerve cells. After the partial or complete severance of a peripheral nerve, the proximal nerve stump responds by sending nerve sprouts towards the distal endoneurial tube stump. These sprouted fibres often grow indiscriminately until some of them attach to the distal tube and that provides a pathway for other fibres to follow. A neuroma can develop at this site. In such a case, the regenerating nerve fibres grow randomly and often into a clumped mass because they cannot penetrate the dense scar tissue that forms at the site of an injury. A neuroma at the end of the proximal nerve stump is referred to as a terminal bulb. This type is associated with amputations or complete severance injuries. In the case of a partial lesion, a neuroma can develop within the nerve itself.

Depending on the type of neuroma formation, it may or may not be symptomatic. Small-fibre, compact neuromas are less sensitive than large, soft ones. It is thought that the fibres that comprise these softer neuromas invade neighbouring tissue, leaving their unmyelinated nerve endings unprotected and more prone to being painful. When the neuroma is symptomatic, the area over the neuroma is extremely sensitive. The client experiences continuous, poorly localized pain , as well as altered sensation in some of the area supplied by the nerve *(Lundborg, 1988)*.

See also Bell's Palsy, median, radial, ulnar and sciatic nerve lesions, diabetes mellitus, HIV, scar tissue, stress reduction and strategies for crush and severance injuries to peripheral nerves.

Painful neuromas are often surgically treated in order to restore continuity to the nerve and to give it another chance to regenerate *(Terzis, Smith, 1990)*. Treatment generally includes a relaxation massage to decrease sympathetic nervous system firing and to provide emotional support to the client. If compression of the neuroma is painful, massage is locally contraindicated. Active free and active assisted movements of proximal and distal joints are encouraged to maintain joint motion and health *(Lundborg, 1988)*.

STRATEGIES:
Crush and Severance Injuries to Peripheral Nerves

Linda Ludwig

Peripheral nerves have the ability to regenerate if the axon is damaged, providing that the cell body of the nerve is intact. If the lesion site is too near the cell body and the cell body is destroyed, regeneration is not possible. In such a case, some permanent functional losses result.

When an injury occurs, the axon of the nerve will degenerate distal to the lesion site. The myelin surrounding the nerve distal to the lesion will likewise degenerate. This process is known as Wallerian degeneration and may occur over several days. In crush or chronic compression injuries (axonotmesis), the endoneurial tube is intact, even through scar tissue that develops at the injury site. This poses a good prognosis for recovery since the nerve fibres will grow from the proximal nerve stump down the intact endoneurial tubes to reinnervate the appropriate distal end organs *(Porth, 1990)*. Generally, regeneration through the lesion site occurs within an average of 10 days *(Terzis, Smith, 1990)*.

Some injuries result in severance of the endoneurial tube and axon (neurotmesis). A gap results between nerve fibres of the proximal stump and the distal connective tissue sheath, part of which is due to the elastic recoil of the tube after it is severed. This is a fifth degree nerve injury according to Sunderland *(Sunderland, 1978)*. In such a case, the factors that will affect regeneration of the nerve are the size of the gap, the speed of axonal regeneration, the amount of scar tissue encountered and the possible presence of a neuroma. In order to ensure the greatest likelihood of successful regeneration, doctors may suture the proximal and distal ends of the perineurium, though frequently only the epineural ends are sutured. If the nerve stumps are too short, a graft *(Figure 61.1)* from another nerve — often the sural nerve from the lower leg — is inserted to bridge the gap *(Stewart, 1993)*. New surgical techniques, known as tension-free coaptation, allow grafting to be performed without undue tension on the epineurial tube and regenerating axons. Following these techniques, it is no longer necessary for the affected limb to be maintained in an exaggerated position to prevent traction on the nerve, after the initial three weeks post-surgery *(Terzis, Smith, 1990)*. But even in this case, it is prudent to be cautious.

761

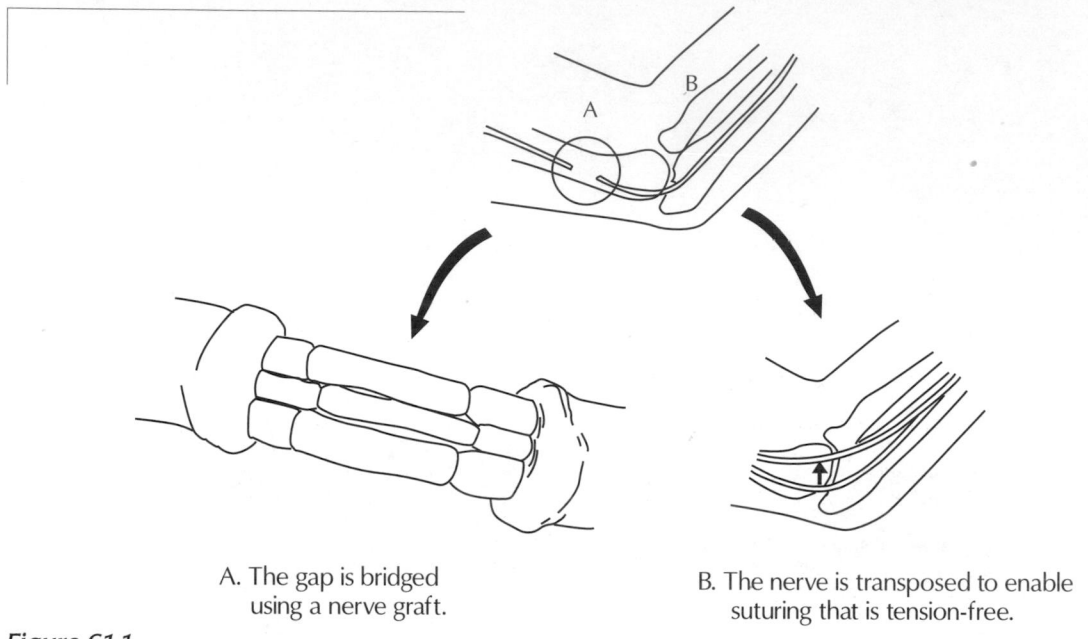

A. The gap is bridged
using a nerve graft.

B. The nerve is transposed to enable
suturing that is tension-free.

Figure 61.1
Repair of a peripheral nerve.

Regeneration of a nerve occurs at a rate of approximately one to two millimetres daily, with the more proximal nerve sections regenerating faster than those at an increased distance from the neuron's cell body. One can measure the distance from the lesion to the end organ and calculate roughly how long recovery might be. An approximate measure of the distance a peripheral nerve has regenerated over time is:

- 7 to 14 mm per week equals 1/2 to 3/4 inches per week
- 28 to 52 mm per month equals 1 1/4 to 2 1/4 inches per month.

Regeneration proceeds more slowly the more distal the axon is to the cell body; for example, in the hands or distal to the knee. There is generally an 18-day delay once the nerve reaches the motor end organ and nerve stimulation produces a contraction. It is another five days before the reflexes are functional *(Terzis, Smith, 1990)*.

Even if regeneration occurs, there are factors that will affect successful functional return. If the reinnervated tissue is severely dystrophic, full functional return is unlikely. In addition, mixed nerve lesions have a lower rate of successful regeneration because it is not unusual for the regenerating fibres to grow to the wrong muscle or sensory receptor. For example, a motor fibre may mistakenly regenerate to a sensory organ. This is known as cross-innervation *(Hopkins, 1994)*. In such cases, the fibres will eventually die; reinnervation from that fibre does not occur.

Ultimately, successful regeneration will be judged by the resulting return of function and sensation for the client *(Hopkins, 1994)*.

A permanent lesion results when the nerve does not regenerate successfully. The cell body may have been damaged or there may be a systemic toxic condition, such as alcoholism or metal poisoning. If surgical intervention was totally or partially unsuccessful, another attempt is usually made within six months *(Terzis, Smith, 1990)*. If this also fails, the functional, sensory and autonomic losses or dysfunctions that occurred upon injury or with only partial regeneration remain.

Causalgia and reflex sympathetic dystrophy (RSD) are severe pain syndromes often associated with traumatic peripheral nerve injuries, frequently with a partial disruption of a peripheral nerve. Causalgia primarily affects the median and sciatic nerves (tibial division). See the Peripheral Nerve Pain section in the chapter Understanding Peripheral Nerve Lesions.

Combination Lesions

Injuries can result in a lesion to a single nerve, namely the median, ulnar, radial, tibial or common peroneal nerves, whereas others result in combination lesions. For example, a severance injury at the wrist could potentially damage the median and ulnar nerves at that level. A sciatic nerve injury may result in lesions in both the tibial and common peroneal nerves, if the injury site occurs proximal to the knee where these two nerves travel together.

A condition known as **Klumpke's paralysis** is a traction injury of the lower brachial plexus. It results in a combination median and ulnar nerve lesion. The traction is extreme and traumatic in nature. In children, poor positioning at birth — breech or legs first — or being pulled from the birth canal by forceps can cause sufficient traction for injury. In adults, falling from a height and grabbing something to break the fall causes traction as the force of the person's body weight stretches the C8 and T1 nerve roots.

Symptoms are similar to those of a median and an ulnar lesion. This includes a "claw hand" presentation combined with the thumb positioned on the same plane as the palm. Atrophy and functional losses primarily affect the muscles of the hand. Severe edema and vasomotor and trophic changes are also evident in the hand. Sensory losses affect the C8 and T1 dermatomes. A dermatome is the area of skin supplied by a posterior root of a spinal nerve; there is considerable overlap among dermatone areas that are adjacent to each other *(Figure 61.2)*. An additional complication to Klumpke's paralysis may be **Horner's syndrome** which manifests on the affected side with constriction of the pupil (miosis), drooping of the eyelid (ptosis), loss of sweating to the face and neck (anhydrosis) and recession of the eyeball into the orbit (enophthalmos).

Erb's paralysis is also a traction injury but involves the upper brachial plexus, namely C5 to C6 nerve roots. In children, a birth trauma can cause this paralysis if the baby is pulled from the birth canal when the neck is extended, rotated and laterally flexed. In adults, the cause is usually a trauma that violently separates the neck and shoulder. This can occur from a motor vehicle or motorcycle accident if the person is thrown and lands on the head and shoulder. Sports accidents can result in a similar violent fall which could traction these nerves. Symptoms include a presentation of the arm and hand called "waiter's tip", with the shoulder adducted and internally rotated, the elbow extended, forearm pronated and the wrist and fingers flexed. Muscle wasting and motor dysfunction affect all muscles above the elbow, especially the shoulder abductors, external rotators and extensors, as well as the forearm supinators and pronators. Sensory loss involves the C5 and C6 dermatomes. Tissue edema and dystrophy are not significant.

With a peripheral nerve injury, it is most likely that the client will be under the care of a neurologist and receive a prescribed course of treatment, including physiotherapy. Contact with this team is important in order to give the client safe and appropriate treatment.

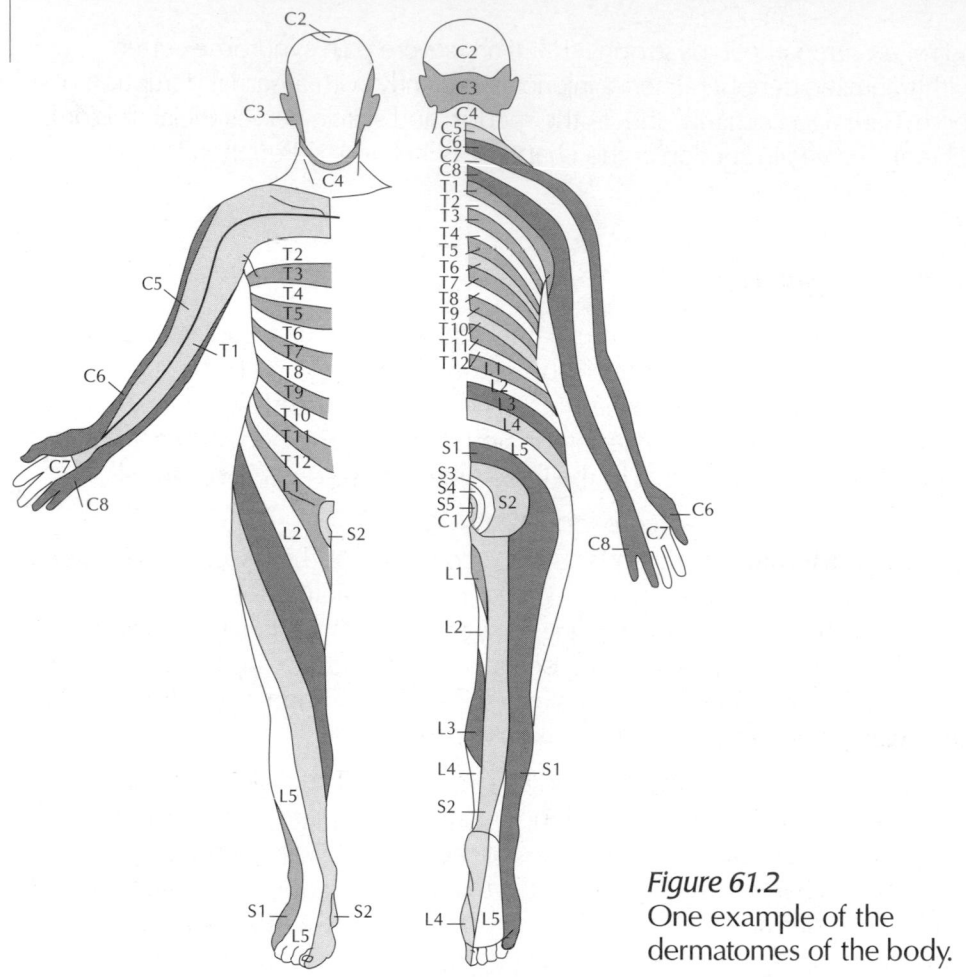

Figure 61.2
One example of the dermatomes of the body.

Symptom Picture

Regenerating Lesions

✦ **Traumatic injuries** resulting in nerve damage will frequently cause damage to other structures, such as skin, bone, muscles and their tendons. Repair and subsequent healing of fractures, severed tendons, etc., is also necessary for recovery of function (*Kline, Hudson, 1995*).

✦ Individual chapters are devoted to the following peripheral nerves: radial, ulnar, median and sciatic. They include details about motor, sensory and autonomic losses. This information is to be used as a guide to treatment. In reality, the therapist must perform his or her own assessment, and consult with the neurologist, to determine the symptom picture for the individual client.

✦ **A complete lesion** is a nerve injury which results in damage to all the fibres within the nerve. A partial lesion results in damage to some fibres within the nerve. Where fascicles are well organized (think of a phone cable) some end organs will suffer more damage than others, depending on which fibres are affected and how severely. Only specific testing will give a clear picture.

✦ **Edema** is present.

- *Complete Nerve Lesions:* Edema will be present initially, due to the injury. If autonomic fibres are affected, the edema will remain until the fibres regenerate and vasomotor function returns; the more autonomic fibres that are affected, the more profound the edema will be. Poor tissue health occurs secondary to edema.

- *Partial Nerve Lesions:* Initially, edema will be present due to the injury. While it will remain present until full function returns to the autonomics, there will be less edema than with a complete lesion. This is because there is still some local muscle function which assists lymphatic return.

✦ There is **altered tissue health**.

- *Complete Nerve Lesions:* Loss of autonomic function will affect skin, hair and nails. The tissue will be fragile, dystrophic and easily injured. If a secondary injury occurs to these structures, a longer healing time is required. Loss of piloerection and loss of sweating will be apparent over the denervated tissue.

- *Partial Nerve Lesions:* Tissue changes will occur, though generally not as severely as with a complete lesion. An increased piloerector response may occur over the area of denervation *(Mumenthaler, 1992)*.

✦ **Motor function** is affected.

- *Complete Nerve Lesions:* Flaccid paralysis results and muscle wasting can occur within three weeks. Fibrillation, a spontaneous contraction of muscle fibres in the denervated tissue, occurs a few weeks after the injury. While these contractions cannot be seen through the skin, their presence is used by neurologists as evidence of peripheral nerve axon damage *(Stewart, 1993)*. Testing will reveal diminished or lost tendon reflexes.

- *Partial Nerve Lesions:* Variable symptoms will result depending on which fascicles were damaged. An interesting example is an injury to the sciatic nerve at the hip. Damage frequently is more severe in the more lateral part of the nerve, that is, the peroneal division. The symptom picture would be weakness in some muscles and possible loss of other peroneal innervated muscles. Fibrillation is present. There will often be diminished deep tendon reflexes *(Stewart, 1993)*.

✦ **Holding patterns** are observed.

- *Complete Nerve Lesions:* Typical holding patterns may be present, such as wrist drop (with a radial nerve lesion) or drop foot (with a sciatic nerve lesion).

- *Partial Nerve Lesions:* Typical holding patterns will generally be less apparent with partial lesions since some muscles are still functional, for example, a partial radial lesion can result in "finger drop" rather than a full wrist drop, or a partial ulnar lesion at the elbow may cause weak intrinsic hand muscles and a less obvious claw hand.

✦ **Contractures** may develop in the unopposed antagonists.

- *Complete Nerve Lesions:* The affected flaccid muscles are unable to exert force on the joints they cross. The intact antagonists are much more powerful in their effect on these joints, even at rest. Contractures will develop in these unopposed antagonists as they draw into a shortened position. This becomes more pronounced if the nerve regeneration and subsequent return of muscle strength in the agonists occur over a prolonged period of time.

- *Partial Nerve Lesions:* Contractures may develop in the unopposed antagonists. These contractures are less severe than with a complete lesion because some opposition to the antagonists is present from the unaffected or less affected agonists.

✦ **Pain** may be present.

- *Complete Nerve Lesions:* There will be an area of anesthesia of the cutaneous division of the nerve. Pain can be variable. There may decreased or altered sensation that may or may not be interpreted by the client as painful.

- *Partial Nerve Lesions:* There will likely be areas of hyperesthesia and possibly dysesthesia which are perceived by the client as painful. Causalgia and RSD may be present, especially in the client presenting with a partial lesion.

✦ **Scar tissue** is present at the lesion site with a complete or partial nerve lesion. It may interfere with the regeneration of the nerve.

✦ Peripheral nerve lesions can have a profound impact on all aspects of a client's life. With some injuries, the prognosis for regeneration is not clear for a few months. If regeneration does occur, it can be several months before function returns. Even if the loss of abilities and sensation is temporary, it can be a fearful and frustrating time.

✦ If the complete or partial lesion regenerates much muscle, sensory and autonomic function will eventually return, though often full recovery is not possible.

Permanent Lesions

✦ If regeneration does not occur, the original functional, sensory and autonomic losses of a complete lesion, or dysfunctions of a partial lesion, will remain.

✦ **Edema** will remain, being more profound with a complete permanent lesion than with a partial permanent lesion.

✦ **Trophic changes** and **muscle wasting** will become more marked with time. The tissue is thin and fragile. Any subsequent injury will result in prolonged healing time of the tissue.

✦ **Holding patterns** will remain. The contractures will develop and become more marked over time *(Thomson et al., 1991)*. A complete permanent lesion will result in a more pronounced pattern compared to a partial permanent lesion. Splints are often used to encourage more functional holding patterns.

✦ **Scar tissue** develops at the lesion site. A neuroma may also develop. Neuromas are usually found just proximal to the lesion site and most often with a complete severance of the nerve. Neuromas are formed at the distal end of a nerve stump, as a result of the attempt to regenerate "gone wrong". Rather than growing towards the distal endoneurial tube, the fibres grow into a tangled mass *(Weiner, Goetz, 1989)*.

✦ **Pain** may be present, especially with a partial permanent lesion. Areas of anesthesia, hypoesthesia or paresthesia may be present.

✦ **Compensatory changes** are present with permanent nerve lesions as other muscles are used to perform lost or weak actions. Secondary conditions, such as tendinitis, may result.

✦ With a permanent peripheral nerve lesion, the client must adjust to permanent functional and sensory losses. Also, disfigurement of a limb may be noticeable.

Subjective Information

HEALTH HISTORY QUESTIONS

✦ Is there any history of a systemic disorder, such as diabetes mellitus?

✦ When and how did the lesion occur?

✦ Is it a complete or partial lesion? Was surgery performed, such as a nerve graft or suturing of the nerve?

✦ Is the client currently under the care of a neurologist? What prognosis has been given?

✦ Is the physician or neurologist aware the client is seeking massage? If splints or supports are being used, has the neurologist given permission to remove them for treatment?

✦ What functions have most been affected in the client's activities of daily life?

✦ Is there any sensory loss or sensory change, such as tingling or burning? Have any hydrotherapy restrictions been imposed by the physician or neurologist?

✦ Does the client experience any pain? What type; where and when does it occur? Has there been a diagnosis of causalgia or RSD?

✦ Is the client on any medication? What type and for what reason?

✦ Is the client receiving any other treatment, such as physiotherapy? If yes, can the client describe the specific treatment being received, such as passive movement and electrical muscle stimulation?

✦ As mentioned earlier, to enable the therapist to develop a safe treatment plan, contact with the neurologist with the client's permission is important. Nerve regeneration can be observed by improvement in muscle bulk and function as well as sensory perception. But the neurologist has access to testing procedures that the massage therapist does not and is able to determine when early muscle contractions, which are not palpable to a therapist, are present.

Objective Information

Observations

✍ Holding patterns typical to the lesion may be evident. For example, a drop wrist holding pattern is present with a radial nerve lesion, due to the loss of the wrist and finger extensors.

✍ Functional losses can be noted as the therapist observes the client before the treatment. These would include the client's inability or difficulty to hold a pen or a sheet of paper, or to remove a coat or undo a button.

✎ Altered gait may result from nerve lesions in the lower limb. For example, with a sciatic lesion, foot drop is present, due to the functional loss of the ankle dorsiflexors.

✎ An antalgic facial expression or posture may be observed if a pain syndrome is present *(Weiner, Goetz, 1989)*.

✎ A decrease in muscle bulk will be evident. The muscle bulk is measured with a measuring tape, at regular intervals so the therapist may chart changes. As reinnervation occurs, muscle bulk increases *(Terzis, Smith, 1990)*.

✎ Edema may be present. Median and tibial nerves have additional autonomic fibres and, in turn, will likely have increased edema, due to the lack of vasomotor control in the blood vessels previously innervated by the fibres.

✎ Trophic changes of the skin, hair and nails often occur. There can be a thickening of the skin immediately under the nail, as well as crossed ridges or a whitish tone on the nail itself *(Mumenthaler, 1992)*. With a complete lesion, skin lines on the fingers, palm of the hand and sole of the foot become less evident *(Pedretti, Zoltan, 1990)*. This results in a smooth, glossy appearance to the skin. In long-standing injuries, the skin can become increasingly dry, scaly and coarse and the nails pitted *(Stewart, 1993)*. Anomalies in hair growth may also be seen. Most commonly, there is an initial decrease in hair growth with possible excessive growth some time after the lesion has occurred *(Weiner, Goetz, 1989)*.

✎ Inflammation or bruising is likely present in the acute and subacute stages of healing. If surgery was performed, the condition of the scar is observed.

✎ Supportive splints or braces may be in use to support the affected limb in a balanced position to allow safe use of the limb while regeneration occurs. Casting of the affected limb may occur in the first few weeks after surgery to promote successful regeneration of a nerve across the lesion site. Skin irritation at splint pressure points can occur if the splint is not properly fitted.

Palpation

✎ **Due to the fragility of the skin and concern for not interrupting the healing process of the nerve, care should be exercised during palpation in the early stages of healing.**

✎ Muscle bulk is likely reduced in the affected tissue. If the lesion is complete, more dramatic muscle wasting will be palpated in the muscles solely innervated by the damaged nerve. These muscles will be flaccid, lacking resiliency.

✎ Loss of local sweating will result in a dry texture to the skin.

✎ Edema results in boggy tissue.

✎ Contractures may be palpated while assessing the tone of the unopposed antagonists.

✎ The amount and mobility of the scar tissue at the lesion site are assessed after the axons have successfully regenerated to the distal endoneurial tube. If the lesion is permanent, increased scar tissue may be assessed. A neuroma may be present.

✎ Tenderness will be variable, depending on the individual lesion. The sensory disturbances may be difficult for the client to classify. For example, an area that is described as feeling like "pins and needles" or "prickly" needs to be documented although the feeling may or may not be considered painful by the client.

✍ Presence of a neuroma or a pain syndrome will usually result in pain when the lesion site is touched. In the case of the latter, movement of the limb distal to the lesion is painful.

✍ The temperature of the skin could be variable, due to the specific lesion and how long-standing it is. If the lesion is permanent, the therapist will palpate coolness of the affected area due to lost or compromised vasomotor function and tissue dystrophy or atrophy.

Testing

✍ Actions that traction the affected nerve are to be avoided until the nerve has regenerated past the lesion site.

✍ **AF ROM** is performed by asking the client to show the movements that can be done easily. A partial lesion will result in difficulty in performing certain actions due to muscle weakness. A complete lesion will result in the loss of function of those muscles solely innervated by the affected nerve. However, the client will only have **difficulty** in performing the action if a muscle has dual innervation or if a muscle's synergists are unaffected. The therapist is alert for substitute movements. See the individual lesions for specific examples of substitution patterns.

✍ **PR ROM** with a complete or partial regenerating nerve is initially performed on the unopposed antagonist muscles only, to assess the amount of contracture present in these muscles. For example, with a complete radial lesion there is a complete loss of extensor function of the wrist and fingers; the unopposed antagonists are the wrist flexors. Therefore, the passive relaxed movement brings the wrist into extension, assessing for muscle spasm end feel or leathery end feel of the forearm flexors. The forearm extensors that are affected by this lesion have lost or diminished protective reflexes to stretching. Therefore, PR range of motion is not performed in any range that stretches the affected tissue until minimal contraction is possible in the muscles crossing the joint being moved.

- With a permanent lesion, there is no concern for tractioning the nerve. However, the protective reflexes in the affected muscles are potentially lost or weakened. PR range of motion is carefully performed on all available planes of movement for that joint, with assessment for the end feel of the unopposed antagonist.

✍ **AR testing** is performed to discern specific lost or weakened functions or to assess what function has returned as the nerve regenerates, with the therapist providing **minimal** resistance to the affected muscles. Muscle strength grading can be useful. Refer to Appendix C for these gradings. The results will vary based on the severity of the lesion, the length of time since the injury occurred and whether the nerve is regenerating or not.

Special Tests

✍ The **sensory testing** performed includes deep and light touch, pain and two-point discrimination, proprioception and piloerector response.

- Peripheral nerve lesions have a very distinct area of sensory impairment, which can be mapped out by the therapist, using the sharp tip of the reflex hammer.

Contraindications

✦ Massage and movement of the affected limb are contraindicated for up to three weeks, if surgical intervention has occurred *(Terzis, Smith, 1990)*.

✦ Massage on the site of the lesion is not advised until the neurologist advises that a trace contraction is present.

✦ Do not traction or excessively move the joints of the affected limb in any way that might affect the regeneration process. This caution should be observed until muscle function has clearly returned.

✦ Hydrotherapy to the limb should not begin until autonomic and vasomotor control have returned, which is often indicated by the return of muscle function and improved appearance of the skin. Initial applications should avoid extremes of temperatures and pressures.

✦ Frictions and deep pressure on the flaccid or compromised tissue must be avoided.

✦ Caution must be used on the flaccid or compromised tissue in the application of all techniques, as well as when grasping the limb to move it or to perform range of motion exercises.

✦ Joint play is not performed on the affected limb until innervation occurs and the joint is stable. At this time it is introduced with caution.

✦ Rhythmic techniques are avoided anywhere on the body until some control of the limb has returned, since the client will likely be apprehensive. Rhythmic techniques are not performed on the affected limb until reinnervation occurs and then they are introduced gradually.

• With a complete nerve lesion, a small area of anesthesia or hypoesthesia will result. There is also likely a larger area of paresthesia *(Mumenthaler, 1992)*.

• Partial nerve lesions often present with hyperesthesia and possibly pain (see Causalgia under Peripheral Nerve Pain in the Understanding Peripheral Nerve Lesions chapter. Pain and temperature awareness return first *(Terzis, Smith, 1990)*.

✍ **Tinel's sign** is positive, resulting in a tingling sensation or similar paresthesia along the course of the nerve up to the most distal point at which it has regenerated. Beyond that point, the Tinel's test will not yield a response. If a pain response is elicited, it will most likely indicate a neuroma *(Mumenthaler, 1992)*.

✍ **Deep tendon reflex testing** is negative with a complete lesion. Deep tendon reflexes are diminished with a partial lesion, in the muscles affected by the injury.

✍ **Upper limb tension, slump** and **straight leg raise tests** may be positive with a peripheral nerve lesion.

Treatment Goals

Treatment Plan

🖐 Treatment aims for regenerating nerves, whether the lesion is complete or partial, are for the most part the same. Initially, all nerve lesions are treated as though they will regenerate. Over time, if motor, sensory and autonomic losses remain, the lesion is referred to as being permanent. If this occurs, the goals and rationale of the treatment are different than those for a regenerating nerve. Therefore, the treatment plan below has been divided into two sections to address these different situations. An oil or lotion enriched with Vitamin E is recommended.

Regenerating Lesions: Early Stages of Healing of a Regenerating Nerve

Do not disrupt the healing process of the regenerating nerve; specifically, be careful not to traction the nerve before there is regeneration past the lesion site.

🖐 Care is taken not to severely traction the limb or stretch denervated tissue. In the consent, the therapist should ask to be kept informed of any pulling or painful sensations in relation to the nerve injury.

🖐 **Positioning** the client supine or seated is the most suitable for treating a nerve lesion in the upper limb. These positions allow for safe and appropriate positioning and pillowing of the affected limb. The prone position is inadvisable and sidelying may be awkward for these types of lesions.

🖐 However, for lower limb lesions, the prone or sidelying position is appropriate. In cases where the upper leg is affected, such as a sciatic nerve lesion, the supine position is best used after reinnervation has occurred in the area.

🖐 If splints or braces are being worn and the neurologist has given permission to remove them, the client should do so just prior to treatment of that specific tissue. The splint is replaced when this work is completed.

🖐 The limb should be gently moved out of its holding pattern and placed in a comfortable and relatively **neutral position**. Pillows are used to support the limb in this position and to ensure client comfort. For example, a radial lesion will result in the elbow, wrist and fingers to be drawn into flexion. The therapist should place a pillow on the client's abdomen and use another pillow under the elbow. The elbow and wrist are brought out of flexion and laid on the abdominal pillow. The fingers can be taken slightly out of flexion and positioned so they are resting over the edge of the pillow or a towel roll could be placed in the palm to open the hand.

🖐 The above pillowing elevates the limb to allow for passive drainage of edema.

🖐 The affected limb may need to be secured while other areas of the body are worked on. The therapist could use a sheet or a large towel, folded to be about one foot wide. It needs to be long enough to tuck

Treatment Goals

Treatment Plan

under the affected arm and supporting pillow, then over the client's torso and finally tucked under the rib cage on the opposite side. This allows for freedom of movement of the unaffected limb and assures the client that the affected limb will not fall off the table or be bumped.

- ✋ **Hydrotherapy,** such as cool compresses, can be used in the acute stage of the healing. This reduces inflammation and edema. A modified temperature is used on fragile or dystrophic tissue.

- ✋ Hydrotherapy is contraindicated to the affected limb if there is loss of dysfunction of the autonomics (since this includes loss of vasomotor control). Hydrotherapy affects the tissue both distal and proximal to where it is applied. Therefore, it should be avoided anywhere on the affected limb, even proximal to the lesion site.

- ✋ As the autonomic and sensory function return, modified applications can be used. Initially, slightly cool or tepid water washes can be applied in a gentle, segmental fashion. Next, mild contrast washes would be appropriate. The temperature differences should be increased gradually, along with the length of time of the application.

General Treatment

- ✋ The treatment is performed in the context of a relaxation massage.

Decrease sympathetic nervous system firing. Provide emotional support. Decrease pain, if present. Address compensatory changes.

- ✋ Nerve regeneration can be a long, uncertain and potentially anxiety-causing process for the client. A calm environment and a supportive touch are important. To decrease the client's apprehension levels, the therapist needs to communicate clearly about what will be done, while avoiding any unexpected techniques or movements. Increasing relaxation will modify the client's pain perception. Swedish techniques are used to address compensatory changes to the contralateral limb.

Specific Treatment

Do not traction the nerve or interfere with the healing process.

- ✋ **Proximal to the lesion site,** the main goal is to decrease edema and treat the overworked but functional muscles for hypertonicity and trigger points.

- ✋ For regenerating nerves, decreasing edema and maintaining tissue health are most important. The therapist is keeping distal tissue healthy so it will hopefully be functional when the nerve reaches it.

Decrease edema.

- ✋ Edema is treated first, using elevation, lymph node pumping and lymphatic drainage techniques. Techniques are applied to the proximal edge of the edema.

Treatment Goals   Treatment Plan

Decrease hypertonicity and trigger points of unaffected proximal muscles.

🖐 When addressing tissue health in the area proximal to the lesion site, segmental applications of petrissage and effleurage are used. In this case, "segmental" means that these techniques are applied at right angles to the direction of the regenerating nerve to minimize the risk of tractioning it. When approaching the lesion site, the therapist may wish to gently place the ulnar border of one hand just proximal to the site. This will stabilize the tissue around the lesion site and assist the therapist in monitoring the amount of drag being placed on the tissue. Trigger points may be treated in any of the functional muscles, proximal to the lesion site providing that post-treatment care is possible. Therefore, heat can only be used if the autonomics are functional and a stretch is only performed if it doesn't traction the injured nerve.

🖐 The therapist is wise not to work on the lesion site before the nerve has regenerated beyond that site. This is at the very least two weeks post-trauma or three weeks post-surgery.

Promote health of denervated tissue.

🖐 **Distal to the lesion site, compromised muscles,** whether flaccid or weak, are treated with light stroking and gentle compressions. It is important to remember that not only is the tissue compromised but there may be a lack of sensory response. In this case, the client is unable to give accurate responses about the depth of techniques used.

Prevent contracture formation of the unopposed antagonist muscles.

🖐 **Distal to the lesion site, the unaffected muscles** are treated using carefully applied Swedish techniques and modified fascial techniques. On the unopposed antagonist muscles, modified fascial techniques are applied in a segmental manner by stabilizing the distal tissue with one hand and applying a gentle moderate pressure in a lateral direction with the other hand. At the edge between the healthy and flaccid tissue, the pressure of the fascial technique is directed towards, but not onto, the flaccid tissue.

Maintain health in all joints of the affected limb.

🖐 If surgical repair has been performed, movement of the affected area is contraindicated for up to three weeks. *Care should be taken when grasping the limb so fragile tissue is not damaged through too much compression. Extreme caution must be taken to avoid any movements that may stretch the affected muscles and nerve.* If the nerve is regenerating, the degree of passive movement applied can increase as reinnervation occurs and the protective muscle reflexes return.

🖐 Initally, **passive relaxed range of motion** is performed in mid- to full ranges to the joints in the direction that **shortens** the affected tissue and nerve. In other words, if a median nerve lesion in the forearm has resulted in lost wrist flexion, the wrist can be moved into flexion. Unless approved by the neurologist, it is contraindicated to perform

773

Treatment Goals

Treatment Plan

any action that will place a stretch on the affected muscles and regenerating nerve distal and immediately proximal to the lesion site. At this stage, in order to maintain joint health, only the innermost ranges should be used at the joints distal to the lesion if the action could traction the nerve.

Encourage motor re-education of the affected muscles.

🖐 It is important to keep the brain conscious of the pathway of the nerve to the affected muscles. For functions that are completely lost, this is achieved by the therapist passively performing the lost actions while at the same time asking the client to mentally focus on the action of these muscles. More specifically, the client is asked to "think into", or visualize, a particular movement as the therapist performs the motion for the client. The action may even be performed by the unaffected side, to reinforce the action.

Maintain the strength of weak muscles.

🖐 The therapist performs active assisted movements with the client, who has weak but not lost actions. For example, with a partial median nerve lesion at the wrist which results in weak wrist flexion accompanied by ulnar deviation, the client is instructed to think into performing the action of wrist flexion while trying to perform this action. The therapist performs an active assisted movement, gently correcting the action where necessary — in this case, assisting full flexion while bringing the wrist midline from its pull to ulnar deviation. This should be performed with each action that is compromised due to the injury.

Later Stages of Healing of a Regenerating Nerve as Function Returns

🖐 The neurologist will be able to advise when motor responses first occur. As reinnervation progresses, tissue health will improve. Gradually, the sensory and autonomic functions will return. A self-care program of motor strength rehabilitation and sensory re-education is also promoted.

🖐 **Positioning** supine and seated are still appropriate, but prone and sidelying positions may be indicated for upper limb lesions. The therapist should avoid letting the client's affected arm hang over the edge of the table.

🖐 For lower limb lesions, any position that is comfortable can be used. The pillowing and limb positioning remain unchanged until the client has the strength to support the affected limb so it does not fall off the table.

🖐 **Hydrotherapy** applications of mild contrast washes are appropriate where the autonomics are functional. The temperature difference is

Treatment Goals

Treatment Plan

increased gradually, along with the length of time of the application. The pressure of the application is also increased and more vigorously applied, according to the health of the tissue. Eventually, compresses can be safely applied, then hydrocollators or thermaphores.

General Treatment

Decrease sympathetic nervous system firing. Continue encouragement of the client. Address compensatory changes.

✋ By charting progress, the client can be made aware of the small gains that may have gone unnoticed. There is an ongoing concern for maintaining tissue and joint health in areas that are still not innervated. Compensatory changes should be addressed, according to the client's needs.

Specific Treatment

Take care with tissue that is not yet fully innervated.

✋ In the tissue that is reinnervated and with functional protective reflexes, tractioning the nerve is not a concern. But, distal to the regeneration site of the nerve, the tissue is still not innervated and is treated as if it were in the early stages of healing.

Reduce edema, if present.

✋ If edema is present, the limb is elevated and lymphatic drainage techniques are applied.

Promote tissue health of unaffected and newly innervated tissue.

✋ General Swedish techniques are applied on tissue proximal to the lesion and tissue distal to the lesion that is reinnervated. Although the affected tissue is still fragile, it will become less so as innervation is restored and muscle function is regained. Working segmentally is still recommended, but the pressure can be gradually increased over a series of treatments. The less aggressive trigger point techniques, such as segmental muscle stripping or mild ischemic compressions, can be used as required.

✋ Fascial techniques to the unopposed antagonists are useful until full strength has been regained by the affected muscles.

Reduce scar tissue formation in the tissue surrounding the lesion site.

✋ Once the nerve has regenerated past the lesion site, effort is made to reduce the scar tissue in the surrounding tissue. As a guide, the therapist can wait until some evidence of muscle function is apparent, indicating that the nerve has reinnervated the tissue. Massage is performed on the soft tissue at the lesion site to promote full function and excursion of the joint and surrounding muscles. Initially the techniques are gently applied, FTK and skin rolling. Over time, deep kneading and, eventually, frictions can be used when addressing the scar tissue at the site of the lesion.

Maintain and improve joint health and range of motion.

✋ The therapist can gradually introduce previously contraindicated techniques, such as rhythmic techniques and joint play.

Treatment Goals   Treatment Plan

🖐 At this stage, **passive relaxed range of motion** is performed on all planes in mid- to full ranges, providing all muscles crossing the joint are functional.

Encourage motor re-education of the affected muscles.

🖐 Maintaining the nerve pathways is only necessary for the functions that are still lost. Active-assisted movement is performed for those actions that are newly recovered and weak.

Perform sensory awareness re-education.

🖐 As motor fibres regenerate, so do sensory fibres. Sometimes sensory fibres may not regenerate to their previous structures. For example, an axon that formerly innervated the distal thumb may regenerate to the palm or index finger, about four to six months following a lesion to the wrist *(Dellon, Jabaky, 1982)*. This leads to unrecognizable or distorted sensory signals after nerve regeneration *(Terzis, Smith, 1990)*. While the client can recognize that something is touching her hand, she is unable to identify the stimulus.

🖐 Re-education of the client's sensory perception is achieved by gradually introducing varied textures to the affected area. This is begun on the upper limb, when regeneration has occurred to the proximal phalanx. The therapist starts by stroking the skin with the eraser on the end of a pencil or with his finger. The pressure is adequate for the client to perceive it but not so much as to cause a perception of pain. The client is directed to observe and think about the sensation. She then closes her eyes and feels the sensation.

🖐 Finally, the client is told to observe once again to confirm the location and the sensation. A variety of textures, such as a feather, a flannel cloth and a washcloth, are gradually introduced.

Permanent Lesions

🖐 A diagnosis of a permanent nerve injury is made by a neurologist. It indicates no hope of regeneration. The therapist is no longer concerned about tractioning the nerve, but rather about dystrophic tissue and compensatory changes.

🖐 **Positioning** includes any positions that are suitable, provided the limb is secure. Care is taken that the client's limbs are not hanging over the table or susceptible to being bumped by the therapist.

🖐 **Hydrotherapy** restrictions must be maintained if there is permanent loss of autonomic function. Modifications in weight, duration and temperature of applications is necessary on denervated and dystrophic tissue.

Treatment Goals

Treatment Plan

General Treatment

Decrease sympathetic nervous system firing.
Provide emotional support to the client.
Treat compensatory changes.

✋ The treatment is performed in the context of a relaxation massage. A calm environment and a supportive touch are important for a client dealing with a permanent loss of function and, potentially, a visible disability. To decrease the client's apprehension levels, the therapist needs to communicate clearly about what will be done, while avoiding any unexpected techniques or movements. Increasing relaxation will reduce the client's pain perception.

✋ Compensatory changes will be more apparent with a permanent lesion and are addressed as necessary.

✋ General Swedish techniques are applied to the tissue proximal to the lesion and to the rest of the body. Hypertonicity and trigger points are addressed.

Specific Treatment

Decrease edema.
Maintain tissue health.

✋ If edema is present, the limb is elevated and lymphatic drainage techniques are applied.

✋ When there is no reinnervation of the affected tissue nutritional feed to the muscles is lost. This can cause a dramatic loss of tissue health.

✋ The therapist maintains the health of the fragile tissue, using gentle segmental effleurage and petrissage techniques. The pressure is modified due to lost or altered sensation, muscle wasting and dystrophic tissue.

Limit the contracture of the unopposed antagonist muscles.

✋ Permanent lesions require more focus on this goal. Passive relaxed full range of motion and segmental fascial techniques are used on the unopposed antagonists to maintain as much function as possible. Eventually, the goal may change to encourage a functional contracture. This is done in conjunction with other professionals working with the client.

Reduce scar tissue formation in the tissue surrounding the lesion site.

✋ At the lesion site, scar tissue is treated using cross-fibre petrissage and frictions. The pressure and duration of these techniques are modified according to the tissue health. With a permanent lesion, a neuroma may be present contraindicating local frictions (*Weiner, Goetz, 1989*).

Maintain joint health.

✋ Joint health is maintained through careful application of passive relaxed movement in full, pain-free ranges. Care needs to be taken when grasping the limb in order not to damage the fragile tissue.

Maintain awareness of the affected limb.

✋ It is important for the client to maintain awareness of the affected limb since the lack of sensation and function can lead to an increased risk of injury. One method of achieving this awareness can be integrated into the range of motion techniques. While the therapist

777

Self-care Goals

Self-care Plan

moves the joints of the affected limb, the client observes this and follows the actions with the unaffected side. Where partial function exists, active assisted movements are performed.

Decrease pain, if present.

✋ Pain perception can be modified by decreasing sympathetic nervous system firing. Direct touch can aggravate causalgia or can cause dysesthesia. If this occurs, the techniques are modified and the pressure altered to within the pain tolerance of the client. If the symptoms persist, direct touch to the area should be stopped.

Self-care Goals

Self-care Plan

Regenerating Lesions: Early Stages of Healing of a Regenerating Nerve

Encourage relaxation.

✍ The client is educated about full diaphragmatic breathing.

Educate the client about tissue health.

✍ The client is encouraged to maintain tissue health. If the affected area is accessible and if there is no open wound, the client can perform self-massage using an enriched cream or oil, such as apricot kernel oil which is high in vitamin A or a vitamin E enriched cream. Sandalwood essential oil has emollient properties (Lawless, 1995); 10 drops of the pure essential oil can be added to 50 ml. of the carrier oil.

✍ When wearing a splint, the client is vigilant for redness and skin irritation at pressure points.

✍ Especially after the splint is removed, the client must protect the affected limb from injury. Injury occurs easily because tissue is fragile and insensitive to many stimuli, such as hot and cold.

Encourage motor re-education.

✍ Passive or active assisted movement is performed to the denervated muscles. With an upper limb lesion, the client should visualize herself performing the impaired actions while moving the elbow, hand or fingers with the unaffected hand. The client is encouraged to perform whatever activities of daily living are possible with the recovering limb once the splints are removed, with care taken not to injure the affected tissue or traction the nerve.

Maintain strength and range of motion.

✍ Three weeks following surgical repair, passive movement **into** shortened ranges is encouraged. Active assisted movement is performed in these same ranges for weak actions. For example, a median nerve lesion would require the hands and fingers to be supported in a slightly flexed position initially and exercises would encourage actions into a flexed position. Gentle, pain-free active resisted isometric contractions of the uninjured flexors maintains their strength.

778

Self-care Goals

Self-care Plan

✍ Progressive splinting is usually used for a few months to gradually support the affected joints into greater ranges that stretch the affected tissue. For example, the above lesion would be splinted into less flexion and eventually extension, with each new splint.

Refer the client.

✍ Biofeedback can assist in motor re-education *(Terzis, Smith, 1990)* as well as facilitating pain reduction.

Later Stages of Healing of a Regenerating Nerve as Function Returns

Educate the client.

✍ The client is encouraged to maintain tissue health. Self-massage with an enriched oil or cream is still beneficial.

Encourage motor re-education.

✍ The client is encouraged to perform activities of daily living with the recovering limb once movement improves. Passive movement with visualization may be necessary only in the distal limb.

Maintain then increase strength and range of motion.

✍ Resisted exercises are introduced. It is extremely important to focus on the specific movements weakened. Initially, gentle resistance is provided by the unaffected hand of the client. The amount of resistance is increased over time. Finally, the strengthening program progresses to isotonic exercises, using light weights or rubber tubing for resistance.

✍ Range of motion progresses from middle to full pain-free ranges in all directions.

Encourage re-education of sensory awareness.

✍ The client introduces a moving stimulus using a variety of textures to the affected area. In the upper limb, this is approximately four to six months after an injury at the wrist. Initially, she starts by stroking the skin with the eraser on the end of a pencil. The client is directed to observe and think about the sensation. She then closes her eyes and feels the sensation. Finally, the client is told to observe once again to connect the location and the sensation. Textures such as a feather, a flannel cloth and a washcloth are gradually introduced. Next, a stationary stimulus is applied in the same procedure as above.

✍ Once moving and stationary pressure can be identified, usually six to eight months after an injury at the wrist, the client retrains the recognition of objects through touch. The client repeatedly handles different objects with her eyes open, then with eyes closed and finally with eyes open again. First, familiar objects are used with a wide variety of shapes, sizes and textures. Then smaller objects of different shapes and sizes but similar textures are introduced. These exercises helps the client memorize the new patterns of sensory input.

Refer the client.

✍ Biofeedback can assist in motor re-education *(Terzis, Smith, 1990)*. At this stage, re-education would be required in only the most distal muscles that are not reinnervated.

779

Permanent Nerve Lesions

Encourage relaxation.

✍ Adjusting to a permanent dysfunction can be very stressful. The client is educated about full diaphragmatic breathing.

Educate the client.

✍ The client is encouraged to maintain tissue health. Self-massage with an enriched cream or oil is beneficial.

✍ Permanent sensory losses will require ongoing vigilance on the part of the client to ensure the affected tissue is not injured.

Maintain strength and range of motion of the affected limb.

✍ The client is encouraged to perform the activities of daily living as much as possible. The client can often develop modified ways to perform the actions of the muscles that have not recovered. A strengthening program is encouraged for the muscles that are still innervated. This could be an isometric or an isotonic program.

✍ Passive movement in all ranges is encouraged, especially those which stretch the antagonist muscles.

Treatment Frequency and Expected Outcome

To maintain tissue health and prevent contracture formation in the earlier stages of healing, ideally, 30-minute treatments a few times a week are suggested.

Clients who are very anxious might prefer a 45-minute treatment with an additional relaxation focus.

As function and sensory perception return, treatments can be weekly, depending on the client's stress levels, compensatory changes and speed of functional return.

If degeneration has occurred, but the endoneurial tube is intact, the prognosis is generally quite good, though full function may not return.

If the degeneration has occurred as a result of a nerve severance, several factors affect the prognosis. The best situation involves a "clean" severance of the nerve, with good apposition, which in turn will lead to the best surgical results. Regeneration also is more favourable in nerves that are not mixed nerves and if the lesion site is close to the effector or receptor organ.

See radial, median, ulnar and sciatic nerve lesions, Bell's palsy and Understanding Peripheral Nerve Lesions for specific details. Also see stress reduction, edema, scars and tendinitis for related treatments.

Finally, the age and general health of the client can be factors that affect the efficiency of the healing of the tissue and the regeneration process of the nerves of severance injuries. Given all of this, even in the most favourable cases, it is unusual to obtain better than a 60 per cent recovery (*Thomson et al., 1991*).

RADIAL NERVE LESIONS

Linda Ludwig

The Path Travelled

The radial nerve is a continuation of the posterior cord (C5 to T1) of the brachial plexus *(Figure 62.1)*. From the posterior axillary wall between the long and medial heads of triceps, the nerve continues to the spiral groove of the humerus, deep to the lateral head of triceps. It winds around the humerus to the lateral side where it travels to the anterior arm. The radial nerve is relatively superficial at this point before it travels between the brachialis and brachioradialis, passing the extensor carpi radialis longus and extensor carpi radialis brevis.

The nerve crosses the elbow joint to the supinator. At this point, the radial nerve divides into two branches. The posterior motor branch enters the supinator muscle, then travels down the lateral aspect of the radius, innervating extensor digitorum, extensor carpi ulnaris, extensor pollicis longus and brevis, abductor pollicis longus, extensor indicis and extensor digiti minimi. This branch terminates at the wrist.

The superficial branch continues down the arm under the brachioradialis, crossing supinator, pronator teres and the radial attachments of the flexor digitorum superficialis and flexor pollicis longus. The radial artery travels on the nerve's medial side. The nerve continues on the dorsal surface of the arm, becoming superficial to abductor pollicis longus and extensor pollicis brevis. After crossing the extensor retinaculum, it divides into more branches. These innervate the dorsal surface of the hand, lateral to a line midway through the fourth digit, including the radial aspect of the thenar eminence distal to the middle phalanx.

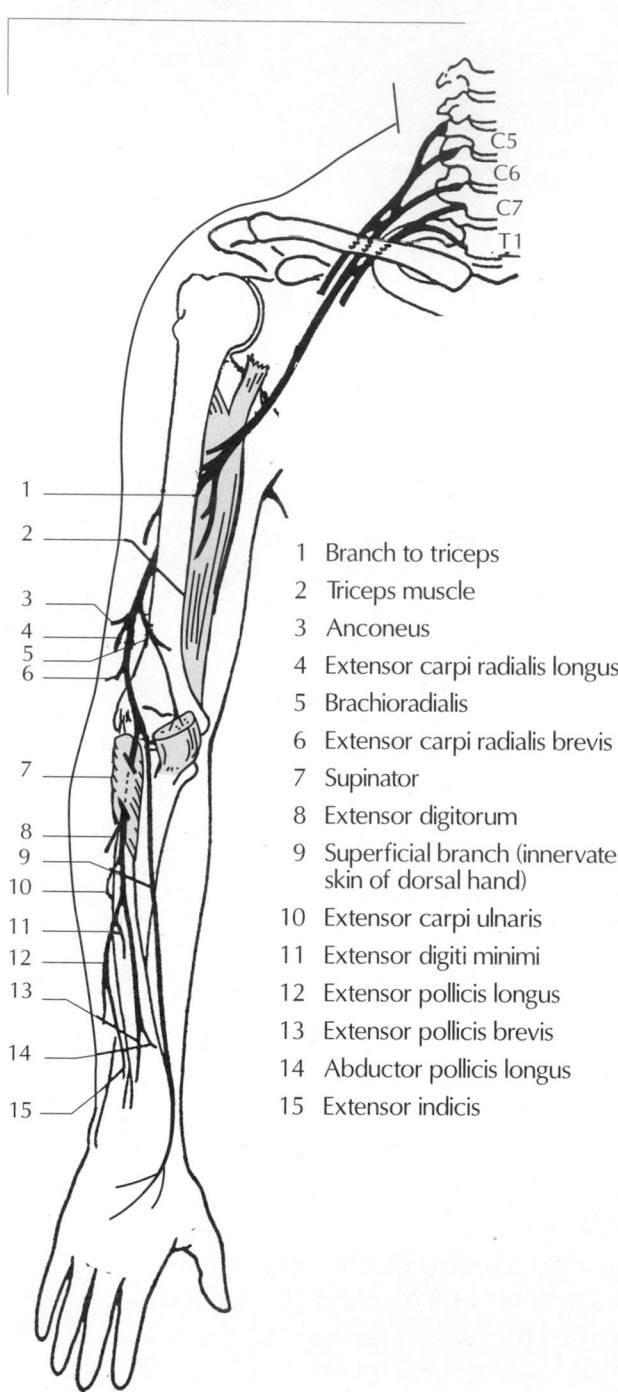

1 Branch to triceps
2 Triceps muscle
3 Anconeus
4 Extensor carpi radialis longus
5 Brachioradialis
6 Extensor carpi radialis brevis
7 Supinator
8 Extensor digitorum
9 Superficial branch (innervates skin of dorsal hand)
10 Extensor carpi ulnaris
11 Extensor digiti minimi
12 Extensor pollicis longus
13 Extensor pollicis brevis
14 Abductor pollicis longus
15 Extensor indicis

Figure 62.1
The radial nerve (C5 to T1).

Muscles Innervated by the Radial Nerve

✦ triceps

✦ anconeus

✦ brachioradialis

✦ extensor carpi radialis longus

✦ extensor carpi radialis brevis

✦ supinator

✦ extensor digitorum

✦ extensor carpi ulnaris

✦ extensor digiti minimi

✦ extensor pollicis longus

✦ extensor pollicis brevis

✦ abductor pollicis longus

✦ extensor indicis

Causes of lesions of the radial nerve are:

➤ **fractures**, primarily at the spiral radial groove — the radial nerve is involved to some degree in 70 per cent of humerus fractures (*Mumenthaler, Schliack, 1991*) and at the supracondylar and upper one-third of the radius;

➤ **dislocation** of the head of the radius, humeroradial and radioulnar joints;

➤ **post-surgical complications**, due to unrelieved pressure on the lateral arm from poor positioning during the surgery;

➤ **compression**, primarily at the axilla from crutch use. A condition known as "Saturday night palsy" occurs when the arm is draped over the back of a chair or table edge, or when the arm is fully abducted and supporting the head against a hard surface — as with an undisturbed sleep resulting from drug use, alcohol intoxication or extreme fatigue.

➤ **Supinator syndrome** compression can occur in the forearm. Fibrosis (usually due to overuse) at the site where the nerve penetrates the supinator muscle leads to the syndrome. The compression may result in a first degree (neuropraxia) or second degree (axonotmesis) nerve lesion.

Generally, the half to lower third of the upper arm is three times as common an injury site as the proximal third.

782

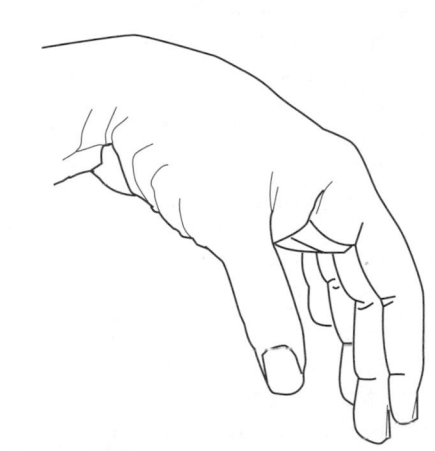

Figure 62.2
Wrist drop in radial nerve injury.

Symptom Picture

◆ Presentation of a complete radial nerve lesion is also known as **wrist drop** (*Figure 62.2*). The hand hangs in flexion because the wrist flexors are unopposed due to the flaccid wrist extensors.

◆ When the injury is proximal to the elbow, before the radial nerve branches, both sensory and motor function are affected. When the injury is distal to the elbow, often only one branch is affected, with the impairment being either motor or sensory.

◆ Muscle wasting is possible depending on the lesion site. The triceps and lateral supracondylar areas over brachioradialis and extensor carpi ulnaris may be wasted. Muscles may also be wasted at the dorsum of the forearm and between the radius and ulna.

◆ There may be swelling on the dorsum of the hand, though the etiology is unknown *(Mumenthaler, Schliack, 1991)*.

Sensory Dysfunction as a Result of a Lesion

◆ Altered sensation is experienced at the posterior arm, forearm and hand, specifically in the thumb, index, middle and one-half of the ring finger, excluding the fingertips (*Figure 62.3*).

◆ Anesthesia occurs at the web between the thumb and second digit.

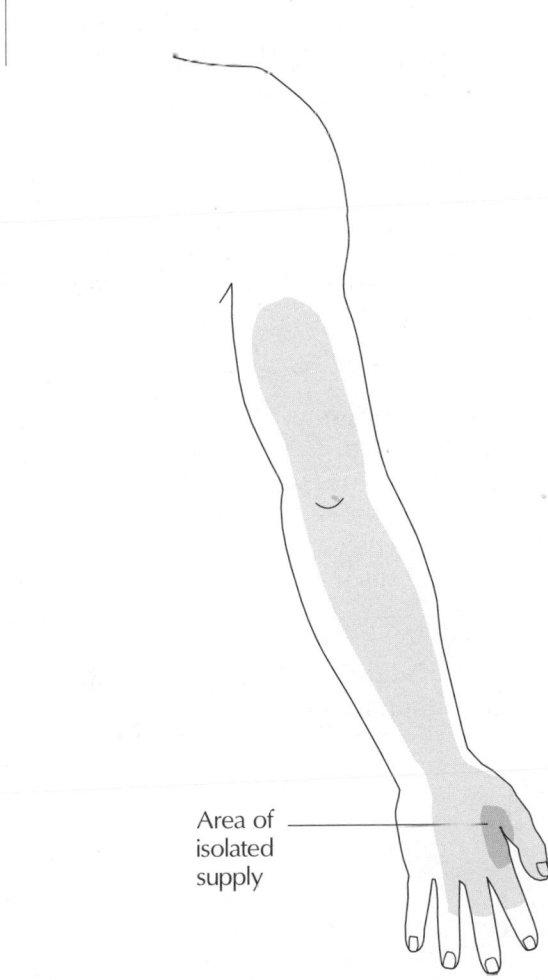

Area of isolated supply

Figure 62.3
Sensory distribution of the radial nerve.

783

Motor Dysfunction Due To a Complete Lesion

LESION SITE Note that "FUNCTIONS AFFECTED" for a specific lesion site include all the muscles involved following from that point on.	FUNCTIONS AFFECTED The function listed is lost unless other muscles supplied by other nerves can perform the action. In this case, the action is weak.
axilla	**extension of the elbow**
upper arm to elbow	**flexion of the elbow in mid-pronated position** (with a complete lesion, this action is only weakened)
elbow to forearm	**supination of the forearm** (with a complete lesion, this action is only weakened)
	extension of the wrist
	adduction of the wrist (with a complete lesion, this action is only weakened)
	abduction of the wrist
	extension of the digits at the MCP joint
	extension of the terminal phalanx at the IP joint of the thumb (with a complete lesion, this action is only weakened)
	extension of the MCP joint of the thumb
	abduction of the CMC joint of the thumb

CMC: carpometacarpal
DIP: distal interphalangeal
IP: interphalangeal
MCP: metacarpophalangeal
PIP: proximal interphalangeal

| MUSCLES INVOLVED | |
| innervated by | |
Radial nerve	*Other nerves*
• triceps • anconeus	
• brachioradialis	• biceps brachii • brachialis *(musculocutaneous nerve)*
• supinator	• biceps brachii *(musculocutaneous nerve)*
• extensor carpi ulnaris • extensor carpi radialis longus and brevis • assisted by extensor digitorum	
• extensor carpi ulnaris	• flexor carpi ulnaris *(ulnar nerve)*
• extensor carpi radialis longus and brevis • abductor pollicis longus • extensor pollicis longus and brevis	
• extensor digitorum • extensor indicis • extensor digiti minimi	
• extensor pollicis longus	• abductor pollicis brevis *(median nerve)*
• extensor pollicis brevis • abductor pollicis longus • extensor pollicis longus	
• abductor pollicis longus	• abductor pollicis brevis (median)

◄ *Substitute Movement Patterns: When testing, the therapist should be aware of the finger extensor muscles (extensor digitorum, indicis and digiti minimi) attempting to substitute for the wrist extensors.*

Substitute Movement Patterns: When testing, the therapist should have the client extend the thumb and fingers before performing the action of abduction to prevent substitute movements. ◄

See also Understanding Peripheral Nerve Lesions, Strategies: Crush and Severance Injuries to Peripheral Nerves, Understanding Compression Syndromes and fractures.

ULNAR NERVE LESIONS

Linda Ludwig

The Path Travelled

The ulnar nerve originates from the medial cord of the brachial plexus (C8 to T1). It follows along the posterior wall of the axilla, under the pectoralis minor *(Figure 63.1)*. In the upper arm, it shares a common neurovascular bundle with the median nerve until it reaches the insertion of coracobrachialis in the mid-upper arm. The ulnar nerve then travels along the medial triceps. Generally, it follows a relatively superficial course in the upper arm.

At the elbow, the nerve goes posterior to the medial epicondyle of the humerus and medial to the olecranon process. The ulnar collateral ligament supports the nerve. There are additional ligamentous fibres which connect the medial epicondyle to the olecranon and under which the ulnar nerve passes. It then follows a path between and deep to the head of the flexor carpi ulnaris muscle. This area can sometimes be a site of compression of the nerve. Continuing to the wrist, the ulnar nerve lies with the flexor carpi ulnaris above it and flexor digitorum profundus below it. The nerve is joined midway by the ulnar artery. There are two main sensory branches: the dorsal branch and the palmar branch. Midway down the forearm, the dorsal branch emerges. It supplies the extensor surface of the fourth digit to the interphalangeal (IP) joint.

At the wrist, the ulnar nerve travels over the flexor retinaculum (carpal tunnel), between the pisiform and the hook of the hamate bone and beneath the volar carpal ligament and the palmaris brevis muscle. This passage is also called Guyon's canal or the ulnar tunnel; it is another site for compression of the nerve.

Here, the ulnar nerve divides into superficial and deep divisions. The superficial branch is primarily sensory and the deep branch is primarily motor. The superficial branch travels deep to palmaris brevis and then divides further into the palmar digital branch, which supplies the ulnar side of the little finger, and another branch for the radial side of the little finger and the ulnar side of the ring finger. The deep division travels with the ulnar artery,

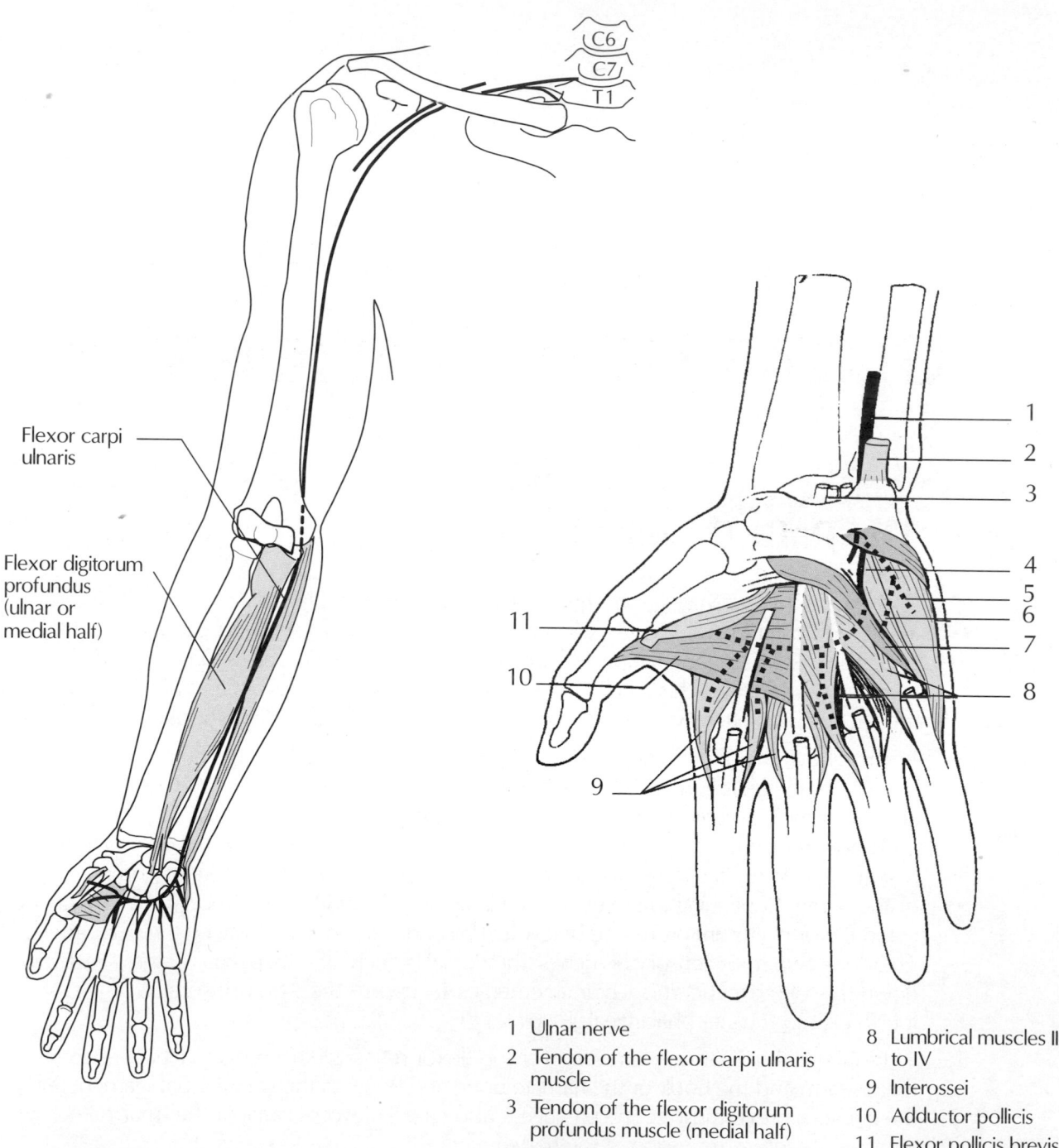

Flexor carpi
ulnaris

Flexor digitorum
profundus
(ulnar or
medial half)

11

10

9

1

2

3

4
5
6
7

8

Figure 63.1
A. The ulnar nerve (C8 to T1).

1 Ulnar nerve
2 Tendon of the flexor carpi ulnaris
muscle
3 Tendon of the flexor digitorum
profundus muscle (medial half)
4 Deep branch of the ulnar nerve
5 Abductor digiti minimi
6 Flexor digiti minimi
7 Opponens digiti minimi

8 Lumbrical muscles III
to IV
9 Interossei
10 Adductor pollicis
11 Flexor pollicis brevis
(may have shared
innervation from the
median and ulnar
nerve)

B. Detail of ulnar nerve innervation of the hand.

going deep between the abductor and flexor digiti minimi. It then pierces the opponens digiti minimi before continuing radially beneath the tendons of the finger flexors to the adductor pollicis.

Muscles Innervated by the Ulnar Nerve

+ flexor carpi ulnaris
+ flexor digitorum profundus (ulnar or medial half) innervation is shared with the median nerve
+ hypothenar muscles:
  • abductor digiti minimi
  • flexor digiti minimi
  • opponens digiti minimi
+ third and fourth lumbricals
+ palmar and dorsal interossei
+ adductor pollicis
+ flexor pollicis brevis (deep head); innervation is shared with the median nerve

Note: approximately one-third of the population shows some variation of innervation of muscles in the hand, such as shared or sole innervation with the median nerve (*Rosenbaum, Ochoa, 1993*).

Causes of lesions of the ulnar nerve are:

➤ **fractures** of the medial condyle of the elbow, mid-forearm or wrist (also called a Colles' fracture);

➤ **dislocation** of the elbow;

➤ **post-surgical complication** such as unrelieved pressure from the arm hanging over the edge of a table or the arm positioned improperly while under anesthesia;

➤ **pathology** such as leprosy; the ulnar nerve is commonly involved (*Sunderland, 1991*);

➤ **prolonged compression** from resting the elbow on a hard surface, from wearing a too-tight wrist band or handcuff or from bicycling;

➤ **repetitive action** causing excessive stress such as pitching a ball or repeated flexion and extension with machine work. Compression syndromes may develop due to fibrosis at specific sites such as the medial elbow or at Guyon's canal. This can result in a first degree (neuropraxia) or second degree (axonotmesis) nerve lesion;

➤ **direct trauma** such as a contusion or laceration at the wrist or hand; this injury is often in combination with a median nerve lesion.

The ulnar nerve is most vulnerable where it is superficial, specifically at the superior posterior elbow. Likewise, the nerve is at risk at the wrist, where it emerges from under the tendon of the flexor carpi ulnaris at the pisiform.

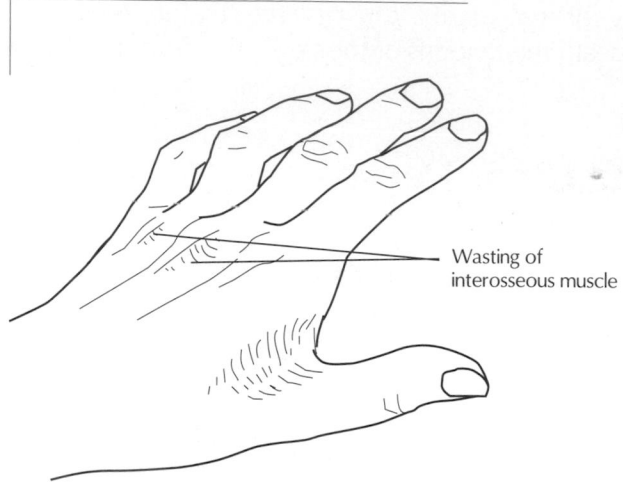

Wasting of
interosseous muscle

Figure 63.2
Claw hand deformity in ulnar lesions.

Symptom Picture

✦ Presentation of a complete ulnar nerve lesion is also known as **claw hand** (*Figure 63.2*). The little finger is hyperextended and abducted at the metacarpophalangeal joint (MCP) as well as flexed at the interphalangeal joint (IP). The ring finger is hyperextended at the MCP joint, with varying amounts of flexion at the IP joint.

✦ The hyperextension is due to the loss of some of the finger flexors, which results in unopposed extensors pulling the fingers back. Flexion at the IP joints combined with extension of the MCP joints is from the loss of the third and fourth lumbricals (and somewhat from loss of the interossei), which usually extend the IP joint and flex at the MCP joint. There is slight abduction of the little finger with loss of function of the adductor digiti minimi.

✦ **Froment's sign** is positive with an ulnar nerve lesion. The client attempts to maintain a firm grip on an object held between the thumb and index finger. This is impossible with loss of the adductor pollicis function. The flexor pollicis longus (innervated by the median nerve) is recruited in order to hold the object better. This results in flexion at the terminal phalanx (*Figure 63.3*).

✦ Muscle wasting is most remarkable at the hypothenar eminence and in the interosseous spaces. It may be present at the ulnar side of the forearm if flexor carpi ulnaris and flexor digitorum profundus are affected by a nerve lesion.

✦ Altered sensation, anhidrosis (diminished or absent sweating) and vasomotor changes may occur.

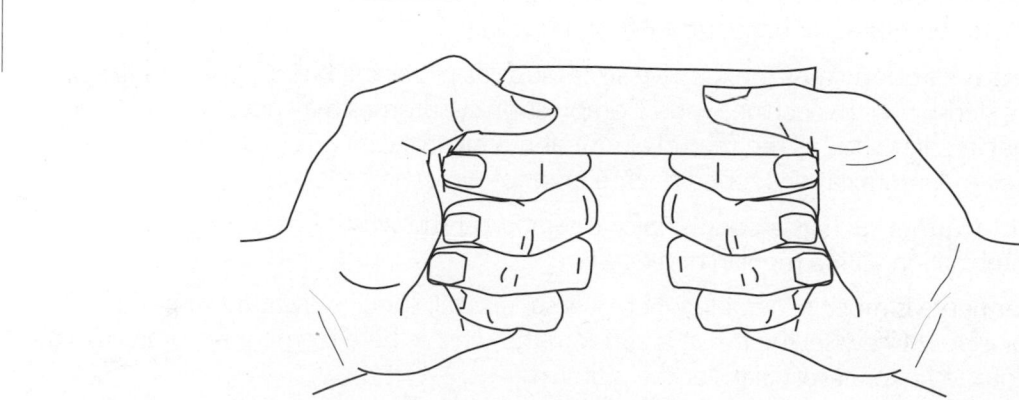

Figure 63.3
Positive Froment's sign in the left hand. Note flexion of the terminal phalanx due to the loss of adductor pollicis function and recruitment of flexor pollicus longus (innervated by the median nerve).

Sensory Dysfunction as a Result of a Lesion

♦ Altered sensation is experienced on the ulnar side of the hand, especially in the little finger and medial half of the ring finger, including the palmar and dorsal aspects of the hand. This extends from a point just above the head of the ulna to the ends of the digits.

♦ Anesthesia occurs along the little finger to the wrist (*Figure 63.4*).

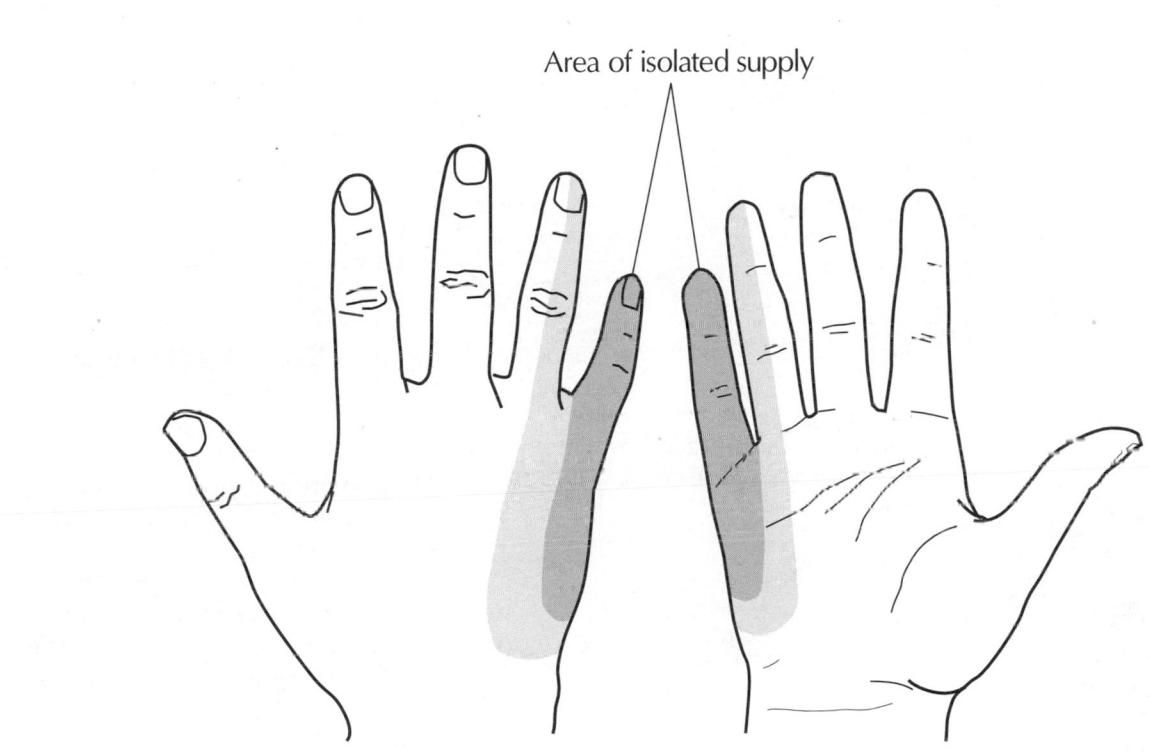

Area of isolated supply

Figure 63.4
Sensory distribution of the ulnar nerve.

Motor Dysfunction Due To a Complete Lesion

LESION SITE Note that "FUNCTIONS AFFECTED" for a specific lesion site include all the muscles involved following from that point on.	FUNCTION AFFECTED The function listed is lost unless other muscles supplied by other nerves can perform the action. In this case, the action is weak.
upper arm to elbow and forearm	**wrist flexion** (with a complete lesion, this action is only weakened)
	wrist adduction (with a complete lesion, this action is only weakened)
	flexion of the ring and little fingers at the DIP joints
wrist Note: It is common for muscles in the hand to share innervation with the median nerve *(Mumenthaler, Schliack, 1991)*	**adduction of the thumb at the MCP joint**
	opposition of the little finger (touching of the pads of the little finger with the thumb)
	flexion at the MCP joint and simultaneous extension of the IP joints of the ring and little fingers
	flexion of the MCP joint of the thumb (with a complete lesion, this action is only weakened)
	abduction of the little finger (with a complete lesion, this action is only weakened)
	abduction of index, middle and ring fingers **adduction of index to little fingers** (with a complete lesion, abduction is only weakened)

CMC: carpometacarpal
DIP: distal interphalangeal
IP: interphalangeal
MCP: metacarpophalangeal
PIP: proximal interphalangeal

MUSCLES INVOLVED	
innervated by	
Ulnar nerve	*Other nerves*
• flexor carpi ulnaris • ulnar half of flexor digitorum profundus	• palmaris longus • flexor digitorum superficialis • radial half of flexor digitorum profundus (*median nerve*) • flexor carpi radialis • abductor pollicis longus (*radial nerve*) 　The latter two muscles will also draw the wrist radially.
• flexor carpi ulnaris	• extensor carpi ulnaris (*radial nerve*)
• ulnar half of flexor digitorum profundus	
• adductor pollicis • first palmar interossei assisted by the first dorsal interossei	
• opponens digiti minimi • third and fourth lumbricals • flexor digiti minimi	
• third and fourth lumbricals • assisted by third and fourth palmar and dorsal interossei	
• flexor pollicis brevis (deep head)	• flexor pollicis brevis (*superficial head, median nerve*)
• abductor digiti minimi	• extensor digiti minimi • extensor digitorum (*radial nerve*)
• dorsal and palmar interossei	• extensor digitorum (*radial nerve*) 　This muscle assists with abduction of the digits.

If innervation is lost, the little finger is unable to move forward (the opponens digiti minimi and flexor digiti minimi are flaccid) and flex at the MCP joint while extending at the DIP and proximal interphalangeal (PIP) joints (the lumbricals are flaccid) to achieve opposition.

See also Understanding Peripheral Nerve Lesions, Strategies: Crush and Severance Injuries to Peripheral Nerves, Understanding Compression Syndromes, dislocations and fractures.

◆64◆

MEDIAN NERVE LESIONS

Linda Ludwig

The Path Travelled

The median nerve innervates primarily the flexor muscles in the forearm and hand. The most notable function of these muscles is their precise performance of hand movements, especially in the thumb and index finger.

The median nerve originates from the medial cord (comprised of fibres from spinal nerves C8 and T1) and the lateral cord (comprised of fibres from spinal nerves C5, 6, 7) of the brachial plexus *(Figure 64.1)*.

Travelling as a neurovascular bundle with the axillary-brachial artery, the median nerve follows a path down the radial aspect of the arm from the axilla to the cubital fossa. The median nerve travels with the axillary artery on its radial side and the musculocutaneous nerve and the coracobrachialis muscle on its ulnar side.

The nerve leaves the cubital fossa and runs between the heads of the pronator teres muscle. From here it penetrates deeper, lying beneath the superficial finger flexors (specifically between flexor pollicis longus and flexor digitorum profundus). In the forearm, the median nerve is well protected from a traumatic injury, though susceptible to compression by the pronator teres, flexor carpi radialis and flexor digitorum superficialis *(Rosenbaum, Ochoa, 1993)*.

Approaching the wrist, the nerve becomes more superficial and is positioned between the tendons of flexor carpi radialis (on the medial side) and palmaris longus. Before it reaches the carpal tunnel at the wrist, the median nerve gives off the palmar cutaneous branch. This branch travels superior to the carpal tunnel, turns radially and supplies sensory innervation to the skin of the thenar area.

The nerve becomes increasingly flat as it enters the carpal tunnel along with the tendons of the flexor pollicis longus, flexor digitorum superficialis and digitorum profundus muscles.

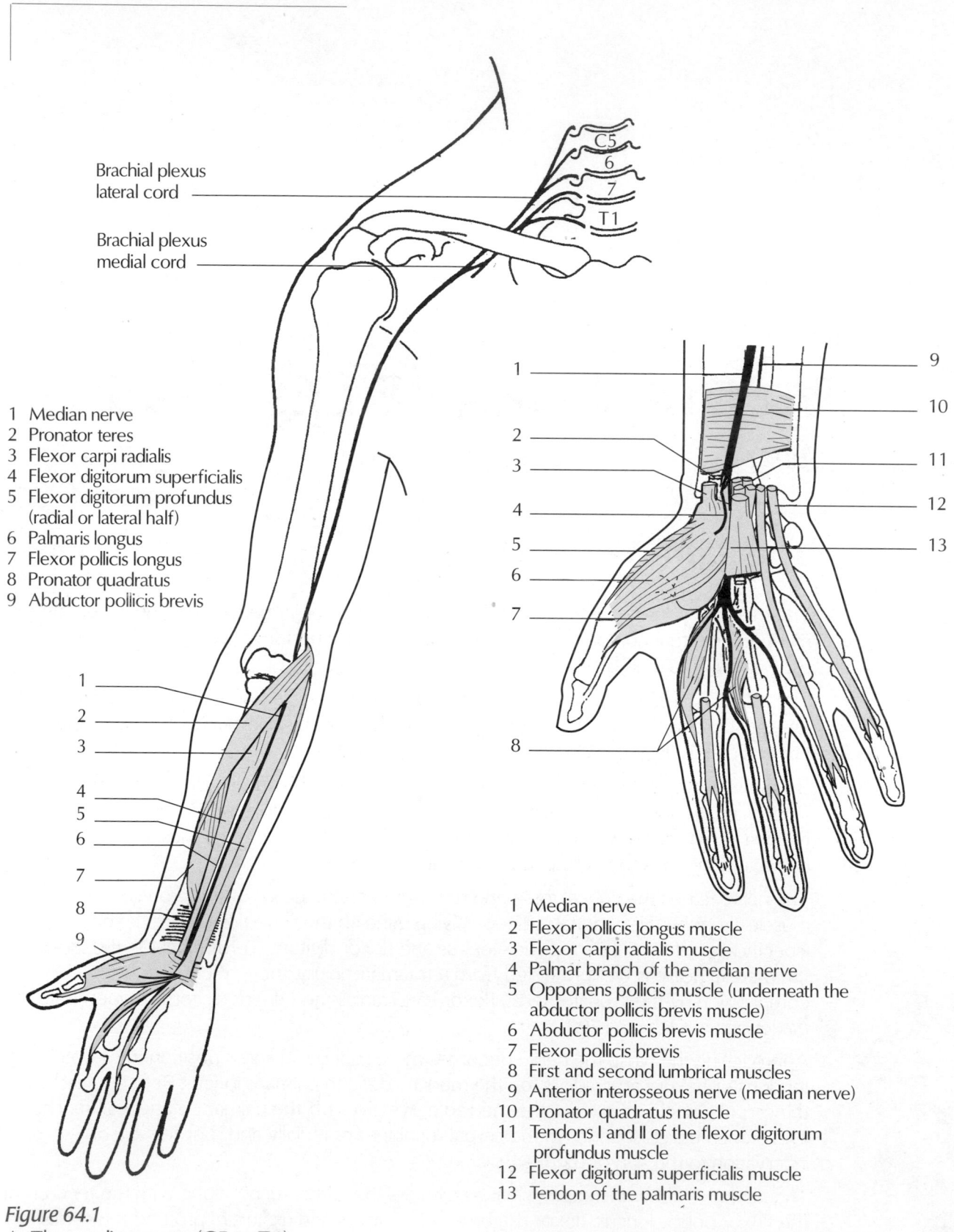

Brachial plexus
lateral cord

Brachial plexus
medial cord

C5
6
7
T1

1 Median nerve
2 Pronator teres
3 Flexor carpi radialis
4 Flexor digitorum superficialis
5 Flexor digitorum profundus
   (radial or lateral half)
6 Palmaris longus
7 Flexor pollicis longus
8 Pronator quadratus
9 Abductor pollicis brevis

1 Median nerve
2 Flexor pollicis longus muscle
3 Flexor carpi radialis muscle
4 Palmar branch of the median nerve
5 Opponens pollicis muscle (underneath the
   abductor pollicis brevis muscle)
6 Abductor pollicis brevis muscle
7 Flexor pollicis brevis
8 First and second lumbrical muscles
9 Anterior interosseous nerve (median nerve)
10 Pronator quadratus muscle
11 Tendons I and II of the flexor digitorum
   profundus muscle
12 Flexor digitorum superficialis muscle
13 Tendon of the palmaris muscle

Figure 64.1
A. The median nerve (C5 to T1).

B. Detail of the median nerve of the hand.

Upon leaving the tunnel, the median nerve passes under the palmar fascia and branches into the hand.

Muscles Innervated by the Median Nerve

✦ pronator teres

✦ flexor carpi radialis

✦ flexor digitorum superficialis

✦ flexor digitorum profundus (radial or lateral half); innervation is shared with the ulnar nerve

✦ palmaris longus — this muscle is absent in up to 20.4 per cent of the population

✦ flexor pollicis longus

✦ pronator quadratus

✦ thenar muscles:

   • abductor pollicis brevis

   • opponens pollicis

   • flexor pollicis brevis

✦ first and second lumbricals

Note: approximately one-third of the population shows some variation of innervation of muscles in the hand, such as shared or sole innervation with the ulnar nerve (*Rosenbaum, Ochoa, 1993*).

Causes of lesions of the median nerve are:

➤ **fractures** at the elbow, wrist and carpal bones. This nerve is rarely injured at the upper arm — only eight per cent of humerus fractures involve this nerve (*Mumenthaler, Schliack, 1991*);

➤ **dislocations** of the elbow, wrist or carpal bones, primarily the lunate and scaphoid;

➤ **compression** from fibrosis and hypertonicity in overused muscles or the carpal tunnel which can lead to entrapment of the nerve and, for example, **pronator teres syndrome** and **carpal tunnel syndrome.** This can result in a first degree (neuropraxia) or a second degree (axontmesis) nerve lesion;

➤ **trauma** such as a traction injury, contusion or laceration, especially at the wrist (possible with a suicide attempt) or hand.

The nerve is most easily injured where it is most superficial, at the elbow and wrist.

Symptom Picture

✦ Presentation of a complete median nerve lesion is also called **ape hand** or **oath hand** (*Figure 64.2*). Ape hand refers to the thumb lying in the same plane as the rest of the hand since there is a loss of opposition. Oath hand presentation is observed as the person attempts to make a fist. The person cannot perform this action because only the third and fourth digits can be flexed. There is a loss of thenar flexors and opponens pollicis, as well as most of the flexors of the index and middle finger.

✦ There is a flaccidity in the opponens pollicis muscle with a complete lesion. If innervation is lost, thumb opposition is severely compromised, especially medial rotation of the thumb. There is difficulty holding a pen or firmly grasping an object between the thumb and finger. True opposition is the touching of the pads of the thumb to the finger. This involves flexion and abduction with some internal rotation of the carpometacarpal joint. Using flexion of the MCP joint of the thumb, a measure of opposition can be gained by the client.

✦ The median nerve is rich in autonomic fibres; therefore, a lesion results in vasomotor and trophic changes. There is edema in the hand, fingers and thumb, nail changes (ridges) and skin changes (skin is thin, glossy, lacking lines).

✦ Depending on the location of the lesion, atrophy of the forearm flexors and thenar muscles is observed.

✦ There is a risk of causalgia with a median nerve lesion (see Understanding Peripheral Nerve Lesions).

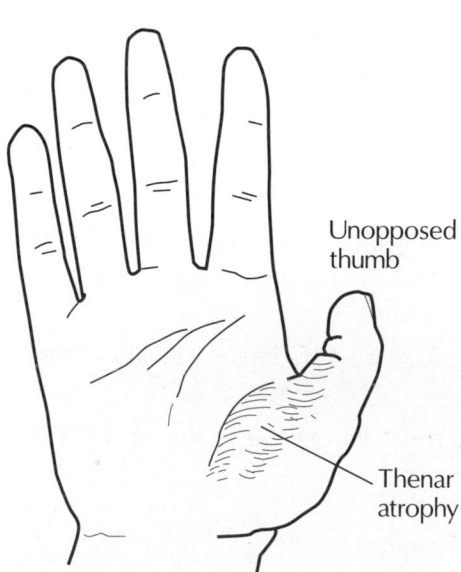

Unopposed thumb

Thenar atrophy

"Ape-hand" deformity in median nerve lesion.

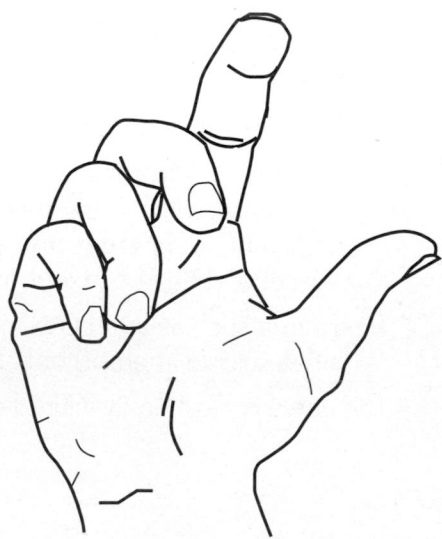

"Oath hand", when the client attempts to make a fist.

Figure 64.2
Presentation of a median nerve lesion.

Sensory Dysfunction as a Result of a Lesion

✦ Altered sensation is experienced on the thumb, index, middle and one-half of the ring finger on the flexor (palmar) surface, including the distal two-thirds of the palm. This extends from the middle to the distal phalanx on the extensor surface.

✦ Anesthesia occurs at the distal interphalangeal joint of the index and middle fingers *(Figure 64.3)*.

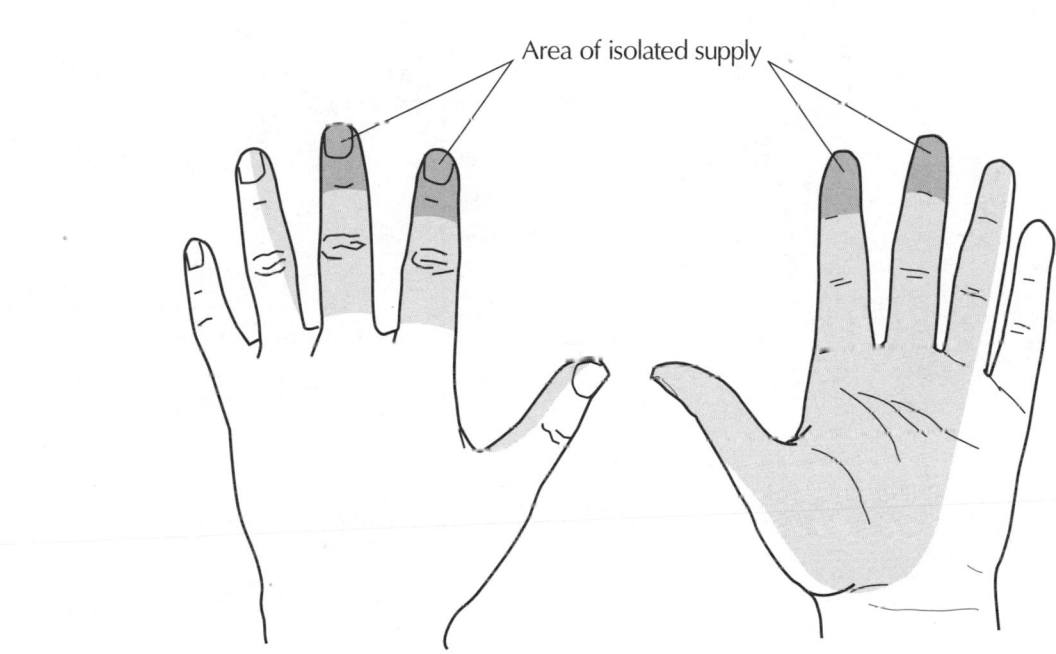

Area of isolated supply

Figure 64.3
Sensory distribution of the median nerve.

Motor Dysfunction Due To a Complete Lesion

LESION SITE Note that "FUNCTIONS AFFECTED" for a specific lesion site include all the muscles involved following from that point on.	FUNCTIONS AFFECTED The function listed is lost unless other muscles supplied by other nerves can perform the action. In this case, the action is weak.
At or proximal to the elbow and in the forearm	**pronation of the forearm**
	wrist flexion (with a complete lesion, this action is weakened)
	wrist abduction
	flexion of the thumb at the terminal phalanx
	flexion of the fingers at the DIP joints of the index and middle fingers
	flexion at the PIP joints of the index to little fingers
At the wrist or hand Note: It is common for muscles in the hand to share innervation with the ulnar nerve *(Mumenthaler, Schliack, 1991).*	**abduction of the CMC and MCP joints of the thumb** (with a complete lesion, CMC joint abduction is weakened, but MCP joint abduction is lost)
	opposition of the thumb (touching of the pads of the thumb and the little finger)
	flexion of the MCP joints and simultaneous extension of the IP joints of the index and middle fingers (with a complete lesion, flexion of the MCP joint is weakened since flexor digitorum superficialis and profundus are intact)
	flexion of the MCP joint of the thumb (with a complete lesion, this action is only weakened)

CMC: carpometacarpal
DIP: distal interphalangeal
IP: interphalangeal
MCP: metacarpophalangeal
PIP: proximal interphalangeal

MUSCLES INVOLVED		
innervated by		
Median nerve	*Other nerves*	
• pronator teres • pronator quadratus	• brachioradialis (*radial nerve*) It can perform pronation when the arm is supinated; this action will not be full pronation but only to mid-position.	*Substitute Movement Patterns: The elbow should be fixed at the client's side to eliminate the appearance of pronation from the client using internal rotation of the glenohumeral joint.*

• palmaris longus
• flexor digitorum superficialis
• radial half of flexor digitorum profundus
• flexor carpi radialis
	• flexor carpi ulnaris (*ulnar nerve*)
	• ulnar half of flexor digitorum profundus
	   Some ulnar deviation of the wrist will be apparent with the above two muscles.
	• abductor pollicis longus (*radial nerve*)
	   Some radial deviation will occur with this muscle.	

• flexor carpi radialis	• extensor carpi radialis • extensor carpi pollicis longus and brevis (*radial nerve*) Some extension of wrist will occur with abduction.	*Substitute Movement Patterns: These can be avoided when testing thumb flexion by placing the thumb in adduction just in front of the index finger on the palmar side and holding the wrist in a neutral position.*
• flexor pollicis longus		
• radial half of flexor digitorum profundus		*Substitute Movement Patterns: The fingers must be stabilized just proximal to the joint being tested to avoid substitute movements.*
• flexor digitorum superficialis • assisted by flexor digitorum profundus for index and middle fingers		
• abductor pollicis brevis	• abductor pollicis longus (*radial nerve*) • extensor pollicis brevis They assist with abduction at the CMC joint.	*Substitute Movement Patterns: Adductor pollicis (ulnar nerve) adducts the thumb and flexes the metacarpophalangeal joint so the thumb moves across the palm of the hand. Flexor pollicis brevis (ulnar nerve) flexes at the CMC and the MCP joints, moving the thumb towards the fingers. This will allow the tips of the fingers and thumb to come together.*
• opponens pollicis • assisted by flexor pollicis brevis		
• first and second lumbricals		
• flexor pollicis brevis (superficial head) • assisted by flexor pollicis longus	• flexor pollicis brevis (deep head) (*ulnar nerve*)	

See also Understanding Peripheral Nerve Lesions, Strategies: Crush and Severance Injuries to Peripheral Nerves, Understanding Compression Syndromes, edema, dislocations and fractures.

SCIATIC NERVE LESIONS

Linda Ludwig

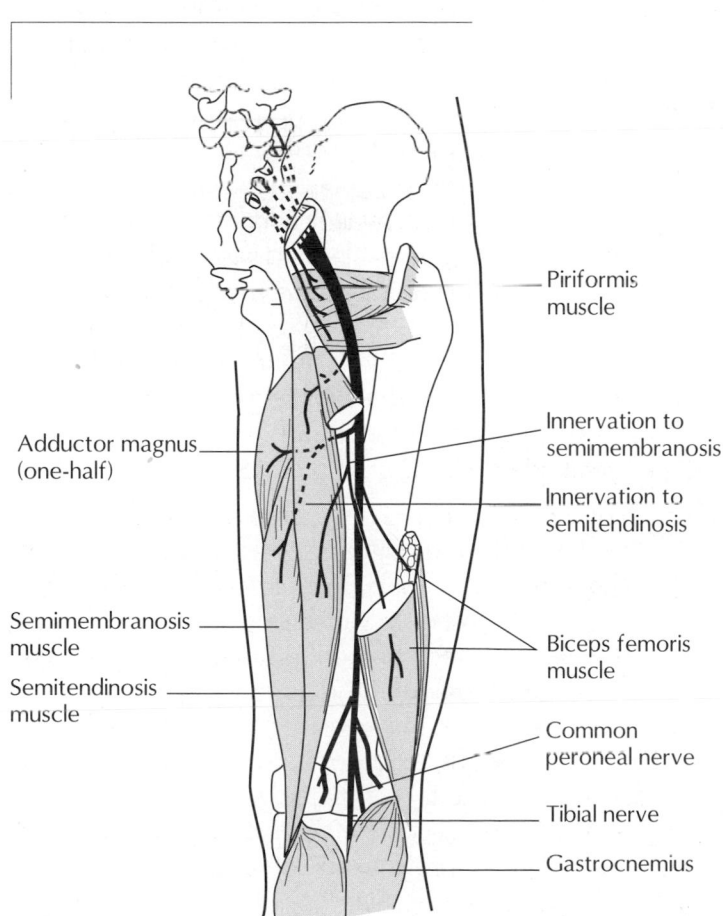

Piriformis
muscle

Innervation to
semimembranosis

Innervation to
semitendinosis

Adductor magnus
(one-half)

Semimembranosis
muscle

Semitendinosis
muscle

Biceps femoris
muscle

Common
peroneal nerve

Tibial nerve

Gastrocnemius

Figure 65.1
The sciatic nerve.

The Path Travelled

The sciatic nerve is the strongest and longest of the peripheral nerves. It primarily provides motor supply to the hamstrings, lower leg and foot, and sensory supply to the posterior leg, most of the anterior and posterior lower leg and the foot. The sciatic nerve (L4 to S1) consists of two independent nerves (the tibial and peroneal divisions) which travel together down the posterior leg as the sciatic nerve until reaching just proximal to the popliteal fossa *(Figure 65.1)*. In 10 per cent of the population, the two nerves remain distinct as they travel down the leg *(Sunderland, 1991)*.

The nerve leaves the sacral plexus, passing through the greater sciatic foramen and usually under the piriformis muscle. It travels midway to one-third of the way between the ischial tuberosity and the greater trochanter. The nerve then goes deep, following the adductor magnus down the leg.

803

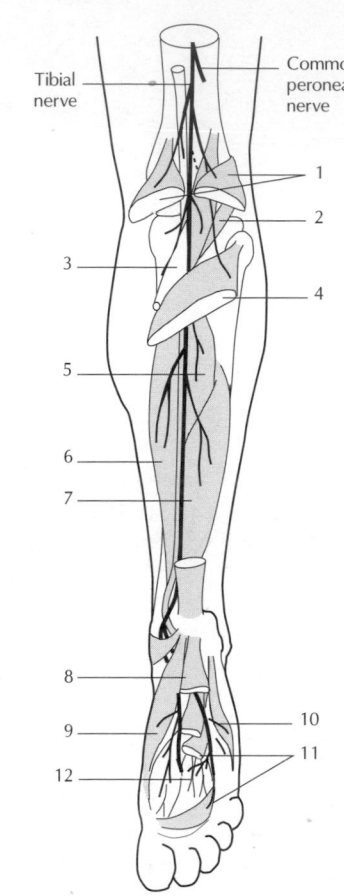

1 Gastrocnemius

2 Popliteus

3 Plantaris

4 Soleus

5 Tibialis posterior

6 Flexor digitorum longus

7 Flexor hallucis longus

8 Flexor digitorum brevis

9 Abductor hallucis

10 Abductor digiti minimi

11 Adductor hallucis

12 Lumbricals and interossei

Figure 65.2
The tibial nerve.

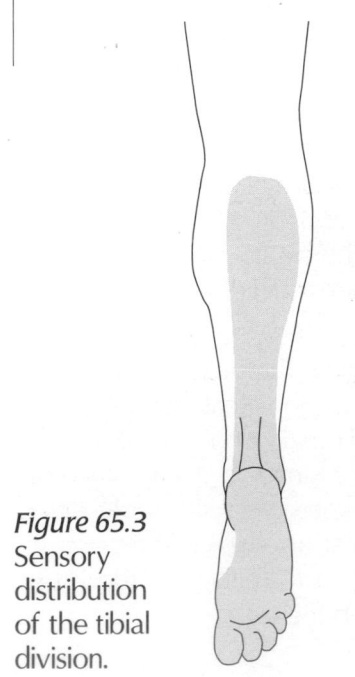

Figure 65.3
Sensory
distribution
of the tibial
division.

At the popliteal fossa, the nerve splits into two branches. The tibial nerve is the larger of the two nerves *(Figure 65.2)*. As it continues its course through the popliteal fossa, it is joined by the tibial vein and artery. They travel as a neurovascular bundle between the heads of gastrocnemius, supplying motor function to this muscle as well as to soleus, plantaris and popliteus, with branches to tibialis posterior, flexor hallucis longus and flexor digitorum longus. At the ankle, the nerve is situated superficially between the medial malleolus and the Achilles tendon. It passes around the malleolus and travels deep to the flexor retinaculum. The tibial nerve divides into the medial and lateral plantar nerves. These supply motor function to the intrinsic foot muscles such as flexor digitorum brevis, abductor hallucis, abductor digiti minimi, adductor hallucis, the lumbricales and interossei. Sensory supply is to the heel of the foot. As well, there are cutaneous branches from both the tibial nerve and the common peroneal nerve which form the sural nerve. This nerve supplies the skin of the lateral and posterior part of the inferior third of the leg and the lateral side of the foot. *(Figure 65.3)*.

The second branch of the sciatic nerve is the common peroneal nerve *(Figure 65.4)*. After passing through the popliteal fossa, it travels around and below the head of the fibula. The nerve is flattened and superficial at this point. It then splits into two divisions: the superficial and deep peroneal nerves. The deep branch travels deep to extensor digitorum longus and continues down to the malleoli, supplying motor function to the extensors of the lower leg, specifically tibialis anterior, extensor digitorum longus, extensor hallucis longus and brevis, and peroneus tertius. In the foot, the nerve is on the dorsal surface. The superficial division is found between peroneus longus and extensor digitorum longus. It provides motor supply to the peroneus longus and brevis. The superficial branch of the common peroneal nerve supplies the skin on the distal anterior surface of the leg, most of the dorsum of the foot and the toes *(Figure 65.5)*.

Muscles Innervated by the Sciatic Nerve

- ✦ hamstrings
  - semitendinosus muscle
  - semimembranosus muscle
  - long head of biceps femoris (tibial nerve)
  - short head of biceps femoris (peroneal nerve)
- ✦ one-half of adductor magnus

Tibial Division

- ✦ gastrocnemius
- ✦ plantaris
- ✦ popliteus
- ✦ soleus
- ✦ tibialis posterior
- ✦ flexor digitorum longus
- ✦ flexor hallucis longus
- ✦ intrinsic foot muscles:
  - flexor digitorum brevis
  - flexor hallucis brevis
  - abductor hallucis
  - abductor digiti minimi
  - adductor hallucis
  - lumbricals
  - interossei

Common Peroneal Division

- ✦ extensor digitorum longus
- ✦ peroneus longus
- ✦ tibialis anterior
- ✦ extensor hallucis longus
- ✦ peroneus brevis
- ✦ peroneus tertius
- ✦ extensor digitorum brevis
- ✦ extensor hallucis brevis

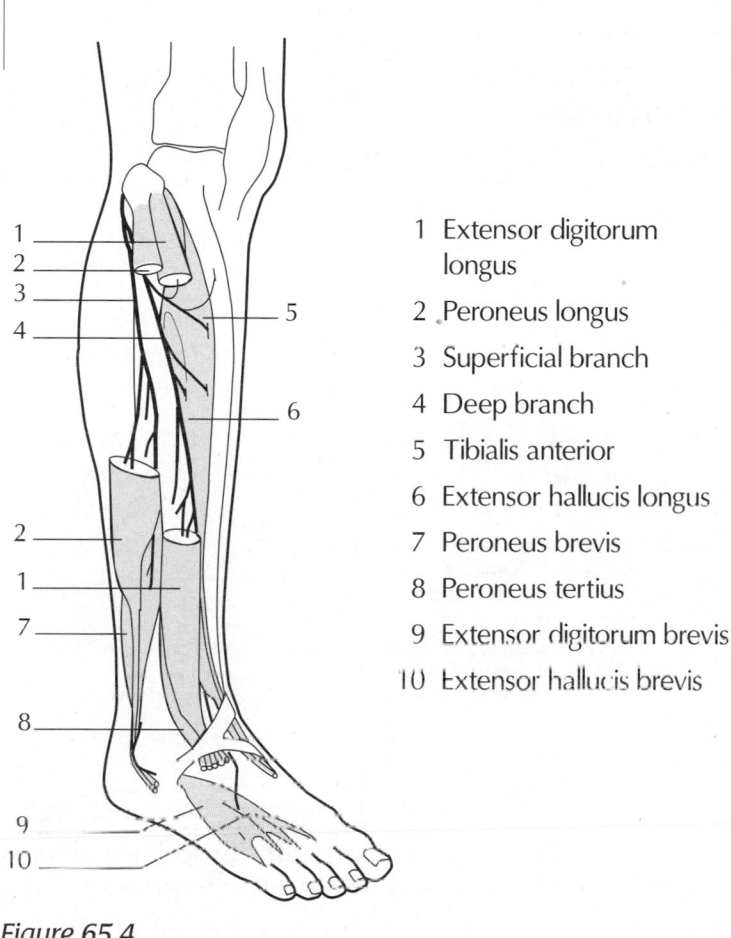

1 Extensor digitorum longus
2 Peroneus longus
3 Superficial branch
4 Deep branch
5 Tibialis anterior
6 Extensor hallucis longus
7 Peroneus brevis
8 Peroneus tertius
9 Extensor digitorum brevis
10 Extensor hallucis brevis

Figure 65.4
The common peroneal nerve.

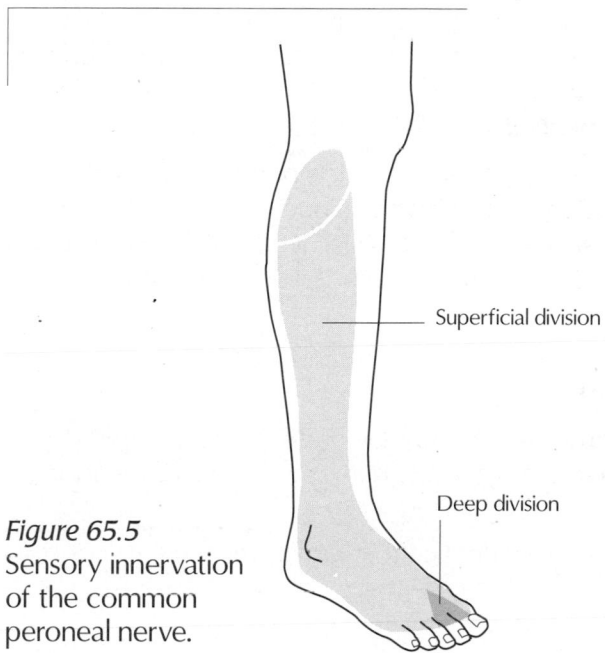

Superficial division

Deep division

Figure 65.5
Sensory innervation of the common peroneal nerve.

Causes of lesions of the sciatic nerve are:

➤ **fractures** at the pelvis, femur, tibia (tibial nerve affected) or fibular head (fibular nerve affected) or ankle (most commonly an inversion fracture);

➤ **dislocation** of the hip, knee (usually affecting the peroneal nerve) or ankle;

➤ **iatrogenic reactions** from injections in the gluteal muscles, hip surgery, meniscal repair (usually to the peroneal nerve), improper positioning during surgery or traction post-surgery;

➤ **compression from internal sources,** such as the piriformis muscle causing **piriformis syndrome** (usually the tibial division), from the flexor retinaculum in the foot leading to **tarsal tunnel syndrome,** from a ganglion or from a **Morton's foot** structure;

➤ **compression from an external source** against the fibular head; for example, a cast or splint, crossing the legs (affecting the peroneal division) or prolonged squatting which compresses the nerve under the tendon of peroneus longus. Compression injuries can result in a first degree (neuropraxia) or second degree (axonotmesis) nerve lesion;

➤ **trauma** such as a contusion in the gluteals.

Symptom Picture

✦ Presentation of a complete sciatic nerve lesion is also known as **foot drop**. Paralysis of dorsiflexors and evertors of the foot cause it to hang limply in plantar flexion and inversion. To walk, the person must lift the leg unusually high so it can be placed on the ground, toe first. This type of walk is referred to as **steppage gait** because of its resemblance to the gait of horses in some dressage movements.

✦ The loss of the intrinsic foot muscles with a tibial nerve lesion may result in **"claw toe"** deformity. This presents as a combination of hyperextension at the MCP joints — since the extensor digitorum brevis and extensor hallucis brevis are intact (common peroneal nerve) and unopposed — and flexion of the IP joints — if flexor digitorum longus (tibial nerve) is not affected by the lesion *(Mumenthaler, Schliak, 1991)*.

✦ Muscle wasting may affect the hamstrings. A common peroneal nerve lesion may cause wasting of the anterior leg between the tibia and fibula due to flaccidity of peronei, tibialis anterior and long extensors of the toes. A tibial nerve lesion may result in wasting of the posterior leg, including the foot, due to the loss of gastrocnemius, soleus and the intrinsic foot muscles.

✦ Injuries that can lead to infection and pressure sores may go unnoticed by the client as a result of sensory loss at the heel and foot.

✦ The tibial portion of the sciatic nerve carries the bulk of autonomic fibres. Lesions involving this nerve result in severe trophic changes and edema in the sole of the foot and the toes.

✦ Causalgia may occur with sciatic nerve lesions affecting the tibial division.

Differential Assessment

✍ An **L4 to L5 radicular lesion** due to a prolapsed disc results in weak inversion of the foot from a weak tibialis posterior muscle. Sensory dysfunction is experienced high on the outer aspect of the leg in the L5 dermatome. In comparison, a peroneal nerve lesion results in weak tibialis anterior, extensor hallucis longus and foot evertors, causing foot drop. Sensory dysfunction is experienced over the entire aspect of the outer lower leg and most of the dorsum of the foot.

Sensory Dysfunction as a Result of a Lesion

Tibial Division

✦ Altered sensation is experienced on the posterior leg, heel and sole of the foot including the toes (*Figure 65.3*).

Peroneal Division

✦ Altered sensation is experienced on the lateral and anterior surface of the lower leg and foot, not including the toes, as well as on the area medial to the medial malleolus and a thin strip at the edge of the foot (this area is supplied by the saphenous nerve) (*Figure 65.5*).

✦ Anesthesia is experienced on the dorsal surface of the foot, at the web space between the great toe and second digit.

Motor Dysfunction Due To a Complete Lesion

LESION SITE Note that "FUNCTIONS AFFECTED" for a specific lesion site include all the muscles involved following from that point on.	FUNCTION AFFECTED The function listed is lost unless other muscles supplied by other nerves can perform the action. In this case, the action is weak.
pelvic region, hip and posterior leg	**extension of the hip** (with a complete lesion, this action is weakened)
	adduction of the hip (with a complete lesion, this action is weakened)
	flexion of the knee (with a complete lesion, this action is weakened)
knee and distal leg	**dorsiflexion of the ankle**
	inversion of the foot (with a complete lesion of the common peroneal nerve, this action is weakened)
	eversion of the foot
	extension of the toes
	plantarflexion of the ankle
	inversion of the foot (with a complete lesion of the tibial nerve, this action is weakened)
	flexion of the toes
	intrinsic foot actions such as adduction and abduction of the toes

TMT: tarsometatarsal
DIP: distal interphalangeal
IP: interphalangeal
MTP: metatarsophalangeal
PIP: proximal interphalangeal

MUSCLES INVOLVED innervated by	
Sciatic nerve	*Other nerves*
• hamstrings	• primary hip extensor, gluteus maximus *(inferior gluteal nerve)*
• adductor magnus (shared innervation with obturator nerve)	• other adductors such as adductor longus and brevis, pectineus, gracilis *(obturator nerve)* and lower fibres of gluteus maximus *(inferior gluteal nerve)*
• hamstrings • assisted by popliteus	• sartorius *(femoral nerve)* • gracilis *(obturator nerve)* Both muscles can produce some weak flexion of the knee.
Common peroneal nerve	*Other nerves*
• tibialis anterior • extensor digitorum longus • peroneus tertius • extensor hallucis longus	
• tibialis anterior • extensor hallucis longus	• tibialis posterior • flexor hallucis longus • flexor digitorum longus *(tibial nerve)*
• the peronei • assisted by extensor digitorum longus	
• extensor digitorum longus and brevis • extensor hallucis longus and brevis	
Tibial nerve	*Other nerves*
• gastrocnemius • soleus • assisted by flexor hallucis longus and flexor digitorum longus and tibialis posterior	
• tibialis posterior • flexor hallucis longus • flexor digitorum longus	• tibialis anterior • extensor hallucis longus *(peroneal nerve)*
• flexor digitorum longus and brevis • flexor hallucis longus and brevis	
• adductor hallucis • abductor hallucis • abductor digiti minimi • interossei • lumbricals	

◄ *Some plantarflexion may accompany the action. If a complete lesion involves both divisions of the sciatic nerve, inversion of the foot is lost.*

◄ *Some dorsiflexion may accompany the action. If a complete lesion involves both divisions of the sciatic nerve, this function is lost.*

See also Understanding Peripheral Nerve Lesions, Strategies: Crush and Severance Injuries to Peripheral Nerves, Understanding Compression Syndromes, decubitus ulcers, edema, contusions, dislocations and fractures.

66

BELL'S PALSY

Linda Ludwig

Bell's palsy is a condition involving a lesion on the facial nerve (CNVII). It results in flaccid paralysis of the muscles of facial expression on the same side as the lesion.

Bell's palsy is one of the most common neurological conditions. It affects at least 25 people out of 100,000 each year *(Hopkins, 1994)*.

The facial nerve leaves the brain stem and passes through the geniculate ganglion before it separates into two divisions (*Figure 66.1*). One division is the motor nerve. It travels through the petrous canal of the temporal bone before exiting at the stylomastoid foramen. Here it travels through the parotid gland where it then gives off five branches to supply motor function to the muscles of facial expression:

+ the temporal branch to the orbital (eye) and forehead muscles except the levator palpebrae superioris, which opens the eye;

+ the zygomatic branch to the muscles of the zygoma, orbital and intraorbital area;

+ the buccal branch to the buccinator and upper lip muscles;

+ the mandibular branch to the lower lip and chin muscles;

+ the cervical branch to the platysma, stylohyoid and posterior digastric muscles.

The other division has mixed sensory and autonomic fibres. It enables taste in the anterior two-thirds of the tongue. It also controls the submandibular and sublingual salivary glands, the lacrimal glands and a small sensory area of the soft palate and around the external auditory meatus.

The cause of Bell's palsy is not entirely understood but may be:

➤ **compression from edema** and swelling from a variety of causes such as pregnancy, middle ear infection or occasionally from diabetes, hypertension, hypothyroidism,

811

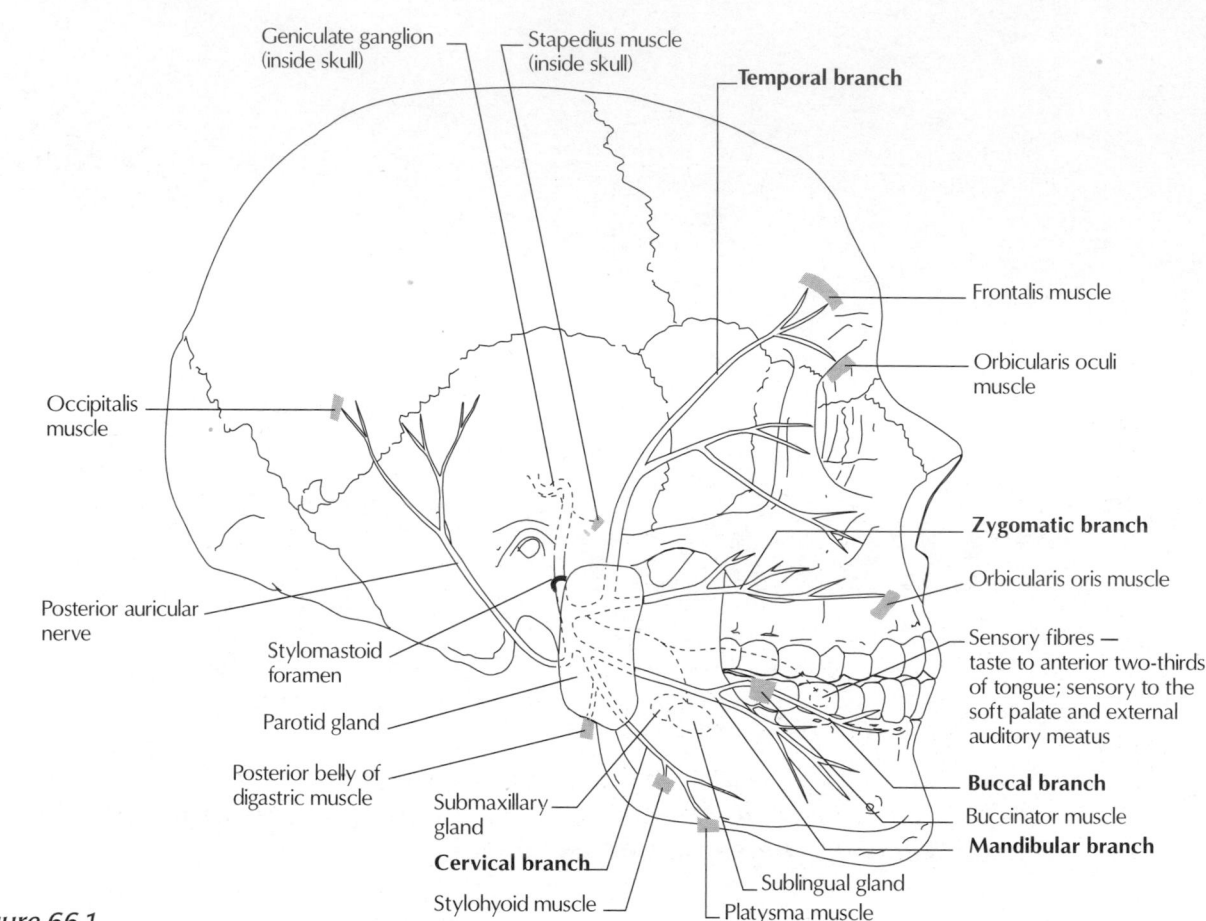

Figure 66.1
Anatomy of the facial nerve.

leprosy or a tumor. It is thought that as the nerve travels down the long, narrow canal in the temporal bone, even minor swelling could cause a compression of the facial nerve which could result in a lesion. In the case of pregnancy, 85 per cent of the women who got Bell's palsy acquired it in the third trimester. It generally resolved in the first few months postpartum. About 45 out of 100,000 pregnant women each year have this condition compared with only 17.4 out of 100,000 women who are of the same age group but not pregnant *(Aminoff, 1995)*;

➤ **conditions affecting the parotid gland**, such as inflammation due to mumps or cancer;

➤ **compression from inflammation secondary to trauma** from a blow or stab wound to the side of the head and neck as well as forceps use during birth. The mastoid process is not present at birth and is not fully developed in young children. While forceps could cause compression at birth, a child lying on a hard object or even a bony surface on his arm could contract Bell's palsy;

➤ **exposure to a chill or draft**, such as experienced while driving or from an open window while sleeping, often precedes this condition.

A **familial tendency** has not been clearly established but is a possibility. This condition can occur at any age but is more likely to strike people between 20 and 50 years of age *(Rowland, 1995)*. The onset of symptoms from weakness to flaccid paralysis is quite rapid.

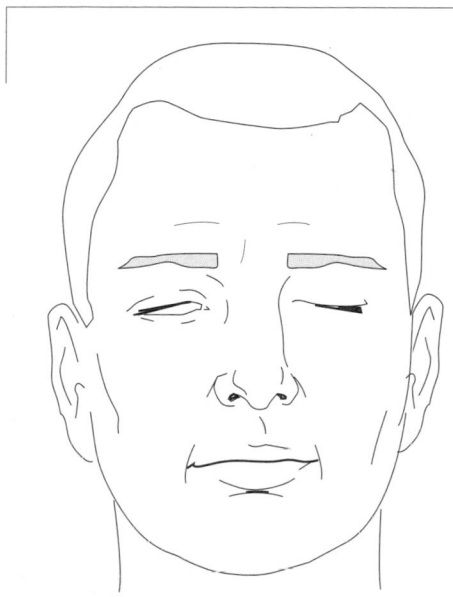

Figure 66.2
An attempt to close the right eye fails.
The eye rolls upward and inward so the
sclera is seen.

The person may go to bed without symptoms but wake up with facial paralysis affecting one side of the face.

The specific symptoms of Bell's palsy will vary depending on the lesion site. If the lesion occurs before the geniculate ganglion, all functions, including motor, sensory and autonomic, will be affected. Onset is often accompanied by pain. If the lesion is along the pathway from this ganglion to the stylomastoid foramen, motor losses are present as well as varying degrees of sensory and autonomic losses. If the lesion occurs after the facial nerve leaves the stylomastoid foramen, generally only motor function is affected. Among the most distinguishing symptoms of Bell's palsy is the eye's inability to close, because this muscle is innervated by the facial nerve (*Figure 66.2*). The muscle responsible for opening the eye is functional because it is innervated by CN III.

Some people initially fear that the paralysis of one side of their facial muscles has been caused by a stroke. In fact, a stroke generally affects the lower muscles of the face, sparing the frontalis and muscles around the eye. With Bell's palsy, all these muscles are weak or flaccid (*Hopkins, 1994*).

The success of recovery will depend on the severity of the damage to the facial nerve. If the lesion resulted from only a segmental demyelination with the axon intact, as would occur with a compression, recovery may be complete in two to eight weeks (*Pedretti, Zoltan, 1990*). If Wallerian degeneration occurred, as with a complete lesion, the prognosis is poorer.

As with any nerve regeneration, the facial nerve may regenerate but in an irregular way. For example, with motor fibres, the neuron that usually supplies the muscle that closes the eye may find its way to a muscle around the mouth. In turn, whenever the person closes the eye, there may be a twitch at the mouth. With autonomic fibres, a neuron originally supplying a salivary gland may regenerate to a lacrimal gland. When the person salivates, his lacrimal glands are also stimulated and tearing occurs. This phenomenon is called "crocodile tears" since the story goes that these reptiles weep while they eat (*Hopkins, 1994*).

Often there is no medical treatment given because spontaneous recovery can occur in up to 70 per cent of cases (*Pedretti, Zoltan, 1990*). An eye patch and antibiotic drops may be prescribed to prevent damage to, and infection of, the affected eye. There is some disagreement about the effectiveness of steroids. These are often prescribed only when there is pain with onset or if the prognosis is considered poor. Ideally, steroids are given within 24 hours of onset (*Rowland, 1981; Taber's Cyclopedic Medical Dictionary, 1981; Hopkins, 1994*). A splint may be used to relieve strain on the facial muscles. It is a prothesis consisting of a rod with a hook on each end, one to fit into the corner of the mouth and the other end to hook around the ear (*Pedretti, Zoltan, 1990*).

Massage has been found useful in maintaining circulation and tissue health on the affected side. Massage also decreases the sensation of pulling and distortion of the unaffected side (*Pedretti, Zoltan, 1990; Wale, 1980*).

Symptom Picture

✦ There is usually a rapid onset of **unilateral** weakness followed by **flaccid paralysis** of the muscles of facial expression. The person experiences:

- an inability to raise the eyebrows; the forehead cannot be wrinkled horizontally (such as with a surprised expression) or horizontally (such as with a concentrating expression);

- incomplete closure of the eye;

- the loss of the blinking reflex which results in tearing from the corner of the eye (usually blinking would move the tears into the lacrimal ducts);

- an inability to actively flare the nostrils;

- an inability to raise the corners of the mouth, to whistle or to pucker;

- difficulty with eating as food collects between the cheek and teeth;

- difficulty articulating some sounds;

- difficulty holding the lower lip to a glass to prevent dribbling.

✦ If **sensory and autonomics** are involved there is:

- a loss of control of lacrimation and usually a decrease of salivation;

- a loss of taste to the anterior two-thirds of the tongue, sometimes with the perception of an unpleasant taste;

- heightened sensitivity of hearing, especially the low tones, called "hyperacusis" *(Chusid, 1985)*, or distortion of sounds, if the fibres to the stapedius muscle in the ear are affected.

✦ There is **sagging of the face** and eyelid, with possible pulling toward the unaffected side of the face. Normal folds around the eye, nose and mouth disappear and the face takes on a smooth appearance.

✦ Attempted **facial expressions** are distorted. For example, attempts to smile result in pulling of the lower facial muscles towards the unaffected side since only the unaffected muscles can perform the action. The combined effect creates a grimace-like expression *(Figure 66.3)*. The distortion of facial expressions can have a profound emotional impact on the person. Often there is embarrassment about appearance as well as anxiety about recovery. The usual sudden onset that lacks an obvious cause is also disconcerting. The client may hold the head down and away in order to hide the face. Sometimes the hand is held over the affected side.

✦ **Pain** is usually not a primary symptom of Bell's palsy, but if pain is present with onset, it is considered a predictor of a poor prognosis for full recovery.

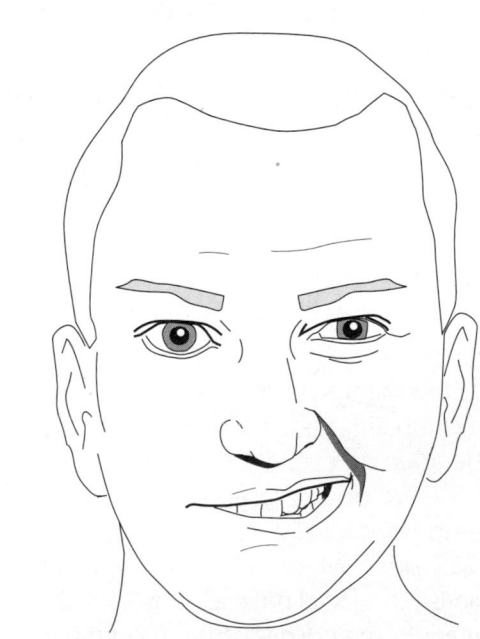

Figure 66.3
Facial expressions attempted by a person with Bell's palsy are distorted. An attempted smile results in the pulling of the lower facial muscles towards the unaffected left side.

✦ For the client, the facial muscles on the unaffected side may feel tense, with a sensation of pulling on the tissue. In severe cases with slow functional return or some permanent losses, there is the risk of contracture formation in the unopposed antagonist muscles.

Subjective Information

HEALTH HISTORY QUESTIONS

✦ Is there any history of a systemic disorder, such as diabetes mellitus, hypertension or kidney disease? Is the client pregnant?

✦ Has a physician diagnosed Bell's palsy? Is it a complete or partial lesion?

✦ What prognosis has been given?

✦ When did the symptoms begin? Does the client know what might have caused the condition? Was pain present with onset?

✦ Has any treatment been prescribed, such as an eye patch, a splint or medication?

✦ Is the physician aware the client is seeking massage? If a patch or splint is being used, has the physician given permission to remove it for treatment?

✦ What functions have been most affected?

✦ Is there sensory loss or sensory change? For example, has the amount of salivation or lacrimation (tearing) increased or decreased?

✦ Does the client experience any pain now? What type of pain is it? Where and when does it occur? Is this the result of altered posture or continuously turning the head away or down to hide the affected side?

✦ Is the client receiving any other treatment, such as physiotherapy? Can the client describe the specific treatment being received?

Objective Information

Observations

✎ There is a pulling of the face downward on the affected side. Especially noticeable are the eye and mouth which droop at the corner. The face may also show a pull towards the unaffected side; this is due to the unopposed antagonist muscles. On the affected side, the face will appear smooth because the folds at the mouth, nose and forehead are gone.

✎ The client's facial expressions appear distorted.

✎ The head may be positioned down and away, in order to hide the affected side.

Sometimes the hand is used to cover the affected side.

✍ Tearing may be seen.

✍ An eye patch or splint may be worn.

Palpation

✍ Palpation is performed with a light touch, especially over the frontal bone where the soft tissue layer is thin.

✍ Flaccidity is palpated in the affected muscles over the forehead, around the eye, nose and mouth, and in the platysma, stylohyoid and posterior belly of digastric muscles.

✍ Edema may be palpated if the condition is caused by systemic or local edema as the result of a trauma.

Contraindications

✦ There is concern about eye infection if the eye cannot close and especially if tearing is diminished.

✦ Pressure applied during massage is modified on the flaccid tissue.

✦ Long dragging strokes and fascial techniques are contraindicated on the affected side.

Testing

✍ **AF ROM testing** of facial expressions includes raising the eyebrows and bringing them together, flaring the nostrils (the client is to imagine smelling something), smiling both with the teeth showing and not showing, making an O shape with the mouth and closing the eyes. The test is positive if the client is unable to make these expressions or has difficulty.

✍ The client is asked to close the affected eye. This is positive for Bell's palsy if the client is unable to close the eye completely and the eye rolls upward and inward so the sclera is seen.

✍ **AR strength testing** of the orbicularis oculi muscle is positive.

Treatment Goals

Ensure that the fragile facial tissues are not compressed.

Treatment Plan

🖐 **Positioning** is supine to allow access to both sides of the face. The prone position is not appropriate because the fragile, flaccid tissue would be compressed. The therapist supports the head in a midline position. While the facial muscles on the unaffected side are treated, the therapist gently supports the opposite side of the head, taking care not to compress the stylomastoid foramen. As an added precaution, a folded towel is placed between the head and the therapist's hand to act as a cushion and ensure that no excessive focused pressure is applied in this area.

🖐 If excessive tearing occurs, another towel or a tissue is kept beside the client to allow the tears to be wiped away. If an eye patch is worn, it may be removed (with permission from the physician) just prior to the

Treatment Goals

Treatment Plan

treatment of the face. The eye can be subject to infection. Therefore, care is taken not to directly touch the eye. It is possible to keep just the patch over the eye, taking the strap from around the head and moving it as necessary to reach the facial muscles.

🖐 **Hydrotherapy** applications consist of cool washes on the affected tissues. Local heat may be indicated over the muscles that are shortened and that contain trigger points due to compensation, such as from turning the head towards the affected side to hide the disability. If there is any risk that the heat application will increase edema in the affected tissues, it should be avoided until some function has returned and there is less chance of compromising healing.

General Treatment

Decrease sympathetic nervous system firing. Provide emotional support.

🖐 The treatment is in the context of a relaxation massage. **Diaphragmatic breathing** is encouraged. A supportive touch is used and slow soothing strokes are applied throughout the massage.

Specific Treatment

Treat compensatory changes and holding patterns. Decrease hypertonicity and trigger points in compensatory muscles of the neck and shoulder.

🖐 Massage is performed on the **unaffected side** first. This is to accustom the client to the therapist's touch and to decrease tone in the unopposed antagonists. If the platysma is affected, care is taken not to traction it in the early stages. The anterior chest (pectoralis major and minor), the posterior neck and shoulder (the suboccipital muscles, trapezius, supraspinatus and levator scapulae) and the anterior neck (the platysma, sternocleidomastoid and scalenes) are treated. The strokes include effleurage and petrissage, such as fingertip kneading, scooping, gentle muscle stripping and pincer grasp compressions.

Reduce edema, if present.

🖐 Lymphatic drainage techniques are used. These are started by pumping at the terminus (at the clavicle) and the axilla. The usual lymphatic techniques, such as a slow stationary circles, are used. The strokes are gently directed to the terminus and axilla. They are applied on the platysma, along the jaw line, down from the zygomatic arch and laterally and inferiorly from the forehead.

🖐 The unaffected facial muscles are treated first. The pressure of the strokes is directed **towards** the lesion site — that is, towards the affected side, going from the lateral side to the midline of the face.

Maintain tissue health. Prevent contracture formation as much as possible. Decrease pain, if present.

🖐 Massage can begin at the platysma or the forehead. Techniques include fingertip kneading, compressions, stroking and vibrations. Short fascial spreading techniques are useful to prevent contractures. The strokes are applied systematically in order to address all the facial muscles.

🖐 The frontalis muscle interdigitates with the orbicularis oculi muscle. It

Treatment Goals   Treatment Plan

attaches to a large tendinous sheath, which begins approximately at the coronal suture. This sheath continues to the occipitalis muscle that attaches below and behind the superior nuchal line of the occipital area. This muscle is sometimes referred to as the occipitofrontalis *(Travell, Simons, 1983)*. Treatment includes addressing the entirety of this muscle by performing a scalp massage from the occiput to the forehead using fingertip kneading. Caution regarding pressure is necessary at the forehead because the tissue is thin and is easily compressed over the bone.

🖐 The muscles around the eyes and those from the eye going down along the nose and encircling the nostrils are addressed. The muscles around the mouth and those going from the mouth to the zygomatic arch are massaged.

🖐 The posterior digastric muscle is treated by working along the mandible to where it inserts at the mastoid. The stylohyoid muscles can be reached at the mandible near the tendon of the posterior belly of the digastric muscle *(Travell, Simons, 1983)*.

🖐 The platysma interdigitates with the orbicularis oris then travels over the mandible and the anterior neck to attach to the thoracic fascia. When the platysma and mandible are massaged, the pressure of fingertip kneading and segmental stroking is directed superiorly, towards the lesion site.

🖐 The **affected side** is addressed in the same manner except that pressure of the strokes is from midline on the face laterally **towards** the lesion site. No fascial techniques are used.

Encourage motor re-education. Maintain client awareness of the affected tissue.

🖐 Massage is followed by **passive movements** performed by the therapist. Initially, these are performed to maintain neuronal pathways as well as to prevent neglect of the affected side. The movements are those that have been compromised by Bell's palsy. The client is instructed to do a particular action, such as wrinkle his forehead by raising the eyebrows. This action will be possible on the unaffected side. The therapist creates this action on the affected side. In this example, the thumb is placed on the eyebrow and the fingers are placed at the hairline. They are then gently brought towards each other.

This is performed for all the lost actions:

• raising the affected eyebrow and bringing the eyebrows together;

• closing the eye (the therapist washes her hands before performing this action or uses a clean tissue over her hands);

• flaring out the nostril;

• smiling with the teeth showing and with the mouth closed (as with a grin);

• making an O shape with the mouth.

Treatment Goals

Maintain range of motion.

Promote whole body integration.

Treatment Plan

✋ **Gentle range of motion** is performed at the temporomandibular joint and cervical spine.

✋ The facial massage is finished with bilateral stroking in a superior and lateral direction.

✋ The therapist may choose to finish the treatment by including the rest of the body. For example, she may wish to perform full-body muscle squeezing followed by a foot massage. This brings the client's awareness to another part of his body and gives a feeling of integration.

✋ As recovery occurs on the affected side, increasingly brisk and stimulating strokes are included, such as gentle tapotement.

✋ Maintenance of neuronal pathways is no longer necessary at this stage but active assisted movements are performed to facilitate and maintain movement of the affected muscles.

Self-care Goals

Encourage relaxation.

Recommend self-massage.

Improve functional ability.

Self-care Plan

✍ Relaxation techniques, such as diaphragmatic breathing, visualization and meditation, are useful.

✍ Self-massage, using an enriched oil such as vitamin E oil, is performed for five to 10 minutes, two to three times each day.

✍ The client performs passive and then active assisted movements of the affected muscles. These initially maintain neuronal pathways and later facilitate functional movement. In the early stages, the client does the movements while lying down, to prevent gravity acting on the muscles. A mirror may be useful to the client. However, he may prefer not to observe the distorted facial expressions.

✍ The actions performed are:

* wrinkling the forehead with the eyebrows pulled upward and towards each other, closing the eye, looking up and looking down;

* flaring the nostril;

* saying vowels, and consonants such as m, n, p, b, blowing through a straw, making an O shape and whistling;

* smiling with and without the teeth showing.

Treatment Frequency and Expected Outcome

In the early stages, shorter, more frequent treatments are appropriate, such as half-hour treatments two to three times per week. Once recovery begins, treatment frequency is reduced to once a week.

See also stress reduction, peripheral nerve lesions, diabetes mellitus, hypertension and pregnancy for related conditions.

Recovery depends on the severity of the lesion. Statistics show full recovery varies from 70 to 85 per cent *(Pedretti, Zoltan, 1990; Hopkins, 1994)*. The remaining 15 to 30 per cent of people will have some residual functional loss. The amount of permanent loss varies; it is severe in two to five per cent of the cases. A poorer prognosis is predicted when the person is of advanced age, has pain with onset, has a complete lesion or has an accompanying alteration in taste and hearing *(Taber's Cyclopedic Medical Dictionary, 1981; Hopkins, 1994)*.

67

UNDERSTANDING COMPRESSION SYNDROMES OF PERIPHERAL NERVES

Linda Ludwig

> *Compression or entrapment injuries, also known as neuropraxia, cause a local conduction block in a peripheral nerve, but with no structural damage to the axon or to tissue distal to the lesion.*

Compression of peripheral nerves can be the result of external or internal forces which impair oxygenation and local neural conduction. Blood vessels within the nerve, as well as those travelling alongside the nerve (called a "neurovascular bundle"), may be compressed along with the nerve.

There are several common compression syndromes. Entrapment syndromes that affect the arm and hand involve compression of the brachial plexus. Potential areas of compression include structures in the neck, shoulder girdle, elbow, forearm and wrist. The most studied and accepted is carpal tunnel syndrome where the median nerve is compressed as it passes through the carpal tunnel at the wrist.

Another syndrome that affects the hand but is more controversial is thoracic outlet syndrome. This syndrome is a broad term encompassing a number of possible compression sites. It could result from compression of the brachial plexus and accompanying vasculature by the anterior scalene muscle, known as anterior scalene syndrome, by the pectoralis minor muscle, known as pectoralis minor syndrome, and by the first rib and clavicle, called costoclavicular syndrome.

In the lower limbs, piriformis syndrome, often referred to as sciatica, describes compression of the sciatic nerve as it passes under or through the piriformis muscle.

Many of these entrapment syndromes seem to be on the rise as people spend longer periods sitting at computers.

Causes of peripheral nerve compression are:

➤ **external forces** such as pressure from casting, crutches, splints, a tourniquet or backpack straps;

➤ **internal forces** which include:

- **hypertonic muscles** that compress the nerve against another structure such as bone or muscle; this can be due to trigger points or postural imbalances. If the nerve penetrates the muscle, it is especially susceptible to compression;

- **structural abnormalities** such as a cervical rib or a poorly developed bony callus at a fracture site;

- **trauma and overuse** that lead to edema and scar tissue which compress the nerve;

- **poor positioning of the limb** while sleeping or during surgery which causes the nerve to be compressed between two structures;

- **systemic conditions** such as pregnancy, hypothyroidism, diabetes mellitus and rheumatoid arthritis, which cause systemic edema.

Symptom Picture

✦ The symptoms likely to occur with nerve entrapment are numbness, tingling, pain and weakness in the affected limb. These are due to a combination of ischemia of the nerve, which impairs the microcirculation within the nerve *(Figure 67.1)*, as well as the local mechanical force of the compression. This is not the same as axon damage and Wallerian degeneration typical of crush (axonotmesis) and severance (neurotmesis) lesions.

✦ When an entrapment occurs, the nerve trunk responds to the trauma as would any

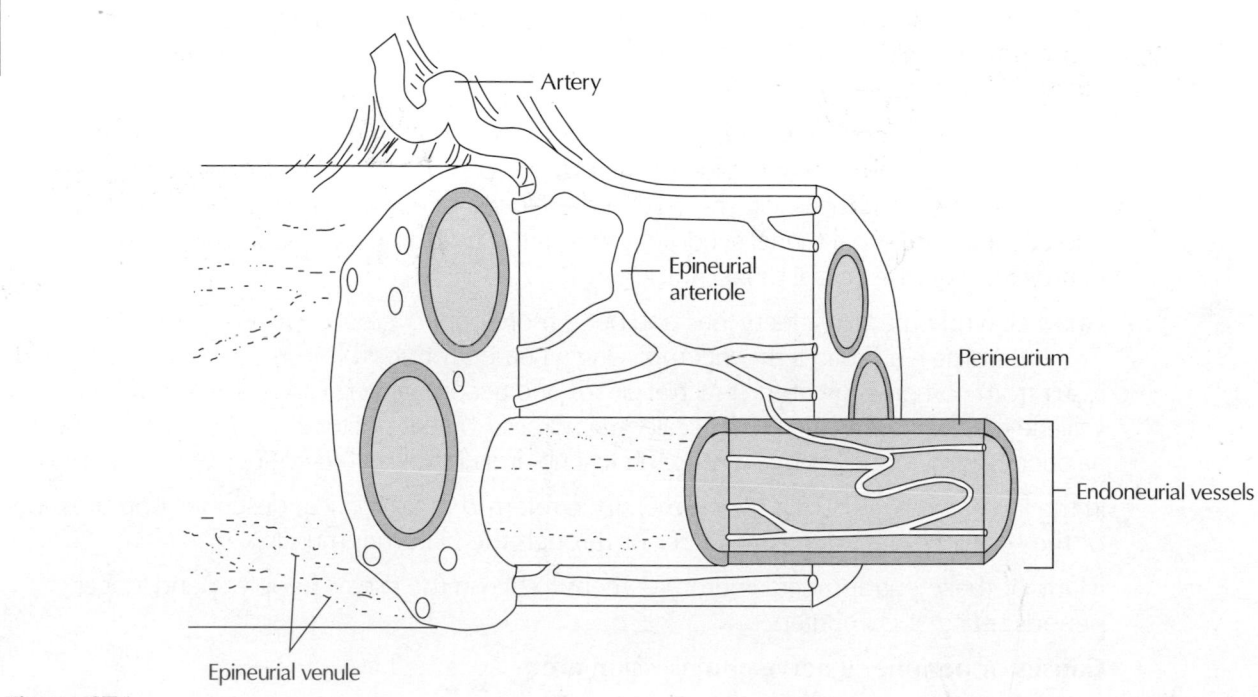

Figure 67.1
Peripheral nerve microcirculation.

other tissue in the body, with an **inflammatory response**. The subsequent increase in vascular permeability and local edema contributes to **impaired nerve transmission**. A common example is when a foot or hand "falls asleep". At first there is numbness and tingling in the hand or foot, followed by anesthesia and paralysis. The compression impairs oxygenation and local neural conduction. When the pressure is released, normal sensation and muscle power return, usually within a few minutes. Intraneural microcirculation is restored to the previously compressed area and conduction recovers. The dysfunction is rapidly reversible.

✦ The longer the disruption of microcirculation, the longer the recovery period. This is due in part to the development of **intraneural edema** during a prolonged compression. Since there are no lymphatic capillaries within the nerve itself to disperse fluid, the edema is difficult to resolve *(Lundborg, 1988)*. In cases where edema develops, the edema is accompanied by mechanical deformation of the nerve fibres and blood vessels. Local myelin is displaced lateral to the compressive force. With such conduction blocks, it may take days, weeks or months for the edema to reduce and the myelin to repair. The more severe the compression, the more extensive the tissue damage to the nerve trunk, with an increasingly poor prognosis. The severity of the lesion is a result of the magnitude and duration of the compression.

✦ The **extent of damage** is also influenced by:

- the structure of the nerve and its location and size within the endoneurium. Because there are varying amounts of protective endoneurium surrounding the fascicles, less endoneurium presents an increased risk of damage;

- fibre size and fascicle location within the endoneurium. Compression lesions often result in a relative sparing of sensation as compared to motor function. This may be explained by the fact that compression affects the large myelinated fibres rather than the small unmyelinated fibres. In addition, a superficial motor fascicle located immediately under a sharp fascial edge will often suffer more injury than deeper, better protected motor or sensory fascicles. Because of these factors, varying amounts of damage will usually occur among a group of fibres in a nerve trunk.

✦ **Recovery time** varies after the compression is relieved. In one case of "Saturday night palsy", where the person was unconscious from alcohol intoxication, recovery of nerve function began in three weeks and was complete in six weeks. In contrast, a compression that was the result of a tourniquet affected the radial, median and ulnar nerves; the first signs of recovery appeared at 10 weeks, with only 50 per cent recovery after four months *(Lundborg, 1988)*.

See also carpal tunnel syndrome, thoracic outlet syndrome — which includes anterior scalene syndrome, pectoralis minor syndrome and costoclavicular syndrome — piriformis syndrome, pregnancy and postural dysfunctions.

✦ The key to treatment is **relief of the compression** on the nerve. Medical treatment is often necessary for a compression that results from systemic conditions or structural anomalies. Massage therapy goes a long way to successfully treat neuropraxia caused by muscle hypertonicity and poor posture. Swedish techniques, trigger point therapy and fascial techniques can relieve the nerve compression. Long-term relief requires client compliance with changes in posture while working, and participating in a stretch and strengthening program.

68

THORACIC OUTLET SYNDROME

Linda Ludwig

Thoracic outlet syndrome (TOS) is a condition that involves the compression of the brachial plexus and its accompanying artery between the anterior and middle scalene muscles (anterior scalene syndrome) or between the coracoid process and the pectoralis minor muscle (pectoralis minor syndrome) or between the clavicle and the first rib (costoclavicular syndrome).

From as early as the 1700s, descriptions can be found of the compression of the thoracic outlet due to a cervical rib. In 1927, Adson and Coffey surgically divided the scalene muscle to relieve compression with anterior scalene syndrome. The costoclavicular region was determined to be a source of compression of the brachial plexus by Falconer and Wenda in 1943. Wright (1945), put forward the pectoralis minor muscle, primarily in hyperabduction, as a cause of thoracic outlet syndrome *(Pecina et al., 1991)*. The compression may be at one or all of these points. This causes numbness and tingling of the fourth and fifth digits and on the ulnar side of the hand and forearm.

In the 1940s, carpal tunnel syndrome (CTS) was named and came to the forefront because of a specific test developed by Phalen in 1954. It was found that many people thought to have thoracic outlet syndrome actually had CTS. In fact, carpal tunnel syndrome is considered the most common of the nerve compression syndromes.

Thoracic outlet syndrome has become somewhat controversial with respect to its etiology and diagnosis. Some sources go so far as to suggest it may not be a true nerve compression syndrome but only a vascular compression *(Szabo, 1989)*. This opinion is due to what some consider often vague symptoms in the arm as well as the difficulty in obtaining objective nerve conduction results *(Dawson et al., 1990)*. Nerve conduction testing is often negative for a nerve lesion because it requires expertise to measure conduction of the ulnar nerve across the thoracic outlet *(Dawson et al., 1990)*.

Unfortunately, this controversy can lead to an overdiagnosis of CTS. In fact, other sources stress that TOS does exist as a nerve compression syndrome, particularly given that numbness and tingling of the lower root of the plexus are often symptoms. Travell, among others, points out that trigger points in the primary muscles involved, especially the scalenes, contribute to muscle hypertonicity which is an important cause of compression of the brachial plexus (Travell, Simons, 1983; Pecina et al., 1991). It may be that the vague symptoms result from the combination of nerve paresthesia from C8, T1 and trigger point referrals.

Surgical examination has demonstrated compression of the brachial plexus by a variety of sources, including soft tissue and osseous structures. It is suggested that diagnosing TOS be a process of eliminating other likely compression syndromes, such as CTS and ulnar compression at the elbow, as these nerve lesions show up more readily with conduction testing (Szabo, 1989).

The brachial plexus is composed of nerve roots C5 to C8 and T1 and provides innervation to the entire upper limb. It travels with the subclavian artery between the anterior and medial scalenes (the intrascalene space). After being joined by the subclavian vein, this neurovascular bundle goes below the clavicle (the costoclavicular space) and travels under the pectoralis minor insertion (the sub-pectoral space) before continuing down the arm.

The condition begins insidiously and progresses slowly.

Causes of the syndrome include:

➤ **internal** (bony callus, cervical rib) or **external** compression (crutches);

➤ **prolonged poor positioning**;

➤ **poor posture**, such as hyperkyphosis and scoliosis, muscle hypertonicity and trigger points;

➤ **systemic immune or metabolic disorders**, such as rheumatoid arthritis, diabetes and hypothyroidism;

➤ **trauma** with inflammation and subsequent scarring as with, for example, whiplash;

➤ **joint subluxation** of the cervical spine;

➤ **pregnancy**, which causes a combination of increased fluid retention and postural changes.

The syndrome causes neuropraxia, which is the loss of conduction at the compression point, with no axonal degeneration (Travell, Simons, 1983). Symptoms of the nerve compression include localized pain, sensory loss and motor weakness (paresis). Vascular compression results in trophic changes in the tissue.

To develop an effective treatment plan, it is essential to accurately identify the location of the compression. A variety of orthopedic tests are used. These tests narrow the space of potential compression sites, enhance the pressure there and then cause an increase in symptoms or a diminishment of the radial pulse at the wrist. These are easy for the massage therapist to perform. However, these tests can yield false positive results. They form only one part of the assessment. It is important that testing be performed in combination with assessment of health history, observation and palpation in order to gain a clearer determination of the client's condition. In some cases, the neurovascular bundle is compressed in more than one location. This situation is referred to as a "double crush syndrome". In one study of 60 cases of shoulder girdle compression, 25 per cent of cases also had a carpal tunnel compression *(Mumenthaler, Schliack, 1991)*.

The Cervical Rib

Some people have an additional rib that forms at C7. This results in symptoms of TOS in about half of those with a cervical rib *(Mumenthaler, Schliack, 1991)*. The transverse process (TVP) is often as broad as T1 and the cervical rib then reaches beyond the C7 transverse process *(Figure 68.1)*. The cervical rib may only be a small cartilaginous projection or may be as long as the first rib. Variations of this rib can include a full cervical rib, with cartilage or with a distinct fibrous band instead of cartilage that connects the rib to the first thoracic rib *(Travell, Simons, 1983)*. It often comes just behind the lateral margin of the tendon of the anterior scalene muscle, frequently on the prominence of the first rib. This narrows the interscalene triangle from below, resulting in the vascular bundle being more or less strung over the cervical rib under tension. This contributes to compression of the bundle, with symptoms varying, depending on the amount of the compression. Such ribs are identified by X-ray and through palpation, at the level of the clavicle, as a bulge in the space between the anterior and middle scalenes.

Anterior Scalene Syndrome

Anatomy

The intrascalene triangle consists anteriorly of the **anterior scalene muscle**, which attaches proximally to the anterior transverse processes of cervical vertebrae three through six and distally to the scalene tubercle on the inner border of the first rib. Posteriorly, it consists of the **middle scalene muscle**, the largest scalene, which attaches proximally to the posterior transverse process of C2 to C7 and distally to the first rib *(Figure 68.2)*. Inferiorly, the first rib forms the base of the triangle. The brachial plexus and the subclavian artery pass through this space *(Mumenthaler, Schliack, 1991)*. At this level, the subclavian vein passes anteriorly to the anterior scalene muscle and is not affected by compression.

A narrowing of the triangle through changes in the muscles or rib, or through space-occupying structures,

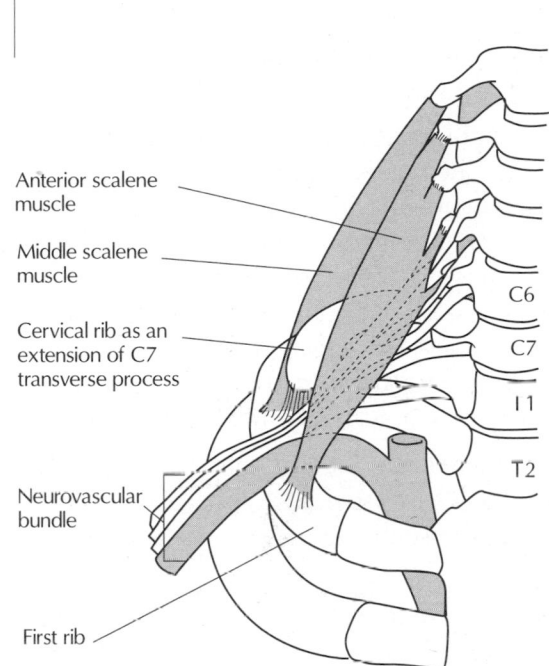

Figure 68.1
The presence of a cervical rib narrows the interscalene triangle.

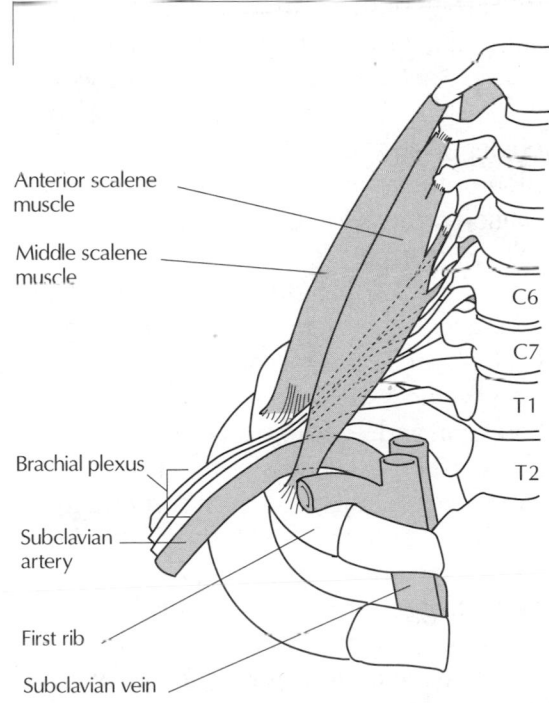

Figure 68.2
Anterior scalene syndrome: Compression of the brachial plexus and subclavian artery by the scalene muscles.

often results in symptoms of compression of the nerves — specifically, the brachial plexus — or of the blood vessels — namely, the subclavian artery *(Szabo, 1989)*.

The medial cord of the plexus is most vulnerable to compression since it lies in an inferior position passing through the triangle *(Szabo, 1989)*. The person experiences predominantly ulnar nerve symptoms because C8 and T1 make up this cord. **Scalene trigger points** will cause pain in the lower lateral neck radiating to the lateral shoulder and arm (over the biceps and triceps), over the upper chest as well as to the medial scapular border. The referral bypasses the elbow and continues down the lateral forearm, thumb and index finger *(Travell, Simons, 1983)*. The trigger points are activated by heavy lifting and carrying as well as through overuse of the respiratory muscles caused by paradoxical breathing or extreme coughing from bronchitis, pneumonia, asthma and emphysema.

➤ **Specific causes of anterior scalene syndrome are** hypertonicity and trigger points in the anterior or middle scalene, or anatomical anomalies such as a cervical rib, a wide C7 TVP or an extra-wide insertion of the anterior scalene. In addition, the general causes of TOS can bring on this condition.

Costoclavicular Syndrome

Anatomy

Costoclavicular syndrome differs from anterior scalene syndrome in that vascular compression plays a larger role *(Pecina et al., 1991; Turner et al., 1990)*. The neurovascular bundle, including both the axillary-subclavian artery and vein, travels through a space created by the clavicle anteriorly and first rib posteriorly. The size of the space is variable, dependent on the shoulder position or anatomical anomalies. Abduction of the arm, retraction of the scapula and elevation of the first rib with inspiration (especially with apical breathing) will lead to narrowing of the space. **Subclavius** inserts on the inferior surface of the lateral clavicle and on the medial first rib and its costal cartilage (*Figure 68.3*). A hypertonic subclavius muscle contributes to compression and leads to fixation of the clavicle. In addition, weakness of the trapezius and levator scapula, muscles which suspend the shoulder, causes drooping of the shoulder, with the clavicle resting on the first rib *(Szabo, 1989)*. **Subclavian trigger points** refer to the lateral arm, bypassing the elbow and wrist, then continuing down the lateral dorsal and palmar sides of the hand as well as into the thumb and index and middle fingers.

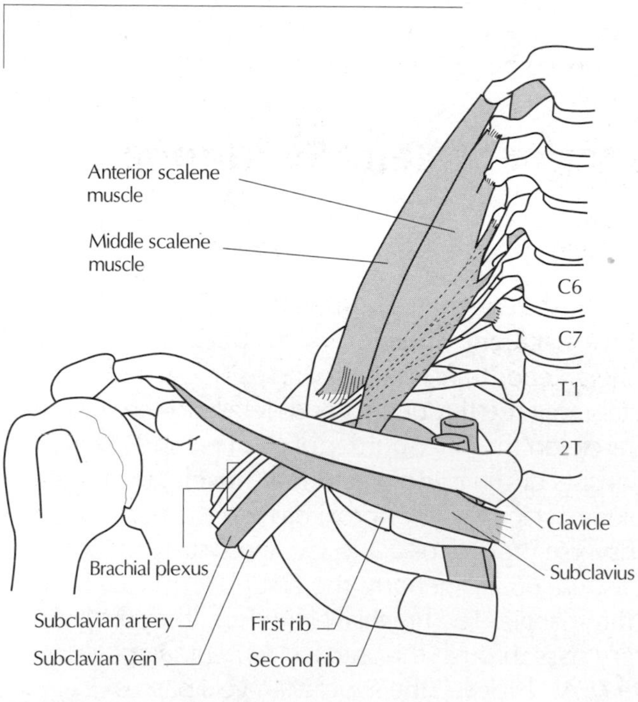

The symptoms of this syndrome are similar to anterior scalene syndrome, which are numbness, tingling and weakness in the fourth and fifth digits

Figure 68.3
Subclavius inserts on the inferior surface of the clavicle. If it is hypertonic, it can contribute to brachial plexus compression.

(Omer, Spinner, 1980). An additional symptom is venous congestion due to impaired venous return because of the compression of the subclavian vein; this leads to temporary or chronic edema *(Pecina et al., 1991).*

➤ **Specific causes of costoclavicular syndrome are** conditions specifically affecting the clavicle and first rib, such as a fracture (particularly if it was poorly set), a marked bony callus, drooping shoulders as are often found in elderly persons, chronic respiratory pathologies such as emphysema, osteoarthritis, carrying a heavy or hard object on the shoulder and hypertrophy and trigger points in the subclavius muscle.

Pectoralis Minor Syndrome

Pectoralis minor syndrome is frequently referred to as **hyperabduction syndrome** because symptoms occur with the raising of the arm into hyperabduction and external rotation.

Anatomy

The sub-pectoral space is formed by the clavicle and the pectoralis minor muscle at its insertion at the coracoid process (the distal attachment is the third, fourth and fifth ribs near the costal cartilages). At this level, the brachial plexus continues to travel with the axillary artery and vein; as the subclavian artery and vein enter the axillary fossa, their names change to axillary artery and vein. The neurovascular bundle enters the axilla under the pectoralis minor muscle. When the arm is extended and maximally abducted (to 180 degrees), the bundle is stretched around, and compressed between, the pectoralis minor tendon and the coracoid process as well as between the clavicle and first rib *(Figure 68.4).*

Pectoralis minor trigger points refer pain primarily over the anterior deltoid muscle, over the pectoral area and possibly to the subclavicular area on the same side. Some pain can extend down the medial side of the arm, to the palm and third to fifth digits.

Symptoms for this syndrome may include those of an entire brachial plexus compression. They usually begin as numbness and tingling in the fingers and progress to the hand. There is also venous compromise resulting in ischemia and edema in the hand. Wright suggests that Raynaud's-disease-like symptoms can appear in over one-third of the people with pectoralis minor syndrome *(Pecina et al., 1991).*

➤ **Specific causes of pectoralis minor syndrome are** primarily positional, especially the arm elevated over the head for a prolonged period during specific activities. This position can be active and repetitive, such as when painting a ceiling or playing an instrument such as a violin or flute. On the other hand, it can be a passive position held for a long time, as in sleeping with the arm above the head, sitting and hanging the arm over a chair back or poor positioning during surgery. Other causes are shoulder dislocation, trauma such as a rib fracture and compression from a backpack or from using a crutch.

Treatment to relieve any of these compressions is recommended for six months to a year, including massage, exercises and activity modification *(Mumenthaler, Schliack, 1991; Szabo, 1989; Dawson et al., 1990; Samii, 1990).* If symptoms persist or if there is evidence of circulatory compromise, surgery may be performed. Resection of a cervical rib, scalenotomy and resection of the clavicle, first rib or scalenes insertion are possible surgical procedures. Success rates vary, with the poorest results relating to surgical correction of the wrong compression site *(Mumenthaler, Schliack, 1991).*

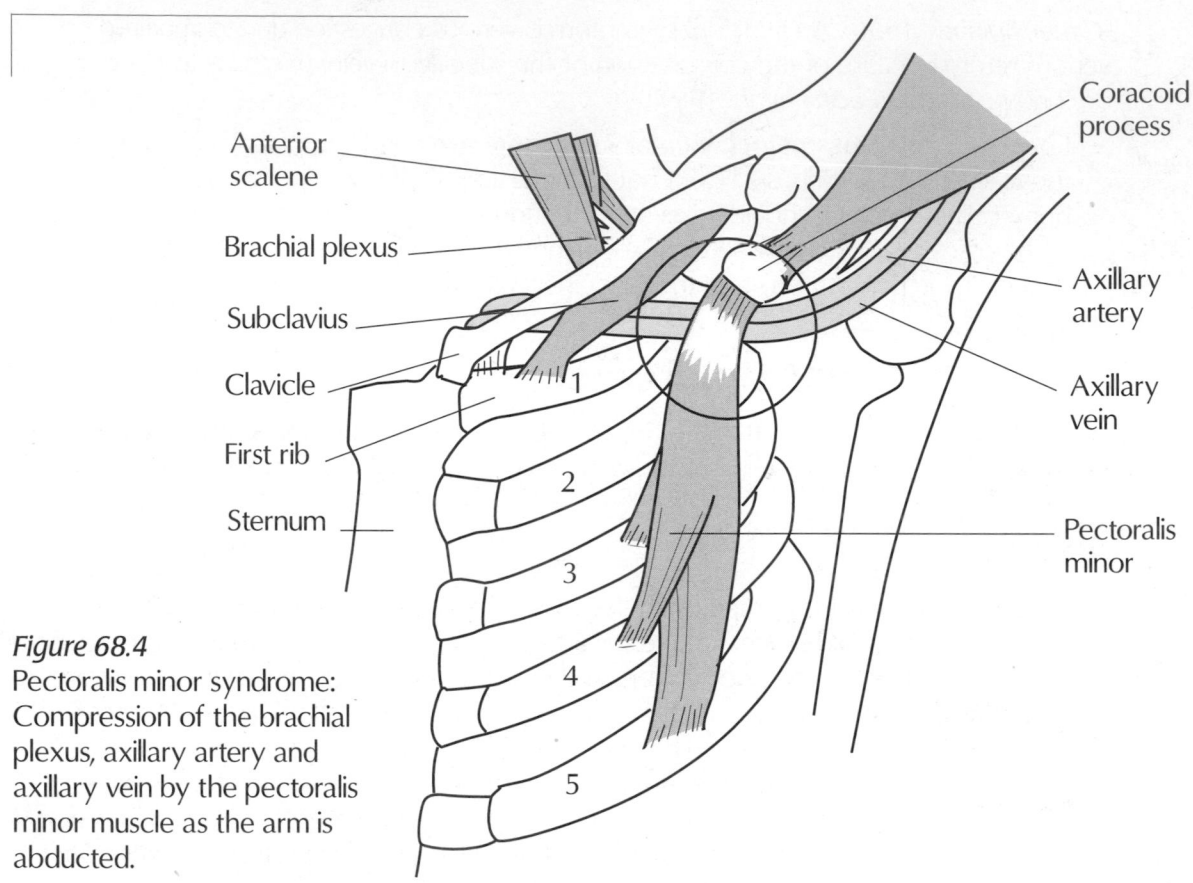

Figure 68.4
Pectoralis minor syndrome:
Compression of the brachial
plexus, axillary artery and
axillary vein by the pectoralis
minor muscle as the arm is
abducted.

Symptom Picture

✦ Symptoms can be unilateral or bilateral. There may be primarily a neurological compression (of the brachial plexus) or a vascular compression (of the subclavian artery and vein and the lymphatic vessel) or a combination of both.

With a Neuronal Compression

✦ Paresthesia and hyperesthesia such as numbness and tingling are primarily on the ulnar side of the hand, especially in the fingers and possibly the forearm *(Turner et al., 1990)* in the C8 to T1 distribution. These lower roots are most susceptible to compression due to their position going through the intrascalene triangle. The altered sensation can spread to the entire hand. A permanent sensory deficit may result if the compression goes untreated.

✦ Sensory symptoms often begin with paresthesia. Pain develops subsequently *(Dawson et al., 1990)*.

• Diffuse, aching or throbbing pain is experienced in the upper limb, predominantly the shoulder, and in the forearm and hand. Less frequently, pain may occur in the neck or chest or as a headache on the side of the head *(Szabo, 1989)*.

- Trigger points are usually present and refer down the arm from the scalenes, pectoralis minor and subclavius. This referral will overlap with the brachial plexus symptoms. Trigger points in latissimus dorsi, serratus anterior and posterior superior can mimic TOS pain patterns.

- Pain is triggered or increased by letting the arm hang down, carrying or lifting heavy objects or raising the arm above the head *(Mumenthaler, Schliack, 1991)* and relieved by lying down.

✦ Gradually, there is increasing motor weakness of the hand and a disturbance of fine motor skills. Clumsiness and a weakened grip result from the compression of C8 and T1 nerve roots, which specifically affect the intrinsic hand muscles. Atrophy is evident in the hypothenar and interossei muscles, with the thenar muscles affected occasionally *(Mumenthaler, Schliack, 1991)*.

With a Primary Vascular Compression

✦ Ischemic changes and compromised circulation cause pain and pallor, possible cyanosis and a sense of coldness in the limb, and blood vessel distention *(Turner et al., 1990)*. Vascular compression may present similar to Raynaud's phenomenon with intermittent ischemic crisis *(Pecina et al., 1991)*. In severe cases, symptoms progress to the development of painful emboli or gangrene in the fingertips as well as trophic changes in the nails and skin.

✦ Compression of the subclavian vein and the subclavian trunk, a lymphatic vessel that travels with it, can result in edema in the hand, especially the dorsal surface. Clients may report stiffness and puffiness on waking *(Travell, Simons, 1983)*.

Subjective Information

HEALTH HISTORY QUESTIONS

✦ Is there a history of a systemic disorder, such as diabetes, rheumatoid arthritis or hypothyroidism? Is the client pregnant?

✦ Does the client have any respiratory conditions, such as bronchitis or asthma?

✦ What parallel therapies, such as physiotherapy or chiropractic treatment, has the client undertaken?

✦ Has the client seen a physician for diagnosis? What tests were performed to determine the diagnosis?

✦ Does the client have a cervical rib? Was it diagnosed by X-ray?

✦ What treatment was prescribed?

✦ Is the client currently taking any medication? Have corticosteroid injections been given? Has an injection been given in the last 10 days?

- How long has the client been experiencing discomfort?

- Can the client describe the sensation? "Numbness and tingling" and "my hand is asleep" are common responses.

- Where does the client experience pain or altered sensation? What is the quality of the pain? How intense is the pain or sensation? How frequent is it?

- What activities or positions aggravate the symptoms? What activities or positions relieve the symptoms?

- Has there been a history of injury to the glenohumeral joint, clavicle or cervical spine?

- Postural questions: What is the client's sleeping position? For example, is the arm above the head, which creates traction and pressure at the pectoralis minor? Are there numerous pillows under the head and shoulders when sleeping supine? Is the head supported in a laterally flexed position when sidelying? Both the latter positions promote shortening of the scalenes.

- What are the client's postural habits, including occupational and recreational sources of stress? Does the client carry a backpack or purse that may compress the pectoralis minor muscle?

Objective Information

Observations

- A postural assessment is performed, observing for drooping shoulders in the anterior or posterior view, head-forward position and hyperkyphosis in the lateral view and scoliosis in the posterior view.

- There may be muscle wasting of the intrinsic hand muscles, including the hypothenar and interossei muscles, with the thenar muscles and long finger flexors occasionally affected.

- Difficulty in gripping and performing other fine motor skills is observed.

- Circulatory compromise results in pallor of the fingers, edema of the hand and, in extreme cases, necrosis of the fingertips (*Mumenthaler, Schliack, 1991*).

Palpation

- Muscle wasting may be palpated in the hand, including the intrinsic hand, hypothenar and, occasionally, thenar muscles.

- Tenderness, hypertonicity and trigger points are present in the scalenes, pectoralis minor and the subclavius muscles.

- Fascial restrictions are found on the anterolateral neck, shoulder and upper arm.

- Edema may be present with vascular and lymphatic compression, more likely occurring with costoclavicular and pectoralis minor syndrome. Some sources suggest edema may occur with anterior scalene syndrome.

✍ The hand may be cool.

Testing

✍ **AF** and **PR ROM** of the shoulder and neck reveal some decreased movement. Specifically for anterior scalene syndrome, there is reduction of rotation and lateral flexion accompanied by pain.

Special Tests

✍ **Adson's test** is positive for anterior scalene compression.

✍ **Travell's variation** is positive for thoracic outlet syndrome with the primary compression at the middle scalene muscle.

✍ **Scalene cramp** and **scalene relief tests** are positive for trigger points in scalenes.

✍ **Costoclavicular** and **Eden's tests** are positive for compression at the first rib and clavicle.

✍ **Wright's hyperabduction test** is positive for pectoralis minor compression.

✍ **Pectoralis minor length test** is positive for a short pectoralis minor muscle.

✍ **Upper limb tension tests** are positive if cervical nerve roots and peripheral nerves are the source of the client's shoulder or arm pain.

Differentiating Conditions with Arm Symptoms

✍ **Cervical spine spondylosis, cervical radiculopathy and cervical tumours** can mimic TOS. Deep tendon reflex tests are positive for these conditions. Spurling's test is positive for facet joint irritation of the cervical spine. Upper limb tension tests are positive with nerve root and peripheral nerve compression.

✍ **Raynaud's disease** results in sensitivity to cold, which is not present with TOS.

✍ **Carpal tunnel syndrome** will yield a positive Phalen's test. Pain and paresthesia are on the thenar side of the hand with thenar muscle wasting with CTS.

✍ **Ulnar nerve compression** at the elbow or at Guyon's canal at the wrist has a similar paresthesia pattern but will not result in atrophy of intrinsic hand muscles. Hypertonicity and trigger points will be palpated in the limb, not the neck and shoulder girdle.

✍ **Tendinitis** of the rotator cuff and forearm muscles will result in a positive active resisted test. Muscle wasting is not present.

✍ **Osteoarthritis** in the glenohumeral joint is diagnosed medically by X-ray and other diagnostic tests.

Contraindications

✦ Do not place deep moist heat over the neck or anterior chest if the client has hypertension or atherosclerosis in the neck vasculature. Do not perform muscle stripping or aggressive techniques in these circumstances.

✦ Avoid frictions if anti-inflammatories are being taken.

✦ If the compression is the result of a pathology, modify positioning, hydrotherapy and techniques accordingly.

✦ Modify techniques and pressure if the tissue is fragile.

✦ Avoid aggressive mobilizations if degenerative disc disease, rheumatoid arthritis or a cervical rib is present.

Treatment Goals

Treat the entire shoulder girdle and neck and any postural contributors.

Treatment Plan

🖐 The treatment strategy considers the actual cause of the compression. If it is a systemic condition or a space-occupying bony structure, massage will not remove the cause but can treat soft tissue and compensatory structures and increase relaxation to give temporary relief. Massage is most effective in treating TOS that has soft tissue causes, such as scalene and pectoralis minor trigger points, hypertonicity and altered posture, such as hyperkyphosis.

🖐 Symptoms may be exacerbated when specific muscles are treated but should decrease with the massage or when pressure is released.

🖐 While a specific muscle may be the main source of compression, the treatment strategy is to treat the entire shoulder girdle and neck as well as any postural compensation or contributors. Edema and ischemia present in the hand will be due to vascular and lymphatic compression. To achieve an effective increase in local circulation and decrease in local edema, these goals are addressed after the source of thoracic compression is treated.

🖐 **Positioning** is flexible. Prone, supine and sidelying positions can be used. While the client is supine, if hyperkyphosis is present, a towel roll is placed under the spine to encourage the chest to open. Sidelying is a particularly efficient position to treat the posterior, lateral and anterior shoulder girdle and neck. If the condition is bilateral, the prone and supine positions are often more comfortable for the client. With pectoralis minor syndrome, sidelying can be made comfortable by rolling the bottom shoulder forward and inferiorly. This opens the costoclavicular space relieving pressure on the neurovascular bundle.

🖐 **Pillowing** for sidelying ensures that the cervical spine is in alignment with the rest of the spine. The client hugs a pillow over the anterior trunk to secure draping as well as to reduce any compressive force on

Treatment Goals   Treatment Plan

the thoracic outlet. If edema is present, the hand and arm are elevated.

🖐 **Hydrotherapy** includes deep moist heat, such as a hot towel wrap, thermaphore, hydrocollator or even wax, on the lateral neck, shoulder or pectoralis minor. If edema is present, cool applications are appropriate providing there is no cold sensitivity in the hand. Contrast hydrotherapy is used to improve circulation in the arm and shoulder, particularly after specific painful techniques.

General Treatment

Decrease sympathetic nervous system firing. Address compensatory structures.

🖐 Throughout the treatment, a relaxation focus is important.

🖐 **Diaphragmatic breathing** is encouraged and soothing circulatory techniques are interspersed with the specific, more painful techniques. In the prone position, a back massage focuses on the postural compensation of hyperkyphosis or scoliosis. The trapezius is addressed for hypertonicity and trigger points. If drooping shoulders are present, trapezius is treated with brisk, segmental circulatory strokes. In the prone or sidelying position, trigger points that radiate to the medial hand and the fourth and fifth digits, imitating the brachial plexus compression referral, are palpated and treated. These include the latissimus dorsi (the trigger point is located at the inferior angle of the scapula), serratus anterior (the trigger point is under pectoralis major at the fifth or sixth rib) and serratus posterior superior (the trigger point is just inferior to the superior angle of the scapula).

🖐 In the supine position, heat is applied to the affected side while the contralateral shoulder and neck are treated using general Swedish techniques.

Specific Treatment

Decrease compression of the neurovascular bundle. Reduce fascial restrictions.

🖐 In the **supine** position, the fascia is treated on the neck, shoulder and anterior chest. Skin rolling is easily applied on the neck because it can be applied to small, discreet areas. A pincer grasp is used around the sternocleidomastoid followed by pulling of the fascia and tissue laterally. If a drooping shoulder is not the cause of the compression, another method to treat the fascia is to place the head in a slightly lateral position away from the side of the compression. The client is asked to depress the affected shoulder by pointing her hand towards her toes. This engages the fascia of the neck. The head position is changed to engage the most prominent fascial restrictions. The position is held for 30 seconds or more until some hyperemia is observed or a burning sensation is felt by the client. The shoulder and anterior chest fascia are treated with crossed-hands spreading, fingertip spreading or skin rolling.

Treatment Goals

Reduce pain, hypertonicity and trigger points.

Treatment Plan

The order that the following muscles are addressed is flexible. Anatomical accuracy is essential for an effective treatment.

Anterior and Middle Scalenes

The **anterior scalene** travels under the sternocleidomastoid. Therefore, the sternocleidomastoid is treated first for hypertonicity and trigger points, which allows easier access to the anterior scalene. Origin and insertion work, Golgi tendon organ release, pincer grasp compression, muscle stripping and fingertip kneading to the muscle belly are used.

The transverse processes of the cervical spine are located. At C3, the therapist rotates his thumb to the anterior aspect of the transverse process to reach the anterior scalene. The bulk of sternocleidomastoid will almost obscure the thumb. If this is not the case, it is possible the therapist is touching lateral fibres of sternocleidomastoid. To help the therapist differentiate between these two muscles, the client is asked to slightly raise the head from the table. This action will contract the sternocleidomastoid, making it prominent.

The anterior scalene is a flat muscle that can be followed down to the first rib (the thumb moves over the clavicular insertion of the sternocleidomastoid as if it were a speed bump). To confirm that the thumb is correctly placed at the first rib, the client is asked to inhale into the chest. The therapist feels the taut tendon and the first rib move upward, towards the thumb.

The **middle scalene** is the largest of the scalene muscles and is dome-shaped. It is located by palpating the transverse processes and moving the thumb posteriorly. This muscle travels in an anterolateral direction to the first rib. The tendon is often cord-like. To confirm that the thumb is on the muscle, the client is again asked to inhale into her chest.

These muscles are treated using the origin and insertion technique along with progressively deeper muscle stripping and fingertip or thumb kneading to the cervical attachments and muscle bellies. This is interspersed with lighter circulatory strokes. Trigger points are treated using ischemic compression or repetitive muscle stripping, followed by the appropriate stretch and heat.

Pectoralis Minor

Pectoralis major is addressed first for hypertonicity and trigger points to allow easier access to pectoralis minor. **Pectoralis minor** is located by placing the client's hand on the abdomen, with the humerus in slight abduction. This creates a space which allows the therapist's

836

Treatment Goals Treatment Plan

relaxed thumbs to be placed against the ribs by pectoralis minor and under the lateral border of pectoralis major. The client is asked to depress the shoulder, making pectoralis minor palpably contract. The two pectoralis muscles can be further distinguished because the pectoralis major fibres travel horizontally in comparison to the pectoralis minor fibres which run vertically.

- A further massage of pectoralis major is performed as the fingers gently form a pincer grasp around the tissue of pectoralis major. The tissue is rolled between the thumb and fingers, proximal to distal. Next, the pectoralis minor muscle is massaged by applying thumb kneading and compressions along the lateral edge of the muscle. The attachments of pectoralis minor are addressed systematically from the sixth to the third rib and then to the coracoid process. The massage may be uncomfortable for the client, especially when the thumbs approach the coracoid process; access to this structure may be limited by fibrosis and muscle hypertonicity. Several treatments may be required before this attachment is actually palpated.

Maintain range of motion.

- Passive range of motion is applied to the cervical spine and shoulder girdle. Joint play is used to mobilize the shoulder girdle and clavicle.
- The recoil technique with breathing mobilizes the upper ribs.
- Passive stretches or PIR is used for the anterior and middle scalenes as well as for pectoralis minor. To stretch the scalenes, first the shoulder is secured by the client placing her hand under her buttock on the side to be stretched. This prevents the shoulder from being elevated by the short scalenes. The *anterior scalene* is lengthened by placing the client's head laterally away from the side to be stretched and then rotating the head by bringing the chin upward and towards the affected side. The *middle scalene* is stretched by bringing the head laterally away from the affected side. No rotation is applied.
- For *pectoralis minor*, the client is asked to slide to the side of the table to allow the affected shoulder to drop off the edge. The therapist applies pressure to the coracoid process with the heel of the hand. The client contracts pectoralis minor minimally against the therapist's resistance. This is followed by stretching the muscle, through pressure on the coracoid process superiorly and posteriorly.
- With PIR, the client gently contracts the muscle for seven to 10 seconds, against resistance, and then relaxes. This is repeated three times. For added effectiveness, the client inhales and holds the breath during the contraction and exhales with relaxation and stretching of the muscle.

Reduce edema, if present.

- Lymphatic drainage techniques to the arm and hand include axillary pumping, unidirectional effleurage and scooping. **Passive movement** is performed at the elbow, wrist and fingers.

837

Treatment Goals

Treatment Plan

Improve tissue health and circulation.

🖐 The affected arm is massaged using Swedish techniques, such as effleurage and petrissage. Trigger points, often found in the forearm muscles, are addressed. In the hand, if the muscles are wasted, strokes are applied gently and in a segmental manner.

🖐 With **sidelying**, there is excellent access to the entire shoulder girdle and lateral neck. Trigger points in latissimus dorsi, serratus anterior and serratus posterior superior are easily palpated from this position. Fascial restrictions of the neck and anterior chest are addressed using skin rolling and spreading techniques.

🖐 The **subclavius** muscle is easily treated with the client in the sidelying position. Facing the head of the table, the therapist puts one arm under the client's arm. The therapist's other arm has access to the back. One hand is placed on the scapula, the other on the anterior chest. The shoulder is internally rotated. While supporting the shoulder position, the thumb of the therapist's anterior hand is positioned under the clavicle. Gentle muscle stripping is applied in a medial to lateral direction along the clavicle; at the same time, the shoulder is brought into external rotation.

🖐 Next, the shoulder is placed in a slightly elevated position. The fingers of the anterior hand are placed in the pocket that is created at the superior aspect of the clavicle. The shoulder is drawn inferiorly while the therapist performs muscle stripping in a medial to lateral direction behind the clavicle. Care is taken to direct the pressure along the clavicle; if pressure is applied more deeply and broadly, the brachial plexus may be compressed, causing the client needless pain. Pectoralis minor is palpated from this position by first rotating the shoulder in an anterior and inferior direction to create a space to place the thumb. The shoulder is then moved in various positions to allow different angles of approach to the muscle fibres.

🖐 The middle scalene is treated with muscle stripping from the clavicle upward to the head. Then, with the therapist sitting or standing at the client's head, the muscle is stripped from the upper transverse processes to the first rib. From this position, a stretch can be applied. The client inhales as the therapist stabilizes the scalene tendon at the first rib; upon exhalation the therapist gently applies a stretch to the muscle by pushing on the rib caudally.

🖐 Pectoralis minor can be stretched in a sidelying position. While facing the head of the client, the therapist places the heel of the right hand securely on the coracoid process. The other hand grasps the scapula. As the client exhales, the hand on the coracoid process pushes superiorly and the hand on the scapula pulls inferiorly, physically pulling the attachment points of the pectoralis minor farther apart. This is repeated for several breathes. While this is an effective stretch, it requires good strength and access to the coracoid process.

838

Treatment Goals

Treatment Plan

✋ As with the supine position, when the client is sidelying, the goals of mobilizing the joints, reducing hypertonicity and trigger points, decreasing edema and improving tissue health apply.

Self-care Goals

Self-care Plan

✍ Remedial exercise is an essential component of treating TOS. Some improvement should be noted after three months. The program should continue for up to 18 months even when the client is symptom-free.

Stretch shortened muscles.

✍ A hot shower spray on the neck muscles is recommended to allow easier stretching.

✍ The sternocleidomastoid is stretched. See the torticollis chapter for details.

✍ An anterior scalene stretch is performed in a supine position. To stretch the right side, the right shoulder is lowered and the right hand is secured under the right buttock. The left arm is drawn over the head so the left hand is touching the right ear. The head is gently drawn towards the left side and the face is turned upward and towards the right side. This is held for 30 seconds.

✍ To stretch the middle scalene, the same positioning as above is used, only there is no rotation of the head. It is simply drawn laterally.

✍ To stretch pectoralis minor, the shoulder is pulled back and the scapula is retracted. This can be performed as part of a pectoralis major stretch. The person positions herself in a doorway, with the hands placed on the doorframe, fingers pointing up. The arms are abducted to 90 degrees or higher as the person leans forward through the door, bringing the scapula into retraction. More fibres of pectoralis minor are stretched as the humerus is increasingly abducted. Care is taken not to hyperextend the lumbar spine when leaning through the doorway.

Educate the client.

✍ Aggravating activities are limited and frequent breaks during activities are encouraged. This is especially important with pectoralis minor syndrome and the action of hyperabduction of the humerus.

✍ Padding is added to straps of a backpack or the straps are shifted so the main stress is placed on the acromion.

✍ The sleep position is modified. For anterior scalene syndrome, Travell suggests elevating the upper end of the bed by 3 to 3.5 inches (8 to 9 centimetres) to keep the chest from riding up and causing compression and to provide gentle traction on the scalenes.

Self-care Goals

Self-care Plan

✎ The pillow should keep the head in a neutral position, avoiding excessive flexion and head-forward positioning, as this further encourages shortening of the scalenes. Foam rubber pillows are often too bouncy and can contribute to trigger points (*Travell, Simons, 1983*).

✎ Applications of deep moist heat over the scalenes and pectoralis minor for 10 to 15 minutes before bed can be helpful. Care should be taken to avoid drafts on the neck and shoulder at night, in air conditioning and on airplanes to prevent activation of trigger points.

Encourage relaxation.

✎ The client should be educated about full diaphragmatic breathing as opposed to apical or paradoxical patterns.

Strengthen weak muscles.

✎ Drooping shoulders require strengthening of the upper trapezius and levator scapulae. Shoulder elevator exercises are found to be helpful even in the presence of a cervical rib (*Mumenthaler, Schliack, 1991*).

✎ Rhomboids are strengthened performing bent-over rowing using handweights or using a rowing machine.

Refer the client.

✎ If symptoms persist or progress, the client is referred to her physician. Referral for chiropractic care or physiotherapy is appropriate.

Treatment Frequency and Expected Outcome

Forty-five minute to one-hour treatments allow a thorough massage of the upper body with a focus on the affected shoulder. Initially, treatments are more frequent — ideally twice a week for two weeks and then once a week for four weeks. This is followed by a thorough reassessment.

See also stress reduction, pregnancy, diabetes mellitus, myofascial trigger points, peripheral nerve lesions (ulnar and median), carpal tunnel syndrome, hyperkyphosis, scoliosis, dislocation, respiratory conditions, whiplash, torticollis, osteoarthritis, degenerative disc disease, inflammatory arthritides and Raynaud's syndrome for related treatments.

Client compliance with therapy for up to six months, including massage, exercises and activity modification, will relieve symptoms of TOS in the majority of people (*Mumenthaler, Schliack, 1991; Szabo, 1989; Dawson et al., 1990; Samii, 1990*). If a systemic pathology is the cause, symptoms are only temporarily relieved.

69

CARPAL TUNNEL SYNDROME

Linda Ludwig

Carpal tunnel syndrome (CTS) is a condition that results from the compression of the median nerve as it passes through the carpal tunnel at the wrist. This results in numbness and tingling in the median distribution — that Is, the lateral three and one-half digits.

CTS is the most common entrapment syndrome in the arm *(Turner et al., 1990)*. During the mid-nineteenth century, cases of median nerve paresis were frequently documented. Causes were linked to nerve compression from callus formation after a distal radial fracture, as well as some occupations such as laundry women, milkers, cigar makers and carpet beaters. During the early part of this century, the flexor retinaculum was considered a source of median nerve compression with the suggested treatment being sectioning of this ligament *(Pecina et al., 1991)*. In the 1940s, this condition was termed "carpal tunnel syndrome". It was associated with compression of the nerve in the carpal tunnel. In 1954, Phalen first demonstrated what is now known as Phalen's test which is used to determine the presence of carpal tunnel syndrome.

This condition is seen in approximately one per cent of the population *(Szabo, 1989)* but is higher in certain populations. Carpal tunnel syndrome is related to highly repetitive flexion and extension actions of the wrist. This leads to numbness and tingling in the distribution of the median nerve, the lateral three and one-half fingers. The condition is aggravated by movement, which causes pain. A distinguishing feature of CTS is the presence of nocturnal symptoms that wake the person up. As the condition persists, there is thenar muscle wasting that can lead to weakness and clumsiness of the thumb and fingers.

Poultry processors, butchers, assembly line workers and keyboard operators are among those who have increased rates of CTS. One study of meat packers found a 15 per cent occurrence of CTS, which seemed related to the repetitive extreme flexion and ulnar deviation of the wrists while holding the knives to cut meat *(Rosenbaum, Ochoa, 1993)*.

Some people are more susceptible to compression of the median nerve due to the presence of other conditions — systemic conditions, such as diabetes mellitus, or a compression proximal to the wrist, such as at the elbow or neck *(Szabo, 1989)*. In case of the latter condition, if CTS is present with another proximal compression it is referred to as a *double crush syndrome (Schaumburg et al., 1992)*.

The Carpal Tunnel

The carpal tunnel is located at the wrist just distal to the wrist creases. It is a fibrosseous canal, with the floor formed by the carpal bones and the roof formed by the flexor retinaculum, also referred to as the *transverse carpal ligament.*

This ligament is a dense fibrous band, approximately 1 to 2 millimetres thick *(Rosenbaum, Ochoa, 1993)* to as much as 3.5 millimetres thick *(Szabo, 1989)*. It attaches to the pisiform and the hook of the hamate bone on the ulnar side of the wrist; on the radial side, it attaches to the scaphoid tubercle and the trapezium. Proximally, the ligament lies at the distal wrist crease and blends with the fascia of the distal flexor surface of the forearm; distally it extends to the base of the metacarpals and into the palmar fascia.

The median nerve becomes increasingly superficial as it approaches the carpal tunnel. Before passing through the tunnel, it gives off a nerve branch called the palmar cutaneous branch. This branch generally travels superior to, *not* through, the carpal tunnel *(Figure 69.1)*. This is significant because the palmar cutaneous nerve supplies the skin over the thenar eminence. In turn, if the median nerve is compressed in the tunnel, the sensation to the thenar area is *not* affected.

✦ Structures that travel through the carpal tunnel *(Figure 69.1)* are:

- the median nerve;
- the four tendons of the flexor digitorum superficialis;
- the four tendons of the flexor digitorum profundus;
- the tendon of the flexor pollicis longus.

Normally, at rest, with the wrist in neutral, the pressure within the carpal tunnel is 2.5 mm Hg. When carpal tunnel syndrome is present, this resting pressure increases to an astonishing 32 mm Hg. The position of the wrist has a dramatic effect on the internal tunnel pressure. Normally, wrist extension and flexion to 90 degrees average about 31 mm Hg. With carpal tunnel syndrome, this pressure increases to an amazing 94 mm Hg with wrist flexion and to 101 mm Hg with

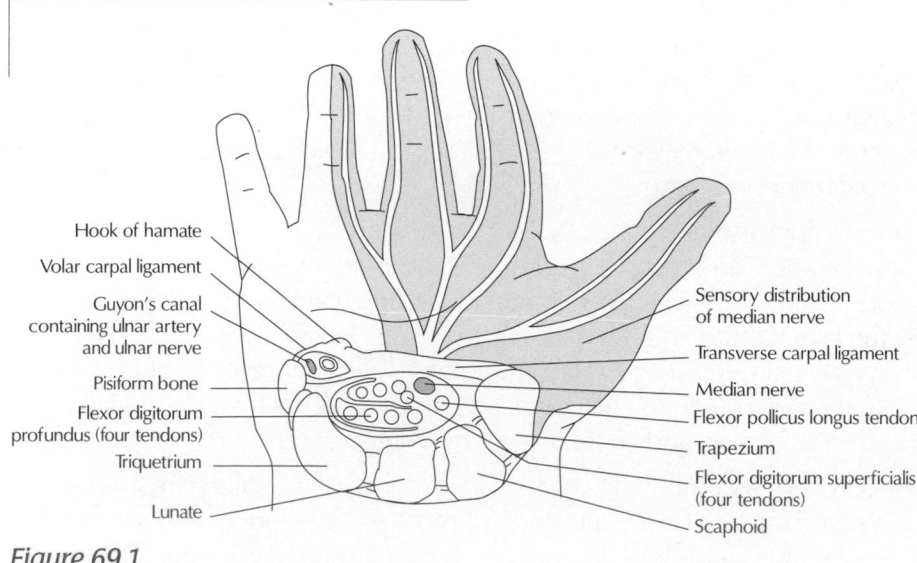

Figure 69.1
A cross-section of the carpal tunnel.

Hook of hamate
Volar carpal ligament
Guyon's canal containing ulnar artery and ulnar nerve
Pisiform bone
Flexor digitorum profundus (four tendons)
Triquetrium
Lunate

Sensory distribution of median nerve
Transverse carpal ligament
Median nerve
Flexor pollicus longus tendon
Trapezium
Flexor digitorum superficialis (four tendons)
Scaphoid

wrist extension (*Szabo, 1989*).

Compression of the median nerve as it passes through the carpal tunnel generally occurs in two basic ways: the size of the tunnel itself decreases or the size of the contents passing through the tunnel increases. It is not unusual that both of these occur in combination. For example, rheumatoid arthritis can result in bony changes of the carpal bones and lead to an increase in fluid within the tunnel itself.

Some causes of CTS are idiopathic.

➤ Causes leading to an **increase in the size of the contents through the tunnel**, that are chronic in nature:

  • repetitive actions of the wrist, primarily flexion and extension. This can lead to edema, followed by chronic fibrosis and thickening of the tendons;

  • thickening of the retinaculum due to scar tissue from repeated trauma;

  • systemic conditions that result in edema and fluid retention or connective tissue degeneration, such as diabetes, hypothyroidism, rheumatoid arthritis and pregnancy.

➤ Causes leading to **decreased canal space** that are chronic in nature:

  • bony callus development after a fracture of a carpal bone or the distal radius;

  • space-occupying lesions such as ganglia, lipomas or cysts;

  • bony changes that occur with rheumatoid arthritis.

➤ Causes that are **acute** in nature:

  • secondary to a trauma, such as a fracture or dislocation (especially of the lunate) of the carpal bones or at the wrist;

  • infection;

  • acute exacerbation of rheumatoid arthritis;

  • new activity requiring repetitive wrist actions;

  • hematoma, which can occasionally occur in people with hemophilia or those on anticoagulants.

Contributing factors:

➤ vitamin B6 deficiency can be present in those with CTS. It is unclear if the deficiency is an actual cause. Supplements of vitamin B6 (pyridoxine) in combination with other conservative treatments, such as splints and drugs, showed a 68 per cent improvement in patients versus only a 14 per cent improvement in a similar group not given the vitamin supplements. This seems to be a controversial area in the medical community. Concern has been expressed over the risk of taking harmful doses of this vitamin (*Rosenbaum, Ochoa, 1993*);

➤ there may be a familial tendency — an inherited systemic condition or a carpal tunnel that is inherently smaller (*Schaumburg et al., 1992*).

The condition is often unilateral, usually affecting the dominant hand. It can be bilateral, though often the non-dominant hand is asymptomatic and the condition is discovered only after electrodiagnosis. While work-related CTS affects women and men equally, women can be additionally affected premenstrually, with pregnancy or with menopause.

Systemic conditions must be considered first and treated by a physician, as appropriate. For example, 14 per cent of those with CTS have diabetes (*Schaumburg et al., 1992*).

Massage therapy focuses on reducing local edema and addressing increased muscle tone in the forearm as well as adhesions and trigger points that contribute to the condition. Through massage and client education, the therapist increases the client's awareness of posture and proper wrist and arm biomechanics.

The Medical Treatment of Carpal Tunnel Syndrome

Medical treatment of CTS may include splinting of the wrist, usually in a neutral position but sometimes in slight extension *(Pedretti, Zoltan, 1990)*. The splint is worn particularly at night to prevent the person from sleeping with the wrist flexed, which would cause compression. In some cases, the client wears the splint during the day. Splint use is prescribed for a three- to six-week period. Oral anti-inflammatories and diuretics may be prescribed. Steroid injections are commonly given in less extreme cases. While providing temporary relief, these injections prove to be less effective over the long term. There are also concerns that frequent injections may damage the tendons and the median nerve *(Stewart, 1993)*. Vitamin B6 may also be prescribed. Surgery is generally used in moderate to severe cases or if the condition has lasted for more than one year or if muscle atrophy has occurred. Before surgery is performed, the diagnosis should be confirmed with electromyography (EMG). Testing will reveal diminished conduction time in the median nerve, if CTS is present.

The surgical procedure involves the complete transection of the flexor retinaculum. This is usually performed employing traditional open surgical techniques which use a longitudinal incision, in line with the ring finger, in order to avoid the median and palmar cutaneous nerves. The wrist is then splinted for several days. It takes up to three months for strength to return. Results vary widely, with an average of 50 to 65 per cent of patients reporting total success *(Rosenbaum, Ochoa, 1993)*. The problems that arise are usually because of a misdiagnosis of the original condition, an incomplete transection of the retinaculum, thickening of the retinaculum from scar tissue, the entrapment of the nerve in developing scar tissue and damage from the surgery to the median or palmar cutaneous nerves, possibly leading to neuroma formation or causalgia. Over the last decade, there has been increasing interest in laser endoscopic surgery. This involves a closed surgery; only two small incisions of 1 to 1.5 centimetres in length are made at the wrist and on the palm above the retinaculum. When this procedure is successful, the person has relief from symptoms and a shorter down-time from activities — only two to three weeks *(Brillhart, 1994)*.

Pronator Teres Syndrome and Median Nerve Compression

With pronator teres syndrome, the median nerve is compressed at the level of the proximal attachment of the pronator teres *(Figure 69.2)*. Compression is usually from the tendons of this muscle, which may be thickened, possibly as a result of local trauma. There is usually a gradual, insidious onset. The person experiences aching (often described as tiredness or heaviness) in the anterior forearm and numbness in the thumb and index finger, with some weakness in the thenar muscles. Dull to sharp pain in the anterior forearm is experienced with repetitive elbow movement rather than wrist movement. Another distinguishing feature is that tenderness is found at the proximal attachment of the pronator teres and pain is present with active resisted testing of pronation of the forearm. There is also no nocturnal pattern to the symptoms *(Schumacher, 1993)*.

Repetitive Strain Injury (RSI)

Repetitive strain injury is a current term used to describe cumulative trauma suffered as a result of highly repetitive and forceful hand movements, often performed in biomechanically unsound positions. It is a more recent name for a combination of conditions that seem to affect white collar workers, often associated with computer work. This condition includes tendinitis, tenosynovitis, carpal tunnel and thoracic outlet syndromes and trigger points *(Pascarelli, Quilter, 1994)*. Whether it be carpal tunnel syndrome or RSI, the condition can lead to chronic pain and disability. Ultimately, if this condition is severe, it may lead to some degree of permanent median nerve damage.

It is not unusual to find the client extremely distressed at not being able to perform his job.

In an effort to help those who suffer from CTS, where computer keyboard work is an aggravating factor, there have been innovations made in wrist and forearm supports. In some cases, voice-activated computers are used. Of course, this has lead to a new repetitive injury referred to as **RSI of the larynx**. If this condition occurs, the person should seek help from a speech therapist, who will assist in voice modulation and other exercises. It seems clear that prevention of overuse syndromes should be the goal of health care. Many of the self-care suggestions in this chapter can be used to this end. See also the tendinitis chapter.

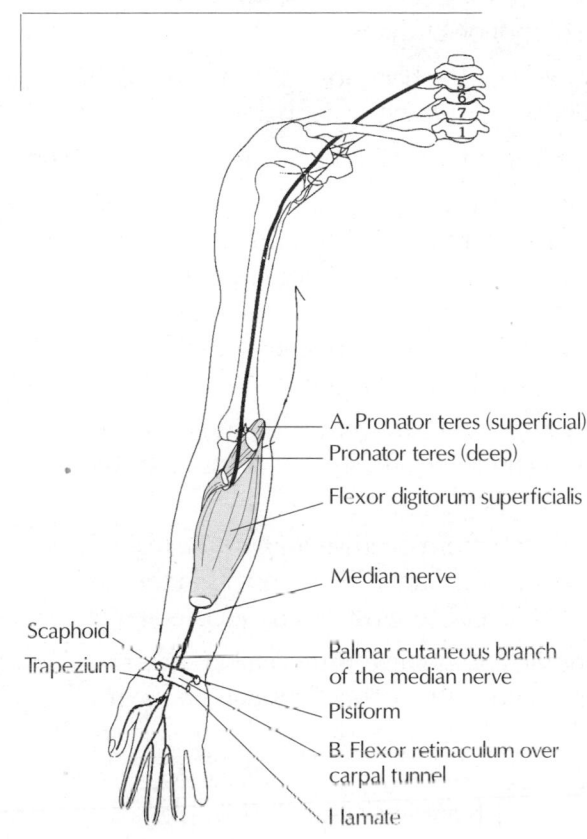

Figure 69.2
The path of the median nerve and common areas of compression: (a) the pronator teres; (b) the carpal tunnel. Note that the palmar cutaneous branch travels outside the carpal tunnel.

Labels in figure:
A. Pronator teres (superficial)
Pronator teres (deep)
Flexor digitorum superficialis
Median nerve
Scaphoid
Trapezium
Palmar cutaneous branch of the median nerve
Pisiform
B. Flexor retinaculum over carpal tunnel
Hamate

Symptom Picture

✦ When CTS has a unilateral presentation, it is usually in the dominant hand. It is often bilateral, however. There is numbness and tingling in a median distribution.

✦ Nocturnal dysthesia is a distinguishing feature of CTS, often waking the person up. Dysthesia may be due to venous stasis or persistent compression from sleeping with the wrists in a flexed position.

✦ These symptoms are accompanied by local pain, which also occurs with wrist activity. In later stages, the pain can be present not only locally in the wrist and hand but in the forearm, elbow and even, rarely, in the shoulder.

+ Movements of the wrist are limited by pain. Space-occupying lesions or bony cysts may also be present, resulting in limited range of motion at the wrist.

+ The person will often shake, massage or exercise the hand for relief of symptoms. Sometimes placing the hand under cool or warm running water helps.

+ Frequently, the person is distressed over the loss of function and the loss of ability to work.

+ Swelling may be present. It may, in fact, be a cause of CTS as it increases pressure on the median nerve. Women may experience an exacerbation of symptoms premenstrually or with menopause. Pregnancy can lead to CTS symptoms in 18 to 31 per cent of women (*Stewart, 1993*). In these cases, it is often bilateral, due to the presence of peripheral edema. CTS will usually begin late in the second trimester, continue into the third trimester and resolve a few weeks to a few months postpartum.

+ The tissue of the forearms may be boggy and fibrous from the build up of metabolic waste. Infrequently, there may be changes in tissue health, such as mottling of the skin. Sometimes there is increased sweating of the hand.

+ Hypertonicity is common in the forearm flexors from overuse and, often, from the presence of trigger points in these muscles and the hand. Trigger points in the subscapularis and scalenes, among others, refer to the wrist, palm and lateral digits.

+ Adhesions can develop at the attachment sites of the flexor retinaculum as well as in the tendons of the forearm muscles that pass through the tunnel. This can be the result of wear and tear due to overuse. Adhesions also develop secondary to rheumatoid arthritis.

+ Atrophy of the thenar muscles occurs as the condition progresses. This leads to clumsy movements of the thumb and index finger, which are apparent with simple tasks such as buttoning clothes or holding a mug. This symptom is often worse in the morning.

Subjective Information

HEALTH HISTORY QUESTIONS

+ Is there any history of a systemic disorder, such as diabetes mellitus, rheumatoid arthritis or hypothyroidism? Is the client pregnant?

+ Has the client seen a physician for a diagnosis? What tests were performed to determine the diagnosis?

+ What treatment was prescribed? Is a splint being used? When?

+ Is the client currently taking any medication? What type and for what reason? Have corticosteroid injections been received? If so, has an injection been given in the last 10 days?

+ How long has the client been experiencing the discomfort?

+ Can the client describe the sensation experienced? "Numbness", "tingling", "like my hand is asleep" are common responses.

+ Where does the client experience the altered feelings, in the entire hand or in specific fingers? If the client is uncertain or vague with this feedback, the therapist should request that he keep track of the location of the dysthesia over the next week.

✦ What are the client's work activities, hobbies and sleeping positions? What functions have most been affected in the client's activities of daily life? What work activities, sports and hobbies may contribute to the condition? When does the discomfort occur? What positions make it occur or make it worse? Are there specific activities that involve prolonged or repeated wrist flexion and extension? Are there nocturnal occurrences?

✦ What relieves the discomfort? Does shaking or massaging the hand help?

Objective Information

Observations

✍ The client's posture is observed as the client demonstrates the actions that aggravate the symptoms.

✍ Unilateral presentation is generally in the dominant hand. CTS often occurs bilaterally.

✍ A splint may be worn.

✍ Edema may be local at the hand and wrist, or more diffuse over the hand and forearm.

✍ In later stages, thenar muscle atrophy occurs, accompanied by decreased tissue health.

✍ In time, weakness of the thenar muscles is revealed by the client's difficulty with holding a pen and writing.

Palpation

✍ Possible signs of inflammation may be found local to the wrist; in chronic cases, ischemia may be present.

✍ Tenderness is reported local to the carpal tunnel at the insertions at the carpal bones and over the median nerve.

✍ Tissue texture may be boggy local to the wrist. The forearm muscles are often dense due to an accumulation of metabolic waste.

✍ There are hypertonicity and fascial restrictions of the forearm muscles due to overuse. Trigger points are also likely in these muscles.

✍ In the later stages, atrophy of the thenar muscles is palpated.

Testing

✍ Occasionally, a therapist may assume too quickly that the client has CTS upon hearing that there is numbness and tingling of the lateral digits. It is important to take a thorough health history and do a full assessment before determining the possible cause of the signs and symptoms.

✍ **AF** and **PR ROM** reveal a decreased range in flexion and extension and, possibly, with ulnar deviation. The end feel is often empty.

✍ **AR strength testing** of the abductor pollicis brevis muscle is positive for weakness if CTS is chronic *(Stewart, 1993)*.

Special Tests

- **Phalen's** and **reverse Phalen's tests** are positive. These tests are thought to be highly indicative of CTS.

- **Cyriax's variation** is positive.

- **Tinel's sign** is positive with paresthesia (often pain and tingling) in the distribution of the median nerve. This test can often result in a false positive as pain and tingling can be elicited in people who do not have CTS (*Schaumburg et al., 1992*).

- The **tourniquet test** (inflating a blood pressure cuff proximal to the elbow) functions to obstruct the venous return and recreate the client's symptoms. It is not considered very accurate, yielding false positives as much as 40 per cent of the time (*Szabo, 1989*).

Differentiating Sources of Wrist Pain

- **C6 and C7 radiculopathies** (conditions affecting the spinal nerves) and disc lesions cause sensory symptoms in the thumb and middle and index fingers, which may radiate along the lateral forearm. They are distinguished by motor weakness in muscles innervated by C6 (biceps brachii) or C7 (triceps brachii). Deep tendon reflexes are decreased. The pain is experienced in the neck and with neck movement. Pain is relieved with cessation of the neck movements, not by shaking the hand. Nocturnal pain is rare.

- **Thoracic outlet syndrome** results in positive results of some of the following tests: Adson's, Travell's variation, costoclavicular, Eden's and Wright's hyperabduction and upper limb tension tests. Numbness and tingling are experienced in the medial forearm and in the medial two digits. Muscle wasting of the hypothenar muscles occurs, specifically over the ulnar border and over the ring and baby fingers.

- **Pronator teres syndrome** is indicated by pain in the anterior forearm with elbow movement, not wrist movement. Tenderness is palpated at the attachments of the pronator teres muscle. No nocturnal pattern is present.

- Any of the above conditions may exist together with CTS. In fact, their presence would cause an increased susceptibility to carpal tunnel syndrome. The term **double crush syndrome** would be used to describe the combined conditions.

Contraindications

- Frictions are not performed if carpal tunnel syndrome is the result of rheumatoid arthritis due to joint instability. They are also not performed if the client has decreased tissue health due to diabetes or if edema is present over the adhered area or if anti-inflammatories are being taken.

- Vigorous joint play is not used if rheumatoid arthritis has resulted in joint hypermobility or if the client is in the third trimester of pregnancy.

- No local massage is performed until 10 days after a corticosteroid injection.

Treatment Goals

Reduce edema, fascial restrictions, hypertonicity, trigger points and stress.

Treatment Plan

✋ The treatment strategies take into consideration the actual cause of the CTS and which massage techniques and other modalities can address this. It is obvious that massage cannot remove bony changes or a space-occupying lesion. But the therapist can address the edema, fascial restrictions, increased muscle tone, trigger points and overall stress the client may be experiencing to give some temporary relief. A systemic condition requires medical attention. With pregnancy, the birth and the passage of time can alleviate the CTS. In both cases, massage offers some temporary relief. Massage treatment is most successful with CTS that is caused by overuse or repetitive activity.

✋ **Positioning** is flexible. The prone position allows access to treat possible subscapularis muscle trigger points. The supine position enables treatment of the arms and easy pillowing for edema. Rather than the arm being held during treatment, pillows are used to support the arm in a neutral or slightly flexed position so both the therapist's hands can be used to apply techniques. Sidelying is possible for unilateral CTS, with the client lying on the unaffected side. This allows pillowing of the arm in an elevated position as well as good access to the shoulder girdle muscles and subscapularis muscle.

✋ If the client is pregnant, positioning will depend on how advanced the pregnancy is. By the late third trimester, most women are unable to lie supine for any period of time. At this stage, bilateral CTS is best treated in a seated position. Sidelying may work but means one arm or the other is compressed during treatment.

✋ **Hydrotherapy** reflects the stage of the condition. Cold applications are used on acute, inflamed or edematous tissue as well as at the end of the massage if deep techniques were used. Contrast hydrotherapy is extremely helpful in creating a vascular flush of the hand and forearm. Heat, especially wax, is appropriate before fascial techniques and frictions. Heat is also used after treating trigger points. All applications are modified if there is atrophy or a decrease in tissue health.

General Treatment

Decrease sympathetic nervous system firing.

✋ Treatment is performed in the context of a relaxation massage. Diaphragmatic breathing is encouraged. If **acute** CTS is present, it is treated like any other acute condition: cold hydrotherapy, no distal work and, likely, no on-site work. The proximal tissue and joints are addressed and the body treated with overall stress reduction techniques.

✋ In **chronic** cases, a relaxation focus is important because treatment can be painful and specific work can temporarily exacerbate symptoms. Soothing circulatory techniques are interspersed with the

Treatment Goals   Treatment Plan

specific, more painful ones. The prone position may be used first to address the shoulder girdle and subscapularis trigger points. In the supine position, the neck, shoulder and arm are treated using general Swedish techniques. Subscapularis trigger points can be treated in this position as well. The arm is abducted to 90 degrees, if possible. The bulk of latissimus dorsi and teres major is palpated and the edge of the scapula is located just above them. The fingers are slipped in the space at the lateral scapula with the subscapularis below and the serratus anterior above. Trigger points are usually palpated on the lateral border of the muscle. Scalenes trigger points can be treated in this position. See the thoracic outlet syndrome chapter for details.

Specific Treatment

Decrease the compression on the median nerve. Reduce fascial restrictions.

If edema is present due to fascial restrictions in the forearm, it is appropriate to treat these restrictions on the proximal non-edematous tissue first. In the supine position, skin rolling, crossed-hands spreading and thumb spreading techniques are applied systematically over the forearm. Both the flexor and extensor surfaces are addressed. This may be painful and is performed within the client's pain tolerance. When hyperemia appears, circulatory strokes are incorporated. Care is taken not to overwork this tissue and cause inflammation. If heat is palpated, a cool wash is applied and the therapist should move on to massage other tissue.

Decrease pain. Reduce hypertonicity and trigger points.

Techniques are applied to pronator teres and the muscles that pass through the carpal tunnel. Specific muscle stripping using the thumb, fist and forearm is applied to the forearm muscles including flexor carpi radialis, brachioradialis, palmaris longus and flexor digitorum superficialis. The full length of the muscle is addressed from the wrist to the elbow. The extensors are treated in a similar manner. Trigger points are treated when they are palpated, followed by heat and stretching. There are numerous trigger points which refer to the thumb and lateral hand. Scalene trigger points refer to the lateral upper arm and forearm and extensor surface of the thumb and index finger. Brachialis trigger points refer to the distal thumb and wrist. Brachioradialis trigger points refer to the thumb at the web and to the radial forearm. Opponens pollicis trigger points refer to the radial palmar wrist and thumb. Adductor pollicis trigger points refer to the thumb and thenar eminence. Palmaris longus trigger points refer to the palm.

Several trigger points refer to the wrist. Subscapularis trigger points refer to the palmar and extensor wrist surfaces. Flexor carpi radialis trigger points refer to the mid-palm and wrist. Pronator teres trigger points refer to the forearm and radial palmar wrist.

Treatment Goals

Reduce edema, if present.

Decrease adhesions.

Maintain range of motion.

Improve tissue health and increase circulation to remove metabolites.

Treatment Plan

☝ Only a few muscles are treated for trigger points in each treatment. As with fascial work, the client may experience tenderness. Therefore, effleurage and broad drainage strokes are interspersed.

☝ If edema is present, the limb is elevated and a cool or cold towel wrap is applied. In order to allow the lymphatic vessels to recover from the deeper work, the contralateral arm is massaged, followed by the neck. Trigger points in scalenes and subscapularis are treated (if these are not treated in the prone position). Axillary pumping is followed by lymphatic drainage techniques, such as unidirectional effleurage and stationary circles, applied down the affected arm to the hand.

☝ The insertions of the flexor retinaculum on the carpal bones and the tendons of the muscles of the forearm are addressed using focused thumb kneading. If adhesions are palpated, they are frictioned. These same techniques are applied to the flexor retinaculum itself, with the pressure modified for the client's pain tolerance. Care is taken not to compress the median nerve.

☝ If muscle tone and tissue health of the hand, especially the thenar area, are good, fascial work is performed on the palm using short spreading strokes. This is followed by specific petrissage techniques, such as thumb or fingertip kneading and muscle stripping, to the palm and fingers. As mentioned earlier, care is taken over the mid palm area since direct work over the median nerve can be painful. If tissue health is compromised, gentle petrissage is performed using vitamin E oil.

☝ Joint play is performed to the elbow, carpal bones and metacarpal joints to normalize joint mechanics and increase successive action of the joints. Rhythmical movements and pain-free passive range of motion of these joints, including the shoulder, are also important for maintaining joint health and mobility.

☝ The treatment to the arm is completed using effleurage and a cool wash. If desired, the effleurage could be performed using a cool cloth.

Self-care Goals

Educate the client.

Self-care Plan

✍ The client is educated about appropriate posture when performing activities that aggravate the condition.

✍ While at the computer, ideally, the wrists are held in a neutral position with the forearm parallel to the floor. The elbow is supported by arm rests that are at a level that allows the shoulders to be supported in a non-elevated position (*Figure 69.3*).

✍ If the client uses a computer mouse, it should be placed so the wrist,

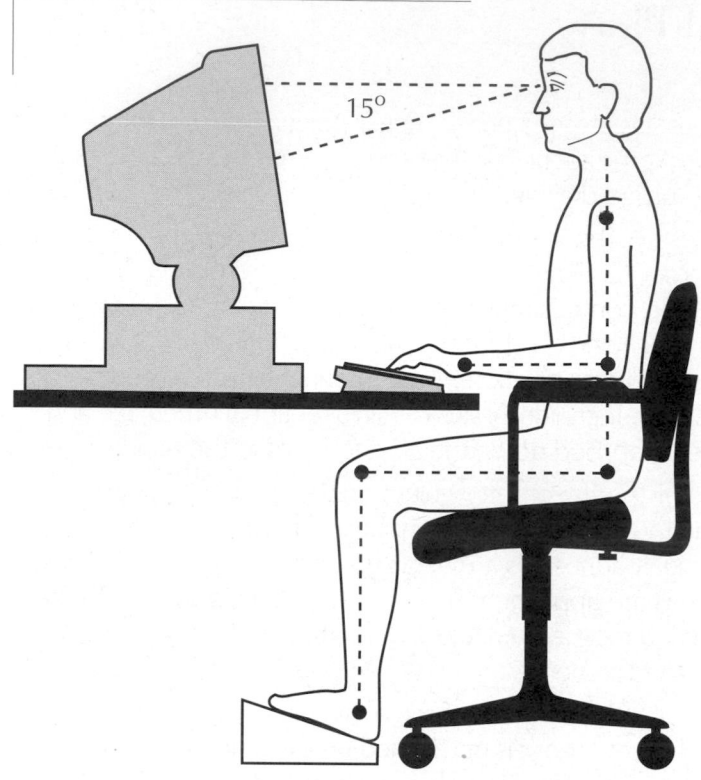

Figure 69.3
Posture when working at a computer.
- The shoulders are relaxed, with the elbows supported by arm rests.
- The wrists are in a neutral position with the forearms parallel to the floor.
- The thighs are parallel to the floor — a foot rest may be necessary to achieve this position.

Self-care Goals	Self-care Plan

forearm and shoulder are positioned as above. The work space is organized so the keyboard and mouse are directly in front of the chair and not to one side. If the keyboard is to one side, the client needs to turn his chair and body so they are aligned with the keyboard. Awkward positioning greatly contributes to stress on the carpal tunnel. Frequent breaks from repetitive activities or other aggravating conditions are encouraged.

Recommend hydrotherapy.

✍ Ice is applied to the wrist and forearm frequently during activity. Contrast arm baths are excellent for flushing out the build up of metabolic waste in the arm and hand. There should be a temperature difference of about 10 degrees between the two arm baths. Temperatures are modified, using less extremes, if tissue health or sensory perception is affected.

Stretch shortened muscles.

✍ Frequent stretching of the forearm flexors maintains range of motion of the wrist. To stretch these muscles, the client stands with the elbows extended and the arms shoulder-width apart. With the hands palm-side down on a table, the person leans the body forward over the hands. This is repeated for the forearm extensors by placing the hands palm-side up and repeating the exercise.

Self-care Goals

Self-care Plan

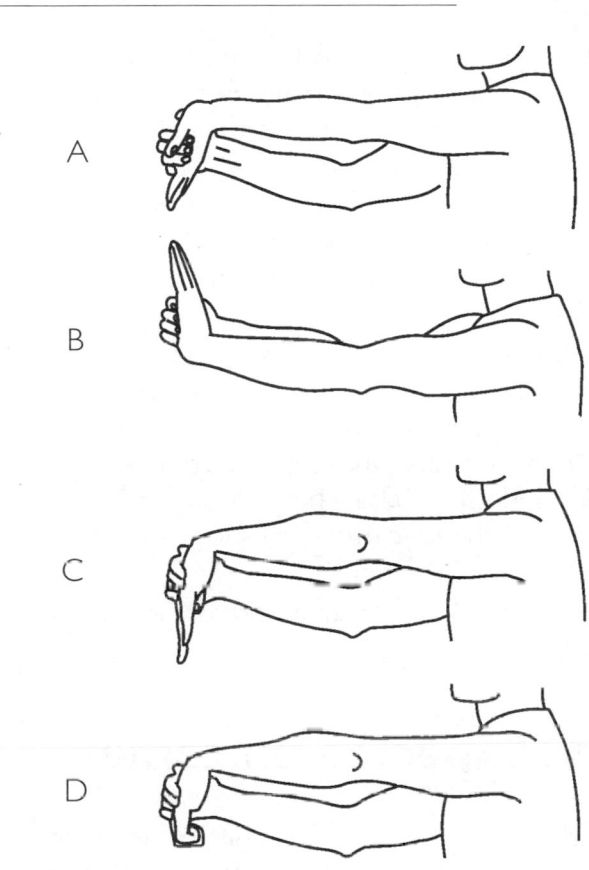

Figure 69.4
Stretching exercises for the forearm flexors (A, B) and forearm extensors (C, D).

✍ In a seated or standing position, the arm is held straight out in front of the client, at 90 degrees forward flexion of the shoulder, and the elbow is extended. The wrist is in extension with the back of the hand towards the floor (this brings the forearm into supination). The client's other hand grasps broadly over the palm and brings the affected hand farther into extension *(Figure 69.4A)*. This is repeated with the fingers towards the ceiling *(Figure 69.4B)*.

✍ With the client still seated, the wrist is held in flexion with the fingers towards the floor *(Figure 69.4C)*. The other hand grasps the affected hand over the metacarpal joints and stretches it farther into flexion. This action is repeated with the affected hand held in a fist *(Figure 69.4D)*.

✍ In all the above stretches, care is taken to keep the shoulder down and to move the affected wrist by supporting the palm and metacarpals, not by pulling the fingers into hyperextension or flexion. These are done pain free. They are initially held for 10 seconds and eventually held for 20 seconds *(Pascarelli, Quilter, 1994)*.

Strengthen weak muscles.

✍ Strengthening exercises are introduced gradually but are performed daily once range of motion of the wrist improves. These exercises focus on the forearm flexors and extensors as well as the thenar muscles.

✍ Initially, resistance can be provided by the unaffected hand. Elastic exercise bands work well to strengthen the thenar muscles. The band is placed around the fingers and the thumb. The client holds the fingers in place while moving the thumb in and out of opposition, into abduction and adduction, and into flexion and extension.

Instruct in self-massage.

✍ Self-massage is recommended for the forearms (the opposite ulnar border and hand is used to perform the massage), at the attachments of the flexor retinaculum on the carpal bones, and for the palms. If tissue health is compromised, vitamin E oil can be used. The therapist can also demonstrate to the client how to treat accessible trigger points.

Self-care Goals

Self-care Plan

Encourage relaxation.

✍ Stress reduction strategies, such as diaphragmatic breathing and meditation, or activities such as yoga or Tai Chi, are recommended. The client is taught to consciously relax the forearm and fingers when performing activities that may aggravate the condition.

Refer the client.

✍ Acupuncture, chiropractic and osteopathic treatments may help the client. Occupational therapists and those specializing in ergodynamics can give the client specific advice about modifying a work or home space.

✍ The client is referred to a physician for a splint. Some clients can become dependent on these supports, which are only meant to be used temporarily, for about four to six weeks unless otherwise indicated by the physician. Ultimately, the client should be encouraged to maintain a stretching and strengthening program so a splint becomes unnecessary. The physician may prescribe physiotherapy for the client for this purpose.

✍ The client is referred to a naturopath or nutritionist for information about supplements, especially vitamin B6.

Treatment Frequency and Expected Outcome

Forty-five minute or one-hour treatments allow time for thorough massage of the entire upper body and affected arm in the context of a relaxation massage. Shorter treatments of 30 minutes require a more focused approach to the affected arm. Treatment duration may be alternated so compensation and possible contributing postural problems in the shoulder and neck can be treated regularly. Treatments are more frequent initially — optimally, they are twice a week for a few weeks. Then they may decrease to once a week for four weeks, followed by a thorough reassessment.

The outcome is dependent on the cause of the carpal tunnel syndrome. Systemic conditions will require additional medical care. If this is successful, the CTS will often resolve.

See also stress reduction, pregnancy, diabetes mellitus, tendinitis, fractures, dislocation, rheumatoid arthritis, myofascial trigger points, thoracic outlet syndrome and peripheral nerve lesions (median nerve) for related treatments.

If CTS is caused by overuse or repetitive action, the prognosis can be good if the client is committed to regular treatments and to following the self-care program. Much of the client's recovery is dependent on his awareness of the contributing factors and his commitment to making the required changes. In some cases, this may require a prolonged leave from a particular job or, perhaps, shorter hours at a certain task.

Surgical treatment has varying results, with a 50 to 65 per cent rate of complete success (*Rosenbaum, Ochoa, 1993*).

70

PIRIFORMIS SYNDROME

Linda Ludwig

> *Piriformis syndrome is the compression of the sciatic nerve by the piriformis muscle.*

Conditions affecting the sciatic nerve that refer pain down the posterior thigh are often referred to by the general public as sciatica. This term is not specific, because it may refer to inflammation of the nerve or compression of the nerve in the lumbar spine, in the gluteals or at another distal point along the pathway of the nerve. It may even refer to the symptoms common to piriformis trigger points. Subjective and objective information will guide the therapist to the area to be treated. With a compression of the nerve by the piriformis muscle, the term "piriformis syndrome" is appropriate.

The sciatic nerve supplies sensory and motor function to the skin and muscles of the posterior thigh, most of the leg and the foot. It is composed of nerve roots L4 to S2 or S3, with sources differing about the latter *(Omer, Spinner, 1980; Dawson et al., 1990)*. The sciatic nerve is comprised of two peripheral nerves: the common peroneal and the tibial nerve which travel as one down to the knee.

The piriformis muscle inserts on the anterior surface of the sacrum (S1 to S4) and runs in a horizontal orientation to attach on the medial superior aspect of the greater trochanter of the femur. Deep to gluteus maximus, the piriformis and upper three lateral rotators spread out from the greater trochanter like a fan. The name "piriformis" actually refers to its appearance, *pirum* meaning pear and *forma* meaning shape. The broader portion of the muscle emerges from the foramen and the muscle narrows at the greater trochanter (*Figure 70.1*).

Functions of piriformis are to:

* restrain rapid or vigorous internal rotation of the hip, such as occurs with running or in the stance phase of walking;

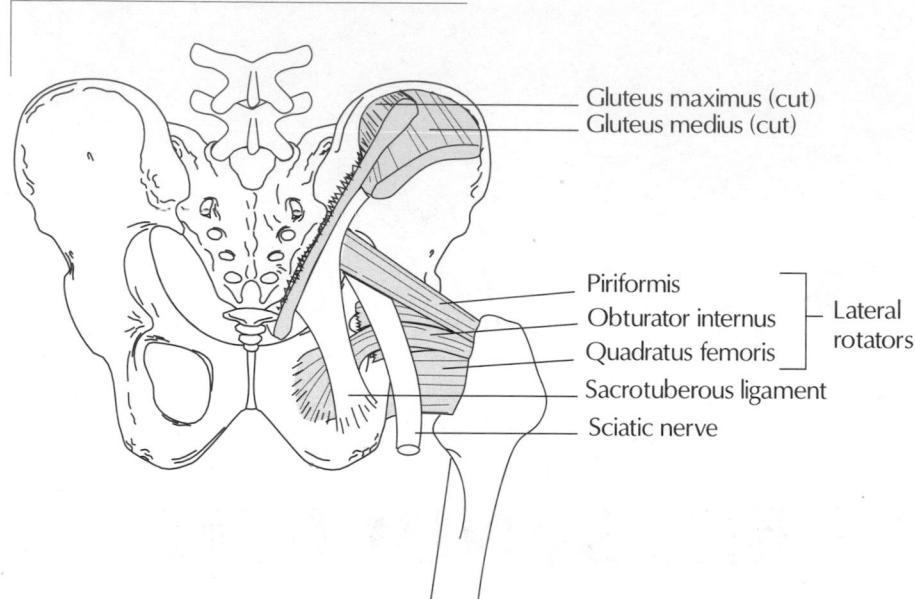

Gluteus maximus (cut)
Gluteus medius (cut)

Piriformis
Obturator internus } Lateral
Quadratus femoris   rotators
Sacrotuberous ligament
Sciatic nerve

Figure 70.1
The sciatic nerve in relation to the gluteals and lateral rotators.

- externally rotate the femur when the hip is extended or in neutral;

- horizontally abduct the thigh when the hip is flexed to 90 degrees;

- internally rotate the femur when the hip is fully flexed.

The sciatic nerve, along with other nerves, exits at the greater sciatic foramen. The pudendal nerve, for example, exits at the foramen then travels anteriorly, where it innervates the skin of the posterior thigh and contributes to sexual function.

Compression of any of the nerves can result here at the greater sciatic foramen. This opening is formed by the osseous greater sciatic notch of the ilium laterally, the sacrospinal ligament inferiorly and the piriformis muscle superiorly. As with other entrapment syndromes, an increase in the size of the contents travelling through this passage can contribute to the compression. Contraction of the piriformis muscle will increase its girth. Therefore, if the piriformis fills the space snugly, any contraction or shortening of the muscle will compress the nerve.

The sciatic nerve then travels under the piriformis muscle before continuing distally. In 10 to 20 per cent of people, the sciatic nerve, or occasionally just the peroneal division (*Figure 70.2*), travels through the piriformis muscle (*Pecina et al., 1991; Szabo, 1989; Travell, Simons, 1992*). In some cases, approximately 18 per cent of the population, the muscle actually separates into two bellies with the nerve travelling between them (*Pecina et al., 1991*). Even sources suggesting that this syndrome is not common agree that the most likely cause of entrapment is the nerve passing through a taut piriformis muscle (*Dawson et al., 1990*). Increased tension in the piriformis muscle leads to displacement of the sacroiliac joint, which, in turn, can lead to trigger points in this muscle.

Piriformis trigger points are located just at the lateral border at the sacrum as well as just under one-third of the way medial from the greater trochanter. They refer to the sacroiliac region, the buttocks and over the hip joint, sometimes extending over the proximal two-thirds of the posterior thigh. When piriformis trigger points are present, the muscle shortens and becomes bulkier, compressing the sciatic nerve. Pain from the nerve entrapment goes down the posterior thigh to the calf and sole of the foot. Therefore, pain can be experienced simultaneously from different sources.

Causes of piriformis syndrome are:

➤ **anomalies in the course of the nerve**, such as penetration of the piriformis muscle;

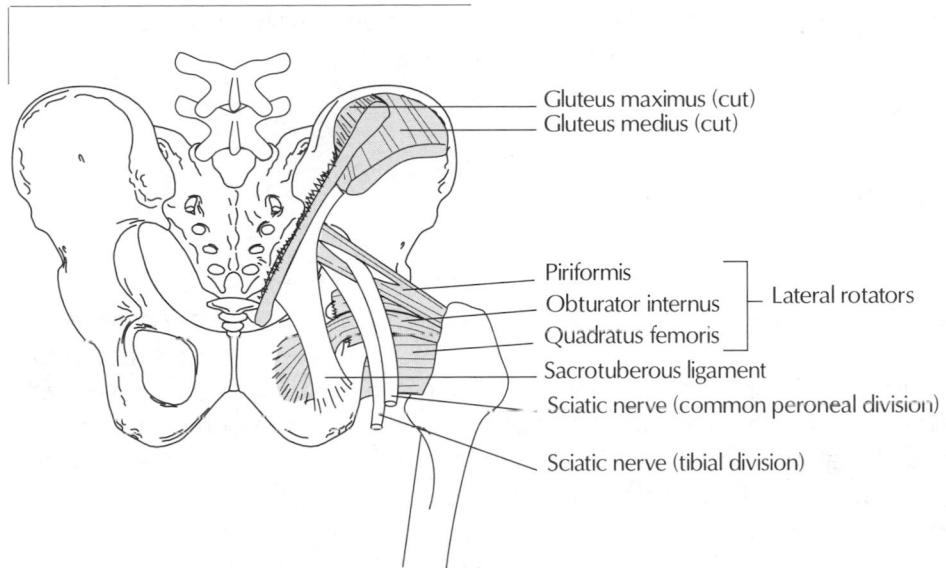

Figure 70.2
A variation of the sciatic nerve position in relation to the piriformis muscle. Here, the common peroneal nerve travels between the tendinous portions of the piriformis muscle.

> **direct and indirect trauma** to the piriformis, such as a fall on the buttocks or a motor vehicle accident. These types of trauma lead to inflammation, ischemia and spasms, eventually resulting in scar tissue, adhesions and trigger points. Travell states that one-third to one-half of passengers and drivers involved in accidents, especially drivers in a side-impact accident, had trigger points in piriformis *(Travell, Simons, 1992)*. Catching oneself from a fall, such as slipping while walking, can overload the muscle and cause trigger points or spasms;

> **inflammation** or degenerative changes of the piriformis muscle, its fascia or adjacent joints. These narrow the foramen and lead to scarring and adhesions. Some examples are arthritis of the hip joint and post-hip-replacement swelling;

> **overuse** of the piriformis muscle with repeated bending and lifting, forceful rotation with the weight on one leg, squatting while holding a weight as when putting down a heavy object or a strong lengthening contraction to restrain vigorous or rapid internal rotation, such as occurs with the thigh when jogging and using step machines;

> **postural and positional concerns**. Hyperpronation tends to increase internal rotation and adduction of the thigh during walking; the piriformis is overworked as it tries to control this excessive rotation. Flexion contracture or hyperlordosis can cause tension in muscles as they try to stabilize the pelvis. The tight, stretched muscles in the buttock push the nerve against the bone. This condition can occur in the third trimester of pregnancy due to the shift in the centre of gravity and the increased external rotation of the hip to accommodate the expanding abdomen. If the muscle is placed in a shortened position for a prolonged time, the piriformis becomes hypertonic and can compress the nerve. Examples of a shortened position are sitting with the knees abducted (often with the ankles together), sitting on one foot or driving a car for prolonged periods with a foot on the accelerator;

> anything that leads to, or aggravates, **trigger points**, which will, in turn, cause shortening of the muscle, such as sitting on a wallet in a back pocket.

Medical treatment includes corticosteroid injections and physiotherapy. Surgery is infrequently used; only in extreme cases is the sectioning of the tendon near the insertion of piriformis performed. Travell feels that, in many cases, trigger points are overlooked in the medical treatment of this condition.

Massage therapy focuses on the reduction of the compression, usually involving treatment of trigger points and a reduction of piriformis hypertonicity.

Symptom Picture

✦ Piriformis syndrome is usually unilateral. Pain is present from a variety of sources. Compression of the sciatic nerve results in pain and paresthesia in the posterior thigh, projecting to the calf and the sole of the foot. This is accompanied by numbness in the foot. There are differing opinions as to the presence of lumbosacral or gluteal pain with a sciatic nerve compression. This location of pain may, in fact, be caused by active piriformis and gluteal trigger points. If the compression is severe, there may be the loss of proprioception or muscle strength in the lower leg which could lead to an ataxic gait or drop foot. Entrapment of other nerves is possible.

✦ Pudendal nerve compression causes perineal and inguinal pain as well as dyspareunia (painful intercourse for women) and impotence in men (*Travell, Simons, 1992*).

✦ Compression of the gluteal nerve causes buttock pain, with possible gluteal atrophy. If sympathetic nerve branches are compressed, there are tissue changes in the skin and swelling in the lower limb.

✦ Active trigger points in piriformis result in pain in the low back, buttocks, hip and posterior thigh. Travell notes that there may occasionally be some pain in the inguinal area and at the greater trochanter.

✦ In cases of both nerve entrapment and active trigger points, the pain is increased by sitting or any position with prolonged hip flexion, adduction and medial rotation, by arising from a seated position or by standing. Symptoms are generally aggravated by activity. Any internal rotation of the hip will exacerbate symptoms, especially if the muscle is split and the nerve passes between its two bellies.

✦ Pain often decreases with external rotation of the hip.

✦ There is weakness in performing abduction, flexion and internal rotation of the affected hip.

✦ Sacroiliac joint dysfunction is often present due to shortening and tension in the piriformis muscle. This type of dysfunction can also be a cause of trigger points and nerve entrapment.

Subjective Information

HEALTH HISTORY QUESTIONS

✦ Is there a history of a systemic disorder, such as diabetes, rheumatoid arthritis or hypothyroidism? Is the client pregnant?

✦ Has the client seen a physician for a diagnosis? What tests were performed to determine the diagnosis?

✦ What parallel therapies, if any, has the client had, such as physiotherapy or chiropractic?

✦ Is the client taking any medication? Have cortisone injections been given? Has an injection been received in the last 10 days?

✦ How long has the client been experiencing discomfort?

✦ What is the sensation? "Numbness and tingling" down the leg is a common response.

✦ Where does the client experience pain or altered sensation? What is the quality of the pain? How intense is the pain or sensation? How frequent is it?

✦ What are the client's postural habits, including occupational, recreational and sleeping? Are there any positions or activities that aggravate the symptoms? What relieves the symptoms?

✦ Is there a history of injury to the hip, sacrum or low back?

Objective Information

Observations

✑ There is guarding of the limb on the affected side.

✑ Possibly an ataxic-like gait may be present due to pain.

✑ Difficulty due to pain with prolonged sitting or standing may be observed; the person may shift position frequently or have difficulty crossing the legs or moving from sitting to standing.

✑ During a postural assessment, torsion of the hips (due to sacroiliac joint dysfunction) and hyperlordosis of the lumbar spine may be noted.

✑ With the client supine, there is an excessive external rotation of the leg on the affected side (the foot is rotated laterally at least 45 degrees).

✑ Swelling may be observed in the lower limb.

✑ Rarely, hypotrophy of the gluteals is apparent with a compression of the gluteal nerves at the greater sciatic foramen (*Mumenthaler, Schliack, 1991*).

859

Palpation

✍ Trigger points are palpated in the piriformis muscle, specifically along the sacrum or just medial to the greater trochanter. They may also be present in the gluteals. Hypertonicity is found in these same muscles. If hyperlordosis is a contributing factor, iliopsoas, quadriceps and quadratus lumborum are hypertonic and may have trigger points.

✍ There is tenderness on palpation of the greater sciatic foramen and piriformis muscle.

✍ Adhesions in, and scarring on, the buttocks may be present.

✍ Swelling may be apparent at the piriformis or in the lower limb.

✍ Rarely, hypotrophy may be palpated in the gluteals.

Testing

✍ **AF and PR ROM** of the hip reveal decreased internal rotation accompanied by pain on the affected side.

✍ **AR strength testing** of piriformis is positive for weakness and pain on the affected side.

Special Tests

✍ **The pace abduction test** is positive.

✍ **The piriformis length test** is positive for a short piriformis on the affected side.

✍ **Sacroiliac joint motion palpation** may reveal restricted movement on the affected side.

Differentiating Sources of Radiating Buttock Pain:

✍ **Compression of the nerve at the lumbar spine** from a herniated disc may also be referred to as sciatica. Sources do not agree as to which location is most common for the nerve compression — the lumbar spine or the piriformis. Symptoms are numbness and tingling which radiate to the lateral foot and the small toe (S1 nerve root compression) or to the dorsum of the foot (L5 nerve root compression) or to the medial calf (L4 nerve root compression). The following tests are likely positive: Valsalva's, Kemp's, Kernig's, slump, straight leg raise or Lasegue's test and deep tendon reflexes. Weakness and difficulty are apparent in the performance of repeated toe walking (S1), heel walking (L5) or one-sided deep knee bends (L3 to 4).

✍ **Lumbar spinal stenosis** results in progressive pain, usually bilateral, in the calf and foot brought on by walking and relieved by lying down.

✍ **Facet joint irritation** will yield a positive Kemp's test. Palpation of the piriformis will not be painful.

✍ **Inflammatory arthritides**, such as ankylosing spondylitis (usually bilateral pain), have similar symptoms to both nerve entrapment and trigger points. Assessment is made medically by X-ray and other diagnostic tests.

Contraindications

✦ Do not massage locally for 10 days after a cortisone injection.

✦ Avoid compression of the sciatic nerve when massaging the buttocks. This precaution is especially of concern when using the elbow at the lateral border of the sacrum. If the client experiences numbness and tingling down the leg to the foot, this could indicate compression of the nerve and the technique is stopped.

✦ Do not perform frictions if the client is on anti-inflammatories.

✦ Joint play, along with hip and sacral mobilizations, are avoided in the third trimester of pregnancy and performed with extreme caution with osteoarthritis or with a degenerative condition affecting the hip or sacrum.

Treatment Goals

Treat soft tissue and compensatory structures.

Treatment Plan

🖑 The treatment strategy considers the actual cause of the sciatic nerve compression. If it is a systemic condition or pregnancy, massage will not remove the cause but will treat soft tissue and compensatory structures and will increase relaxation to give temporary relief. Massage is very effective when treating piriformis syndrome that results from soft tissue causes, such as hypertonicity and trigger points, and from altered posture, such as hyperlordosis.

🖑 Although the piriformis muscle is the main source of the compression, the treatment strategy is to address the lumbar spine and entire pelvic girdle, including any postural compensation or contributing factors. Edema or ischemia in the foot and leg is more effectively treated after the compression is relieved in the buttocks.

🖑 This is a potentially painful treatment which may recreate symptoms temporarily. Symptoms should decrease as the massage proceeds or when pressure is released.

🖑 The therapist should take care in using the elbow on the gluteal area because of the possibility of injuring the sciatic nerve. Prolonged pressure from the elbow could result in nerve damage (*Travell, Simons, 1992*). Using the elbow should not cause problems near the greater trochanter but if numbness and tingling occur below the knee, pressure should be removed. Tingling could signal compression of the nerve.

🖑 **Positioning** is in the prone or sidelying position for the specific treatment. The client is pillowed for comfort, with additional pillows under the ankles if edema is present. If possible, the leg should be placed in a neutral position and not in excessive external rotation. This can be done by grasping the ankle and gently tractioning the leg while bringing it into alignment. A towel can be tucked in on the lateral side of the thigh to secure the position. If sidelying is used, a pillow is

861

Treatment Goals Treatment Plan

placed between the thighs and knees to keep the leg and hip in a neutral position.

✋ When treating the piriformis, **draping** over the gluteals should allow access to as much of the buttock as is comfortable for the client. When the therapist obtains consent to treatment, it can be proposed that the client not wear underwear during the treatment. In such a case, extremely precise and secure draping is required. The gluteal cleft is never exposed. A towel can be used just distal to the iliac crest to secure the sheet from slipping down.

✋ **Hydrotherapy** includes deep moist heat over the affected buttock while massaging the lumbar region. If edema is present, cool towel wraps are used over the affected area. Contrast applications can be used post-treatment to improve circulation and flush metabolites.

General Treatment

Decrease sympathetic nervous system firing. Treat any compensatory structures.

✋ Throughout the treatment, a relaxation focus is important. This is achieved through encouragement of **diaphragmatic breathing** and use of soothing circulatory strokes interspersed with the more specific and painful techniques.

✋ If hyperlordosis is a contributing factor, the treatment is started with the client **supine**. The therapist addresses the hypertonic iliopsoas and rectus femoris before turning the client prone. Joint play is used on a hypomobile sacroiliac joint. If hyperlordosis is not a concern, the treatment is started in the **prone** or **sidelying** position. The latter position is obviously used if the client is in the third trimester of pregnancy. The lower back is massaged using effleurage and petrissage as well as mobilization techniques to the lumbar spine. The quadratus lumborum is treated thoroughly for hypertonicity and trigger points, especially if hyperlordosis is present. If pes planus is a contributing factor, specific treatment of this condition is incorporated. See the hyperlordosis or pes planus chapter for details.

Specific Treatment

Decrease compression on the sciatic nerve. Reduce fascial restrictions.

✋ Over the gluteals, skin rolling can be attempted. A technique that works well in this area is using one hand to form a C-shape, while the fingers of the other hand drag the fascia into the concave part of the C in short strokes. The fascial techniques are systematically applied over the entire buttock.

Reduce pain, hypertonicity and trigger points.

✋ The buttock is massaged using petrissage, such as scooping and fingertip kneading. The strokes are applied along the iliac crest and the sacrum and around the greater trochanter. The gluteals, especially the gluteus maximus, are treated thoroughly so the piriformis can be

Treatment Goals   Treatment Plan

reached through it. Trigger points in gluteus maximus refer locally into the buttock, along the sacroiliac joint and superior to the ischial tuberosity. Trigger points in the posterior fibres of gluteus medius refer over the sacrum, along the sacroiliac joint and the posterior crest of the ilium and into the mid-gluteal area. The minimus trigger points refer locally and to the posterolateral thigh *(Travell, Simons 1992)*.

The piriformis muscle is palpated deep to gluteus maximus. To landmark the attachments, the posterior superior iliac spine is palpated on the unaffected side and a line is imagined between it and the greater trochanter on the affected side. The piriformis will lie along this line. To ensure that the muscle is being reached, the therapist places his fingertips where the piriformis is thought to be and the client is asked to resist external rotation of the hip. The therapist should feel the piriformis muscle contract. The muscle is treated using the origin and insertion technique, scooping and progressively deeper fingertip kneading and muscle stripping. Trigger points are palpated near the insertion at the sacrum and one-third of the way medially from the greater trochanter. These are treated using ischemic compression or other appropriate techniques. The massage is followed with an application of heat and a stretch to the piriformis muscle.

The sacrotuberous ligament is treated with muscle stripping and cross-fibre fingertip kneading, starting at the ischial tuberosity and moving superiorly towards the sacrum.

Maintain range of motion.

Passive movement in external and internal rotation is performed on the hip, with the knee flexed to 90 degrees. A stretch to the external rotators, which includes piriformis, can be incorporated into this movement. The therapist's hand is formed into a loose fist. Short, specific strokes are applied around, and medial to, the greater trochanter. A slow, rhythmical internal and external rotation of the hip is performed. Moderate pressure is applied to the muscles as the leg is brought towards the therapist (into internal rotation) and released when the leg is moved away from the therapist (external rotation). The therapist takes care not to torque his wrist and not to apply pressure on the greater trochanter laterally and the sciatic nerve medially.

PIR is also used. The piriformis muscle may be difficult for the client to focus on. For a more effective stretch, the muscle is palpated and the client is educated about its location and action. With the knee flexed, the client is asked to inhale and contract the muscle against the therapist's resistance. After six to 10 seconds the client exhales and relaxes the muscle. The muscle is then stretched by picking up the slack and drawing the hip into internal rotation. This is repeated three times. If there is a history of knee or hip injury, the stretch is performed supine or an easily controlled self-stretch is prescribed.

Treatment Goals

Treatment Plan

- • **Eye movement** can be incorporated by having the client look up with inhalation and contraction, and look down with exhalation and relaxation. Intermittent applications of cold can be added to the relaxation phase.

- An **agonist contraction** stretch has the client contract the internal rotators against resistance, allowing no movement. After the muscles are relaxed, the hip is pulled into internal rotation.

- **A supine stretch** used with an otherwise healthy client requires the hip and knees to be flexed. The client's anterior thigh of the affected side rests on the abdomen. This knee is then slowly extended and adducted. A more gentle supine stretch has the hip and knee extended on the unaffected side. On the affected side, the hip and knee are flexed and the foot is placed on the lateral side of the opposite extended knee. The therapist stands on the side to be stretched. While stabilizing the hip on the same side with one hand, the thigh is abducted — pushed away from the therapist — with the other hand.

Reduce edema, if present.

- Lymphatic drainage techniques are applied to the leg, including sacral and popliteal pumping, unidirectional effleurage and stationary circles.

Improve tissue health and circulation.

- The entire lower limb and buttock are massaged using effleurage and petrissage techniques. Passive movement is performed at the knee and ankle.

Self-care Goals

Self-care Plan

- Remedial exercise is an essential component to treating piriformis syndrome.

Stretch tight, short muscles.

- The client can perform a self-stretch for the piriformis muscle using a belt or rope (*Figure 70.3*). The client lies supine on the floor with the rope looped around the foot of the affected side. The ends of the rope are held in the opposite hand. On the side to be stretched, the knee is extended and the hip is flexed to approximately 90 degrees. The hips are kept stable on the floor while the leg is drawn away from the side to be stretched towards the opposite hip. The stretch is held for 30 seconds. The leg is then drawn farther towards the opposite hip, placing an additional stretch on the piriformis muscle.

- For a standing self-stretch, the client places the foot of the affected side on a chair, with the hip flexed to 90 degrees and the thigh parallel to the floor. The client

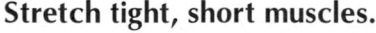
Pull leg to left side

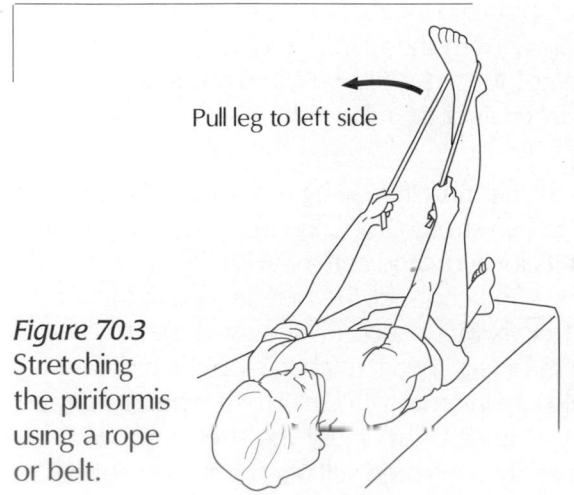

Figure 70.3
Stretching the piriformis using a rope or belt.

Self-care Goals

Self-care Plan

bends at the waist with the arms loosely reaching towards the floor. The stretch is held for 30 seconds. Then the muscle is stretched farther by bending deeper at the waist and increasing the reach towards the floor.

✎ A tennis ball is used on gluteal and piriformis trigger points. While lying on the floor or standing against a wall, the ball is placed over the trigger point and the client leans into it. She will experience tolerable discomfort. The referral pattern appropriate to the specific trigger point will likely occur. This position is held until the discomfort resolves. The client is advised to avoid compression of the sciatic nerve. This is indicated by numbness and tingling down the back of the leg to below the knee.

Strengthen weak muscles.

✎ To strengthen a weak muscle in a sidelying position on the unaffected side, the client flexes the hip and knee 90 degrees. If possible, someone assists with the exercise by passively abducting the leg. Then the client lowers the thigh slowly to the floor. This is an eccentric or lengthening contraction. It is followed with a concentric or shortening contraction by actively abducting the thigh against gravity.

Educate the client.

✎ Sitting positions are modified. The client should avoid sitting on the foot and rolling the knees out to the side but instead should keep the knees and feet in midline. Frequent changes of position are encouraged; a rocking chair is recommended.

✎ Sleeping positions are modified. A pillow is placed between the knees when the client sleeps sidelying to avoid excessive adduction of the hip, which can aggravate the shortened muscle and wake the person.

✎ Frequent breaks, during any aggravating activity, are taken with stretching or a brief walk performed every hour. Frequent breaks and stretching or walking are also necessary when driving long distances.

✎ Activities such as tennis, volleyball, running and using a stairmaster require pre- and post-stretching of piriformis, since these sports can easily activate trigger points. If symptoms are acute, the client may require a prolonged break from the specific sport until symptoms are less severe.

Refer the client.

✎ Chiropractic adjustments may be necessary if there is sacroiliac joint dysfunction. Orthotics may be required if pes planus and hyperpronation are present.

Encourage relaxation.

✎ Educate the client about full diaphragmatic breathing. Yoga and Tai Chi may help with relaxation and stretching.

Treatment Frequency and Expected Outcome

A one-hour treatment allows a thorough treatment of the lower body. The treatment focus is alternated between the piriformis syndrome and aspects of a contributing condition, such as hyperlordosis or pes planus. Initially, treatments are more frequent, ideally twice a week for a few weeks. Otherwise, once a week for four to six weeks is recommended, followed by a thorough reassessment.

See also pregnancy, diabetes mellitus, myofascial trigger points, peripheral nerve lesions (sciatic nerve), inflammatory arthritides, hyperlordosis and pes planus for related conditions.

If pregnancy is the cause, the condition will often resolve postpartum. Only temporary relief is possible if a systemic pathology is present.

If the cause involves soft tissue, the prognosis is good, providing the client is compliant with the self-care program.

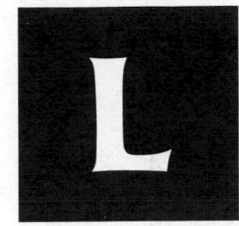

RESPIRATORY PATHOLOGIES

71

SINUSITIS

Fiona Rattray

Sinusitis is an acute or chronic inflammation of the paranasal sinuses.

The nasal passage twists around the nasal turbinates, a series of baffles that mix and warm the air as it is inhaled. Before curving down to the pharynx, the passages open into sinuses in the frontal, ethmoid, sphenoid and maxillary bones. The sinuses are air-filled continuations of the nasal passages, lined with mucous membranes. These membranes are thinner than the rest of the nasal membranes and are loosely attached to the bones.

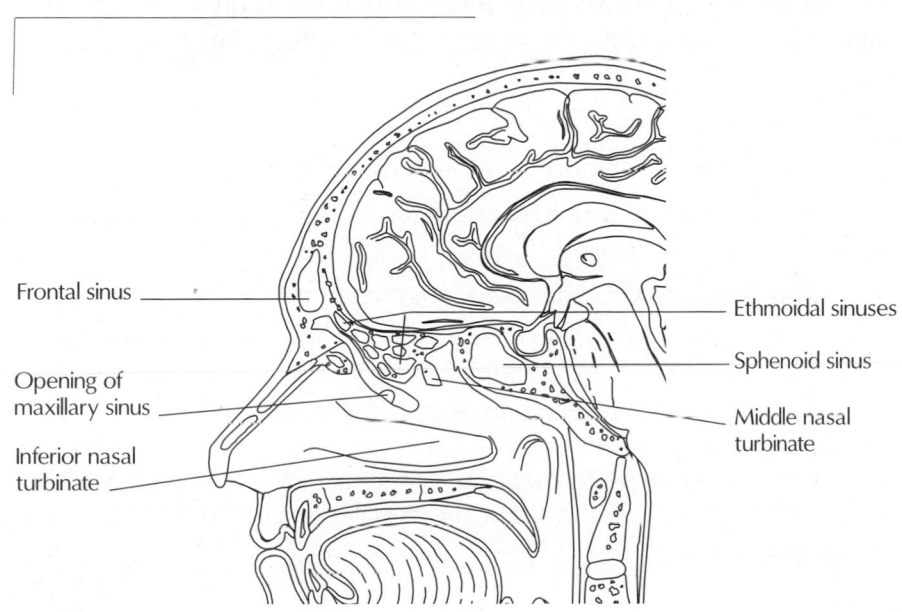

Frontal sinus

Opening of maxillary sinus

Inferior nasal turbinate

Ethmoidal sinuses

Sphenoid sinus

Middle nasal turbinate

Figure 71.1
Frontal, ethmoidal and sphenoid sinuses.

The sinuses, which develop mostly after birth, are outgrowths of the nasal cavities (*Figure 71.1*). They continue to enlarge into adulthood. The frontal sinuses appear on X-rays by seven years of age (*Moore, 1985*). They vary from five millimetres (pea-sized) to larger hollows that stretch almost to the sphenoid bones. The frontal sinuses drain into ducts that empty into the top of the nasal cavity. The ethmoidal sinuses are a variable number of small cells that empty into the lateral portions of the nasal

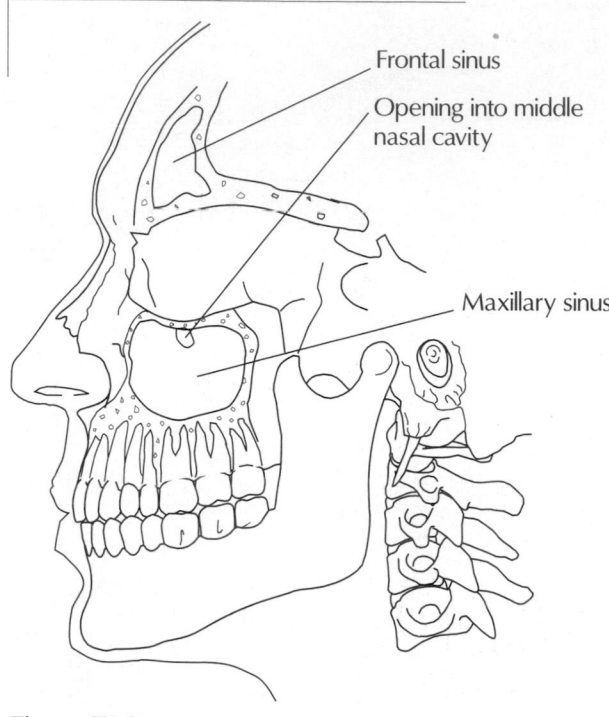

Figure 71.2
Maxillary sinus, lateral view.

Labels: Frontal sinus; Opening into middle nasal cavity; Maxillary sinus

cavity. These sinuses appear between two and eight years of age. The two sinuses in the sphenoid bone are relatively large, making the walls of the sphenoid bone itself thin. They drain into posterior portions of the nasal cavity. Sphenoid sinuses appear after two years of age.

The largest sinuses are the maxillary ones. These sinuses are present at birth and continue growing up to 25 years of age, when all the permanent teeth have erupted. The roots of the upper molars are close to the floor of the maxillary sinus. This sinus drains superiorly to the nasal cavity (*Figure 71.2*). If the head is held upright it is impossible for the sinus to drain until it is full. The head must be horizontal to completely drain the maxillary sinus.

With acute sinusitis, there is inflammation and swelling of the sinus mucosa. The sinus openings become blocked. A mucopurulent discharge is produced, which fills the affected sinus. Chronic sinusitis occurs as a result of persistent or recurrent infection. The mucosal lining thickens and may form into elongated masses called polyps. In rare cases, due to the proximity of the meninges, complications of sinusitis may occur, such as meningitis or a brain abscess.

Causes of sinusitis are:

➤ **viral infection** from a cold virus, **bacterial infection** from the extraction of upper molars or a molar root abscess, or an **increase in pressure,** such as during an airplane flight or underwater diving, which causes the forcible entry of infected material into the sinuses *(Cawson et al., 1989)*.

Predisposing factors are:

➤ **deviation of the nasal septum** which obstructs the sinus outlets;

➤ **dairy and wheat products** which may predispose to an overproduction of mucus in people who have sensitivities to these foods *(Davis, 1988)*;

➤ an **upper molar abscess** which may spread infection to the maxillary sinus.

Medically, sinusitis is treated with analgesics and decongestants. However, prolonged use or overuse of medication, including over-the-counter remedies, can lead to worsening of the symptoms. Prolonged use of medication can damage the tissues and the mucosa may respond to overmedication by producing more mucus in a rebound effect *(Kunz, Finkel, 1987)*. In chronic cases, surgery may be performed. An additional opening may be made to drain the sinus, the mucous lining may be removed or the deviated septum may be corrected to open the passage.

Symptom Picture

✦ The symptoms of acute sinusitis are pain, often severe, and tenderness over the affected sinus. Pain from frontal infections is above the eyes and it increases when the person bends forward. Pain from maxillary infections is across the cheeks. Pain from sphenoidal or ethmoidal infections is referred to the side or back of the cranium. There may be a headache or the sensation of a toothache.

✦ There is a feeling of fullness and pressure in the affected sinus and the person has difficulty breathing through the nose. The person feels ill and may have a low-grade fever. Nasal discharge changes from clear and runny to yellow or green and thick. Infection may spread from one sinus to another because the nasal mucosa is continuous.

✦ With chronic sinusitis, the pain is dull. The discharge may stop entirely as the sinuses remain blocked.

Contraindications

✦ Massage is contraindicated with fever.

✦ Local lymphatic drainage is contraindicated with acute infection.

Treatment Considerations

Assessment

✎ **Palpation** of the frontal sinuses is made by the therapist gently pressing superiorly at the medial angle of the superior orbital margin. The maxillary sinuses are palpated under the zygomatic arch. Tenderness and, possibly, heat are present. The lymphatic nodes in the neck may be enlarged.

✎ **Testing** by transillumination of the sinuses may reveal blockage.

Massage

🖐 The treatment is a half hour in duration to avoid exhausting the client. The treatment is in the context of a relaxation massage including unforced **diaphragmatic breathing.**

🖐 The **pre-treatment hydrotherapy** is a five-minute facial steam. This makes the mucus more liquid and aids in drainage. Adding five drops of pure, undiluted essential oil to the water is beneficial. Suggested essential oils are eucalyptus, cajeput, tea tree or thyme to treat infection, while lavender may also help to reduce pain *(Lawless, 1995; Davis, 1988).* When essential oils are used in an inhalation, the client closes the eyes to avoid irritation from the oils. Plenty of disposable facial tissues and a wastebasket should be on hand for the client throughout the facial steam and treatment.

🖐 **Positioning** may be prone, sidelying or supine. The prone position allows draining of bilaterally affected maxillary sinuses. Sidelying, with the affected sinus uppermost, is the best position for draining a single infected maxillary sinus. The supine position may allow the other sinuses to drain.

🖐 The **prone** position is a good drainage position but pressure on the affected sinuses from a face cradle may be painful; it may be necessary for the client to turn the head to one side. The treatment includes general soothing Swedish work to the shoulders and upper thoracic area. Trigger points in upper trapezius refer into the temporal region.

- **Supine** treatment for chronic sinusitis may incorporate lymphatic drainage techniques on the neck. This is performed for a short period of time and the client is monitored for signs of an acute flare-up of symptoms. If this occurs, the technique is discontinued. However, if there is no flare-up, the time spent doing drainage techniques is slowly increased over several treatments and the site of the infection is gradually included (*Kurz, 1990*).

- Soothing Swedish techniques, such as effleurage, stroking and fingertip kneading, are used on the pectorals and posterior neck muscles to reduce hypertonicity. Petrissage is used on the muscles of mastication, facial muscles, scalp and suboccipitals. Trigger points are treated with muscle stripping and gentle ischemic compressions.

- Trigger points in sternocleidomastoid refer pain across the forehead and around the eyes and ears. Trigger points in masseter refer into the maxilla and frontal bone. Trigger points in temporalis refer into the teeth and above the eyes and ears. Lateral pterygoid trigger points refer into the zygoma and anterior to the ear (*Travell, Simons, 1983*).

- After the facial steam and positioning have allowed some drainage to occur, gentle static fingertip compressions to the client's pain tolerance are used over the affected sinuses. These compressions may give relief from the feeling of congestion. Light fingertip tapping may also be used. Care is taken as the area may be tender.

- The head, neck and shoulder massage is finished with passive range of motion, gentle long-axis traction or Golgi tendon organ release to the occiput.

- Although it is part of a regular routine following any treatment, it is especially important with this treatment to spray and wipe down the table and face cradle with antiseptic cleanser, and for the therapist to thoroughly wash the hands with antiseptic soap.

Self-care

- Self-care includes facial steams (up to five a day) and vaporizers.

- The client should be taught how to blow the nose properly. Using a clean tissue or handkerchief, the client clears the nostrils one at a time. The other nostril is kept shut by pressing on that side of the nose. Holding both nostrils partially shut at the same time should be avoided, as this prevents a clear passage. The client should not blow too hard, as this may spread the infection through the eustachian tubes to the ears (*Kunz, Finkel, 1987*). Self-massage of the facial muscles and pressure points over the sinuses is also indicated.

See also tension headache for a related treatment.

- The client is **referred** to a physician or dentist for assessment if the infection worsens or does not resolve. A naturopath can help with strengthening the immune system and reducing the infection.

72

CHRONIC BRONCHITIS

Fiona Rattray

Chronic bronchitis is a condition that results in the production of purulent sputum for at least three months in a row over two consecutive years.

Chronic bronchitis is more common in males and in individuals over 40 years of age. Between 10 and 25 per cent of adults are affected with the disease (Irwin, Tecklin, 1995). Although there is a significant association with cigarette smoking, not all people with chronic bronchitis smoke.

There are two sources of bronchial mucus: the bronchial glands and the epithelial goblet cells which line the bronchial walls. In chronic bronchitis, there is an enlargement of the mucus-secreting bronchial glands and an increase in the number of epithelial goblet cells (Irwin, Tecklin, 1995). There is also a decrease in the number of ciliated epithelial cells which help to mobilize and remove mucus.

Airways become chronically inflamed from ongoing irritation, such as from cigarette smoke which leads to edema and thickening, or hyperplasia, of the bronchial walls. Airways become obstructed due to an increase in bronchial mucus and the increase in size of the bronchial glands. This results in decreased expiratory airflow rates and prolonged expiration. The person may wheeze. Severe productive coughing, dyspnea (laboured, distressed breathing) and bouts of respiratory infection develop. As the disease progresses, the person has less and less tolerance for exercise and eventually has no physical reserve left for times of stress. Even eating becomes exhausting.

Blockage of the airways leads to insufficient oxygenation in the alveoli. Cyanosis (a bluish tinge to the skin) occurs due to reduced oxygenation and general peripheral edema results from ventricular failure. The person with chronic bronchitis tends to retain weight, in contrast to those with emphysema, who tend to be thin. A person with combined cyanosis, edema and weight retention is called a "blue bloater". Another term is "non-fighter", since the person with chronic bronchitis does not compensate for obstructed airways by increasing ventilation or fighting for air *(Porth, 1990)*. For reasons not clearly understood, the ends of the fingers become bulbous or clubbed. Over time, severe chronic bronchitis can lead to pulmonary hypertension, right-sided heart failure (cor pulmonale) and death.

Chronic obstructive pulmonary disease (COPD) is a combination of chronic bronchitis and emphysema. This most commonly occurs in people who smoke.

A person with chronic bronchitis may be taking different medications. Various antibiotics may be prescribed with bacterial infections. Robitussin and Benylin E are expectorants. Bronkosol is a bronchodilator. Beclovent is a corticosteroid used to suppress the inflammation present with COPD.

Causes of chronic bronchitis are:

➤ **smoking**, which results in airway inflammation that is thought to trigger the specific pathological changes seen in the airway goblet cells and epithelium;

➤ **environmental factors** including air pollution and occupational exposure to inhaled particles or fumes.

The Respiratory Tract and Lungs

In the upper respiratory tract, air flows through the nasal cavity and pharynx where it is warmed and humidified. The air is filtered and particles are removed by mucosa and cilia. In the lower respiratory tract, air is transported to the alveoli where gas exchange takes place. Ventilation is the air exchange from atmosphere to alveoli, as opposed to respiration, which is the blood transport and exchange of gases at the alveolar capillary membrane *(Vander et al., 1994)*.

The trachea branches into the left and right main bronchi at the level of the second rib anteriorly and T5 posteriorly *(Figure 72.1)*. The bronchi supply the left and right lungs through a further division into lobar and segmental bronchi. The bronchi divide into bronchioles, then into terminal bronchioles, respiratory bronchioles and finally alveoli. The trachea and bronchi are well supplied with mucus-producing cells and ciliated cells, which line the airways to the level of the respiratory bronchioles *(Vander et al., 1994)*.

The left lung is divided into two lobes. The division or fissure between the left upper and lower lobes runs obliquely from the fifth rib anteriorly to T3 posteriorly. The right lung is divided into three lobes, the upper, middle and lower. The fissure between the upper and middle lobes runs obliquely from the third rib anteriorly to T3 posteriorly. The fissure between the smaller middle lobe and the lower lobe runs obliquely from rib six anteriorly to rib five at the level of the lateral border of the scapula.

When the diaphragm is relaxed, the left dome of the diaphragm is at the level of rib five, while the right dome is slightly higher, at the level of the intercostal space between ribs four and five.

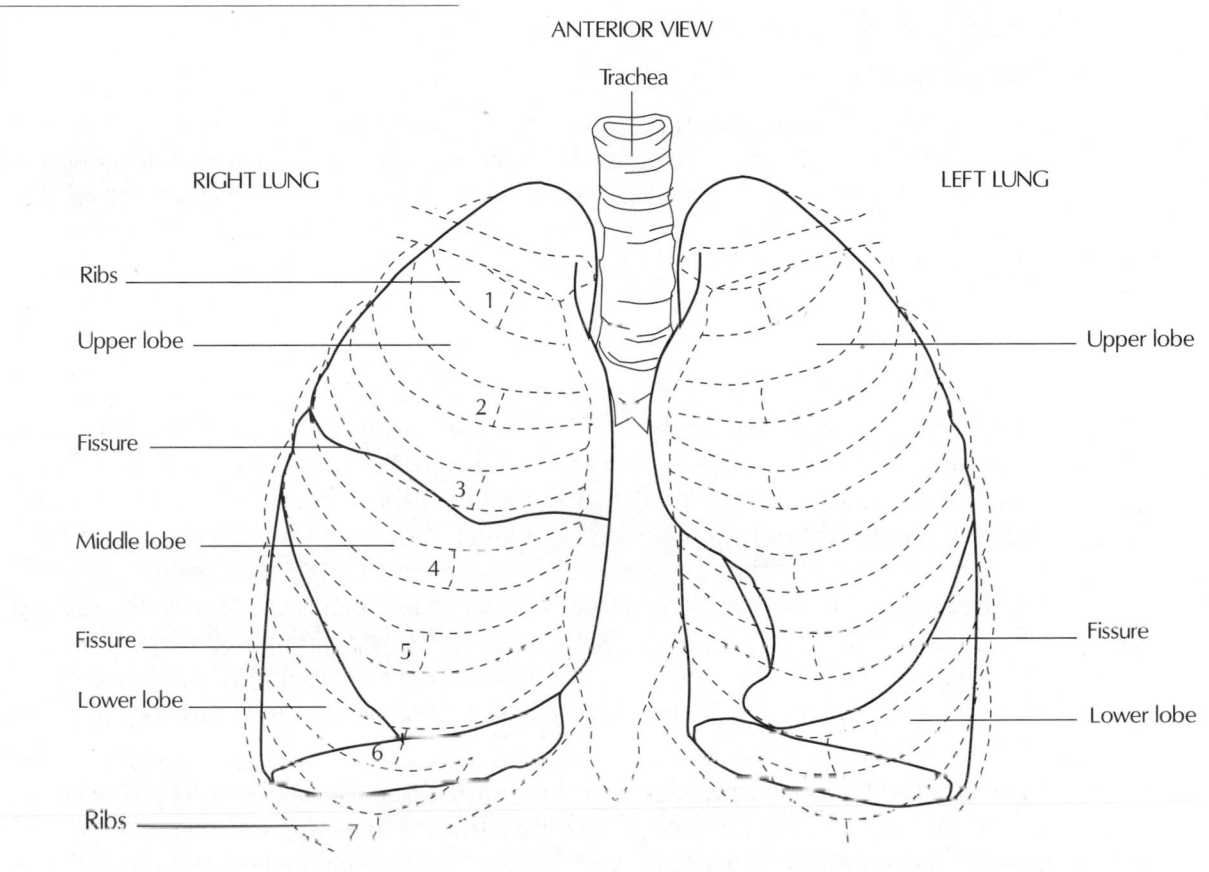

ANTERIOR VIEW

Trachea

RIGHT LUNG

LEFT LUNG

Ribs

Upper lobe

Upper lobe

Fissure

Middle lobe

Fissure

Fissure

Lower lobe

Lower lobe

Ribs

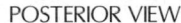

POSTERIOR VIEW

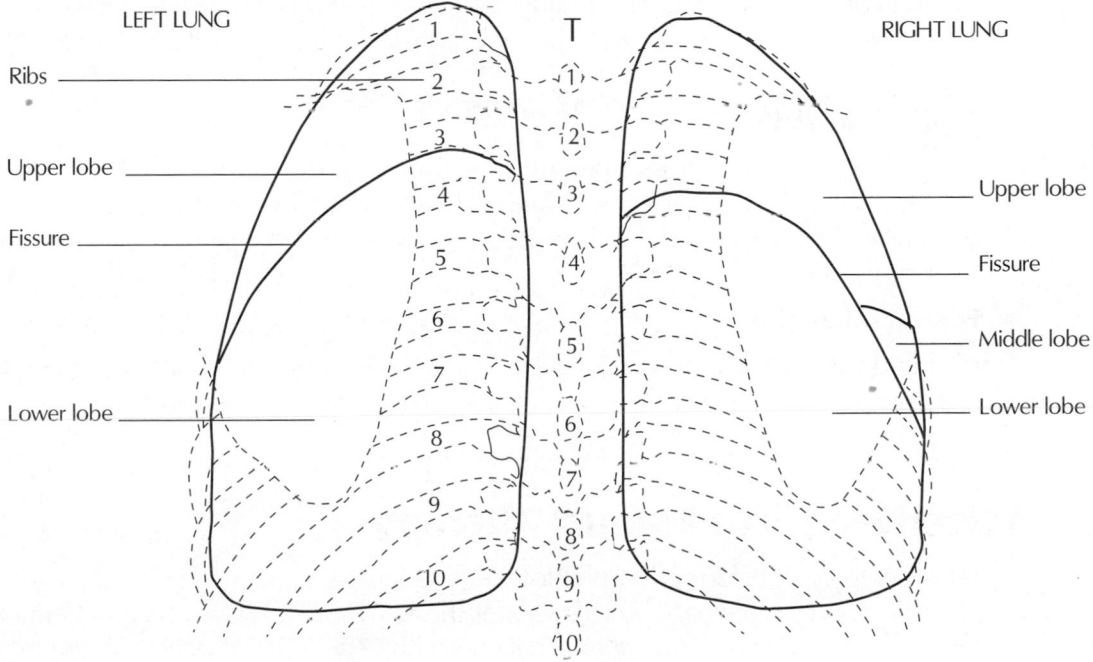

LEFT LUNG

RIGHT LUNG

T

Ribs

Upper lobe

Upper lobe

Fissure

Fissure

Middle lobe

Lower lobe

Lower lobe

Figure 72.1
Lobes and fissures of the lungs. Sternum, ribs and vertebrae are dotted lines.

Muscles of Respiration

✦ **Resting Inhalation**

During resting inhalation, the diaphragm contracts and flattens. The external intercostals contract, lifting the ribs. This increases the anteroposterior and transverse dimensions of the thorax. The thoracic volume increases and the pressure in the lungs decreases. This causes air to move into the lungs. The scalenes elevate the first two ribs, becoming active towards the end of resting inhalation and increasingly so with deep or forced inhalation *(Basmajian, 1985)*. The average adult breathes 10 to 12 times per minute at rest *(Zadai, 1992)*.

✦ **Forced Inhalation**

With forced inhalation, the diaphragm descends at least three to four intercostal spaces *(Irwin, Tecklin, 1995)*. With deep or forced inhalation, the accessory muscles of inhalation are recruited. The sternocleidomastoids lift the sternum only when the head and neck are upright or hyperextended, not when they are flexed *(Basmajian, 1985)*. Subclavius elevates the first rib when the clavicle is fixed. Levator costarum muscles lift the ribs posteriorly and superiorly. Serratus posterior superior muscles raise the second through fifth ribs, while latissimus dorsi fibres raise ribs nine through 12 *(Kendall et al., 1993)*. Pectoralis major raises the sternum and second to sixth ribs, while pectoralis minor lifts the third through fifth ribs. With activity, the average adult breathes 50 times a minute *(Zadai, 1992)*.

Some sources *(Kisner, Colby, 1990; Pansky, 1979)* assign an accessory inhalation function to upper trapezius, stating that it fixes the scapula, allowing the pectoral muscles and serratus anterior to move the ribs. Others question this function *(Basmajian, 1985; Travell, Simons, 1992)*. Nevertheless, upper trapezius is tight in those suffering from respiratory dysfunctions, especially asthma *(Lewit, 1993)*. The respiratory function of serratus anterior is similarly disputed *(Kendall et al., 1993)*. Iliocostalis lumborum become active with both forced inhalation and exhalation *(Travell, Simons, 1983)*.

✦ **Relaxed Exhalation**

Relaxed expiration is a passive process. The diaphragm relaxes upward into a domed shape and the external intercostals and scalenes relax, allowing the ribs to drop. This decreases the thoracic volume. The pressure in the lungs increases, pushing air out of the lungs.

✦ **Forced Exhalation**

In forced exhalation, as when coughing, the internal intercostals contract, pulling the ribs downward. Rectus abdominus, internal and external obliques and quadratus lumborum are also recruited.

Effectiveness of Manual Therapy

Manual therapy, as performed by physiotherapists, includes joint manipulation, mobilizations and stretching. Combinations of these techniques have proven effective in increasing peak expiratory flow rates in patients with COPD. Seven patients were treated for 30 minutes, twice a week for three weeks. Mobilization of the thoracic spine and costovertebral joints, as well as stretching of the intercostals, resulted in improved lung function after one treatment. The forced expiratory volume in one second (FEV1) is a measurement used to determine the reversibility in COPD. While manual therapy did not produce an increase in FEV1, the maximum oxygen uptake showed an increase of 20 per cent *(Pryor, 1991)*. High-velocity, low-amplitude thrust manipulation techniques are outside the scope of practice for massage therapists. However, joint play techniques (mobilizations) and stretching are part of the therapist's mandate and can be effectively used to mobilize the thorax.

Effectiveness of Respiratory Physical Therapy

Respiratory physical therapy, as performed by physiotherapists, has two groups of techniques. Five modalities designed to improve mucociliary clearance, to increase the volume of expectorated sputum and to improve the function of the airways are *postural drainage, cough, tapotement* (called "percussion" by physiotherapists), *vibrations* and *shaking*. Modalities designed to relieve dyspnea and improve efficiency of ventilation and respiratory function are *diaphragmatic breathing, segmental breathing* and *pursed-lip breathing*.

In the past few years, physiotherapists have debated the effectiveness of various techniques *(Kisner, Colby, 1996; Rochester, Goldberg, 1980)*. Part of this debate seems to stem from inconsistencies within the literature due to inconsistent terminology, comparison of one technique to a series of techniques and diverse populations (healthy, unhealthy, young, elderly) used in various studies. Also, mechanical devices ranging from vibrating machines to padded anesthesia masks (used for cupping tapotement) have been used to perform techniques in various studies, along with manual tapotement, making comparisons difficult *(Zadai, 1992)*.

✦ **Postural drainage** aligns the affected bronchial segment with gravity to assist in removing secretions. It has been extensively studied both as a technique by itself and in combination with tapotement. It appears that postural drainage combined with tapotement and cough enhances mucociliary transport better than drainage alone *(Irwin, Tecklin, 1995)*. Postural drainage is described in the treatment plan section of this chapter.

✦ **Productive cough** produced a greater amount of sputum than postural drainage or exercise alone in a study of eight patients with chronic bronchitis *(Oldenberg et al., 1979)*. The rate of airflow in a cough can be as high as 115 kilometres per hour. Productive cough and its variations (huffing and the forced expiratory technique) are described later in the self-care section.

✦ **Percussion (tapotement)** is used to loosen mucus secretions so they can be expectorated more easily. In one study, the technique has been associated with a minor bronchospasm that lasts for 20 to 30 minutes. This transient brochospasm can be alleviated by the person using her regularly prescribed bronchodilator medication 30 to 60 minutes before percussion *(Irwin, Tecklin, 1995; Dettenmeier, 1992)*. The study in question found a small (130 ml.) decrease in forced expiratory volume after percussion in seven of 17 patients with chronic bronchitis. The decrease spontaneously corrected in 20 minutes *(Campbell et al., 1975)*. This study is contrasted with results of percussion on 11 children with mild to moderate asthma where the forced expiratory volume *increased* 10.3 per cent half an hour after treatment *(Rochester, Goldberg, 1980)*.

When viewed with fibre optic bronchoscopy, percussion showed a "spattering of plugs" which blocked the bronchi *(Barnes, 1988)*. **Vibrations and shaking** were noted as increasing peripheral secretion clearance in some studies, as well as increasing sputum production *(Zadai, 1992)*.

✦ The **combination** of postural drainage, cough and tapotement was shown in another study to clear five times the mucus from the central and peripheral regions than was cleared on days when this therapy was not administered *(Bateman et al., 1979)*. It is often concluded that postural drainage is more effective with abundant secretions (more than 30 ml. per day) than with scanty secretions *(Irwin, Tecklin, 1995; Rochester, Goldberg 1980)*. However, even in patients with stable chronic bronchitis and lower production of secretions, 5.5 ml. of sputum were produced during postural drainage and percussion *(May, Munt, 1979)*. While a relationship between increased volume of sputum produced and improvement in airway function has not been proven *(Rochester, Goldberg, 1980)*, there is a decreased chance for infection if mucus is removed promptly *(Hough, 1996; Irwin, Tecklin, 1995)*.

✦ **Diaphragmatic breathing** reduces the work involved in breathing and alleviates dyspnea. It potentially eliminates accessory muscle activity and decreases the respiratory rate. In the past, it had not been thought to increase diaphragmatic mobility, but recent research shows improved excursion of the diaphragm *(Irwin, Tecklin, 1995)*. The ability of diaphragmatic breathing to increase lower lung zone ventilation (oxygenation) in healthy individuals has been documented. While diaphragmatic breathing has not been shown to increase alveolar ventilation in chronically obstructed persons *(Irwin, Tecklin, 1995)*, it does improve respiratory muscle endurance in these individuals *(Rochester, Goldberg, 1980)*. Diaphragmatic breathing is described in the chapter on non-Swedish techniques.

✦ **Segmental breathing** is used to increase thoracic excursion in cases of hypomobility. This hypomobility can result when hypoventilation of specific lung areas occurs in response to pain and muscle guarding *(Kisner, Colby, 1996; Persing, 1994)*. Segmental breathing has been described as breathing into a particular segment of the lung while the other areas are kept quiet. Resistance or mobilization techniques may follow segmental breathing, applied specifically to hypomobile areas. Segmental breathing is described in the treatment plan of this chapter.

✦ **Pursed-lip breathing exercises** have been proven to decrease respiratory rate and increase tidal volume (amount of air entering and leaving the lungs) even during exercise. They also improved performance and enhanced the ventilation of previously under-ventilated areas of the lungs in persons with severe COPD. Pursed-lip breathing exercises bring symptomatic relief from dyspnea and reduce the effort of breathing by shifting the work from the diaphragm to the intercostal muscles *(Irwin, Tecklin, 1995; Hough, 1996)*. They are described in the self-care section of this chapter.

✦ Diaphragmatic breathing alone has not been shown to increase ventilation in persons who have COPD. However, the **combination** of diaphragmatic breathing, segmental breathing and pursed-lip breathing (and general physical exercise) increases the function, strength and endurance of the muscles of respiration. This does not reverse lung damage, but modifies the disability that arises from it *(Hough, 1996)*, helping to decrease the effects of chronically obstructive respiratory diseases *(Rochester, Goldberg, 1980)*. In addition, people report a sense of well-being and control over breathlessness.

Symptom Picture

- There is an increase in mucus production from the bronchial glands and an increase in the number of goblet cells due to chronic irritation.
- The airways narrow due to chronic inflammation, thickening of the bronchial airways and accumulated mucus.
- There is decreased mobility of the thoracic joints *(Pryor, 1991)*.
- Respiratory infections may be present.
- A chronic productive cough is present, which worsens in the morning and evening and in the winter months. The cough begins slowly, worsening over weeks or months until it is productive. The mucus is purulent.
- Over time, cyanosis occurs due to hypoxemia. The finger ends are clubbed or bulbous. The person tends to retain weight. Peripheral edema results from venous stasis and right-sided heart failure.

Subjective Information

HEALTH HISTORY QUESTIONS

- When was the onset of the chronic bronchitis? Has it been diagnosed by a physician?

- Does the client have any other respiratory conditions such as emphysema or asthma, or cardiac conditions such as right-sided heart failure?

- What are the client's occupation and recreational activities?

- Does the client smoke? If yes, how much and how frequently?

- Does the client know which lobes are affected?

- Does the client have dyspnea? Is the client's sleep interrupted by breathlessness?

- Is the cough productive? Is it severe? What times of day or year is the cough worse?

- What is the colour of the sputum? Mucoid (clear or whitish) sputum is common. With acute exacerbation of chronic bronchitis, yellow or greenish sputum indicates infection. Blood-streaked sputum (hemoptysis) may also be present. If it is severe, postural drainage is contraindicated.

- What is the quantity of the sputum?

- Has the client ever been hospitalized for chronic bronchitis? When and for how long?

- Does the client have a fever now? If so, massage is contraindicated.

- Is the client taking any medication? How frequently?

- Is the client taking other parallel therapies such as physiotherapy?

Objective Information

Observations

✍ The seated client may lean forward, stabilizing the shoulder girdle to assist with inhalation.

✍ The accessory muscles of respiration are likely hypertrophied.

✍ There may be dyspnea or tachypnea (rapid, shallow breathing). The breathing pattern may be apical (using the upper chest only).

✍ A barrel chest (increased anteroposterior thoracic dimensions) may be present.

✍ Hyperkyphosis, hyperlordosis or scoliosis may be present. See the appropriate chapters for postural assessment.

✍ In severe cases, the client may breathe through pursed lips. There may be signs of anxiety.

✍ Cyanosis may be observed at the nail beds or the lips.

✍ Clubbing of the fingers, weight retention and peripheral edema may be present in advanced cases.

Palpation

✍ The muscles of respiration and accessory muscles including the diaphragm, intercostals, scalenes, sternocleidomastoids, pectoralis major, pectoralis minor and abdominals are tender and hypertonic. The axillary attachments of pectoralis major and latissimus dorsi as well as the costal margins are frequently tender.

✍ Trigger points are likely present in the above muscles and they may feel ropey and fibrosed.

✍ In advanced cases, peripheral edema is palpated.

Testing

✍ **AF ROM** of the thoracic and cervical spine and the shoulder girdle reveals reduced ranges, especially in the thoracic spine.

✍ **PR ROM** including **static** and **motion palpation** of the thoracic and cervical spine reveal areas of hypomobility, especially in the thoracic spine.

✍ **AR strength testing** for muscles of the shoulder girdle and the abdominals may be performed, assessing for possible weakness.

Special Tests

✍ **Vocal fremitus** and **mediate percussion tests** will be positive for areas of congestion due to mucus. These tests help to locate the affected lobes for postural drainage.

✍ **Measurements** of the thoracic circumference at full inhalation and full exhalation are taken using a tape measure and recorded. Measurement is at two levels, the axilla and the xiphoid process *(Pryor, 1991)*. The measurement at exhalation is subtracted from the measurement at inhalation to give the amount of thoracic expansion. Normal differences in adults are between 3 to 7.5 centimetres *(Magee, 1992)*.

✍ The **rib motion test** is positive when the client shows larger areas of restricted motion, while the **rib palpation test** and **first rib mobility test** reveal specific restricted ribs. The **levatores costarum test** is positive with rib fixation due to shortened levatores costarum muscles. **Anterior** and **lateral spinous challenges** reveal areas of hypomobility. With hyperkyphosis, **pectoralis major** and **minor** are short.

Contraindications

✦ Do not exhaust the client with overtreatment or the prolonged application of painful techniques.

✦ Joint play techniques for the ribs and rib springing are contraindicated with rib hypermobility and a history of rib subluxation.

✦ Postural drainage is contraindicated with severe hemoptysis (copious amounts of blood in sputum), severe pulmonary edema, congestive heart failure, pulmonary embolism, severe hypertension or hypotension, recent myocardial infarction and recent neurosurgery *(Kisner, Colby, 1996; Hough 1996)*.

✦ Do not use postural drainage directly after the client has eaten.

✦ Tapotement is contraindicated over bony prominences, floating ribs and breast tissue.

✦ The prolonged tapotement that accompanies postural drainage is contraindicated with chest-wall pain, unstable angina, anticoagulation therapy, osteoporosis, rib fracture, prolonged steroid therapy, hemoptysis, untreated lung abscesses, pulmonary embolism and open thoracic wounds or burns *(Irwin, Tecklin, 1995)*.

✦ Thyme essential oil is contraindicated (see treatment goals) with pregnant clients or those with hypertension *(Lawless, 1995)*.

✦ A client with cardiac or renal disorders should not increase the daily intake of water (see self care) to thin mucus secretions *(Bach, 1996)*.

✦ Chronic airflow obstruction may lead to pulmonary hypertension and, in occasional cases, to right-sided heart failure. Treatment modifications are listed in the chapter on hypertension and congestive heart failure.

Treatment Goals   Treatment Plan

Spread treatment over several appointments.

🖐 The therapist may choose several or all of the following techniques. However, particularly if the client is debilitated, these may be spread over several treatments, rather than all being performed in one appointment.

🖐 If the client has long-standing, severe chronic bronchitis where there is a possibility of hypertension, the therapist should monitor the client's blood pressure before and after the treatment. With hypertension, modifications to the treatment plan may be required. See the chapter on hypertension for details. If the therapist is in doubt about the proposed treatment plan, with the client's permission, the physician should be contacted.

🖐 **Positioning** of the client depends on the structures to be treated, the location of affected lobes and the client's general health.

- Prone, supine, sidelying or seated are all options. The position of the client for specific postural drainage is discussed later in this chapter.

- Positioning choices during the massage are increasingly important with more severe cases of bronchitis. The time that the client spends in the supine position is reduced or the client is placed only in a sidelying position, avoiding supine entirely.

- In general, the prone position was shown to improve ventilation and oxygenation, while the supine position decreased these factors. With unilateral lung diseases, lying on the unaffected side provides better oxygenation than lying supine. When the disease is bilateral, lying on the right side increases oxygenation. In the seated position, leaning forward has been clinically observed to help reduce the work of breathing (Irwin, Tecklin, 1995).

Thin secretions.

🖐 **Hydrotherapy,** such as a facial steam for five minutes prior to the massage, will help to thin the mucus. Five drops of pure, undiluted essential oil can be added to the bowl of hot water before the client covers the head and bowl with a towel. The client should close the eyes during a steam, to avoid possible eye irritation by the oils. Eucalyptus, benzoin and frankincense are expectorants. Thyme has antibacterial and antiseptic effects on the respiratory tract, but may irritate mucous membranes in some people (Lawless, 1995).

General Treatment

🖐 This treatment addresses a moderate chronic bronchitis presentation where modifications for hypertension or ventilation are not needed.

🖐 The treatment begins in the **supine position,** with pillows under the client's knees. If hyperkyphosis is present, a small towel roll is placed along the client's spine to flatten the curve. The client is later turned prone.

Treatment Goals

Decrease sympathetic nervous system firing. Encourage diaphragmatic breathing.

Reduce fascial restrictions.

Stretch shortened muscles.

Reduce hypertonicity. Reduce trigger points. Reduce pain.

Increase local circulation to flush out metabolites.

Mobilize the thorax.

Treatment Plan

- **Hydrotherapy** applications are pre-treatment heat applied over one pectoralis major muscle before treating the fascia. The heat is then moved to the other side during treatment. Heat may also be applied to the posterior lower intercostals before fascial work.

- It is important to perform this treatment in the context of a relaxation massage, including **diaphragmatic breathing** to help reduce stress and eliminate accessory respiratory muscle activity.

Specific Treatment

- Anteriorly, fascial techniques including skin rolling, fascial spreading and connective tissue cutting are used on the pectoral fascia, sternum, costal margins, lower intercostals and abdominal attachments (*Ebner, 1980*). A towel is used to cover the client's chest while working on the costal margins. See the chapters on asthma and hyperkyphosis for details.

- PIR or stretching is applied to the cervical muscles including the scalenes and the accessory muscles of respiration such as the pectorals (*Pryor, 1991*).

- Swedish techniques for pectoralis major, pectoralis minor, subclavius, serratus anterior, the anterior intercostals and the abdominals include effleurage, fingertip kneading, muscle stripping and the origin and insertion technique. The diaphragm is treated with costal border scooping and specific muscle stripping under the costal border, working with the client's breathing. For more details, see the chapter on asthma. Trigger points in pectoralis major refer into the chest, shoulder and medial arm. The sternalis muscle is not found in all people. It may be unilateral or bilateral, overlying the sternum and medial attachments of pectoralis major. Trigger points in this muscle refer pain over the sternum and are associated with pectoralis major trigger points. The serratus anterior muscle refers pain to the lateral ribs. Symptoms of breathlessness and reduced tidal volume due to restricted thoracic expansion are attributed to trigger points in this muscle (*Travell, Simons, 1983*).

- The scalenes, sternocleidomastoids, upper trapezius, levator scapulae, suboccipitals and posterior cervical muscles are treated with petrissage, including muscle stripping, fingertip kneading and Golgi tendon organ release.

- Repetitive effleurage is used on the shoulder and neck muscles.

- To develop strength and flexibility in a restricted area of the thorax, the therapist places both hands on the restricted area and asks the

Treatment Goals   Treatment Plan

client to breathe diaphragmatically. As the client inhales, a gentle resistance is applied to the ribs. A combination of resisted breathing and thoracic joint play is sometimes called **segmental breathing** or thoracic expansion (*Kisner, Colby, 1996; Bach, 1996*).

🖑 Joint play techniques are used on the thorax to create movement at the costal articulations. With the client supine, the therapist positions one hand under one side of the lower ribs, fingertips touching the transverse processes. The other hand is placed on the anterior costal margin on the same side, with the heel of the hand near the sternum. The hands are brought together in an alternating, kneading motion, taking up the elastic recoil in the tissue only. The technique is repeated all the way up the thorax (*Irwin, Tecklin, 1995*). Rib springing and rhythmic techniques are also indicated for areas of hypomobility.

🖑 Anterior-posterior and lateral challenge joint play are used on hypomobile cervical vertebrae.

🖑 The client is turned **prone.** Folded towels are placed under the client's shoulders if they are protracted.

Reduce fascial restrictions.

🖑 Fascial techniques are used on the lower intercostals and quadratus lumborum attachments.

Reduce hypertonicity.
Reduce trigger points.
Reduce pain.
Encourage circulation in overused structures.

🖑 Swedish techniques such as effleurage and petrissage are applied to serratus posterior superior, erector spinae, multifidi, posterior intercostals and quadratus lumborum. Trigger points in these muscles are addressed.

Mobilize the thorax.

🖑 Anterior and lateral challenge and spinous process oscillation joint play are used on hypomobile thoracic vertebrae. Thoracic mobilization and rib springing are indicated for areas of hypomobility. Rhythmic mobilizations for the shoulder girdle are also used.

Postural Drainage

Remove secretions.

🖑 Prior to postural drainage, the client should practise diaphragmatic breathing and productive coughing if copious amounts of mucus are being produced. The therapist should have tissues and a plastic-lined wastebasket available for the client to expectorate into.

🖑 The positioning is based on the location of the affected lobe and bronchi (*Figure 72.2*). Gravity drains the mucus into the main bronchi where it can be more easily expectorated by coughing. For the lower lobes, the client's hips must be elevated above the head. A wedge of pillows is created so the client's thorax is placed at an angle between 30 and 45 degrees. For the right middle lobe, the client lies one quarter turn from supine on the left side, supported on the right side

884

Lower Lobes

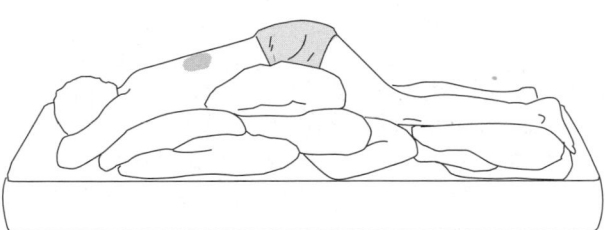

Pillows built into a wedge under hips.
Sheets not shown for clarity.

Right Middle Lobe

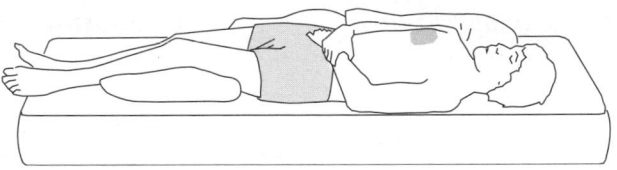

Pillows under right thorax and knees.
Sheets not shown for clarity.

Upper Lobes

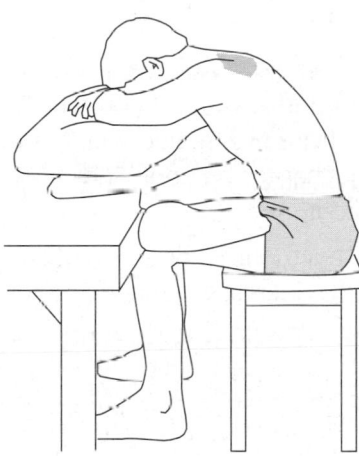

Pillows piled up in lap and on table to support thorax.

Figure 72.2
Postural drainage positioning. Client is always securely draped; only the area to be tapoted is uncovered.

Treatment Goals   Treatment Plan

posteriorly by pillows. For the upper lobes, most commonly affected if the person is bedridden, the client is seated. Postural drainage positioning is maintained for three to five minutes or longer if the client can tolerate it *(Brannon et al., 1993; Dettenmeier, 1992; Frownfelter, 1987)*. Although the client could be left in this position while resting and some drainage could also occur, the addition of tapotement makes drainage more efficient.

🖐 Before tapotement begins, the therapist should arrange a signal with the client so tapotement is stopped if the client needs to expectorate. The client should practise diaphragmatic breathing and pursed-lip breathing during postural drainage and tapotement.

885

Treatment Goals

Treatment Plan

Remove secretions.

✋ Tapotement is performed at a slower rather than faster rate to achieve maximum relaxation and to avoid possible bronchospasm *(Frownfelter, 1987)*. The techniques are applied in a pattern — for example, moving from the bifurcation of the trachea at T5 towards the affected lobe. One method of tapotement should not be applied continuously in one area for an extended time. A sequence of pincement, loose fingertip hacking, cupping and pounding is indicated to avoid problems. The order is reversed to end the tapotement sequence. If the therapist loses the rhythm, or the client or therapist fatigues, coarse vibrations can be used. Tapotement is continued for three to five minutes *(Frownfelter, 1987)*.

✋ The therapist should wear vinyl or latex gloves to dispose of the used tissues and wastebasket plastic liner after the treatment. Any spills of body fluids are treated with the bleach and water solution mentioned in the chapter on contraindications for specific conditions and medications.

✋ The treatment is ended with soothing effleurage and stroking to the back to decrease sympathetic nervous system firing.

Treat other conditions.

✋ Other conditions, such as hyperlordosis or scoliosis, are addressed in subsequent treatments.

Self-care Goals

Self-care Plan

Practise breathing exercises.

✍ To practise **pursed-lip breathing,** the client is comfortably relaxed, with both hands placed on the abdominals to monitor how relaxed they stay during pursed-lip breathing. Inspiration is slow and deep. The client then loosely purses the lips and exhales. Exhalation must be relaxed. The client should not contract the abdominal muscles to exhale, since this may cause airway turbulence and further constriction of the small bronchioles *(Kisner, Colby, 1996)*.

✍ To practise **productive coughing,** the client is seated, leaning forward on the arms. Diaphragmatic breathing is practised first. The client then places both hands on the abdominals and makes two or three coughs. The client is asked to take a deep breath, contract the glottis, then rapidly contract the abdominal muscles to increase the intrathoracic pressure. The client should feel the abdominal muscles contract under her hands. The glottis is then released to expel the air. The client performs relaxed diaphragmatic breathing again. This entire cycle, thought to remove more secretions from the peripheral airways than coughing alone, is called the **forced expiratory technique** *(Irwin, Tecklin, 1995)*.

Self-care Goals

Self-care Plan

✍ In clients with COPD, high intrathoracic pressures can close off small airways. For these people, the cough to clear mucus is then modified to a huff. **Huffing** uses the same coordinated steps as coughing, except that the glottis is not closed. A medium-sized inhalation is followed by forced exhalations through an open airway, as if the client were saying "ha, ha, ha" *(Brannon et al., 1993)*.

✍ **Diaphragmatic breathing** is practised in a comfortable position — for example, lying supine with pillows under the shoulders, head and knees. This allows the accessory muscles of respiration to relax *(Bach, 1996)*.

✍ Postural drainage combined with breathing and productive coughing should be practised at home for 10 to 20 minutes twice daily *(Thomson et al., 1991)*.

Encourage relaxation strategies.

✍ Relaxation techniques for the muscles of the neck and shoulder girdle are important. See the chapter on stress reduction for details.

Thin secretions.

✍ Inhalation of steam in a hot shower helps to thin secretions, as does drinking six to eight glasses of water per day *(Bach, 1996)*.

Mobilize the thorax.

✍ The seated client inhales and bends the thorax away from the restricted side to lengthen the muscles. Using the right side as the restricted side, the client bends towards the left, then makes a fist with the right hand and pushes the hand into the lateral aspect of the right thorax. At the same time, as she exhales, the client changes position and bends to the right side as far as possible to mobilize the ribs inferiorly. The exercise is repeated several times *(Kisner, Colby, 1996)*. The chest can also be mobilized. First, the seated client clasps the hands behind the head. On inhalation, the client extends the thoracic and cervical spine. On exhalation, the client flexes the spine *(Bach, 1996)*. Stretching once a day maintains the range of motion; stretching more often increases the range *(Irwin, Tecklin, 1995)*.

Stretch short muscles.

✍ Stretching the muscles of the shoulder girdle and neck is important. See also remedial exercises for hyperkyphosis if appropriate.

✍ Self-massage to the costal margins, intercostals and scalenes is indicated.

Strengthen weak muscles.

✍ Breathing exercises will strengthen the muscles of respiration. Overall conditioning exercises, such as walking, are indicated with the physician's approval. The client should pace any physical activities so dyspnea does not occur.

Reduce or eliminate perpetuating factors.

✍ The client is encouraged to stop smoking if this is a factor, joining a smoking cessation program if necessary.

✍ Airborne pollutants in the home can be reduced with air conditioning or other filtering mechanisms.

Self-care Goals

Self-care Plan

- ✍ Avoidance of people with respiratory infections is also helpful.
- ✍ The client should attempt to reduce consumption of mucus-producing foods such as dairy products.

Refer the client.

- ✍ The client's physician or a smoking cessation program can help with stopping smoking. A naturopath or nutritionist can help with diet modifications.

Treatment Frequency and Expected Outcome

Treatments should be 45 minutes to one hour in length, once a week while cough and dyspnea are present.

See also stress reduction, emphysema, asthma, hypertension, hyperkyphosis, hyperlordosis, scoliosis and frozen shoulder chapters for related conditions.

Outcome is variable, depending on the presence of perpetuating factors and the length of time the disease has been present.

Chronic bronchitis is likely to be an ongoing condition but massage can modify the symptoms. Massage can reduce dyspnea, increase thoracic mobility and facilitate mucus expectoration. The more severe the condition, the less of an impact treatment will have.

EMPHYSEMA

Fiona Rattray

Emphysema is a disease that causes enlargement of air spaces distal to the terminal bronchioles and destruction of the alveolar walls.

Emphysema is defined according to the portion of the primary lobule of the lung (acinus) that is affected. The acinus is the lung section that is supplied by an individual bronchiole. The two most common forms are centrilobular and panlobular emphysema.

Centrilobular (centriacinar) **emphysema** destroys the central portion of the acinus and is the form most associated with smoking. Abnormal, enlarged air spaces are surrounded by normal tissue. They are most frequently found in the upper lobes. **Panlobular** (panacinar) **emphysema** destroys the lobules uniformly throughout the lungs. This form is most associated with an inherited enzyme deficiency disorder. **Paracicatrical emphysema** is an irregular form that is associated with a previous lung pathology, such as tuberculosis. Enlarged air spaces are formed due to the fibrosis and scarring that follow the healing process.

In all forms of emphysema, the destruction of the alveolar walls leaves large air spaces. The largest of these are called "bullae". These air spaces cause inefficient gas exchange due to the reduced surface areas. As the elastic tissue in the alveolar walls is destroyed, normal elastic recoil of the lungs is lost. This contributes to early airway collapse on exhalation and air trapping. Over the long term, emphysema can lead to congestive heart failure and death.

Some studies have found emphysema in as many as two-thirds of men and one-seventh of women autopsied. The most severe forms of emphysema are found in smokers *(Irwin, Tecklin, 1995)*.

Medically, diagnosis of emphysema is made easier using computerized tomography rather than X-rays *(Vermeire et al., 1988)*. Medications used with emphysema include: Beclovent

889

and Azmacort, which are used to control the inflammation; and theophylline (Theo-Dur), which helps to relieve bronchospasm and increase the diaphragm's force of contraction *(Irwin, Tecklin, 1995)*.

Causes of emphysema are:

➤ **an overabundance of proteolytic enzymes** caused by an inflammatory response to an airway irritant. This irritant is most commonly cigarette smoke. When neutrophils and basophils have finished participating in the inflammatory response in the airway walls, they necrose. This releases proteolytic enzymes that digest the lung tissue;

➤ **an inherited lack of proteolytic enzyme inhibitors** which allows naturally occurring enzymes to destroy elastic tissue in alveolar walls. This causes larger-than-normal air spaces.

Either or both of these mechanisms can exist in the person with emphysema.

Symptom Picture

✦ Symptoms include dyspnea (difficult breathing) on exertion in the early stages of the disease. In later stages, dyspnea is also experienced at rest.

✦ Cough, wheezing, prolonged expiration and physical inactivity leading to deconditioning are present.

✦ Hyperinflation of the lungs leads to an increased anteroposterior dimension of the thorax called "barrel chest". The ribs and muscles of inspiration are virtually at a position of constant maximum inspiration. The diaphragm is flattened and the accessory muscles of respiration are overused.

✦ The person often assumes a seated position, leaning forward on the arms to give the accessory muscles of respiration mechanical advantage. However, the hyperinflated thorax has little respiratory reserve.

✦ Although hypoxia occurs with emphysema, for some reason the person is able to struggle and overventilate, maintaining blood gas levels until later in the disease. The terms "pink puffer" or "fighter" may be used *(Porth, 1990)*.

✦ The person with emphysema is often thin. Tachypnea (rapid, shallow breathing) is present and the person exhales through pursed lips. Breathlessness when lying supine may be caused by pulmonary or cardiac pathologies. Pressure on the diaphragm from the viscera can compromise breathing. Breathlessness may also result from a poorly functioning left ventricle, which may be unable to tolerate the increase in blood returning to the heart.

✦ As the disease progresses, pulmonary hypertension is followed by enlargement of the right ventricle, right-sided heart failure (cor pulmonale) and death.

✦ Emphysema can occur by itself or with other respiratory diseases. When combined with chronic bronchitis or other respiratory infection, there is a productive cough.

Chronic Obstructive Pulmonary Disease

Chronic obstructive pulmonary disease (COPD) describes a spectrum of diseases, most frequently some combination of emphysema and chronic bronchitis. Cystic fibrosis (CF) is also a COPD. Asthma, due to its episodic nature, is not a classic chronic obstructive disease but may be listed with other COPDs.

Tobacco smoke is the most common cause of COPD, although pollution or hereditary factors play a part. About 20 per cent of smokers have accelerated decline of lung function. If they continued to smoke, this decline would result in COPD. The first signs of breathlessness occur at 40 to 50 years of age in susceptible smokers. This may progress to respiratory failure and cor pulmonale. It may be difficult to differentiate COPD from undiagnosed chronic asthma in adults *(Cochrane et al., 1996).*

Cystic fibrosis is a genetic disorder of the apocrine glands. There is an increase in size and number of the bronchial mucous glands. Increased secretions also occur from the salivary, sweat and pancreatic glands. The bronchial mucous glands produce copious quantities of mucus that is exceedingly sticky. Over time, airway obstruction occurs, with coughing becoming less productive. Secondary respiratory infections develop. Bronchiectasis, an irreversible dilation and thickening of the bronchi, takes place. Hyperinflation of the lungs results from the increased secretions. Atelectasis, or loss of lung inflation, takes place when obstruction is complete. Pulmonary complications are the cause of death.

Cystic fibrosis is managed throughout the person's life by diet, medication, pancreatic enzyme replacement and chest physical therapy, including tapotement and postural drainage. The person with cystic fibrosis is typically thin, barrel chested and lethargic due to bouts of coughing, dyspnea and hypoxia.

CF was first recognized as a specific disease in 1936. The majority of children with cystic fibrosis in the early years of CF care died in infancy. Today, with ongoing comprehensive care, the lifespan has increased and adulthood is common for people with CF *(Irwin, Tecklin, 1995).*

Treatment Considerations

HEALTH HISTORY QUESTIONS

✦ When was the onset? What is the cause of the emphysema?

✦ Does the client have dyspnea? When does this happen? Is there a productive cough indicating chronic bronchitis?

✦ What medication is the client taking? Has the client been hospitalized for complications resulting from emphysema? Is oxygen being used?

✦ What are the client's functional abilities? Does the client fatigue easily? Is the client able to go up stairs? How many?

✦ Does the client smoke?

✦ Does the client eat well, live alone? If the client lives alone, household tasks may become impossible as the disease progresses.

✦ Is the client depressed? Is the client's motivation reduced?

✦ Has the client been advised not to take very hot showers or baths by the physician, indicating a more severe cardiopulmonary condition?

✦ Is the client taking other parallel therapies such as physiotherapy?

Further Assessment

✍ **Observations:**

- A postural assessment reveals elevated shoulders, a barrel chest, horizontal ribs and head-forward posture.

- Exhalation is prolonged. The breathless client will lean on his elbows so the shoulder girdle muscles can work as accessory muscles of respiration. Pursed-lip breathing may be used on expiration.

- Accessory muscles of respiration are prominent. The client is likely thin and fatigued-looking. The skin may be rosy or pink.

- The fingertips may be clubbed or enlarged.

✍ In terms of **palpation,** thoracic rigidity occurs with emphysema *(Lewit, 1993).* The muscles of respiration are hypertonic, including the diaphragm, intercostals, scalenes and sternocleidomastoids.

✍ **Testing:**

- Testing for emphysema includes the same tests that are used for chronic bronchitis. See chapter on chronic bronchitis for details.

- **AF** and **PR ROM** are reduced in the thoracic and cervical spine.

- **AR strength testing** of the shoulder girdle may reveal weaker and overused muscles.

- **Vocal fremitus** and **mediate percussion tests** will be either very hollow-sounding with emphysema alone or positive for areas of congestion with associated chronic bronchitis. This helps to locate the affected lobes if postural drainage is indicated.

Contraindications

◆ Do not exhaust the client with overtreatment or use of prolonged painful techniques. This is increasingly important as the severity of the emphysema increases.

◆ Avoid placing the client with severe emphysema in a supine or prone position.

◆ Postural drainage is contraindicated with severe hemoptysis (copious amounts of blood in sputum), severe pulmonary edema, congestive heart failure, pulmonary embolism, severe hypertension or hypotension, positional dyspnea in the head-down position, recent myocardial infarction and recent neurosurgery (Kisner, Colby, 1996; Hough 1996).

◆ Do not use postural drainage directly after the client has eaten.

◆ Tapotement is contraindicated over bony prominences, floating ribs and breast tissue.

◆ The prolonged tapotement that accompanies postural drainage is contraindicated with chest-wall pain, unstable angina, anticoagulation therapy, osteoporosis, rib fracture, prolonged steroid therapy, hemoptysis, untreated lung abscesses, pulmonary embolism and open thoracic wounds or burns (Irwin, Tecklin, 1995).

◆ Joint play techniques for the ribs and rib springing are contraindicated with rib hypermobility and a history of rib subluxation.

◆ A client with cardiac or renal disorders should not increase the daily intake of water as is sometimes recommended as self-care (Bach, 1996).

◆ Chronic airflow obstruction may lead to pulmonary hypertension and, in occasional cases, to right-sided heart failure or cor pulmonale, necessitating treatment modifications. See the chapters on hypertension and chronic congestive heart failure for details.

Massage

🖐 In treating a client with emphysema, the therapist must take into account the severity of the client's symptoms. A milder presentation of emphysema may allow for more vigorous techniques such as fascial work and careful mobilization of the thorax. The treatment of a severe presentation is likely limited to promoting relaxation and encouraging improved breathing patterns. A reduced treatment duration of half an hour may be indicated. Cardiac pathologies will require treatment modifications in terms of positioning and the use of segmental petrissage. The client's use of a portable oxygen tank will require the therapist's awareness to avoid pulling on the line or becoming entangled in it. If the therapist is in doubt about the proposed treatment plan, with the client's permission, the physician should be contacted.

🖐 The primary goals are to reduce sympathetic nervous system firing, promote relaxation of accessory muscles of respiration, encourage diaphragmatic breathing to minimize shortness of breath and mobilize the thorax (Kisner, Colby, 1996). Other goals include removing accumulated mucus, if chronic bronchitis is present, and treating postural dysfunctions such as hyperkyphosis over a series of appointments.

🖐 Since there is a possibility of hypertension with emphysema, the therapist should monitor the client's blood pressure before and after the treatment.

🖐 **Positioning** for relaxation has the client lying in a semi-supine position with the trunk, arms and head well supported by pillows. The client with severe emphysema is treated in a propped-up, sidelying position or in a seated position, leaning forward.

🖐 **Hydrotherapy** modifications, such as avoiding heat applications, may be necessary with hypertension. Facial steams that help to mobilize secretions may be appropriate with associated chronic bronchitis. See the chronic bronchitis chapter for more information.

🖐 It is important to perform this treatment in the context of a relaxation massage, including diaphragmatic breathing to help reduce stress and eliminate accessory respiratory muscle activity.

🖐 With mild to moderate emphysema, muscle stripping and fascial techniques for the upper and lower intercostals are performed within the client's pain tolerance. Less aggressive techniques, such as fascial spreading, and slower speeds for techniques are recommended with debilitated clients. The chapter on asthma has more details on fascial work for the thorax and diaphragm attachments.

🖐 Mobilization of the thorax, if indicated, is done gently, especially with debilitated clients. Techniques include rhythmic techniques, anterior and lateral spinous challenge joint play, thoracic joint play and gentle rib springing.

🖐 Swedish techniques, such as effleurage, vibrations, slow rocking or rhythmic techniques and gentle petrissage, are used on the muscles of respiration including the scalenes and pectoralis major. The work is light, soothing and repetitive. Trigger points are addressed with muscle stripping and intermittent ischemic compressions. The client's shoulders, neck, head, back, arms, legs and abdomen may also be treated.

🖐 Postural drainage, breathing exercises and tapotement are used to remove mucus secretions with associated chronic bronchitis. These techniques may all need to be modified for the debilitated client. Huffing is indicated instead of productive coughing.

Self-care

✍ Self-care goals include decreasing or moderating the severity and frequency of the symptoms through correct breathing patterns (Lewit, 1993), pursed-lip breathing and productive coughing, described in the chronic bronchitis chapter. With moderate and severe presentations of emphysema, it is important to have the client's physician approve the remedial exercise plan and hydrotherapy application before the client begins the self-care program.

✍ Shortness of breath can be relieved by having the client sit, leaning forward with his elbows on his knees. In a standing position, the client can place both hands on a table, then lean forward. In either of these positions, the client then practises relaxed exhalation or pursed-lip breathing (Irwin, Tecklin, 1995).

✍ If not contraindicated, postural drainage combined with diaphragmatic breathing is used with associated chronic bronchitis.

> ✍ Self-massage to the scalenes, intercostals and costal margins is indicated.
>
> ✍ Stretching for the shoulder girdle muscles and accessory muscles of inhalation is helpful.
>
> ✍ In mild to moderate emphysema, exercise tolerance is gradually increased — for example, from walking around the house to walking around the block.
>
> ✍ If the client smokes, he is encouraged to stop.

See stress reduction, chronic bronchitis, asthma, hyperkyphosis, frozen shoulder, hypertension and congestive heart failure for related treatments.

ASTHMA

Fiona Rattray

Asthma is a chronic inflammatory disorder characterized by bronchospasm (narrowing of the airways in the lungs), which is reversible over time either spontaneously or following treatment (Clark, Rees, 1996; Cochrane et al., 1996).

Asthma disease has been known and described for at least 2,000 years. The word asthma comes from a Greek word meaning panting. In 1698, Sir John Floyer wrote, "I have assigned the immediate cause of asthma to the straitness, compression or constriction of the bronchi", which is an accurate description of an acute asthma attack *(Kaliner et al., 1990)*.

The prevalence of asthma varies in different parts of the world, with an estimated five per cent of the world's population suffering from the disease. There has been a recent increase in both the number of cases reported and in the mortality rate *(Cochrane et al., 1996; Kaliner et al., 1990)*.

Most people with asthma have mild symptoms. This accounts for about 60 per cent of asthmatics. Studies in several countries have shown that the cost of treating these individuals is 15 per cent of the national expenditure on asthma. Severe and very severe asthma affect 20 per cent of asthmatics, who may account for up to 60 per cent of the total asthma health care costs, mostly resulting from emergency care and hospital treatments. One source suggests that, worldwide, 40,000 deaths per year can be attributed to asthma *(Cochrane et al., 1996)*.

New cases of asthma usually appear either in childhood or in middle age. Between 10 and 20 per cent of children up to 10 years of age acquire the condition. At this age, remissions are common. Those with less frequent symptoms are the most likely to experience remission. Boys are more prone to developing asthma than girls by a ratio of 3:2. From the late teens to 30 years of age the prevalence drops. With people over 40 years of age, the prevalence again increases, though there are fewer cases than in childhood. At this age, the asthma is more persistent and remissions are less frequent. The ratio of asthma in adults is equal between males and females, because young women are less likely to lose their asthma during adolescence *(Clark, Rees, 1996)*.

Causes of asthma are:

➤ **underlying airway inflammation** and an **abnormal bronchospasm response** to triggers that would not normally provoke such a response.

- Asthma is more common in urban than in rural locations. There is an increase in the incidence of asthma in migrant populations moving to urban environments. This suggests that **environmental factors** override genetic factors predisposing to asthma, although whether the increase is due to allergens, air pollution or changes in diet is not known.

- Exposure to **dust mites** present in bedding and house dust is likely a major causative factor in both severity and prevalence of asthma. An allergen is found in the fecal pellets of the house dust mite, *Dermatophagoides pteronyssinus*.

- Bronchoconstriction is provoked by **cigarette smoking,** especially in asthmatics, yet approximately one-fifth of asthmatics continue to smoke *(Clark, Rees, 1996)*. As well as the other harmful effects of cigarette smoke, the persistent inhalation of irritants makes asthma symptoms more difficult to control. Asthmatic smokers may go on to develop chronic airflow obstruction and accompanying chronic bronchitis.

- **Occupational factors** are responsible for five per cent of adult-onset asthma *(Clark, Rees, 1996)*. Repeated exposure to chemicals, such as isocyanates and epoxy resins present in the manufacture of adhesives, polyurethane foam, paint and plastics, can lead to asthma. Wood, grain and flour dusts may also cause occupational asthma.

- Asthma can result from **food allergies.** The 1840-41 edition of the British Medical Journal, *The Lancet*, reported a case of asthma resulting from eating veal, salted meat and pastry, while in 1855 a detailed account was given of a wheat allergy causing asthma *(Speer, 1983)*.

- **Exercise-induced asthma** is believed to be triggered by the cooling and drying effect of inhaled air on the respiratory epithelium. The exact mechanism producing the bronchoconstriction is not clearly understood *(Rupp, 1996)*.

As early as 1885 it was noted that asthma, hay fever, eczema and hives (urticaria) have a common origin *(Speer, 1983)*. A tendency to develop an allergy can be inherited, but not the specific allergy itself. This tendency is called "atopy". Relatives of asthmatics are more likely to develop asthma, as well as hay fever and eczema. It is believed that atopic status (a positive skin test for eczema and hay fever) is inherited separately from a predisposition to asthma. However, when the two coincide, atopy increases the likelihood that the person will be susceptible to asthma *(Clark, Rees, 1996)*. Persons with both asthma and eczema often note that one condition or the other is prevalent. When the asthma is particularly bothersome, the eczema will be mild or non-existent *(Chapman, 1995; Cochrane et al., 1996)*.

Types of Asthma

✦ **Extrinsic:** Irritating substances from outside the body cause an immune system or allergic response. There is a release of inflammatory mediators from mast cells within the airways. The immune system responds to irritating agents such as pollens, animal dander, foods and cigarette smoke.

  • Attacks are related to exposure to the irritating substances. Skin tests for allergens are positive.

  • Most childhood-onset asthma is extrinsic. There is usually a personal or family history of asthma, hay fever and eczema.

✦ **Intrinsic:** This type of asthma is characterized by a lack of clearly defined precipitating factors such as an allergic response.

  • Skin tests are negative.

  • Factors within the body, such as respiratory infections, may cause an attack. Other factors are weather changes, emotional stress and bronchial irritants including air pollution and fumes found in the workplace.

  • Adult-onset asthma is usually intrinsic. There is less reversibility and more long standing airflow obstruction *(Cochrane et al., 1996)*.

✦ **Exercise-induced asthma** can be either extrinsic or intrinsic.

Other Terms Used with Asthma

✦ **Inducers** of asthma act by causing airway inflammation. They include allergies, genetic factors, infections and occupational and environmental influences.

✦ **Triggers** of asthma are factors that cause airway smooth muscle contraction in conjunction with pre-existing airway inflammation and airway hyperresponsiveness *(Cochrane et al., 1996)*. Usually several of these factors can trigger an attack.

✦ **Triggering Factors**

  • *Inhaled allergens* such as dust mite feces, cat dander, pollens and spores

  • *Cigarette smoke*

  • *Respiratory infections*, including viral and bacterial infections

  • *Environmental pollution*, including ozone, particulate matter and nitrogen oxide *(Vermeire et al., 1988)*

  • *Exercise*

  • *Food intolerances or allergies*; for example, to peanuts, milk, eggs, tartrazine and sulphur dioxide

  • *Drugs* such as beta blockers, Aspirin and tetracycline

  • *Occupational factors*; for example, exposure to epoxy resins, grain or flour dust and laboratory animals

  • *Psychological factors* such as emotional stress or anxiety associated with the breathlessness of acute asthma attacks, although emotional factors are not believed to produce asthma on their own

- *Hormonal factors* during pregnancy and menstruation, which have variable effects on asthma

- *Gastro-esophageal reflux* which irritates the bronchi, producing bronchoconstriction

✦ **Other Risk Factors**

- *Genetic predisposition:* asthma, hay fever and eczema are more prevalent among relatives of those with atopic asthma *(Kaliner et al., 1990)*.

- *Climatic factors:* epidemics of severe asthma attacks following abrupt weather changes, such as thunderstorms, have been reported. This may be due to the increase in atmospheric pollen and spore counts, or an increase in dust particles. It has not been substantiated that asthma and other respiratory complaints are more prevalent in cold or wet climates. Children in temperate New Zealand had a similar prevalence of asthma to children in southern Ontario, where there are greater climatic extremes *(Kaliner et al., 1990)*.

The Medical Treatment of Asthma

The medical perception of asthma has recently changed. For many years, asthma was described as acute episodes of airflow obstruction (bronchospasm); the medical approach was to relieve the bronchospasm. Mast cells were thought to be the principal mediators of the attack. Now it is recognized that asthma is a complex, chronic disease with inflammatory changes in the airways. Numerous inflammatory cells release a variety of mediators causing mucus secretion, edema and bronchospasm, amplifying the ongoing inflammatory process *(Cochrane et al., 1996)*. The approach is to control the inflammatory process.

Two approaches are used to treat asthma — one is prevention, the other is treatment during an attack. Prevention involves avoidance of known triggers, including allergens, and suppression of the inflammatory response with medication. Stress reduction and controlled breathing help to reduce anxiety that aggravates respiratory difficulties. Treatment during an attack focuses on relieving the bronchospasm.

The main categories of drugs used to treat asthma are sympathomimetics and corticosteroids. *Beta-2 sympathomimetics* influence the sympathetic nervous system, causing bronchodilation. Ventolin (albuterol) is an example of this type of drug. Sympathomimetics also increase both blood pressure and heart rate. *Corticosteroids* are used to reduce bronchial inflammation. Azmacort and Beclovent are corticosteroids *(Irwin, Tecklin, 1995)*.

These medications are usually administered by a metered dose aerosol inhaler, although dry powder inhalers (Diskhalers) may be used.

Corticosteroids may also be taken in oral form. There are side effects to long-term steroid use, including skin atrophy, episodes of bruising and hyperkyphosis associated with osteoporosis *(Cochrane et al., 1996)*.

Since asthma is a variable disease, the medical treatment is adjusted to the frequency and severity of the symptoms. Attacks occurring more than once a month are treated with regular medication and avoidance of precipitating factors, whereas attacks occurring three or four times a year are treated as they occur. Bronchodilators are used with mild episodic symptoms as primary therapy and with more severe symptoms as relief therapy. Many adult asthmatics are now also treated with inhaled or oral steroids to control the underlying inflammatory process (Clark, Rees, 1996).

By self-monitoring with a portable peak-flow meter, a person with asthma can record her maximum air-flow levels at various points during the day. Moderate changes in these levels become apparent. The person can avoid an acute attack by stepping up medication usage as symptoms worsen and reducing medication as symptoms improve (Cochrane et al., 1996). However, a decreased response or lack of response to an inhaled bronchodilator signals the onset of a severe attack, which requires more therapy than can be taken at the time. This necessitates prompt medical referral (Vermeire et al., 1988).

Asthma is considered under control if the symptoms are minimal, activities of daily living are normal, inhalant medication is needed no more than twice daily (ideally not at all) and air-flow rates are normal (Clark, Rees, 1996).

Massage Therapy and Asthma

In one study, the parents of asthmatic children were taught to give therapeutic massage to their children. The children then received 10 minutes of daily massage for a one-month period. Measurements of the children's anxiety and depression levels, stress hormones, cortisol and epinephrine levels and respiratory peak-flow readings were taken before and after the study. The parents were assessed for stress levels and coping skills. Results indicated that the children's self-reported anxiety and depression decreased and their stress hormone levels decreased. Fewer asthma attacks were experienced and several of the children's peak air-flow readings had improved, indicating that they could breathe more easily. The parents felt less anxiety and had decreased feelings of being controlled by their children's needs (Field et al., 1995a).

Another study found that forced expiratory volume in children with asthma increased after tapotement (Rochester, Goldberg, 1980). Massage therapy, including fascial techniques and joint play, helps to decrease asthma symptoms (Chapman, 1995; Ebner, 1980).

Anatomy of Respiration in Asthma

In all types of asthma, there is an abnormal response of the airways or bronchospasm. This airway hyperresponsiveness probably occurs as a consequence of chronic underlying inflammation. Environmental and genetic influences likely act by provoking the underlying inflammation of the airways, rather than by directly stimulating hyperresponsiveness.

With extrinsic asthma, an immune response occurs to the irritating stimuli. Active substances such as histamines are released from mast cells in the airways. An inflammatory chain of events leads to edema of the airways and thickening of the bronchial walls. Inflammatory cells, usually eosinophils, invade the walls, resulting in edema. Between attacks, these changes are reversible. However, in the long term, the goblet cells enlarge and the bronchial smooth muscles may become thickened.

There is increased mucus production. Mucus in asthma is abnormally sticky and inhibits ciliary action in the airways, leading to mucus retention and plug formation. Air trapping occurs when mucus plugs trap air in the lungs. Over time, this trapped air causes increased lung volume.

During forced inhalation, the diaphragm, external intercostals and scalenes are assisted by numerous muscles: serratus posterior superior, pectoralis major and minor, levator costarum, and subclavius. These muscles become shortened due to air trapping and increased lung volume. During forced exhalation, as when coughing, the internal intercostals, the abdominals and quadratus lumborum are recruited. These muscles shorten and tighten. The shoulder girdle stabilizers and elevators are also involved with the typical asthmatic posture, including hypertonic upper trapezius, levator scapulae, serratus anterior, rhomboids and the cervical muscles. For more details, see the chapter on chronic bronchitis.

Control of the bronchial airways is by the autonomic nervous system, through the vagus nerve and fibres from the thoracic ganglia. Nerves supply airways down to the level of the respiratory bronchioles. In addition to regulating smooth muscle tone, the autonomic nervous system may influence secretion from the submucosal glands, permeability and blood flow in the bronchial circulation and release of mediators from inflammatory cells *(Kaliner et al., 1990)*.

Symptom Picture

✦ Asthma symptoms are episodic and range from wheezing and chest tightness to an acute attack with breathlessness and coughing. Between attacks the person may be asymptomatic.

✦ There are varying degrees of severity of asthma:

• **Mild asthma** is indicated by occasional wheezing or a cough that does not cause major impairment of physical activity, by sensitivity to triggers including allergens and cold air and by symptoms that restrict activity two or three times a week.

• **Moderate asthma** is indicated by daily symptoms, occasional nocturnal symptoms and avoidance of exercise.

• **Severe asthma** is indicated by daily wheezing, severe nocturnal symptoms, absence from work or school several times a year or more, poor quality of life and occasional hospital admissions.

✦ Nocturnal symptoms of breathlessness and coughing are usually at their worst between 2 a.m. and 4 a.m. when the person has been lying down, which narrows the airways and allows mucus secretions to build up.

✦ With exercise-induced asthma, a cough is noticed about five or 10 minutes after exercise begins. Maximal symptoms occur usually three to 15 minutes after the exercise ceases *(Rupp, 1996)*.

✦ Airway obstruction in all types of asthma is reversible, especially with the use of bronchodilator medication. Over time, with some asthmatics, airway obstruction gradually becomes irreversible. This is usually associated with poorly controlled severe asthma and a long-standing condition. These persons may also suffer from chronic bronchitis or emphysema.

✦ With chronic uncontrolled asthma, air trapping eventually leads to lung hyperinflation and changes in the shape of the thorax. Persistent airflow obstruction may lead to pulmonary hypertension and, in occasional cases, to right-sided heart failure resulting from primary lung disease (also called cor pulmonale).

✦ In children, asthma is initially characterized by paroxysmal coughing, especially at night. Chest tightness, wheezing and breathlessness occur in mid-childhood.

✦ Warning signs of an **acute asthma attack** are sleep disturbance, an increase in symptoms, an increasing need for bronchodilator treatment combined with decreasing medication effectiveness and a fall in the peak air-flow *(Clark, Rees, 1996)*.

• During an acute asthma attack, expiration becomes prolonged due to the airway obstruction. The amount of air that can be exhaled forcefully from the lungs with each breath decreases. Air that cannot be exhaled becomes trapped in the lungs, resulting in hyperinflation. The anteroposterior dimension of the thorax increases and there is limited movement of the ribs on inhalation. The diaphragm becomes flattened due to hyperinflation, preventing the lower ribs from moving up and out. The person must work harder to exhale, recruiting the accessory muscles of respiration. Coughing to clear the mucus becomes unproductive during the attack and productive afterwards, when gelatinous mucus plugs may be coughed up. Wheezing is audible on both inhalation and exhalation. The person is visibly anxious and may be sweating. The most comfortable position is sitting upright. Dyspnea, or distressed, laboured breathing, and tachypnea, or rapid, shallow breathing, may be severe.

• Acute severe asthma occurs when an attack becomes persistent and intractible. This requires immediate emergency medical attention. The person cannot complete a sentence in one breath; respiration is more than 25 breaths per minute and the pulse is more than 110 beats per minute. Life-threatening indicators are cyanosis, feeble respiratory effort, exhaustion, confusion and coma *(Clark, Rees, 1996)*. "Status asthmaticus" is an imprecise term that is sometimes used interchangeably with "life-threatening acute severe asthma". When used correctly, "status asthmaticus" describes an asthma attack that lasts over 24 hours, leading to dehydration and exhaustion *(Hough, 1996)*.

Subjective Information

HEALTH HISTORY QUESTIONS

✦ When was the onset of the asthma? Has it been diagnosed by a physician? Has the client had skin tests for allergies?

✦ Does the client have any other respiratory conditions such as emphysema or chronic bronchitis?

✦ Does anyone else in the client's family have asthma, hay fever or eczema? Does the client have hay fever or eczema?

✦ Has the client ever been hospitalized for asthma? When and for how long?

- What kind of asthma does the client have?

- What triggers an attack? Does the client wheeze or have chest tightness? When was the last attack?

- Is the client under continuous stress or increased amounts of stress at home or at work?

- Does the client have pets that could trigger attacks? If not, does someone in the client's life have pets or engage in a sport such as horseback riding that could expose the client to allergens?

- Does the client smoke? If yes, how much and how frequently?

- Is the client's living space insulated, sealed or dusty? Is the asthma worse at home, work or with recreational activities?

- Does the client have immediate symptoms on exposure to smoke, cold air, exercise or dust? This indicates airway hyperresponsiveness.

- Does the client have nocturnal symptoms of cough or waking with shortness of breath? Is the quality of sleep impaired?

- Is the client taking any medication? How frequently? How effective is the medication?

- What is the colour of the sputum? Expectorated mucus secretions may be clear, yellow or green. The colour is produced by degenerating eosinophils in asthma or by purulent sputum in superimposed respiratory infections such as bronchitis.

- What are the client's activity levels?

- Does the client self-monitor for severity of asthma symptoms using a peak-flow meter?

- If the client has an inhaler, where is it? What would the client like the therapist to do if an acute attack happens during the treatment?

- Is the client taking other parallel therapies such as physiotherapy or stress reduction techniques?

Objective Information

Observations

✍ The accessory muscles of respiration are likely hypertrophied.

✍ There may be dyspnea or tachypnea. The breathing pattern may be apical (using the upper chest only).

✍ Hyperkyphosis, head-forward posture or scoliosis may be present. See the appropriate chapters for postural assessment.

✍ A barrel chest (increased anteroposterior thoracic dimensions) may be present with chronic, poorly controlled asthma.

✍ During an attack, the seated client may lean forward, stabilizing the shoulder girdle to assist with inhalation. Exhalation is rapid, laboured and incomplete. There may be signs of anxiety.

Palpation

✍ The muscles of respiration and accessory muscles including the diaphragm, intercostals, scalenes, sternocleidomastoids, pectoralis major, pectoralis minor and the abdominals are tender and hypertonic. The axillary attachments of pectoralis major and latissimus dorsi, as well as the costal margins, are frequently tender (Ebner, 1980).

✍ Trigger points are likely present in the above muscles and they may feel ropey and fibrosed.

Testing

✍ **AF ROM** of the thoracic and cervical spine and the shoulder girdle reveals reduced ranges, especially in the thoracic spine.

✍ **PR ROM** including **static** and **motion palpation** of the thoracic and cervical spine reveal areas of hypomobility, especially in the upper and lower thoracic spine.

✍ **AR strength testing** for muscles of the shoulder girdle and the abdominals may be performed, assessing for possible weakness.

Special Tests

✍ **Vocal fremitus** and **mediate percussion tests** will be positive for areas of congestion due to mucus. This helps to locate the affected lobes for postural drainage if indicated.

✍ **Measurement** of the thoracic circumference at full inspiration and full expiration is taken with a tape measure and recorded. Measurement is at two levels, at the axilla and at the xiphoid process (Pryor, 1991). The measurement at exhalation is subtracted from the measurement at inhalation to give the amount of thoracic expansion, with normal differences in adults between 3 to 7.5 centimetres (Magee, 1992).

✍ The **rib motion test** is positive with larger areas of restricted motion, while the **rib palpation test** and **first rib mobility test** reveal specific restricted ribs. Rigidity of the ribs at T7 to T10 is common with asthma (Lewit, 1993). The **levatores costarum test** is positive if there is a rib fixation due to shortened levator costarum muscles. **Anterior** and **lateral spinous challenges** reveal areas of hypomobility.

✍ With hyperkyphosis, **pectoralis major** and **minor** are short.

Contraindications

✦ Determine the client's asthma triggers. If the triggers are allergens, such as dust or mould spores, these may exist in the treatment room. The room should be kept clean and dust-free. If strong smells trigger an attack, the therapist should detemine if the client is sensitive to any essential oil and avoid using it in the treatment.

✦ Do not exhaust the client with overtreatment or prolonged painful techniques.

✦ Avoid direct compression on the xiphoid process and the floating ribs. Joint play techniques for the ribs and rib springing are contraindicated with rib hypermobility and a history of rib subluxation.

✦ Massage therapy, lymphatic drainage and hydrotherapy are contraindicated during an acute attack.

✦ Postural drainage is contraindicated with severe hemoptysis (copious amounts of blood in sputum), severe pulmonary edema, congestive heart failure, pulmonary embolism, severe hypertension or hypotension, recent myocardial infarction and recent neurosurgery (Kisner, Colby, 1996; Hough 1996).

✦ Do not use postural drainage if the client has recently eaten.

✦ Tapotement is contraindicated over bony prominences, floating ribs and breast tissue.

✦ The prolonged tapotement that accompanies postural drainage is contraindicated with chest-wall pain, unstable angina, anticoagulation therapy, osteoporosis, rib fracture, prolonged steroid therapy, bronchospasm, untreated lung abscesses, pulmonary embolism and open thoracic wounds or burns (Irwin, Tecklin, 1995).

✦ Bronchodilator medication taken recently may indicate treatment modifications. Long-term steroid use may lead to osteoporosis. This condition requires treatment modifications. See the chapters on contraindications to massage therapy and osteoporosis.

✦ Chronic air-flow obstruction may lead to pulmonary hypertension and, in occasional cases, to right-sided heart failure or cor pulmonale, necessitating treatment modifications.

✦ Avoid an increase in daily water intake self-care if client has cardiac or renal disorders.

Treatment Goals

Reduce stress.
Mobilize the thorax.

Treatment Plan

Between Attacks

🖐 The therapist may choose several or all of the following techniques, focusing on the client's presenting symptoms. For example, stress reduction is a major component for a client who is under increased stress, while thoracic mobilization is a focus for someone with thoracic rigidity.

🖐 If the client has frequent asthma attacks, she should bring her inhaler with her to the treatment. Some clients may need to use a

Treatment Goals

Treatment Plan

bronchodilator before tapotement *(Hough, 1996)* and others may find this unnecessary.

✋ **Positioning** of the client will depend on the structures to be treated and the client's general health. Prone, supine, sidelying or seated positions are all options.

- During the massage, positioning choices are increasingly important with more chronic, severe cases of asthma. The time the client is in the supine position is reduced or the client is placed in sidelying, avoiding supine entirely.

- In general, the prone position was shown to improve ventilation and oxygenation, while the supine position decreased these factors *(Irwin, Tecklin, 1995)*. For more information on positioning for ventilation and postural drainage, see the chapter on chronic bronchitis.

Thin secretions.

✋ **Hydrotherapy** includes a facial steam five minutes prior to the massage to help thin the mucus. Five drops of pure, undiluted essential oil can be added to the bowl of hot water before the client covers her head and the bowl with a towel. The client should close her eyes during a steam, to avoid possible eye irritation by the oils. Eucalyptus, benzoin and frankincense are expectorants *(Lawless, 1995)*. Frankincense also helps to slow and deepen respiration, inducing relaxation *(Sellar, 1992)*.

General Treatment

✋ This treatment addresses a moderate asthma presentation where modifications for hypertension or ventilation are not needed. The treatment begins in the **prone position,** with pillows under the client's abdomen and ankles. Folded towels are placed under the client's shoulders if they are protracted. The client is later turned supine.

✋ **Hydrotherapy** applications are pre-treatment heat applied over the lower posterior intercostals before treating the fascia. When the client is supine for fascial work, heat may be applied to one pectoralis major muscle, then moved to the other side during work.

Decrease sympathetic nervous system firing. Encourage diaphragmatic breathing.

✋ It is important to perform this treatment in the context of a relaxation massage, including **diaphragmatic breathing** to help reduce stress and eliminate accessory respiratory muscle activity.

Specific Treatment

Reduce fascial restrictions.

✋ Fascial restrictions over the posterior thorax are treated first, including latissimus dorsi *(Ebner, 1980)*, the lower intercostals and quadratus lumborum attachments. Skin rolling, fascial spreading and the

905

Treatment Goals Treatment Plan

connective tissue cutting technique are indicated, working within the client's pain tolerance.

Reduce hypertonicity and trigger points. Reduce pain. Encourage circulation in overused structures.

Swedish techniques such as effleurage and petrissage are applied to upper trapezius, levator scapulae, serratus posterior superior, erector spinae, multifidi, posterior intercostals and quadratus lumborum. Trigger points in these muscles are addressed.

Mobilize the thorax.

Anterior and lateral challenge and spinous process oscillation joint play are used on hypomobile thoracic vertebrae. Thoracic mobilization and rib springing are indicated for areas of hypomobility. Rhythmic mobilizations for the shoulder girdle are also used.

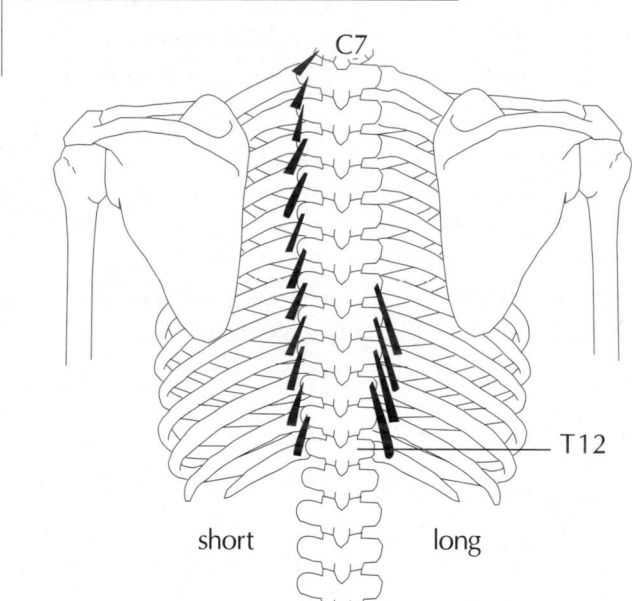

Tight levator costarum muscles are treated with the recoil technique. Levator costarum muscles run from the transverse process of one vertebra to the angle of the next inferior rib (*Figure 74.1*). They are found from C7 and rib 1 to T11 and rib 12. When short, these muscles fix ribs posteriorly. The rib is hypomobile to palpation in an anteriolateral direction. The therapist places one thumb on the angle of the posteriorly fixed rib. The other thumb slides medially to the nearest spinous process, which is the other attachment of the muscle. The spinous process is challenged laterally only to elastic end feel, placing a stretch on levator costarum. The thumbs maintain the end feel between the rib and spinous process while the client inhales. On exhalation, the therapist smoothly releases the spinous process and rib, allowing elastic recoil to mobilize levator costarum (Barral, 1991).

Figure 74.1
Levator costarum muscles. The short levatores costarum run from the C7 transverse process and rib 1 through to T11 and rib 12. The long levatores costarum run from the T7 transverse process and rib 9 through to T10 and rib 12.

The client is turned **supine** with pillows placed under the knees. If hyperkyphosis is present, a small towel roll is placed along the client's spine to flatten the curve.

Reduce fascial restrictions.

It is important to work within the client's pain tolerance. Anteriorly, fascial techniques including skin rolling, fascial spreading and connective tissue cutting are used on the pectoral fascia and sternum.

Before treating the costal margins and abdominal attachments, a towel is used to cover the client's chest. Skin rolling is performed over the

Treatment Goals   Treatment Plan

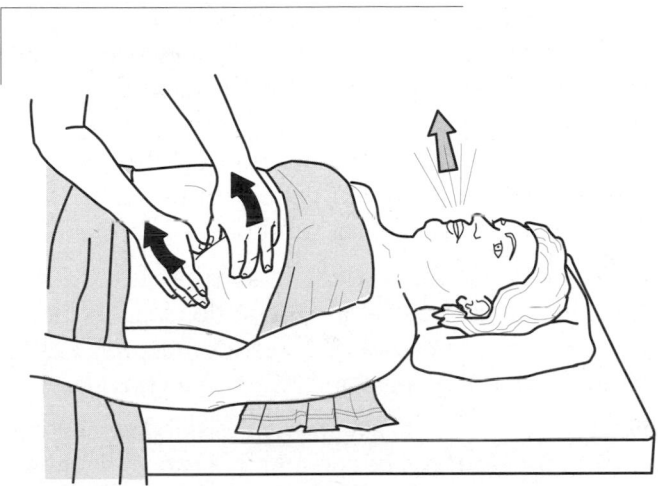

The lateral ribs are pulled medially as the client exhales to create slack. The therapist's thumbs move slowly under the costal margin.

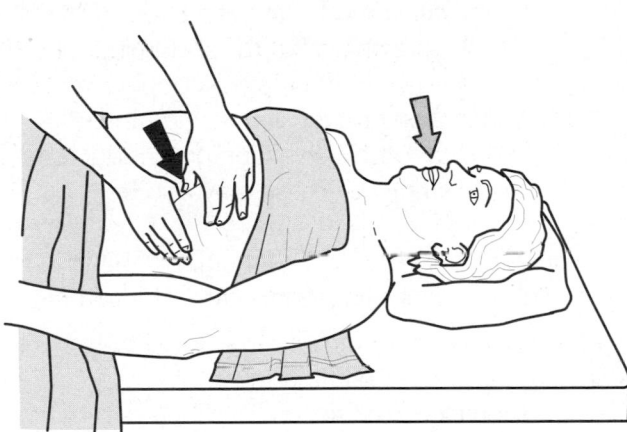

As the client inhales, the therapist keeps the thumbs in place, preventing them from being pushed out.

Figure 74.2
Treatment of diaphragm attachments.

lower anterior ribs and abdominal attachments.

🖐 Skin rolling is also performed over the abdominals, starting several centimetres above the pubic bone and moving superiorly to the costal margins in parallel strips.

🖐 The connective tissue cutting technique is used on the lower intercostals and inferior to the costal margin from the xiphoid process to the lateral ribs. Fascial spreading is applied on the abdominal attachments. The therapist stabilizes over the lower ribs with one hand. With the other hand, short fingertip spreading is used. The pressure is directed inferiorly on the attachments just below the costal margins. Dyspnea is relieved by this approach (*Ebner, 1980*). The tissue may be dense and restricted.

🖐 The diaphragm attachments are treated next. There are a few ways to approach this muscle. One method is used here. Another approach is described in the chapter on stress reduction. If the therapist is standing on the client's right side, the diaphragm attachments on the left anterior side are treated. The therapist places both thumbs together just under the costal margin, several centimetres down from the xiphoid process. The fingers of both hands are placed on the lateral ribs. Slack is created by pulling the lateral ribs medially as the client exhales. At the same time, the therapist's thumbs slowly move under the costal margins (*Figure 74.2*). As the client inhales, the therapist's thumbs stay in place. Working with the client's breathing, the therapist slowly moves the thumbs onto the attachment of the diaphragm, which can be visualized as an inverted bowl. To help accurately locate the diaphragm, the client is asked to inhale and hold her breath for a few seconds. The diaphragm should tighten up underneath the therapist's thumbs. Again working with the client's breathing, the therapist makes short spreading strokes from the underside of the costal margin up towards the muscle fibres of the diaphragm. Cross-fibre kneading may also be used. The diaphragm attachments are treated systematically from near the xiphoid process

Treatment Goals   Treatment Plan

to the lateral ribs, allowing the client breaks as necessary. This technique is not performed in an invasive or abrupt manner, and should be pain free. The technique is repeated on the right attachments. All anterior attachments of the diaphragm need not be treated in one appointment. The therapist may choose to treat the medial third of the right and left attachments at one time, progressing to the lateral portions of the attachments at subsequent treatments.

Reduce hypertonicity.
Reduce trigger points.
Reduce pain.

ᗡ Swedish techniques for pectoralis major, pectoralis minor, subclavius, serratus anterior, the anterior intercostals and the abdominals include effleurage, over-handed palmar kneading on the abdomen, fingertip kneading, muscle stripping and the origin and insertion technique.

ᗡ The intercostals are worked systematically from medial to lateral using repetitive slow muscle stripping. Pressure is gradually increased with each repetition, working within the client's pain tolerance. The intercostals between the first, second and third ribs, as well as those between the lower ribs, are most likely to be hypertonic. The intercostals may be treated over a series of appointments. The therapist does not work through breast tissue.

ᗡ The diaphragm may also be treated with Swedish techniques such as costal border scooping and specific muscle stripping under the costal border, working with the client's breathing. Rectus abdominus and the abdominal obliques are addressed with effleurage, scooping, muscle stripping and fingertip kneading along the costal margins and iliac crest. Specific consent is required to treat the suprapubic attachments of the abdominals with muscle stripping. These may also be addressed by massaging through the client's hand. The client places her fingers at the suprapubic attachments. The therapist's hand is placed over top and moves the client's fingers in a cross-fibre direction.

ᗡ Trigger points in pectoralis major, sternalis (if present) and the intercostals are treated. Symptoms of breathlessness and reduced tidal volume due to restricted thoracic expansion are attributed to trigger points in serratus anterior *(Travell, Simons, 1983)*.

ᗡ The scalenes, sternocleidomastoids, upper trapezius, levator scapulae, suboccipitals and posterior cervical muscles are treated with petrissage including muscle stripping, fingertip kneading and Golgi tendon organ release.

Increase local circulation to flush out metabolites.
Mobilize the thorax.

ᗡ Repetitive effleurage is used on the shoulder and neck muscles.

ᗡ Joint play, resisted breathing and rib springing are indicated to treat areas of hypomobility on the sternum and ribs. See the chapter on chronic bronchitis for details.

ᗡ Anterior and lateral challenge joint play are used on hypomobile cervical vertebrae.

Treatment Goals

Treatment Plan

Stretch shortened muscles.

👋 PIR is applied to the cervical muscles, including the scalenes, and the accessory muscles of respiration, such as the pectoral muscles (*Pryor, 1991*).

Remove secretions.

👋 If postural drainage is required, the client is placed in the appropriate postural drainage position. This may be **prone** or **sidelying**. Postural drainage, breathing exercises and tapotement are indicated to remove mucus secretions. Prior to postural drainage, the client should practise diaphragmatic breathing and productive coughing or huffing. The client may find it easier to expectorate using a huff instead of a cough (*Pryor, 1991*). The therapist should have tissues and a plastic-lined wastebasket for the client to expectorate into. For specific drainage positions, productive coughing or huffing and tapotement sequence and duration, refer to the chapter on chronic bronchitis.

👋 Coughing can relieve or exacerbate asthma. Depending on the client's presentation, cough suppression techniques may be necessary. These include voluntarily inhibiting the cough, avoiding the supine position, swallowing, nose-breathing, taking sips of cold water, taking repeated short sniffs or slow, shallow breaths and breathing through pursed lips (*Hough, 1996*).

Treat other conditions.

👋 Hyperkyphosis, hyperlordosis and other conditions are addressed in subsequent appointments.

Self-care Goals

Self-care Plan

Encourage relaxation strategies.

✍ Relaxation techniques for the muscles of the neck and shoulder girdle are important. See the chapter on stress reduction for details.

✍ Relaxation exercises and yoga reduce stress and may help people with asthma (*Thomson et al., 1991*).

Instruct the client to control an acute attack.

✍ While the effectiveness of breathing exercises in controlling asthma is debated (*Clark, Rees, 1996*), the following exercise has been found helpful. The supported, seated client assesses the quality of her breathing, including any wheeze. The client then inhales slowly through the nose, so the wheeze is eliminated. Breathing is temporarily deepened to compensate for the slow breath. The rate is slowed as breathing becomes more comfortable. As the hunger for air decreases, the client feels more in control. Muscle tension in the neck and thorax is observed by the client and modified. The depth of breathing is gradually increased, with the client breathing into the diaphragm, then into the lateral ribs and then the upper chest. She reverses the order to exhale. The client reassesses the tension of the muscles of respiration. She progresses to unsupported sitting, then standing (*Hough, 1996*).

Self-care Goals

Self-care Plan

Instruct in breathing exercises. Strengthen weak muscles.

✍ Diaphragmatic breathing, pursed-lip breathing and productive coughing are important breathing exercises. See the chapter on chronic bronchitis for details.

Reduce or eliminate triggering factors.

✍ *Dust mites* are widespread and thrive in damp, warm conditions. It is impossible to eradicate them entirely from a house, so the client is advised to focus on controlling them in the bedroom. Regular changing of bed linens, the use of synthetic rather than feather pillows and comforters, and gore-tex mattress covers that are impervious to mites are suggested. Regular vacuuming of the floors, curtains and mattress is indicated. The vacuum cleaner can be fitted with a filter over the exhaust to remove the mite's fecal products rather than redistributing them around the room. Bedroom rugs should be regularly vacuumed or removed entirely. With children, stuffed toys should be cleaned regularly.

✍ *Pollens and spores* are also impossible to avoid. Air conditioning may provide some relief, as may closing the windows when pollen counts are highest. Face masks may be helpful at these times.

✍ *Exercise-induced asthma* can be lessened by breathing warm, moist air during exertion (using a face mask) or by inhaling beta-2 sympathomimetic medication before exercise. Controlled, paced breathing may help. The choice of activity may also reduce the symptoms. Short bursts of activity decrease exercise-induced asthma while prolonged activity increases it. Swimming is less of a stimulus to asthma than long-distance running or cross-country skiing. The client should gradually increase her exercise tolerance. Overall physical conditioning can reduce medication requirements and decrease the incidence of attacks *(Rupp, 1996)*.

✍ *Occupational-related asthma triggers* may be reduced by using masks or air filters.

Stretch short muscles.

✍ Stretching for the scalenes and shoulder girdle muscles is important. See chapters on whiplash and hyperkyphosis for more information.

Teach self-massage.

✍ Self-massage to the intercostals, scalenes and costal margins and suprapubic attachments of the abdominals is indicated.

Mobilize the thorax.

✍ For exercises to mobilize the thorax laterally and anteriorly, see the chapter on chronic bronchitis. Stretching once a day maintains the range of motion. Stretching more often increases the range *(Irwin, Tecklin, 1995)*.

Thin secretions.

✍ Inhalation of steam in a hot shower helps to thin secretions, as does drinking six to eight glasses of water per day. However, a client with cardiac or renal disorders should not increase the daily intake of water *(Bach, 1996)*.

Self-care Goals

Refer the client.

Self-care Plan

✍ The client is referred to a physician for a self-assessment plan using a peak-flow meter.

✍ The client is encouraged to recognize the need for medical attention if there is a change in symptoms or new symptoms *(Hough, 1996)*.

✍ The client's physician or a smoking cessation program can help with stopping smoking.

✍ A self-help group, such as the Asthma Association, may be helpful.

✍ Movement therapy, such as the Mitzvah, Feldenkrais or Alexander technique, may be helpful for retraining the client's posture.

Treatment Frequency and Expected Outcome

Treatments should be one hour in length, once a week until posture and breathing improve. Ongoing treatment may be required during periods of increased stress and to maintain thoracic and cervical mobility.

See also stress reduction, chronic bronchitis, emphysema, hyperkyphosis, hypertension and myofascial trigger points for related treatments.

Outcome is variable depending on the type of asthma, the length of time the disease has been present, monitoring of the client's peak-flow readings, medication use, stress reduction and the client's exposure to known triggers.

Asthma may be well controlled if the client complies with necessary modifications and self-care plans.

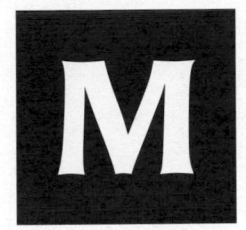

CIRCULATORY PATHOLOGIES AND DYSFUNCTIONS

HYPERTENSION AND CONGESTIVE HEART FAILURE

Linda Ludwig

Hypertension is the elevation of blood pressure above the normal range for a prolonged period of time. It can increase the risk of stroke or heart attack.

Congestive heart failure (also known as heart failure) reflects the heart's inability to pump sufficient blood to supply the body's needs.

Understanding Blood Pressure

When the heart beats it pushes blood through the arteries to supply all areas of the body. **Blood pressure (BP)** is the pressure or force of the circulating blood against the blood vessel walls *(Heart and Stroke Foundation of Canada, N.d.b.)*.

A person's blood pressure is determined by the amount of blood ejected into the aorta **(stroke volume)** combined with the number of contractions of the heart **(heart rate)** while taking into account the resistive factors in the circulatory system that affect the ease of blood flow **(peripheral resistance).** The peripheral resistance is influenced by the tone of the blood vessels and the viscosity of blood; if the blood vessels constrict and the blood viscosity increases, the total peripheral resistance is increased.

✦ The formula reads:
$$BP = \frac{\text{cardiac output (stroke volume x heart rate)}}{\text{total peripheral resistance}}$$

The body maintains healthy blood pressure by adjusting any of the above variables. If the total peripheral resistance is high, the body alters cardiac output to compensate for it. If cardiac output is altered, the total peripheral resistance changes to maintain appropriate blood pressure.

In established hypertension and severe hypertension cases, there is often an increase in peripheral resistance, with the cardiac output lower than normal *(Hickey, Graham, 1988)*.

Measuring Blood Pressure

By the early part of this century, physicians were beginning to take a patient's blood pressure using the sphygmomanometer, also known as a blood pressure cuff. This instrument consists of an inflatable blood pressure cuff and mercury manometer which are used with a stethoscope for measuring the systolic and diastolic blood pressure. The clinical usefulness of this measurement was not clear at that time. In the 1920s, benign and malignant hypertension were recognized. Interest in these conditions began to rise and continues to this day.

In some cases, massage therapist training includes instruction in taking blood pressure. Only therapists who have education in blood pressure measurement should use it in their practice.

When the blood pressure is measured, the cuff is placed around the upper arm, level with the heart, and a stethoscope is placed just under the cuff over the brachial artery to monitor sounds. The blood pressure cuff is inflated until its pressure is higher than the arterial pressure; this temporarily impedes blood flow and no sounds are heard. The cuff is then deflated very slowly while the first sound (a thumping or whooshing noise) of the blood flowing back into the arteries is monitored and this point is measured on the manometer. This is the systolic pressure (SP). The cuff continues to be slowly deflated until there are no more sounds, suggesting the vessels are no longer compressed by the cuff. The point at which the sounds cease is noted on the manometer. This reflects the diastolic pressure (DP). Subsequent readings of the same client's pressure should be taken from the same arm, with the client in the same position.

+ **Systolic pressure** denotes the maximum pressure reached during the ejection of blood into the aorta with contraction of the ventricles of the heart. When blood pressure is recorded, SP is the first and highest number. It reflects the tension placed on the wall of the blood vessel that occurs with the ejection of blood. The pressure is influenced by the amount of blood ejected (stroke volume), the speed of ejection and the amount of elasticity in the walls of the blood vessel itself. If the volume or speed of ejection is increased or the aorta is less elastic, it is reflected as an increase in SP.

+ **Diastolic pressure** is the term used to reflect the minimum amount of pressure maintained in the walls of the aorta between contractions of the heart. When blood pressure is recorded, DP is the second or lower number. Therefore, a measurement, written as SP over DP might be 120/80 mm Hg. Diastolic pressure is influenced by the elastic qualities in the walls of the arterial blood vessels, the competency of the aortic valve and the resistance of the arterioles into which the "run off" of the arterial blood flows. An increase in total peripheral resistance, through an increased sympathetic response or from rigid arteries (atherosclerosis), can increase DP. A decrease in diastolic pressure results if the aortic valve is unable to close properly, allowing back-flow of blood into the left ventricle of the heart.

+ **Pulse pressure** is the difference between the systolic and diastolic pressure. It can be palpated as a rhythmical throbbing over the arteries in the wrist or neck.

From infancy onwards, a person experiences a steady rise in blood pressure. At five years old, a child's systolic pressure averages 97 mm Hg; by 19 years of age, the SP raises to 129 mm Hg in women and 131 mm Hg in men. It then stabilizes between ages 25 and 44. In Western cultures, those with the higher-end blood pressures seem to have the highest readings after middle age. Diastolic pressure averages 60 to 70 mm Hg in adults. Its increase over a lifetime is less dramatic than with systolic pressure. Currently, a normal blood pressure is considered to be 140 or less, for the systolic pressure, and 90 or less, for the diastolic pressure.

Factors in Maintenance of Healthy Blood Pressure

Blood pressure changes continuously with daily physical activity, positional changes (such as standing to sitting, lying to standing and so on) and emotions. Over the short term, as this pressure fluctuates up or down, the body uses nerves and hormones to restore "normal blood pressure".

✦ **Baroreceptors** are receptors within the walls of blood vessels that are sensitive to pressure changes. These are located in the neck at the division point of the carotid arteries, referred to as the "carotid sinus", and at the arch of the aorta. Other baroreceptors are contained in the large veins, pulmonary blood vessels and heart. Through the afferent nerves, input about changes in the stretch of a vessel wall is relayed to the brain and its cardiovascular centres so adjustments to heart action and vascular tone are made. These are short-term changes that require only seconds to occur.

✦ **Chemoreceptors** are receptors, located in the carotid sinuses and the aorta, monitoring the concentration of oxygen, carbon dioxide and hydrogen in the blood. While primarily influencing one's breathing rate, these receptors also communicate with the vasomotor centres in the brain and can change vascular tone.

✦ **The autonomic nervous system** modifies heart rate and peripheral resistance to influence blood pressure over the short term. Both sympathetic and parasympathetic nerves innervate the heart. The parasympathetic nervous system, through stimulation of the vagus nerve, can slow the pulse rate. Sympathetic nervous system stimulation increases heart rate. It also controls vascular tone and, therefore, peripheral resistance.

✦ The **central nervous system** uses massive vasoconstriction to raise blood pressure to the extreme in a situation where there is insufficient blood flow to the brain; this prevents ischemia of brain tissue.

✦ The **renin-angiotensin-aldosterone mechanism** uses salt retention or salt loss to influence blood pressure. Renin, an enzyme from the kidneys, is released with sympathetic nervous system firing. It begins a chemical cycle that causes vasoconstriction and salt and water retention which will then affect blood pressure.

✦ **Hormones** such as renal prostaglandins and vasopressin influence vasoconstriction of blood vessels.

✦ Over the long term, the **renal body-fluid pressure control system** uses water and salt excretion through the kidneys to maintain blood pressure *(Porth, 1990)*.

Hypertension

Hypertension is the elevation of blood pressure above the normal range for a prolonged period of time. It can increase the risk of stroke or heart attack.

Classification of Blood Pressure

According to the American Joint National Committee on Detection, Evaluation and Treatment of High Blood Pressure, 1993:

	Systolic BP (mm Hg)	Diastolic BP (mm Hg)
Normal	less than 130	less than 85
High normal	130 to 139	85 to 89
Hypertension		
Stage 1 (mild)	140 to 159	90 to 99
Stage 2 (moderate)	160 to 179	100 to 109
Stage 3 (severe)	180 to 209	110 to 119
Stage 4 (very severe)	210 or more	120 or more

(National Institute of Health, 1993)

Ten to 30 per cent of the population is affected by high blood pressure or hypertension. It is surprising that the body often seems able to tolerate elevated blood pressure for many years, before detrimental effects on the heart are detected *(Porth, 1990)*. With hypertension, the heart (specifically, the left ventricle) works harder to pump blood against increased arterial pressure. As with other muscles, as the heart performs more, it develops more mass and requires more oxygen. Initially, this adaptation works but, over time, the heart's ability to function as a pump can be affected, leading to heart failure.

Hypertension is often called the "silent killer" because the transition from health to illness is often asymptomatic with few signs clinically detected in the heart or kidneys. Occasionally, people may experience headache, shortness of breath or dizziness. Over time, the excessive arterial pressure of hypertension can lead to damage of the arterial walls. Untreated hypertension can lead to pathological changes to the blood vessels such as atherosclerosis ("hardening" of the arteries), stroke (the rupture of blood vessels in the brain), heart attacks (the presence of blood clots or the narrowing of the arteries that supply the heart) and peripheral vascular disease (affecting the blood vessels of the limbs, especially the legs) as well as problems with the heart (heart failure) and the kidneys (kidney failure). These complications of hypertension often develop over years or decades. The risk of cardiovascular disease and stroke also increases with a person's age, as blood vessels lose their elasticity and the body experiences other changes associated with aging *(Hickey, Graham, 1988)*. In the elderly, hypertension is blood pressure with a systolic pressure of 160 mm Hg or over. For this age group a systolic pressure of 140 to 160 mm Hg and diastolic of 90 mm Hg or less is considered within normal limits *(Kart et al., 1992)*. Despite the expectation that hypertension is inevitable with aging, this is not necessarily the case.

Risk Factors for Hypertension

Hypertension should always be seen in the context of risk factors that may influence blood pressure. For example, high BP may be considered more of a concern when the person smokes or has diabetes.

✦ **Those most at risk of developing hypertension are:**

- anyone over 45 years old; over half the population over 65 has hypertension;

- those with a family history of premature cardiovascular disease, hypertension, stroke or hyperlipidemia;

- Blacks, who are affected one-third more than Caucasians especially those between the ages of 24 to 44, (the former group is 18 times more likely to have kidney failure from hypertension);

- men more than women until after women reach menopause, when the numbers become more even.

✦ **Pregnant women also have an increased risk** of elevated blood pressure, **especially**:

- teenagers or women over 35;

- Black women;

- women in their first pregnancy;

- women with a history of hypertension, diabetes, kidney disease or heart problems;

- women whose mother had a high blood pressure disorder in pregnancy.

Hypertension affects five to 10 per cent of pregnant women. In this case, the definition of hypertension is slightly different and includes a combination of hypertension, proteinuria and edema, especially in the face and hands *(Knuppel, Drukker, 1993)*. It is classified as pregnancy induced hypertension (PIH), referred to as "pre-eclampsia" (mild or severe) or "eclampsia". It usually disappears after the birth of the baby.

✦ **Hypertension is often associated with:**

- heart disease (a narrowing of blood vessels that supply the heart; an additional risk develops with angioplasty or bypass surgery to correct this narrowing);

- myocardial infarction (heart failure) and post infarction; often hypertension is related to a higher mortality rate in the case of a second infarction *(Hickey, Graham, 1988)*;

- angina pectoris (heart pain due to a reduction of the blood supply to the heart, especially when the heart must do more work);

- left ventricular hypertrophy;

- transient ischemic attacks and stroke;

- arteriosclerosis;

- kidney disorders;

- diabetes (one to two per cent of the population has this condition) *(Hickey, Graham,*

919

1988). A person with diabetes seems to be more likely to have hypertension than someone without the condition, especially in the systolic levels. With this condition, there is an increase in the mortality rate from cardiovascular disease and, specifically, atherosclerosis;

- metabolic disorders such as hyperthyroidism. These disorders have been correlated with a predisposition to lipid and blood pressure abnormalities;

- adrenal tumours *(Balch, Balch, 1997)*.

✦ **Lifestyle risk factors for hypertension are:**

- smoking, which causes plaques to build up in the arteries. Smokers are at twice the risk for a heart attack or stroke *(Heart and Stroke Foundation of Ontario)*;

- stress, which, through the sympathetic nervous system, constricts the walls of the arteries. Ongoing stressors may result in chronically elevated blood pressure and hypertension *(Porth, 1990)*;

- high sodium intake in those genetically predisposed *(Vander et al., 1994)*;

- oral contraceptive use;

- obesity;

- excessive alcohol intake;

- physical inactivity.

✦ **Risk factors can be cumulative.** For example, with a family history of hypertension, a person is twice as likely to develop hypertension; but the addition of another risk factor, such as obesity, increases the risk by three or four times *(Porth, 1990)*.

Types of Hypertension

There are two main categories of hypertension: **primary hypertension** (also known as idiopathic or essential hypertension) and **secondary hypertension.**

Primary hypertension is a silent, long-term condition that is not associated with any underlying disease. In over 95 per cent of those with hypertension, the cause of the arteriolar constriction is unknown, though it is associated with the risk factors listed.

Secondary hypertension is the result of an underlying pathology such as kidney disease, vascular disease or alterations in adrenal functions (often from a tumour). Malignant hypertension is an accelerated and potentially fatal form of secondary hypertension that can develop in a small number of people. It can affect younger people, usually Black men, women with toxemia in pregnancy and those with renal and collagen diseases *(Porth, 1990)*. Diastolic pressure in someone with this condition can rise above 120 mm Hg. Immediate medical treatment is needed.

The Medical Treatment of Hypertension

Generally, if a person's blood pressure is elevated, his physician will monitor the BP on two to three occasions over a four-week period.

If the BP goes below a SP of 180 mm Hg or a DP of 105 mm Hg, the BP will simply be monitored over a three- to six-month period. If the BP remains elevated, treatment will often be through lifestyle changes rather than drug therapy to lower the BP over a three-month period. Lifestyle changes include moderate-intensity aerobic exercise, weight loss (if necessary), cessation of smoking, reduction of alcohol intake and diet modifications (*Buschbacher, 1994*).

According to the 1993 American Joint National Committee on High Blood Pressure, if a person's blood pressure remains above 140/90 mm Hg over a three- to six-month period despite strong recommendations to make lifestyle changes, antihypertensive medication is usually started, especially if heart or kidney damage or other risk factors exist.

A 1993 World Health Organization Report along with the International Society of Hypertension suggests drug therapy if the diastolic pressure is 95 mm Hg or above, as well as for those in the 90 to 95 mm Hg range who have additional risk factors (*Kaplan, Ram, 1995*).

If DP is 100 mm Hg or above, or SP is 160 to 180 mm Hg with DP at 95 mm Hg or above, usually both lifestyle changes and drug therapy are used, whether or not additional risk factors exist. At these levels the possibility of complications increases dramatically (*Kaplan, Ram, 1995*).

Prescription hypertensive medications include diuretics to reduce sympathetic nervous system effects on vascular smooth muscle, angiotensin-converting enzyme inhibitors to reduce vasoconstriction, beta blockers to inhibit the action of the sympathetic nervous system on vascular smooth muscle and, in turn, vasoconstriction, calcium channel blockers to reduce tone in venous and arterial smooth muscle and to reduce cardiac output, and vasodilator drugs to decrease peripheral resistance through the relaxation of the smooth muscle of the arterioles (*Kart et al., 1992; Porth, 1990*).

The Effects of Massage on Circulation

Massage affects circulation in a few ways. It mechanically assists in emptying blood and lymph vessels and facilitating forward movement of the blood and lymph. Blood vessels collapse and refill as massage techniques are applied. The vasomotor nerves supplying the blood vessels are also stimulated, resulting in visible hyperemia after prolonged massage in an area. Animal studies have shown that deep stroking and kneading techniques result in "consistent, and definite increases in the blood flow of the...extremities" (*Basmajian, 1985*). Petrissage was found to cause an initial increase in arterial pressure, which was then followed by a decrease in pressure as the result of peripheral vasodilation (*Basmajian, 1985*). Considering these effects, as hypertension is more severe or complicated with other circulatory or organ conditions, it may be prudent to begin the massage to the client's limbs to encourage peripheral vasodilation and a decrease in peripheral resistance, which would then lower the blood pressure.

The therapist must also consider the effect of dramatically increasing venous and lymphatic fluid return to the heart. Full-body lymphatic drainage techniques and other full-body applications of techniques can cause a sudden increase in the volume of lymphatic fluid or venous return through the body to the heart (*Wittlinger, Wittlinger, 1990*).

To address both concerns, the therapist begins the massage by treating the limbs using segmental or short effleurage and petrissage techniques to increase peripheral vasodilation but avoids long stroking and full-limb effleurage to control the amount of venous return to the heart.

Treatment Considerations

HEALTH HISTORY QUESTIONS

◆ When was the hypertension diagnosed?

◆ What treatment was given? Were lifestyle changes encouraged such as dieting, exercise and smoking cessation? Did the client make these changes? Was medication prescribed? If so, which drugs? Does the client take the medication? Is the blood pressure stable now?

◆ Has the client or the physician imposed any lifestyle restrictions such as no hot baths, a reduction in the vigour of exercise or alteration of the sleeping position (to avoid sleeping on the stomach or lying flat on the back)?

◆ Is this the client's first massage experience? If so, does the client's physician know he is receiving massage? If not, what was the client's response to previous massage experiences?

◆ Does the client consent to the therapist contacting his physician to get more information about his condition?

◆ Is there a history of: heart disease; treatment including angioplasty or bypass surgery; arteriosclerosis; kidney disorders; myocardial infarction (heart failure); angina pectoris; left ventricular hypertrophy; transient ischemic attacks and stroke; familial hyperlipidemia; diabetes; metabolic disorders such as hyperthyroidism or adrenal tumours.

Further Assessment

✍ **Measuring Blood Pressure:**

◆ *With any new client,* blood pressure should be taken at the beginning of a treatment. Even if the pressure is normal, it is still recommended that blood pressure be taken periodically. The more risk factors in the health history, the more regularly the blood pressure should be monitored.

  • If the blood pressure has changed from previous readings, the therapist asks about recent activities that may have temporarily increased the blood pressure. BP is monitored over the next few treatments. If it remains changed, the client is referred to a physician.

  • As a guide, the client should be referred to a physician if:

    — there are changes in the BP from the person's normal range; or

    — the BP is measured twice on two different occasions with a value of 140 to 180 mm Hg (SP) or 90 to 105 mm Hg (DP).

◆ *With a client who is diagnosed with hypertension,* the blood pressure is measured before each treatment. The client is asked specific question to ascertain his compliance with lifestyle changes and medication use:

  • Does the client smoke?

  • Does the client exercise?

922

- Has the client's diet been modified since the diagnosis?
- Is the client on medication? If so, is the blood pressure stable now?
- Does the client take medication as prescribed?

✍ In any case, if the blood pressure is elevated, modifications are made to the massage treatment and the blood pressure is taken again after the treatment to gauge the client's response.

Guidelines for the Accurate Measure of Blood Pressure

✍ Blood pressure readings can be temporarily elevated when the following guidelines are not observed.

✍ Blood pressure should be measured when the client is relaxed and has rested for at least 15 minutes.

✍ There should be no smoking or consumption of caffeine (coffee, tea, chocolate or cola) as well as no performance of heavy physical activity within a minimum of 30 minutes of taking the BP.

✍ The urinary bladder should be emptied because a full bladder can increase blood pressure.

✍ The client should not talk while the BP is being taken.

✍ Any medications taken before the BP measurement should be noted, such as cold remedies, nicotine gums or patches, or pain medications.

✍ Ideally, the pressure should be taken at the same time of day each time *(Heart and Stroke Foundation of Canada, N.d.b.)*.

✍ The therapist should be aware that, for some clients, the simple process of taking the blood pressure may elevate the BP. This is referred to as "white coat syndrome." *(Hickey, Graham, 1988)*.

Contraindications

✦ In the case of clients with severe hypertension, those with a severe complicating pathology or those who have moderate hypertension but appear uncompliant with medical treatment (based on the health history questions), their physician should be contacted (with their consent) to determine the appropriateness and safety of massage therapy, as well as the extent of the treatment modification required.

✦ Increasing sympathetic nervous system firing will elevate the blood pressure. Prolonged painful techniques are avoided.

✦ Potentially painful techniques, such as trigger point therapy or fascial techniques, are applied to a limited area interspersed with gentle, soothing techniques. Stimulating techniques such as vigorous tapotement — cupping, hacking and pounding — are avoided.

✦ There are concerns regarding the neck and the associated vasculature, especially the carotid artery. The client's neck should not be rotated for prolonged periods of time as this could occlude the blood flow through the blood vessels in the neck. Bilateral treatment (especially with deep techniques) of the sternocleidomastoid muscles is contraindicated for the same reason.

✦ The therapist should avoid techniques and modalities that would contribute to the return of large volumes of venous and lymphatic fluid to the heart, especially in the case of severe hypertension and with clients who have complicating cardiovascular conditions. The full-body application of repetitive long and broad strokes is modified by using short, segmental strokes. Repetitive, passive, large limb movements in mid- and full ranges should be avoided (*DeLisa, Gans, 1993*).

✦ Prolonged elevation of the legs above the level of the heart is not recommended.

✦ Full-body lymphatic drainage is contraindicated (*Wittlinger, Wittlinger, 1985*).

✦ Full-body hydrotherapy applications or prolonged heat applications over the back or over the pectoral region are avoided.

✦ Hypertensive essential oils such as camphor, hyssop, rosemary, sage and thyme, as well as vasoconstricting essential oils such as cypress, geranium and rosemary, should not be used (*Sellar, 1992*).

Massage for Hypertension

🖐 The number of modifications made within the treatment will relate to the severity of the hypertension and the client's compliance with medical advice. A client with mild, stable hypertension, who is compliant with medical treatment, will generally not require modifications. Even in such a case, the therapist must remain vigilant for any signs of distress during the treatment.

🖐 If the client has moderate, stable hypertension, some modifications are made to the treatment, such as reduced treatment time in the prone position and some elevation of the upper body while the client is supine. Painful techniques are performed over a series of treatments with only a limited use of long strokes.

🖐 Because no two people are the same, the therapist needs to exercise some judgement based on a thorough assessment of the client. When in doubt, the therapist should contact the client's physician and may choose not to give a massage that day. If a massage is given the therapist should take a very conservative approach that includes modifications, until the physician is consulted.

🖐 **Positioning:** In determining a safe treatment position, the therapist enquires as to the client's sleeping position or for any other restrictions a physician has given for positioning. If the client is able to sleep on his stomach, the prone position may be used during the treatment. Because of the pressure on the abdominal aorta, the therapist may choose to reduce the time the client is in the prone position. Sidelying is appropriate, though it is thought that left-side lying can place additional stress on the heart. Time in this position may be reduced or the position avoided in the case of moderate to severe hypertension. The preferred position is supine, with pillows supporting the trunk in a semi-seated posture. It places less stress on the cardiovascular system. The seated position is excellent for clients with moderate to severe hypertension as it puts the least stress on the cardiovascular system.

✋ A key goal of massage treatment is to reduce sympathetic nervous system firing, which will reduce blood pressure. Soothing, less vigorous techniques are used. Slow, relaxed breathing is encouraged. Visualization is effective if the client is comfortable with this technique.

✋ With moderate hypertension or where there are complicating cardiovascular conditions, rather than starting with techniques to the trunk, the therapist should begin by massaging the limbs, using short, segmental strokes. Essential oils such as marjoram, ylang ylang, lavender and lemon can be used to enrich the massage lotion and facilitate decreased sympathetic nervous system firing (Lawless, 1992). Twenty-five drops of pure essential oil are used in 50 ml. of vegetable oil. Other treatment goals will relate to the client's specific requests, with attention paid to contraindications.

✋ Throughout the treatment, the therapist must be alert for changes in the client and signs of cardiovascular distress, such as increased heart rate or dizziness reported by the client, increased respiratory rate, shallow breathing, sweating or facial flushing. If any of these are observed, the therapist should ask how the client is feeling and make appropriate modifications.

- These may include a change into the semi-seated supine position and a switch to segmental techniques on the limbs. If the client is in agreement, the therapist can continue the treatment, observing for a decrease in distress symptoms. If the distress symptoms do not diminish, the treatment is stopped and the client is put in a sitting position until the symptoms pass.

Self-care for Hypertension

✍ Relaxation training, meditation and biofeedback have been shown to reduce blood pressure (Hickey, Graham, 1988). Herbert Benson, a Harvard physician who developed the Relaxation Response technique, has studied meditation for its effect on blood pressure. The technique consisted of two 20-minute periods each day of quiet meditation with the person comfortably positioned, taking slow, easy breaths. This practice decreased the sympathetic response. In a study of hypertension, people performed the Relaxation Response (RR). Their blood pressure decreased and stayed down for as long as they continued the daily meditation. Before the study, their average systolic BP was 146 mm Hg but after several weeks of RR it dropped to an average of 137 mm Hg. Their average diastolic pressure went from 93.5 to 88.9 mm Hg (Benson, Klipper, 1975).

✍ Essential oils can be used by the client at home.

✍ Moderate aerobic exercise has been found to improve cardiovascular health and reduce blood pressure. The best exercise results are combined with other lifestyle changes, such as improvements to diet and cessation of smoking (Heart and Stroke Foundation of Canada, N.d.b.). A specific stretch and strengthening regime may be prescribed, as determined by the client's needs.

> See stress reduction, hemiplegia, diabetes mellitus and pregnancy for related treatments.

✍ The client is encouraged to maintain physician-prescribed lifestyle changes.

Congestive Heart Failure

Congestive heart failure (also known as heart failure) reflects the heart's inability to pump sufficient blood to supply the body's needs.

This condition may be acute or chronic. It may be secondary to heart disease, chronic high blood pressure, valvular disease and other conditions that place excessive stress on the heart, as well as viral infection and alcoholism. Each year in Canada, 40,000 people are diagnosed with congestive heart failure. Statistically, the prognosis suggests about half of those diagnosed will not survive five years past diagnosis. With medical treatment and adaptations to their routines, the other half will survive well past five years (*Heart and Stroke Foundation of Canada, N.b.a.*).

There are often both systolic and diastolic dysfunctions relating to problems with the contractile properties of the ventricles of the heart *(Figure 75.1)*. Usually, about two-thirds of the blood volume in the heart is ejected with ventricle contraction. With heart failure, the volume of blood ejected becomes progressively less. In severe cases, this volume may be as low as one-quarter to one-fifth the volume of blood in the heart. The remaining fluid causes the dilatation of the faulty ventricle and passive congestion of the organs proximal to it. Left ventricle problems cause lung congestion whereas right ventricle difficulties cause congestion in the liver and limbs. Secondary to ventricular enlargement is the fact that the heart must work harder to elicit contractions that will eject the blood in this ventricle. Circulation will become sluggish.

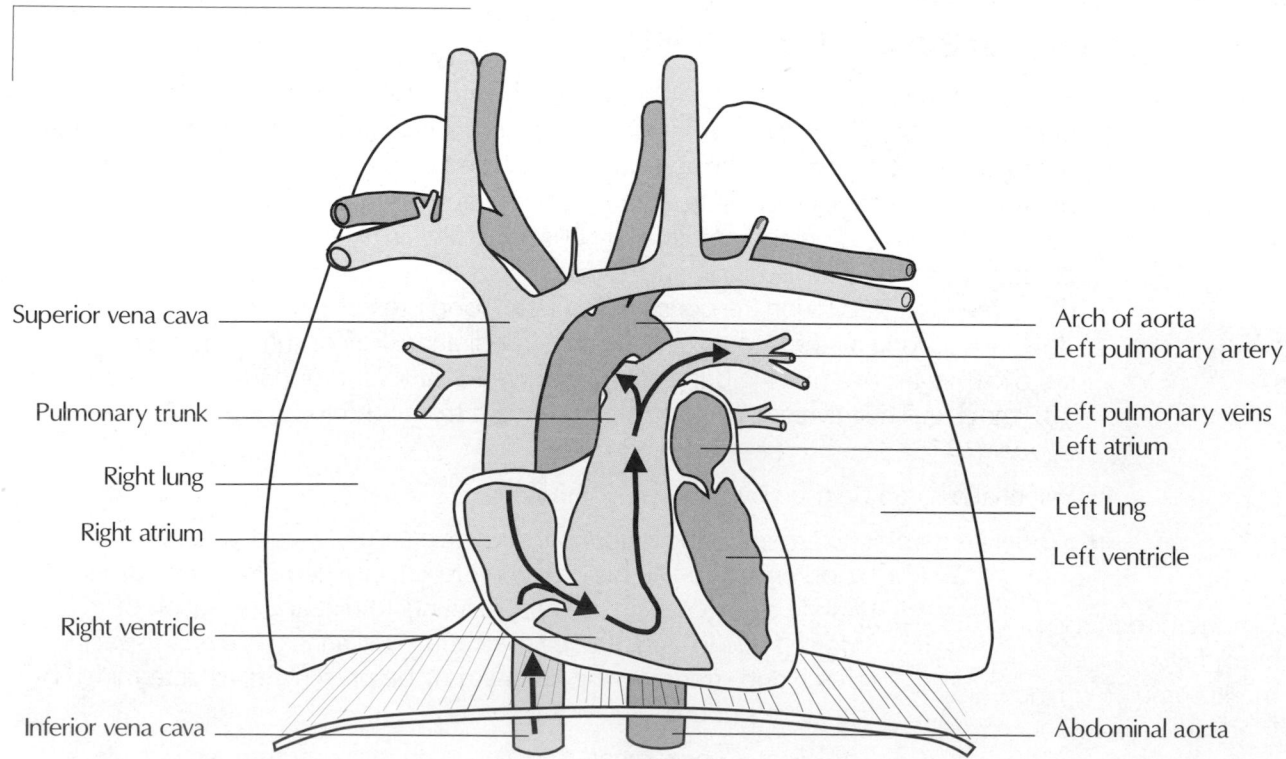

Figure 75.1
Chambers of the heart.

Early decreases in heart function often go undetected because of the system's ability to compensate for the problems. The body has a cardiac reserve through which the cardiac output is maximized. The heart rate and the force of contractions are increased, as well as hypertrophy of the heart. As the heart failure progresses, this initial compensation will eventually result in observable signs and symptoms.

Chronic Congestive Heart Failure

✦ Risk Factors:

- pre-existing heart disease;
- exacerbating factors such as physical and emotional stress, dysrhythmia, fever, infection, anemia, thyroid disorders, pregnancy, Paget's disease, pulmonary disease, poor renal function or medications such as steroids (*Goodman, Snyder, 1995*).

A client with congestive heart failure may have several of the following symptoms or none of them. Over time, the symptoms may change, appearing, reappearing or disappearing. There may be acute periods during which they get worse. Eventually, either because the disease progresses or because there is poor control of the condition, there may be an increase in symptoms

Symptoms of Left Ventricular Failure

✦ Left-sided heart failure is characterized by pulmonary congestion and edema. Another primary symptom is dyspnea — laboured or difficult breathing — which is influenced by the client's position, activity and stress levels. Orthopnea (advanced dyspnea) and paroxysmal nocturnal dyspnea (PND), the feeling of suffocation when lying supine, may be experienced. In this position, there is an increase in blood returning to the heart from the legs causing increased congestion in the lungs and breathing difficulties. Orthopnea is relieved in time (up to 30 minutes) when the person is placed in an upright position (*Goodman, Snyder, 1995*). With PND, a semi-supine position is necessary, with the trunk and head elevated by pillows during sleep.

✦ Pulmonary edema may cause feelings of anxiety, tachypnea (very rapid breathing), noisy, wet breathing and profuse sweating; the accessory breathing muscles may be engaged resulting in muscular hypertension and trigger points.

✦ A hacking cough with frothy, bloody sputum is the result of the irritating nature of the fluid in the lungs.

✦ Fatigue, drowsiness and muscular weakness are caused by tissue hypoxia. These symptoms progress as the day wears on. There is a decreasing tolerance for exercise.

✦ In advanced cases, a decrease in blood supply to the brain results in cerebral hypoxia. This causes anxiety, irritability, restlessness, confusion, loss of concentration, impaired memory and insomnia.

Symptoms of Right Ventricular Failure

✦ With right-sided failure, there is generalized edema distal to the heart, including ascites (edema in the peritoneal cavity) and weight gain; breathing is less affected than with left ventricular failure.

✦ Edema is most marked in the lower limbs, beginning at the ankles, the sacral area and the backs of the thighs; chronic and pitted edema develop.

✦ Liver function may be impaired and the spleen enlarged.

✦ Abdominal pain, intestinal problems and anorexia are secondary to the ascites.

✦ With severe right-sided failure, distension of the jugular veins is observable when the person is standing.

✦ The other symptoms, which may be present with both types of failure, are decreased renal function or frequent nocturnal urination, cyanosis of the digits and the nail beds, and coldness and pallor of the limbs.

Contraindications

✦ With chronic congestive heart failure, full-body lymphatic drainage techniques are avoided, as is elevation of the limbs above the level of the heart. Lymphatic drainage is absolutely contraindicated with cardiac edema, since a sudden increase in the volume of lymphatic fluid or venous return through compromised tissues and organs has potentially serious results, such as pulmonary edema (Wittlinger, Wittlinger, 1990).

✦ See also Hypertension for additional contraindications.

The Medical Treatment of Congestive Heart Failure

✦ Treatment of this condition includes:

• dietary modification such as reductions in the intake of salt (to make the diet salt free, or low in salt, containing only 2,500 to 4,000 milligrams of salt per day) and water (no more than 1.5 litres per day);

• regular progressive physical activity, which may stabilize or even reverse the process;

• rest after a meal or after physical activity;

• stress reduction techniques to control anxiety.

✦ Medications are used to improve heart function and to control heart failure. These include diuretics, vasodilators and cardiotonics which improve the strength and efficiency of the heart and regulate the heartbeat.

Massage for Congestive Heart Failure

🖐 Permission is obtained from the client's physician before performing massage.

🖐 The client's sleeping position is a good guide for positioning during massage; likely seated or semi-seated and supported by pillows will be most comfortable for a client who has dyspnea.

See stress reduction, tension headache, migraine, hemiplegia, diabetes mellitus and pregnancy for related treatments.

🖐 A relaxation massage is performed; it may be advisable to only massage the head, neck and limbs, avoiding the trunk. Short, segmental strokes are used. Essential oils mentioned under hypertension for relaxation may be appropriate.

OTHER CIRCULATORY CONDITIONS

Linda Ludwig

Raynaud's Phenomenon

> *Raynaud's phenomenon is a peripheral vascular disorder, which means it affects blood vessels outside the heart and thorax. It occurs secondary to another underlying condition.*

Raynaud's phenomenon is characterized by intense spasms of the arteries and arterioles that supply the fingers and, sometimes, of the vessels that supply the feet. The vasospasms impair blood supply to the digits. This causes colour changes and sensory symptoms. Eventually, tissue dystrophy is observable in the affected digits.

➤ **The cause of Raynaud's phenomenon is cold or emotional stress.**

➤ **Raynaud's phenomenon is secondary to:**

- occlusive arterial disease;

- arteriosclerosis;

- connective tissue diseases such as systemic scleroderma (Raynaud's phenomenon is frequently the earliest symptom) and lupus erythematosus *(Cawson et al., 1989)*;

- thoracic outlet syndrome and other compression syndromes;

- pulmonary hypertension;

- myoedema;

- Buerger's disease (thromboangiitis obliterans) — a chronic inflammation of the blood vessels in the limbs and extremities (especially the legs and feet) that causes thrombus formation; it is related to smoking;

- previous vessel injury through frostbite or trauma;

929

- occupational causes such as the use of vibrating tools or continuous exposure to hot and cold temperatures (such as with butchers and kitchen preparation staff).

Medical treatment of Raynaud's phenomenon includes the treatment of any underlying conditions. If attacks are frequent, vasodilator drugs, such as calcium channel blockers, are often prescribed to reduce the vasospasm and, ultimately, to avoid the risks secondary to compromised tissue health.

Raynaud's Disease

Raynaud's disease is a term used to denote arterial spasms and symptoms similar to Raynaud's phenomenon, when there is no underlying, related condition and the blood vessels appear normal (Balch, Balch, 1997; Porth, 1990).

Raynaud's disease may begin unilaterally but will usually become bilateral within four to six months of onset. This peripheral vascular disorder usually affects women between 18 and 30 years of age. It is characterized by symptoms similar to Raynaud's phenomenon; that is, intermittent attacks of pallor followed by cyanosis in the digits due to abnormal vasoconstriction in the extremities. It is brought on by exposure to cold or emotional stress. There appears to be some risk of rheumatoid arthritis, as well as reduced tissue health and gangrene in the skin at the fingertips *(Porth, 1990; Taber's Cyclopedic Medical Dictionary, 1981).*

Treatment is similar to that given for Raynaud's phenomenon.

Symptom Picture

- ✦ Vasospasm of the blood vessels supplying the hands and, sometimes, the feet constitute an "attack". During an attack:
  - digits appear white and shiny, often going numb. They then turn red, which is accompanied by a burning sensation before returning to normal;
  - slight swelling may occur.
- ✦ Over time, tissue health is affected. Muscles may atrophy, the nails may become brittle, and the skin at the fingertips may thicken.
- ✦ Ulcers may result in chronic infection or, infrequently, gangrene around the nail and fingertips.

Contraindications

✦ Cold hydrotherapy applications should not be used on the affected tissue.

✦ Stimulating or painful techniques should be used judiciously to avoid stimulating sympathetic nervous system firing and precipitating an attack.

✦ Deep techniques are avoided on affected tissue, if the tissue health is poor.

Treatment Considerations

Assessment

✦ **Health history questions** are asked that include the following: How is the client's general health? What underlying condition is related to the Raynaud's phenomenon? How frequent are the attacks? What specifically triggers the attacks? What treatment is the client receiving? Are any medications being taken?

✐ **Observations** are made of tissue and nail health for colour, thickness and ulceration.

✐ **Palpation** reveals decreased skin temperature in the affected area compared with an unaffected area. Some edema may be present.

Massage

✋ The therapist should ask permission to speak with the client's physician regarding the risk of thrombus formation and tissue health concerns such as gangrene.

✋ Full-body relaxation massage is performed.

✋ Where connective tissue and fascial restrictions are palpated, fascial techniques such as connective tissue cutting are used over a limited area per treatment. Slow, short strokes are used over the low back and gluteals. Over a series of treatments the proximal limb may be included *(Ebner, 1980)*.

✋ Fascial work is interspersed with soothing techniques. Likely this will include treatment of tissue local to and just proximal to the affected digits *(Thomson et al., 1991)*.

✋ Essential oils such as lemon and ginger may be used to promote circulation; benzoin has the added benefit of promoting relaxation *(Lawless, 1992; Sellar, 1992)*. These oils are used alone or blended, with a total of 25 drops added to 50 ml. of vegetable oil.

Self-care

✐ The client is encouraged to reduce stress, through relaxation strategies such as meditation and diaphragmatic breathing. Biofeedback may be used as a relaxation strategy; it seems to be particularly helpful in controlling the vasospasm associated with Raynaud's disease *(Porth, 1990)*.

✐ The client is educated about avoiding the cold by wearing gloves in cool weather and always wearing shoes. The client is also educated about vasoconstricting substances such as stimulants in foods (caffeine), smoking and drugs such as birth control pills, migraine medication and decongestants *(Balch, Balch, 1997; Porth, 1990)*. Their intake should be restricted, if possible.

✐ A nutritionist or naturopath can be consulted for nutrition recommendations which may include vitamin E, calcium, magnesium and zinc supplements *(Balch, Balch, 1997)*.

See also
inflammatory
arthritides,
compression
syndromes,
hypertension and
stress reduction.

✍ Aerobic exercise is recommended to improve general circulation. The client can be taught the McIntyre manoeuvre which is used in the early stages of an attack to bring blood to the fingers. With the arms straight at the elbows, the client swings the arms up in front of the body and over the head then down and behind the body quickly and repeatedly until the hands are warm. The suggested speed is about 180 movements per minute *(Porth, 1990)*.

✍ Modified contrast baths, where warm and cool applications are alternated, may be helpful. The temperatures are modified so they do not trigger an attack. Cool water is used instead of cold.

Thrombophlebitis

Thrombophlebitis is the inflammation of a superficial or deep vein that leads to the formation of a thrombus.

Thrombophlebitis or deep vein thrombosis (DVT) is **not** a condition that can be treated with massage and the massage therapist's role is to refer cases of suspected DVT. Information here is to instruct the massage therapist in detection so the client can be referred and in educating the client about prevention.

A thrombus is a clot which is fibrin-based and enmeshed in red blood cells; it is attached to the wall of the blood vessel. Once it has developed, coagulation in the slow-moving blood can cause an extension of the thrombus much like a tail. The thrombus may extend for as much as 20 inches along the wall of the vein. A thrombus forms because of a combination of factors that includes the increased coagulation of venous blood, stasis of the blood and injury to the wall of the blood vessel. The presence of a thrombus can lead to occlusion of the lumen of the blood vessel *(Cawson et al., 1989)*. The majority of thrombi, almost 95 per cent, develop in the veins of the leg. Commonly, the condition is referred to as superficial vein thrombosis or deep vein thrombosis (DVT), depending on the vein affected. The presence of a deep vein thrombosis is of greatest concern.

Superficial vein thrombosis is caused by irritation to the walls of the vein. This condition presents with localized redness and warmth, and a cord-like swelling along the course of the superficial vein. Pain is experienced at rest and worsens with movement. As the condition resolves the skin may develop a brownish pigmentation along the course of the affected vein.

Treatment of superficial vein thrombosis is similar to deep vein thrombosis.

The remainder of this section deals with thrombus development in the deep veins (DVT).

➤ **The cause of deep vein thrombosis is venous stasis.** While this is the biggest culprit, any increase in blood coagulation may contribute to DVT formation.

➤ **Contributing factors are:**

• age: generally those over 40 and especially the elderly (particularly with a fractured femur or pelvis) are affected, but a venous thrombus can form in a fit, young person or an athlete;

• prolonged immobilization;

• cardiac failure or stroke and heart disease;

- anesthesia and surgery;
- trauma, especially to the leg or pelvis; burn patients are especially susceptible to pulmonary embolism (PE);
- previous history of a venous disorder, especially a thromboembolism;
- pregnancy and the postpartum state;
- oral contraceptive use;
- diabetes mellitis;
- cancer: certain malignancies are associated with an increased tendency for clotting, such as lung or pancreatic cancer *(Porth, 1990; Alexander, 1995a);*
- clotting disorders.

Medical Detection and Prevention

Several medical tests can be performed to determine venous flow or to detect the accumulation of fibrinogen in a thrombus. They allow for monitoring of those susceptible to a DVT and PE as listed above.

Prevention of thrombus formation is the preferable course. After pregnancy or surgery, ambulation is encouraged as soon as possible. The patient can exercise the legs in bed or while sitting, taking care to avoid sudden and extreme movements. Diaphragmatic breathing is encouraged as it assists the venous return from the legs. Special stockings are worn to improve venous flow and to prevent pooling of the blood in the lower leg. The legs are elevated to 20 degrees whenever possible. Care is taken that there is no excessive knee and hip flexion that can slow blood flow. The prevention of venous stasis is actively encouraged with anyone who is sitting for long periods of time such as during long car rides or plane travel.

If the person has already developed a DVT, treatment includes a brief period of bedrest in order to stabilize the thrombus. Elevation of the legs is encouraged. Anticoagulants, such as heparin and coumadin, are used to prevent and to treat the condition.

Special Concerns for Therapists in a Hospital or Nursing-Home Setting

Extreme caution must be exercised in light of the possibility of DVT when massaging people who have undergone any general surgery. Particularly at risk are those with hip replacement, femoral fracture and pneumatic calf compression and those who have undergone major knee surgery, prostate surgery, gynecological surgery (which entails long bedrest afterward), neurosurgery and cesarean section. It is possible for thrombi to develop bilaterally with a femoral fracture *(Alexander, 1992).* As a preventative measure, those at highest risk are often given small doses of heparin.

As a precaution, massage to the legs is contraindicated if there is calf cramping, especially if this occurs before the person is active, post-surgery *(Goodman, Synder, 1995).* There is documentation in a hospital setting of a family member, who was *not* a massage therapist, causing a pulmonary embolism by massaging a thrombophlebitic calf *(Alexander, 1992).* The therapist is strongly advised to get the physician's permission before massaging the legs of a client after surgery.

933

Symptom Picture

+ DVT can happen in any vein — for example, in the arm — however, they are most common in the legs.

+ The most common signs of deep vein thrombosis are those of the inflammatory process: heat, redness, swelling and deep muscle pain as well as fever and general malaise. The pain is often described as localized, deep, aching, cramping and throbbing, and is exacerbated by activity such as walking. The amount of swelling found distal to the occlusion (swelling is often in the ankles) varies, depending on the amount of blockage in the affected vein. The risk of thrombus formation, often the result of increased frequency of attacks of inflammation, indicates the need for physician consultation regarding the possibility of an embolus occurring with leg massage.

+ Unfortunately, the condition may be symptomless, in 30 to 50 per cent of the cases *(Goodman, Snyder, 1995; Alexander, 1992).*

+ In some cases the thrombus is securely attached to the wall of the vein. However, a serious concern with the development of a deep venous thrombus is the risk that it will break free and become an embolus — a mobile clot. If the embolus enters the circulatory system it can become entrapped in the pulmonary vasculature. This can lead to a serious situation, with the obstruction of blood flow to an area of the lung. The risk of a pulmonary embolism (PE) from a deep vein thrombus is very high; most frequently the thrombus originates in the ileofemoral vein. Pulmonary embolism is the cause of 10 to 20 per cent of hospital mortalities *(Cawson et al., 1989).*

+ If a pulmonary embolism is present, the client will feel extreme distress and dyspnea. Sharp, localized pain may be experienced in the chest and behind the sternum, along with general chest discomfort. There may be distention of the veins in the neck. The person may collapse or go into shock *(Thomson et al., 1991; Goodman, Snyder, 1995).*

Contraindications

+ If the therapist suspects a DVT, local massage and massage to the affected limb are contraindicated.

+ With a femoral fracture, both legs are contraindicated. The client is referred to a physician, especially if DVT is previously undiagnosed. It is useful to all concerned if the therapist writes a note for the client offering the reasons for suspecting a circulatory problem.

+ Passive and active movements are contraindicated in the acute stage of DVT *(Kisner, Colby, 1996).*

+ If a DVT is suspected in a client already receiving treatment, treatment is discontinued. The client is referred for immediate medical attention. As the condition resolves, massage treatment may resume with consent from the physician but the affected limb is avoided.

+ Treatment of DVT with coumadin or heparin leads to the risk of hemorrhage from any tissue or organ *(Canadian Pharmaceutical Association, 1996).* With a client on one of these medications, consultation with a physician is necessary to establish the safety of massage therapy. Appropriate modifications should be discussed, such as shorter treatments, avoiding the legs and lower body and using less aggressive techniques on the upper body to avoid bruising. These precautions are observed for as long as the person is on the medication.

✦ The therapist must remain aware that once a person has a history of DVT or PE, she is more susceptible to developing it again. Caution is advised regarding aggressiveness of the massage to the legs. The therapist must be vigilant for symptoms of DVT or PE recurrence.

✦ Extreme temperature contrast hydrotherapy should be avoided to the limb affected with the DVT.

✦ Heat is contraindicated distal and immediately proximal to the DVT to avoid further congestion of the area.

Treatment Considerations

Assessment

✦ **Health history questions** include the following: Is there a history of recent surgery, accident, injury to blood vessels (bruising), heart disease, DVT or PE? Has the client been be immobilized for a prolonged period; this could include a recent plane trip or uninterrupted drive? Is the client pregnant or postpartum? Does the client take oral contraceptives?

✦ What is the location of pain or cramping? Is it localized? What aggravates the pain? Active dorsiflexion of the ankle can be aggravating; the ankle may be achy at rest.

✦ If the client has been diagnosed with DVT, has massage therapy been approved by the client's physician? Is the client taking anticoagulant medication? These are taken for two to three months after an uncomplicated DVT and up to six months following a pulmonary embolism *(Porth, 1990)*.

✎ **Observation** may reveal signs of inflammation. Edema is present distal to a partial or complete obstruction; this is most likely observed in the distal leg, especially around the ankle. Leg pallor may be noted. Distal veins may be distended in the lower leg.

✎ With deep **palpation**, there can be local tenderness when a thrombus is present. A diminished or absent dorsalis pedis pulse may be palpated.

See also spasm, edema, hypertension, diabetes mellitus, cancer, wounds and burns, fractures and pregnancy for related conditions.

✎ **Testing** may be positive with **Ramirez's test** and **Homan's sign**. The therapist must keep in mind that only about half of those with a DVT experience pain as a symptom. Therefore, a negative result will not necessarily rule out the presence of a thrombus.

• Specific medical testing is required to detect the presence of a thrombus and its effect on blood flow.

Varicose Veins

"Varicose" means distended or dilated. Therefore, varicose veins are abnormally large and bulging veins. They are caused by the impaired function of the venous valves.

Blood is circulated through the body by the arteries and veins. Nutrients and oxygenated blood are transported to tissues in the body by the arteries; blood is propelled by the pumping actions of the heart. The veins return the deoxygenated blood to the heart; movement of blood through the veins occurs via the contraction of muscles. To prevent backflow of the blood, there are valves in the veins. Varicose veins develop when there is an increase in venous pressure. The result is prolonged venous dilation that causes the valves to become incompetent. The valves are unable to prevent back-flow which leads to impaired circulation and regurgitation of blood *(Figure 76.1)*.

The veins stretch and dilate further. A vicious cycle is created. Once the veins experience repeated periods of increased venous pressure, they become permanently stretched. At this point, little can be done to return the venous tone and valvular competence. Standing aggravates the condition as the full weight of the venous blood is in the legs. In fact, standing increases the venous pressure in the legs to five times the pressure experienced in the supine position *(Cawson et al., 1989)*. Gravity compounds the effects, further increasing venous pressure.

Varicose veins should not be confused with spider veins. Spider veins are chronically dilated capillaries near the skin surface. While some people consider them cosmetically unappealing, they are harmless.

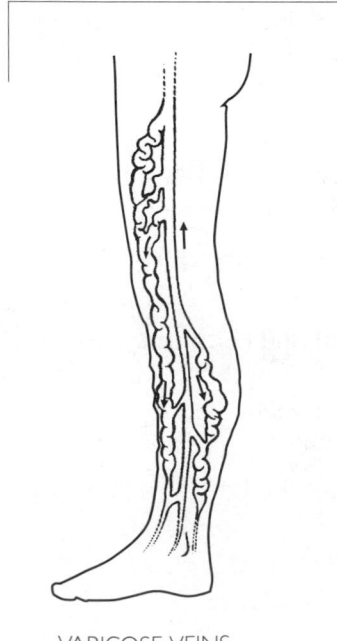

VARICOSE VEINS

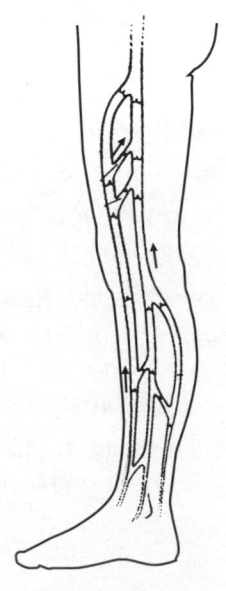

NORMAL VEINS

Figure 76.1
Varicosities in the leg.

Causes of varicose veins are:

➤ **habits that impair circulation** and increase venous pressure such as prolonged sitting or standing in one position, sitting with the legs crossed and a sedentary lifestyle, tight garters or girdles;

➤ **increased pressure on pelvic veins** from excess weight, heavy lifting, chronic constipation or pregnancy;

➤ **secondary to impaired or blocked blood flow** from:

- deep vein thrombosis

- congenital venous malformation

- heart failure

- liver dysfunction

- abdominal tumours;

➤ **vitamin C deficiency** which can weaken the collagen structure of the veins *(Balch, Balch, 1997)*.

Two primary concerns about varicose veins are: first, the increased risk of developing superficial venous thrombosis; and, second, with ongoing edema and impaired circulation, the resulting poor tissue health which can lead to sores or ulcers on the legs.

Medical treatment may include injections into the affected veins of solutions such as tetradecyl sulfate (saline); this procedure is followed by compression to the area. The solutions act to close the affected vein by fusing its walls so blood cannot pass through. The body will then find an alternate route for the blood.

In cases where extreme pain is experienced, surgery may be used to remove the dilated veins. This surgery is followed by elevation of the legs, active foot and ankle movements and walking. Support bandages or stockings are worn for several weeks *(Thomson et al., 1991)*.

The most commonly known varicosities are those in the legs but varicose veins can also occur in the esophagus and the rectal and anal areas. Esophageal varicosities are a common complication of portal hypertension which is secondary to cirrhosis of the liver. Rupture of these veins can lead to bleeding, which can be fatal. Rectal or anal varicosities are referred to as hemorrhoids. They are often secondary to constipation, pregnancy and, occasionally, tumours. Bleeding and pain occur on defecation and there is a risk of infection with severe cases.

Contraindications

+ Deep, specific techniques are contraindicated over varicosities and on any local tissue that appears dystrophic.

+ If the varicosities are painful and sensitive to the touch, local massage may be contraindicated.

+ Massage is contraindicated over esophageal varicosities *(College of Massage Therapists of Ontario, 1991)*.

+ Local massage is contraindicated for 24 hours after the medical treatment of saline injections in the affected veins; after surgery, local massage is contraindicated until approved by the physician.

+ Massage to the affected legs is contraindicated if there is no previous diagnosis of varicosities or thrombophlebitis but the client presents with DVT symptoms.

Symptom Picture

+ While they can occur at any age, varicose veins are most common in people between 40 and 50 years of age, affecting more women than men.

+ There is a familial tendency to developing varicose veins.

+ Varicosities result in enlarged and bulging veins; they are often bluish and lumpy. The veins can become tortuous — that is, twisting and knotted. This is easily observed when superficial veins are affected.

+ In some cases, the affected veins are relatively asymptomatic but in others, dull, achy pain is experienced. Swelling may be observed around the ankles. A feeling of heaviness and fatigue in the legs is reported; walking may be difficult.

+ Leg cramps, especially in the calf muscles, often occur at night. The pigment of the skin over the leg may be variable, appearing to be a shiny bluish-brown.

Treatment Considerations

Assessment

✍ The symptoms associated with varicose veins are similar to thrombophlebitis. Therefore, a thorough assessment for the possibility of deep vein thrombosis is carried out and referral to a physician is suggested for a diagnosis.

Massage

✋ The client is positioned with the legs elevated. If the client is in the prone position, a few pillows are placed under the shin and foot; when the supine position is appropiate, several pillows are used to raise the legs above the heart.

✋ When a client who has varicose veins is massaged, the pressure of the techniques applied on the affected leg should be modified. A lighter pressure is used and its purpose is promoting lymphatic and venous return. The direction of pressure is towards the core of the body, with care taken not to direct the pressure towards the feet. Lymphatic drainage techniques are generally beneficial.

✋ Passive movement of the joints in the leg, including the hip, knee and ankle, is interspersed throughout the massage.

✋ Cypress essential oil may be used on the legs. Twenty-five drops of pure essential oil are added to 50 ml. of vegetable oil *(Lawless, 1992; Sellar, 1992)*.

Self-care

✍ To improve venous return, support stockings are worn to support the veins and prevent swelling.

✍ Clothing that is restrictive at the waist or legs should be avoided.

✍ Prolonged periods of standing or sitting, and crossing the legs and heavy lifting are minimized or avoided.

✍ Care is taken not to scratch or injure the skin over varicosities since this may cause ulceration and bleeding.

✍ Standing in a bathtub of cold water and walking on the spot (water treading) can improve circulation *(Bruggemann, 1982)*. The legs are dried off thoroughly afterward and warm socks are put on.

✍ Foot and ankle exercises are encouraged as is daily activity such as walking. Buerger's exercises, described in the edema chapter, are useful.

✍ Clients are encouraged to take regular breaks — to sit and elevate the legs above the heart. Breaks may be taken as often as three times a day for 10 minutes at a time.

✍ The end of the client's bed can be raised slightly to encourage venous drainage during sleep *(Thomson et al., 1991)*.

✍ Self-massage for the legs is recommended, using specific techniques to increase lymph and venous return. The key is to direct the pressure towards the heart. Essential oil of cypress can be used to promote venous health. Twenty-five drops of pure cypress essential oil are diluted in 50 ml. of vegetable oil. The solution is lightly stroked over the affected leg. Cypress should not be used by clients who are pregnant *(Sellar, 1992)*.

See also edema, pregnancy and spasm.

938

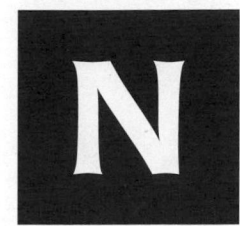

GASTROINTESTINAL CONCERNS

CONSTIPATION

Linda Ludwig

Constipation is the slow, difficult or infrequent movement of feces through the bowel.

Constipation is considered a symptom rather than an actual condition. It may be due to a physiological cause or a perception that the elimination process is not happening with normal frequency.

Up to 25 per cent of the population feel they suffer from constipation. This high number reflects the many and varied definitions of constipation. Historically, there were varying opinions on what constituted "normal" bowel regularity. In fact, some physicians seemed to regard the functions of the bowel as a necessary evil that, in turn, required regular (daily) clearing by any means, in order to keep it empty. This included regular enemas containing turpentine and castor oil. In the early 1900s, Sir Arbuthnot Lane, an English physician, went so far as to suggest colonectomy for the treatment of chronic constipation, feeling that the colon was a "cesspool" responsible for a host of conditions ranging from "sagging breasts and premature senility, to rheumatoid arthritis" *(Thompson, 1979)*. Some of his followers went further to suggest that the large intestine and appendix should be removed at the age of two or three years as a matter of course *(Thompson, 1979)*. Today, some of this thinking prevails as is evidenced by the multimillion dollar laxative industry.

Generally, medical sources agree that a comfortable bowel movement daily or as little as three times a week fall within normal limits for the average western population *(Kamm, Lennard-Jones, 1994; Wexner, Bartolo, 1995)*. This seems largely based on diet. In other cultures, with higher fibre diets, an increased frequency of bowel movements results. In some cases, this may be up to three bowel movements a day. Some sources consider size and weight of stools to be an indicator of constipation; that is, a smaller, light-weight stool would indicate constipation. Generally, a stool weight of 125 to 200 grams is considered within normal limits. Here again, this will vary with different cultures. Those with high fibre

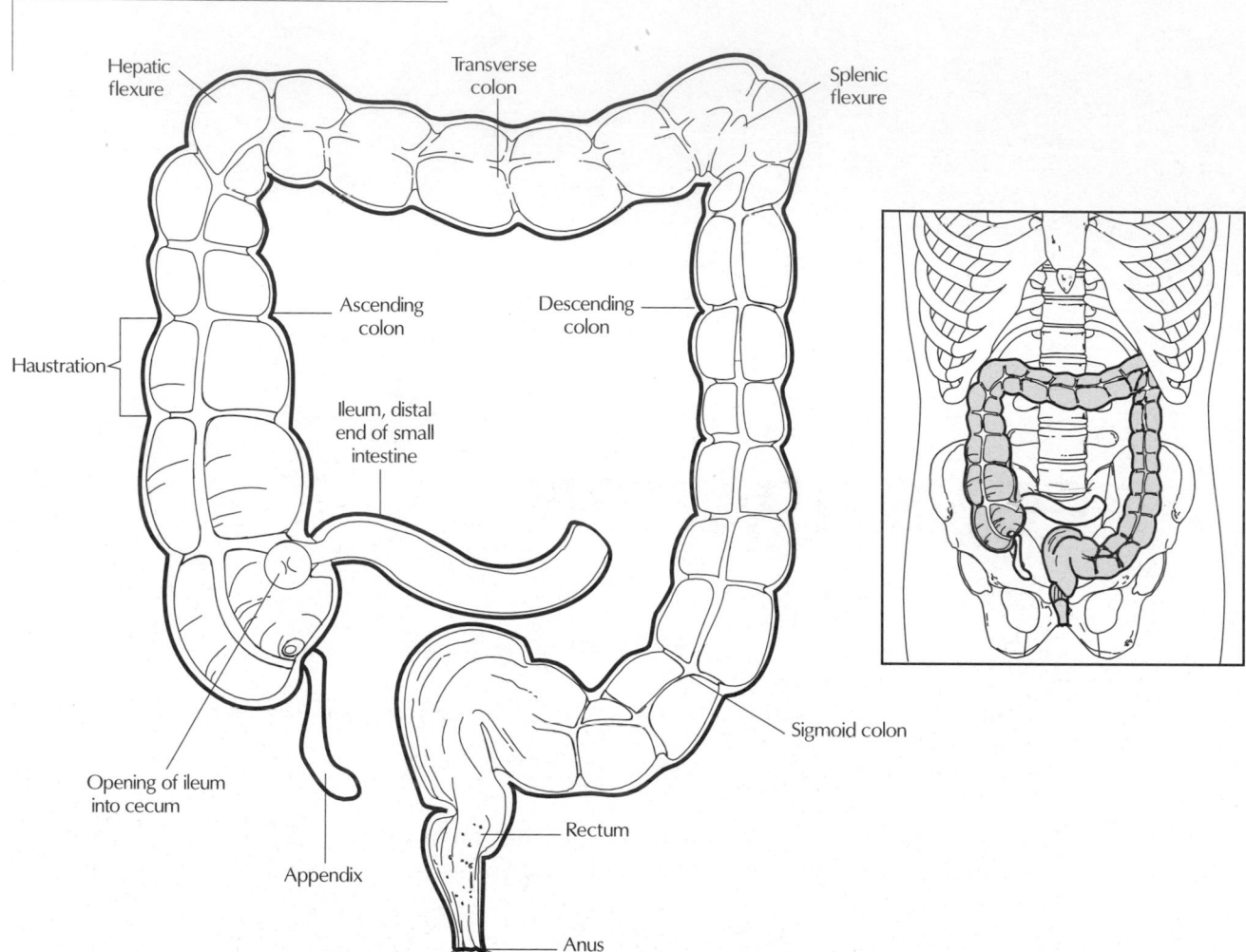

Figure 77.1
The large intestine. The tucked-in sections of the colon are referred to as haustrations.

diets produce heavier stools, approximately 300 to 400 grams in weight *(Wexner, Bartolo, 1995)*. This chapter is written in the context of what are considered Western "norms".

The digestive process functions to break food down into basic components. These are absorbed into the bloodstream through the walls of the small intestine. The unusable and undigested food, referred to as chyme, has a fluid consistency and moves from the small intestine, through the ileocecal valve, to the large intestine, also referred to as the colon *(Figure 77.1)*. The large intestine functions to absorb water, to develop a soft, formed feces and to store the feces until it can be expelled from the body. The **large intestine** is comprised of:

- the cecum, to which the appendix is attached;
- the colon which is divided into the ascending, transverse, descending and sigmoid sections;
- the rectum which lies just anterior to the sacrum and coccyx; the distal portion of the rectum is called the anal canal which terminates with the anus.

Movement in the Digestive System

Movement through the intestines is governed by an intrinsic nervous system that lies within the gastrointestinal wall. This network includes the enteric nervous system and the autonomic nervous system. The enteric nervous system controls the muscular contraction of these structures. The autonomic nervous system is comprised of the sympathetic and the parasympathetic systems, both of which innervate the gastrointestinal tract. The parasympathetic system functions to support the digestive process through the vagus nerve and the sacral nerve plexus; these nerves primarily terminate in the enteric system. On the other hand, the sympathetic system has an inhibiting effect on the digestive process through the nerves from the thoracic and lumbar portions of the spinal cord. These terminate in the enteric system as well as directly in the intestinal wall *(Guyton, 1984)*. A decrease in the digestive process is appropriate if stimulation of the sympathetic nervous system occurs because of a life-threatening situation. Unfortunately, stimulation of this part of the system is often secondary to emotional upset or stress. Digestive problems result with the change in movement of the fecal matter through the gastrointestinal tract.

✦ Movements in the colon:

- **Segmental movements**, sometimes referred to as mixing movements, "contain" the fecal matter so absorption of substances can occur through the intestinal walls and into the bloodstream. In the small intestine nutrients are absorbed and in the large intestine water and electrolytes are absorbed.

- The **propulsive contractions** are those which move the fecal matter through the colon towards the anus.

- **Peristalsis** refers to smaller, more frequent propulsive contractions.

- **Mass movements** refer to infrequent but powerful propulsive contractions in the large intestine. Over a 24-hour period, an average of four to six mass movements occurs in the large intestine — some of the forces of contractions have been measured at up to 200 mm Hg *(Kamm, Lennard-Jones, 1994)*.

Movement in the colon is influenced in various ways. Primarily, the colon responds to increases in intraluminal pressure — that is, the sense of pressure created by the volume of fecal matter. This stimulates receptors of the smooth muscle in the intestinal wall and causes a contraction. Hormones and emotions also play roles and are discussed later in the chapter.

Transit Times

The speed with which the fecal matter moves through the large intestine is referred to as the transit time. An optimal transit time will result in a soft, formed stool. The average time is from 24 to 48 hours from ingestion of food to defecation *(Thompson, 1979)*. A harder, more difficult-to-pass stool is the result of an increased transit time, since this allows more water to be absorbed. Transit time may be longer due to an increase in segmenting movements and a decrease in propulsive movements. In those with severe constipation, it was found that mass movements were 50 per cent less frequent and of a shorter duration than in those not experiencing constipation. Another reason for large, bulky and difficult-to-pass fecal matter is its retention in the rectum for a long period of time *(Kamm et al., 1994)*.

A faster transit time reduces the time available for water to be absorbed. This results in a less formed, more liquid stool as is found with diarrhea. This may be caused by a decrease in segmenting movements and an increase in mass movements, sometimes referred to as hyperperistalsis.

Hormones, emotions and diet are some of the factors that can influence transit time. Hormones and emotions can decrease or increase colon movement. Fear and anxiety seem to increased motility, especially segmentation. In some cases, there is disordered activity, rather than the organized, alternating contractions, which interferes with movement through the colon. Depression results in reduced bowel activity, which increases in severity as the depression is more severe.

An example of the effect of hormones on transit time is demonstrated by the hormone enterogastrone. It slows down stomach contractions which, in turn, slows down movement through the intestines. Other hormones, such as gastrin or secretin, which facilitate digestion in the stomach, reflexively cause increased mass movements in the large intestine. This is one reason why the "urge to defecate" is frequently experienced after meals. Therefore, the use of artificial hormones or abnormalities in hormonal levels can affect transit time.

Transit time is also influenced greatly by diet. High fibre and adequate water intake result in bulkier but soft stools. Low fibre, high fat, highly processed foods and diuretic foods result in longer transit times and hard, often difficult-to-pass stools. A high saturated fat diet is also considered a major risk factor for developing colorectal cancer, whereas a protective factor appears to be an adequate intake of dietary fibre. Researchers also suggest increased fruit and vegetable consumptions combined with low fat intake and regular physical activity will provide some protection against this type of cancer (*Canadian Cancer Society, 1996f*).

Autointoxication

Over the centuries, "autointoxication" due to chronic constipation has been blamed for many illnesses. It is a fact that many of those experiencing constipation also suffer a multitude of other symptoms, such as headaches, nausea and irritability. These symptoms are considered to be due to the toxic effect of retaining the fecal matter. Thompson, in his book **The Irritable Gut**, reports a study done in 1922 by Dr. Donaldson to disprove the autointoxication theory. "Five healthy men were required to eat normally but refrain from defecating for 90 hours. All complained of symptoms associated with autointoxication such as foul breath, irritability, depression and headache. All experienced immediate relief following an enema" (*Thompson, 1979*). Such prompt relief would seem to contradict a toxicity theory; it is suggested that the symptoms are actually the result of distention and mechanical irritation of the colon and rectum. In fact, Donaldson did a subsequent study which involved packing the rectum of subjects with cotton wool and this elicited identical symptoms to those listed above (*Thompson, 1979*).

Elimination

The normal process of eliminating fecal matter is a combination of coordination of reflexes with conscious effort. At the distal colon, the rectum is followed by the anal canal. There are two sphincters in this section of the colon. The first is the internal anal sphincter which opens when pressure occurs on the walls of the distal colon and on the sphincter, itself. About 100 to 200 grams of feces are needed to initiate the reflex, which is governed by the parasympathetic nervous system (*Thompson, 1979*). The fecal matter then moves further into the rectum, just proximal to the external anal sphincter. Sensory receptors perceive the pressure and signal the brain with the "urge" to defecate. If the place and time are appropriate, the person consciously relaxes this sphincter. This action is coordinated with a voluntary contraction of the diaphragm and abdominal muscles to increase the intrapelvic pressure. At the same time, the pelvic floor muscles along with the anus and the surrounding muscles relax. The result is defecation. This "urge" to defecate can be ignored. In such a case, there is a retrograde movement of the fecal matter into the rectum and possibly the colon. This is accompanied by a general slowing of the transit of fecal matter throughout the colon (*Kamm, Lennard-Jones, 1994*).

There are numerous causes of constipation.

➤ **Lifestyle factors include:**

- **poor diet** due to low fibre and low water intake or low food intake. The result is decreased bulk of the fecal matter. Movement of the fecal matter through the colon relies, in part, on the reflexes stimulated when the colon walls are distended. Distention does not occur if fecal matter is too small. Therefore, transit time through the colon is slower;

- **sedentary lifestyle** by choice or due to illness;

- **resisting the urge** due to poor or inadequate toilet facilities, travel or lack of an appropriate opportunity to defecate;

- **stress**;

- **postural imbalances** that contribute to the inability of the abdomen, diaphragm, low back and gluteal muscles to contract effectively. Pain in these muscles can also lead to muscle guarding and, in turn, constipation (*Goodman, Snyder, 1995*).

Constipation from any of the above causes is sometimes referred to as simple constipation (*Goodman, Snyder, 1995*).

➤ **Physiological factors include:**

- **poor muscle control or muscle tone or lack of coordination** such as would cause weak abdominal and diaphragm contractions, inability of the pelvic floor muscles to relax with defecation or the co-contraction of the gluteal muscles and the external sphincter when defecating;

- **psychological factors** such as depression, eating disorders (anorexia), obsession with "inner cleanliness", denial of the actions of the bowel or addiction to laxatives and other purgatives such as enemas;

- **medication side effects** as occur with opiates, anticholinergics (these block parasympathetic nerve impulses), antidepressants and anticonvulsives;

- **post-surgery effects,** especially abdominal surgery, which results in paralytic ileus. This refers to the absence of motor activity in the large intestine for approximately 72 hours and incoordination of the stomach and small intestine function for 24 hours;

- **gastrointestinal conditions** such as irritable bowel syndrome, diverticular disease, megacolon, obstruction, colorectal cancer and Hirschsprung's disease;

- **physiological and structural disorders** such as rectal prolapse or internal and external sphincter abnormalities (*Kamm, Lennard-Jones, 1994*);

- **pregnancy and early postpartum** — the first six weeks after childbirth;

- **underlying disorders** such as hypothyroidism, hypercalcemia and diabetes as well as neurological disorders such as Parkinsons, multiple sclerosis and sacral lesions.
➤ Some causes have variable effects on the colon, with constipation a secondary effect from an obstruction, colon stasis, hypotrophy or hypertrophy of the colon. In some cases, a condition leading to pain in the colon or pain upon defecation (such as hemorrhoids) can result in constipation.

Laxatives

Many people experiencing constipation do not seek medical attention. Commonly, laxatives are self-prescribed and may be taken regularly to establish what that person perceives as a "normal" bowel frequency.

✦ *Bulk laxatives* increase the ability of fecal matter to hold water. This increase in fluid is limited but adequate to facilitate normal colon movements. An example of this type of laxative is psyllium, which is a plant-based substance (it is found in Metamucil). These laxatives require an increase in water intake of two to three litres per day in order to prevent constipation developing from too much fibre and not enough water *(Wexner, Bartolo, 1995)*. This form of laxative may take several days to be effective but will usually result in a soft, formed, easily passed stool. Caution needs to be exercised by people who may be vulnerable to an obstruction (such as those who are bedridden) or those whose constipation is from a neurological disorder, as the use of bulk laxatives may result in further difficulty.

✦ *Laxatives containing salts such as magnesium hydroxide or sulphates* (as is found in Milk of Magnesia) act by osmosis. They retain water in the stool. This leads to hyperperistalsis because of increased pressure in the colon. The stools are often watery. This type of laxative is disruptive to the normal bowel processes and should only be used temporarily.

✦ *Laxatives containing unabsorbed sugars and polyhyrialcohols* make use of the intestinal bacteria. Fermentation by the bacteria, which are 80 per cent water, results in increased bulk of the stool *(Kamm, Lennard-Jones, 1994)*. This increase in bulk allows a more efficient transit time. There is some concern that this type of laxative alters the bacterial population in the colon.

✦ *Laxatives such as senna, cascara and aloe,* also called arthraquinone laxatives, are from plants (senna and aloe) or bark (cascara). They stimulate colon motility. Dosages are carefully monitored until a soft, formed stool results (too high an amount can result in hyperperistalsis, cramping and a watery stool).

Certainly, some people can develop a psychological reliance on laxatives for regular bowel movement. While there is no consensus, some physicians suggest that with chronic laxative use there can be a thickening and fibrosis of the colon accompanied by atrophy of the mucous layer. Long-term use can lead to what is sometimes called a "cathartic colon". This can affect nervous transmission and can cause ongoing constipation, electrolyte imbalances and seepage of fecal fluid from the anus. This does not occur as a result of long-term use of **all** laxatives, but more likely with those that alter rather than facilitate "normal" bowel function.

Considered a *"natural" laxative, fibre* is an important component of the diet. Its benefit to those experiencing constipation has been documented since the early part of the twentieth century. A diet consisting of as little as 35 grams of bran a day can reduce transit time by half. Fibre acts as a bulking agent, increasing colon motility and decreasing transit time. Fibre should be introduced gradually to the diet to prevent bloating, flatulence and possibly diarrhea. It may take a few weeks before results are achieved. Bran fibre is popular but for those with a wheat intolerance, corn bran or a bulk laxative such as psyllium may be effective.

With the **treatment** of constipation, the therapist must first clearly establish what the client considers to be constipation. A medical examination will determine whether the symptoms relate to a medical or to a psychological disorder. Causes that relate to lifestyle are effectively treated with massage therapy as well as being addressed through education about diet, exercise, postural imbalances and relaxation strategies.

Symptom Picture

◆ Straining, pain or discomfort may be experienced when passing stools.

◆ Infrequent bowel movements occur. These will be different for each person depending on his usual pattern; from every day up to three times a week is considered within normal limits.

◆ Hard stools, which may be small "rabbit" or "pellet" stools, are passed. These types of stools may be interspersed with softer stools, even diarrhea. This is referred to as irritable bowel syndrome (IBS).

◆ Abdominal pain, cramps or discomfort may occur intermittently.

◆ Low back pain or discomfort can result. Stimulation of the rectum from the presence of fecal matter can cause pain referral to the sacrum.

◆ Bloating and flatulence are experienced.

◆ Hemorrhoids can result from straining due to large or hard stools.

◆ A bad taste in the mouth, bad breath (halitosis), nausea and a lack of appetite can result due to the slowing of gastric emptying which results with constipation *(Kamm, Lennard-Jones, 1994).*

◆ Headaches, irritability and malaise seem to result reflexively from the distention of the rectal wall *(Thompson, 1979).*

Subjective Information

HEALTH HISTORY QUESTIONS

✦ How is the client's general health? For example, hypothyroidism and diabetes can lead to constipation.

✦ What indicates to the client that he is constipated? Is there straining, pain or small stools?

✦ Is the client taking any medications that could result in constipation as a side effect?

✦ Has the client consulted a physician?

✦ Does the client have any idea what may be causing the constipation?

✦ How long has this been present?

✦ How frequently is the person having a bowel movement? How is this different from his usual pattern?

✦ What is the consistency of the fecal matter? Is it soft (normal), hard (slow transit time), thin (increased tone in the colon), lumpy (spasm in the colon) or variable (alternating diarrhea and constipation can indicate irritable bowel syndrome).

✦ What is the colour of the stools? Black could indicate distal colon bleeding; red could indicate intestinal bleeding or hemorrhoids; a light colour could indicate bile and a hepatic disorder; a whitish coating indicates mucus from an intestinal disorder such as IBS.

✦ Is there any pain present? What type is it; where and when does it occur?

✦ What aggravates the pain? What relieves the pain?

✦ Has the client done anything to relieve the constipation?

✦ Are laxatives used? If so, what kind and how frequently?

✦ What is the client's general lifestyle? What are the stress levels? Does the client exercise frequently? Does the client allow himself time to have a bowel movement when the urge is present?

Objective Information

Observations

✎ There is bloating of the abdomen.

✎ A postural assessment is performed to check for imbalances. For example, hyperlordosis leads to a shortened psoas muscle. This muscle is in contact with the colon. Trigger points in psoas can cause irritation of the colon (Travell, Simons, 1992). Abdominal muscles that are stretched and weak can lead to difficulty bearing down to facilitate defecation. Posterior pelvic tilt results in shortened diaphragm and abdominal muscles. This results in compression to the abdominal contents. Pelvic tilt also occurs with scoliosis. In both cases, constipation can result because the shortening of these muscles can affect their ability to be recruited for bearing down for defecation.

Palpation

✍ The distended abdomen may feel firm, often in the distal colon. Tenderness is often palpated along the colon, especially distally.

✍ Hypertonicity or hypotonicity of abdominal muscles is possible. Hypertonicity may also be present in the diaphragm and the gluteals. These muscles are often contracted to control the urge to defecate. Trigger points can develop.

Testing

✍ **AF and PR ROM** is done on the muscles that the postural assessment indicated were shortened. Testing will show decreased range of motion.

✍ **AR strength testing** is done on the muscles that the postural assessment indicated were affected, such as the abdominal muscles. Testing will reveal weak muscles.

Special Tests

✍ The **rebound test** will be negative for general constipation.

Differentiating Other Conditions

✍ **Inflammatory bowel disease,** such as ulcerative colitis, results in frequent bloody and loose stools. Crohn's disease, another inflammatory bowel disease, results in periods of abdominal, hip and low back pain which is often relieved after a bowel movement or passing gas. The disease is accompanied by transient arthritis in 25 per cent of cases (*Goodman, Snyder, 1995*). In any case, the client should be referred to a physician if such a condition is suspected.

✍ **Appendicitis** may be indicated by a positive rebound test. Symptoms of appendicitis are nausea and vomiting, low-grade fever and pain in the lower right quadrant. This condition is a potential medical emergency and the client is sent immediately to the hospital. Some conditions that are mistaken for appendicitis are Crohn's disease, a gall bladder attack, a kidney infection (right sided), a ruptured ectopic pregnancy, an ovarian cyst or a hemorrhaging ovarian follicle at the middle of the menstrual cycle. In any case, a referral to a physician is necessary.

✍ An **obstruction of the colon** is a medical emergency especially in the very young and elderly. Symptoms include an absence of defecation, distention of the abdomen, vomiting and pain. Most frequently, the block occurs at the rectum (98 per cent), which often results in leakage of fecal matter around the blockage and fecal soiling (*Jones, 1972*).

✍ A client with constipation who has a sudden, unexplained change in bowel patterns which lasts over two weeks, or who has blood in the stools, should be referred to a physician. These symptoms may indicate a serious medical condition such as an obstruction, an inflammatory bowel disease or a tumour (*Canadian Cancer Society, 1996f*).

Contraindications

✦ Hydrotherapy applications of heat on the abdomen should not be used if the client has any history of increased blood pressure or cardiovascular problems. Also, heat would not be used if the client has an inflammatory bowel disease that is flaring up.

✦ Diarrhea is a contraindication to abdominal massage.

Treatment Goals   Treatment Plan

Reduce stress.

☝ Stress can be a cause of constipation and it can be caused by constipation. Therefore, this treatment is done within the context of a relaxation massage.

☝ **Positioning** includes prone with a pillow under the abdomen and placed under the ankles. The abdominal pillow acts to reduce the lordotic curve and to prevent lumbar hyperextension with the application of deep pressure. An abdominal massage is done with the client in the supine position. This requires adequate pillowing under the knees to maintain the hips in almost 90 degrees of flexion. An alternative is to have the client bring the knees and hips into flexion, keeping the feet flat on the table and placed close together. Then, the bottom sheet is folded over the feet and tucked under the heels. Another possibility is for the client to place the knees together but keep the feet apart. The option that is most comfortable for the client is used.

☝ When the abdominal massage is completed, the usual supine positioning for the legs can be used, with a pillow under the client's knees.

☝ **Hydrotherapy** can range from warm to cool applications. Warm applications, such as a heating pad, may be placed on the abdomen to increase local circulation. Cool or cold applications act to stimulate the colon. They include a cool wash or a heating compress. The hydrotherapy applications will also reflexively decrease sympathetic nervous system firing.

General Treatment

Decrease sympathetic nervous system firing. Decrease pain.

☝ A smooth, rhythmic pace is used. Full-body rhythmic techniques and effleurage are used throughout the massage.

Specific Treatment

Address contributing postural imbalances. Decrease hypertonicity and trigger points in the lumbar spine and gluteals.

☝ With the client in a **prone** position, the entire back is massaged. Techniques are focused on the lumbar area, sacrum and gluteal muscles. If the fascia is restricted, skin rolling and crossed-arm fascial techniques are used. Heat applied beforehand will make the fascial work easier.

☝ Effleurage and petrissage techniques, such as reinforced fingertip kneading, palmar kneading, scooping and muscle stripping, are applied systematically along the iliac crest (inferior and superior to the crest), spine and twelfth rib. This addresses the quadratus lumborum and lumbar erector spinae. Trigger points are treated using ischemic compression, heat and lengthening of the affected muscles

Treatment Goals

Treatment Plan

🖑 Fingertip and thumb kneading followed by vibrations are applied over the sacrum. This is followed by sacral pumping.

🖑 The gluteal muscles are treated using similar techniques to the ones above. The therapist massages systematically along the inferior edge of the iliac crest, along the sacrum and around the greater trochanter. A loose fist can be used to apply static compressions as well as muscle stripping to the gluteal muscles. Trigger points are treated using ischemic compressions or repetitive petrissage, followed by heat and lengthening of the affected muscles.

🖑 To treat the lateral rotators, the leg is used as a lever to lengthen and shorten these muscles. The therapist is positioned facing the gluteal muscles. The leg is flexed at the knee and loosely held by the therapist below the ankle. As the therapist rotates the ankle and leg into internal rotation — this stretches the lateral rotators — pressure is applied into the lateral rotators with a loosely made fist. Care is taken not to press into the greater trochanter. The pressure is released as the leg and ankle are brought into external rotation, shortening the lateral rotators.

🖑 The hamstrings are treated using a variety of petrissage techniques. If these muscles are short, passive stretching or contract-relax stretching is performed when the client is supine.

Encourage diaphragmatic breathing. Decrease congestion in the abdomen. Increase circulation to the abdomen.

🖑 **Supine** work includes attention to the abdomen and the head, neck and shoulders. The latter group is addressed to decrease sympathetic nervous system firing and facilitate relaxation. Diaphragmatic breathing is encouraged throughout the treatment. Specific instruction in appropriate breathing may be necessary.

🖑 For work to the abdomen, the hips and knees are flexed. Techniques are performed in a clockwise direction, the same direction as peristalsis. The therapist may find it easier to position herself on the client's right side.

🖑 The massage begins with overhanded palmar kneading. A modified effleurage may be used. The effleurage stroke is applied by moving both hands in a superior direction, from the lower abdomen to the xiphoid process. At this point, the hands rotate and separate so pressure is now applied through each thumb. The thumbs glide firmly along each of the costal borders and move towards the back. Care is taken to release the pressure over the floating ribs and to simply glide around the waist to the back. The hands are repositioned with the fingertips at the base of the spine. Each hand now draws along the superior edge of the iliac crest towards the anterior hips. These four movements are performed in one fluid motion. This can be followed by vibrations at each "corner" of the large intestine, namely the ileocecal area, the hepatic flexure, the splenic flexure and the sigmoid colon area.

Treatment Goals   Treatment Plan

🖐 Specific work to the diaphragm is focused bilaterally, with kneading and static pressure applied just under the costal border. The pressure is applied up and under the border; downward pressure is avoided so as not to compress the liver and gall bladder on the right side and the stomach on the left side. Long strokes are performed from the xiphoid process to the lateral costal border.

🖐 The abdominal muscles are treated with slow skin rolling to release any fascial restrictions. Abdominal obliques are addressed by specific muscle stripping along the iliac crest. These are most easily performed if the therapist works across the body, directing the techniques from the posterior attachments to the anterior lateral attachments. With the therapist massaging on the same side, muscle stripping is applied superiorly to inferiorly, from the costal border to the iliac crest. This is followed by scooping along the lateral thorax.

Decrease hypertonicity and trigger points in iliopsoas, if present.

🖐 If hyperlordosis is contributing to the constipation, the iliopsoas and quadriceps are treated for trigger points. A variety of petrissage techniques are used to lengthen these shortened structures. Psoas trigger points, in particular, can be irritated if hard feces move over the muscle, since it lies next to the colon. Ischemic compressions are applied to psoas, with referral pain to the low back temporarily evoked. This is followed by heat and lengthening of the iliopsoas. Passive stretches to the quadriceps are also appropriate. See also the chapter on hyperlordosis for more details.

Move fecal matter.

🖐 The colon is specifically addressed using reinforced fingertip kneading. First, to move the fecal matter through the colon, the techniques are applied from the distal colon to the proximal colon **but** pressure is always applied in a clockwise direction. By imagining the haustrations of the large intestine *(Figure 77.1)*, the therapist applies slow short specific kneading strokes to the colon from the sigmoid colon, superiorly along the descending colon, to the splenic flexure, across the transverse colon to the hepatic flexure and inferiorly to the cecum. This process is repeated a few times with increased pressure, provided the client is comfortable.

🖐 The therapist now applies the same techniques, beginning at the proximal colon and moving towards the distal colon. That is, the cecum is the starting point and fingertip kneading moves towards the sigmoid colon. Again, this is repeated a few times.

🖐 The therapist will possibly palpate hard areas that may be tender to the touch. Pressure may need to be lightened and the technique slowed. Repetition of the technique will often bring some relief for the client, especially if the area contains trapped gas. Overhanded palmar kneading and modified effleurage are repeated.

Maintain range of motion.

🖐 Rhythmic movements of the hips are performed by placing the hands

952

Treatment Goals Treatment Plan

loosely at each side of the waist and gently rocking back and forth. **Passive relaxed range of motion** of the hips and knees is interspersed in the treatment.

Self-care Goals Self-care Plan

Educate the client.

✍ Hydrotherapy used in the treatment, such as hot or cold compresses, is recommended. Epsom salt baths are useful. Self-massage to the abdomen is demonstrated for the client to use at home. A lotion enriched with an essential oil can be used. See irritable bowel syndrome chapter.

Promote an exercise regime.

✍ A general exercise program, such as walking or swimming as well as Tai Chi or yoga, can be helpful. Physical activity after eating reflexively increases mass movements and has been found to be helpful for those with constipation (*Wexner, Bartolo, 1995*).

Refer the client.

✍ A referral to a naturopath or nutritionist for diet counselling is appropriate. Increased intake of water and fibre is encouraged. Biofeedback can be learned to retrain the bowels, especially when problems of poor coordination of muscle contractions cause the constipation.

Design a stretch and strengthening program as indicated.

✍ Exercises will depend on the specific results of the postural assessment. If the client has weak abdominal muscles, AR strengthening exercises, such as curl-ups, are recommended. If hyperlordosis is apparent, quadriceps and psoas stretches are given. If a C-curve scoliosis is compressing unilaterally on the abdomen, heel-sitting exercises are suggested. See the appropriate chapters for details.

Encourage relaxation.

✍ Diaphragmatic breathing is encouraged to facilitate bearing down and to increase overall relaxation. Relaxation techniques such as meditation are important. The use of lavender essential oil may also facilitate relaxation. Twenty-five drops of pure essential oil are mixed in 50 ml. of carrier oil (*Lawless, 1995*). The mixture can be massaged into the abdomen or put in the bath.

Educate about bowel retraining.

✍ The bowel can be retrained over time. This is especially important for clients who have chronically resisted the urge. First thing in the morning, the client eats a piece of fruit and drinks a glass of warm water. He then sits on the toilet for 10 to 15 minutes. This is repeated at the same time each day. Eventually, the bowel is trained to move at this time. If the morning is not convenient, then another time is chosen, usually following a meal.

✍ Because squatting with the hips flexed is the optimal position for defecation, the client may wish to place a stool in front of the toilet to put his feet up on, increasing hip flexion and facilitating bearing down.

Treatment Frequency and Expected Outcome

Treatments should be twice a week for two weeks, then once a week for two weeks. If there is a postural cause, it will need to be addressed in order to relieve the constipation. If the cause is a chronic pathology or medication, treatment will be ongoing. Resisting the urge or dietary causes will require client compliance in order to deal with the constipation.

See also stress reduction, irritable bowel syndrome, hyperlordosis, scoliosis , diabetes, Parkinsons, multiple sclerosis and pregnancy.

IRRITABLE BOWEL SYNDROME

Linda Ludwig

Irritable bowel syndrome (IBS) is also known as spastic colon, spastic constipation, irritable colon and nervous indigestion. It is a motility disorder which is strongly associated with anxiety, stress or depression in over half the cases (Porro, Read, 1990).

Irritable bowel syndrome is the most common gastrointestinal disorder in Western society. It has been referred to as the "common cold of the stomach" *(Goodman, Snyder, 1995)*. It often occurs in women, starting in childhood or early adulthood *(Kamm, Lennard-Jones, 1994)*. There is generally no underlying organic cause or physical abnormality in the gastrointestinal (GI) tract.

Contributing Factors:

➤ With IBS, there are **disruptions and incoordination of the natural peristaltic actions and mass movements of the colon.** This may be caused by autonomic dysfunction, notably with the stress response.

➤ **There may be autonomic dysfunction, notably with response to stress.** This disturbs the transit time of the fecal matter and results in alternations between constipation and diarrhea.

➤ **Food intolerance** affects those with irritable bowel syndrome; figures vary from 6 per cent to 60 per cent *(Read, 1985; Goodman, Snyder, 1995)*. Common food intolerances include wheat, coffee, dairy products, yeast and citrus fruit. Such allergies cause motor and secretory dysfunctions in the GI tract.

Symptom Picture

✦ Symptoms are brought on by emotional stress, fatigue, alcohol and eating, especially consuming meals high in fat, roughage or fruit.

✦ Some people will experience mainly constipation with regular bouts of diarrhea, while others will have the reverse symptoms.

  • **Constipation** results in hard stools due to decreased propulsive movements and an increase in the segmental movements in the colon. Small "unit" or "pellet" stools result when there is increased tone in the distal colon accompanied by segmenting contractions. There is then a breakdown of the hard stool into small pieces.

  • **Diarrhea** results from an increase in propulsive movements and a decrease in segmental movements. This reduces the amount of water the body can reabsorb and accounts for a watery stool.

✦ Accompanying this altered bowel function is steady or intermittent pain in the lower abdomen. Pain can be dull with sharp cramps occurring after eating or in the morning. Pain is the result of increased pressure from the fecal matter in the colon accompanied by gas build-up *(Thompson, 1979)*. It is thought that those with IBS have particularly sensitive visceral pain receptors. Frequently this pain is relieved with a bowel movement *(Read, 1985)*.

✦ Other symptoms include the feeling of incomplete evacuation of the feces — eliminating pellet stools is difficult for anyone, even those without IBS — bloating, nausea, vomiting, anorexia and halitosis. Straining with defecation may occur if the stool is hard or soft, possibly due to an inability to relax the anal sphincter. IBS is often accompanied by anxiety and depression *(Porro, Read, 1990)*.

Contraindications

✦ Hydrotherapy applications of heat on the abdomen should not be used if the client has any history of increased blood pressure or cardiovascular problems. Also, they would not be used if the client has a flare-up of an inflammatory bowel disease.

✦ Diarrhea is a contraindication to abdominal massage.

✦ Many symptoms of IBS are common to inflammatory diseases such as ulcerative colitis. These are distinguished from IBS by the presence of rectal bleeding and through a medical examination, which will reveal GI inflammation common to these diseases *(Porro, Read, 1990)*.

✦ The prognosis for ridding the client of IBS is not particularly good. It is considered a chronic and recurring condition. Client compliance with diet modifications and relaxation strategies has been shown to improve the symptoms *(Kamm, Lennard-Jones, 1994)*.

Treatment Considerations

Assessment

✦ **Health history questions** are asked about the client's symptoms. These include: Can the client describe her usual bowel movement frequency and consistency? What is the colour of the stool? Is there pain? Where is it located? What are the quality, frequency and duration of the pain? What relieves the pain? Pain is often reduced after having a bowel movement.

✍ **Testing** includes performance of the **rebound test**. It will be negative for irritable bowel syndrome.

✍ **Differentiating Types of Abdominal Pain:**

- A positive **rebound test** can indicate appendicitis. Symptoms of appendicitis are nausea and vomiting, low-grade fever and pain in the lower right quadrant. This condition is a potential medical emergency and the client is sent immediately to the hospital.

- Some conditions that are mistaken for appendicitis are Crohn's disease, a gall bladder attack, a kidney infection (right sided), a ruptured ectopic pregnancy, an ovarian cyst or a hemorrhaging ovarian follicle at the middle of the menstrual cycle. In any case, a referral to a physician is necessary.

- A client with constipation who has a sudden, unexplained change in bowel patterns which lasts over two weeks or who has blood in the stools should be referred to a physician. These symptoms may indicate a serious medical condition such as an obstruction, an inflammatory bowel disease or cancer (*Canadian Cancer Society, 1996f*).

Massage

✋ Because this syndrome is the alternation of constipation and diarrhea, the treatment for constipation is appropriate during the constipation stage. Somewhat less pressure may be appropriate if the client is sensitive. At all times, there is an emphasis on the relaxation component of the treatment because stress can play such a significant role in exacerbating symptoms.

✋ Abdominal massage is effective in promoting movement of fecal matter and gas contained in the bowel. Essential oils that promote the release of gas are fennel, lemon, peppermint and basil. Those that combine gas release and the promotion of relaxation are bergamot, marjoram and chamomile. In all the above cases, 25 drops of essential oil are diluted in 50 ml. of vegetable oil (*Lawless, 1992*). The oil is used for the abdominal massage during the treatment and at home by the client for self-care.

Self-care

See also stress reduction, inflammatory bowel disease and constipation.

✍ Self-care is similar to that given for constipation and stress reduction treatments. One notable exception to the self-care recommendations is the increase of fibre in the diet in the form of wheat. Wheat fibre may cause irritation in some clients with IBS. If, after three weeks, the omission of wheat fibre is not helpful, a referral to a naturopath is suggested. In any case, nutrition counselling is usually necessary, because caffeine, alcohol and smoking can often increase the symptoms of the syndrome.

INFLAMMATORY BOWEL DISEASE

Linda Ludwig

> *Inflammatory bowel disease is used to identify two conditions: ulcerative colitis and Crohn's disease.*

Ulcerative colitis and Crohn's disease commonly begin to affect people between the ages of 15 to 20 and other people in their mid-fifties to sixties *(Porth, 1990)*. Both diseases can affect multiple systems in the body and cause peripheral arthritis, arthralgia, myalgia and obstructive pulmonary disease *(Porth, 1990)*.

➤ **The cause of these conditions is unknown, although there is a familial tendency.**

✦ **Ulcerative colitis** results in a broad area of ulceration in the mucosa of the left colon and rectum. Periods of pain and bloody diarrhea, up to 20 to 30 times per day, alternate with remission. Other symptoms include nausea, vomiting, anorexia and weight loss. There are varying degrees of severity, from mild to severe. The majority of people (about 60 per cent) have the mild form. Serious complications can occur, such as toxic megacolon which is dilation of the colon that leads to systemic toxicity. Over the long term, there is an increased risk of colon cancer associated with ulcerative colitis. **Medically**, management of this condition is through medication and possibly surgery to remove ulcerated areas.

✦ **Crohn's disease** results in multiple, patchy ulcerative lesions which may affect any part of the gastrointestinal (GI) tract. These cause scarring and thickening of the bowel. If the lesion penetrates the bowel, abscesses result. The ileum of the small intestine and ileocecal area of the colon are most commonly affected. All layers of the intestinal wall may be affected. The recurrent inflammation results in scarring and thickening of the affected areas. With Crohn's disease, rectal bleeding is less common initially. Symptoms are more painful compared to ulcerative colitis. Pain may diminish after a bowel movement or release of gas. Intermittent diarrhea, weight loss, malaise, low-grade fever and nutritional deficiencies occur. Complications include intestinal obstruction and

Contraindications

- During a flare-up, any treatment of the abdomen or low back is contraindicated.

- Vigorous or deep work to the abdomen or low back is generally contraindicated, due to the ulcerative and inflammatory nature of these diseases.

- Arthralgia and myalgia may be more severe if medication to control intestinal inflammation is suddenly reduced. Modification of pressure and vigour of techniques may by necessary.

- See also inflammatory arthritides for related contraindications.

abdominal abscesses. Eventually, the majority of those with Crohn's disease require surgical intervention to address complications. **Medically**, management is through nutritional supplements, diet modification, stress management and medication.

- Although periods of relative quiescence occur, neither disease heals completely. Periods of stress are thought to increase the client's symptoms.

- In longstanding cases of inflammatory bowel disease, with the client's permission, his physician should be consulted for an assessment of tissue fragility and possible complications.

Treatment Considerations

Assessment

- **Health history questions** include the following: Has the condition been diagnosed by a physician? How long has the client had the condition? Are there any complications or are other areas of the body affected? What treatment has been received? Is the client on any medications? Has the client had surgery? What symptoms are experienced and what exacerbates them? What relieves the symptoms?

- **Testing** includes the **rebound test,** which will be negative for an inflammatory bowel disease.

Massage

- The focus of the massage treatment is on stress reduction and relaxation. Gentle vibrations and rocking to the sacrum will help to decrease sympathetic nervous system firing. If the client is not experiencing a flare-up, gentle and soothing abdominal techniques are performed.

- An enriched lotion using essential oils such as chamomile or neroli can be used for the abdominal massage. Ten drops of essential oil are added to 50 ml. of vegetable oil *(Sellar, 1992).*

- Indirect connective tissue techniques may be helpful if the therapist is well trained in such techniques *(Barral, 1989).*

Self-care

See also stress reduction, cancer and inflammatory arthritides.

- The client may be referred to the Bowel Disease Association. A nutritionist or naturopath can assist in dietary modifications.

- The therapist may encourage stress reduction techniques such as full diaphragmatic breathing and meditation.

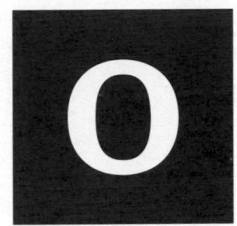

SYSTEMIC CONCERNS AND OTHER CONDITIONS

INFLAMMATORY ARTHRITIDES

Fiona Rattray

> *Inflammatory arthritides are a group of inflammatory diseases affecting connective tissue including the joints.*

There are numerous arthritides. Some of the more commonly encountered are described below. A pathology text should be consulted for conditions not covered. The therapist may need to confer with the client's physician, with the client's written permission, to determine the specific diagnosis and contraindications. It is important to have enough information in order to select appropriate treatment goals.

Ankylosing Spondylitis

> *Ankylosing spondylitis (AS) is a chronic, systemic inflammatory disorder that involves specific areas of the body, primarily the spine.*

✦ Peripheral joints such as the knees and finger joints are also affected. Ankylosing means immobility and fixation of a joint, while spondylitis is inflammation of the vertebrae.

➤ **The cause of ankylosing spondylitis is idiopathic**, but is associated with HLA-B27 antigen and may be genetic. Ankylosing spondylitis was thought to be more common in males than females, but it now appears that the frequency is about the same, with men being more severely affected. The onset of AS is insidious, usually beginning in early adulthood, with the inflammatory stage of the disease usually ending by age 40 (*The Arthritis Society, 1996a*). The development of AS is highly variable, with spontaneous remissions and periods of flare-up. A flare-up is when the disease is active or when

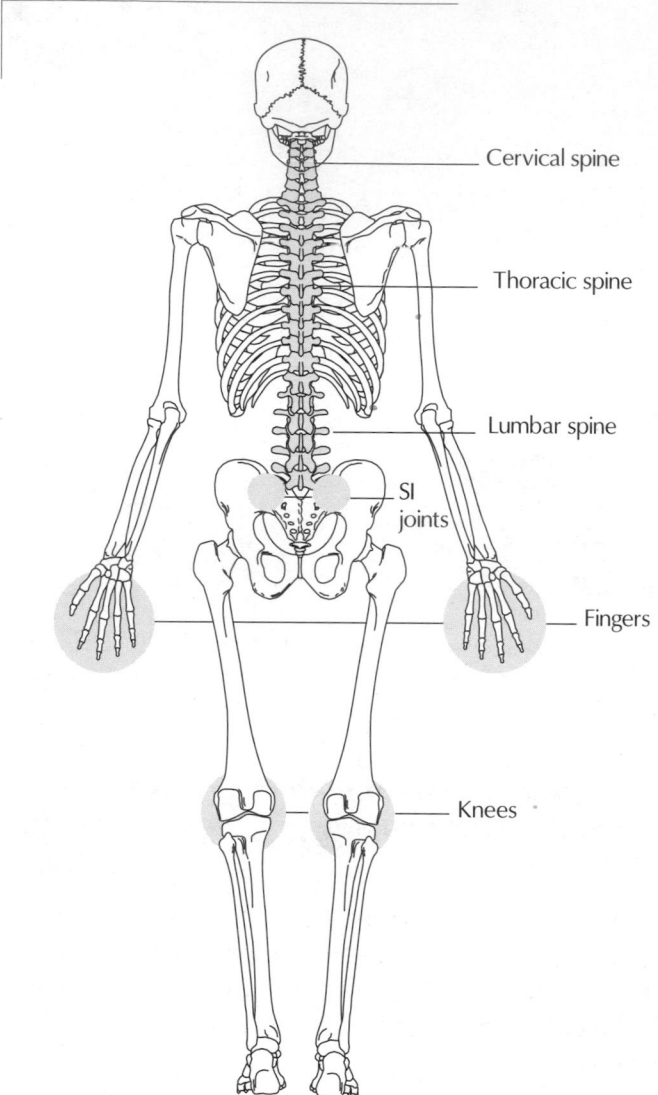

Figure 80.1
Ankylosing spondylitis: Joints affected.

Labels on figure: Cervical spine, Thoracic spine, Lumbar spine, SI joints, Fingers, Knees

symptoms are exacerbated. The course of AS is generally favourable, although in some cases severe deformities occur.

✦ The disease begins with synovitis at the sacroiliac joints — sacroiliitis *(Hertling, Kessler, 1996; Schumacher, 1993)* — and, over many years, proceeds gradually up the spine *(Figure 80.1)*. Inflammation at the junctions of ligaments and vertebrae results in fibrosing of the ligaments, bone erosion and later its replacement with new bone. Ankylosing occurs first at the sacroiliac joints, then in the ligaments, intervertebral discs, facet joints and intervertebral foramina of the lumbar and later thoracic spine. The vertical bone growths replacing the intervertebral discs are called "syndesmophytes".

✦ With severe, longstanding AS, the vertebrae take on a fused appearance, termed "bamboo spine", when viewed on an X-ray. Inflammation of the iris (uveitis) leading to pain, blurred vision and edema is present in up to 30 per cent of people with AS. Cardiovascular involvement such as aortic valve incompetence occurs in rare cases *(Schumacher, 1993)*.

✦ In the early stages, the client experiences fatigue, morning stiffness in the lumbar spine and pain in the buttocks, low back and, occasionally, down the posterior thighs. The lumbar lordosis is lost due to spasm; flexion contractures occur in the hips. The symptoms are worse after a period of immobility, such as prolonged sitting.

✦ In later stages, movement in the spine is severely reduced and muscle wasting due to disuse atrophy may be present. With the loss of the lumbar lordosis, the thoracic curve becomes more evident. The chest becomes fixed and flattened, and the thoracic muscles atrophy. Chest expansion is reduced as a result of costovertebral joint involvement; breathing becomes primarily diaphragmatic. As the disease progresses to the cervical spine, neck movements are lost and a head-forward posture develops.

✦ Ankylosing of the spine occurs at variable rates and in different patterns. Sometimes only the sacroiliac joints and lumbar spine are affected whereas in extreme cases the whole spine is fused into flexion, causing the person to look down instead of ahead while walking. Pain may diminish over the years with fusion.

- **Medically**, AS is managed with anti-inflammatories. While there is no cure for AS, spinal deformity is prevented or minimized by regular therapeutic exercises such as stretching and diaphragmatic breathing *(Schumacher, 1993)*. Surgery is rarely used as treatment, except with severe hip involvement.

- One study found that 26 people were able to maintain a significant improvement in mobility and function for four months after participating in a home physiotherapy program for AS *(Walker, Helewa, 1996)*.

- There is a relationship between large and small bowel disease and arthritis. For example, up to 20 per cent of those with Crohn's disease develop sacroiliitis, spondylitis and transient non-destructive arthritis, usually in the legs or feet. Pain is present in the low back, similar to AS. In one study, 62 per cent of people with active ulcerative colitis also had arthritis in large and small joints *(Schumacher, 1993)*.

Gout

Gout is a group of disorders in which crystals of monosodium urate are deposited in the tissues, accompanied by attacks of acute arthritis.

- The metatarsophalangeal joint of the big toe is the area most commonly attacked by gout, with the tarsal area and ankle also frequently involved. The other joints are less commonly affected.

- **Pseudogout**, a similar condition, is caused by calcium pyrophosphate dihydrate crystals. Joints attacked are usually ankles, knees, shoulders and wrists, with the big toe rarely affected.

- Up to 90 per cent of those affected by gout are men, usually between the ages of 40 and 50 years. Women who develop gout are usually post-menopausal. Children are rarely affected *(The Arthritis Society, 1996b)*.

- **The cause of gout is a malfunction of the normal chemical process that breaks down purines.** These substances are found in all the body's cells, as well as in certain foods such as meat and fish. People who develop gout have either an overproduction of uric acid, an underexcretion of uric acid or, in some cases, both abnormalites. High levels of blood uric acid are termed "hyperuricemia".

- The excess uric acid accumulates in the extracellular fluid, eventually changing to needle-shaped urate crystals. These crystals collect in synovial tissue and eventually precipitate into the synovial fluid where they trigger an acute attack of gout. It is possible that gout primarily affects the peripheral tissues because the extremities are slightly cooler than the body's core, and sodium urate is less soluble at temperatures lower than 37 degrees *(Porth, 1990)*.

- An acute attack usually affects a single joint. The initial onset is sudden and extremely painful. It may occur at night after a day of more than usual activity. The gnawing, intense pain may be such that the person is unable to bear the weight of the bed sheets on the joint *(Schumacher, 1993)*.

✦ The affected joint is obviously red, hot and swollen. The skin over the joint is shiny and taut. While gout can be an inherited condition, attacks can also be precipitated by excessive alcohol consumption, obesity, certain foods and medications, trauma, surgery and "crash" diets.

✦ In the early stage, an acute attack may last for a few days, followed by a symptom-free period of several months or years. If untreated, attacks are more frequent and severe as the disease progresses. Repeated flare-ups cause joint stiffness and reduced range of motion and, eventually, cartilage and subchondral bone destruction leading to joint deformation.

✦ In the chronic stage, inflammation spreads to other peripheral joints. This stage, termed "chronic tophaceous gout", occurs on average 10 years after the initial attack. It is marked by subcutaneous deposits of urate crystals called "tophi". These lumps occur outside the joints. Tissues commonly affected include the olecranon bursa, subcutaneous tissue along the forearm extensors, skin over joints, the helix of the ear and tendon sheaths in the hands and around the Achilles tendon. If left untreated, tophi can break through the skin and lead to infection or carpal tunnel syndrome or trigger finger. Over time, uric acid crystals may form kidney stones. Renal impairment, hypertension and diabetes mellitus are also associated with chronic gout.

✦ **Medically**, gout is diagnosed through identification of urate crystals in synovial fluid. The inflammation and pain of acute attacks are treated with NSAIDs and colchicine. Uric acid production is reduced using allopurinol. Some foods such as liver and sardines can raise blood levels of uric acid, while alcohol can trigger attacks. A person with gout may initially be advised to avoid these substances. Once medication stabilizes uric acid levels, most people with gout can consume these substances in moderation. In addition, obese people with gout may be placed on a physician-directed weight-reduction plan.

Infectious Arthritis

Infectious arthritis is joint inflammation resulting from infection by bacteria, viruses or fungi.

✦ In most cases, infectious arthritis involves one joint, such as the knee, hip, shoulder, elbow and small joints in the hand or foot. However, 20 per cent of infectious arthritides *(Schumacher, 1993)* are polyarticular (affecting more than one joint). Infectious arthritis is more common among people with prosthetic joints, immunosuppression and chronic illnesses.

✦ The affected joint is red, hot and swollen with reduced range of motion due to pain. During the inflammatory response, fibrin is deposited on the cartilage and synovial lining, leading to ischemia and necrosis. If untreated, as the inflammation resolves, relative capsular fibrosis, or a reduced flexibility of the joint capsule, is present.

➤ **Infectious arthritis may be caused by a number of organisms.** Bacteria reach joints both directly and indirectly: directly as a result of trauma, surgery and arthrocentesis and from nearby abcesses and wounds; and indirectly through the bloodstream from other sites of infection such as in the gastrointestinal tract, the respiratory system or the urinary tract. Bacterial causes include staphylococcus, streptococcus, pneumococcus, gonococcus and tuberculosis infections. The onset is usually sudden. Fever, shaking and chills may or may not be present.

✦ Bacteria multiply rapidly in synovial fluid. They are either killed by the synovial lining cells or form abscesses in the synovial membrane. Both the toxins produced by the bacteria and enzymes released during phagocytosis have a destructive effect on the cartilage.

✦ **Medically**, it is important to treat bacterial arthritis quickly with a full course of antibiotics. Unfortunately, the normal compressive forces at a joint reduce the diffusion of medication from the bloodstream into the joint, perhaps allowing bacteria to remain dormant even in the presence of medication. Moreover, medication does not remove the bacterial toxins in the joint, allowing for the possibility of chronic inflammation (*Walker, Helewa, 1996*).

✦ Arthritic reactions may follow a viral infection. Viral causes include rubella, hepatitis and parvovirus. Joint inflammation usually lasts one or two weeks and resolves on its own.

✦ Fungal arthritis develops very slowly, over weeks or months. The fungi enters the skin through cuts. Fungi that cause arthritis are found in soil and bird droppings. Antifungal medications such as fluconazole are used to treat this arthritis.

Lyme Disease

Lyme disease is a complex rheumatic disease that affects many systems of the body.

✦ The illness mimics other diseases including the flu and several other rheumatic conditions.

➤ **Lyme disease is caused by the spirochete *borrelia burgdorferi,*** which is transmitted to humans by tick bites. In western North America, the tick species is *Ixodes pacificus*, while in eastern and central North America, *Ixodes dammini* is the vector. These ticks are quite small and hard to observe: an immature tick is about the size of a period on this page *(Arthritis Foundation, 1993)*.

✦ Ticks live outdoors in wooded or marshy areas, and are most active in the spring and summer months. They spend part of their life cycle living on birds and other animals such as white-footed mice, then develop to their next stage, where they bite humans.

✦ Lyme disease begins after an incubation period of up to 32 days. In 80 per cent of those affected, a large, expanding skin rash (erythema migrans) is noticed around the site of the tick bite, although the person may not have noticed the bite itself. In some people the rash is ring-shaped. In others there is a raised, vesicular area in the centre *(Schumacher, 1993)*. The rash is hot to the touch, but not painful.

✦ Several days after the onset of erythema migrans, severe headache, fever, chills, stiff neck, swollen lymph nodes, fatigue, muscle ache and joint pain occur. These symptoms are typically intermittent and changing. Brief, sporadic attacks of arthritis may affect large joints, especially one knee. These episodes may become longer after the second year of Lyme disease, lasting for months instead of weeks.

✦ Other more serious manifestations of Lyme disease are neurological abnormalities developing months after the initial symptoms, including meningitis, bilateral facial palsy, memory impairment and distal paresthesia. Cardiac involvement can include irregular or slow heartbeat.

✦ **Medically**, Lyme disease is treated with antibiotics and is curable if treatment is begun early. Preventative measures to avoid tick bites include wearing protective clothing that covers the legs and arms — for example, when in a tick area, tucking pant legs into socks prevents ticks climbing onto the skin. After being in wooded areas, people should check for ticks on themselves, children and pets. Typically, ticks are attracted to warmer skin areas such as the axilla, inguinal area and trunk. If a tick is found attached to the skin, tweezers are used to carefully remove the tick without squeezing the tick's body. After wiping the skin over the tick bite with an antiseptic, the tick may be saved in a jar for later identification *(Arthritis Foundation, 1993)*.

Reiter's Syndrome

Reiter's syndrome is a triad of arthritis, non-gonococcal urethritis and conjunctivitis, following inflammation of the intestine or urinary tract.

✦ Reiter's syndrome is only one manifestation of reactive arthritis, an inflammatory joint response to an infection distant to the inflamed joint(s). While the bacteria that caused the infection are not directly found in the inflamed joint, antigens and RNA from the bacteria are present.

➤ **The cause of Reiter's syndrome is idiopathic**, but is associated with an initial infection of a genetically susceptible person by salmonella, shigella, campylobacter or yersinia bacteria in the gastrointestinal tract or by chlamydia trachomatis in the urinary tract. There may be a connection to the HLA-B27 antigen in some persons who develop Reiter's syndrome. Most cases are seen in adults after an episode of gastroenteritis. Reiter's syndrome was thought to be 20 times more common in males than females, but it is now believed that the male to female ratio is 5:1 *(Schumacher, 1993)*.

✦ Early symptoms include joint stiffness, myalgia and low back pain. Arthritis develops up to three weeks after the initial infection. Typically, joint involvement is asymmetric. The feet, ankles, knees and wrists are commonly affected. Those with severe or chronic Reiter's syndrome are more likely to have the spine affected as well, including the sacroiliac joints (sacroiliitis).

✦ Inflammation occurs mostly at the insertion of a tendon to a bone, rather than, or in addition, to the synovium. For example, the plantar fascia and the Achilles tendon attachments at the calcaneus are commonly inflamed. In the toes and fingers this presents as a uniformly swollen digit, termed "sausage digit". In the majority of cases, the arthritis does not lead to permanent disability or joint deformity.

+ Some people with Reiter's syndrome have repeated attacks of arthritis lasting from three to six months. Successive flare-ups are similar in terms of severity, although different joints may be affected each time. However, more than half of those affected will not experience another flare-up *(Arthritis Foundation, 1992)*.

+ Conjunctivitis is experienced by 40 per cent of those with Reiter's syndrome, while urethritis and cystitis affect both men and women who have the syndrome. Associated skin problems are a rash on the plantar surface of the foot and small, painless sores in the mouth or on external genitalia. These symptoms fluctuate and are not experienced by all persons with Reiter's.

+ **Medically**, Reiter's syndrome is difficult to diagnose. Medications such as NSAIDs and remedial exercises are used to control the arthritis, combined with treatment of other presenting symptoms as needed. Reiter's syndrome is associated with human immunodeficiency virus (HIV), the arthritis predating symptoms of HIV infection. It is thought that certain drugs, such as methotrexate, used to treat Reiter's syndrome may increase the suppression of the body's immune response, provoking the AIDS symptoms in those with the virus *(Schumacher, 1993)*.

Rheumatoid Arthritis

Rheumatoid arthritis (RA) is an inflammatory, destructive, chronic autoimmune disease of multiple joints and connective tissue throughout the body.

➤ **The cause of RA is unknown.** It is possible that there is more than one cause of the disease; in genetically predisposed individuals, a diminished immune response to bacteria and viruses may play a part. The immune system likely plays a role in this disease, since rheumatoid factor (an antibody) is present in 70 per cent of those with RA *(Porth, 1990)*.

+ Severe rheumatoid arthritis may be a disease with modern origin, as it cannot be isolated in ancient skeletons, nor is it represented in literature or art from a few hundred years ago, as is gout *(Walker, Helewa, 1996)*.

+ RA affects one per cent of the population, with women affected more than men in a ratio of 3:1. Although RA can affect people of all ages, the prevalence increases with age; those between 25 and 50 years are most commonly affected *(The Arthritis Society, 1998a)*.

+ The onset is often gradual over several months, with symptom-free periods following for several months or years. There are periods of flare-up and remission. There may be complete remission in the first two years of the disease *(Hellman, 1995)*; this is less likely in later stages.

+ Prognosis is uncertain. The disease can be mild, attacking a few joints for brief periods. After the first year, in 90 per cent of the cases studied, joints initially involved are those which are ultimately affected *(Schumacher, 1993)*. In three per cent of those with RA, it

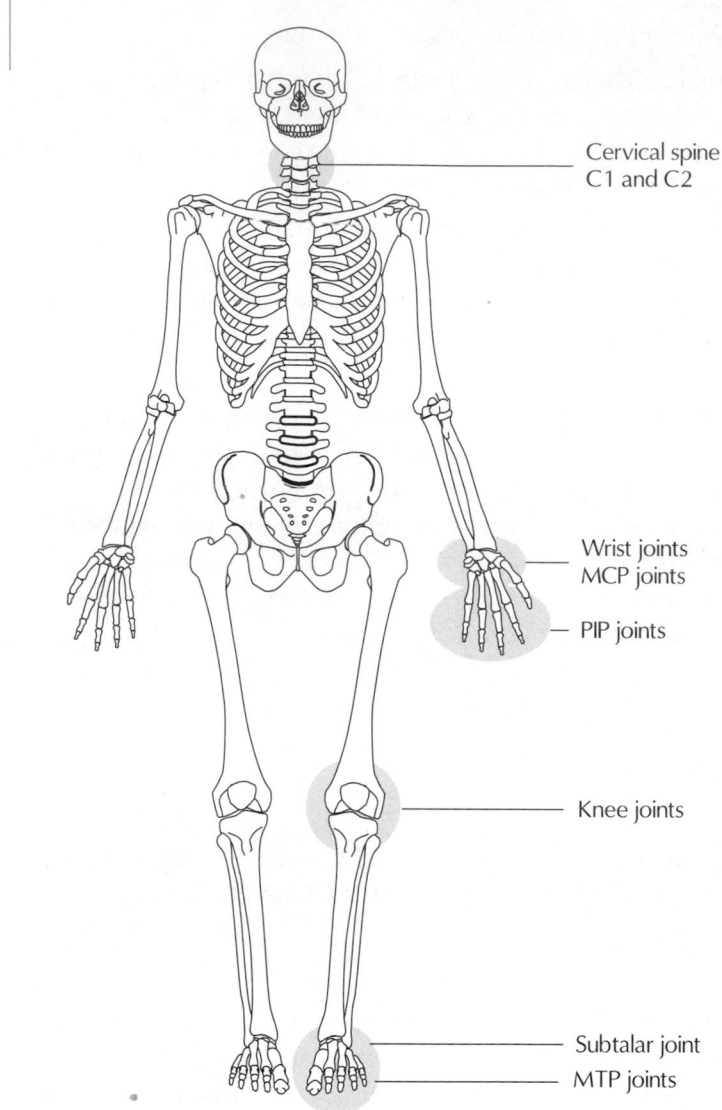

Cervical spine
C1 and C2

Wrist joints
MCP joints

PIP joints

Knee joints

Subtalar joint

MTP joints

Figure 80.2
Joints affected with RA.

has an unremitting and progressive course, rapidly leading to severe disability. Occasionally, with severe RA, death results from pulmonary and renal disease.

✦ RA begins with activation or injury of the synovial microvasculature of the endothelial cells. Edema and inflammation result and the synovial cells multiply and grow; capillaries proliferate among the newly grown synovial cells within a few weeks. The affected joints are hot, puffy and swollen; the skin over the joint is shiny and tight. The range of motion is reduced due to pain and stiffness, especially after a period of immobility such as sleeping. The stiffness persists for at least one hour and may be relieved by a hot shower. The duration of morning stiffness gives an indication of the severity of the inflammation *(Walker, Helewa, 1996)*.

✦ The disease often starts in the hands and wrists; joints are usually affected symmetrically. Most commonly involved are the proximal interphalangeal (PIP) joints, metacarpophalangeal (MCP) joints, wrists, knees, metatarsophalangeal (MTP) joints, subtalar joints and C1 to C2 in the cervical spine *(Figure 80.2)*. The person also experiences systemic symptoms such as generalized aching, stiffness, fatigue and weight loss.

✦ As RA progresses, synovitis occurs and the synovial membrane thickens and folds in a process similar to granulation which occurs with wound healing. This vascularized membrane (or pannus) extends from the synovium to involve the articular cartilage. The inflammatory process liberates proteolytic enzymes, which attack and erode the cartilage, eventually exposing subchondral bone. Pannus develops between the joint margins, forming adhesions which restrict range of motion. Over the long term, fibrous ankylosis may form bony ankylosis.

✦ The surrounding joint capsule, ligaments, bursae and bones are affected as the joint structure erodes and crumbles. Joint deformities occur as the joint capsule swells and thickens. The fingers may become spindle-shaped. The tendons and muscles crossing the affected joints develop spasms leading to imbalances which move the joint further out of alignment. Subluxations may develop; the joint capsule and surrounding tendons can rupture.

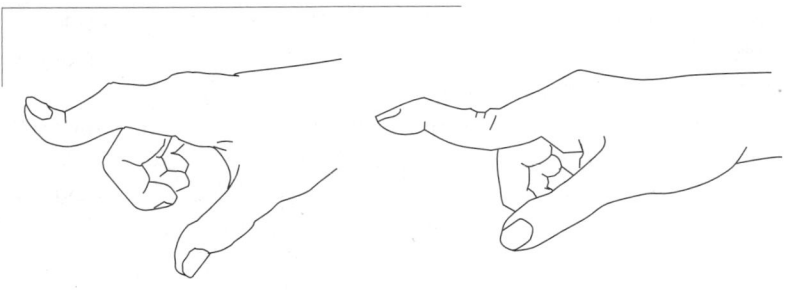

Boutonniere deformity   Swan-neck deformity

Figure 80.3
Common joint deformities.

✦ In the hand *(Figure 80.3)*, common joint deformities include: **swan neck deformity** due to intrinsic hand muscle contracture (proximal interphalangeal joint hyperextended, distal interphalangeal joint flexed); and **boutonniere (buttonhole) deformity** resulting from ruptures of the central slip of the extensor tendons (proximal interphalangeal joint flexed, distal interphalangeal joint hyperextended). Severe loss of function occurs with a swan neck deformity, as the person can no longer make a fist. In addition, ulnar deviation may occur with subluxed metacarpophalangeal joints. Disuse atrophy, tenosynovitis and carpal tunnel syndrome may also be present.

✦ Knee valgus deformity is quite common. Swelling is pronounced and the normal contours of the patella disappear. A Baker's cyst, enlargement of the posterior knee bursa, may form in the popliteal space. Knee flexion contractures may eventually develop if the person is unable to weight bear and uses a wheelchair. If ankle flexion and extension are reduced, gait and postural problems may result. Entrapment neuropathies can occur at peripheral nerves such as the femoral nerve.

✦ Neck pain is common. In severe cases, erosion of the alar ligaments and the odontoid process of C2 may lead to cervical instability and neurological symptoms.

✦ As RA is a systemic disease, there are several extra-articular symptoms. During flare-ups, pain, fatigue, low-grade fever, weight loss and anemia are likely experienced. Rheumatoid nodules, present in 25 per cent of those with RA, develop where skin and subcutaneous tissues are subject to pressure — for example, at the extensor surface of the forearm *(Walker, Helewa, 1996)*. These granulomatous lesions are variable in size; they may or may not move, and may be tender or not. The nodules may be permanent unless surgically removed or may spontaneously resolve.

✦ Sjorgren's syndrome of dry eyes and dry mouth is present in up to 15 per cent of those with RA. The eyes may feel gritty and the person feels thirsty *(Porth, 1990)*. This is often treated with artificial tears and liquids to moisten the mouth.

✦ More serious symptoms include pericarditis, pleurisy and eye lesions. Renal complications result from prolonged medication use (gold salts or penicillamine).

✦ **Medically**, diagnosis of RA is made with laboratory tests and X-rays and in the presence of the following: morning stiffness for at least one hour; involvement of at least three joints for six weeks; symmetrical joint swelling; and rheumatoid nodules.

✦ NSAIDS, methotrexate (an immunosuppressive), antimalarial drugs, penicillamine or gold salts (chrysotherapy) may be prescribed. A short course of corticosteroid treatment will dramatically improve the joint symptoms but will not alter the course of the disease. Splints and orthotics may be prescribed. Joint replacement is becoming more common, especially for the knees. Severe cases affecting C1 and C2 may require vertebral fusion.

✦ Persons with RA are often referred for physiotherapy to maintain range of motion and strength. One study showed that isometric exercise can increase strength in quadriceps muscles of RA patients *(Walker, Helewa, 1996)*. However, with respect to most studies that demonstrate the effectiveness of physiotherapy techniques in treating RA, physiotherapists are in a situation similar to that of massage therapists. While literature is available on the effectiveness of medication, literature on the physiotherapy management of RA, which includes exercise and hydrotherapy modalities, is lacking. Those resources that do exist often neglect to mention which specific exercises (passive or active) or the number of repetitions that are used. Frequently, studies show a lack of consistency in approach, so comparisons are difficult to make. As there has been little research on the effectiveness of physiotherapy and RA, physiotherapists are asked to employ research methods that encompass the science as well as the art of physiotherapy to evaluate its effectiveness *(Stewart, 1996)*, directives which also apply to massage therapists and massage therapy.

Scleroderma

Scleroderma is a systemic disorder affecting collagen, characterized by slowly spreading fibrosis and collagen deposits throughout the body.

✦ Scleroderma is an autoimmune disorder.

➤ **The cause of scleroderma is unknown.** However, occupational exposure to vinyl chloride, silica and organic solvents may be connected to scleroderma-like diseases. Scleroderma is a rare disease, usually affecting adults between ages 30 and 50, with women affected more commonly than men in a ratio of up to 5:1 *(Arthritis Foundation, 1997)*.

✦ Often the first symptom is Raynaud's phenomenon, swelling or puffiness of the digits and arthritis of the digits. The skin thickens and indurates.

✦ There are two forms of scleroderma: *localized* and *generalized.*

✦ **Localized scleroderma** affects the skin, fascia, muscle and sometimes bone. It strikes children and young adults, mostly females. Fibrotic lesions, composed of abnormal fibroblasts, form hard oval patches on the skin's surface (morphea scleroderma) or extend from the skin deep into muscles and bones of the limbs and forehead (linear scleroderma). Range of motion is reduced in the affected joints and collagen deposits in the synovial lining give rise to joint pain. On the face, the lips pucker and there is difficulty in opening the mouth, termed "Mauskopf" (mouse-headed appearance).

✦ **Generalized scleroderma** affects multiple systems of the body: the skin, capillaries, gastrointestinal tract, lungs, heart and kidneys. It is further divided into two categories: *limited* and *diffuse.*

• The onset of limited generalized scleroderma is over a period of five to 10 years. The skin is affected first, followed later by contractures of the digits (sclerodactyly) and dilated superficial skin capillaries (telangiectasia).

• The onset of diffuse generalized scleroderma is more sudden, with the skin affected first. Later, stiffness, flexion contractures, tendon involvement (a leathery, rubbing sensation with range of motion), carpal tunnel syndrome and arthritis of large and small joints are present. Muscle weakness occurs due to restricted range of motion. More serious symptoms result from visceral involvement. Collagen build-up can narrow the esophagus and small intestine, causing reflux, diarrhea or constipation. Congestive heart failure, restrictive lung disease, malignant hypertension and renal failure may also occur.

✦ **Medically**, although there is no cure for scleroderma, certain drugs such as penicillamine may slow its progression. NSAIDs are also used to treat arthritis pain. Raynaud's phenomenon is treated by keeping the extremities warm. Other symptoms are controlled as they arise.

✦ Scleroderma varies considerably in its course and outcome from person to person. The survival rate 10 years after diagnosis is 65 per cent. Disability and death are most common early on with the development of diffuse scleroderma, especially for those with pulmonary, cardiac or renal complications *(Schumacher, 1993)*.

Still's Disease and Juvenile Rheumatoid Arthritis

Still's disease and juvenile rheumatoid arthritis (JRA) are conditions of chronic synovial inflammation in children.

➤ **The causes of these conditions are unknown.** JRA may develop at any stage of childhood; girls are generally more affected than boys.

• *Pauciarticular onset* describes arthritis of four or fewer joints, that usually manifests during the first six months of the disease. This condition comprises about half of the children affected with JRA. The knee is commonly affected.

• *Polyarticular onset* is arthritis of more than four joints. Onset is between one and three years of age as well as between eight and 10 years of age. The hands, feet and temporomandibular joints are often affected, usually symetrically. Mild fever, malaise, adenopathy, anemia and stunted growth may occur. This onset affects about 40 per cent of children with JRA. Growth disturbances that may result with JRA are made worse by corticosteroids.

• *Still's disease*, affecting up to 10 per cent of those with juvenile arthritis, has a systemic onset. Symptoms include a high, spiking fever, pink rash, hepatosplenomegaly and anemia. Later, polyarthritis develops. Symptoms usually diminish after 12 months.

✦ The prognosis for most children with JRA is good, with up to 75 per cent experiencing remission with little or no residual disability. Aspirin is the most common medication. Exercise programs are important, as is encouraging the child to lead as normal a life as possible *(Walker, Helewa, 1996)*.

• *Adult onset Still's disease* can affect young adults of both genders. It is a polyarthritis identical to childhood-onset Still's disease, with additional symptoms of lymphadenopathy and, less commonly, pericarditis. In some cases infections and adrenal insufficiency can be fatal.

Systemic Lupus Erythematosus

Systemic lupus erythematosus (SLE) is one type of chronic, attack-remitting autoimmune inflammatory disease that can affect any system or organ in a variable manner.

➤ **The cause of lupus is unknown,** although there may be a genetic component that is triggered by factors outside and inside the body.

✦ In Canada, SLE affects 15,000 people *(The Arthritis Society, 1998d)*. People of all ages can be affected; however, women of childbearing age are most at risk. Generally, more women than men get SLE.

✦ Aggravating factors that can trigger an attack include prolonged and severe stress, medications such as chlorpromazine and methyldopa, viral infections and sun exposure. Certain foods such as plant protein found in soy beans and corn may also act as triggers to attacks *(Bullard-Dillard et al., 1993)*.

✦ The symptoms of SLE are variable from person to person, ranging from mild to severe. There may be periods of remission and exacerbation. Some of the more common symptoms include fatigue, joint and muscle pain, fever, headache, anemia, loss of appetite, nausea, diffuse abdominal pain, skin rash (especially a butterfly-shaped rash across the cheeks and chin), sun sensitivity and hair loss. Ulcers may form in the mouth and throat and the skin may bruise easily.

✦ Arthritis flare-ups, whether transient or chronic, can affect any joint, but usually the hands and knees are involved. Joint deformities may develop in the fingers.

✦ More serious symptoms include hypertension, pericarditis, recurring pleuritis and renal dysfunction varying from mild dysfunction to renal failure.

✦ Central nervous system involvement is less common, but may include cranial neuropathies (causing visual defects or blindness), peripheral neuropathies (causing motor and sensory impairments), seizures and psychosis.

✦ SLE is the most common form of lupus. Other milder types include discoid lupus erythematosus (DLE) and subacute cutaneous lupus erythematosus (SCLE). Whereas DLE symptoms are fixed, chronic, thickened, scaly skin lesions, SCLE presents as distinct skin lesions, usually in areas exposed to sunlight. SCLE lesions are migratory, with periods of remission and exacerbation. Up to 10 per cent of those with DLE and SCLE develop symptoms of SLE *(The Arthritis Society, 1998d)*.

✦ **Medically**, diagnosis may be difficult; it is made through laboratory tests and observation of symptoms over time. Although SLE has no cure, many of the symptoms are controllable. Anti-inflammatories and corticosteroids are commonly prescribed. In earlier studies, 50 per cent of patients died within six months of diagnosis; now 95 per cent are functioning 10 years after diagnosis *(Walker, Helewa, 1996)*.

Contraindications for Inflammatory Arthritides

✦ Testing, except for active free range of motion, is contraindicated on acutely inflamed joints.

✦ Hot hydrotherapy applications are contraindicated during acute inflammation.

✦ General massage is contraindicated with significant fever (38.5° C, 101.5° F).

✦ Lymphatic drainage techniques proximal to the affected joint are avoided with acute infectious arthritis.

✦ Local massage is avoided on acutely inflamed joints or over open lesions. Avoid distal techniques that will painfully increase circulation through the joint.

✦ Do not fatigue the client with a prolonged or overly vigorous treatment.

✦ Joint play is contraindicated on acutely inflamed joints to prevent aggravation of the condition. Gentle, progressive grades of joint play may be cautiously used with restricted tissue between flare-ups. Forceful techniques may rupture connective tissue and joint capsules, creating instability (Kisner, Colby, 1990). With severe RA progression that creates C1 and C2 instability, tractioning and range of motion of the cervical spine are contraindicated.

✦ In treatment and self-care, passive or active range of motion used as remedial exercise is avoided on acutely inflamed joints.

✦ Between flare-ups, deep, vigorous techniques such as frictions and direct fascial techniques may provoke inflammation in some clients (Boyling, Palastanga, 1994).

✦ With joint laxity and hypermobility, stretching techniques are used with caution, if at all. Vigorous passive stretching may also cause inflammation (Walker, Helewa, 1996).

✦ Strengthening exercises should not be painful and should not fatigue the muscles.

Treatment Considerations

HEALTH HISTORY QUESTIONS
(For all inflammatory arthritides)

✦ How is the client's general health?

✦ What specific inflammatory arthritide does the client have?

✦ When was the onset?

✦ Is there a history of this arthritide in the client's family?

✦ What is the frequency of acute attacks? When was the most recent flare-up?

♦ What are the client's current symptoms? What are the client's activities of daily living? How did the client feel first thing in the morning?

♦ Which joints are affected? Is range of motion affected? Are there any associated systemic concerns, such as cardiopulmonary, neurological or gastrointestinal symptoms?

♦ Is the client using specific medication for the arthritide or other medication? How frequently is it taken? When was it last taken? Is it effective? Are there any side effects from the medication?

♦ Has there been any surgery for affected joints, or prostheses to replace affected joints?

♦ Are any other therapies used, such as physiotherapy?

Further Assessment: Ankylosing Spondylitis

♦ Additional **health history** information needed from the client includes: Has the onset of the low back pain been insidious and has stiffness occurred for more than three months? Is there a family history of AS? Are the symptoms worse with rest and better with exercise?

✍ **Observations:**

• **Gait assessment** reveals a rigid gait with some knee flexion due to hip flexion contractures.

• **Postural assessment**, lateral view reveals decreased lordotic curve, increased hyperkyphosis and head-forward posture. With increasing severity of the condition, the hyperkyphosis worsens, rib movement is reduced or absent with breathing, and the abdomen may protrude.

✍ **Testing:**

• **AF ROM** of the hips and sacroiliac joints and lumbar, thoracic and cervical spine may be reduced due to stiffness and pain. All ranges may be affected, most commonly trunk flexion.

• **AF ROM** of the spine and **AF trunk and hip flexion tests** are positive.

• **PR anterior** and **lateral spinous challenges** reveal hypomobility of the affected vertebrae, while **rib motion** and **rib palpation tests** reveal hypomobility of the affected ribs.

• **PR ROM** of other affected joints is also assessed revealing reduced range and either muscle spasm or leathery end feel.

Massage

🖐 **Massage** treatment goals include decreasing pain, hypertonicity and trigger points, maintaining thoracolumbar mobility and respiratory function, preventing or reducing postural changes and educating the client about correct posture and exercises.

🖐 Positioning is prone and supine. Hot hydrotherapy applications are used on affected tissues between flare-ups.

🖐 The massage is a combination of stress reduction and hyperkyphosis treatments. Fascial techniques are used on the anterior thorax, especially on the intercostals and pectoral muscles. Swedish massage is used on the hip flexors, pectoralis major and minor, scalenes, sternocleidomastoids, intercostals and rotator cuff muscles. Back extensors, quadratus lumborum and scapular retractors are treated as in the hyperkyphosis treatment. Work is also performed on compensating structures such as hamstrings and lateral rotators of the hip.

🖐 PIR is used to lengthen shortened muscles such as hip flexors and pectorals. Joint play techniques are indicated to maintain mobility in hypomobile joints, such as hips, sacroiliac joints, vertebrae, ribs, scapulothoracic articulations and sternoclavicular joints.

Self-care

✍ **Self-care** includes exercises to maintain mobility and strength of the hips, entire spine and shoulders. Although the client may become bored with repetitive exercises that are aimed at prevention, it is important that the client be encouraged to continue with them. Active free back muscle extension and rotation, as well as stretches for the hip flexors, pectoral muscles, scalenes and sternocleidomastoids, are indicated.

✍ Posterior pelvic tilt exercises and strengthening for the back extensors and scapular retractors are also useful. Swimming is an excellent exercise that does not stress the affected joints.

✍ Diaphragmatic breathing exercises with an emphasis on lateral rib motion and sternal lifting help to maintain thoracic mobility. See hyperkyphosis treatment for details.

✍ Several 15-minute rest periods during the day are recommended, where the client can lie prone with the arms above the head to prevent hyperkyphosis. A pillow can be placed under the thorax and a towel roll under the forehead (*The Arthritis Society, 1996a*).

✍ Sleeping on a firm mattress with no pillow and sleeping supine instead of curled up in sidelying to prevent flexion deformities are also suggested (*Schumacher, 1993*). Movement therapy, such as the Mitzvah, Feldenkrais or Alexander technique, may be helpful for retraining and monitoring the client's posture. The client may be referred to the Arthritis Society for more help.

Further Assessment: Rheumatoid Arthritis and Other Inflammatory Arthritides

✦ Additional **health history questions** are: Which inflammatory arthritide does the client have? At what stage is the disease? Is the condition physician-diagnosed. It is also important to differentiate an inflammatory arthritide from osteoarthritis, as the treatments are different; see osteoarthritis for more information.

✍ **Observations:**

• Guarded movement to prevent pain and a possibly pained or medicated facial expression may be noted. Depending on the affected joints, gait and postural

977

dysfunctions are likely present due to pain.

- Aids such as splints, canes and wheelchairs may be used. A **postural assessment** may be performed to determine sources of muscle imbalance.

- Affected joints are red and swollen, more so during flare-ups. The skin may be taut and shiny over the joint and joint deformities may be visible. Contractures may occur at affected joints. With lupus and scleroderma, skin lesions and rashes may be noted. Persons with scleroderma who have Raynaud's phenomenon may exhibit blanching or cyanosis in the affected extremities.

✎ **Palpation:**

- Heat and tenderness of affected joints are palpated, which are worse during flare-ups.

- Affected joints have a spongy, soft feel due to synovitis.

- There may be spasm in muscles crossing affected joints. Between flare-ups, hypertonicity, trigger points, crepitus, adhesions and disuse atrophy may be palpated.

- Dense contractured tissue may be present with scleroderma. Rheumatoid nodules may be present with RA, frequently around the elbow.

✎ **Testing:**

- During flare-ups, only **AF ROM** is used, with affected joints having reduced range of motion due to pain and swelling. Crepitus may be present in tendons crossing the joint. Each actively affected joint is recorded on a chart. It is important to reassess the client after a flare-up to determine joint stability and any tissue changes.

- Between flare-ups, **AF ROM** of affected joints is also reduced due to pain and swelling, but not as much as during an attack.

- **PR ROM** is restricted due to pain. With synovitis, a muscle spasm combined with capsular restriction end feel is noted *(Hertling, Kessler, 1996)*. Contractures have a leathery end feel.

- **AR isometric testing** is weak and possibly painful for muscles crossing the affected joint. A modified blood pressure cuff is used to accurately record strength. See Appendix C for details.

✎ **Differentiating Sources of Joint Pain:**

- **Trigger point** pain is in the referral pattern for the muscle that contains the taut band and trigger point.

- **Tendinitis** pain is positive with the tendinitis differentiation test.

- **Bursitis** pain is positive with the bursitis differentiation test.

Massage

✎ **Massage** treatment goals depend on the specific arthritide and whether the client is in remission or active flare-up. They include stress reduction and relaxation, decreasing pain, edema and spasm, maintaining joint mobility, maintaining and increasing strength and preventing or reducing postural changes and joint deformities. Reducing contractures is especially important with JRA to prevent flexion deformities at the elbow, the hip and the knee. Encouragement is provided for the client. Massage techniques, including self-massage, are recommended for arthritis pain management *(Lorig, Fries, 1995)*.

- On the initial visit, before the client and therapist understand the client's post-treatment reaction to massage therapy, a gentle, conservative treatment of shorter duration is prudent.

- **During flare-ups**, massage, if tolerated by the client, is to the unaffected areas of the client's body. The treatment is a half hour in duration to avoid exhausting the client. The focus is on relaxation including unforced **diaphragmatic breathing**.

- **Hydrotherapy** is cold applications to the client's tolerance at the affected joint. **Positioning** may be prone, sidelying or supine, as is comfortable for the client. A head, neck and shoulder massage is appropriate for relaxation. Techniques include stroking, muscle squeezing, light circular kneading and static kneading. AA ROM of the affected joints, or AF ROM if symptoms are controlled by medication, and gentle isometric contractions may be interspersed in the treatment (*Kisner, Colby, 1996*).

- **Between flare-ups**, the treatment is initially a half hour, increasing to 45 minutes according to the client's tolerance. Treatment is again in a relaxation context, including diaphragmatic breathing. Positioning is again for the client's comfort. **Hot hydrotherapy** may be used with chronically arthritic joints, as it controls pain and spasm, providing relief for one or two hours (*Walker, Helewa, 1996*). A warm room is especially important if the client has active Raynaud's phenomenon associated with scleroderma.

- Pure essential oils added to the massage oil or lotion may help with the treatment of inflammatory arthritides. Sandalwood is an emollient (skin moisturizer). Lavender can help reduce pain and roman chamomile has anti-inflammatory properties. A 2.5 per cent solution, or 25 drops total of pure essential oil in 50 ml. of carrier oil, is suggested (*Lawless, 1992*).

- **Specific treatment** begins with pain-free rhythmic techniques, rocking and shaking. Contralateral and compensatory structures are treated to reduce hypertonicity and trigger points, especially in muscles that cross the affected joint. Working proximal to distal on the affected limb, soothing Swedish techniques, such as effleurage, stroking and various petrissage techniques, are used to reduce hypertonicity. Trigger points are treated with muscle stripping and gentle ischemic compressions.

- Gentle fascial techniques are employed if soft tissue contractures are present (*Souza, 1997*).

- For gout, rheumatoid arthritis, infectious arthritis (once the infection is under control), juvenile rheumatoid arthritis, and Reiter's syndrome, gentle, passive movements of the affected joints are indicated. These are interspersed throughout the treatment to maintain range of motion (*Souza, 1997*). With scleroderma, short treatments of fascial techniques starting on the posterior trunk and moving towards the affected extremities are indicated (*Ebner, 1980*). Passive and active movements may help to keep joints flexible, to maintain blood flow and to prevent contractures (*Walker, Helewa, 1996*).

- Gentle joint play techniques may be used with caution on the affected joint capsule to reduce adhesions present with gout and RA (*Kisner, Colby, 1996*). Other conditions, such as postural dysfunctions, are also addressed during the massage.

- Treatments are of an ongoing nature as most inflammatory arthritides (unless spontaneously remitting) are chronic degenerative conditions.

Self-care

✍ **Self-care** includes exercise to the client's pain tolerance. Between flare-ups, self-stretching is used to prevent contractures. Submaximal isometric exercise to maintain strength of muscles crossing affected joints is progressed to low-impact or water aerobics, if possible. Control of inflammation and swelling is important before the client progresses to cardiovascular exercise. Submaximal isometric exercise is preferred for inflamed or unstable joints. If pain persists one or more hours after treatment, including self-care, the intensity or frequency should be reduced. Short periods of rest, including one or two hours of bedrest, can help those with multiple joint involvement. Pain during activity is a warning to reduce activity levels *(Kisner, Colby, 1996; Walker, Helewa, 1996).*

✍ Stress reduction exercises and diaphragmatic breathing are important, especially with SLE and scleroderma. Self-massage between flare-ups is also useful as a pain management tool for all arthritides. Scleroderma skin protection is important and includes keeping affected skin moisturized; lotions can be applied during self-massage.

✍ Splints to protect joints, orthotics and devices to help with activities of daily living may be helpful. The client is referred to a physician for more details.

✍ Larger objects are easier to grip than small ones, so some specialized kitchen implements have oversized handles. If the client has to go up and down stairs, tasks can be organized so fewer trips need to be made.

See also stress reduction, edema, trigger points, tendinitis, hyperkyphosis, hypermobility and hypomobility, osteoarthritis, inflammatory bowel disease, migraine, diabetes mellitus, HIV infection and AIDS, carpal tunnel syndrome, peripheral nerve lesions, hypertension and the chapter on other circulatory concerns for related treatments.

✍ During flare-ups, cool hydrotherapy applications may relieve pain. Between flare-ups, heat is used on affected joints. Instead of using home hot wax applications for the hands which can be dangerous unless the client has a wax bath, the client can apply mineral oil to the hands, put on rubber dishwashing gloves and soak the hands in hot tap water for five or ten minutes *(Walker, Helewa, 1996).*

✍ Keeping the extremities warm is important. Movement therapy, such as the Mitzvah, Feldenkrais or Alexander technique, may be helpful for retraining and monitoring the client's posture. The client may be referred to the Arthritis Society for more help. A naturopath can help with strengthening the immune system and nutrition information.

81

FIBROMYALGIA AND CHRONIC FATIGUE SYNDROME

Linda Ludwig

Fibromyalgia

Fibromyalgia (FM) is a painful non-articular rheumatic condition of at least three months' duration, characterized by widespread muscular achiness and specifically the palpation of tender points at 11 of 18 prescribed locations on the body.

Generalized muscular aches and pains described as muscular rheumatism were discussed in literature from the seventeenth century. In 1904, the term "fibrositis" was coined. In the 1960s and 70s, fibrositis was used interchangeably with fibromyalgia to describe the symptoms of generalized muscular aching, multiple tender points, poor sleep and pain. These two terms are, in fact, quite distinct since fibrositis suggests inflammation of the muscle tissue, whereas fibromyalgia indicates pain in the tissue. The existence of both conditions was put in doubt when studies of the tissue of people with these symptoms showed no evidence of inflammation. It was not until the late 1980s and 90s that fibromyalgia became accepted in the medical community as a legitimate condition. During this time, controlled studies were carried out which demonstrated that the symptoms of pain and specific tender points were more common in those with "fibromyalgia syndrome" than in age-, sex- and race-matched control groups. The mechanism for the symptoms is still not clearly understood *(Pillemer, 1994)*.

Fibromyalgia is a systemic disorder that affects an estimated two to six per cent of the adult population *(The Arthritis Society, 1998b)*. Two-thirds of those diagnosed state they "hurt all over" *(Rachlin, 1994)*. There is no obvious origin of the pain. FM affects points above and below the waist including the low back, shoulders, including the trapezius muscle, neck, back of the head, upper chest, arms, hands, thighs and legs. Other areas such as the temporomandibular region and anterior chest may also be affected *(Rachlin, 1994)*.

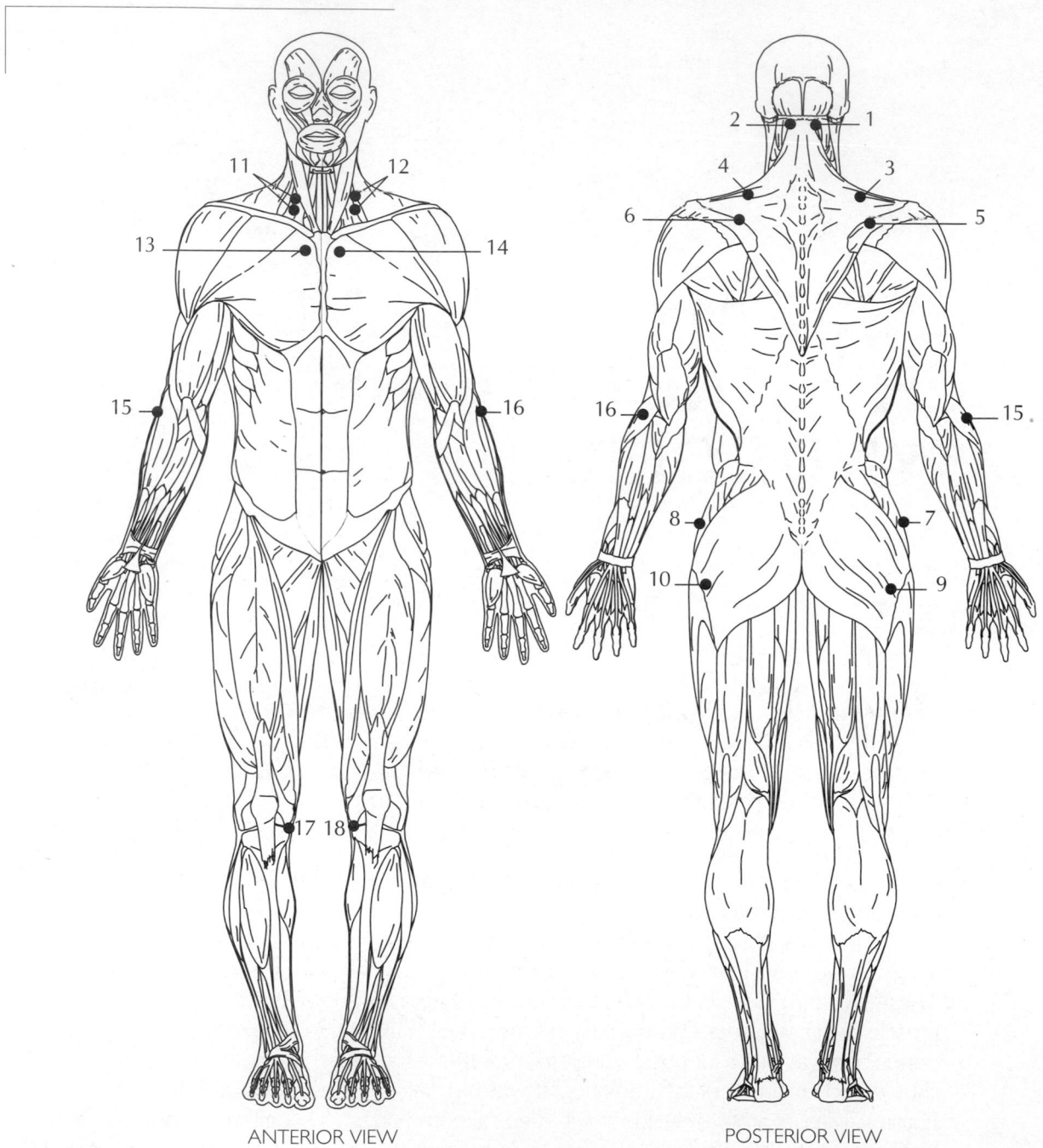

ANTERIOR VIEW   POSTERIOR VIEW

Figure 81.1
Bilateral abnormal tender points with fibromyalgia. Control sites at the forehead, the flexors of the fingers, the lateral epicondyle and the insertion of the deltoids should not be tender.

There are 18 symmetrical tender points of which at least 11 need to be found on examination *(Figure 81.1)* to confirm fibromyalgia. This distinguishes fibromyalgia from other conditions such as chronic fatigue syndrome, myofascial pain syndrome (trigger points), myalgic encephalomyelitis or various forms of arthritis and lupus.

Abnormally tender points are:

Posterior view

1,2   suboccipital muscle insertion, just inferior to the occiput

3,4   upper trapezius, just at midpoint on the upper border of the muscle

5,6   supraspinatus origin, at the medial border near the spine of the scapula

7,8   gluteus medius, at the anterior portion of the muscle

9,10   greater trochanter, at a point 2 cm. posterior to it, specifically at the trochanteric prominence

Anterior view

11,12   cervical region, at the anterior aspect of the TVPs of C5 to C7

13,14   second rib, at the costochondral junction

15,16   extensor digitorum, at a point 2 cm. distal to the lateral epicondyle

17,18   knee, at the medial collateral ligament proximal to the joint line

➤ **Causes of fibromyalgia are not clear** but there seem to be connections with **immune abnormalities** and a **genetic predisposition** which causes **neuroendocrine dysfunction** *(Rachlin, 1994)*.

➤ There is some evidence of a deficiency of serotonin due to abnormalities of serotonin binding to platelets *(Bennett, 1990)*. This results in a negative effect on the pain inhibitory pathways of the nervous system *(McCain, 1990)*.

➤ **Symptoms can be triggered or aggravated** by overexertion, lack of exercise, stress, anxiety, depression, lack of or poor quality of sleep, trauma, extremes of temperature or humidity (especially cold and wet weather) and infectious illness.

➤ Some sources suggest two types of fibromyalgia: post-traumatic fibromyalgia is thought to develop after a fall, whiplash or back strain; whereas primary fibromyalgia has an uncertain origin *(Goldberg, 1998)*.

Approximately four women are affected for every man *(The Arthritis Society, 1998b)*. Fibromyalgia can occur at any age, even in children and the elderly *(Jamer, N.d.; Rachlin, 1994)*. Most commonly it begins in young adulthood with symptoms developing slowly, and gradually increasing in intensity as the person reaches between 30 and 50 years of age *(Balch, Balch, 1997)*. The course of this syndrome is unpredictable; it may be chronic, go into remission or become cyclical with periods of flare-up alternating with periods of remission.

While FM is not life-threatening or progressive, it can affect the person's quality of life. For many people it is possible to continue working. Others become quite debilitated and have difficulty keeping a job or participating in physical activity. Outcomes may be improved by seeking treatment as soon as possible after the onset of symptoms *(The Arthritis Society, 1998b)*.

Psychological factors are present in some cases of fibromyalgia, with anxiety scores significantly higher for those with fibromyalgia compared to control groups. The concept of a "fibrositic personality" has been discounted. Rather than being a cause, psychological disturbances are related to an increased severity of pain experienced by a small group of those with fibromyalgia. In fact, more psychological disturbance was experienced by people who had increased severity of pain due to other chronic pain disorders such as rheumatoid arthritis *(Rachlin, 1994)*. People with fibromyalgia have often been treated with doubt by the medical profession regarding their symptoms. Once diagnosed, the person is often glad of no longer being perceived as a hypochondriac and having a name for the pain and other symptoms that have affected her life for possibly years.

Medically, a three-month history of generalized symmetrical pain is diagnostic. After palpating 11 out of 18 tender points, bilaterally, the physician will often use blood tests and X-rays. Because the secondary symptoms are also common to arthritis, these tests are performed to confirm the diagnosis of FM rather than arthritis.

There is no cure for fibromyalgia. The condition is frequently treated with medication, physical therapy and development of lifestyle management skills. Low doses of antidepressants (tricyclic and tetracyclic antidepressants) are found most effective in increasing deep sleep, improving serotonin levels and decreasing pain *(The Arthritis Society, 1998b)*. Exercise is encouraged, though it must be introduced gradually. The focus is to improve posture, encourage stretching and increase endurance. Initially, the person experiences increased muscular achiness post-exercise, but gradually seems to improve and feel better about herself *(Jamer, N.d.)*.

Lifestyle management involves learning to listen to the body for pain and fatigue levels and then reorganizing activities accordingly.

Massage and Fibromyalgia

Massage treatments help to reduce stress levels but have also been found to reduce pain and to result in overall improvement in the client. A Swedish study demonstrated a relationship between pain levels and myoglobin (the oxygen-carrying protein in muscle tissue). The pain may be the outcome of myoglobin leaking from the muscles. Along with pain reduction after massage, there was a gradual decline in the high levels of myoglobin in the client's blood *(Goldberg, 1998)*.

A study on 30 persons with fibromyalgia compared the effects of massage therapy and TENS machines. The group receiving massage therapy had more improvement in tender-point pain, reported less anxiety, depression, stiffness and fatigue and had fewer nights of interrupted sleep *(Sunshine et al., 1995b)*.

Symptom Picture

✦ The most common and characteristic symptom of fibromyalgia is generalized **pain** which occurs in 100 per cent of those with this syndrome. Stiffness is also common, affecting 80 per cent of those with fibromyalgia, and it is usually worse in the morning and the evening.

✦ A moderate or severe level of **fatigue** is experienced in approximately 85 per cent of people with fibromyalgia *(Rachlin, 1994)*. Fatigue can lead to feelings of weakness. It is aggravated by physical activity and can, therefore, affect the person's ability to perform activities of daily living.

✦ **Poor sleep** is commonly experienced with up to 80 per cent of those with fibromyalgia. They experience morning fatigue which may aggravate pain (*Rachlin, 1994*). The sleep disturbances common to fibromyalgia are specifically referred to as alpha-EEG anomaly. This lack of restorative sleep results in the interruption of deep sleep with periods of waking-type brain activity (*Balch, Balch, 1997*). Other sleep disturbances such as sleep apnea, restless leg syndrome and bruxism contribute to ongoing fatigue in people with fibromyalgia.

Contraindications

✦ Avoid very deep work or techniques that overstretch the client's muscles. Deep or invasive techniques will frequently result in increased pain post-treatment.

✦ Treatments should not be so long and vigorous as to fatigue the client. Massage of over one-hour duration should be avoided (*Brooks et al., 1996*).

✦ Frequently muscle relaxants, analgesics and antidepressants will be prescribed to help the client cope with the symptoms. Techniques should be modified accordingly.

✦ **Other symptoms** that may be experienced by those suffering from fibromyalgia are intolerance to cold, a swollen feeling in tissue, dysmenorrhea, anxiety, palpitations, altered sensation (such as numbness, tingling or pins and needles) usually in the extremities but maybe in other areas, dry eyes and mouth, skin sensitivities and cognitive disorders such as problems with memory and concentration.

✦ **Other conditions** associated with FM include premenstrual syndrome, depression, chronic headaches, migraine, insomnia, temporomandibular joint dysfunction, myofascial pain syndrome, irritable bowel and irritable bladder syndromes and chronic fatigue syndrome (*Cady, Fox, 1995*).

Treatment Considerations

HEALTH HISTORY QUESTIONS

✦ How is the client's general health?

✦ Has fibromyalgia been diagnosed by a physician? What method of diagnosis was used? Were specific tender points palpated throughout the body?

✦ What other symptoms are experienced?

✦ Has the client received massage since the diagnosis? How did she respond? Was post-treatment soreness experienced?

✦ What other therapies has the client tried or is currently having? How did she or is she responding?

✦ What is the client's activity level?

✦ Is the client taking any medication, for pain, depression or sleep disturbances?

Further Assessment

✍ **Observation and Palpation:**

- A **postural assessment** is performed. Antalgic postures are often evident. Hyperkyphosis with head-forward posture may be observed. There may be an imbalance of the anterior tilt of the pelvis.

- Apical or paradoxical breathing patterns may be observed.

- Pain is present bilaterally on palpation, above and below the waist.

- Trigger points are palpated. These should not be confused with tender points.

✍ **Testing:**

- **AF ROM** may result in reduced ranges in affected areas due to pain and weakness of the muscles crossing the joints.

- **AR strength testing** may result in pain and weakness in affected muscles.

- Pain will be experienced by the client in 11 of the 18 tender points, which must include the control areas (see *Figure 81.1*). Approximately 4 kg. of pressure are applied to each point. It is important to remember that it is not in a massage therapist's scope of practice to diagnose a client. If the above test of tender points is positive the client should be referred to her physician for confirmation of the results.

✍ The **differential assessment** for fibromyalgia is that palpation of these tender points causes pain local to the area palpated. Unlike myofascial trigger points, there are no referral patterns of pain or taut bands present with fibromyalgia tender points (*McCain, 1990*).

Massage

✋ Initially, the treatment is a half hour in duration to avoid exhausting and overworking the client. Shorter, more frequent treatments are the ideal, with two to three half-hour massages per week. This may not be practical for the client; therefore, if the client feels no ill effects from a short treatment, the time can be extended to one hour, once a week. Regularity of treatment is important for more lasting benefits.

✋ No two clients will respond the same so the treatment must be tailored to the individual.

✋ **Positioning** and **pillowing** are for comfort; prone, sidelying or supine may be possible.

✋ Pre-treatment **hydrotherapy** of heat is applied for a generally relaxing effect. Cold hydrotherapy is appropriate in areas experiencing acute tenderness.

✋ The treatment is in the context of a relaxation massage including unforced **diaphragmatic breathing**. Ideally, the full body is addressed for maximum relaxation, even if some areas are only massaged briefly. Treatment of postural imbalances and secondary syndromes is addressed over a series of massages so the client is not overworked. Throughout the massage, the therapist provides a respectful and caring touch as a way of offering support to the client. Vigilance must be maintained for the person's body language, facial expression and tensing of areas in response to techniques applied. Modifications should be made accordingly.

- Initially, the treatment includes general soothing Swedish techniques such as effleurage, stroking, scooping and fingertip and palmar kneading over the entire body. Lymphatic drainage techniques which are slow, light and rhythmical may be used if there is diffuse tenderness or a specific area of severe tenderness (*Tucker et al., 1998*).

- A light to moderate pressure is often used in the first few treatments to gauge the client's tolerance to manual therapy. The level of pressure may vary from area to area and from treatment to treatment. Some clients may tolerate some deep pressure, while others require only the lightest of touch. The therapist should be cautious with clients who wish deeper pressure to painful tender points (not to be confused with trigger points); while it may feel good to them at the time, post-treatment achiness and pain may result. The client must be informed of this possibility in the consent to treatment as well as at the time any changes to pressure are made during the treatment.

- If an area cannot tolerate touch, areas distant to the painful site are massaged. This may still provide the client with an overall feeling of decreased pain (*Rachlin, 1994*). For example, if the client's trapezius and upper back are too painful for massage, the pectoral region, neck, lower back and arms can be massaged. If the client has severe low back pain, the feet, legs, psoas muscle, abdomen, head, neck and shoulders are treated. With continued treatment the client's tolerance to massage and increased pressure may improve.

- Interspersed with Swedish techniques are gentle rhythmical mobilizations, stretching, joint play and trigger point therapy over the entire body.

- Trigger point techniques such as muscle stripping and gentle ischemic compressions are used to treat active trigger points. For those experiencing headaches or temporomandibular joint dysfunction, likely areas include upper trapezius trigger points which refer into the temporal region and trigger points in sternocleidomastoid which refer pain across the forehead and around the eyes and ears. Trigger points in masseter refer into the maxilla and frontal bone. Temporalis trigger points refer into the teeth and above the eyes and ears. Lateral pterygoid trigger points refer into the zygoma and anterior to the ear (*Travell, Simons, 1983*).

- Key relaxation areas should be included, such as the head, neck and shoulders, the abdomen, hands and feet.

- Specifically, petrissage is used on the muscles of mastication, facial muscles, scalp and suboccipitals as well as the muscles of respiration, scalenes, sternocleidomastoid, the intercostals and diaphragm. The head, neck, shoulder and abdominal massage is finished using stroking or lymphatic drainage techniques. This is followed by passive range of motion to the cervical spine and gentle long-axis traction or Golgi tendon organ release to the occiput.

- The therapist teaches diaphragmatic breathing and should encourage the client to use this style of breathing as part of a pain relief strategy.

- When treating clients with chronic pain syndromes, it is more reasonable for a therapist to expect a diminishment of pain rather than an end to pain. For clients suffering from chronic pain, any gain in comfort is appreciated. Some decrease in pain often occurs after four to six treatments (once a week for one to one-and-a-half months), though changes may be noticed after just one or two treatments (*Rachlin, 1994*).

987

Self-care

- Warm or hot hydrotherapy, such as Epsom salt baths, whirlpools and heating pads, may offer temporary relief *(The Arthritis Society, 1998b)*.

- Essential oils, such as chamomile (German or roman), lavender, marjoram or rosemary, have analgesic and relaxation properties *(Sellar, 1992)*. A dilution of 10 drops of pure essential oil mixed with 50 ml. of vegetable oil can be used by the client to massage accessible tender areas.

- Self-massage to the abdomen with an oil enriched with essential oils will assist in relaxation.

- Referral to a naturopath may help with strengthening the immune system and support for the system taxed by chronic pain.

- Relaxation strategies, such as diaphragmatic breathing and meditation, Tai Chi and yoga, may also be helpful.

- The client is encourage to perform daily exercise at the time of day that she feels most energetic. This program should include a stretch and strengthening regime as well as gentle to moderate aerobic activity such as walking or swimming to increase the client's stamina. The client may be discouraged because pain is often experienced while performing exercises and up to 24 to 48 hours post-exercise *(The Arthritis Society, 1998b)*. This is especially common at the beginning of a new program.

- Initially, mild exercise is recommended. If the client can be motivated to continue, after six to eight weeks the pain on exercising will usually be decreased and improvements may be noticed. If pain is severe and lasts more than 48 hours, the exercise regime should be re-evaluated for appropriateness.

See also stress reduction, trigger points, edema, headaches, migraine, temporomandibular joint dysfunction, inflammatory arthritides, osteoarthritis, irritable bowel syndrome, hyperkyphosis, hyperlordosis and HIV infection and AIDS for related treatments.

- Referral to a group, such as the Ontario Fibromyalgia Association, for those who suffer from this condition may be helpful in offering information and support.

- Referral for movement therapy such as the Mitzvah, Feldenkrais or Alexander technique may be helpful to improve body awareness and posture.

- Optimal postural patterns need to be learned. The therapist can design an exercise program to encourage these.

Chronic Fatigue Syndrome

Chronic fatigue syndrome (CFS) is a condition distinguished by persistent fatigue that does not resolve and severely reduces activity levels for at least six months (Balch, Balch, 1997).

Chronic fatigue syndrome seems to be widespread in North America, though it is often misdiagnosed as a flu or viral infection, hypochondria or depression. A number of reports have documented outbreaks of flu-like symptoms associated with fatigue over the past 50 years *(Davidoff, 1995)*.

➤ **The cause of CFS is not well understood.**

- It was linked to the Epstein-Barr virus (a part of the herpes virus group which causes mononucleosis) but is now thought to be related to some other viral or infective source. There is a deficiency of T-lymphocytes or natural killer cells *(Davidoff, 1995)*.

- There is a link to fibromyalgia, which is frequently found in people with CFS; but how the two are connected is unclear.

Symptom Picture

✦ The syndrome may be **chronic or recurrent**. A primary symptom is **disabling fatigue** that does not resolve with rest. Other symptoms include aching muscles and joints (the pain is migratory), spasm, weakness, fever, sore throat, swollen lymph nodes, recurrent upper respiratory tract infections, loss of appetite, intestinal problems, jaundice, memory loss, an inability to concentrate, confusion, anxiety, depression, mood swings, sensitivity to light and heat, and sleep disturbances *(Yehuda, Mostofsky, 1997)*.

✦ Up to 90 per cent of those affected complain of **persistent daily headache or migraine**. Some people are completely disabled by the fatigue, pain and muscle weakness *(Davidoff, 1995)*.

✦ Chronic fatigue syndrome is three times more common in women than men, generally occuring between the ages of 20 and 40.

✦ While not life-threatening, this condition has no cure. Some people recover spontaneously; for others the condition may improve but recur following periods of stress or illness.

Massage

✋ A study of 30 persons with chronic fatigue syndrome who were treated with massage therapy revealed that their total hours of sleep increased while anxiety and depression were reduced *(Sunshine et al., 1995a)*.

✋ Massage can help to relieve muscular pain and reduce stress levels but care must be taken not to fatigue the client *(Klimas, Patarca, 1995)*. Treatments are usually of shorter duration and not vigorous in nature with a relaxation focus.

Self-care

✍ The person affected with CFS must organize her day carefully, assigning priority to activities and allowing for rest periods. It is important to balance activity and rest. Exercise should include strengthening, initially using isometric contractions. The program progresses gradually. In the beginning, the person may only perform three contractions held for six seconds each for one set, with a rest period of six seconds between each contraction *(Klimas, Patarca, 1995)*.

✍ Flexibility is also maintained through stretching.

See also fibromyalgia, stress reduction, trigger points, edema, headaches, migraine, irritable bowel syndrome, spasm and respiratory pathologies for related treatments.

✍ Walking is encouraged, beginning with only five to 10 minutes of the activity. By adding a few minutes each week, the client will gradually build up to 30 minutes of walking daily. If excessive fatigue is experienced, the length of time spent walking is decreased slightly and maintained there for a few weeks longer *(Klimas, Patarca, 1995)*.

✍ Additional self-care suggestions from fibromyalgia may be recommended for clients with CFS.

82

DUPUYTREN'S CONTRACTURE

Fiona Rattray

Dupuytren's contracture is a contracture of the palmar fascia, resulting in a flexion deformity of the fingers.

The metacarpophalangeal (MCP) and interphalangeal (IP) joints of the fourth and fifth digits are the most frequently affected (Hueston, Tubiana, 1985). Due to the contracture, a client with this condition is unable to extend the affected digits voluntarily or by force.

In 1831, the French surgeon Guillaume Dupuytren thoroughly documented this flexion contracture, although nine years earlier Dr. Astley Cooper had described the condition in medical literature and suggested fasciotomy as a medical treatment. Currently, surgical intervention may still be used to reduce the contracture in advanced stages of the condition.

In order to understand Dupuytren's contracture, it is important to understand the anatomy of the palmar fascia. The skin, subcutaneous tissue, including cushioning fat lobules, and the strong palmar fascia of the hand are relatively fixed together in a manner that does not appear in any other part of the body with the exception of the plantar surface of the foot. The purpose of this fixation appears to be to absorb pressure and to limit the mobility of the skin, functions that are needed on both the palms of the hands and the soles of the feet. While being relatively fixed to the skin — in anatomy textbooks this tissue often appears as an inert mass of fibres — the dense connective tissue of the palmar fascia is actually organized into groups of fibres that allow for a small but important amount of functional movement between the fibre groups.

There are three fibre directions to the palmar fascia: longitudinal, transverse and vertical. These various fibre directions are necessary to counteract the forces applied to the palm of the hand. Longitudinal and transverse fibres counteract the forces acting on the palm when the hand is gripping something.

The longitudinal fibres are on the most superficial plane and run from the palmaris longus tendon to the skin midway between the proximal and distal palmar creases. Some of these fibres also continue to spiral around the metacarpophalangeal joints and insert on the lateral portions of the phalanges. The longitudinal fibres function to prevent longitudinal shear forces. In other words, they control rotational forces on the palm, such as those that arise when applying palmar wringing techniques to a limb or when gripping a baseball bat or golf club.

The transverse fibres are the deeper layer of the palmar fascia. They run from the anterior portions of the flexor tendon sheaths to the thenar and hypothenar eminences. These fibres stabilize against transverse forces, such as those created by C-scooping techniques applied to a limb or by sliding down a firefighter's pole.

The vertical fibres have a slightly different function from the previous two fibre groups. These fibres run from the skin down to the tendon sheaths and the metacarpal bones. Their function is to bind the layers of the palmar fascia to the skin and the bones of the hand.

If the fibres were not organized in this fashion, the shearing forces that occur when gripping something would tear the skin off the palm of the hand. If tearing does occur, it is due to extreme forces, which rupture the fibres. This injury is referred to as a palmar degloving injury.

Dupuytren's contracture begins with a shortening and fibrosing of some of the longitudinal fibre bundles, which ascend into the palmar skin. When the fibres that spiral around the phalanges become involved, joint flexion contractures develop *(Hueston, Tubiana, 1985)*.

The palmaris longus muscle functions to flex the wrist and is the only muscle that tenses the palmar fascia *(Figure 82.1)*. Palmaris longus has no antagonist, perhaps predisposing it to flexion deformity. It is interesting that the muscle may show variations in its attachments or may be absent altogether. One study reports that the muscle is absent in up to 20.4 per cent of the population and that this absence is slightly more common in women and in people of European descent. It also is more often bilaterally absent than unilaterally absent *(Travell, Simons, 1983)*. Flexor carpi ulnaris may act as a flexor of the palmar fascia when palmaris longus is absent. Dupuytren's contracture is known to occur even if palmaris longus is absent *(Hueston, Tubiana, 1985)*.

Dupuytren's contracture does not fit clearly into one specific pathological category because it overlaps several of them, including genetic disorders and abnormal tissue response.

At present, it is thought that a proliferation of fibroblasts in the palmar fascia produces new collagen which forms into nodules. This collagen infiltrates the loose connective tissue of

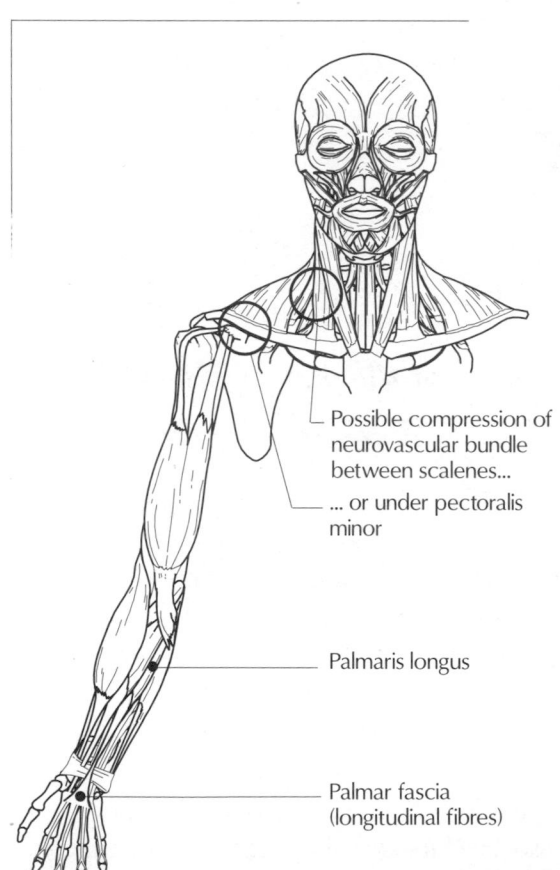

Possible compression of neurovascular bundle between scalenes...

... or under pectoralis minor

Palmaris longus

Palmar fascia (longitudinal fibres)

Figure 82.1
Dupuytren's contracture affects the palmar fascia. Trigger points in palmaris longus and compression of the neurovascular bundle supplying the arm may also diminish circulation to the palm.

the palmar fascia. Myofibroblasts, the cells that play a role in granulation tissue contraction, are also found in the nodules. However, there is **no** inflammation present in Dupuytren's contracture: the myofibroblasts develop spontaneously *(Hueston, Tubiana, 1985)*. These nodules produce flexion deformities by causing an intrinsic shortening of the fibres of the palmar fascia. The fibres become cord-like adhesions, eventually producing flexion contractures as the longitudinal fibres contract around the metacarpophalangeal joints. Although the palmar skin is fixed to the fascia by Dupuytren's contracture, there are no direct adhesions infiltrating the muscles, tendons or tendon sheaths, or within the joints of the hand itself *(Schumacher, 1993)*.

It is possible that this change or metaplasia of the connective tissue is in response to certain intrinsic or extrinsic factors *(Hueston, Tubiana, 1985)*.

✦ **The intrinsic theory** holds that the shortening occurs due to changes **within** the palmar fascia itself, leading to the nodules and then the contractured bands of tissue.

✦ **The extrinsic theory** holds that the shortening occurs due to changes in the tissue **between** the dermis and the palmar fascia. The nodules are found subcutaneously, anterior to the palmar fascia. For reasons that are not clearly understood, the tension created on this tissue by the nodules (perhaps by the myofibroblasts within the nodules) anterior to the palmar fascia results in a secondary shortening of the fascia itself. Contractured bands of tissue then develop.

➤ **Dupuytren's contracture is idiopathic in nature.**

  • **Heredity — inheritance of a dominant gene — appears to be a factor.** Although anybody may develop Dupuytren's contracture, it occurs most frequently in people of northern European and Japanese descent. There is often a family history of the condition. Of those affected, 85 per cent are men.

  • **There is an association between Dupuytren's contracture and epilepsy**, prolonged immobilization of the hand, alcoholism and possibly diabetes mellitus, although the nature of these associations is not clear.

  • It is believed that recurrent microtrauma to the hand is **not** the primary cause. The condition appears equally in manual workers and clerical workers. Although the condition may appear following an isolated injury to the hand, the injury itself does not induce Dupuytren's contracture *(Hueston, Tubiana, 1985)*.

➤ Other **contributing factors** include hyperkyphosis and thoracic outlet syndrome, leading to reduced circulation, trigger point referral and reduced tissue health in the client's arms. An increase in overall sympathetic nervous system firing may also be a contributing factor *(Travell, Simons, 1983)* and there is an apparent connection to tennis elbow, frozen shoulder, ulnar nerve lesions *(Hueston, Tubiana, 1985)* and shoulder-hand syndrome, also called reflex sympathetic dystrophy *(Travell, Simons, 1983)*. All these conditions may lead to trophic disturbances of the palmar fascia and, perhaps, Dupuytren's contracture.

This condition is most likely to occur in people in their 40s and 50s, although it may appear earlier *(Hueston, Tubiana, 1985)*. Dupuytren's contracture usually progresses slowly, over a period of many years, with stages of remission and progression.

It is more frequently bilateral than unilateral in presentation. Associated fibrosing may also occur in other parts of the body, including the plantar surface of the foot and the skin over the extensor surface of the proximal interphalangeal joints *(Hueston, Tubiana, 1985)*.

Massage therapy can address many of the possible contributing conditions. Dupuytren's contracture responds best to treatment when the nodules are initially noticed and the palmar skin becomes thickened and fibrosed, before flexion of the digits occurs and the palmar fascia has become severely contractured.

Symptom Picture

✦ The condition is often bilateral. In one study, 55 per cent of people with Dupuytren's contracture were affected bilaterally. When the condition was unilateral, 16 per cent had the left hand affected and 29 per cent had the right hand involved (*Travell, Simons, 1983*). However, it was not found to affect the dominant hand more frequently (*Hueston, Tubiana, 1985*).

✦ Initially, the palmar fascia becomes tender, thickened and nodular. There may be a small dimple or pucker just distal to the palmar crease, visible when the MCP joints are extended and the IP joints are flexed, and disappearing when the hand is relaxed.

✦ As the condition progresses, the palmar fascia contracts, drawing the affected digits into flexion. The affected flexor tendons appear thickened and raised. The skin over them becomes ridged.

✦ Dupuytren's contracture may stop at any stage of progression.

✦ Initially, the palmar surface is diffusely tender. Over time, the tenderness may diminish.

✦ A decrease in local circulation occurs due to the dense tissue of the contractures and the fibrous bands. The temperature in the affected fingers is lowered by three to five degrees Celsius (*Hueston, Tubiana, 1985*).

✦ There is an increase in tone of the wrist flexors. Trigger points that refer to the palm, especially in palmaris longus, latissimus dorsi and serratus anterior, may contribute to compromised tissue health and pain (*Travell, Simons, 1983*).

✦ Active free extension of the affected interphalangeal joints is not possible due to the flexion contractures.

✦ Contributing factors such as hyperkyphosis and thoracic outlet syndrome lead to diminished tissue health in the arm and hand.

Subjective Information

HEALTH HISTORY QUESTIONS

✦ How is the client's general health? Does the client have any associated conditions, such as epilepsy or diabetes mellitus?

✦ Does anyone in the client's family have this condition?

✦ When was the onset? If the onset was more recent, the treatment may take less time and be more effective.

✦ What is the type and location of the pain? It may be described as a tenderness or achiness in the palm.

✦ What activity aggravates the condition? The use of tools, such as scissors, a screwdriver or a trowel, may be mentioned. Walking with a cane or using a golf club or tennis racquet may also aggravate the contracture.

Objective Information

Observations

✍ A postural assessment will indicate possible contributing factors, such as hyperkyphosis and a head-forward posture.

✍ The palmar aspect of the affected hand is assessed for dimpling of the palmar skin immediately distal to the palmar crease, ridging of the palmar skin and, usually, fixing of the fourth and fifth fingers in flexion at the metacarpophalangeal or interphalangeal joints. The affected flexor tendons may be raised.

Palpation

✍ Discrete, palpable nodules in the palmar fascia and, possibly, over the proximal phalange are indicators of Dupuytren's contracture. They are usually adjacent to the flexor tendons. Thickening of the palmar skin is evident.

✍ Tenderness is present around the nodules and contractures, and diffuse tenderness is present in the palm.

✍ Increased tone in the cervical muscles, rotator cuff and flexor muscles of the wrist may be present. Palpation may be done for trigger points that refer into the palm. There may also be increased tone in the intrinsic hand muscles.

✍ To differentiate whether the palmar tenderness is a result of a trigger point in palmaris longus or the contracture itself, the muscle is specifically palpated. A trigger point here refers a prickly sensation to the palm, whereas the contractured tissue is diffusely tender (*Travell, Simons, 1983*).

✍ Coolness due to ischemia is possible in the palm and affected fingers.

Testing

✍ **AF ROM** of the cervical spine, shoulder girdle, elbow, wrist and each of the joints of the affected digits is performed. The client will be unable to fully extend the affected wrist and fingers. Pain on extension may be present.

✍ **PR ROM** of the affected wrist and each of the joints of the affected fingers will reveal decreased extension, with a leathery end feel and possible pain on attempted forced extension.

✍ **AR testing** reveals possible reduced strength of the wrist and finger flexors and extensors of the affected hand.

Contraindications

✦ Friction techniques are contraindicated if the client is taking anti-inflammatory medication.

✦ Following the surgical treatment of Dupuytren's contracture, with the client's permission, the client's physician and physiotherapist should be contacted before specific massage treatment to the wrist and hand occurs. The incision site must be completely healed prior to any massage, fascial work or stretching of the tissue.

Special Tests

✍ The severity of the condition is measured with a **degrees of Dupuytren's contracture test**. A positive **Adson's test**, **costoclavicular syndrome test** or **Wright's hyperabduction test** indicates the presence of thoracic outlet syndrome, which could be a contributing factor.

Treatment Goals

Treatment Plan

🖐 **Positioning** is prone and supine.

🖐 **Hydrotherapy** is a pre-treatment application of wax (using a wax bath) applied to the affected hand to soften the fascia. The hand is then wrapped in plastic wrap and a towel to retain the heat. Contrast is used after the treatment to increase local circulation.

General Treatment

Decrease sympathetic nervous system firing.

🖐 The treatment is performed in the context of a relaxation treatment. However, there is some degree of discomfort or pain possible with the treatment of this condition. This is clearly stated by the therapist in the consent to treatment statement, so the client may alter or stop the

Treatment Goals   Treatment Plan

treatment at any point if he wishes. The therapist must ensure that the discomfort or pain is tolerable for the client at all times, working with the client rather than pushing past his pain limits. To facilitate this, the client is directed to do **diaphragmatic breathing** during any deep and painful techniques. The therapist also intersperses the deeper fascial techniques with effleurage and lighter techniques.

Reduce hypertonicity and trigger points. Reduce pain if present.

With the client **prone,** the muscles of the upper back and rotator cuff are treated with effleurage and petrissage to reduce hypertonicity and trigger points. Latissimus dorsi and serratus anterior trigger points can refer into the palm *(Travell, Simons, 1983).*

The client is turned **supine.** The muscles of the cervical spine, the pectoral muscles and the unaffected arm are treated. In this position it is easy to reach any trigger points present in the scalenes and pectoralis major and minor on the affected side, which may refer pain into the arm and hand.

Treat other conditions.

See the hyperkyphosis and thoracic outlet syndrome chapters for specific work if these conditions are present.

Specific Treatment

The flexors and extensors of the affected arm are treated next, using progressively deeper petrissage, skin rolling, muscle stripping and ischemic compressions. Any trigger points in both the forearm flexors and extensors are treated to prevent possible shortening activation from trigger points in the extensors.

Alternate thumb kneading to the wrist, palm and intrinsic hand muscles is followed by progressively deeper kneading of the palmar surface from the wrist to the metacarpophalangeal joints.

Reduce fascial restrictions.

Fascial techniques to treat the contractured tissue include fascial spreading, C- and S-bowing techniques and the J-stroke to individual contractures. These techniques are applied in different directions to reduce the contractures.

Reduce adhesions.

The adhesions and thickening in the palmar fascia and around the tendons are treated using frictions, followed by ice.

Maintain or increase the range of motion

Massage, fascial techniques and frictions are interspersed with **passive relaxed extension**, progressing to slow **passive forced extension** of each of the affected joints. Sufficient pressure is used to stretch the contractures **without** tearing the tissue. In order to have more control over the applied passive movement, the client's hand is placed in pronation. The therapist uses one hand to first stabilize the metacarpal bone while the other hand slowly flexes and then extends as far as possible the proximal phalange. The process is repeated,

Treatment Goals

Treatment Plan

stabilizing the proximal phalange while slowly flexing and then extending the middle phalange and, finally, stabilizing the middle phalange while moving the distal phalange. This is followed with **passive relaxed extension** of the wrist and elbow.

Increase local circulation to improve tissue health.

The treatment is finished with repetitive effleurage and **contrast hydrotherapy** to the entire arm to increase local circulation.

Post-Surgical Treatment

◆ There are several surgical approaches to removing the nodules and contractures, including palmar fasciotomy and the "open palm" technique. A palmar fasciotomy consists of a longitudinal incision following the course of the affected tendon. With the open palm technique one or several lateral incisions are made in the fascia and the affected digits are splinted in extension. Granulation tissue then heals the gaps. The open palm method seems to offer more effective correction of the flexion deformity, with less possibility of post-surgical hematoma and edema; the average complete healing time is 24 days. With either method, the person is usually on a physiotherapy follow-up program. Recurrence of the contracture years after the surgery is most likely in people with an early onset of the condition *(Hueston, Tubiana, 1985).*

In terms of massage, applied techniques are appropriate to the stages of healing of the incision site. In the acute and subacute stages, care must be taken not to infect the incision site. In the acute stage, local work is contraindicated. In the early subacute stage of healing, caution is used so as not to traction the incision. Lymphatic drainage, vibrations, stroking and gentle kneading around the site are used to facilitate circulation and drainage. In the late subacute stage, more specific techniques to reduce adhesions are employed. The treatment is progressed gradually to the specific treatment outlined above. See Strategies: Massage and the Inflammatory Process for more details.

Self-care Goals

Self-care Plan

Maintain tissue health.

✍ The client can use a wax bath followed by self-massage consisting of skin rolling and muscle stripping, applied to the flexors and palmar fascia. Contrast baths are helpful to maintain local circulation.

If possible, restore range of motion.

✍ The focus of stretching is on extension of the wrist, metacarpophalangeal and interphalangeal joints. The client can use one hand to slowly stretch the fingers of the affected hand into extension. With the affected hand in pronation and the fingers on a flat surface such as a table, the client tries to extend the wrist, while pushing down slowly on the affected metacarpophalangeals and interphalangeals. The stretch is done slowly so a rebound spasm does not occur. The client should be cautioned not to use excessive force when applying the stretch, to avoid damaging the tissue.

✎ Specific stretches for the cervical and pectoral muscles are recommended if this is indicated by the assessment.

Treatment Frequency and Expected Outcome

Treatment should be given for half an hour, once a week for six weeks. The client is then totally reassessed, including the remedial exercise self-care plan.

The earlier this condition is treated, especially before flexion occurs and the fascia becomes severely contractured, the better the prognosis.

See also stress reduction, trigger points, tendinitis, frozen shoulder, ulnar nerve lesions, hyperkyphosis, thoracic outlet syndrome, Strategies: Massage and the Inflammatory Process and scar tissue chapters.

The condition may be more severe and tend to recur when it is bilateral or has an early onset, where there is a family history and where other areas of the body are affected (Hueston, Tubiana, 1985).

The treatment may take several weeks to months, depending on the longevity and severity of the contracture. Full extension of the affected joints may not be obtained.

The treatment of Dupuytren's contracture may not be a focus for the client unless the condition significantly alters the quality of the client's daily life.

83

OSTEOPOROSIS

Linda Ludwig

> *Osteoporosis is a progressive disease in which the bones become gradually weaker and thinner, causing changes in posture and posing an increased risk of fractures.*

Osteoporosis is a potentially debilitating condition affecting 1.4 million Canadians, with another 2 million people at risk for developing the disease *(Osteoporosis Society of Canada, 1997)*.

Bone is living tissue. It undergoes a continuous process whereby old bone breaks down and is then replaced by new bone. Specifically, osteoclast cells erode the bone, creating cavities in it; osteoblast cells form bone and fill in the cavities. In a healthy person, the osteoblasts replace all the lost bone resulting in optimal strength. In the case of someone with osteoporosis, there is an imbalance between the breaking down and restoring processes resulting in thinner, more porous and brittle bones over time.

Osteoporosis is often referred to as the "silent thief" because bone mass is lost continuously, over many years, often without the person experiencing any signs or symptoms until a fracture occurs. The pain, debility, deformity and fractures that are common with osteoporosis are a major health concern, with hip fractures especially serious in the elderly population resulting in death in 12 to 20 per cent of cases.

➤ **The cause of osteoporosis is not related to any one problem, but certain risk factors have been identified.**

➤ **Risk Factors:**

- Gender: Woman are affected almost twice as often as men due to differences in physiology, nutrition and hormones *(Balch, Balch, 1997)*. In fact, one in four women over the age of 50 has osteoporosis *(Osteoporosis Society of Canada, 1997)*.

➤ Along with aging, **other concerns for women are:**

- post-menopause situation (due to loss of the hormone estrogen);
- prolonged sex hormone deficiencies;
- ovaries removed before the age of 45;
- family history of osteoporosis;
- Caucasian or Eurasian ancestry;
- thin, small bones;
- primary hyperparathyroidism, hyperthyroidism, rheumatoid arthritis, liver or kidney disease and diabetes mellitis *(Goodman, Snyder, 1995)*;
- excessive use of medications such as cortisone, prednisone, anticonvulsants, thyroid hormone, heparin and aluminum in antacids;
- calcium deficiency;
- limited exposure to sunlight or inadequate vitamin D intake;
- caffeine consumption of more than three cups per day;
- alcohol consumption of two drinks or more per day;
- limited exercise or weight bearing;
- cigarette smoking.

➤ One or more of these factors puts one at risk; four or more factors suggest referral to a physician for further assessment. It is important to keep in mind that even those with no risk factors may develop osteoporosis.

Why Women Are Affected More than Men

Bone mass usually reaches a peak when a woman reaches the age of 30 to 35 years. Normally a loss of bone occurs at a rate of one per cent of bone per year after age 35; by the time many women reach between the ages of 55 and 60 years, a 30 to 40 per cent bone loss may be experienced *(Balch, Balch, 1997)*.

Why are women more at risk? Normally, the hormone estrogen slows the pace of bone breakdown. While aging itself will result in some bone loss, the change in estrogen levels accelerates this rate of loss. With the natural onset of menopause, estrogen levels decrease; women can lose as much as two to five per cent of bone density each year during the five to 10 years following menopause. This loss is called post-menopausal osteoporosis.

Women generally need 35 to 40 years of reproductive hormone levels for optimal bone health. There are several ways in which young women experience amenorrhea (a disruption of the menstrual cycle) and a resulting deficiency in optional hormone levels. Early menopause can be natural or the result of chemotherapy or surgery. Occurring before the age of 40, it results in a loss of as many as 10 years of the effects of naturally produced estrogen. Hormone levels can also be disrupted due to extreme levels of exercising or eating disorders *(Osteoporosis Society of Canada, 1997)*.

Osteoporosis is less common, though not unheard of, in men. This lower risk is due to a greater peak bone mass in men compared to women and a slow gradual decline of sex hormones rather than the relatively fast loss of sex hormones experienced by women in menopause. Men with very low levels of male hormones, known as hypogonadism, are at greater risk for osteoporosis *(Osteoporosis Society of Canada, N.d.)*.

Disuse Osteoporosis

Disuse of the long bones, specifically the lower limbs, can lead to osteoporosis. This may be secondary to any trauma or musculoskeletal or neuromuscular pathologies that affect the person's ability to weight bear. Those who experience prolonged immobilization, who have decreased use of limbs or who require a wheelchair are susceptible. This includes people with lower limb fractures, long term rheumatoid arthritis, spinal cord injuries, cerebral palsy and advanced multiple sclerosis.

The condition can develop relatively quickly. In one study it was found that, a year after a spinal cord injury, osteoporosis may be sufficient for a pathological fracture to occur *(Pedretti, Zoltan, 1990)*. If a person is able to weight bear at all, it is important for her to be assisted into a standing position regularly to delay the onset of disuse osteoporosis.

Prevention and Medical Treatment

Standard X rays will only reveal osteoporosis if at least one quarter of the bone density is lost. There is a specific X-ray, densitometry, which will most accurately reveal bone density problems in the low back or hip; unfortunately, this technology is not always available in smaller communities. A more affordable and transportable method for testing bone density is a heel ultrasound. This technology is currently being evaluated in a number of countries.

The results of current bone density tests of an individual are compared to the bones of an average young adult between the ages of 30 and 45 years. Taking into account the normal bone loss that occurs with aging, this comparison helps determine whether the person is losing bone more rapidly than expected for her age. Classification of osteoporosis is:

- **low bone mass**, sometimes called "osteopenia", which includes a low to moderate risk of fracture and may be treated with diet and lifestyle changes depending on the amount of bone loss and the person's age;

- **osteoporosis**, which includes a moderate to high risk of fracture; medical treatment is advised through diet and lifestyle changes;

- **severe osteoporosis**, which includes a very high to extremely high risk of fracture; medical treatment is strongly recommended.

Medical treatment focuses on ensuring adequate calcium and vitamin D levels, regular weight bearing exercises and resistance training, and the use of medication. Drugs, known as bisphosphonates, prevent bone loss and help the rebuilding of the bone.

For many women, hormone therapy is recommended. Estrogen is the hormone needed to treat osteoporosis but if taken alone it can increase the chance of developing uterine cancer. To reduce this risk, progesterone is combined with the estrogen. There are some concerns about increased risk of breast cancer with hormone therapy use. At present, it appears that short-term hormone therapy, up to five years, may increase the risk only slightly. Studies continue to evaluate these risks. Those at high risk for osteoporosis and experiencing menopause must also consider the possible resulting health problems if no treatment is taken. Risk of fractures is high; hip fractures can result in death from complications in up to 20 per cent of individuals. Of those who survive a hip fracture, up to

Contraindications

✦ Overpressure testing procedures are best avoided with clients who are either at risk for, or who have, osteoporosis.

✦ Any mobilization technique that creates stress on the bones, such as rib springing, aggressive joint play and some rhythmic mobilization techniques, is contraindicated for clients with osteoporosis. Caution is exercised if the client has not been tested for her bone density but has a number of risk factors. With severe osteoporosis it is safest to avoid joint mobilization techniques.

✦ Avoid giving flexion exercises, such as bending from a standing position or full sit-ups, if the client has a history of compression fractures. Such exercises have been associated with an increase in spinal compression fractures compared to extension exercises (*Canadian Medical Association Journal, 1996a*).

✦ High impact exercises, such as jogging on pavement or high impact aerobics, are used with extreme caution since they may cause stress fractures.

✦ Immobilization should be avoided, if possible, in people with osteoporosis or at risk for osteoporosis.

50 per cent have a permanent disability from the injury. Clients should be advised to talk to their physicians about specific benefits as well as risks and side effects of any prescribed treatment.

Prevention is achieved through good nutrition and regular exercise in the first 20 years of life in order to achieve maximum bone density. Calcium in the diet or as supplements functions to maintain bone strength. Exercise has been found to reduce bone loss, even in post-menopausal women (*Basmajian, Wolf, 1990*).

Consultation with a nutritionist or naturopath is helpful for information about food sources of calcium and proper supplements.

Symptom Picture

✦ Many women with osteoporosis do not experience any symptoms for years.

✦ Periodic acute low thoracic or high lumbar pain may be present.

✦ Often women only become aware of the problem when a minor injury results in a fracture of a wrist or hip; even a strong cough or hug could cause a rib to crack or break.

✦ As the osteoporosis continues, vertebrae start to wedge or fracture; this causes compression of the nerves and a loss of height of more than an inch. It can also result in hyperkyphosis and the "dowager's hump" often seen in women as they age.

Treatment Considerations

HEALTH HISTORY QUESTIONS

✦ What is the client's general health? Is there a diagnosis of primary hyperparathyroidism, which has been shown to be a high predictor of osteoporosis?

✦ Is there a family history of osteoporosis?

✦ Is the woman menopausal or post-menopausal?

✦ Has she ever experienced amenorrhea over a period of time especially in her teens and twenties?

✦ Does the client experience back pain in the mid- to lower spine? This may be a sign of osteoporosis or osteoarthritis.

✦ Has the client noticed a loss of height of more than one inch or increased stooping or rounding of the shoulders?

✦ Has the client taken any of the following medications over a long period of time: cortisone, prednisone, anticonvulsants, thyroid hormone, heparin or antacids?

✦ Does the client experience any pain? Is this acute pain (from a possible fracture or a muscle spasm) or chronic pain (achy, deep in the bone which may be a micro-fracture or muscular compensation from altered posture)?

Further Assessment

✍ **Testing:**
  • Testing is performed to rule out other possible causes of back and joint pain. This includes testing for degenerative disc disease, osteoarthritis and rheumatoid arthritis. If any of these conditions are suspected, the client is referred to her physician for diagnosis.
  • **AF ROM** and **PR ROM testing**, as well as weight bearing, are painful in the groin or hip region if a hip fracture is present. This is accompanied by shortening of the external rotators on the affected side. This type of fracture can occur with a sudden twisting motion, with the head of the femur most at risk *(Kisner, Colby, 1990)*.

Massage

🖐 The client may not be aware that she is developing this condition, unless it has been diagnosed by a physician.

🖐 The therapist may want to contact the client's medical doctor, with the client's permission, to obtain more information about the client's degree of osteoporosis.

🖐 Positioning is for client comfort. In the prone position, a pillow should be placed lengthwise under the truck, if there is a pronounced humping of the back. In the supine position, the trunk may need to be supported by a few pillows under the trunk and cervical spine so the spine is not stressed. In cases of a less severe stooping of the back, a towel roll supporting the neck or a pillow under the head and neck may be adequate.

✋ The massage is performed in the context of a relaxation treatment, including the use of **diaphragmatic breathing**.

✋ Depending on the severity of the osteoporosis and the age of the client, a hyperkyphosis treatment may be performed with modifications to the pressure and the intensity of the massage techniques.

✋ Passive movement of the joints is incorporated throughout the massage to facilitate joint health.

✋ If a client is at risk for osteoporosis, the first clinical manifestations are often pain accompanied by skeletal fracture *(Spake, 1995)*. If the client is being treated with massage for back or hip pain of a musculoskeletal nature but does not show any improvement in four to six weeks, a referral to a physician for bone scan is recommended. If a client is diagnosed with osteoporosis and massage treatment for musculoskeletal complaints does not resolve symptoms in four to six weeks, or symptoms increase after treatment, referral for X-ray is recommended. This will determine if there is another cause for the pain such as osteoarthritis or a fracture.

Self-care

✍ Education about relaxation strategies will help those experiencing pain. Diaphragmatic breathing is encouraged as well as meditation and visualization techniques.

✍ Referral to a naturopath or nutritionist is recommended for guidelines to appropriate levels of calcium and vitamin D, as well as for other appropriate nutrition advice for strong bones.

✍ Exercise involves a multifaceted program which includes weight bearing exercises, muscular strength building exercises and activities to address balance and coordination. These activities aim to decrease the risk of falling, to improve balance, muscular strength, range of motion and endurance, to improve posture, to lessen pain and to improve overall quality of life. The activities and level of intensity are chosen to minimize the potential for injury. Specific activities should be discontinued if pain is experienced or existing pain is aggravated.

✍ Weight bearing exercises include walking, cycling, dancing or low impact aerobics. These are introduced gradually and maintained at a moderate level of intensity. Walking has proven to be especially appropriate and shown to be associated with a decreased risk of hip fractures and falling *(Canadian Medical Association Journal, 1996a)*.

✍ Weight training or resistance exercises can be performed using weight training machines, therabands or free weights. Strong back and abdominal muscles are needed to support an erect posture. Pelvic tilt, isometric abdominal strengthening exercises and gentle back extension exercises should be performed regularly *(Canadian Medical Association Journal, 1996a)*. For those clients inexperienced at such exercise, consultation with a fitness trainer or physiotherapist may be appropriate.

✍ Activities, such as Tai Chi, that encourage balance and coordination help to prevent falls.

✍ Referral to a local association for osteoporosis is useful for gaining more education about the condition.

See also stress reduction, hyperkyphosis, inflammatory arthritides, central nervous system pathologies and fractures for related treatments.

DIABETES MELLITUS

Linda Ludwig

Diabetes mellitus is a chronic condition that results in problems with carbohydrate, protein and fat metabolism.

The metabolism problems associated with diabetes mellitus result from an imbalance caused by the body's inability to make or to use insulin. Normally, the hormone insulin is produced in the pancreas and helps to utilize glucose, the body's main source of fuel. With diabetes, the body is unable to transport glucose into fat and muscle cells; this results in very high levels of glucose in the blood (hyperglycemia) and, ultimately, the starvation and increased breakdown of the fat and muscle cells.

There are several types of diabetes, the most common being diabetes mellitus. Millions of people are being treated for diabetes mellitus in North America, with as many cases going undetected. In Canada, an estimated 1.5 million people recognize that they have this disease and another 750,000 people have diabetes that is undiagnosed (*Canadian Diabetes Association, 1997b*). The metabolic imbalances that are present with diabetes can affect almost all systems and tissues of the body. Complications include small- and large-vessel vascular problems causing atherosclerosis and hypertension, poor tissue health and gangrene, impotence, problems in pregnancy, kidney disease, eye disease that can lead to blindness and peripheral neuropathies that frequently decrease sensation in the hands and feet.

Insulin Production and Glucose Levels

Normally, insulin and blood glucose levels rise within minutes of a meal, peak about 30 minutes after eating and return to baseline within three hours. Some glucose is used by skeletal muscles or fat cells and large amounts are taken up by the liver for storage. Between meals, insulin levels are low. Sources of stored glucose and amino acids are mobilized to supply the energy needs of glucose-dependent tissue such as the brain *(Porth, 1990)*. When insulin production is impaired the glucose remains in the blood. Since the liver has taken in no new glucose, it releases more into the circulation; this goes to further increase the blood sugar levels, which results in hyperglycemia.

In 1921, through the discovery of insulin by physicians Banting and Best, diabetes was changed from a frequently fatal condition to the chronic health problem that it is today *(Porth, 1990)*. The control of diabetes mellitus is through the control of insulin levels in the blood. This is achieved by diet modification, exercise and, when necessary, the administration of insulin by injection. At present, an inhaler dispensing insulin is being experimented with *(Balch, Balch, 1997)*.

Types of Diabetes Mellitus

Type 1 Diabetes Mellitus

✦ **Type 1 insulin-dependent diabetes mellitus** (IDDM) (sometimes called "juvenile" diabetes) is usually associated with a dysfunction in the pancreas resulting in an absolute deficiency of insulin. Approximately 10 per cent of people with diabetes have IDDM *(Goodman, Snyder, 1995)*.

✦ **Those at Risk of Having Type 1**

  • While it may occur at any age, it mostly affects children or young adults (before age 25).

  • There is some suggestion that the cause may be viral, such as with exposure to coxsackie B, or autoimmune in nature.

  • There is usually a family history of diabetes.

  • Diabetes mellitus is more prevalent in people of Black, Aboriginal and Latin American descent.

Symptom Picture of Type 1 Diabetes Mellitus

✦ The onset is often abrupt with extreme symptoms including:

  • frequent urination (polyuria);

  • glucose and ketones in urine (glycosuria and ketonuria);

  • excessive thirst (polydipsia);

  • extreme hunger (polyphagia);

  • unusual weight loss with normal or increased eating;

  • extreme fatigue;

  • irritability;

  • sweet-smelling breath;

  • nausea or vomiting.

✦ The blood sugar levels fluctuate often and include very high levels (hyperglycemia) and very low levels (hypoglycemia); either extreme can have potentially serious medical consequences, such as a tendency to develop ketoacidosis. Unfortunately, it is often difficult to stabilize this type of diabetes mellitus *(Taber's Cyclopedic Medical Dictionary, 1981)*.

Type 2 Diabetes Mellitus

✦ **Type 2 non-insulin-dependent diabetes mellitus** (NIDDM) is when the pancreas produces inadequate insulin or when the body is unable to utilize the insulin produced. This type of diabetes is often linked to poor diet.

✦ **Those at Risk of Having Type 2**
  • Adults (usually after age 45).
  • People who are overweight *(Balch, Balch, 1997; Porth, 1990)*.
  • People with a family history of diabetes mellitus *(Aminoff, 1995)*.
  • Physically inactive people.
  • Certain racial origins such as people of Black, Aboriginal and Latin American descent.
  • Those with a previous diagnosis of impaired glucose tolerance (IGT).

Symptom Picture of Type 2 Diabetes Mellitus

✦ As this type has a gradual onset, many people are often asymptomatic and the diabetes remains undetected. Symptoms that do manifest include:
  • any symptoms of IDDM;
  • frequent infections;
  • slow-healing cuts and bruises;
  • tingling or numbness in the hands or feet;
  • recurring skin, gum or bladder infections;
  • blurred vision.

✦ Type 2 diabetes is fairly stable and easy to control *(Taber's Cyclopedic Medical Dictionary, 1981)*.

Other Types of Diabetes

✦ **Impaired glucose tolerance** is another classification of diabetes mellitus. It is considered a latent form of diabetes that may ultimately lead to diabetes mellitus. In this case, levels and utilization of glucose are not quite that of a person with diabetes, yet not quite healthy.

✦ **Gestational diabetes mellitus** (GDM) is a temporary diabetes with the onset during pregnancy. It affects one out of every 20 women and creates an increased risk for perinatal complications. While it resolves after delivery, 40 per cent of those with GDM will develop Type 2 NIDDM in the following five to 10 years *(Canadian Diabetes Association, 1997b)*.

Complications of Diabetes Mellitus

✦ **Ketoacidosis** is a complication of Type 1 IDDM and gestational diabetes which often occurs before a diagnosis of the diabetes has been made. It has a gradual onset and a prolonged recovery. Ketoacidosis occurs when sodium, potassium and ketones are lost in the urine.

 • It begins with a state of **hyperglycemia** which builds over a period of hours or a day. This often occurs secondary to an emotional or physical stress such as pregnancy, infection, illness, surgery, trauma or extreme anxiety; these are times when the body's requirement for insulin is high. Because the need of the body cannot be met, the blood sugar levels increase. Dehydration and electrolyte imbalance follow; fats are broken down to liberate glucose and ketones are produced in the process. Ketones form in the blood very rapidly, resulting in the potentially serious condition of ketoacidosis. The symptoms include warm, dry skin, tachycardia, hypotension, the characteristic fruity smell of ketones on the breath, depression of the central nervous system, lethargy, vomiting, abdominal pain, stupor and coma.

✦ **Hyperosmolar nonketotic coma** is another complication. The onset is often insidious, taking from one day to two weeks. An initial hyperglycemia episode occurs, brought on by a resistance to the effects of insulin and an excessive carbohydrate intake (in one case the person had consumed nine quarts of milk in one day)*(Porth, 1990)*. The resulting blood serum is "hyperosmotic" or highly concentrated with glucose. It draws fluid from the interstitial tissue, which is then lost through the kidneys with increased urination. Glucose often is excreted in the urine as well. As serious amounts of fluids are lost the person becomes extremely thirsty, drinking copious amounts. Therefore, the initial symptoms include extreme thirst, excessive urination, severe dehydration, dry skin and lethargy progressing to coma and seizures. In the elderly, this type of coma may be mistaken for a stroke.

✦ **Hypoglycemia**, or an insulin reaction, usually occurs in insulin-dependent diabetes or may be an early sign of diabetes. It is precipitated by error in the insulin dose, failure to eat, increased exercise, decreased insulin need following the removal of a stressful situation or a change in the insulin injection site.

 • Hypoglycemia can cause central nervous system problems such as headache, numbness of the lips and tongue, blurred vision, slurred speech, confusion, euphoria, difficulty problem solving and impaired motor function. Autonomic symptoms are also experienced. Initially, there is hypotension and feelings of hunger leading to emotional changes, nervousness and irritability, tachycardia, shaking, sweating and constriction of the peripheral vasculature causing cool, clammy skin. Ultimately, convulsions and coma may result. Different numbers of symptoms are experienced by each person; one must recognize one's individual pattern. Treatment should be given at the first sign of hypoglycemia; usually this involves the ingestion of a concentrated carbohydrate source such as sugar, honey, candy or orange juice. Most people with diabetes carry a fast-acting source of carbohydrate for ready use in an attack of hypoglycemia.

 • *In those without diabetes,* hypoglycemia results from an oversecretion of insulin which then causes a reduction of glucose in the blood. The condition may be inherited or secondary to adrenal, thyroid, pituitary, kidney and pancreatic disorders. Many people have hypoglycemia from a poor diet, high in simple carbohydrates, sugar, alcohol and caffeine, but inadequate in complex carbohydrates *(Balch, Balch, 1997)*. Increased stress levels likely play a role. Symptoms are similar to those with hypoglycemia as part of diabetes but also include pain in different parts of the body (especially the eyes), insomnia and increased aggressiveness. The symptoms usually appear a few hours after eating sweets or fats; severity increases the longer the time between meals. People with this condition are recommended to eat many small meals a day, cutting back on simple carbohydrates. In the case of a severe attack, ingestion of a fast-acting carbohydrate is useful.

Long-Term Complications in Other Body Systems

The incidence of complications seems to increase with the severity of the hyperglycemia and the duration of the disease, with a critical level being reached 10 to 15 years following onset *(Aminoff, 1995)*. While secondary to diabetes, complications can, in time, become primary. Some of these complications indirectly make diabetes the third leading cause of death in the United States *(Balch, Balch, 1997)*.

Infection

Over time, there is a decrease in the individual's tissue health. There is poor healing time, decreased peripheral sensation due to nerve damage, infection and tissue breakdown leading to ulcers and gangrene. If the blood sugar levels are not controlled, those with diabetes have an increased risk of infection in the lower extremities, mouth, gums, urinary tract and incisions after surgery. Of the over 1.5 million Canadians who have diabetes mellitus, it is estimated over 100,000 experience some form of foot ulceration. In many cases, dermagraft, a new skin replacement treatment, is used. This dermal replacement is made up of fibroblast cells in a mesh structure which aids closure of the area. Its use has resulted in a 60 per cent improvement in healing wounds of those with diabetes versus the conventional methods *(Muggeridge, 1997c)*.

Peripheral Neuropathy

Diabetic neuropathy affects about 40 to 50 per cent of those with diabetes *(Canadian Diabetes Association, 1997c)*. The feet are often at risk; unfortunately, lower extremity amputation is 11 times more likely in people with diabetes than in those without.

There are various theories about why the distal peripheral and cranial nerves are affected by diabetes; the main hypothesis is that microcirculation in the nerves is affected as the axon travels increasingly distal from the cell body. The nutrition to the fibres is affected, resulting in increasing necrosis of fibres as the nerve travels distally. For example, the sciatic nerve travels from the sacral area and gives off two divisions, the peroneal and tibial, as it reaches the knee; if the person is affected by diabetes there would be increased nerve fibre loss at this division point due to increased ischemia compared with the more proximal nerve *(Aminoff, 1995)*.

✦ **Distal symmetrical neuropathy** is the most common form of neuropathy. With impaired circulation and sensory losses, an injury to the foot may be painless and then ulcerate. In other cases, the ankle joint may collapse. Weakness may begin in the most distal muscles such as the toe dorsiflexors or the intrinsic hand muscles and then progress proximally (though rarely proximal to the knee or elbow).

+ **Diabetic radiculopathy and polyradiculopathy** are common in long-standing cases of diabetes mellitus. They may be confused with a nerve root compression. Usually thoracic and lumbar roots are affected. Acute burning pain and supersensitivity of the skin occur unilaterally in the trunk. Generally, minimal sensory loss and weakness are experienced. The pain reaches a maximum level within weeks of onset, persists for several months and then gradually resolves completely. In some cases, the radiculopathy occurs in episodes separated by months or years.

+ **Plexopathy** usually affects older people. It sets in rapidly over days to a few weeks. Pain is in the anterior thigh with minimal sensory loss. This is followed by reduced or absent knee flexion and buckling of the knee due to quadriceps weakness and atrophy. The maximum weakness is reached in a few weeks then stabilizes for weeks to years and improves over months to years.

+ **Compression syndromes**, such as carpal tunnel syndrome, ulnar neuropathy at the elbow and peroneal neuropathy at the fibular head, are more common in those with diabetes. Carpal tunnel syndrome affects from five to 16 per cent of those with diabetes *(Goodman, Snyder, 1995)*. Treatment is the same as for those without diabetes, with tissue health and sensory loss concerns taken into consideration. Surgical treatment is considered a last resort.

+ **Retinopathy** is a loss or impairment of vision due to damage of the microcirculation to the eyes. It is the sole cause of blindness in approximately 86 per cent of people with onset of diabetes under 30 years of age and in 33 per cent of those with onset over 30. Diabetes is the leading cause of adult blindness *(Canadian Diabetes Association, 1997c)*.

Problems Associated with Vascular Damage

+ **Cardiac problems** such as hypertension, heart disease and stroke result secondary to damage to the macro- and microvasculature. **Kidney disease** such as nephropathy is common as microvascular changes occur in the capillaries of the kidneys.

+ **Hand stiffness**, with limited hand and finger mobility and diabetic contractures, is common in about 75 per cent of the people with diabetes mellitus of both types *(Goodman, Snyder, 1995)*. The severity of symptoms is dependent on the amount and severity of vascular damage. Both **flexor tenosynovitis** and **Dupuytren's contracture** are associated with diabetes.

+ **Reflex sympathetic dystrophy** may also develop.

Diabetes, Exercise and Massage

While exercise has long-term benefits of improving hyperglycemia after eating, it may induce delayed hypoglycemia *(Basmajian, Wolf, 1990)*. Massage therapy is thought to create a similar effect of predisposing the person with diabetes or those with a tendency to hypoglycemia to potentially experiencing a hypoglycemic attack secondary to the treatment. In the case of increased stress and exercise, the person is advised to monitor his blood sugar levels and adjust both diet and insulin accordingly; blood sugar levels should be good before the massage. The client will often carry a readily available source of carbohydrates in case of an attack; it should be kept available during the massage. As a precaution, the therapist should also have some form of carbohydrate available to the client, to be given either before the treatment or at the first sign of hypoglycemia (the person should know his usual symptoms). The client should also be encouraged to be vigilant for such symptoms immediately after the massage.

Medical treatment of the disease will often cause anxiety in the person with diabetes because of the need for regular food monitoring, blood sugar testing and insulin injections. Many people with diabetes experience depression about the lifelong impact it will have on their social lives and about the almost inevitable physical complications 10 to 15 years after onset. This is particularly evident in situations where parents are helping children with this disease. One preliminary study demonstrated that when parents massaged their child, both parents and children felt less anxious and depressed. At the end of one month, the children's insulin and food regulation scores improved and the children's blood glucose levels decreased to almost normal *(Field et al., 1997b)*.

Contraindications

✦ If a client with diabetes arrives for a treatment in a confused or lethargic state or exhibits changes in mental function, massage is contraindicated. An immediate referral to his physician is necessary *(Goodman, Snyder, 1995)*.

✦ If a client has a hypoglycemic attack during the treatment, rapidly utilized carbohydrates are administered and the massage is discontinued. If the client loses consciousness, emergency care must be called immediately.

✦ Care must be taken when doing slow, deep diaphragmatic breathing with those who have IDDM and with anyone with diabetes who is susceptible to ketoacidosis. To compensate for a tendency towards acidosis, the person may need to breathe more rapidly. Diaphragmatic breathing may actually change insulin levels. A physician should be consulted, with consent from the client, before any changes in breathing pattern are attempted *(Fried, 1990)*.

✦ If the client has hypertension or cardiac complications, see the hypertension chapter for contraindications.

✦ If a peripheral nerve lesion or compression syndrome is present, see the appropriate chapter for contraindications.

✦ If a decubitus ulcer or gangrene is present, local and distal massage is contraindicated. Tissue health, especially of the feet, should be checked for red or blistered areas from shoe pressure, the first sign of a potential decubitus ulcer. See the decubitus ulcer chapter for other appropriate contraindications.

✦ If deep cracks are observed on the heels of the feet, the therapist should avoid using oil in this area; it may provide an avenue for infection.

✦ Tissue health throughout the body must be considered, with technique pressure modified accordingly. Techniques such as frictions or deep cross-fibre petrissage are contraindicated if tissue health is compromised or sensory losses are present.

✦ Hydrotherapy extremes are contraindicated in light of the possibility of decreased tissue health and sensory losses.

✦ Avoid using eucalyptus essential oil, which may lower blood sugar levels *(Davis, 1988)*.

Treatment Considerations

HEALTH HISTORY QUESTIONS

✦ What is the person's general health, particularly heart, vascular system and kidney health?

✦ When was the diabetes diagnosed? What type is it?

✦ How is the diabetes controlled? If through insulin use, where are both old injection sites (scarring is present) and new sites (fragile skin)?

✦ For all types of diabetes:

• Is the client stable?

• Does the person have a tendency to hypoglycemia? If so, what are his specific symptoms? How frequent are the episodes? Are there any usual precipitating factors to an episode of hypoglycemia? Does the person carry a ready supply of carbohydrates in case of an attack? If so, is it accessible to the therapist if needed?

• Are blood sugar levels checked regularly?

• When was the client's most recent crisis?

• Does the client have a stable diet and regular sleeping habits? Is there any alcohol consumption?

• Does the client exercise and does exercise change the insulin requirements?

• How are the client's tissue health and gangrene risk?

• Is there any indication of peripheral neuropathy? Are there any motor problems (weakness in fine and gross motor activities such as turning a key and going up stairs), sensory problems (tingling, numbness especially in a sock pattern on the foot or glove pattern in the hands) and autonomic abnormalities (sweating changes in particular areas or dry, cracked skin, particularly over the feet)?

• Is fainting or postural light-headedness experienced that may be a concern for the client getting off the massage table safely?

• Just prior to the treatment: Has the client not eaten within the last hour, experienced a stressful situation, recently changed injection site or performed exercise or strenuous activity, any of which may increase the risk of hypoglycemia?

Massage

🖐 If the diabetes is long standing with cardiac and kidney complications, if the client's insulin levels are unstable (often with IDDM) or if the client is not compliant with medication use or food and alcohol intake restrictions, a physician consultation with the client's consent is appropriate and recommended before treatment with massage therapy.

🖐 **Positioning** is according to client comfort. The client may need help getting on and off the massage table or changing positions if he experiences faintness or postural light-headedness.

🖐 Appropriate **hydrotherapy** is modified according to complications such as cardiac or tissue health problems. If a peripheral neuropathy results in poor tissue health or altered sensation, milder temperatures and gentler applications are used.

🖐 If the client's insulin levels are stable, a relaxation treatment is appropriate because stress can destabilize blood sugar levels. Diaphragmatic breathing may be helpful to a person with diabetes, but the therapist must check with the physician first. See the contraindications section.

🖐 The therapist must consider any complications and modify the treatment accordingly.

🖐 Unhealthy tissue and edema are addressed if present. Improving circulation and drainage to susceptible tissue such as in the feet and legs is important. Pressure is modified over areas that have sensory losses. Elevation of an edematous limb, nodal pumping and lymphatic techniques are used to reduce edema. The therapist is vigilant for tissue health changes and possible decubitus ulcers.

See also stress reduction, edema, other circulatory concerns, hypertension, congestive heart failure, decubitus ulcers, headaches, migraine, pregnancy, conditions of the peripheral nervous system, tendinitis, Dupuytren's contracture and compression syndromes for related treatments.

Self-care

✍ Relaxation strategies such as deep breathing, meditation and visualization are given.

✍ Referral to the local diabetes association, such as the Canadian Diabetes Association, is appropriate. Thirty per cent of people with Type 1 diabetes and 70 per cent of people with Type 2 diabetes never receive appropriate education about the disease and about appropriate self-care strategies (*Canadian Diabetes Association, 1997a*).

✍ The client should be educated about tissue health and decubitus ulcer concerns.

CANCER

Linda Ludwig

Cancer is a general term used for the abnormal, uncontrolled growth of cells (Dollinger et al., 1995).

Unlike normal cells, cancer cells do not respond to the normal restraints on proliferation. Once growth has commenced, these cells divide in an uncontrolled way. The terms "tumour" and "neoplasm" are used to describe these new growths. Neoplasms fuel their growth by using the nutrients and blood supply of their hosts. After the abnormal growth has started, there is frequently a "silent" period which follows. During this time the tumour is too small to detect. It may be many months and often many years, even decades, before the tumour has grown to a size that will show up on an X-ray or cause enough pressure to result in symptoms such as pain or bleeding.

Not all tumours are a concern. A benign tumour is an encapsulated growth comprised of slowly proliferating cells. Benign tumours are not considered serious unless they compress vital structures. On the other hand, a malignant tumour is a type that can destroy other tissues. Malignant tumours have two important qualities: they are invasive — without an encapsulated structure, malignant tumours spread into neighbouring tissue — and they are able to move to new sites. Referred to as "metastasizing", the movement of cancer cells to other areas of the body occurs by way of the circulatory system or the lymphatic system. Fortunately, not all cancer cells that metastasize result in an invasion of other tissue. Most are destroyed by the body's immune system *(Dollinger et al., 1995)*.

Naming Types of Cancer

✦ The suffix "oma" is used to designate a tumour and is added to the name of the tissue type from which the tumour originated: a benign tumour such as osteoma (a benign tumour of the bone); or a malignant tumour such as a glioma (a malignant tumour of the glial nerve cells).

✦ "Carcinoma" is a term used for a malignant tumour that originates in epithelial tissue. An example is squamous cell carcinoma (a malignant cancer of the skin).

✦ "Sarcoma" is the term used for a tumour that develops in connective tissue such as cartilage, bone, muscle and fat. It is often highly malignant though, fortunately, not common. An example is osteosarcoma (a malignant bone cancer).

Cancer Rates

In Canada, approximately 130,000 new cases of cancer and 63,000 deaths from cancer occur in a year *(National Cancer Institute of Canada, 1998)*. The most frequently diagnosed remains breast cancer for women and prostate cancer for men. Cancer rates in Canada are similar to those in the United States and Europe. In North America, the top three cancers affecting men are lung, colorectal and prostate; and affecting women are lung, colorectal and breast cancers.

On a positive note, mortality rates for prostate and breast cancers are slowly declining. In fact, the leading cause of cancer deaths for both men and women is lung cancer. While for men the mortality rate from lung cancer is declining slowly, unfortunately, for women this rate is actually increasing; a woman's current risk of being diagnosed and dying from lung cancer is four times greater than the rate of 30 years ago.

Causes of Cancer

Cancer is not one disease but more than 200 different diseases. For many cancers the cause is not known and for any specific cancer there is not one single cause. Recently, it has been discovered that genes in healthy cells can be transformed into genes that promote cancer growth. These genes are called "oncogenes". If the body's suppressor genes are missing or fail to stop this transformation, cancerous growth occurs. Research into these genes is ongoing.

Cancer development is the result of a cumulative process with many different effects on the cells that interact over many years *(National Cancer Institute of Canada, 1998)*. Therefore, while cancer can strike at any age, this disease primarily affects older people. Over 70 per cent of new cases and over 80 per cent of deaths from cancer occur in those 60 years of age and older.

It is thought that cancerous growth results if the genes are changed in at least two different ways. Chronic irritation from exposure to carcinogens results in these cell changes.

➤ **Carcinogens are chemical and environmental agents known to cause cancer. These include:**

• cigarette smoke;

• radiation from UV rays of sunlight;

• certain drugs and hormones such as some immunosuppressors and estrogen;

• industrial agents or toxic substances such as asbestos, chromium, coal tar, benzene, cadmium, radon, uranium and nickel;

- excesses or deficiencies in diet, particularly low fibre and high fat.

➤ Heredity plays a role with some types of cancers such as breast cancer, retinoblastoma (eye cancer affecting children) and polyposis of the colon.

Contributing Factors:

➤ Weakness of the immune system secondary to excessive or chronic stress, disease or immunosuppressor drugs can contribute to the development of cancer.

➤ Alcohol plays a role in four per cent of cancers of the head, neck and liver.

The Medical Treatment of Cancer

The main types of medical treatment for cancer are surgery, radiation and chemotherapy. A relatively new way of treating cancer is through biological therapy. Treatment often involves a combination of therapies for the best effect.

Surgery

Surgery is primarily used to excise localized tumours. To optimize success in removing the cancer, other forms of treatment are frequently used in conjunction with surgery. This is due to the fact that most cancers will metastasize, even microscopically, into neighbouring tissue. In some cases, the cancer has invaded the tissue such that its removal would require the removal of a significant organ. Again, surgery may be used to partially remove the cancer and another therapy used to treat the remaining cancer.

Side Effects: These are the same following any surgical procedure including risks from anesthesia use, respiratory complications, bleeding, deep vein thrombosis, infection of the incision, pain and fatigue. Later complications can include movement restrictions from scarring and, in the case of abdominal surgery, possible bowel obstruction or other blockage.

Chemotherapy

Chemotherapy is the use of chemical agents to destroy the cancer cells. This therapy differs from radiation therapy or surgery because the chemotherapy drugs travel through the bloodstream and affect the entire body. The drugs are administered orally, by injection or intravenously, depending on the type of cancer and drugs to be used. Chemotherapy is used with metastasizing cancers, bone marrow and blood cancers (leukemias) as well as lymphatic cancers (lymphomas). The drugs interfere with the cancer cells' ability to reproduce and thereby prevent the development of a new tumour. Unfortunately, because these agents target rapidly dividing cells, chemotherapy results in the destruction of healthy, quickly growing non-cancerous cells such as hair, blood and skin cells as well as those lining the digestive tract and reproductive system.

Over 50 different drugs are used in chemotherapy with varying side effects. It is important that the person try to maintain a relaxed attitude during treatment, because stress can make a person's physical reaction worse (*Canadian Cancer Society, 1996a*).

Side Effects: The most common side effect of chemotherapy is nausea and vomiting after treatment. This is short term and usually resolves quickly. Often anti-emetic medication is taken to decrease nausea, though it too has side effects such as drowsiness and fatigue.

Chronic side effects include hair loss, mouth sores, nausea, diarrhea or constipation and low blood counts. Low blood counts may cause malaise, fatigue, anemia, increased susceptibility to infections as well as easy bruising and bleeding. Some chemotherapeutic drugs, anti-viral agents or vincristine (a drug used to interfere with cell division) can result in a peripheral neuropathy. With such a neuropathy, the person often experiences burning in the hands and feet.

Radiation Therapy

Radiation therapy is used with approximately half of those who develop cancer. It is frequently used to destroy localized cancer. External radiation is similar to receiving X-rays; internal radiation involves implanting radioactive material in the body near or into the tumour, or at the site where the tumour was removed. The latter form of radiation has fewer side effects and damages fewer normal cells during treatment. Radiation is also used to shrink tumours to give relief from symptoms during palliation—care given when no cure is possible and quality of life is the focus of treatment.

General Side Effects: Fatigue is common, especially if a large area is treated, such as the entire abdomen.

Since technology has improved, the skin is usually not seriously affected with radiation treatments. Most skin reactions are temporary and appear similar to a sunburn, including redness, tenderness, slight swelling and, eventually, peeling. Permanent skin changes can occur, with some people experiencing thickening and deep tanning of the affected tissue.

Localized Side Effects: Head, face and neck radiation may result in irritation of the mucosa of the mouth and dry mouth; taste may also be affected. Hair loss can occur.

Chest radiation may cause irritation of the esophageal lining resulting in heartburn-like symptoms, difficulty chewing or swallowing and coughing. Acute-radiation pneumonitis is lung inflammation occurring one to three months post-treatment. It is caused by immunosuppression due to bone marrow damage. Symptoms are dyspnea, cough, low-grade fever and edema.

Aggressive treatment involving chest radiation and strong chemotherapy drugs can cause cardiopulmonary dysfunction especially with Hodgkin's disease and breast and lung cancers. It may result in exercise dyspnea, pericardial fibrosis and constrictive pericarditis.

Radiation-related fibrosis is extensive scarring which may occur from nine months up to two years post-treatment. When nerves are involved in the fibrosis, neuropathic pain may be experienced. Fibrosis secondary to chest radiation can result in restrictions of the chest leading to reduced pulmonary function (*Dollinger et al., 1995; Goodman, Snyder, 1995*).

Breast radiation causes tenderness of the breast or axilla. Local edema may be observed up to four to six weeks post-treatment. Over the long term, the breast may change in size, becoming larger or smaller. Abdominal radiation can cause nausea or diarrhea.

Biological Therapy

Biological therapy destroys cancer cell by exploiting the immune system and its ability to eliminate and destroy foreign substances in the body. It involves highly purified proteins that help activate or generally enhance the immune system. This type of therapy has been found useful in treating melanoma, kidney cancer and some cancers of the blood. It has also shown evidence of being helpful with breast, ovarian and colon cancers (*Dollinger et al., 1995*).

Massage and Cancer

A diagnosis of cancer has a tremendous emotional impact on people. There is fear of the disease as well as of the medical treatments and their side effects. This anxiety and stress will often worsen symptoms, especially pain (*Dollinger et al., 1995*). Support systems and relaxation strategies including massage are recommended to the client to promote psychological wellness. Massage cannot treat cancer; rather it can reduce some of the symptoms such as pain or muscular tension associated with the disease. Relaxation, or stress reduction, will also support the immune system. In this respect, massage is recognized by health care professionals as a complimentary therapy, benefiting those with cancer.

It is not clear if massage can promote the metastasizing of cancer (*Curties, 1994*). Within the massage therapist community, it is suggested that the therapist inform the client regarding the uncertainty about massage increasing the risk of metastasizing the cancer. Generally, exercise for those with cancer is encouraged by the Cancer Society and physicians. The Swedish massage techniques that affect circulation are considered to have a similar impact on the circulatory system as exercise or a full-body heat application. Therefore, if the client exercises regularly and has no hydrotherapy restrictions or physician restrictions to activity, massage could be considered. If there are any concerns on the part of the therapist or client, the physician can be consulted and the treatment modified. For example, circulatory strokes could be avoided but specific local massage to other areas of the body not affected by the cancer would be appropriate.

WARNING SIGNS OF CANCER

✦ While these symptoms could occur with many other conditions, it is prudent for the therapist to refer a client to her physician if she answers "yes" to any of the following questions (*Goodman, Snyder, 1995*).

✦ These questions are especially relevant for any client with a personal or familial history of cancer. The most common cancers, namely of the breast, colon and lung, frequently show a genetic predisposition:

- Has the client noticed any changes in bowel movements or flow of urination?

- Has the healing time of injuries increased (especially a sore that has not healed in six weeks)?

- Is there any unusual bleeding including prolonged menstruation or any bleeding in a woman who is menopausal or prolonged discharge from any part of the body?

- Has any thickening or lump in the breast or elsewhere be palpated?

- Have there been any changes in digestion, such as increased episodes of indigestion or unusual constipation?

- Does the client have difficulty swallowing or eating? Is there chronic coughing, recurrent laryngitis, hoarseness or difficulty speaking?

- Are there any obvious changes, such as size, shape or colour, in a wart or mole? See Appendix E in this text for more details.

- Has there been an unexplained sudden loss of weight such as 10 or 15 pounds in two weeks?

- Has the client experienced unusual headaches or changes in vision? Are they accompanied by vomiting?

- Is there a noticeable proximal muscle weakness for no apparent cause? Is it accompanied by one or two decreased deep tendon reflexes?

WARNING SIGNS OF ADVANCED STAGES OF CANCER

✦ Is the client experiencing unexplained chronic pain? Does the pain feel like bone pain that is not related to movement?

✦ Has there been any unexplained bleeding? This can be due to ulcerations; these ulcerations occur at the location of the tumour or in surrounding tissue. As the tumour continues to grow, it overwhelms the specific tissue's nutrient supply and invades neighbouring areas placing pressure on, or rupturing blood vessels. Moreover, it is possible that the tumour may grow beyond the capacity of the surrounding tissue to support it. This ultimately leads to local tissue necrosis, secondary infection, severe hemorrhage and pain.

✦ Does the client experience persistent fatigue?

Contraindications

✦ Post-surgical massage is contraindicated locally. Massage may be appropriate to the hands and feet for relaxation. If the cancer is not local to the back or head and neck, stroking to the spine or a head and neck massage may be an appropriate modification. Contact with the physician is advised, before performing post-surgical massage, to discuss deep vein thrombosis risk.

✦ Radiation frequently creates local burns and loss of epithelial cells. Creams, powder, ointment, lotion, essential oil or salve should not be used over the affected area during the radiation treatment period. In some cases these products should be avoided for several weeks post-treatment; the physician is consulted before any products are used over the affected area (Canadian Cancer Society, 1998b). Radiated tissue is often sensitive to touch. Therefore, all massage techniques are contraindicated on the affected tissue for a few days after treatment; extremes of temperature are also avoided locally during this time. Massage is safe to be performed on other areas of the body for the purpose of relaxation.

✦ Chemotherapy and radiation can often result in nausea. Massage may or may not be tolerated by the client. Some people do not want to be touched if they feel ill; others may find stroking to the back, as well as foot and hand massage, helps them feel better.

◆ Lymphatic drainage techniques are contraindicated with untreated or metastasizing neoplasms, including melanomas *(Wittlinger, Wittlinger, 1990; Kurz, 1990)*. However, with edema that is a result of medical treatment (for example, following lymph node removal or radiation therapy), lymphatic drainage and massage techniques may proceed with a physician's approval.

◆ Hot hydrotherapy applications are contraindicated with lymphedema *(Kurz, 1990)*.

◆ It is possible that, in the clinically latent period (weeks or years) following surgery, especially where the lymphatics have been removed, the distal limb may be in a state of "edemic readiness" *(Harris, 1996)*. The heavy pressure technique of frictions, which relies on the inflammatory process, should, therefore, be avoided at the scar or in the distal limb, so as not to provoke a lymphedema.

◆ Full-body massage may need to be modified by restricting massage to more discrete areas that are not affected by the cancer. Deep techniques over known or likely tumour sites are contraindicated. They serve no purpose — one cannot friction away a tumour.

◆ Vigorous or stimulating techniques or treatments of long duration are contraindicated for debilitated clients, especially those receiving palliative care.

Treatment Considerations

HEALTH HISTORY QUESTIONS

(After diagnosis)

◆ When was the client's cancer diagnosed? How has it progressed? Does the client know the location of tumours and the risk of metastasis?

◆ What symptoms are being experienced from the cancer?

◆ If surgery has been performed, what tissue or organ was removed? Was the surgery successful?

◆ Is further treatment currently being received? What is the treatment and its schedule? What side effects are being experienced? If treatment is finished, how long ago was the last treatment received?

◆ What is the prognosis?

◆ Is any pain being experienced? What are the location, quality, duration and frequency of pain? What are the aggravating and relieving factors?

◆ Is the client taking any medication, prescribed or over-the-counter? Are any side effects being experienced? In the case of breast cancer the client may be taking tamoxifen for two and up to five years post-treatment. Hot flashes, mild nausea, weight gain and menstrual irregularities are possible side effects *(Canadian Cancer Society, 1997b)*.

◆ Is edema present? If so, since when? There is a greater possibility of fibrosis and hardening of the tissue with resultant tissue dysfunction the longer the edema has been present *(Harris, 1994)*.

◆ Is the client's physician aware she is seeking massage?

◆ Does the client consent to the therapist contacting the physician? This must also be obtained in written form. The physician can elaborate on the stage, metastasizing concerns and the prognosis of the cancer.

◆ Is the client exercising regularly or is she generally physically active? What specifically does the client do, how vigorously, for how long and how often?

◆ Have any restrictions been placed on the client by herself or the physician?

Further Assessment

✍ **Observation and Palpation:**

- Tissue health is observed. Redness and warmth may be noticed after radiation treatments. Tissue wasting and disuse atrophy may be present if the client is bedridden or in later stages of terminal cancer.

- Edema due to local lymphatic obstruction or removal involves the whole limb distal to the lesion site. The limb will be puffy and congested. Ascites, an abnormal edema found in the abdomen, may result from cancer.

- Scars from surgery should be noted; secondary fascial restrictions are very likely. These can lead to reduced range of motion in nearby joints as well as creating postural dysfunction. For example, frozen shoulder may occur secondary to mastectomy.

- Tenderness and pain may be present post-surgery. Pain is also a symptom that can increase as the cancer progresses or if it is terminal.

Massage During Medical Treatment

👋 Frequently, clients with cancer want massage for its stress-reducing effects. In obtaining consent from the client, the therapist must be clear that the effects of massage on the spread of cancer are not known.

👋 Relaxation massage is beneficial for clients with cancer. It offers comfort and support during a particularly stressful and uncertain time. Pain relief and symptom relief are achieved through the decrease of sympathetic nervous system firing. A full-body massage may not be possible because tumour sites, new surgical sites and recently radiated sites must be avoided. Omission of some areas will not detract from the stress-reducing effect of the treatment. Slow stroking down the spine and massage to the hands and feet are recommended if the client is post-surgical or after chemo- or radiation therapy.

🖐 Pure essential oils to promote relaxation are lavender, bergamot or cedarwood in a 2.5 per cent dilution, or 25 drops per 50 ml. of carrier oil. Essential oils that help with grief are rose and neroli essential oils in a one per cent dilution, or ten drops per 50 ml. of carrier oil *(Davis, 1988)*.

🖐 The diluted oils can be applied on the skin or five to 10 drops of the pure essential oil can be put in a diffuser with water.

🖐 Diaphragmatic breathing and positive visualization are encouraged.

Massage After Medical Treatment

🖐 Stress-reduction massage is continued. Frequently, people who have experienced cancer have had to face the fact of their mortality. Lifestyle changes may be made which include improving the quality of life. Massage therapy plays a role in reducing stress on the body and mind. A further component in the treatment is positive touch to improve the client's self-image and body awareness.

🖐 On a functional level, treatment of edema, scar tissue and fascial restrictions is appropriate, if requested or consented to by the client. The therapist must keep in mind that the client may need the emotional support of the massage and not the specific treatment of surgical scars. If the client experiences painful restrictions or postural dysfunction, and the therapist thinks they could be addressed with massage, then a clear explanation of the rationale and treatment expectation is included in the consent to treatment.

🖐 Edema may be present local to a surgical site. With breast cancer surgery and lymph node removal, edema of the limb is quite likely. Sometimes, edema will occur weeks or years after the surgery following an apparently insignificant injury or with overuse of the arm. Lymphatic drainage techniques are performed first in the unaffected axilla. This allows the functioning lymphatics of the healthy side to begin draining the edematous side through the lymphatic capillary anastomoses. For example, with a right arm lymphedema, the left axillary nodes and skin over the pectorals are treated first. The edematous limb is then treated, again starting proximally and working distally; pumping at the terminus is followed by unidirectional effleurage and stationary circles. See the chapter on edema for more details *(Foldi et al., 1985; Casley-Smith, Casley-Smith, 1986)*.

🖐 It is appropriate to treat the secondary fascial restrictions surrounding the affected area in an attempt to regain good joint movement and reduce postural imbalances. For example, secondary to mastectomy or lumpectomy, women may develop frozen shoulder or hyperkyphotic posture. For more details, see the chapters on these treatments in the text.

🖐 Fascial work is recommended before performing deep Swedish techniques to the scar site. The techniques used to address the scar are applied peripherally first to the least adhered area, progressing to the more restricted areas slowly. See the appropriate chapter for the specific treatment to scars.

🖐 The therapist should observe for emotional responses to the treatment. If they occur, the specific work is usually stopped for that day. If the client wishes to continue the massage, breathing and relaxation techniques are used to complete a full-body treatment. Treatment of the scar and fascia is followed by stretching the involved soft tissue. Passive movement of proximal and distal joints and joint play are also recommended.

Palliative Care

- Palliative care involves providing the best emotional and physical quality of life for a terminally ill person. Each person will react in her own way, often experiencing a variety of emotions during this time. There may be feelings of disbelief, shock or fear. These emotions may give way to anger at the situation or acceptance that one's time has come. As a person becomes more debilitated, there are concerns about the future of loved ones, about being a burden. People question the meaning of their lives; they may feel alone in their experience facing death. Some people find this a time of growth and inner peace.

- Any or all of these feelings are natural. Frequently, the therapist's role goes beyond providing only touch to include passive listening and acknowledgement of the client's feelings.

- It is important that the client is not pushed to talk about this experience if she chooses not to. There are many way to explore one's mortality in addition to talking about it, including, for example, keeping a diary or meditating to music. The therapist should take his cue from the client. Moreover, each therapist must examine his own emotions to discover if he is comfortable with the idea of dying; this is necessary in order to support the client. For some therapists, palliative massage may not be something they can comfortably give for a variety of reasons, including unresolved grief issues of their own. In such circumstances it is appropriate to refer these clients to another therapist.

- A relaxation massage is given, with extra focus on those areas the client requests. Diaphragmatic breathing and visualization are useful for relaxation and pain control.

- The client's tissues and organ systems will be deteriorating and fragile. The treatment approach should be modified accordingly. The use of gentle and soothing techniques and local massage to the face, neck and hands may be all that can be done.

- Pure essential oils are particularly beneficial at this time, either blended with a carrier oil or in a diffuser. Rose and neroli may be useful for their calming and centring effects. A one per cent dilution, or 10 drops per 50 ml. of carrier oil, is used. Bergamot and frankincense are also indicated for their comforting effects. A 2.5 per cent dilution, or 25 drops per 50 ml. of carrier oil, is used (Davis, 1988).

- Family and friends will benefit from massage and essential oils during this time of palliation as well.

Self-care

- Referral for nutrition counselling by a naturopath or nutritionist is recommended for building the immune system secondary to receiving treatment.

- Relaxation strategies such as ongoing massage, meditation and diaphragmatic breathing are encouraged.

✍ Essentials oils, such as lavender, can be used post-radiation for burns and all the oils listed above for relaxation and calming are appropriate. Oils are applied on the skin, after dilation in a carrier oil or "neat" in a diffuser.

✍ Some form of exercise such as regular walking is advised. A general stretch and strengthen program is also appropriate. Clients with lymphedema, especially of the upper limb, should be encouraged to perform moderate active free range of motion exercises without overexercising. Isometric resisted exercises are also indicated *(Stillwell, 1969)*.

✍ Women who have been treated for breast cancer should be encouraged to follow a program to prevent shoulder dysfunction. Daily exercises include wall walking, the pendulum and general active free shoulder range of motion. See the chapter on frozen shoulder for more details about self-care.

See also stress reduction, scars, edema, hyperkyphosis, constipation, peripheral nerve lesions, other circulatory concerns, inflammatory bowel disease, frozen shoulder and Appendix E.

✍ Clients with lymphedema may also be referred to a manual lymphatic drainage specialist such as someone trained and certified in Vodder's Manual Lymph Drainage and Combined Decongestive Therapy.

✍ Ideally, the client is urged to alter contributing behaviours by quitting smoking or eating a healthier diet.

✍ Support groups for people with cancer are available in most areas of the country. The Cancer Society offers information about different cancers, treatment and support groups.

Common Types of Cancer

Breast Cancer

Who Is Affected?

✦ Breast cancer risk increases with age. Eighty per cent of those diagnosed are 50 years of age or older *(Canadian Cancer Society, 1996e)*.

Causes and Contributing Factors

✍ There are associated factors which increase risk:

- a familial or personal history of breast cancer before menopause;
- a woman's hormonal history — that is, her increased exposure to estrogen such as an early age onset of menstruation, first pregnancy at a late age, few or no pregnancies, a limited breast-feeding period and menopause at a late age;
- a familial history of cervical, uterine or colon cancer;
- increasing age; (in Canada) by age 40, one in 262 would develop cancer; by age 50,

one in 58 would develop cancer *(Dollinger et al., 1995)*;

- a high-fat diet and sedentary lifestyle.

Symptom Picture

- ✦ Breast lumps are palpated by the woman or may be detected during a mammogram. The lump may feel hard and have an irregular shape. Sometimes a thickening of breast tissue is palpated: generally it feels different from the rest of the breast tissue. Fibrocytic breasts (small lumps found in the breasts) are not related to an increased risk of breast cancer.

- ✦ Enlarged lymph nodes may be palpated in the axilla.

- ✦ Pain is more common with a benign lump, but should be investigated.

- ✦ Changes in the nipple or breast appearance may be observed. The nipple may become retracted. Tissue scaling around the nipple may indicate Paget's disease, a form of local nipple cancer. Discharge from the nipple is usually benign, except for bloody or serous discharge which is often a warning sign of cancer. All discharge should be investigated.

- ✦ The skin of the breast may appear irregular or retracted in an area. Differences in the size or shape of one breast to the other may occur. In advanced cases of cancer, swelling is observable. The surface may appear similar to that of an orange, called "peau d'orange" due to the increased edema. This may be accompanied by redness or increased heat.

- ✦ Sometimes, due to metastasizing, pain or swelling may be present in other areas, such as pain in an area of bone metastasis, swelling in the neck or liver enlargement.

Medical Treatment

- ✦ Surgery may involve a lumpectomy or a mastectomy. A lumpectomy removes the lump and a small amount of normal tissue. Removal of the axillary lymph nodes is also performed due to the risk of cancer metastasis. A modified radical mastectomy is the removal of the entire breast and lymph nodes of the axilla.

- ✦ Radiation therapy is used with surgery. Usually the armpit, breast and chest wall are irradiated.

- ✦ Chemotherapy is usually used with cancer that is thought to have metastasized. It is used along with surgery or radiation therapy, or a combination of both.

- ✦ Hormonal therapy is used with breast cancer. With some types of tumours, growth is facilitated by the hormone estrogen. Suppression of this hormone can be achieved by surgery (removal of hormone-producing organs such as the ovaries) or drugs (tamoxifen suppresses hormone production in relevant estrogen-producing organs).

Post-treatment Complications

- ✦ Obstruction of the lymphatic flow may occur because of surgical removal of the lymph nodes, radiation treatment or scarring secondary to mastectomy. Obstruction of the lymphatics in the upper limb leads to a retention of plasma proteins, which, in turn, attracts more fluid. This chronic edema is called lymphedema. The edematous tissue becomes stretched and is unable to return to its original shape. It will be puffy and congested (following a lymphectomy). The temperature may be cool due to ischemia or warm due to congestion.

✦ With lymphedema resulting from surgery, there may be a latent period following the operation where the tissue appears to return to normal. Weeks or years after the surgery, an apparently insignificant injury — a bruise, a cut, a sprained ankle, the pinprick of a diabetes blood sugar test or even an insect bite *(Brennan, Weitz, 1992)* — may provoke lymphedema distal to the scar.

Massage

With full-limb lymphedema resulting from mastectomy and removal of the lymph nodes or radiation, massage techniques are started in the contralateral quadrant. For example, with a right arm lymphedema, the left axillary nodes and skin over the pectorals are treated first. This allows the functioning lymphatics of the healthy quadrant to begin draining the edematous quadrant through the anastomoses across the watershed. The edematous limb is then treated, again starting proximally and working distally *(Foldi et al., 1985; Casley-Smith, Casley-Smith, 1986).*

Colorectal Cancer

Who Is Affected?

✦ This cancer seems to affect men and women equally. It is unusual for it to occur before the age of 50 unless the person has a predisposing factor such as chronic ulcerative colitis, a history of colorectal cancer, a strong family history of this cancer or familial polyposis coli — a rare disease resulting in multiple benign tumours early in life. With treatment of colon cancer, the five-year survival rate is 70 per cent; if the cancer has metastasized to the lymph nodes, the survival rate is reduced to 30 per cent. Fortunately, with those surviving five years, it is likely that the cancer is cured. Rectal cancer prognosis is not as good, unless the tumour is in the distal colon; in this case the five-year survival rate is about 60 per cent *(Canadian Cancer Society, 1996f).*

Causes and Contributing Factors

✦ The cause is unknown. Diet appears to play a role. Too much fat, especially saturated fats, in the diet is a major risk factor.

✦ Preventative factors are an adequate intake of fibre, fruits and vegetables as well as vitamins C and E.

Symptom Picture

✦ Early symptoms include changes in bowel habits lasting over two weeks, such as increasing constipation or alternating constipation and diarrhea.

✦ Polyps, benign intestinal tumours, are precursors to cancer, though they take years to change. A sign of polyps is blood in the stools as a result of bleeding from the intestine; this may appear bright or dark red in the stool. Anemia may result (paleness, shortness of breath and being easily fatigued).

✦ Crampy abdominal pain and swelling may be present.

✦ A tumour in the rectum may be indicated by a ongoing desire to have a bowel movement but with little success at passing stool.

Medical Treatment

✦ Surgery is most commonly used to remove the localized cancer of the colon or rectum. Because the colon's function is primarily to convert waste to solid stool, with colon cancer, large sections can be removed with little change in function, though looser stools result when greater sections of the colon are removed. Rectal cancer requires rectal surgery often involving the removal of the sphincters (muscles that control the action of the bowel) along with the anal canal in order to remove the tumour. In such cases, a colostomy is necessary; this involves the creation of an opening in the wall of the abdomen through which the stool can be excreted.

✦ Radiation therapy, if used, is given in combination with surgery or chemotherapy, though tumours of the anus are especially easily treated with radiation only. Chemotherapy may be given in combination with surgery or with surgery and radiation. Chemotherapy is also useful after surgery, if the cancer has spread.

Massage

🖐 Massage therapy is used for relaxation and client support. If a colostomy has been performed, abdominal massage is not recommended. Some positional modifications may be necessary, such as prone positioning being replaced with three-quarters prone.

Lung Cancer

Who Is Affected?

✦ Lung cancer is the leading cause of death from cancer in both men and women. It is frequently preventable by avoidance of smoking. The risk of lung cancer is related to the total amount of exposure to cigarette smoke. The duration of smoking, the number of cigarettes smoked and the depth of inhalation all determine the actual risk. Therefore, those at greatest risk have smoked for many years (for example, over 20 years), averaged over 20 cigarettes a day and inhaled freely. With such a person the risk is increased 15 to 30 times compared with a non-smoker. Those who smoke only pipes or cigars tend to do so less frequently and "puff" rather than inhale freely. The risk of developing lung cancer from pipes or cigars is less than with cigarette smoking but higher than someone who does not smoke. Exposure to second-hand smoke can increase anyone's risk of lung cancer.

Causes

✦ Carcinogens such as asbestos, chromium, benzene, cadmium, nickel, radon and coal tar products can cause lung cancer, though the majority of cases, 85 per cent, are related to cigarette smoking *(Canadian Cancer Society, 1996g)*.

Symptom Picture

✦ Chronic coughing occurs as the person attempts to dislodge the tumour in the lungs. Mucus production increases in response to the lung irritation, and the mucus must be coughed up. If the coughing damages the tumour, blood may appear in the sputum.

✦ Over time, airway obstruction may result as the tumour grows. Secondary to the obstruction, infections and pneumonia can develop, leading to increased coughing, chest pain and fever.

Medical Treatment

✦ Surgery is performed if the tumour is localized, with 30 to 35 per cent of people doing well five years post-treatment *(Canadian Cancer Society, 1996g)*.

✦ Radiation is used if the tumour cannot be safely removed or the person is unable to tolerate surgery.

✦ Chemotherapy is most often used if the cancer is thought to have metastasized. It has been found to be especially helpful with a small-cell variant of lung cancer.

Massage

✋ Massage therapy is used for stress reduction. Post-treatment postural changes secondary to surgery may be treated using appropriate Swedish techniques to address fascial restrictions.

✋ If the cancer is terminal, stress reduction and client support are the focus of the massage.

Prostate Cancer

Who Is Affected?

✦ One in nine men will develop prostate cancer in their lives. It frequently tends to affect men over 70 and is rare under the age of 50 *(Canadian Cancer Society, 1998a)*. This cancer is often slow growing and, if it remains within the prostate, will result in few or no symptoms and will not affect the length of the man's life. The prostate is a small organ located just below the bladder and in front of the rectum. It surrounds the urethra, the duct through which urine flows from the bladder.

Causes and Contributing Factors

✦ The cause is unknown, though diet is thought to play a role. Fats, in particular animal fats, may contribute to an increased risk.

Symptom Picture

✦ The following symptoms may signal a benign enlarged prostrate or may be a sign of cancer. Occasionally, there are no symptoms in the prostate and the cancer is only detected after it has metastasized to another area.

✦ Incomplete emptying of the bladder can lead to bladder infections and pain or burning with urination.

✦ Men may have difficulty starting urination and may notice a weak stream.

✦ There may be an increased frequency in urination or leakage. In the case of a complete blockage, urination is impossible.

Medical Treatment

✦ In men over 70, with a slow growth type of prostate cancer, the physician will regularly observe the progress of the disease.

✦ Surgery may be used to remove the prostate completely or it may be partially removed to relieve symptoms.

✦ Radiation is frequently used to destroy the cancer cells.

✦ Hormone treatment is used if the cancer has metastasized or is very advanced locally. In such cases, the release of testosterone must be stopped in order to slow the cancer growth. This is achieved by the removal of the testes or by the use of hormones or chemicals to counteract the testosterone.

✦ Impotence may be a side effect of all treatments for prostate cancer.

Massage

✋ Massage is used for stress reduction and client support.

HIV INFECTION AND AIDS

Fiona Rattray

> **HIV (human immunodeficiency virus) is the virus that causes AIDS (acquired immune deficiency syndrome).**

The Immune System

The immune system is composed of specialized organs and cells that protect the body against infection and the growth of malignant cells. Lymphocytes are small white blood cells, the primary cells of the immune system. They are divided into T-lymphocytes (T-cells), so named because they originate in the thymus, B-lymphocytes (B-cells, which mature in the bone marrow), and the remaining lymphocytes which are called natural killer cells. T-cells control viral infections by recognizing antigens on the surface of macrophages; a subset of these cells is called T-4, T-helper or CD4 cells. B-cells eliminate bacteria and their toxins by producing antibodies. Natural killer cells rapidly identify and destroy virus-infected cells and tumour cells.

HIV/AIDS

First recognized in 1981, HIV is the most common acquired immune deficiency condition in the world today. The virus selectively infects the T-helper cells, destroying them. HIV may also be present in the brain. After the initial infection, there is a latent period where the person is asymptomatic.

Over time, the weakened immune system is vulnerable to opportunistic infections and other conditions. A person is diagnosed with AIDS when one or more "AIDS-defining" diseases or cancers develops (*National AIDS Awareness Campaign Resource Guide, 1998/9*). These include:

• **cervical cancer** which occurs in HIV-infected women at a rate five times higher than in other women. Symptoms include vaginal bleeding between periods or after menopause;

- **cryptococcus neoformans** which is a yeast that causes meningitis, fever and severe secondary headache *(Davidoff, 1995)*. It may also affect the skin, lungs and kidneys;

- **cryptosporidium** which is an infection by a protozoa. It produces severe diarrhea which may last for months; death may occur from massive fluid loss;

- **cytomegalovirus (CMV)** which is an opportunistic infection causing fever, sore throat, fatigue, muscle pain and swollen lymph nodes. Severe CMV infection can cause pneumonia, hepatitis, colitis, retinitis and even blindness;

- **Kaposi's sarcoma (KS)** which is cancer of the capillaries. Lesions start as small, purple, raised patches, often on the legs. Initially, they are usually only mildly painful. The lesions may infiltrate the skin, growing down into the tissue. Over time, they become thicker and grow into each other; they may ulcerate. While KS lesions often appear simultaneously in many locations, suggesting a causative factor, perhaps blood-borne, the lesions may also spread through the lymphatic system. KS lesions may appear: in the eyes; inside the mouth, causing discomfort; in the gastrointestinal tract, leading to an inability to eat; and in the lungs, causing difficulty in breathing and eventually death. Lesions in the lymphatics lead to edema in the affected part. KS is not considered curable *(Dollinger, et al., 1995);*

- **lymphoma** which is cancer of the lymphatic system. With HIV, the lymphoma often involves the central nervous system;

- **mycobacterium avium intracellulare (MAI)/mycrobacterium avium complex (MAC)** is an opportunistic infection that causes diarrhea, weight loss and fevers;

- **nervous system manifestations** which include AIDS dementia, also called subacute encephalitis. Subtle behavioural and cognitive changes such as memory loss occur over several months, eventually leading to severe dementia with tremor, spasticity, motor loss and ataxia. Peripheral neuropathies may develop in 30 to 50 per cent of those with AIDS. These neuropathies consist of numbness, weakness and pain;

- **pneumocystis carinii pneumonia (PCP)** which is a fungal infection that grows rapidly in the lungs. It is commonly found in soil and inside buildings;

- **toxoplasma gondii (toxoplasmosis or "toxo")** which is a common organism that causes lung and central nervous system infections. Commonly, central nervous system symptoms of fever, severe secondary headache, altered mental status and seizures are experienced *(Davidoff, 1995);*

- **tuberculosis (TB)** which is an opportunistic bacterial infection affecting the lungs and different areas of the body. Coughing, malaise, fatigue and night sweats may occur;

- **wasting syndrome** which is diarrhea, fever, chronic weakness, severe weight loss and loss of muscle mass in the absence of other infections. In Africa, this aspect of AIDS gave rise to the name "slim disease".

HIV Transmission

HIV is a fragile virus that does not survive outside the body. It is not transmitted through casual contact such as touching, hugging or sharing eating utensils, nor is it airborne. The virus cannot pass through skin that has no cuts or abrasions. It is not passed along through a mosquito bite.

A person must perform certain actions that allow sufficient quantities of HIV into the bloodstream from the body fluids of someone who has HIV. These actions include unprotected sexual intercourse, sharing of intravenous needles and transfusion of unscreened, infected blood and blood products. In Canada since 1985, all donated blood has been tested for HIV *(AIDS Committee of Toronto, 1998)*. Before this precaution was taken, large numbers of hemophiliacs were infected with the virus. HIV may also be transmitted from mother to baby during pregnancy, labour or breast-feeding.

There are four body fluids that contain HIV in sufficient quantities to cause infection. These are blood, semen, vaginal secretions and breast milk. Urine, sweat, tears and saliva do not contain enough of the virus to infect a person *(AIDS Committee of Toronto, 1998)*.

HIV/AIDS Statistics

✦ More than 95 per cent of HIV-infected people live in developing countries. The United Nations Programme on HIV/AIDS estimates that, world-wide, 33.4 million people are infected with HIV; the cumulative number of deaths since the pandemic began in 1981 is 13.9 million persons. Since the deaths are occurring primarily among young adults, the reproductive and economic impact of HIV/AIDS is enormous.

✦ Globally, women comprise 43 per cent of all adults living with HIV *(Interagency Coalition on AIDS and Development, 1998)*. If a mother has HIV, there is a 25 per cent chance that her baby will be infected *(AIDS Committee of Toronto, 1998)*. Approximately half of all new infections with HIV in 1998 occurred in young people between the ages of 15 and 24.

✦ While HIV is commonly thought of in North America and Europe as affecting primarily gay or bisexual men, in most of the developing world it primarily affects heterosexual men and women.

  • Africa: Perhaps two-thirds of those infected world-wide live in Sub-Saharan Africa. Many are children and young adults.

  • Asia and the Pacific: Over 7 million people are infected, especially in southeast Asia.

  • Eastern Europe and the Commonwealth of Independent States: There are 270,000 persons infected with HIV; the highest rate of infection is among injection drug users.

  • Industrialized Countries of Australia and New Zealand, Europe and North America: These countries have 1.4 million HIV-infected people. While gay and bisexual men and injection drug users comprise the largest population, HIV can be found in the heterosexual population also. In Canada, gay and bisexual men comprise the largest group of those living with HIV/AIDS; women comprised 19 per cent of those with HIV in 1995; Aboriginals made up 17 per cent of new cases of HIV infection in 1997; injection drug users comprized 33 per cent of new cases. HIV infection is on the rise among young gay men and young people in general *(National AIDS Awareness Campaign Resource Guide 1998/9)*. Although medication is reducing the number of deaths, the numbers of people living with HIV are increasing as people live longer and new infections continue at a stable rate.

  • Latin America and the Caribbean: 1.7 million people are living with HIV/AIDS. In Latin America, most infections occur in gay and bisexual men and injection drug users. In the Caribbean, heterosexual transmission is the primary route *(Interagency Coalition on AIDS and Development, 1998)*.

The Potential Stigma of HIV/AIDS

Because the origin of HIV and how it causes AIDS is not completely understood, and perhaps due to its method of transmission and who gets it, a lot of misinformation has surrounded HIV/AIDS. The search for a cure has lead to myths of blame, guilt and denial.

People with HIV/AIDS may feel isolated, afraid and lonely. Because the prognosis is uncertain, and because of its association as a terminal illness, the person living with HIV/AIDS may feel depressed and angry. It may not be possible for the person to talk about the illness. He may suffer rejection and discrimination from family, friends, neighbours and employers. During periods of severe illness he may be unable to work, causing economic hardship. There may be periods of hospitalization or a hospice stay. The person may make arrangements to settle his financial affairs or get rid of his accommodations, believing that death is imminent. Where HIV-fighting drugs are available, a person may recover from a serious, formerly life-threatening illness only to have to start over again in terms of living accommodation and income.

HIV/AIDS are illnesses; nobody deserves an illness. Instead people with HIV/AIDS deserve understanding and support in whatever manner they choose it. Education about the disease is a key in this process.

➤ **The cause of HIV infection/AIDS is a retrovirus.**

➤ **Contributing factors** to the rate of HIV infection include infections such as hepatitis B, stress and poor nutrition.

Medically, HIV is diagnosed through laboratory tests which assess for antibodies to the virus. A person who tests positive for the antibodies is termed HIV-positive; someone who tests negative for antibodies is termed HIV-negative. A positive test result does not indicate whether the person will develop AIDS; it only shows infection by the virus. A diagnosis of AIDS is made when secondary opportunistic infection occurs.

If an HIV-positive status is revealed, a series of tests are recommended to determine the person's baseline of health. These tests include assessment of exposure to various infections, eye examinations and blood tests for viral loads. Retesting is performed periodically and medication is started or adjusted according to test results.

In terms of medication, anti-HIV drugs inhibit the ability of the virus to replicate itself. If the drug affects the beginning of the replication process, it is a reverse transcriptase inhibitor. Some examples of these drugs are AZT, ddl, ddC, d4T and T3C. Other anti-HIV drugs affect the end of the replication process and are called protease inhibitors. Some examples are ritonivir and saquinivir (AIDS Council of New South Wales).

Medication such as vinblastine is used to control KS lesions. These lesions also respond to radiation therapy; however, these therapies further depress the immune system (Dollinger et al., 1995).

Numerous other medications are used prophylactically to prevent the different opportunistic infections. Proper nutrition is important. For those who can afford it, these drugs are often combined with antiviral medication in what is termed a "drug cocktail". It is important that the person strictly adhere to the specific medication schedule. There can be side effects of both the drugs individually and in interaction with each other.

Increasingly people are using complimentary therapies such as acupuncture, vitamin supplements and herbs to reduce stress, improve immune function and reduce side effects of medication.

1036

While HIV/AIDS is fully preventable, no cure exists. HIV treatment and clinical science are constantly changing; there is still a lot that is not known about HIV/AIDS. Even a dedicated health care practitioner has difficulty keeping up with the changes.

Massage and HIV

Massage therapy is often recommended as a therapy for those people with HIV/AIDS for relaxation, stress reduction, a heightened sense of well being and treatment of peripheral neuropathies *(AIDS Committee of Toronto, 1999; Carrol, 1995)*.

There are other benefits. One study on the effects of massage therapy and HIV/AIDS showed that one month of daily massage increased the number and activity of natural killer cells in people who were HIV-positive, stimulating immunity. Although the volunteers' T-cell counts were unaffected, meaning that the progression of the virus was unchanged by massage, the study shows that massage may have helped fight some of the secondary infections associated with AIDS. Anxiety levels were also decreased during this period *(Ironson et al., 1995)*.

Another study examined the effects on HIV-exposed babies of massage three times daily for a two-week period. It reported that these babies had significant weight gain and showed improvement in behaviour such as responsiveness over babies in a control group *(Scafidi, Field, 1995)*.

Lymphatic drainage is recommended for treatment of edema that develops secondary to Kaposi's sarcoma *(Steinberg, 1990)*.

Finally, a person's beliefs and emotions have an effect on the body's ability to fight off illness. Several psychoneuroimmunology studies have revealed how grief and depression can suppress the immune system through the stress response *(Carroll, 1995)*. As HIV/AIDS may be seen as an "untouchable" disease, touch itself can be healing. It indicates support and acceptance. Massage therapy may help the HIV-positive person deal with feelings of loneliness, isolation and guilt *(Steinberg, 1990)*.

Symptom Picture

+ Initial HIV infection is often symptomless. Some people may experience a short, initial period of **flu-like symptoms** such as night sweats, sore throat, muscle pain, headache and swollen lymph nodes when antibodies to the virus are being created.

+ The infected person may continue to be **asymptomatic** for a long time. In some cases people with HIV continue to feel healthy for 10 or 15 years *(AIDS Committee of Toronto, 1998)*. During this period, the person with HIV is capable of infecting others.

  • During this asymptomatic period, T-helper cells are attacked by the virus. After a certain point the immune system is overwhelmed and no longer able to control the virus. Blood tests at this point show that the T-cell count (CD4 count) is decreasing and the amount of virus in the blood (or viral load) is increasing. The immune system is also no longer able to fend off opportunistic infections. Some of the organisms that cause these opportunistic infections are quite common; they are often already in the person's body and were formerly controlled by a healthy immune system.

- When the immune system is overwhelmed, the person begins to experience symptoms such as swollen lymph nodes, fatigue, recurrent fever, night sweats, diarrhea, decreased appetite, rapid weight loss, mouth sores, vaginal yeast infections and changes in the menstrual cycle.

✦ Over time, more **serious infections and cancers** such as pneumocystis carinii pneumonia and KS are experienced; at this point the person is described as having AIDS. The symptoms that the person experiences will depend on which opportunistic infection, cancer, or combination of the above, the person has.

✦ **AIDS dementia** may occur.

✦ **Peripheral neuropathies** may result from HIV itself or from medication use. HIV does not infect neurons directly. Instead it affects the insulating myelin sheath, creating a distal painful neuropathy. These neuropathies are often bilateral. Certain medications such as D4T and AZT can also damage axons. In addition, vitamins B1, B6 and B12 deficiencies may cause a neuropathy.

- Neuropathies affect six to eight per cent of those in the asymptomatic stage of HIV disease. Most commonly neuropathies strike those with AIDS. One or several nerves may be affected, often in the feet and hands. The sensations vary from constant mild pain to a deep burning; this can be very exhausting for the person. Painful burning and numbness may progress to paralysis in some people.

Contraindications

✦ Do not massage over open lesions or over a tumour.

✦ General massage is contraindicated with significant fever (38.5° C, 101.5° F).

✦ Avoid working over the insertion site of an indwelling medication catheter if the client has such a device; it is often located on the upper chest.

✦ Vinyl gloves are worn as usual if there are any cuts, sores or abrasions on the therapist's hands or the client's body.

✦ Do not overtreat a debilitated client with too long or vigorous a treatment.

✦ If the therapist has a contagious illness, treating the client is likely contraindicated until she is better. This protects the client from getting the illness. Clarify the situation over the phone with the client before the treatment; reschedule if necessary.

✦ **Rheumatic manifestations** of severe joint and muscle pain may be present. HIV-associated arthritis may intermittently affect knees, shoulders and elbows. In 10 per cent of cases, the arthritis pain is unresponsive to analgesic medication. HIV-induced transient muscle pain is also common. Reiter's syndrome, spondylarthritis and medication-induced (AZT) myopathies may be present. Fibromyalgia and other soft tissue involvement such as tendinitis may occur (*Schumacher, 1993*).

✦ There may be **periods of relatively good health between bouts of serious illness.** Although HIV/AIDS is described clinically as following a certain progression and increasing severity of symptoms, not all persons experience these stages in the same way. Symptoms may come and go and vary in discomfort and severity.

✦ Although AIDS was once thought of as a fatal illness, not every person infected with HIV will become ill or die from AIDS-related illnesses. This depends on the person's geographical location, socioeconomic situation and the availability of good nutrition and medication to control the opportunistic infections.

Treatment Considerations

Assessment

✍ **Observation and Palpation:**

- Tissue health is observed. The client may appear healthy in the asymptomatic stage. Tissue wasting and disuse atrophy may be present with wasting disease or if the client is bedridden.

- Edema due to local lymphatic obstruction from KS lesions may be present, involving the whole limb distal to the lesion site. The limb will be puffy and congested.

- Tenderness, numbness and pain may be present with neuropathies; joint and muscle pain may also occur.

Massage

✋ Because the symptoms and medical treatment protocols are constantly changing, it is important for the therapist to update herself on the client's current symptom status and medication usage. Often the client himself is an expert on treatment protocols. The therapist may need to consult with the client's physician or other specialist, with the client's written permission.

✋ It is also important for the therapist to examine herself for biases or prejudices that may hinder the therapeutic process. Ongoing education is part of this process. A non-judgemental presence on the part of the therapist is key for treatment.

✋ Because the symptoms of HIV/AIDS vary depending on whether the person is asymptomatic, suffering an opportunistic infection, in remission or in the terminal stages of AIDS, the treatment is directed to the client's presenting symptoms.

✋ **Positioning** may be prone, sidelying or supine, as is comfortable for the client.

✋ **Hydrotherapy** applications also depend on the client's symptoms. The duration of the treatment is also variable, ranging from a half hour to a full hour of relaxation massage. **Diaphragmatic breathing** is important.

✋ Stress reduction is the basic treatment, whether in the asymptomatic stage or later in the illness. Slow, soothing and predictable techniques are used, such as effleurage, petrissage, rocking and shaking. See the chapter on stress reduction for details.

✋ Pure essential oils may be added to the massage oil in a 2.5 per cent solution; 25 drops of essential oil in 50 ml. of carrier oil are indicated. Lavender and roman chamomile can reduce pain; bergamot and frankincense are helpful for depression (*Lawless, 1995*). Pre-treatment facial steams of five drops of tea tree or thyme oil are useful with respiratory conditions; the client should close the eyes to avoid mucous membrane irritation.

✋ Edema is reduced using lymphatic drainage techniques.

✋ Massage to a limb that is experiencing a peripheral neuropathy may initially feel uncomfortable for the client. The pressure is adjusted to the client's pain tolerance (*Kaiser, 1997*).

✋ Treatment can end with a head, neck and shoulder massage.

🖐 In later stages of the disease, when the person has opportunistic infections or KS, treatments may be shorter in duration to avoid fatiguing the client.

🖐 If the client is in a wheelchair or is bedridden, the therapist should be alert for the possibility of decubitus ulcers and postural changes.

Palliative Massage

🖐 If the illness progresses into a terminal stage, palliative massage is used. Palliative care is the concept that, even though a cure or long-term control of an illness is not possible, the person's quality of life should be paramount. A person who is dying is entitled to the best physical, emotional, spiritual, vocational and social life possible. The goals of palliative care are pain reduction and support of the client. Each person will react in his own way, often experiencing a variety of emotions during this time. There may be feelings of disbelief, shock or fear that it is happening, anger at the situation or acceptance that one's time has come. Any or all of these feelings are natural.

🖐 Frequently, the therapist's role goes beyond providing only touch but includes passive listening and acknowledgement of the client's feelings. It is important that the client is not pushed to talk about this experience if he chooses not to.

🖐 A relaxation massage is given, with extra focus on those areas the client requests. Diaphragmatic breathing is useful for relaxation and pain control. Pure essential oil of rose helps with stress and grief reduction; a one per cent solution is made using 10 drops of essential oil in 50 ml. of carrier oil. Bergamot helps to reduce anxiety; 25 drops of essential oil in 50 ml. of carrier oil give a 2.5 per cent solution.

🖐 The client's tissues and organ systems will be deteriorating and fragile. The treatment approach should be modified accordingly. The use of gentle and soothing techniques and local massage to the face, neck and hands may be all that can be done.

🖐 The client's partner, family and friends may also benefit from massage.

🖐 Each therapist must look into herself to discover if she is comfortable with the idea of dying; this is necessary, in order to support the client. For some therapists, palliative massage may not be something they can comfortably give for a variety of reasons, including unresolved grief issues of their own. In such circumstances it is appropriate to refer these clients to another therapist. See the chapter on cancer for more details on palliative care.

Self-care

✍ HIV-positive people are advised to avoid exposure to organisms that cause illness. Some guidelines include prophylactic medication usage and vaccinations (*D'Amico, 1998; PI Perspective, 1997b*). Those HIV-positive people whose baseline tests reveal no antibodies for toxoplasmosis should thoroughly cook meats, wash fruits and vegetables, wash hands after gardening and avoid changing cat litter boxes or petting stray cats who may harbour the disease.

✍ Peripheral neuropathies resulting from medication are controlled by the physician reducing the dose or changing medication. Self-massage of the limbs affected with peripheral neuropathies may help to relieve pain. The client can experiment with differing pressures to find the one that helps to manage pain *(Bowers, 1997; PI Perspective, 1997a)*. Avoiding extreme temperature changes may reduce the pain; wearing warm socks and boots in the winter may help, as may wearing sandals in hot summer weather. Removing the shoes for several minutes several times a day is also suggested. Nightly hydrotherapy applications of cool foot or arm baths are also recommended *(Bowers, 1997)*.

See also stress reduction, edema, cancer, tendinitis, inflammatory arthritides, migraines, decubitus ulcers, ambulation aids and peripheral nerve lesions for related treatments.

✍ Stress-reduction classes and aerobic exercise are important to maintain the health of the immune system.

✍ The client is referred to a physician for immediate assessment if new symptoms occur. A naturopath, acupuncturist and nutritionist may also be recommended.

✍ Self-help and support groups can provide emotional support and an opportunity to learn more about the disease and how others are dealing with similar problems.

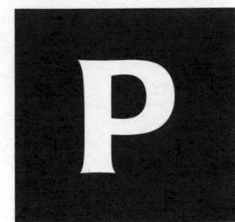

APPENDICES

Appendix A:

ANATOMICAL DIRECTIONAL TERMS

Fiona Rattray

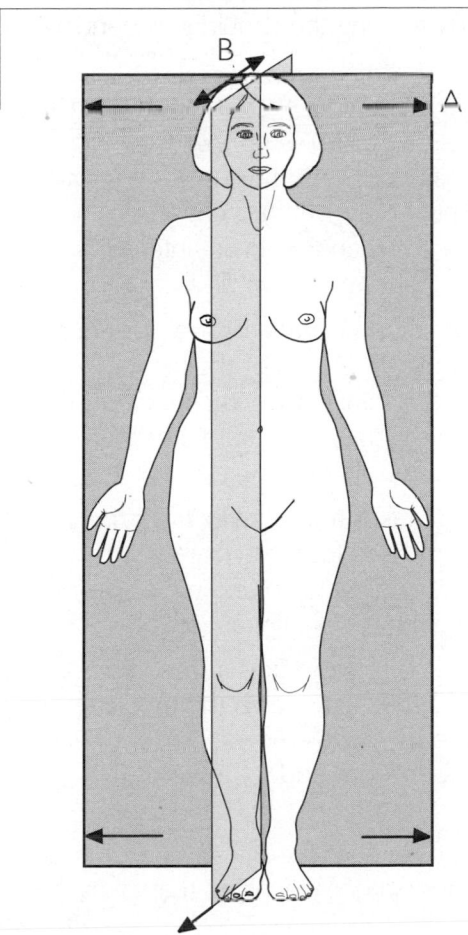

Figure A.1
The coronal (A) and median (B) planes.

Anatomical directional terms are used to clearly describe specific directions and the numerous positions a person's body can assume *(Kapit, Elson, 1977)*. The terms relate to the basic posture known as the anatomical position: the person is standing, the feet are parallel and slightly apart, the arms are relaxed and at the sides with the palms facing forward.

Planes of the Body

The body is divided into planes *(Figure A.1)*. The coronal plane, also called the frontal plane, divides the body into anterior (front) and posterior (back) portions.

The median, midsagittal or midline plane divides the body into left and right halves. It is at right angles to the coronal plane. A sagittal plane can appear in variable locations parallel to the median plane. A sagittal plane divides the body into unequal left and right parts.

The horizontal plane divides the body into upper and lower segments. This plane is at right angles to both the coronal and median planes. An exception is in the foot. In order to divide the foot into upper and lower segments, the plane is not at right angles to the coronal and median planes. In this case the plane is referred to as a transverse plane.

The coronal, median, horizontal and transverse planes are collectively called the cardinal planes.

Positional and Directional Terms

Positional and directional terms describe structures relative to one another.

Anterior or ventral locates a structure more in front relative to another. Posterior or dorsal refers to a structure more behind.

Superior and cephalad indicate a structure that is higher or closer to the head than another structure. Inferior or caudal indicates a structure lower or closer to the feet than another structure.

Medial places a structure closer to the median plane than another structure. Lateral locates the structure further away from the median plane.

In terms of the limbs, proximal means closer to the trunk or root of the limb. Distal locates structures that are further away from the trunk or root of the limb.

Describing Movement

Movement of the limbs at a joint are described relative to the planes of reference (*Calais-Germain, 1993*). It is easier to describe the movement of a limb which combines several planes of reference by breaking down the movements into the cardinal planes. For example, a person who is reaching in front of herself with one arm is either flexing and externally rotating the shoulder or flexing and internally rotating the shoulder depending on which direction she reaches.

The term flexion describes movement on a sagittal plane that takes a body part in an anterior direction away from the anatomical position, as in flexion of the hip, trunk or shoulder. Flexion of the knee (where the leg moves posteriorly) and flexion of the ankle (called dorsiflexion) are exceptions to this concept. The term protraction describes movement on a sagittal plane that takes the scapula or the mandible in an anterior direction away from the anatomical position.

Extension describes movement on a sagittal plane that takes a body part in a posterior direction away from the anatomical position. For example, extension of the hip moves the leg to a posterior position. Extension of the ankle (called plantarflexion) is an exception to this rule. The term retraction describes movement on a sagittal plane that takes the scapula or mandible in a posterior direction away from the anatomical position.

Abduction describes movement on a coronal plane that takes a limb away from the median plane, as in abduction of the shoulder. In the hand and foot, the planes of reference are the middle fingers and the second toes, respectively. For example, the little finger, ring finger and index finger all abduct away from the middle finger.

The term adduction describes movement on a coronal plane that takes a limb towards the median plane. For example, adduction of the hip moves the leg towards the median plane. Again, in the hand and foot, the planes of reference are the middle fingers and the second toes. For example, the little finger, ring finger and index finger all adduct towards the middle finger.

Eversion describes movement on a coronal plane that takes the hindfoot away from the median plane. The term inversion describes movement on a coronal plane that takes the hindfoot towards the median plane.

Radial deviation describes movement on a coronal plane that takes the hand at the wrist joint away from the median plane. The term ulnar deviation describes movement on a coronal plane that takes the hand at the wrist joint towards the median plane.

Elevation describes movement on a coronal plane that takes a body part superiorly, as in elevation of the scapula or mandible. The term depression describes movement on a coronal plane that takes a body part inferiorly, as in depression of the scapula or mandible. Lateral flexion or sidebending describes movement on a coronal plane away from the median plane, such as lateral flexion of the neck and trunk.

The term external rotation or lateral rotation describes movement on a transverse plane that rotates the limb outward or laterally. An example of this is external rotation of the shoulder. Internal rotation or medial rotation describes movement on a transverse plane that rotates the limb inward or medially. An example of this is internal rotation of the hip.

The term pronation is an internal rotation of the hand and forearm from the anatomical position, so the palmar surface faces posteriorly or backwards. In the foot, pronation is abduction of the forefoot, eversion of the hindfoot and some dorsiflexion at the subtalar joint, so the medial longitudinal arch is flattened.

Supination is an external rotation of the hand and forearm towards the anatomical position, so the palmar surface faces anteriorly or forward. In the foot, supination is adduction of the forefoot, inversion of the hindfoot and some plantarflexion at the subtalar joint, so that the medial longitudinal arch is raised.

The term rotation, whether left or right, is a movement of the head, neck or trunk around the median axis of the body.

Circumduction is a circular motion of a body part in a cone-shaped action. A complete circle is made by the distal end of the limb, while the apex of the cone is the joint at the proximal end. In the anatomical position, circumduction of the hip occurs through the coronal and sagittal planes; circumduction of the shoulder occurs through the sagittal plane; and circumduction of the thumb occurs through the coronal and sagittal planes.

Appendix B:

POSTURAL AND GAIT ASSESSMENT

Fiona Rattray

Postural Assessment

The following information provides a protocol for objective assessment of posture and gait. First, a static postural assessment is performed, followed by gait assessment. Posture is defined as a synthesis of the positions of all the body's joints at any given time. This may be the client's habitual position or the position taken during an activity (Kendall et al., 1993; Kisner, Colby, 1990).

Gravity places stress on the structures that maintain the body's upright posture. A weight bearing joint maintains its stability either by having the body mass fall exactly through its rotational axis or by maintaining a muscular or structural counterforce to the effects of gravity. The body is supported by structures such as fascia, ligaments, joints and bones, and is moved by the muscles and tendons that attach to these structures.

In normal posture, gravity acts in a balanced line on the physiological curves of the spine. Shifting the body's weight away from this line means that another region of the spine or body must compensate to regain postural equilibrium or stability.

Postural pain has various causes. Faulty posture causes pain due to mechanical stresses on well-innervated joint capsules and ligaments (Kisner, Colby, 1990) and stretched nerve fibres within muscles (Mumenthaler, 1992; St. John, 1994). Initially, pain is felt in tissues that are experiencing a prolonged stretch. This pain is usually relieved by reducing the mechanical stresses placed on the affected structures, by changing position or by performing a different activity.

Over time, if these postural imbalances continue, an adaptive shortening of the muscles and fascia elsewhere in the body occurs in response to the stretched tissues. This adaptive shortening occurs to stabilize the body's posture.

There are other reasons why muscles and fascia shorten: following trauma, surgery or prolonged inactivity such as bedrest. Here the contractured scar tissue or shortened connective tissue limits the normal stretch of the soft tissues. In these cases, the pain is also a result of stress being placed on shortened tissues.

The combined tissue stretching and compensatory tissue shortening are called postural dysfunctions *(Kisner, Colby, 1990)*. Postural dysfunctions often contribute to secondary painful conditions. For example, a hyperkyphosis can contribute to adhesive capsulitis or bronchitis. Eventually, if these dysfunctions remain, the mechanical stresses will exceed the tissue's capabilities to accommodate them, resulting in tissue breakdown and overuse syndromes. At this stage, inflammation is present within the joints, tendons or muscles.

Postural Assessment Strategies

A thorough **postural assessment** by the therapist will help to indicate any imbalances and misalignments of the body. During the assessment, the bony prominences and joint positions provide landmarks for bilateral comparison. Relative muscle bulk and muscle outlines are observed bilaterally for symmetry. The source or contributing factors of a client's problem will frequently be revealed by this process. By combining the results of a postural assessment and specific muscle length and strength testing, a treatment plan can be formed to correct any imbalances, using both massage techniques and a remedial exercise plan.

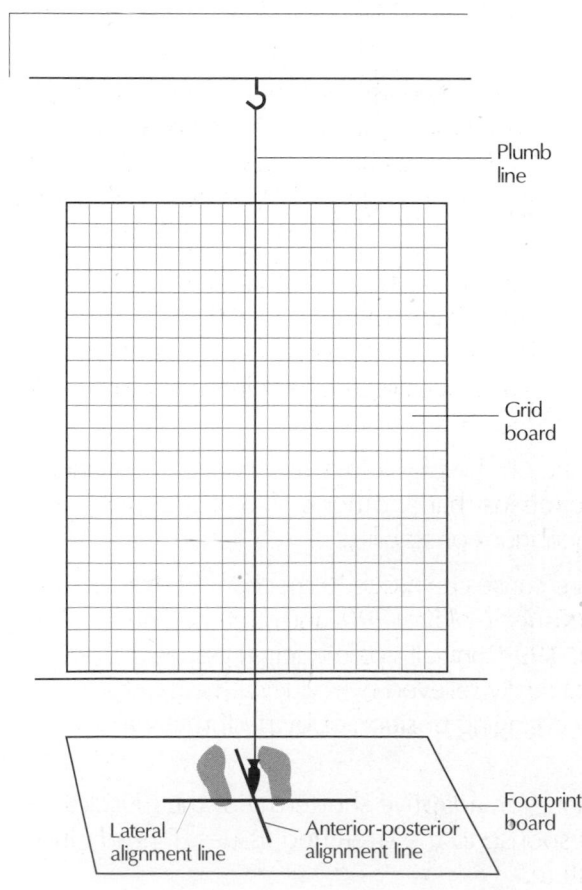

Plumb line

Grid board

Footprint board

Lateral alignment line

Anterior-posterior alignment line

Figure B.1
Plumb line set up in a clinical space.

Postural Assessment Equipment and Technique

The therapist uses a **plumb line** with plumb bob (or other suitable weight) as a reference line to check alignments in the client's body. The plumb line should be long enough to reach from the clinic ceiling to the floor. The plumb bob is suspended so it almost, but not quite, touches the floor *(Figure B.1)*.

A grid board — a background with a grid marked on it — is another tool for detecting postural imbalances *(Kendall, McCreary, 1983)*. The squares of the grid should be large enough to be easily seen, at least 5 centimetres square. The grid board should be larger than an average adult client — for example, 200 by 100 centimetres. The grid board is attached to the clinic room wall, so the grid lines are accurately horizontal and vertical. The bottom of the grid should touch the floor. The horizontal lines are useful for assessing the relative levels of pairs of bony landmarks.

A footprint board — a board with footprints marked on it — indicates where the client should stand relative to the plumb line *(Kendall, McCreary, 1983)*. Two intersecting reference lines for aligning the plumb bob may be marked on the footprint board.

One line is from front to back (on the median plane) equidistant between the two marked footprints. This is the plumb bob alignment for the anterior and posterior views. The other line is from left to right (on the coronal plane) through the footprints at the level of the lateral malleoli. This is the plumb bob alignment for lateral views.

The plumb line is suspended from the ceiling so it hangs about 100 centimetres from the wall in front of the grid board. The footprint board is also positioned on the clinic floor in front of the grid. The footprint board can be moved for different postural views, aligning the reference lines with the plumb bob.

✦ A **goniometer** is needed for more accurately measuring pelvic angles. A **measuring tape** is also useful, especially if the goniometer does not have a ruler marked on one arm.

✦ The therapist can ask the client to bring a bathing suit for the assessment so observation will not be limited by clothing. The client can also wear underwear only or a clinical gown, whichever is the most comfortable. The client is asked to stand comfortably with weight on both feet and the toes aligned on the coronal plane, arms at the sides and the head facing forward.

✦ The therapist should begin the assessment at the feet, moving towards the head, to understand how gravity is acting on the client's body and to note as many indicators of imbalances as possible. Both the posterior and anterior views are assessed, as well as the left and right lateral views.

✦ One strategy is to begin by marking the symmetry of the **bony landmarks** with the grid board, working inferiorly to superiorly. It is important for the therapist to **palpate** for the location of the bony landmarks rather than guessing their locations. For example, the superior aspects of both greater trochanters are located with the palpating index fingers of both hands. The levels of the two landmarks are compared using the nearest horizontal line on the grid board. In a posterior view, the therapist compares the levels of both lateral malleoli, fibular heads, greater trochanters, iliac crests and so on. This is followed by a visual scan for differences in the soft tissue: bilateral muscle bulk, skin creases and the orientation of the limbs.

✦ Another possibility is to assess the bony landmarks and the soft tissues together in the order that they occur, inferiorly to superiorly. For example, in a posterior view, a comparison is made of the height of the malleoli, the orientation of the Achilles tendons, the bulk of the gastrocnemius, the level of the fibular heads and so on.

Recording the Results

The findings are recorded on a body chart, as part of the regular health history, for later reference. The chart provides a baseline for charting the client's progress and the effectiveness of the therapist's plan. A body chart is a blank outline of the body, showing anterior, posterior and both lateral views *(Figure B.2)*. One sample of a body chart has various bony landmarks as well as vertical and horizontal register lines that pass through these landmarks for more accurate recording of information *(St. John, 1991)*.

✦ All findings, including asymmetrical ones, are recorded. For example, the client's right acromioclavicular joint is 3 centimetres higher than the left, according to the horizontal reference lines on the grid board. On the body chart, a diagonal line is drawn through the acromioclavicular joints, with the line slightly higher on the right side. The notation "3 cm. superior" or "⬆3 cm." is written beside the right acromioclavicular joint.

Body Chart

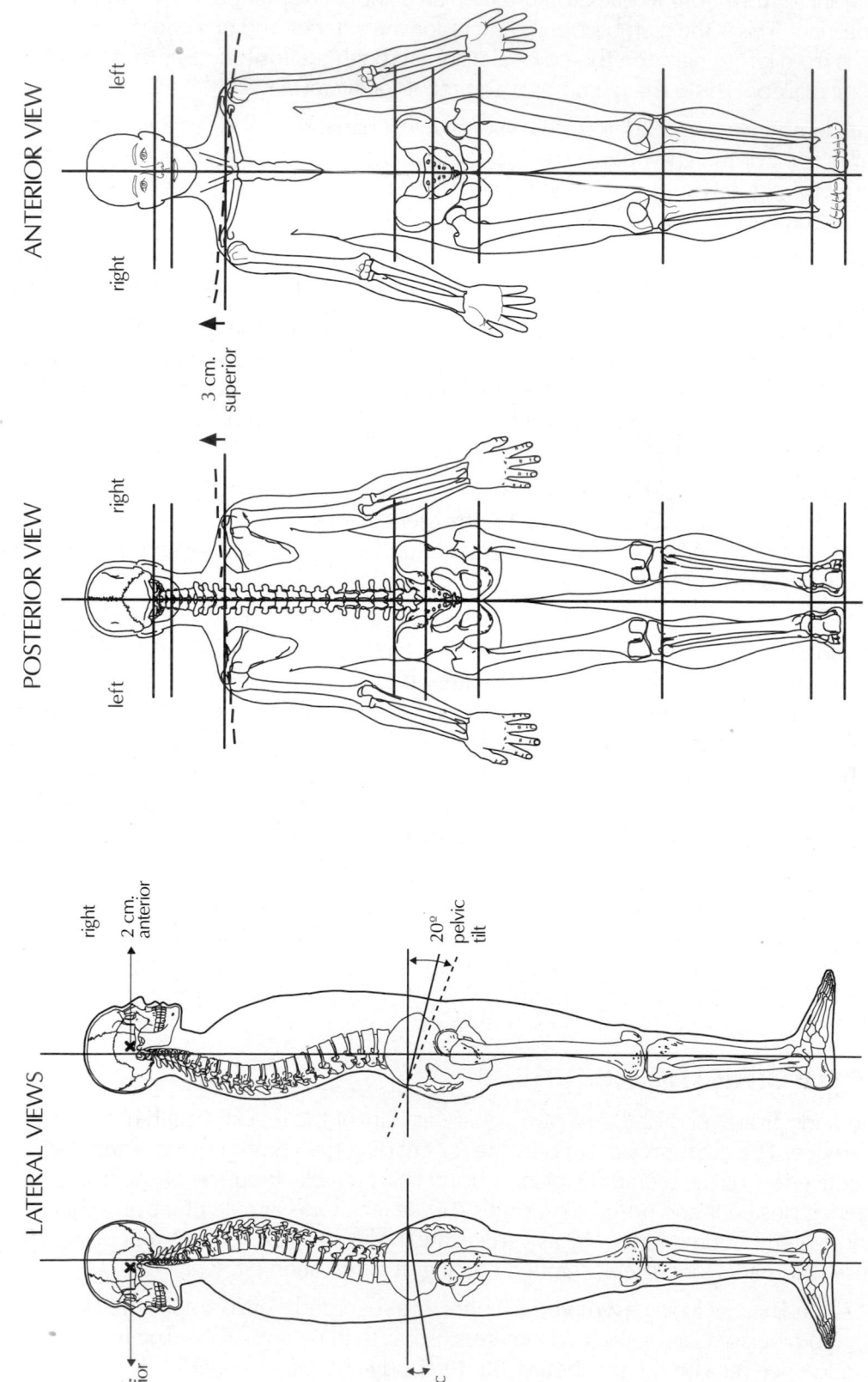

Figure B.2
Body Chart

Solid lines are included in the body chart to indicate the bony landmarks used for a postural assessment. Dotted or coloured lines are drawn onto the chart by the therapist to indicate the results of a postural assessment. For example, this assessment shows the right shoulder 3 cm. higher than the left, and 20° of anterior pelvic tilt on the right; head 2 cm. anterior. Arrows or words are used with the measurement to indicate the position of a structure out of alignment.

+ The therapist should regularly reassess the client's posture, especially if treatment occurs over several months or if it is concerned with altering a postural imbalance.

+ If a postural imbalance is noted, with the client's consent, polaroid photos may be taken of the appropriate posterior, lateral or anterior views *(Kendall, McCreary, 1983)*. The grid board and plumb line are included for reference. When the client's posture is reassessed after several treatments, new photos can be taken. This is useful for record keeping, educating the client and research purposes. The usual precautions for maintaining the confidentiality of the client's records applies to the postural assessment photos. For example, the photos are named, dated and kept in an envelope attached to the client's records. Any third party reporting or publishing research that includes the photographs requires the client's written consent to release them.

Posterior View

Position the client behind the plumb line with the plumb bob centred between the client's heels.

+ Assess the heights of the medial longitudinal arches of both feet: are they symmetrical; are the arches high or flat?

+ Compare the levels of both medial malleoli. A lower malleolus may indicate foot pronation.

+ Look for asymmetries in the orientation or width of both the Achilles tendons. Does one tendon and calcaneus have a valgus orientation, indicating foot pronation, or a varus orientation, indicating foot supination? Is one Achilles tendon wider than the other, indicating possible overuse?

+ Bilaterally assess for the relative muscle bulk of the gastrocnemius, soleus, hamstring and gluteal muscles. Compare the symmetry of the outline of the space between each leg. This space between body parts is called negative space. It can be used to make asymmetries more obvious to the therapist.

+ Palpate for, then using the grid board compare, the levels of the fibular heads.

+ Check for possible varus or valgus orientation of the knees.

+ Assess the skin fold levels at the knees and gluteals: if present, are they symmetrical? For example, asymmetry in the levels or lengths of the gluteal folds indicates postural imbalances, such as a lateral pelvic tilt or different leg lengths.

+ Palpate for, then using the grid board compare, the levels of both greater trochanters, both iliac crests and both posterior superior iliac spines (PSIS).

+ Observe the spinous processes for possible lateral rotation or scoliosis.

+ Check the symmetry of any skin folds present on the torso. Increased skin folds on one side could indicate a scoliosis or a lateral tilting of the torso towards that side.

+ Observe the orientation of the client's arm relative to the trunk by comparing the negative space between them.

+ Assess the levels of the inferior borders of both scapulae. Palpate for, and compare, the levels of the inferior angles of the scapulae. Compare the distance from the medial borders of the scapulae and spinous processes of the spine. Do the scapulae lie flat against the rib cage or are they winged posteriorly at the medial borders?

✦ Assess for the relative muscle bulk of the trapezius and erector spinae.

✦ Check the levels of the acromioclavicular joints using the grid board as a reference.

✦ Observe the head position for a possible lateral tilt by comparing the levels of the angles of the mandible, the levels of both external auditory meatus and the level of the occiput.

✦ Record any scars observed, since these may contribute to adhesions or fascial restrictions.

Anterior View

Position the client behind the plumb line with the plumb bob centred between the client's feet.

✦ Observe the orientation of the feet for pes varus ("pigeon toe", indicating internal femoral rotation) or pes valgus ("splay foot", indicating external femoral rotation).

✦ Check for pronation or supination of the medial longitudinal arches.

✦ Assess the knees for a possible valgus or varus orientation.

✦ Compare the levels of the superior surfaces of both patellae.

✦ Compare the relative bulk of the quadricep muscles.

✦ Palpate for, and using the grid board compare, the levels of both anterior superior iliac spines (ASIS) and then both iliac crests. Is a lateral pelvic tilt or unilateral anterior tilt present?

✦ Compare the levels of the fingertips with the grid board lines. Check the orientation of the hands to the thighs. Compare the distance each hand is from the thighs which may indicate a rotation of the spine or protraction or retraction of the scapulae. The direction the palms are facing can also indicate a possible rotation of the humerus.

✦ Assess the shape of the rib cage. Is one side flatter than the other? Is the rib cage depressed anteriorly? Is there a "barrel chest" (a superior and lateral flare of the rib cage)?

✦ Check the levels and angles of the clavicles for symmetry.

✦ Assess the position of the head. Is the head in midline, tilted laterally or rotated?

✦ Observe the position of the mandible. Is it in midline or deviated laterally?

✦ Check the levels of both external auditory meatus for symmetry.

✦ Record any scars observed.

Lateral Views

Assessment must be done for both left and right sides. It is essential for the therapist to observe both the left and right lateral views, since asymmetries are possible, as in the degree of pelvic tilt or in the rotation of one shoulder or hip.

Position the client behind the plumb line. Place the plumb bob slightly anterior to the lateral malleolus. With ideal posture, the plumb line will coincide with the following bony landmarks (*Kendall, McCreary, 1983*):

✦ slightly anterior to the lateral malleolus

✦ slightly anterior to the head of the fibula

♦ at the greater trochanter

♦ at the acromion

♦ at the external auditory meatus.

♦ Note if any of these bony landmarks are anterior or posterior to the plumb line, which is on the coronal plane. The greater trochanter may have to be palpated to locate it. If the landmarks are not in alignment with the plumb line, measure and note this on the body chart. With a ruler, measure from the plumb line either anteriorly or posteriorly to the landmark. For example, a client with shortened tibialis anterior and gluteus maximus muscles will be projected anteriorly to the coronal plane (St. John, 1991; Kendall, McCreary, 1983). The head of the fibula could be 1 centimetre anterior, the greater trochanter 2 centimetres anterior, the acromioclavicular joint 2.5 centimetres anterior and the external auditory meatus 3.5 centimetres anterior to the plumb line. Note these measurements on the body chart by, for example, putting a dot at the level of the head of the fibula, anterior to the coronal plane and recording "1 cm. anterior" or "1 cm. ➡" and so on for each landmark.

♦ Assess the orientation of the knees, checking for hyperextension, where the lateral epicondyle of the femur is posterior to the plumb line. Is only one knee visible or can both be seen? For example, in a left lateral view, if the right knee is visible anterior to the left one, the client's pelvis is likely rotated to the left.

♦ Check the levels of the ASIS and PSIS for the pelvic angle, also referred to as the pelvic tilt. To assess the pelvic tilt with a goniometer, first find the PSIS. (If the left lateral view is being assessed, the left PSIS is used.) Sit on a stool at the client's left side. Using the right hand, palpate for the inferior lip of the PSIS, hooking the palpating finger underneath the landmark. Hold the goniometer in the right hand against the client's left side, with the axis of the goniometer aligned with the palpating fingertip at the PSIS. Using the left hand, palpate for the left ASIS, hooking the palpating finger underneath the landmark. The arms of the goniometer are positioned so one arm is aligned with the fingertip at the ASIS and the other arm is aligned with the horizontal. (The horizontal lines on the grid board are useful for this.) Read the degree of pelvic tilt from the goniometer (Figure B.3). Record this on the left lateral view of the body chart in front of the ASIS as, for example, "3 degrees". This method of pelvic angle measurement has been found to be extremely accurate (Alviso et al. 1988).

• Assess the pelvic tilt approximately by marking the ASIS and the PSIS on the same side, using both hands held horizontally as marking points. Draw an imaginary line

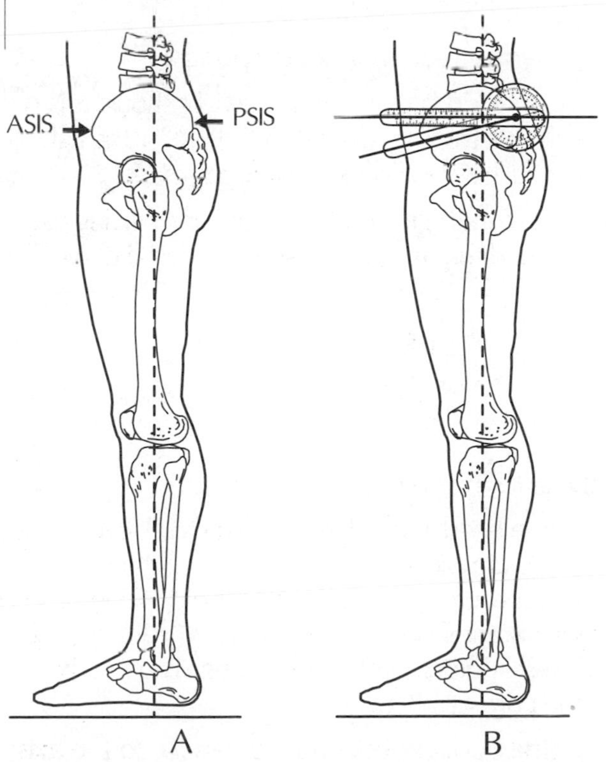

Figure B.3
(A) Landmarks and (B) goniometer placement for measuring pelvic tilt.

1055

between these points and compare the angle between this line and the horizontal.

- The normal position for the female pelvis is from five to 10 degrees of anterior pelvic tilt, while the normal position for the male pelvis is from zero to five degrees of anterior pelvic tilt *(St. John, 1991)*. Assess and compare both sides, to note if one side is more tilted than the other or if an anterior or posterior tilt is present bilaterally. An anterior pelvic tilt occurs when the anterior superior iliac spines have moved anteriorly and inferiorly. This is due to tight hip flexors and lumbar extensor muscles, which flex the hip, tilt the pelvis forward and increase the lumbar lordotic curve. With a posterior pelvic tilt, the anterior superior iliac spines move posteriorly and superiorly. Tight hip extensors and trunk flexors tilt the pelvis backwards and extend the hip *(Kisner, Colby, 1990)*.

- Health care professionals who have access to X-ray assessment determine the pelvic tilt in a different manner. The pelvis, in a neutral position, has the ASIS and the symphysis pubis in the same vertical plane. An anterior pelvic tilt means that a vertical plane drawn through the ASIS is anterior to a vertical plane drawn through the symphysis pubis. A posterior pelvic tilt means that the vertical plane through the ASIS is posterior to the vertical plane through the symphysis pubis *(Kendall et al., 1993)*.

✦ Assess for rotation of the pelvis. For example, in a left lateral view, if the right ASIS is visible anterior to the left one, the client's pelvis is rotated to the left.

✦ Check for possible lumbar hyperlordosis (an increase in the normal lumbar curve), lumbar hypolordosis (a decrease in the normal lumbar curve) or thoracic hyperkyphosis (an increase in the normal thoracic curve).

✦ Assess whether the shoulder is in a protracted, retracted or neutral position.

✦ Assess for rotation of the trunk. For example, in a left lateral view, if the right shoulder is visible anterior to the left one, either the client's trunk is rotated to the left or the right shoulder is protracted. See the superior postural view to confirm this assessment.

✦ Check for a cervical hyperlordosis (an increase in the normal cervical curve, giving rise to a head-forward posture) or hypolordosis (a decrease in the normal cervical curve, resulting in a head-retracted posture).

✦ Record any scars observed.

Superior View

Standing on a chair and looking down on the standing client:

✦ Confirm any laterally observed rotation of the head, shoulders and hands relative to the axis of the body and the coronal plane. For example, the position of the acromioclavicular joints is compared to the coronal plane to indicate the position of the shoulders. If the right acromioclavicular joint is anterior to the plane and the left is posterior to the plane, a right rotation of the shoulder girdle is occurring. The head may also be rotated to the left or right from the coronal plane.

✦ Confirm any laterally observed rotation of the pelvis, knees and feet relative to the axis of the body and the coronal plane. For example, the positions of both ASIS are compared to the coronal plane to indicate the position of the pelvis.

Gait Assessment

An understanding of the gait cycle aids the therapist in interpreting observations of the client's gait *(Buschbacher, 1994; Magee 1992)*. The normal gait cycle is viewed from the perspective of one foot or the other. The distance from the point of first contact of one foot to the point of first contact of the opposite foot is termed the step length. The distance from the point of contact of one foot to the next point of contact of the same foot is called the stride length. Two steps, for example a left and a right step, equal one stride.

The gait cycle *(Figure B.4)* is divided into a **stance phase,** when the foot is in contact with the ground and bearing weight, and a **swing phase**, when the foot is not fixed to the ground and is non-weight-bearing. Both the stance and stride phases are further divided into subphases, or instants.

At the beginning of the stance phase, one foot is coming off the ground, while the other foot begins weight bearing. This is called **initial contact**, or heel strike, since the heel is usually the first point of contact. The weight of the trunk is aligned between the two limbs. Next comes **load response**, or foot flat, as the person instinctively assesses whether the foot will bear the weight of the body. The foot is in pronation to allow it to adapt to

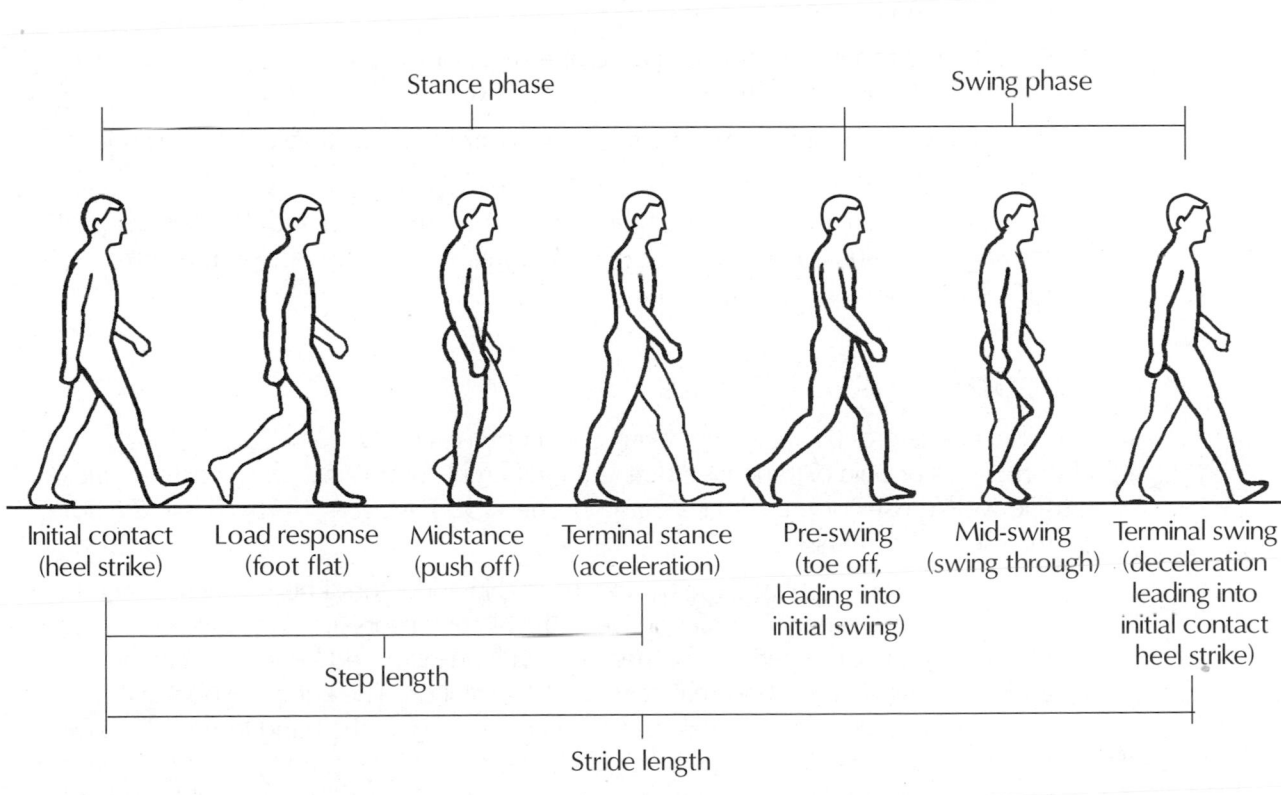

| Initial contact (heel strike) | Load response (foot flat) | Midstance (push off) | Terminal stance (acceleration) | Pre-swing (toe off, leading into initial swing) | Mid-swing (swing through) | Terminal swing (deceleration leading into initial contact heel strike) |

Figure B.4
The gait cycle of the right foot.

different terrain and posture, while the trunk is aligned over the stance leg. **Midstance**, or push off, occurs next. As the foot supports the body, the hip and knee move into extension. The trunk is still aligned over the stance leg and the pelvis drops slightly over the swing leg. This is followed by the **terminal stance**, or the acceleration phase, when the hip, knee and ankle begin to flex and the heel comes up off the ground. The trunk now shifts towards the new stance leg. The last part of the stance phase is **pre-swing**, or toe off. Here only the toes are in contact with the ground.

The gait cycle next moves into the swing phase. During **initial swing**, the hip continues to flex and medially rotate as the knee flexes. The ankle moves into dorsiflexion to clear the ground, while the trunk is aligned with the new stance leg. In **mid-swing**, the hip, knee and ankle continue to flex. In **terminal swing**, or deceleration, the hip flexes and medially rotates and the knee moves into maximum extension. The ankle dorsiflexes and supinates, while the trunk weight remains over the stance leg.

Technique

+ The therapist makes observations of the client's gait to further locate any postural imbalances. The client is barefoot and dressed in a clinical gown, underwear or bathing suit for the assessment so the observation will not be limited by clothing. The therapist instructs the client to walk at a normal pace, while the motion of the toes, feet, legs, pelvis and trunk are noted.

+ Anteriorly, the therapist observes for the foot position during the gait cycle, any lateral pelvic tilt and the position of the trunk.

+ Laterally, the relative position and ease of motion of the ankle, knee, hip and low back are noted during all the subphases of the gait cycle.

+ Posteriorly, the therapist observes for the foot and heel positions, and the motions of the knees, pelvis and trunk.

+ The client is then asked to walk in the footwear usually worn and the therapist makes the same anterior, lateral and posterior observations. This may assist in determining how the client's shoes affect the gait pattern.

Recording the Results

Specific muscle groups are active during the subphases of the gait cycle. Gait abnormalities or pain experienced during the different subphases may reveal specific muscle weaknesses or pathologies *(Buschbacher, 1994; Magee, 1992)*. These are noted on the client's health history.

+ In the initial contact phase, the hip extensors, hip adductors, knee extensors and flexors and the foot dorsiflexors are all active. If the hip extensors are weak, allowing the trunk to lurch forward, the person compensates with an increased lordosis. Weak hip adductors result in an abnormal pelvis and leg rotation. The knee will buckle if its extensors and flexors are weak and the person may use the hand to push the knee into extension. This weakness may be caused by reflex inhibition, an L2 through L4 nerve root lesion, internal knee derangement or poliomyelitis. Weak foot dorsiflexors will allow the foot to drop or slap down on heel strike. This weakness may be due to a peroneal neuropathy or an L4 nerve root lesion. Pain in the heel on initial contact may be due to a heel spur, a bruise or bursitis.

✦ During midstance, the hip abductors and foot plantarflexors are active. A lesion of the L5 nerve root results in gluteus medius weakness, and a Trendelenburg gait or lurch occurs as the pelvis on the non-weight-bearing side is allowed to drop. Weakness in the plantarflexors from an S1-S2 nerve root lesion results in a short step on the unaffected side. Pain in the weight bearing ankle or foot may be due to osteoarthritis, pes planus or plantar fasciitis.

✦ In the terminal stance, the hip flexors and knee extensors are active. Weak hip flexors cause the person to compensate by moving the trunk posteriorly to passively swing the leg. This is called gluteus maximus gait. Weak knee extensors allow the knee to buckle.

✦ During the pre-swing phase, the hip adductors are active. Weakness of these muscles allows the leg to rotate. Hallux rigidus will cause the person to push off from the lateral aspect of the foot instead of the great toe.

✦ In the initial swing and mid-swing phase, the foot dorsiflexors are active. An L4 nerve root lesion results in foot drop or steppage gait.

✦ During terminal swing, the knee flexors are active to slow the knee extension. An S1-S2 nerve root lesion allows the knee to snap out excessively at the end of the swing.

Other common gait abnormalities are as follows.

• A person with antalgic gait is attempting to protect against further injury to the foot, ankle, knee, hip or low back. The stance phase on the affected leg is shorter as the person attempts to quickly remove weight from the affected leg.

• Ataxic gait is seen with poor sensation in the extremities or loss of muscle coordination. The person keeps the feet farther apart for balance and may exaggerate all movements.

• A person with hemiplegic gait swings the affected leg into abduction and flexion. Frequently, the affected arm is held in some degree of shoulder adduction, elbow and wrist flexion and pronation of the forearm.

• Parkinsonian gait, also called festinating gait, is characterized by short, shuffling steps. The person holds the knees, trunk and neck in flexion and the arms move stiffly (Magee, 1992).

• At this point, other orthopedic tests including active free range of motion, passive relaxed range of motion, overpressure, muscle length tests and active resisted strength tests are performed on joints and muscles where imbalances are observed. The client's symptom picture will also help to indicate where these tests are necessary to determine the tissues affected by the client's complaint.

Appendix C:

SPECIAL ORTHOPEDIC TESTING

Linda Ludwig, Fiona Rattray

The following standard orthopedic tests assist the therapist in assessing the client's condition. The most common tests and methods of performing them are described, with some variations included. They are listed under names most frequently used in source textbooks, although some tests may be known by other names. This appendix covers all the tests named in the treatment chapters. There are many other orthopedic tests and it is recommended that the reader refer to additional sources on orthopedic testing for further information as needed.

The basic principles regarding assessment are reviewed in the Assessment chapter. Ranges of motion definitions, end feel interpretations and suggested testing progressions are found there. It is useful to remember that the range of motion that causes the client pain is performed **last**.

This appendix is arranged into tests that pertain to specific body regions, starting with the head and progressing to the feet. General and sensory tests that are used on any part of the body are listed at the end. For each body region, the tests are generally arranged to start with active free tests, then passive relaxed tests and, finally, active resisted tests.

The client's usual and expected responses to an orthopedic test, when experiencing a particular condition, are given in the section on assessment in each treatment chapter. If a test result is different from what is expected, the therapist should repeat the testing procedure, since it is possible that it was not performed correctly. However, due to variances in human anatomy — the absence of some muscles (such as palmaris longus); variations in the locations of specific muscle attachments; and differing degrees of flexibility, strength and hypermobility — it is possible for the results of tests to be inconclusive or falsely negative or positive even when they are correctly performed (*Gerard, Kleinfield, 1993*).

Quick Reference for Appendix C

Head and Neck Tests:

Shoulder Tests:

Arm, Wrist and Hand Tests:

Trunk, Low Back and Abdomen Tests:

Head and Neck Tests

Vertebral Artery Test

To assess for circulation deficiency of the vertebral artery at the transverse foramen:

- Place the client in a seated position.
- Instruct the client to rotate the head fully to one side and then extend the neck and hold for 30 seconds.
- Repeat the test on the other side. Instruct the client to rotate the head fully and then extend the neck.
  - The test is **positive** for ischemia or circulation deficiency of the vertebral artery if the client complains of a feeling of dizziness or of nystagmus (an involuntary,

repetitive, circular motion of the eyes) or both (*Gerard, Kleinfield, 1993*). Common causes of vertebral artery occlusion are arteriosclerosis, atheroma, severe cervical osteoarthritis and rheumatoid arthritis of the cervical spine.

A variation:

- Place the client in a supine position.

- Passively fully extend the head and neck, then fully rotate the head to one side, holding this position for 30 seconds.

- Repeat by rotating the client's head to the other side while maintaining the neck in extension.

  ✦ The test is **positive** for circulation deficiency of the vertebral artery if the client reports vertigo and nausea, and the eyes show signs of nystagmus.

  ✦ If the test is **positive**, with either version, the client's head is smoothly and quickly returned to the neutral position. Do not perform further testing (*Magee, 1992*). Refer the client to a physician for **medical assessment**.

Temporomandibular Joint, AF ROM

To assess for the motion of the mandible at the temporomandibular joint:

- Place the client in a seated position.

- Stand behind the client.

- Place the index fingers of both hands just anterior to each of the client's external auditory meatus, with the pads of the fingers resting on the posterior portion of the mandibular condyles, allowing the motion of both the temporomandibular joints to be palpated simultaneously.

- Instruct the client to open and close the mandible slowly and fully.

- Assess the quality of motion at the condyles of the mandible. This motion should feel bilaterally symmetrical and smooth.

  ✦ **Positive** signs of temporomandibular dysfunction are clicking, crepitus, asymmetry of motion and pain.

Further assessment of mandibular motion:

- Place the client in a supine position.

- Sit at the head of the table, observing the client's upside-down face.

- Instruct the client to part the lips with the jaw closed.

- Note the alignment of the upper and lower incisors relative to each other.

- Instruct the client to open and close the mandible slowly and fully, keeping the lips parted. In the first centimetre of mandibular depression, observe for a pivoting of the mandible before it slides anteriorly. The mandible should depress and elevate in a straight line.

- As an alternative, place the client in a standing position.

- Stand face to face with the client and instruct the client to open and close the mandible slowly and fully, keeping the lips parted, as above. Observe for pivoting.

✦ **Positive** signs of temporomandibular dysfunction are asymmetrical motion, hesitation in motion and a lateral deviation or wobble in the movement of the mandible. An S-shaped wobble indicates a muscular source of the dysfunction. A C-shaped wobble indicates a capsular source, with the mandible deviating to the side that is capsularly restricted *(Magee, 1992; Hertling, Kessler, 1996)*.

Three-Knuckle Test

To demonstrate the available active range of depression of the mandible:

- Instruct the client to open the jaw and insert as many of her own flexed proximal interphalangeal joints of the non-dominant hand *(Travell, Simons, 1983)* between the upper and lower incisors as is possible. The functional width of mandibular opening is two or three knuckles wide.

  ✦ A **positive** test for temporomandibular joint hypomobility is indicated if the client can get only one knuckle or no knuckles at all between the incisors.

Swallowing Test

To determine whether pain on swallowing is due to referred pain from a sternocleidomastoid muscle trigger point:

- Place the client in a seated position.
- Palpate the sternocleidomastoid muscle in a pincer grasp. When the most tender point in the muscle is found, maintain firm pressure on the muscle belly while the client swallows.

  ✦ If the pain diminishes while the client swallows, the test is **positive** for trigger points as the cause of the pain *(Travell, Simons, 1983)*.

To determine if pain is due to another pathology:

- If pain is experienced on swallowing **without** the sternocleidomastoid muscle being compressed, the pain may be due to throat infection, hematoma, bony protuberance of the cervical spine or tumour.

  ✦ If this variation of the swallowing test is **positive** following a trauma to the cervical spine, refer the client to a physician, since a hematoma may be present *(Hoppenfeld, 1976)*.

Scalene Cramp Test

To reproduce the pain of active scalene trigger points:

- Place the client in a seated position.
- Fully rotate the head to the affected side. By contracting the affected scalenes the neck is flexed to the same side. Pull the chin inferiorly into the hollow just posterior to the clavicle.

  ✦ A **positive** test for active scalene trigger points is indicated by pain in the referred pattern for the scalene muscles *(Travell, Simons, 1983)*.

Scalene Relief Test

To assess for the presence of active trigger points in the anterior scalene muscle:

- Place the client in a seated position.

- Instruct the client to place the forearm on the affected side across the forehead, as close to the elbow as possible.

- Instruct the client to elevate and protract the shoulder, which lifts the clavicle, relieving any compression of the scalenes and brachial plexus.

  ✦ A **positive** test for the presence of active trigger points in the anterior scalene muscle is indicated by the reduction of pain within a few minutes. Pain due to a cervical radiculopathy is not affected by this test *(Travell, Simons, 1983)*.

Atlanto-occipital Articulation, PR ROM

To assess movement (flexion and extension, coupled with sidebending) at the atlanto-occipital joints:

- Place the client supine on the table.

- Stand at the head of the table and grasp the client's head in both hands, placing the hands on the occipital region.

- To assess the **flexion and sidebending components** of this articulation, flex the client's cervical spine to end range. This locks the lower cervical spine in flexion, eliminating any movement from these vertebrae.

- Using small movements, apply a laterally directed pressure to the head, from left to right, and then from right to left. The client's eyes are kept on the horizontal plane during this slight lateral motion.

  ✦ A **positive** result, indicating a flexion and sidebending restriction at the atlanto-occipital articulation, is palpated as a subtle leathery end feel in either left or right flexion and sidebending *(Hertling, Kessler, 1990; Greenman, 1989)*.

- To check the **extension and sidebending components**, slightly extend the head, without bringing it off the table. This action rotates the head on the sagittal plane around an imaginary axis drawn through both external auditory meatus.

- Apply a laterally directed pressure to the head, from left to right and then from right to left. The motion is subtle. The client's eyes are kept on the horizontal plane during this lateral motion.

  ✦ A **positive** result, indicating an extension and sidebending restriction at the atlanto-occipital articulation, is palpated as a subtle leathery end feel in either left or right extension and sidebending *(Greenman, 1989)*.

Note: The flexion-sidebending and extension-sidebending tests can be performed one after the other.

Atlanto-axial Articulation, PR ROM

To evaluate the movement (mostly rotation) present at the atlanto-axial articulation:

- Place the client in a supine position.

- Stand at the head of the table and grasp the client's head in both hands at the temporal region, while flexing the cervical spine to end range. This locks the lower cervical spine in flexion, eliminating any rotation from these vertebrae.
- While flexion is maintained, rotate the head fully to both sides.
  - ✦ A **positive** result, indicating a rotational restriction, is palpated as a leathery end feel in either left or right rotation *(Greenman, 1989)*.

Spurling's Test

To assess for compression of a cervical nerve root or for facet joint irritation in the lower cervical spine:

- Place the client in a seated position.
- Stand behind the client.
- Instruct the client to slowly extend, sidebend and rotate the head to the affected side.
- Carefully apply compression downward on the client's head. The combined action of the client's head position and the downward pressure compresses the intervertebral foramen, the nerve root and the facet joints on that side.
  - ✦ A **positive** test is indicated by radiating pain or other neurological signs in the arm on the affected side. The distribution of the pain indicates which nerve root is involved. Pain remaining local to the neck or shoulder indicates cervical facet joint irritation on the side being tested *(Gerard, Kleinfield, 1993)*.
- **Do not** perform this test if the vertebral artery test is positive.

Cervical Compression Test

A variation, the **cervical compression test**, is used when the client cannot rotate or extend the head:

- Position the client as above.
- Stand behind the client.
- With the client's head in a neutral position, carefully apply compression downward on the client's head.
  - ✦ A **positive** test is indicated by radiating pain or other neurological signs in the affected arm. Pain remaining local to the neck or shoulder indicates cervical facet joint irritation on the side experiencing pain *(Hoppenfeld, 1976)*.

Cervical Distraction Test

To relieve pressure on the cervical nerve roots (particularly following Spurling's or cervical compression test):

- Place the client in a seated or supine position.
- Grasp the client's head at the occiput and temporal areas.
- Return the head to the anatomically neutral position.
- Apply a slow traction in a superior direction, maintaining traction for at least 30

seconds to allow the cervical muscles to relax.

✦ A reduction of the client's pain is a **positive** finding for this test and may be due to opening the intervertebral foramina, reducing pressure on the facet joints or relieving muscle spasm *(Magee, 1992)*.

First Rib Mobility Test

To assess the mobility of the first rib:

- Place the client in a seated position.

- Instruct the client to rotate the head fully away from the affected side and then flex the head forward to the chest as far as possible.

  ✦ A **positive** test for first rib hypomobility is indicated by limited flexion. Scalene hypertonicity or fascial restrictions may cause the hypomobilty.

First variation:

- Place the client in a supine position.

- Place one hand immediately inferior to the medial clavicle, on the first rib.

- Place the other hand on the posterior aspect of the neck, just lateral to the spine at the level of the first rib.

- Apply alternating pressure, directed anteriorly and posteriorly on the rib.

Second variation:

- Place the client in a supine position.

- Place the index or second finger in the hollow just posterior to the clavicle, where the first rib is palpated.

- Instruct the client to inhale and exhale while the motion of the rib is assessed.

  ✦ A **positive** test for either variation is indicated by hypomobility of the rib *(Buschbacher, 1994)*.

Anterior Neck Flexors Strength Test, AR

To assess the strength of the sternocleidomastoids, anterior scalenes, suprahyoids, infrahyoids, longus capitis, longus colli and rectus capitis anterior muscles:

- Place the client in a supine position with the arms abducted to 90 degrees, elbows flexed and the back of the hands resting on the table. This position reduces the effects of shoulder muscle recruitment.

- Instruct the client to tuck in the chin, and then to lift the head off the table, flexing the cervical spine. If the client can maintain the head position against gravity this indicates three on the strength scale (see muscle strength grading in General Tests).

- If the head position can be maintained against gravity, apply posteriorly directed pressure to the client's forehead, instructing the client not to let the head be pushed posteriorly.

  ✦ The test is **positive** for anterior neck muscle weakness if the client is unable to hold this position *(Kendall et al., 1993)*.

Anterolateral Neck Flexors Strength Test, AR

To assess the strength of the sternocleidomastoid and the scalene muscles on one side:

- Place the client in a supine position on the table with the arms abducted to 90 degrees, the elbows flexed and the back of the hands resting on the table, reducing shoulder muscle recruitment.

- Stabilize the shoulder on the side to be tested and instruct the client to rotate the face away from the side to be assessed.

- Instruct the client to lift the head into slight flexion and hold it in this position against gravity.

- If the client can hold this position against gravity, this indicates three on the strength scale (see muscle strength grading in General Tests).

- Push against the temporal region on the side being tested, in an oblique posterolateral direction away from the side being tested.

  + The test is **positive** for anterolateral neck muscle weakness if the client is unable to hold this position *(Kendall et al., 1993)*.

Posterolateral Neck Flexors Strength Test, AR

To assess the strength of splenius capitis, splenius cervicis, semispinalis capitis, semispinalis cervicis and cervical erector spinae on one side:

- Place the client in a prone position with the arms abducted to 90 degrees, the elbows flexed and the palms of the hands on the table, reducing the ability to recruit shoulder muscles.

- Instruct the client to extend the neck, rotate the head **towards** the side being tested and hold the head in this position against gravity.

- If the client can hold this position against gravity, this indicates three on the strength scale (see muscle strength grading in General Tests).

- Stabilize the shoulder on the side being tested.

- Apply pressure against the posterolateral head and attempt to push the head obliquely anterior, away from the side being tested.

  + The test is **positive** for weakness of the posterolateral neck muscles if the client is unable to hold the head in this position *(Kendall et al., 1993)*.

To assess the strength of the upper trapezius:

- Position the client as above, except that the head is rotated **away** from the side being tested.

- Instruct the client to hold the head in this position against gravity.

- If the client can hold this position against gravity, this indicates three on the strength scale (see muscle strength grading in General Tests).

- Stabilize the shoulder on the side being tested.

- Apply pressure on the posterior head, attempting to push the head obliquely anterior, away from the side being tested.

✦ A **positive** sign of muscle weakness is the client's inability to hold the head against pressure *(Kendall et al., 1993)*.

Orbicularis Oris Strength Test, AR

To confirm Bell's palsy:

- The client can be seated or supine.
- Instruct the client to keep her eyes closed.
- Gently try to open the eyes. Because the eyes are a sensitive area, have clean hands and do not use excessive force.
    - ✦ The test is **positive** if the client is unable to resist this action and the eye on the affected side is opened.

Sinus Transillumination Test

To test for infection of the frontal and maxillary sinuses:

- Perform the test in a dark room using a very bright, small flashlight. Place a clear plastic bag over the flashlight and dispose of the bag after the test for sanitary purposes.
- To assess the maxillary sinus, instruct the client to place the flashlight against the roof of the opened mouth. A normal maxillary sinus shows as a bright red glow in the area occupied by the sinus on the anterior aspect of the client's cheek.
- Remove the plastic bag from the flashlight and discard, then assess the frontal sinus. Instruct the client to close the eyes and hold the flashlight against the medial aspect of the superior orbital margin (just below the medial aspect of the eyebrow). A normal frontal sinus shows as a red glow on the forehead over the vertical part of the sinus.
    - ✦ A blocked and infected sinus does not transilluminate (glow red), which is a **positive** test result *(Moore, 1985)*.

Shoulder Tests

Adson's Test

To assess for thoracic outlet syndrome caused by the anterior scalene muscle:

- Place the client in a seated position.
- Stand behind the client.
- Extend and slightly externally rotate the client's affected arm.
- Monitor the radial pulse of this arm.
- Instruct the client to rotate the head **towards** the affected side, to slightly elevate the chin and to take a deep breath, holding it for at least 15 to 20 seconds. This action elevates the first rib, compressing the neurovascular bundle against the tight anterior scalene muscle.
    - ✦ A **positive** test is indicated by a diminished radial pulse or recurrence of the client's symptoms *(Travell, Simons, 1983)*.

Travell's Variation on Adson's Test

To assess for the middle scalene muscle as the possible cause of a client's thoracic outlet syndrome:

- Place the client in a seated position, as in Adson's test.
- Stand behind the client.
- Extend and slightly externally rotate the client's affected arm.
- Monitor the radial pulse of this arm.
- Instruct the client to rotate the head **away** from the affected side and to take a deep breath, holding it for at least 15 to 20 seconds. The first rib is elevated, compressing the neurovascular bundle against the tight middle scalene muscle.
  - ✦ Diminishment of the pulse or recurrence of the symptoms indicates a **positive** test for the middle scalene muscle involvement (*Travell, Simons, 1983*).

Wright's Hyperabduction Test

To assess pectoralis minor muscle as the possible cause of thoracic outlet syndrome:

- Place the client in a seated position.
- Stand behind the client.
- Passively fully abduct the client's affected arm to 180 degrees and then slightly extend the arm. This places a stretch and torsion on the brachial plexus and axillary artery as they pass inferior to the pectoralis minor muscle.
- Monitor the radial pulse as the arm is held in hyperabduction.
  - ✦ A diminishment of the radial pulse or recurrence of the client's symptoms is **positive** for a tight pectoralis minor muscle (*Travell, Simons, 1983*).

Costoclavicular Syndrome Test

To assess for thoracic outlet syndrome caused by compression of the neurovascular bundle between the clavicle and the first rib:

- Place the client in a seated position.
- Stand behind the client and monitor the affected arm's radial pulse.
- Passively depress and retract the shoulder of the affected arm.
  - ✦ A **positive** test is indicated by a diminished pulse or an increase in symptoms.

Eden's Test

To further assess compression of the neurovascular bundle between the clavicle and the first rib:

- Place the client in a standing position with arms at the side.
- Stand behind the client and monitor the affected arm's radial pulse.
- Instruct the client to bring the shoulders as far into retraction and depression as possible.

✦ A **positive** test is indicated by a diminished pulse or an increase in symptoms (*Gerard, Kleinfield, 1993*).

Upper Limb Tension Tests

Four tests determine whether cervical nerve roots and peripheral nerves are the source of the client's shoulder or arm pain. The peripheral nerves and the nerve roots are stretched in these tests, similar to the straight leg raise test. Depending on the position of the arm, elbow and wrist, specific nerves can be stressed. These tests can be performed adequately when restricted range of motion at the shoulder makes tests requiring full range of motion — such as Adson's and Wright's — difficult to perform.

• Place the client in a supine position for all four tests, with the side to be tested close to the edge of the table.

• With one hand, grasp the client's shoulder and apply a constant depressive force to it. With the other hand, hold the client's wrist and move the arm into the various positions described below.

Upper Limb Tension Test 1 (ULTT1)

To assess C5, C6, C7 and the median nerve as the source of the client's painful shoulder or arm:

• First, abduct the humerus to approximately 110 degrees. Extend the arm to 10 degrees below the coronal plane and to 60 degrees of external rotation. A stretching sensation is normally experienced across the anterior shoulder.

• Second, slowly extend the client's wrist, then the fingers. Tingling is normally experienced in the lateral three digits.

• Third, fully supinate the forearm, then slowly extend the elbow. A stretching sensation is normally experienced in the anterior elbow.

✦ Reproducing the client's original shoulder or arm pain is a **positive** sign for C5 to C7 nerve roots or the median nerve as the source of the pain.

If this position does not reproduce the pain, a fourth step (the sensitizing test) is added:

• Sidebend the client's neck to the side opposite the one being tested.

• Repeat the test from steps one to three. The neck position places a further stretch on the nerve roots.

✦ A **positive** test is reproduction of the client's symptoms.

• If the symptoms are reproduced, bend the client's neck back towards the side being tested. The symptoms should diminish.

Note: The sensitizing test can be added to the following tests.

ULTT2

To assess the median, musculocutaneous and axillary nerves:

• Depress the client's shoulder and abduct the humerus to 10 degrees.

- Slowly extend the wrist and fingers.
- Fully supinate the forearm and extend the elbow. Tissue tightness in the shoulder or elbow, or tingling in the fingers is a normal response.
  - ✦ A **positive** test is reproduction of the client's symptoms.

ULTT3

To assess the radial nerve:

- Depress the client's shoulder and abduct the humerus to 10 degrees.
- Slowly flex the wrist and fingers and deviate them ulnarly.
- Fully pronate the forearm and extend the elbow. As before, tissue tightness and tingling are normal.
  - ✦ A **positive** test is reproduction of the client's symptoms.

ULTT4

To assess C8 and T1 nerve roots and the radial nerve:

- Depress the client's shoulder and abduct the humerus to 90 degrees.
- Flex the elbow, bringing the hand towards the client's ear.
- Supinate the forearm.
- Slowly extend the wrist and fingers and deviate them radially. As before, tissue tightness and tingling are normal.
  - ✦ A **positive** test is reproduction of the client's symptoms (*Magee, 1997*).

Neer Impingement Test

To assess for overuse injury to the supraspinatus tendon:

- Place the client in a seated position.
- Passively flex the client's humerus forward through its range, compressing the tendons against the acromion.
  - ✦ Pain indicates a **positive** test.

Hawkins-Kennedy Impingement Test

A variation, the **Hawkins-Kennedy impingement test:**

- Flex the client's arm forward to 90 degrees, then internally rotate the humerus. This compresses the supraspinatus tendon against the coracoid process.
  - ✦ Pain indicates a **positive** test (*Magee, 1997*).

Painful Arc Test

To assess for subacromial impingement of supraspinatus tendon and subacromial bursa:

- Instruct the client to abduct the humerus through full range.

    - ✦ A **positive** test is pain starting at about 70 degrees of abduction, which eases off after about 130 degrees of abduction *(Bunker, Wallace, 1991)*. In this range the soft tissues are compressed by the humerus against the acromion. Before and after the range the tissues are no longer compressed. The pain must lessen above 130 degrees.

- When the client cannot actively move beyond this range, assist the client to 130 degrees and then ask the client to continue if possible *(Souza, 1997)*.

Apley's Scratch Test

To assess combined movements at the shoulder:

- Place the client in a seated position.
- Stand behind the client to observe the range of motion.
- Instruct the client to reach behind the head to touch as far down the spine as possible with the fingertips. This assesses external rotation and abduction of one glenohumeral joint.
- Instruct the client to reach up, at the same time, behind the back with the other hand, touching as far up the spine as possible. This action checks internal rotation and adduction of the other glenohumeral joint.
- Note the location of the fingertips of each hand according to the thoracic vertebral level.
- Instruct the client to reverse the position of arms.
- Repeat the test to assess the full range of motion of both glenohumeral joints.
- Compare the available ranges of both shoulders.
- As motions are combined in this test, it is important to correctly assess which individual movements are restricted and which are not. Therefore, it may be necessary to follow this test with the individual cardinal planes of shoulder motion to track down the specific limited range.

Shoulder Apprehension Test, AF

To explore a previous glenohumeral dislocation only when the injury has progressed to the chronic stage:

- Instruct the client to **slowly** move the arm and joint into the position in which the dislocation took place; for example, abduction with extension and external rotation.

    - ✦ A look of apprehension on the client's face or an unwillingness to complete the range of motion indicates a **positive** test and means that the glenohumeral joint capsule is probably unstable.

- With a positive result, **do not** perform PR range of motion testing, to avoid further injuring the joint capsule; progress instead to AR isometric testing of the muscles that cross the glenohumeral joint.
- If the AF apprehension test is **negative**, progress to the PR apprehension test.

Shoulder Apprehension Test, PR

To passively assess the integrity of the glenohumeral joint capsule following a chronic dislocation:

- **Slowly** move the arm and joint towards the position in which the injury took place.

- With an anterior glenohumeral joint dislocation, stand slightly behind and to one side of the client, placing one hand on the back of the client's affected shoulder to stabilize it.

- **Slowly** abduct the client's arm.

- Monitor the client's face for signs of apprehension that the joint may redislocate, while slowly externally rotating the humerus.

    ✦ A **positive** result is indicated if the client has a look of apprehension or pulls away from the therapist to stop the motion. The end feel is empty. This positive result indicates that either the joint capsule has not fully healed or the severity of the dislocation has compromised the joint's stability.

- If the test is **negative**, carefully challenge the joint in an anterior direction to further assess its integrity. Use the stabilizing hand on the client's posterior shoulder to create overpressure. If it is possible to apply this overpressure to the joint without apprehension on the client's part, the joint is considered stable, despite the previous injury.

Adhesive Capsulitis Abduction Test, PR

To test for restricted motion at the shoulder resulting from fibrosing and adhesion of the axillary fold of the inferior glenohumeral joint capsule:

- Place the client in a seated position.

- Stand behind the client.

- Palpate the inferior angle of the scapula and with one hand monitor its position throughout the test.

- With the other hand just proximal to the client's elbow, slowly, passively abduct the client's humerus, noting when the inferior angle of the scapula begins to move. In a normal shoulder, a leathery end feel is encountered at greater than 90 degrees of abduction of the humerus. The axillary fold is stretched and the scapula begins to move along with the humerus at greater than 90 degrees of abduction.

    ✦ A **positive** result for a frozen shoulder has a painful, leathery end feel encountered anywhere before 90 degrees of abduction. Since the axillary fold is fibrosed, the scapula begins to move before 90 degrees of abduction *(Donatelli, 1991)*.

Acromioclavicular Shear Test

To assess the integrity of the acromioclavicular joint:

- Place the client in a seated position.

- Stand behind the client.

- Place cupped hands over the client's shoulder, the fingers interlaced, with one palm on the clavicle and the other on the spine of the scapula.

- Slowly squeeze the heels of the hands together.
    - ✦ A **positive** test, resulting in pain or excessive movement of the joint, indicates joint pathology, including acromioclavicular joint sprain *(Magee, 1992)*.

Drop Arm Test

To assess the integrity of the rotator cuff, especially the supraspinatus muscle and tendon:
- Place the client in a seated position.
- Abduct the arm to 90 degrees and instruct the client to hold the arm in this position.
- Instruct the client to slowly adduct the arm back to the starting point.
    - ✦ The test is **positive** if the client is unable to return the arm smoothly and slowly to the side or if there is pain on the attempt.

Supraspinatus Strength Test, AR

To assess for supraspinatus tendinitis, strain or weakness:
- Place the client in a seated position
- Instruct the client to abduct the humerus to 90 degrees, then to adduct the humerus horizontally to 30 degrees.
- Instruct the client to internally rotate the humerus, as if the client were holding a can full of liquid, then emptying it.
- Apply pressure to the humerus in the direction of adduction, instructing the client not to let the arm be adducted.
    - ✦ Pain or weakness is a **positive** result.

Note: This is also called the **empty can test** *(Magee, 1997)*.

A variation:
- With the client's humerus by the side of the body, apply pressure to the humerus in the direction of adduction, while the client attempts to abduct the humerus.
    - ✦ Pain along supraspinatus or weakness is a **positive** test result. This test does not distinguish between supraspinatus or deltoid muscle strength, since both abduct the humerus *(Kendall et al., 1993)*.

Infraspinatus Strength Test, AR

To assess the infraspinatus muscle for tendinitis, strain or weakness:
- Place the client in a seated or prone position.
- Abduct the humerus to 90 degrees and flex the elbow to 90 degrees.
- Apply pressure to the client's wrist in the direction of internal rotation, while the client attempts to externally rotate the humerus.
    - ✦ Pain along infraspinatus or weakness is a **positive** sign. This test does not distinguish between infraspinatus or teres minor strength, since both externally rotate the humerus *(Kendall et al., 1993)*.

A variation:

- With the client's humerus by the side of the body and the elbow flexed to 90 degrees, apply pressure to the client's wrist in the direction of internal rotation, while the client attempts to externally rotate the wrist *(Bunker, Wallace, 1991)*.

  ✦ Pain or weakness is a **positive** result.

Subscapularis Strength Test, AR

To assess the subscapularis muscle for tendinitis, strain or weakness:

- Place the client in a seated or supine position, with the humerus by the side of the body and the elbow flexed to 90 degrees.

- Apply pressure to the client's wrist in the direction of external rotation, while the client attempts to internally rotate the wrist *(Bunker, Wallace, 1991)*.

  ✦ Pain along subscapularis or weakness is a **positive** sign. This test does not distinguish between subscapularis, pectoralis major, latissimus dorsi and teres major strength, since all internally rotate the humerus *(Kendall et al., 1993)*.

Speed's Test

To assess for biceps tendinitis:

- Place the client in a seated position.

- Instruct the client to completely extend the elbow while supinating the arm.

- Resist flexion of the arm by placing one hand on the shoulder and the other hand distal to the client's elbow.

  ✦ Pain at the tendon on resistance indicates a **positive** test.

Yergason's Test

Sources differ on the results and efficacy of this test. To assess the stability of the biceps tendon in the bicipital groove *(Hoppenfeld, 1976)* or the presence of biceps tendinitis *(Magee, 1992)* or both *(Gerard, Kleinfield, 1993; Hartley, 1995a)*:

- Place the client in a seated position, with the elbow of the affected arm flexed to 90 degrees and the forearm pronated.

- Stabilize the client's elbow against the client's thorax with one hand.

- With the other hand, apply resistance while the client actively supinates the forearm, extends the elbow and externally rotates the humerus, all at the same time.

  ✦ A **positive** test for biceps tendon instability and the loss of integrity of the transverse humeral ligament is indicated by pain and the sensation of the tendon popping out of the bicipital groove. Pain along the course of the tendon may indicate biceps tendinitis; however, motion of the tendon along the groove is required for a true positive tendinitis test *(Magee, 1992)*.

Pectoralis Minor Length Test

To assess pectoralis minor muscle length:

- Place the client in a supine position.

- Sit at the head of the table.

- Observe for shoulder protraction on the affected side, since pectoralis minor protracts the scapula *(Kendall et al., 1993)*.

A variation:

- Place the client in a supine or seated position.

- Apply the palmar surface of one hand to the anterior surface of the shoulder on the side that pectoralis minor muscle length is to be tested on.

- If the client is supine, compress the affected shoulder posteriorly into the table.

- If the client is seated, stabilize the client's mid-thoracic spine with the other hand. Then push the client's affected shoulder into retraction.

    ✦ A **positive** sign of a shortened pectoralis minor muscle is reduced range of motion in retraction. Be aware of possible compensatory rotation of the client's torso on the unaffected side.

Pectoralis Major Length Test

To assess the length of the pectoralis major muscle.

- Place the client in a supine position.

- To assess the length of the superior or clavicular fibres, instruct the client to abduct the affected arm to 90 degrees.

    ✦ A **positive** sign of shortened pectoralis major clavicular fibres is if the arm does not drop below the level of the table into extension and external rotation.

- To assess the length of the inferior or sternal fibres, instruct the client to abduct the affected arm to about 150 degrees.

    ✦ A **positive** sign of shortened pectoralis major sternal fibres is if the arm does not drop below the level of the table into extension and external rotation.

Shoulder Adductors Length Test

To assess the length of latissimus dorsi and teres major muscles:

- Place the client in a supine position.

- Instruct the client to flex the hips and knees with the plantar surface of both feet flat on the table. The pelvis is in posterior pelvic tilt so the low back is held flat on the table.

- Instruct the client to raise both arms above the head, through full flexion at the glenohumeral joints, allowing the posterior surface of both arms to contact the table.

    ✦ If the glenohumeral joints cannot be fully flexed, the arms will not rest on the table above the client's head. This is **positive** for latissumus dorsi and teres major shortness *(Kendall, McCreary, 1983)*.

Rhomboids Strength Test, AR

To assess the strength of the rhomboid muscles:

- Place the client in a prone position, with the affected humerus abducted to 90 degrees and internally rotated.
- Ask the client to lift the arm into extension. If the client can hold this position against gravity this indicates three on the strength scale (see muscle strength grading in General Tests).
- Stabilize the unaffected shoulder with one hand.
- With the other hand, apply pressure to the distal end of the humerus in an anterior direction.
  - ✦ The test is **positive** for weakness of the rhomboid muscles if the client is unable to hold the arm in the original position.

Middle Trapezius Strength Test, AR

To assess the strength of the trapezius muscle:

- Place the client in a prone position, with the affected humerus abducted to 90 degrees and externally rotated.
- Ask the client to lift the arm into extension. If the client can hold this position against gravity this indicates three on the strength scale (see muscle strength grading in General Tests).
- Stabilize the unaffected shoulder with one hand.
- With the other hand, apply pressure to the distal end of the affected humerus in an anterior direction.
  - ✦ The test is **positive** for weakness of the middle fibres of the trapezius muscle if the client is unable to hold the arm in the original position.

Arm, Wrist and Hand Tests

Degree of Dupuytren's Contracture

To record the flexion contractures found in Dupuytren's contracture:

- Add together the degrees of active free flexion present at the metacarpophalangeal joint, the proximal interphalangeal joint and the distal interphalangeal joint of **each** affected digit. This will give a total number of degrees of flexion deformity for each finger, from 0 degrees (complete extension) to 200 degrees (the finger is fixed into the palm).
  - ✦ **Stage 0** has no flexion deformity, only thickening of the palmar fascia, and nodules are present.
  - ✦ **Stage 1** is a total deformity from 0 to 45 degrees, mostly occurring at the metacarpophalangeal joint.
  - ✦ **Stage 2** is a total deformity from 45 to 90 degrees, also including flexion of the proximal interphalangeal joint.

✦ **Stage 3** is a total deformity from 90 to 155 degrees, also including flexion of the distal interphalangeal joint.

✦ **Stage 4** is a total flexion deformity greater than 135 degrees, where the terminal phalange becomes **hyperextended,** while the other joints are flexed *(Hueston, Tubiana, 1985).*

Phalen's Test

To assess for the presence of carpal tunnel syndrome or compression of the median nerve:

- Place the client in a seated position.

- Instruct the client to put the backs of the hands together. The client's wrists are flexed, the elbows are held horizontally and the shoulders are not elevated.

- Instruct the client to strongly compress the backs of the hands together for one minute. This position produces maximum compression on the structures within the carpal tunnel.

  ✦ Tingling or pain reported in the thumb, index finger, middle finger and lateral half of the ring finger are **positive** for carpal tunnel syndrome.

Reverse Phalen's Test

A variation of this is the **reverse Phalen's test**:

  ✦ Instruct the client to put the palms of the hands together and to strongly compress the palms together for one minute. Tingling or pain reported as in the test above are **positive** for carpal tunnel syndrome.

Cyriax's Variation on Phalen's Test

To assess for the presence of carpal tunnel syndrome or compression of the median nerve:

- Place the client in the same position as in Phalen's test.

- For this variation, after the full minute of bilateral wrist hyperflexion, instruct the client to add sudden wrist extension.

  ✦ The reproduction of the client's symptoms is a **positive** result *(Cyriax, 1991).*

Finger Flexion Test

To assess for the presence of active trigger points in the scalene muscle group:

- Place the client in a seated position.

- Instruct the client to hold the metacarpophalangeal joints of the affected side in full extension throughout the test.

- Instruct the client to flex the interphalangeal joints, attempting to touch the fingertips to the palmar surface over the metacarpophalangeal joints. (Do not allow the client to make a fist.)

  ✦ If all four fingertips cannot touch the metacarpophalangeal joints, a **positive** test for active scalene trigger points is recorded.

A variation on this test: active trigger points in extensor digitorum will prevent full index finger flexion only (*Travell, Simons, 1983*).

Finkelstein's Test

To determine the presence of deQuervain's tenosynovitis:

- Place the client in a seated position.
- Instruct the client to make a fist of the affected hand, with the thumb firmly held in flexion **inside** the flexed fingers.
- Stabilize the arm proximal to the client's wrist with one hand.
- With the other hand, ulnarly deviate the wrist.
  - ✦ Pain along the abductor pollicis longus and extensor pollicis brevis tendons at the wrist is **positive** for tenosynovitis.
- Because this test can be painful even if tendinitis is not present, perform the test bilaterally, comparing affected and unaffected sides.

A variation:

- Instruct the client to actively ulnarly deviate the wrist, keeping the thumb and fingers flexed in a fist as in the first version of the test.
  - ✦ Pain along the tendon sheath is a **positive** result.

Froment's Sign

To assess for an ulnar nerve lesion:

- Instruct the client to grasp a piece of paper between the extended thumb and index finger.
- Try to pull the paper away from the client.
  - ✦ The test is **positive** if adductor pollicis weakness or paralysis will allow the terminal phalanx of the client's thumb to flex.

Wrist Extension Ligamentous Stress Test, PR

To assess for sprain of the palmar wrist ligaments or strain of the wrist flexor muscles:

- Place the client in a seated position with the affected hand in pronation.
- Stabilize the client's hand proximal to the wrist with one hand.
- Place the other hand against the client's affected hand so that the two palms are in opposition.
- Passively move the client's wrist into extension, applying overpressure at the end of the passive range.
  - ✦ Pain and hypermobility at the joint are **positive** for a sprain of the palmar radiocarpal ligament.

✦ Pain local to the flexor muscles or tendons is **positive** for a strain. A muscle spasm end feel may be present with a subacute strain.

✦ Pain with dysesthesia into the palm and from the wrist proximally along the flexor surface may indicate carpal tunnel syndrome.

✦ Pain on PR wrist extension, which is noted on the dorsal surface of the joint, may indicate extensor tenosynovitis *(Gerard, Kleinfield, 1993)*.

Wrist Flexion Ligamentous Stress Test, PR

To assess for sprain of the dorsal wrist ligaments or strain of the wrist extensors:

• Place the client in a seated position.

• Pronate the client's affected hand and stabilize it proximal to the wrist.

• With the other hand, passively move the client's wrist into flexion, applying overpressure at the end of the passive range.

    ✦ Pain and hypermobility at the joint are **positive** for a sprain of the dorsal radiocarpal ligament.

    ✦ Pain local to the extensor muscles or tendons is **positive** for a strain. A muscle spasm end feel may be present with a subacute strain.

    ✦ Pain with dysesthesia into the palm and from the wrist proximally along the flexor surface may indicate carpal tunnel syndrome *(Gerard, Kleinfield, 1993)*.

Radial Ligamentous Stress Test, PR

To assess for sprain of the ulnar collateral ligament or strain of the wrist adductor muscles:

• Place the client in a seated position, with the affected hand in supination.

• Stabilize proximal to the wrist with one hand.

• With the other hand, passively move the client's affected hand into radial deviation, applying overpressure at the end of the passive range.

    ✦ Pain and hypermobility at the joint are **positive** for a sprain of the ulnar collateral ligament.

    ✦ Pain local to extensor carpi ulnaris or flexor carpi ulnaris muscles or tendons is **positive** for strain of either or both of these muscles *(Gerard, Kleinfield, 1993)*. A muscle spasm end feel may be present with a subacute strain.

Ulnar Ligamentous Stress Test, PR

To assess for sprain of the radial collateral ligament or strain of the wrist abductor muscles:

• Place the client in a seated position, with the affected hand in supination.

• Stabilize proximal to the wrist with one hand.

• With the other hand, passively move the client's affected hand into ulnar deviation, applying overpressure at the end of the passive range.

    ✦ Pain and hypermobility at the joint are **positive** for a sprain of the radial collateral ligament.

✦ Pain local to extensor carpi radialis longus and brevis or flexor carpi radialis muscles or tendons is **positive** for strain of these muscles *(Gerard, Kleinfield, 1993)*. A muscle spasm end feel may be present with a subacute strain.

Mill's Test

To assess for tendinosis of the common extensor tendon:

- Place the client in a seated position.
- Passively flex the client's wrist with the elbow extended.
   - ✦ A **positive** test result is pain local to the common extensor tendon *(Souza, 1977)*.

Reverse Mill's Test

To assess for tendinosis of the common flexor tendon:

- Place the client in a seated position.
- Passively extend the wrist with the elbow in extension.
   - ✦ Pain is a **positive** test result local to the common flexor tendon *(Souza, 1997)*.

Extensor Tendinosis Test

To assess for tendinosis:

- Place the client in a seated position, with the elbow in extension and the wrist in pronation and slight extension.
- Instruct the client to hold the wrist in this position.
- Attempt to flex the wrist.
   - ✦ Pain at the common extensor tendon and weakness are **positive** signs for tendinosis.

Note: This is also called **Cozen's test** *(Souza, 1997)*.

To isolate extensor carpi radialis brevis, which is often the source of extensor tendinosis pain:

- Place the client in a seated position in front of a table.
- Instruct the client to lean forward, fully flexing the elbow and resting the forearm on the table. The test proceeds as above with the client resisting wrist flexion *(Kendall, McCreary, 1983)*.

Flexor Tendinosis Test

To assess for tendinosis:

- Place the client in a seated position, with the elbow in extension and the wrist in supination and slight flexion.
- Instruct the client to hold the wrist in this position.
- Attempt to extend the wrist.
   - ✦ Pain at the common flexor tendon and weakness are **positive** signs for tendinosis.

Abductor Pollicis Brevis Strength Test, AR

To assess for the strength of abductor pollicis brevis:

- Place the client in a seated position, with the affected arm supinated and the thumb fully abducted.

- Instruct the client to hold this position.

- Place opposing pressure on the **proximal phalanx** of the thumb, attempting to adduct it.

    ✦ The test is **positive** for weakness of the abductor pollicis brevis muscle if the client is unable to hold the thumb in abduction.

Trunk, Low Back and Abdomen Tests

Vocal Fremitus Test

To assess for areas of bronchial congestion, due to emphysema or chronic bronchitis:

- Place the client in a prone position.

- Place both relaxed hands symmetrically on the thorax and move them over the various aspects of the thorax.

- At the same time, instruct the client to repeat words containing nasal sounds, such as "ninety-nine", which will cause the thorax to vibrate in a palpable manner. The vibrations are most noticeable over the lungs and bronchi, tissue containing air spaces that transmit the vibration of the client's voice. As an example, this palpable vibration increases over the superior aspect of the right lung and decreases over the heart and inferior to the diaphragm.

- Assess the areas over the lungs and bronchi for the presence of vocal fremitus or vibrations in the various lobes.

    ✦ If the vibrations are decreased over the lungs and bronchi, the test is **positive** for congestion due to infected mucus, serum or lymph, indicating which pleural lobe is affected *(Taber's Cyclopedic Medical Dictionary, 1981).*

- Repeat the test with the client lying supine.

- Do not place the hands over the client's nipples while performing this test.

Mediate Percussion Test

To assess the lung density, specifically for the presence of mucus congestion in specific lobes as in chronic bronchitis, or hyperinflation as in emphysema:

- Begin with the client in a prone position, and then supine.

- Place the middle finger of the non-dominant hand flat on the thorax along an intercostal space.

- With the tips of the first and second fingers of the dominant hand, tap firmly on the finger positioned on the thorax.

- Repeat the tapping over various aspects of the thorax. The tapping produces a sound that varies with the density of the underlying tissue.
  - ✦ The sound is **duller** over areas of congestion, and more **resonant** over hyperinflated lungs *(Kisner, Colby, 1996)*. The sound is also duller over solid areas, such as over the heart or abdomen.

Spine, AF ROM

To assess the active free range of motion in the spine:

- Place the client in a standing position.

- From the posterior view, examine the entire spine and instruct the client to move slowly through the available range of flexion, extension and lateral bending of the spine.

- Instruct the client to move through the range of rotation of the spine. The lumbar spine has little rotational capabilities, the thoracic spine has more and the cervical spine rotates the most.

- Observe the relative motion of the individual vertebrae and ribs.
  - ✦ **Positive** results include hypomobile segments, which move as one unit, and hypermobile segments, which move more than the segments above or below them.

- Note any visible lateral shift of the spinous processes and possible posterior unilateral rib humping.

- One method to record the available range of motion of the client's spine is to use the Maigne diagram *(Neumann, 1989)*. Specify which part of the spine the diagram represents, such as lumbar, thoracic or cervical spine *(Figure C.1)*.

- Note any restriction by drawing a short line through the corresponding range line. Write the degree of restriction beside it. Another notation method uses from one to three short lines across the range line, each short line indicating increasing restriction of motion. Pain within a range or at the end range can be designated with a capital letter "P".

Trunk and Hip Flexion, AF ROM

To assess the length of gastrocnemius, hamstring and lower and upper back extensor muscles:

- Instruct the client to sit on the floor with both knees in extension and to bend forward from the hips to touch the toes.

- Observe the client in a lateral view. Normal length of all the above muscles is indicated when the client touches the toes with the fingertips, with the pelvis in a relatively neutral position and the ankles neither dorsiflexed nor plantarflexed. The contour of the lower and upper back is a smooth curve.
  - ✦ **Shortness** of gastrocnemius muscle is indicated when the client is unable to touch the toes due to ankle plantarflexion.
  - ✦ **Shortness** of hamstring muscles shows up as an inability to touch the toes, along with a more posterior pelvic tilt.
  - ✦ **Excessive length** of hamstring muscles is indicated when the client reaches past the toes and exhibits a more anterior pelvic tilt.

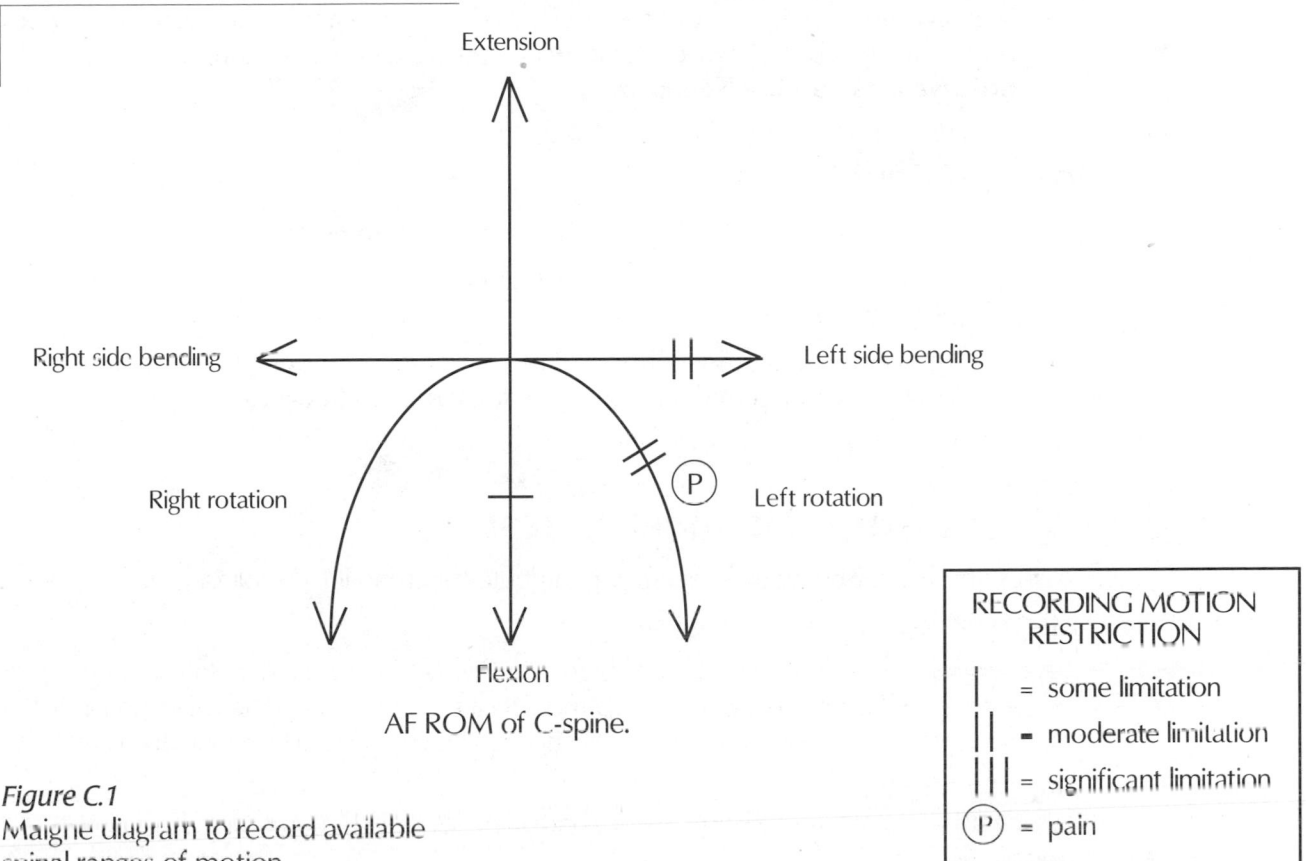

Figure C.1
Maigne diagram to record available
spinal ranges of motion.

- ◆ **Shortness** of lower back extensor muscles is indicated when the client cannot reach the toes and the lower spine remains vertical.
- ◆ **Excessive length** of lower back extensor muscles is indicated by an increase in the curve of the lumbar area.
- ◆ **Excessive length** of upper back extensor muscles shows as an increase in the curve of the thoracic spine (Kendall, McCreary, 1983).

Functional or Structural Scoliosis Test

To help determine whether spinal curves are functional or structural in nature:

- Place the client in a standing position.
- Stand or sit behind the standing client and observe the spinous processes for any visible curves.
- Instruct the client to perform active free range of motion of the spine in lateral bending to both sides and in flexion.
  - ◆ Lateral bending is **positive** for **functional scoliosis** if the curve corrects or reverses as the client bends towards the convex side. If the curve does not correct and the lateral bending is asymmetrical, the test is **positive** for **structural scoliosis.**

✦ Flexion is **positive** for **functional scoliosis** if the curve and rib humping correct or reverse as the client slowly bends forward. If there is no correction, the test is **positive** for **structural scoliosis.**

Forward Bending Test

A combination of these two tests is called the **forward bending test:**

- Instruct the standing client to bend forward, allowing the arms to hang, and then to laterally bend the torso to both sides.

    ✦ If the curve or rib humping corrects or reverses, the test is **positive** for **functional scoliosis.** A lack of correction is **positive** for **structural curves** *(Hoppenfeld, 1976).*

Scoliosis Small Hemipelvis Test

To assess for a small hemipelvis that may contribute to a functional scoliosis:

- Place the client in a seated position.

- A hemipelvis, or one side of the pelvis, may be smaller in the superior to inferior dimension, between the iliac crest and the ischial tuberosity, than the other hemipelvis. Observe the iliac crest and acromioclavicular joint levels bilaterally, noting any lateral tilt and scoliotic curve.

- Place an ischial lift (a thin book will do) under the lower side, correcting the lateral pelvic tilt.

    ✦ If the curve neutralizes, the test is **positive** for functional scoliosis due to the small hemipelvis. If the lift is placed under the high side, the curve in a functional scoliosis will worsen *(Travell, Simons, 1992).*

Scoliosis Short Leg Test

To assess a short leg that contributes to a functional scoliosis:

- Place the client in a standing position.

- Observe the iliac crest and acromioclavicular joint levels bilaterally, noting any lateral tilt and scoliotic curve.

- Place a foot lift (a thin book will do) under the apparently short leg, correcting the pelvic tilt.

    ✦ If the curve neutralizes, the test is **positive** for functional scoliosis due to the short limb. If the lift is placed under the long limb, the curve in a functional scoliosis will worsen *(Travell, Simons, 1992).*

Motion Palpation of the Spine

To assess the ranges of motion of the spine, identifying hypomobile or hypermobile segments:

- Place the client in a standing position.

- Place the fingertips in the laminar groove immediately lateral to the spinous processes or place the palm of the hand over the spinous processes with the fingertips oriented superiorly.

- Instruct the client to move slowly through flexion, extension, sidebending and, finally, rotation.

  ✦ **Positive** results include hypomobile segments that move as one unit, with a leathery end feel, and hypermobile segments that move more than the segments above or below them.

- Perform this motion palpation on the entire spine, checking segment by segment from the lumbar to the cervical spine or vice versa.

Static Palpation of the Spine

To explore for minor rotation, flexion or extension of the vertebrae in the cervical, thoracic and lumbar spine:

- The direction of the initial assessment may be from the lumbar to the cervical spinous processes or vice versa. It is important to thoroughly assess each vertebral segment.

- Place the client in a prone position to assess the **thoracic** and **lumbar** spine.

- Palpate along the spinous processes, moving from T1 to L5. Use the index and middle fingers of one hand, one finger on each side of the tips of the spinous processes.

- Use a moderate downward pressure, sliding the palpating fingers along the skin.

- Outline each spinous process as the fingers slide inferiorly, in order to assess the position of each relative to the spinous process above it. Count each vertebra from T1 down or from L5 up as it is palpated to accurately locate a possible minor positional dysfunction.

  ✦ The test may be **positive** if the spinous processes are not symmetrical. If the spinous process of T8 appears to be to the left of T7 and T9, the vertebral body of T8 may be rotated to the right. If there is a larger apparent space between the spinous processes of T4 and T5, as well as a smaller apparent space between T5 and T6, the vertebral body of T5 may be in **extension** (backward bent) relative to T6. If there is a smaller apparent space between the spinous processes of T4 and T5, as well as a larger apparent space between T5 and T6, the vertebral body of T5 may be in **flexion** (forward bent) relative to T6.

- Place the client in a supine position to assess the **cervical** spine.

- Lean your elbows on the table, hands supinated.

- Use the fingertips to palpate both sides of the spinous processes, stroking from T1 up to C1. (C1 has a posterior tubercle, not a spinous process.)

- Again, count the vertebrae to determine the location of the dysfunction, using T1 as a reference point.

  ✦ The test may be **positive** if rotation, flexion or extension of a spinous process is noted.

Note: This palpation assessment may not be entirely accurate, since an oddly shaped spinous process — one that is short or slightly curved to one side — may create the appearance of a deviation (*Basmajian, Nyberg, 1993*). Following this palpation assessment, passive relaxed anterior and lateral spinous challenge tests may help to confirm the findings.

Anterior Spinous Challenge Test, PR

To determine the location of a minor vertebral derangement — either hypomobility or hypermobility of a vertebral segment of the cervical, thoracic or lumbar spine on the **sagittal** plane:

- The direction of the initial assessment may be from the lumbar to the cervical spinous processes or vice versa. It is important to thoroughly assess each vertebral segment.

- Place the client in a prone position to assess the **thoracic** and **lumbar** spine.

- Be thorough and assess each vertebral segment. The lateral spinous challenge and the anterior spinous challenge may be performed one after the other on the lumbar and thoracic spine with the client prone. They may then be repeated on the cervical spine with the client supine for a complete assessment of the spine.

- Place your thumbs or hypothenar eminences over an individual spinous process, applying slow pressure in an anterior direction.

- Count each vertebra from T1 down or from L5 up, as it is palpated to accurately locate a dysfunction.

  - ✦ The test is **positive** if the client reports local mild pain with the pressure at a specific vertebral level. A **hypomobile** segment is indicated during palpation by its decreased mobility relative to the adjacent vertebrae; this may be perceived as blocked or decreased movement, almost a bony end feel. A **hypermobile** segment is identified by its increased mobility relative to the adjacent vertebrae.

- Place the client in a supine position to assess the **cervical** spine.

- Lean your elbows on the table, hands supinated.

- Use the fingertips to anteriorly challenge the spinous processes. Again, count the vertebrae to determine the location of the dysfunction, using T1 as a reference point.

  - ✦ The test is **positive** if the client reports local mild pain with pressure at a specific vertebral level *(Basmajian, 1985)*.

- The direction of the initial assessment may be from the lumbar to the cervical spinous processes or vice versa. It is important to thoroughly assess each vertebral segment.

Lateral Spinous Challenge Test, PR

To determine the location of a minor intervertebral derangement — either hypomobility or hypermobility of a vertebral segment of the cervical, thoracic or lumbar spine on the **coronal** plane:

- The direction of the initial assessment may be from the lumbar to the cervical spinous processes or vice versa. The initial lateral challenge may be from left to right, or right to left.

- Place the client in a prone position to assess the **thoracic** and **lumbar** spine.

- Be thorough and assess each vertebral segment. The lateral spinous challenge and the anterior spinous challenge may be performed one after the other on the lumbar and thoracic spine with the client prone. They may then be repeated on the cervical spine with the client supine for a complete assessment of the spine.

- Place the thumbs together on the lateral border of the spine and apply slow pressure to an individual spinous process. Pressure is directed to the opposite side. For example, the thumbs are placed on the left side of the spinous process and pressure is to the right.

- Begin, for example, on the lumbar spine at L5 and move superiorly to T1, laterally challenging each vertebra from left to right.

- To accurately locate a dysfunction, count each vertebra from L5 as it is palpated.

  ✦ The test is **positive** if the client reports local mild pain with pressure at a specific vertebral level — at T8, for example. A **hypomobile** segment is indicated during palpation by its decreased mobility relative to the adjacent vertebrae; this may be perceived as blocked or decreased movement, almost a bony end feel. A **hypermobile** segment is palpated by its increased mobility relative to the adjacent vertebrae.

- When a dysfunction is located, apply a lateral challenge to this painful vertebra's spinous process in the opposite direction. In the above example, the direction of opposing pressure is from right to left. This opposing pressure is usually reported by the client as painless.

- Place the client in a supine position to assess the **cervical** spine.

- Use the fingertips to laterally challenge the spinous processes.

- Count the vertebrae to determine the location of the dysfunction, using T1 as a reference point.

  ✦ The test is **positive** if the client reports local mild pain with pressure at a specific vertebral level

A modification to locate the minor vertebral derangement — at the facet joints between the vertebrae immediately **superior** to or immediately **inferior** to the affected segment:

- Apply the lateral pressure that caused pain. In the example above, this pressure is from left to right at T8.

- Then apply counterpressure from right to left at the spinous processes superior and inferior to the affected vertebra.

  ✦ An increase in the pain reported by the client is a **positive** sign. In the example above, right to left counterpressure at T9 does not change the pain at T8. But right to left counterpressure at T7 increases the pain at T8. This locates the dysfunction at the facet joints between T7 and T8 *(Basmajian, 1985)*.

- The direction of the initial assessment may be from the lumbar to the cervical spinous processes or vice versa. The initial lateral challenge may be from left to right, or right to left.

- Be thorough and assess each vertebral segment. The lateral spinous challenge and the anterior spinous challenge may be performed one after the other on the lumbar and thoracic spine with the client prone. They may then be repeated on the cervical spine with the client supine for a complete assessment of the spine.

Rib Motion Test

To assess the motion of the ribs:

- Place the client in a prone or supine position.

- Place your relaxed hands symmetrically over the various aspects of the thorax, moving systematically from superior to inferior ribs during the assessment.

- Palpate for rib motion on the left and right sides, as the client inhales and exhales, noting any imbalances.

- Following specific movement patterns, ribs 2 through 5 move anteriorly and superiorly on inspiration and posteriorly and inferiorly on expiration. This is described as a pump-handle motion. Ribs 7 through 10 move laterally and superiorly on inspiration and medially and inferiorly on expiration, or in a bucket-handle motion. Ribs 5 to 7 are transitional and show characteristics of both movements. Ribs 11 and 12 move laterally on inspiration and posteriorly on expiration, or in a calliper-like motion. The 11th and 12th ribs are frequently restricted by quadratus lumborum *(Greenman, 1989; Edmond, 1993)*. Likewise, the first rib may be restricted by the scalenes.

- Assess for any asymmetry in the rib movement.

  ✦ On inhalation, a rib that stops moving relative to the other ribs is a **depressed** rib. On exhalation, a rib that does not move relative to the others is described as an **elevated** rib *(Magee, 1992)*.

- If a group of ribs is restricted, assess for the key rib that is primarily responsible for the restriction. This is the rib at the superior or inferior end of the dysfunctional group.

  ✦ With an **inhalation** rib-group dysfunction, the key rib is at the **superior** end of the group. With an **exhalation** rib-group dysfunction, the key rib is at the **inferior** end of the group *(Greenman, 1989)*.

Rib Palpation Test

To assess the position of individual ribs:
- Place the client in a prone position.
- Palpate the rib angles bilaterally with flat hands.

  ✦ A rib that is subluxed or fixed in a **posterior** direction has a **more** prominent rib angle contour than the other ribs. A rib that is subluxed or fixed in an **anterior** direction has a contour that is **less** prominent. In both cases, there is restriction of rib motion on inhalation and exhalation, and the iliocostalis muscle is point tender and hypertonic.

- Turn the client to a supine position.
- Palpate the anterior extremities or aspects of the ribs with flat hands, avoiding the nipples.

  ✦ A **posteriorly** subluxed rib has a **less** pronounced contour, while an **anteriorly** subluxed rib has a **more** pronounced contour when palpated anteriorly *(Greenman, 1989)*.

Levatores Costarum Fixation

To assess the length of individual levatores costarum muscles, which may be affected following thoracic injury, restricting rib motion:
- Place the client in a prone position.

- Assess rib motion and locate the affected rib (see Rib Palpation Test).
- Rotate the head to the unaffected side.
- Stabilize the spinous process immediately superior to the affected rib with pressure that is directed anteriorly and towards the opposite side.
- With the palm of the other hand, apply pressure, inferolaterally directed, to the posterior angle of the rib.
  - ✦ The test is **positive** for levator costarum restriction if the end feel is leathery and the client reports tenderness. A **negative** test has an elastic end feel and the client reports no tenderness.

A variation:

- In a seated position, the client clasps both hands behind the head, elbows as close together as possible.
- Stand behind the client.
- With one hand, elevate the client's elbows while using the elbows to rotate the client's thorax towards the unaffected side in a smooth motion.
- Place the other hand so the thumb contacts the posterior angle of the affected rib. Apply pressure interolaterally, away from the spinous process of the vertebra immediately superior to the affected rib.
  - ✦ A **positive** test is indicated by difficulty in moving the rib angle inferolaterally (*Greenman, 1989*).

Valsalva's Test

To asses for a space-occupying lesion, such as a herniated disc, osteophyte or tumour, which would increase the pressure within the spinal cord:

- Place the client in a seated position
- Instruct the client to take a breath and hold it while bearing down, as if moving the bowels.
  - ✦ The result is **positive** if the client reports pain, which is experienced local to the lesion site or as a radiating pain in a dermatomal pattern. This same pain may be reproduced by coughing or sneezing. Pain is the result of increasing the venous back-pressure, within the spinal column (*Buschbacher, 1994*).

Note: Use this test cautiously with clients who have cardiac disorders. Here, the temporarily decreased blood supply to the brain may result in post-test dizziness and syncope.

Kemp's Test

To assess for nerve root compression, usually due to a discal lesion or to facet joint irritation in the lumbar spine:

- Place the client in a standing position.
- Instruct the client to slowly extend, sidebend and rotate the thorax and lumbar spine to the affected side. This can be accomplished by having the client run the fingertips of the hand on the affected side down the posterolateral aspect of the affected leg as far as

possible. The combined action of the client's torso movement and the shifting weight of the client's body compresses the intervertebral foramen, the nerve root and the facet joints on that side.

✦ A **positive test** is indicated by radiating pain or other neurological signs in the affected leg. The distribution of the pain indicates which nerve root is involved. Pain remaining local to the back indicates lumbar facet joint irritation. A **false positive** Kemp's test may occur with severe unilateral lumbar muscle spasm; the presence of radicular symptoms is needed to confirm a nerve root compression *(Gerard, Kleinfield, 1993)*.

Quadrant Test

A variation of this is the **quadrant test**:

• Instruct the standing client to extend, sidebend and rotate the lumbar spine to the affected side.

• Apply an inferiorly directed overpressure to the shoulder on the affected side *(Magee, 1992)*.

• The assessment may also be performed with the client seated *(Gerard, Kleinfield, 1993)*.

Note: This test performed at the cervical spine is called **Spurling's test.**

Kernig's Test

To stretch the dural tube and spinal cord to reproduce pain caused by nerve root involvement, meningeal irritation or dural irritation:

• In a supine position, the client cups the hands behind the head.

• Instruct the client to flex the head to the chest and indicate if pain is present.

• Next, instruct the client to flex one hip with the knee in extension.

✦ A **positive** test is indicated if the client feels pain along the spine and sometimes in a referral pattern to a limb. The pain is experienced at the level of the lesion. When pain is experienced, the client flexes the knee, sometimes involuntarily, reducing the stretch on the dural tube and diminishing the pain.

Note: Sources differ as to the name of this test, which may also be called the **Kernig's/ Brudzinski test** *(Hoppenfeld, 1976; Magee, 1992; Chusid, 1985)* or **Soto/Hall test** *(Foreman, Croft, 1995)*.

Slump Test

If the client is seated for this test, it is called the **slump test** *(Magee, 1992)*.

• Place the client in a seated position, allowing the lumbar and thoracic spine to slump through full flexion.

• Instruct the client to flex the head to the chest.

• Next, instruct the client to extend one knee, followed by ankle dorsiflexion.

The other knee is then extended and the ankle dorsiflexed. If the client was experiencing symptoms in one leg, the unaffected leg is positioned *first*.

✦ A **positive** test is indicated if the client feels pain along the spine and sometimes in a referral pattern to a limb at any point in the test. The pain is experienced at the level of the lesion *(Hertling, Kessler, 1996)*.

Straight Leg Raise or Lasegue's Test
(includes Bragard's Test, Fajerztajn's Test and Freiburg Sign)

To help to determine the cause of low back pain:

• Place the client in a supine position, with the affected leg in adduction and internal rotation.

• Raise the affected leg by grasping it around the calcaneus and flexing the hip. The knee must be in extension; one hand can apply pressure on the anterior aspect of the knee to ensure this.

• Flex the hip until the client indicates pain is felt, which is usually at about 70 to 80 degrees of flexion.

• Slowly lower the leg until no pain is reported by the client.

• Then, dorsiflex the client's foot, stretching the sciatic nerve (this portion of the test is also called **Braggard's test**).

   ✦ Pain reported in the posterior thigh and knee on hip flexion **only** is **positive** for hamstring tightness.

   ✦ Pain reported down the leg on forced dorsiflexion is **positive** for sciatic nerve involvement.

   ✦ Pain reported down the opposite leg is **positive** for a space-occupying lesion or disc herniation. This last test result is called the **well leg straight leg raising test** or **Fajerztajn's test**.

   ✦ Pain reported in the low back after 70 degrees of hip flexion **without** ankle dorsiflexion to stretch the sciatic nerve is **positive** for lumbar or sacroiliac joint dysfunction only.

   ✦ Pain reported in the buttock and potentially radiating down the leg combined with limited range of motion with internal rotation of the extended thigh, or the **Freiburg sign**, are **positive** for a short piriformis muscle.

   ✦ With a straight leg raise test, flexing the hip less than 30 degrees does not move the nerve root within the intervertebral foramen and, with a lesion, no pain is produced. Between 30 degrees and 90 degrees, the greatest amount of traction through the sciatic nerve occurs to the lumbosacral nerve roots at the L4 to L5 level, where the motion of the nerve root is up to three to five millimetres. Some sources feel traction is minimal at the L3 to L4 level and, therefore, the test may yield inaccurate results. At the L2 to L3 level, traction may not occur at all. It is, therefore, possible that a **false negative** test may result if the lesion is superior to L4 *(Caillet, 1988)*.

Rebound Tenderness Test

To assess for the possibility of appendicitis:

• Place the client in a supine position, with the knees and hips flexed.

• The appendix is located in the lower right quadrant of the abdomen, two-thirds of the distance inferiorly along an imaginary line drawn from the umbilicus and the right ASIS. This area is called McBurney's point. Slowly apply pressure over McBurney's point and then quickly release the pressure.

✦ A **positive** test for rebound tenderness and possible appendicitis is indicated if the client feels severe pain when the pressure is released usually in the presence of low-grade fever and nausea. A positive test necessitates an **emergency medical referral.** A lack of pain on release of pressure is a **negative** result *(Porth, 1990)*.

Quadratus Lumborum Length Test

To assess the length of quadratus lumborum muscle:

- Place the client in a seated position to stabilize the pelvis *(Travell, Simons, 1992)*.
- Stand behind the client and landmark both iliac crests.
- Instruct the client to laterally bend the torso away from the side to be tested and then towards the side to be tested.
- Note the available range of motion on both sides.
  - ✦ If restriction in the range is noted on laterally bending away from the side being assessed, the test is **positive** for quadratus lumborum muscle shortness.

A variation:

- Place the client in a sidelying position on the side to be tested.
- Stabilize the client's pelvis and instruct the client to raise the shoulders up from the table.
  - ✦ The test is **positive** for shortness of quadratus lumborum muscle if there is reduced lateral bending when compared to the unaffected side.

Quadratus Lumborum Strength Test, AR

To assess the strength of quadratus lumborum muscle:

- Place the client in a prone position.
- Place the lower limb on the side to be tested in 30 degrees of abduction and slight extension, so the fibres of quadratus lumborum are in alignment with the limb. Instruct the client to hold the limb and the pelvis in this position.
- Traction the leg directly against the line of pull of the quadratus lumborum fibres.
  - ✦ The test is **positive** for weakness if the client is unable to hold the pelvis in the given position and the ilium is pulled inferiorly *(Kendall, McCreary, 1983)*.

Abdominals Strength Test, AR

To assess abdominal strength:

- Perform this test after the strength of neck and hip flexors is determined and the length of the hamstrings and back extensors is assessed to be sure that extensor muscle shortness is not confused with abdominal weakness.
- Place the client in a supine position with the knees in extension.
- Do not hold down the feet.

- Instruct the client to complete a slow curled-trunk sit-up by tilting the pelvis posteriorly and flexing the spine. The head, shoulders and trunk are raised in sequence and then the trunk is flexed towards the thighs, flexing the hips.

   + **Grade five** or normal strength: the client is able to complete the trunk flexion to a sitting position with the hands clasped behind the head.

   + **Grade four** or good strength: the client is able to complete the flexion to a sitting position with the forearms crossed against the chest.

   + **Grade three** or fair-plus strength: the client is able to complete the flexion to a sitting position with the arms held out in front.

   + **Grade two** or fair strength: the client is able to only flex the trunk with the arms held out in front.

To assess the strength of the **abdominal obliques:**

- Stabilize the client's legs, which are extended.

- Instruct the supine client to raise the right shoulder off the floor to test the right external obliques and left internal obliques, and raise the left shoulder off the floor to test the left external obliques and right internal obliques. The client's hands are clasped behind the head.

   + **Grade five strength:** the client is able to hold the test position with the hands behind the head.

   + **Grade four strength:** the client is able to hold the position with the arms crossed over the chest.

   + **Grade three strength:** the client is able to hold the position with the arms held out in front.

   + **Grade two strength:** the client is able to hold the position with the arms held in front and only the scapula held off the table *(Kendall, McCreary, 1983)*.

Pelvic Tests

Supine to Sit Test

To assess for a functional leg length discrepancy:

- Place the client in a supine position with the knees in extension.

- Compare the level of both malleoli.

- Instruct the client to sit up.

- Note whether the affected limb appears to lengthen when comparing the malleoli levels.

   + If the affected limb appears longer when the client is supine, but shorter when sitting up, this is **positive** for functional leg length difference on the affected side due to anterior innominate rotation.

   + If the affected limb appears shorter when the client is supine, but longer when sitting up, this is **positive** for functional leg length difference on the affected side due to posterior innominate rotation *(Magee, 1992)*.

Sacroiliac Joint Motion or Gillet's Test

To assess the mobility of the sacroiliac joint:

- Place the client in a standing position, using her outstretched hands against a wall for stability, if necessary.
- Kneel behind the client and, with one thumb, palpate for the posterior superior iliac spine on the affected side.
- With the other thumb, mark the S2 spinous process on the sacrum.
- Instruct the client to stand on the unaffected leg and, flexing the hip and knee on the affected side, slowly raise the knee as high as possible.
- At the same time, palpate for the relative motion of the posterior superior iliac spine. Normal sacroiliac joint motion is indicated if the thumb on the posterior superior iliac spine moves inferiorly as the knee lifts.
  - ✦ A **positive** sign for sacroiliac joint hypomobility is indicated by the thumb on the affected side moving superiorly as the knee lifts.
- Compare the unaffected side for sacroiliac joint mobility.

Sacroiliac Joint Gapping or Transverse Anterior Stress Test

A stress test to assess the anterior ligaments that cross the sacroiliac joints:

- Place the client in a supine position
- Apply a crossed-arm pressure to the medial aspects of the anterior superior iliac spines, attempting to push the spines laterally and inferiorly at the same time.
- Be careful not to painfully compress the soft tissue lying medial and anterior to the anterior superior iliac spines.
  - ✦ The test is **positive**, indicating an anterior sacroiliac ligament sprain, if the client reports unilateral gluteal or posterior leg pain.

Sacroiliac Joint "Squish" or Transverse Posterior Stress Test

A stress test to assess the posterior ligaments that cross the sacroiliac joints:

- Place the client in a supine position.
- Place one hand on the lateral side of each anterior superior iliac spine and apply pressure from lateral to medial and then posteriorly towards the sacroiliac joints at a 45 degree angle, stressing the posterior ligaments.
  - ✦ The test is **positive**, indicating a posterior sacroiliac ligament sprain, if the client reports pain local to the sacroiliac joint *(Magee, 1992)*.

A variation:

- Place the client in a sidelying position.
- Apply pressure to the uppermost iliac crest in a medial direction.

✦ Pressure or pain reported by the client local to the sacroiliac joint is a **positive** sign for posterior sacroiliac ligament sprain.

Hip Quadrant or Scouring Test

To assess for joint capsule tightness or other pathology at the hip:

- Place the client in a supine position.
- Flex and adduct the affected hip, so the knee is positioned towards the client's opposite shoulder.
- When you feel resistance to the movement, maintain minimal resistance and move the flexed hip through an arc into abduction.
- Palpate the quality of hip motion throughout the range.
  - ✦ A **positive** test for capsular tightness, osteophyte formation or other pathology is indicated by early leathery end feel, bumpiness or crepitus in the movement and pain or client apprehension to the motion.

Faber Test
(also called Patrick's Test or Figure 4 Test)

Faber stands for **f**lexion, **ab**duction and **e**xternal **r**otation. To assess the hip and psoas muscle:

- Place the client in a supine position with the legs extended.
- Place the client's foot of the affected side on the knee of the uninvolved side, making the shape of the number four. The affected hip is now abducted, flexed and externally rotated.
  - ✦ If the affected knee remains above the unaffected knee, the test is **positive** for a possible hip joint pathology or shortened or spasmed psoas muscle.

To assess the sacroiliac joint:

- With the client in a supine position, stabilize the unaffected anterior superior iliac spine with one hand and gently push the affected knee in a posterior direction.
  - ✦ Pain reported by the client local to the sacroiliac joint is **positive** for sacroiliac joint dysfunction *(Hoppenfeld, 1976)*.

Gaenslen's Test

To assess for hip or sacroiliac joint dysfunction:

- Place the client in a sidelying position on the unaffected side.
- Instruct the client to flex the unaffected hip and knee to the chest, holding them there.
- Stand behind the client and stabilize the pelvis with one hand.
- With the other hand, hyperextend the client's affected leg at the hip.
  - ✦ The test is **positive** for sacroiliac joint or hip dysfunction if the client reports pain in these areas.

A variation:

- Place the client in a supine position, with the affected hip just off the edge of the table.
- Instruct the client to flex the unaffected hip and knee, holding the knee to the chest, while allowing the affected leg to slowly drop into hyperextension.
    + Pain reported in the sacroiliac joint is a **positive** sign *(Gerard, Kleinfield, 1993).*

Thomas Test

To assess for hip flexor muscle shortness or contracture:

- Place the client in a supine position, with the legs flexed at the knee over the end of the table. For a client experiencing low back pain, a variation is to place the client in a supine position with the legs flexed at the knee with heels resting at the edge of the table.
- First, check for the increased hyperlordosis usually present with tight hip flexors by sliding one hand between the client's lumbar curve and the table, then flexing the client's unaffected hip and knee so the anterior thigh is brought towards the chest. The vertebrae of the client's lumbar spine will touch the therapist's hand. At this point, the lordotic lumbar curve is flattened, the pelvis is stabilized and further flexion can occur only at the hip.
- While maintaining the unaffected hip and knee in flexion, instruct the client to flex the affected hip and knee, and to hold the leg in this position with both hands.
- Have the client then slowly lower the affected leg as far into extension as it will go.
    + A **positive** sign of hip flexor shortness or contracture is indicated if the leg will not touch the table at the posterior knee. If the leg does touch the table at the knee, the test is **negative.**

To assess rectus femoris muscle shortness or contracture using a modification of the Thomas test:

- Place the client in a supine position, with the legs flexed at the knee over the end of the table. For a client experiencing low back pain, a variation is to place the client in a supine position with the legs flexed at the knee with heels resting at the edge of the table.
- Flex the unaffected hip and knee towards the chest as in the Thomas test.
- Observe the affected leg.
    + If the knee extends, the test is **positive** for rectus femoris shortness or contracture. If the knee stays flexed, the test is **negative.**

Ely's Test

Another method of assessing for rectus femoris muscle shortness or contracture:

- Place the client in a prone position.
- Flex the affected knee, attempting to bring the heel to the gluteus maximus, ensuring that the leg does not abduct.
- Observe the client's pelvis.

✦ If the pelvis on the affected side flexes as the knee is flexed, the test is **positive** for shortened rectus femoris muscle.

Hip Adductor Length Test

To assess the length of the adductor muscles:

- Place the client in a supine position.
- Place the plantar surface of the client's foot of the affected side on the medial aspect of the knee of the uninvolved side. The affected hip is now abducted, flexed and externally rotated, and the knee is flexed.
- Stabilize the unaffected anterior superior iliac spine with one hand.
- With the other hand, apply posterolaterally directed pressure at the medial aspect of the affected knee.
    - ✦ Using bilateral comparison, the test is **positive** for a shortened adductor group when there is reduced range of motion of the hip in abduction and extension.

Piriformis Length Test

To assess the length of piriformis muscle:

- Place the client in a prone position with the knees together.
- Keeping the client's feet together, flex the client's knees to 90 degrees.
- Then allow the feet to separate from the midline as far as is comfortable, which internally rotates both femurs, stretching both the piriformis muscles.
    - ✦ Using bilateral comparison, a **positive** sign of a shortened piriformis muscle is indicated by a reduced range of motion of the affected femur in internal rotation. The foot of the affected leg stays closer to the original position at midline, while the foot of the unaffected leg moves farther from the original position.

Ober's Test and Modified Ober's Test

(According to Kendall *et al.* (1993), this test, and the normal range of hip adduction, have been incorrectly described in numerous texts.)

Original Ober's test to assess the length of the iliotibial band and tensor fascia lata by stretching these structures and observing adduction at the hip:

- Place the client in a sidelying position, with the affected leg uppermost. The client's lateral torso on the unaffected side remains on the table.
- Slightly flex the unaffected leg (on which the client is lying) at the hip and knee to flatten the lumbar spine. This removes the lordosis, preventing any anterior pelvic tilt that would allow shortening of the tensor fascia lata.
- Stand behind the client, with the client close to the edge of the table so you do not have to reach over the table.
- Using either the proximal hand (the hand closer to client's head) or the ulnar border of the proximal arm, stabilize the client's pelvis by pressing the uppermost iliac crest into

1101

the table **and** slightly upwards. The pelvis must be kept perpendicular to the table (on the coronal plane) **and** be prevented from tilting laterally downward on the side being tested. Otherwise a false negative test may result. If the pelvis is allowed to move off the coronal plane and hip flexion occurs, or if the pelvis tilts laterally downward due to the weight of the leg, the tensor fascia lata will be able to shorten *(Kendall et al., 1993; Magee, 1992)*.

- With the distal hand (the hand farther from the client's head) at the medial aspect of the affected leg, passively hyperabduct and extend the femur of the affected leg at the hip. This position aligns the iliotibial band over the greater trochanter on the coronal plane.

- Prevent the femur from internally rotating at the hip, which would once again allow the tensor fascia lata to shorten.

- With the affected knee in 90 degrees of **flexion**, support the leg at the ankle.

- Instruct the client to relax the leg fully.

- Allow the leg to lower on the coronal plane without internally or externally rotating.

  ✦ A **positive** test, revealing a shortened tensor fascia lata and iliotibial band, is indicated if the leg remains strongly abducted. A **negative** test, indicating a normal length of the muscle and fascia, has the leg adducting slightly below the horizontal.

In the **modified Ober's test:**

- Position and stabilize the client as above, but with the affected knee in full **extension.** This prevents undue stress on the knee and interference from a tight rectus femoris muscle.

- Instruct the client to relax the leg fully.

- Allow the leg to lower on the coronal plane without internally or externally rotating.

  ✦ A **positive** test, revealing a shortened tensor fascia lata and iliotibial band, is indicated by the leg remaining strongly abducted. A **negative** test, indicating a normal length of the muscle and iliotibial band, has the leg adducting 10 degrees below the horizontal. Note that a greater stress is placed on the iliotibial band when the knee is extended *(Magee, 1992)*. Therefore, if the test is performed with the knee extended, the length of iliotibial band itself is assessed; with the knee flexed (slackening the iliotibial band) the length of tensor fascia lata is assessed.

Iliopsoas Strength Test, AR

To test for iliopsoas weakness:

- Place the client in a supine position, with the knee in full extension.

- Stabilize the opposite anterior superior iliac spine with one hand.

- Instruct the client to put the hip into 30 degrees of flexion and slight external rotation, holding the leg up off the table. If the client can hold this position against gravity, this indicates three on the strength scale (see muscle strength grading in General Tests).

- Apply pressure against the medial tibia, in a posterior and lateral direction, attempting to push the leg towards the floor.

  ✦ The test is **positive** for iliopsoas weakness when the client is unable to hold the hip in flexion.

Trendelenburg's Sign

To assess the strength of the gluteus medius muscle:

- Place the client in a standing position.
- Stand behind the client, observing the relative heights of the client's posterior superior iliac spines and iliac crests.
- Instruct the client to stand on the affected leg.
- Observe the non-weight-bearing side of the pelvis.
    - ✦ If the pelvis on the unsupported side stays level or drops, the test is **positive** for gluteus medius weakness. A nerve root lesion or poliomyelitis may be the cause of the weakness. However, if the pelvis on the unsupported side rises slightly, the test is **negative.**

Gluteus Maximus Strength Test, AR

To assess gluteus maximus muscle strength:

- Place the client in a prone position, with the knee of the side to be tested in 90 degrees of flexion.
- Stabilize the client's pelvis with one hand over the iliac crest and instruct the client to place the affected hip in as much extension as possible, holding this position. If the client can hold this position against gravity, this indicates three on the strength scale (see muscle strength grading in General Tests).
- Apply anteriorly directed pressure to the distal femur.
    - ✦ The test is **positive** for gluteus maximus muscle weakness when the client is unable to resist this pressure.

Piriformis and Other Lateral Rotators Strength Tests, AR

To assess the strength of piriformis and other lateral rotator muscles:

- Place the client in a prone position, with both legs together, flexing the knee of the affected side to 90 degrees.
- With one hand, stabilize the pelvis at the iliac crest of the unaffected side.
- With the other hand, move the affected foot across the midline, positioning the femur in external rotation. Instruct the client to hold the leg in this position.
- Apply pressure to the medial aspect of the ankle in a lateral direction.
    - ✦ A **positive** sign of weakness is the client's inability to hold the leg in position.

A variation:

- Place the client in a seated position, with the knees flexed over the edge of the table.
- Externally rotate the femur of the affected leg by bringing the foot in an arc medially and then past the midline. Instruct the client not to let the foot and leg rotate from this position. If the client can hold this position against gravity, this indicates three on the strength scale (see muscle strength grading in General Tests).

- Stabilize the lateral aspect of the knee with one hand and apply a laterally directed pressure to the medial ankle, so the femur goes into internal rotation.
  - ✦ A **positive** sign is weakness of the piriformis and other lateral rotator muscles..

Pace Abduction Test

To assess the strength of piriformis muscle:

- Place the client in a seated position, with the hips in 90 degrees of flexion and the knees together.
- Instruct the client to place both hands on the lateral knees and apply resistance, holding the knees together.
- Then instruct the client to abduct the hips by pushing the knees apart against the resistence.
  - ✦ Piriformis muscle weakness is a **positive** sign; pain indicates piriformis trigger points (*Travell, Simons, 1992*).

Hamstring Strength Test, AR

To differentiate between a strain of the **medial hamstrings** (semitendinosus and semimembranosus) and the **lateral hamstring** (biceps femoris) muscles:

- Place the client in a prone position, with the affected knee in less than 90 degrees of flexion.
- Stabilize at the pelvis on the affected side with one hand and at the distal posterior tibia with the other hand.
- To assess the medial hamstrings, rotate the femur slightly internally. Instruct the client to hold the leg in this position against gravity. If the client can hold this position against gravity, this indicates three on the strength scale (see muscle strength grading in General Tests).
- Apply pressure in the direction of knee extension.
  - ✦ Pain located deep in the tissue is **positive** for semimembranosus muscle, while pain felt superficially is **positive** for semitendinosus muscle. Pain may also be felt at the tendinous attachment at the ischial tuberosity.
- To assess the lateral hamstring, rotate the femur slightly externally. Again, instruct the client to hold the leg in this position against gravity. If the client can hold this position against gravity, this indicates three on the strength scale (see muscle strength grading in General Tests).
- Apply pressure in the direction of knee extension.
  - ✦ Pain located more laterally is **positive** for biceps femoris strain. Weakness is present in all cases (*Kendall et al., 1993*).

Hip Adductor Strength Test, AR

To differentiate among strains of the **adductor longus, pectineus** or **adductor magnus** muscles:

- Place the client in a supine position, with the knee of the affected leg in extension and the hip in a neutral position.
- Stabilize at the medial knee of the uninjured limb with one hand and at the proximal medial tibia of the affected leg with the other hand.
- To assess **adductor longus** muscle, place the femur in a neutral position, with no internal or external rotation. Instruct the client to hold the leg in this position.
- Apply pressure in the direction of abduction.
- To assess **pectineus** muscle, rotate the femur internally. Again, instruct the client to hold the leg in this position.
- Apply pressure in the direction of abduction.
- To assess **adductor magnus** muscle, rotate the femur externally. Once more, instruct the client to hold the leg in this position.
- Apply pressure in the direction of abduction.
  - ✦ Pain and weakness in one of the above tests are **positive** results for a strain of that muscle *(Brukner, Khan, 1993)*.

Knee Tests

True Tibia and Femur Length Test

To assess tibia and femur length:
- Place the client in a supine position, with the hips and knees flexed and the plantar surfaces of the feet on the table. The malleoli are even and the knees are together.
- Stand at the foot of the table and compare the heights of the tibial plateaus, looking for the shorter tibia.
- Move to the side of the table and compare the positions of the patellas, looking for the shorter femur *(Magee, 1992)*.

Noble's Test

To assess for the presence of iliotibial band friction syndrome:
- Place the client in a supine position, with both the affected hip and knee flexed to 90 degrees.
- Firmly yet tolerably compress the iliotibial band two centimetres proximal to the lateral femoral condyle.
- Instruct the client to extend the knee and hip slowly while compression is maintained.
  - ✦ If the client complains of pain over the lateral femoral condyle at about 30 degrees of knee extension, the test is **positive** for iliotibial band friction syndrome.

Q (Quadriceps) Angle

The Q angle is the angle between the quadriceps tendon and the patellar tendon. It is formed by two intersecting lines, one from the anterior superior iliac spine through the middle of the patella and the other from the tibial tubercle through the middle of the patella. Measurement of the Q angle reveals whether the client is prone to patellar tracking problems. There is debate as to whether the angle is measured with the knee in full extension and with *(Hertling, Kessler, 1990)* or without *(Magee, 1992)* the quadricep muscles contracted, or whether the knee should be partially flexed to measure the functional angle *(Fox, Del Pizzo, 1993)*.

To measure the Q angle with the knee in extension:

- Place the client in a standing position, with the knees in extension and the feet in a neutral position with no pronation or supination. The femur is also in a neutral position with no internal or external rotation. Due to the biomechanics of the ankle, knee and hip, different positions of these joints can alter the Q angle. For example, the Q angle is increased during internal rotation of the femur (anteversion) coupled with external rotation of the tibia.

- Place the central pivot of a goniometer over the centre of the patella. The proximal arm lies over the quadriceps tendon, aligned with the anterior superior iliac spine. The distal arm of the goniometer lies over the patellar tendon, aligned with the middle axis of the tendon itself *(Fox, Del Pizzo, 1993)*.

  ✦ A **normal Q angle** with the knee extended and the quadriceps muscle relaxed is 18 degrees for women and 13 degrees for men *(Hertling, Kessler, 1990)*.

  ✦ A Q angle of less than 13 degrees allows the patella to track medially between the femoral condyles, placing extra stress on the medial articulating facets of the patella and leading to chondromalacia patellae.

  ✦ A Q angle of greater than 18 degrees allows the patella to track laterally, stressing the lateral facets. This is associated with patellar tracking dysfunction, chondromalacia patellae and patellar subluxation *(Magee, 1992)*.

To measure the **functional** Q angle:

- Place the client in a seated position, with the affected knee held between 30 and 40 degrees of flexion. This places the knee in a functional (as opposed to a static) position for measurement. The same landmarks as above are used *(Fox, Del Pizzo, 1993)*.

Posterior "Sag" Sign
(also called the Gravity Drawer Test)

To assess the integrity of the posterior cruciate ligament:

- Place the client in a supine position, with the hips flexed to 45 degrees and the knees flexed to 90 degrees with the feet flat on the table. In this position, the tibia is able to drop or sag posteriorly on the femur if the posterior cruciate is torn.

- Observe the profile of both knees from the side of the table.

  ✦ A **positive** test is indicated if the affected tibia sags posteriorly compared to the unaffected knee *(Magee, 1992)*.

Waldron's Test

To assess for patellofemoral syndrome:

- Place the client in a standing position.

- Palpate the affected patella while the client performs a number of slow deep knee bends.

  ✦ The test is **positive** when pain, crepitus and poor patellar tracking are present.

Ballottable Patella or Major Effusion Test

To assess for a major increase in the synovial fluid within the knee joint capsule following an acute knee injury:

- Place the client in a supine position, with the affected knee in as much extension as possible. When swelling is present in the knee, the client will likely hold the knee in slight flexion. Large amounts of effusion will cause the patella to float on the synovial fluid between it and the femoral condyles.

- Gently but firmly extend the knee. Compress the patella down on to the condyles and then release it.

  ✦ If the patella clicks onto the femur and then rebounds to the floating position, the test is **positive** for major swelling. Torn cruciate ligaments, meniscal tearing or osteochondral fracture may be the cause *(Magee, 1992)*.

- With a positive test, immediately refer the client for **emergency medical attention.**

  ✦ The swelling could be a hemarthrosis. Blood in the joint capsule is irritating and erosive to the articular cartilage and must be aspirated. A hemarthrosis develops one to two hours after the injury occurs. Joint effusion due to synovial fluid usually develops over eight to 12 hours.

  ✦ However, a **negative** test does not indicate the absence of major intracapsular damage, since a severe injury may allow the synovial fluid to leak outside the knee joint capsule into the surrounding soft tissue.

- If this test is negative, yet swelling is still present, the **brush or minor effusion test** for swelling may be performed.

Brush or Minor Effusion Test

To assess for lesser amounts of synovial fluid within the knee joint after an acute injury:

- Place the client in a supine position.

- With the client's knee in as much extension as possible, attempt to slowly brush or sweep the effusion from the superior lateral aspect of the knee and suprapatellar pouch.

  ✦ If excess fluid is present, it may take one or two seconds to appear in a bulge inferior to the patella. This **positive** test will indicate from four to eight millilitres of extra synovial fluid within the joint *(Magee, 1992)*, possibly resulting from cruciate or meniscal damage.

- A positive brush test also indicates immediate **emergency medical attention.**

  ✦ Swelling that does not move — indicating a **negative** result — is likely an extracapsular interstitial edema. This may be due to a medial collateral ligament injury, for example.

Valgus Stress Test, Knee

To assess the integrity of the structures that prevent a medial instability at the knee:

- Place the client in a supine position.
- Stabilize the affected leg in slight external rotation with one hand on the medial malleolus and the other hand at the lateral aspect of the knee, and with the knee in full extension.
- Apply a valgus, or medially directed, stress on the lateral knee.
- As you apply this pressure, you are assessing the joint capsule, medial collateral ligament and both cruciate ligaments.
- With the knee in 20 to 30 degrees of flexion, you are assessing the medial collateral ligament.
  - ✦ A **positive** test in either full knee extension or in 20 to 30 degrees of flexion is indicated by pain in the injured tissues and excessive movement or gapping at the medial aspect of the knee *(Magee, 1992).*

Varus Stress Test, Knee

To assess the integrity of the structures that prevent lateral instability at the knee:

- Place the client in a supine position.
- Stabilize the affected leg in slight external rotation with one hand on the lateral malleolus and the other hand on the medial aspect of the knee, and with the knee in full extension.
- Apply a varus, or laterally directed, stress on the medial knee.
- As you apply this pressure, you are assessing the joint capsule, lateral collateral ligament and both the cruciate ligaments.
- With the knee in 20 to 30 degrees of flexion, you are assessing the lateral collateral ligament.
  - ✦ A **positive** test in either full knee extension or 20 to 30 degrees of flexion is indicated by pain in the injured tissues and excessive movement or gapping at the lateral aspect of the knee *(Magee, 1992).*

Lachman's Test

This test is considered to be the most accurate for assessing the integrity of the anterior cruciate ligament. There are several positions for performing this test, two of which are described here *(Larson, Grana, 1993):*

- Place the client in a supine position, with the affected knee in 30 degrees of flexion. This places the knee in the position where the anterior cruciate ligament plays the maximum functional role. This position also reduces the stabilizing effect of the menisci and the bony lip at the posterior aspect of both tibial condyles.
- Stabilize the distal femur with one hand and grasp the proximal tibia in the other hand.

If the client's leg is large or heavy, the ankle of the leg being tested can be placed between your torso and elbow, adducting your humerus to clamp the lower leg against your body.

- Apply an anteriorly directed stress to the tibia.

A variation:

- Place the client in a seated position, with the affected leg over the edge of the table.
- Sit in front of the client, supporting the client's ankle on your thigh and placing the client's knee in 30 degrees of flexion.
- Stabilize the distal femur with one hand.
- Apply an anteriorly directed stress on the proximal tibia with the other hand.
    - ✦ In either variation, the test is **positive**, indicating damage to the anterior cruciate ligament, when there is pain with an acute injury, an excessive anterior motion of the tibia and a disappearance of the infrapatellar tendon slope.

Anterior-Posterior Drawer Test, Knee

While it is agreed that the cruciate ligaments are assessed, sources differ as to which other specific structures might also be assessed with this test *(Hertling, Kessler, 1990; Magee, 1992).*

To assess anterior and posterior stability at the knee:

- Place the client in a supine position, with the affected knee flexed to 90 degrees, the hip flexed to 45 degrees and the foot flat on the table. This places the anterior cruciate ligament almost level with the tibial plateau and allows the hamstrings to relax, not stabilizing the tibia.
- Sit on the table, anchoring the client's foot under your thigh.
- Grasp the tibia with both hands, placing the thumbs over the tibial plateau. Take care not to compress the common peroneal nerve.
- Assess the integrity of the anterior cruciate ligament by pulling the tibia towards you. Six millimetres is the normal amount of movement.
    - ✦ If the tibia moves anteriorly more than 6 millimetres, the test is **positive** for anterior cruciate ligament and posterior joint capsule damage. Pain may or may not be present. If the anterior movement is accompanied by a snapping or jerking motion, there may also be meniscus damage *(Magee, 1992; Gerard, Kleinfield, 1993).*

To test the posterior cruciate ligament:

- With you and the client in the same position as above, push the tibia posteriorly on the femur.
    - ✦ Excessive posterior motion of the tibia may be **positive** for posterior cruciate injury.
- The tests can be combined in a back and forth rocking motion.

Patellar Apprehension Test, PR

To assess whether the patella is likely to dislocate laterally:

- Place the client in a supine position, with the knee in extension.
- Use a slow, moderate pressure against the medial aspect of the patella, moving it in a

lateral direction while observing the client's face.

✦ A **positive** test is indicated by an expression of apprehension and, perhaps, the client's attempt to move the knee away from the pressure.

Helfet's Test

To assess the dynamic rotary function of the tibia:

• Place the client in a seated position, with the legs hanging over the edge of the table and the knees flexed to 90 degrees. In this position, the tibial tuberosity is perpendicular to the midline of the patella.

• Slowly extend the client's knee.

• Observe the relative alignment of the tibial tuberosity to the midline of the patella or palpate the movement of the tibial tuberosity. The medial femoral condyle is approximately one centimetre longer than the lateral femoral condyle. Because of this, as the tibia moves into extension, it first moves over the available lateral condyle surface and then must rotate laterally to use the remaining medial condyle surface. This lateral tibial rotation in the last few degrees of extension locks the knee into full extension.

✦ An absence of this slight lateral tibial motion, indicating a **positive** test, means that a torn meniscus or injured cruciate ligament is physically blocking extension.

Note: It is not possible to perform this test if knee joint effusion restricts full extension.

McMurray's Test

To assess for injury to the menisci:

• Place the client in a supine position, with the hip and knee in flexion.

• Cup one hand over the client's knee, with the palm over the patella and the fingers and thumb over the joint line.

• With the other hand, grasp the client's heel.

• Slowly extend the client's knee, while applying different stresses to check both menisci. With external rotation of the tibia and a valgus stress placed on the knee, the medial meniscus is assessed. With internal rotation of the tibia and a varus stress placed on the knee, the lateral meniscus is assessed.

✦ In either case, a **positive** test, meaning meniscal injury, is indicated by a click or catch in the extension of the knee. However, a **negative** test does not completely rule out a meniscal tear *(Buschbacher, 1994)*.

Bragard's Sign

To assess for meniscal tearing:

• Place the client in a supine position, with the hip and knee flexed.

• Externally rotate the tibia with one hand while extending the knee.

• With the other hand, stabilize proximal to the knee.

✦ A **positive** sign of pain or tenderness along the medial aspect of the joint line indicates medial meniscus injury. Internal rotation of the tibia should decrease the pain.

✦ The test is **positive** for lateral meniscus damage if internal rotation of the tibia with knee extension gives rise to lateral joint line pain. External rotation of the tibia should decrease the pain *(Magee, 1992)*.

Apley's Compression Test

To assess for meniscal injury:

• Place the client in a prone position, with the affected knee flexed to 90 degrees.

• Compress the flexed knee joint and the menisci by pushing the client's foot and tibia down into the table, followed by internal and external rotation of the tibia.

✦ If the client reports pain on the medial aspect of the joint, the test is **positive** for medial meniscus damage, while pain on the lateral side means lateral meniscus injury.

Apley's Distraction Test

To assess the integrity of the collateral knee ligaments:

• Place the client in a prone position, with the knee flexed to 90 degrees.

• Stabilize the client's leg by placing your knee on the client's posterior thigh.

• Grasp the client's leg proximal to the ankle.

• Apply traction to the tibia towards the ceiling, which distracts the knee joint.

• Then apply internal and external rotation to the tibia.

✦ If the client reports pain on the medial side of the knee, the test is **positive** for medial collateral ligament damage, while lateral knee pain indicates lateral collateral ligament injury.

Coronary Ligamentous Stress Test, PR

To assess the coronary ligament:

• Place the client in a seated position, with the knee flexed to 90 degrees.

• Passively externally rotate the tibia on the femur.

✦ Pain on external rotation of the tibia is **positive** for coronary ligament sprain. With a sprain of this ligament, there is no pain with a **valgus stress test**.

Clarke's Patellofemoral Grind Test

To assess for patellofemoral syndrome:

• Place the client in a supine position, with the knees extended.

• Compress the patella posteriorly onto the femoral condyles and then, with moderate pressure, move the patella distally.

• Instruct the client to contract the quadricep muscles, which pulls the patella proximally.

✦ If apprehension, pain and crepitus are present as the irritated surfaces of the patella move over the femur, the test is **positive.** This test may be uncomfortable even for asymptomatic clients if force is used to compress the patella. Therefore, the test should be repeated several times, using gradually increasing pressure.

McConnell's Test

To assess for patellofemoral tracking problems:

- Place the client in a seated position, with the legs hanging free over the end of the table.

- Sit in front of the client.

- Instruct the client to externally rotate the femur of the affected leg while performing active resisted isometric contractions with the quadricep muscles of the affected knee at 0, 30, 60, 90 and 120 degrees of flexion.

- Note the painful ranges.

- Then passively bring the client's knee to full extension, resting the heel on your knee to allow the client to relax the quadricep muscles fully.

- Glide the affected patella medially and hold it in this position.

- Instruct the client to perform isometric contractions at the knee ranges that were painful before.

  ✦ The test is **positive** for patellofemoral lateral tracking problems if the pain **decreases** significantly.

To assess for medial tracking problems:

- Repeat the above test, gliding the patella laterally and holding it there for the second part of the test.

  ✦ The test is **positive** for medial tracking problems if there is a significant **decrease** in pain *(Fox, Del Pizzo, 1993).*

Ankle and Foot Tests

Homan's Sign

To assess for deep vein thrombosis:

- Place the client in a seated or supine position, with the knee of the affected leg extended.

- Passively dorsiflex the client's ankle.

  ✦ Pain deep to the calf indicates a **positive** test. In addition, you may palpate tenderness or heat local to the thrombophlebitis. The dorsalis pedis pulse is diminished or absent and the affected leg is swollen and has a pallor.

- Massage is locally contraindicated with a positive test; refer the client for **medical assessment.**

Ramirez's Test

To assess for deep vein thrombosis:

- Place the client in a supine position, with the affected knee in flexion and the foot on the table.
- Wrap a blood pressure cuff around the thigh and inflate it to 40 mm Hg.
- Maintain this pressure for at least two minutes.
  - ✦ The resulting venous pressure will cause pain in the calf at the site of the thrombosis. If the client experiences both an increase in pain and an inability to tolerate cuff inflation and sustained pressure for two minutes, the test is **positive** for venous thrombosis.
- Massage is locally contraindicated with a positive test; refer the client for **medical assessment.**

Functional or Structural Pes Planus Test

To determine whether a pes planus is functional or structural:

- Observe the orientation of the client's medial longitudinal arch while the client is weight bearing.
- First, instruct the client to stand with both heels and toes on the ground, and then to stand on the toes only.
- Then instruct the client to sit on the table.
- Observe the medial arch when the client is not weight bearing.
  - ✦ If the medial longitudinal arch is restored when the client is either standing on the toes or seated, the test is **positive** for **functional pes planus**. This is due to muscular or ligamentous weakness. If the arch remains flat when the client is standing on the toes and when seated, the test is **positive** for **structural pes planus.**

Thompson's Test

To assess for third degree strain or rupture of the Achilles tendon:

- Place the client in a supine position, with the feet over the edge of the table and the leg muscles relaxed.
- Squeeze the affected gastrocnemius and soleus muscles.
  - ✦ A **positive** test is the absence of plantarflexion when the muscles are squeezed.
- Note that the client may still be able to plantarflex the affected foot while not weight bearing by using flexor hallucis longus and flexor digitorum longus.

Babinski's Test

To test for the spasticity present with central nervous system lesions:

- Place the client in a supine position.
- Run a pointed object along the plantar aspect of the client's foot. The end of a reflex hammer may be used.

+ Any extension of the big toe and abduction of the other toes is **positive** for a central nervous system lesion. The test is normally positive for infants up to a few weeks old but is negative after five to seven months *(Chusid, 1985).*

Anterior Drawer Test, Ankle

To evaluate the stability of the anterior talofibular ligament:

- Place the client in a seated or supine position.
- With one hand, stabilize the anterior surface of the distal tibia and fibula, superior to the ankle joint.
- With the other hand, grasp the calcaneus.
- Distract the calcaneus from the tibia and fibula by pulling the calcaneus inferiorly.
- With the foot in 20 degrees of plantarflexion, place an anteriorly directed pressure on the calcaneus and talus, applying overpressure at the end of the passive range. This stresses the anterior talofibular ligament.

  + Excessive anterior translation of the talus, sometimes accompanied by an audible thunking, indicates a **positive** test, or ligamentous laxity or rupture *(Buschbacher, 1994).*

Anterior Talofibular Ligamentous Stress Test, PR

To assess the integrity of the anterior talofibular ligament:

- Place the client in a seated position with the affected leg flexed at the knee, hanging over the end of the table.
- With one hand, stabilize the anterior surface of the tibia and fibula proximal to the ankle.
- With the other hand, grasp the dorsal surface of the foot and apply a combined movement of plantarflexion, inversion and adduction applying overpressure at the end of the passive range.
- Minimize the protective muscle splinting of an early subacute sprain by gradually increasing pressure until the ligament is fully stressed.

  + A **positive** test for a subacute, mild to moderate anterior talofibular ligament sprain is pain local to the ligament and some excessive movement with a muscle spasm end feel. However, a subacute total ligament rupture may present either as hypermobility or as a false negative result due to protective muscle spasm. A chronic total ligament rupture is painlessly hypermobile.

Calcaneofibular Ligamentous Stress Test, PR

To assess the calcaneofibular ligament:

- Place the client in a seated position as in the previous test.
- With one hand, stabilize the anterior surface of the tibia and fibula proximal to the ankle.
- With the other hand, grasp the calcaneus and invert the hindfoot, applying overpressure at the end of the passive range.
- Keep the ankle in a neutral position with no plantarflexion or dorsiflexion.

✦ A **positive** result for acute calcaneofibular ligament sprain is pain local to the ligament and some excessive movement, as in the previous test. Muscle spasm end feel may be present with a subacute injury.

Calcaneocuboid Ligamentous Stress Test, PR

To assess the integrity of the calcaneocuboid ligament:

- Place the client in a seated position as in the previous tests.
- With one hand, stabilize the calcaneus.
- With the other hand, supinate and adduct the affected forefoot, applying overpressure at the end of the passive range.
    - ✦ Pain and hypermobilty local to the ligament are **positive** results for calcaneocuboid sprain. Muscle spasm end feel may be present with a subacute injury.

Deltoid Ligamentous Stress Test, PR

To assess this ligament using three separate passive movements:

- Place the client in a seated position, with the leg flexed at the knee and hanging over the table.
- With one hand, stabilize the anterior surface of the tibia and fibula proximal to the ankle.
- To assess the anterior fibres of the deltoid ligament, use the other hand to grasp the dorsal surface of the foot, combining eversion and plantarflexion of the foot and applying overpressure at the end of the passive range.
- To assess the middle fibres, reposition the hand so you are grasping the calcaneus so the hindfoot can be taken into eversion with overpressure.
- To assess the posterior fibres, reposition the hand again along the plantar surface of the foot, combining eversion and dorsiflexion of the foot with overpressure.
- To perform a general, non-specific assessment of the deltoid ligament, evert the hindfoot only.
    - ✦ As with the previous three ligaments, pain and hypermobility local to the ligament are signs of a **positive** test. Muscle spasm end feel may be present with a subacute injury.

Morton's Neuroma Test

To assess for the presence of Morton's neuroma:

- Place the client in a seated position.
- Compress the foot by applying pressure to the medial and lateral aspects of the foot at the metatarsophalangeal joints. A hypermobile forefoot, or one that has become hypermobile through repeated injury, may compress or pinch one of the interdigital nerves. The most commonly affected nerve is between the third and fourth metatarsal bones. Pressure compresses the neuroma.
    - ✦ A **positive** test is indicated by a sharp pain at the location of the neuroma. The pain is worsened by activity *(Booher, Thibodeau 1989)*.

Gastrocnemius Length Test

To assess the length of gastrocnemius muscle:

- Place the client in a supine position with the knee fully extended and the heel over the edge of the table.
- Grasp the calcaneus with one hand and place the other stabilizing hand on the lateral plantar surface along the metatarsals.
- Apply traction inferiorly to the calcaneus, moving the foot into dorsiflexion.
- Use the stabilizing hand to prevent the foot from inverting or everting.
- The ankle should be able to dorsiflex to 20 degrees *(Janda, 1984)*.

A variation:

- Perform this test with the client in a prone postition.
    + The test is **positive** for a shortened gastrocnemius muscle with reduced dorsiflexion.

Soleus Length Test

To assess soleus muscle length:

- Place the client in a seated position, with the knee in flexion and the heel over the edge of the table.
- Grasp the calcaneus with one hand and place the other stabilizing hand on the lateral plantar surface along the metatarsals.
- Apply traction inferiorly to the calcaneus, moving the foot into dorsiflexion.
- Use the stabilizing hand to prevent the foot from inverting or everting.
- The ankle should be able to dorsiflex to 20 degrees.

A variation:

- Perform this test with the client in a prone position.
    + The test is **positive** for soleus muscle shortness with reduced dorsiflexion.

To perform a functional length test:

- Place the client in a squatting position, with the elbows resting on the thighs. The knees are parallel, but not touching.
    + The test is **positive** for soleus muscle shortness if the heels do not touch when the client is squatting. If the soleus is of normal length, the client is able to squat with the heels touching the floor *(Janda, 1984)*.

Gastrocnemius Strength Test, AR

To assess the strength of the gastrocnemius muscle:

- Place the client in a prone position, with the knee of the leg to be tested in extension and the foot extending over the end of the table. The ankle is in a neutral position with no dorsiflexion or plantarflexion.
- Apply pressure in a superior direction to the plantar surface of the foot, at the heads of the metatarsals.

- Instruct the client not to let the foot be pushed in this direction.
    - ✦ The test is **positive** for gastrocnemius weakness if the client is unable to resist the pressure.

To assess the strength of gastrocnemius and soleus muscles in a functional test:

- Instruct the standing client to walk on the toes for several seconds.
    - ✦ The test is **positive** for muscle weakness if the client is unable to perform this function.

Soleus Strength Test, AR

To assess the strength of the soleus muscle:

- Place the client in a prone position, with the knee of the leg to be tested in 90 degrees of flexion.
- Place the ankle in plantarflexion and instruct the client to hold this position.
- Apply pressure to the plantar surface of the foot, attempting to push the foot into dorsiflexion.
    - ✦ The test is **positive** for a weak soleus if the client cannot hold the ankle in plantar flexion.

Tibialis Posterior Strength Test, AR

To assess the strength of tibialis posterior muscle:

- Place the client in a supine position, with the knee in extension.
- Place the ankle in plantar flexion and inversion, stabilizing with one hand the anterior surface of the tibia and fibula proximal to the ankle.
- Instruct the client to hold the ankle in this position.
- With the other hand, apply pressure over the navicular and cuneiform bones at the medial and plantar surface of the foot. The direction of pressure is into dorsiflexion and eversion.
    - The test is **positive** for tibialis posterior muscle weakness if the client is unable to resist this pressure *(Kendall et al., 1993)*.

Tibialis Anterior Strength Test, AR

To assess the strength of the tibialis anterior muscle:

- Place the client in a supine or seated position.
- With one hand, stabilize the anterior surface of the tibia and fibula proximal to the ankle.
- Dorsiflex the client's ankle and invert the foot.
- Instruct the client to hold this position.
- With the other hand, apply pressure over the cuneiform and navicular bones on the dorsal and medial surface of the foot, in the direction of plantarflexion and eversion.
    - ✦ The test is **positive** for tibialis anterior muscle weakness if the client is unable to resist this pressure.
- To avoid including extensor hallucis longus and brevis, instruct the client not to extend the great toe and do not apply pressure over the metatarsophalangeal joint or the toe itself.

To assess tibialis anterior muscle strength in a functional test:

- Instruct the standing client to walk on the heels for several seconds.
    - ✦ An inability to maintain this posture indicates a **positive** test for tibialis anterior muscle weakness.

Peroneus Longus and Brevis Strength Test, AR

To assess the strength of peroneus longus and brevis muscles:

- Place the client in a supine position.

- With one hand, stabilize the anterior surface of the tibia and fibula proximal to the ankle.

- Place the client's ankle in plantarflexion with the foot everted. Instruct the client to hold this position.

- With the other hand, apply pressure over the fifth metatarsal bone on the dorsal and lateral surface of the foot, in the direction of dorsiflexion and inversion.
    - ✦ The test is **positive** for weakness of the peroneus longus and brevis muscles if the client is unable to resist this pressure.

General Tests

Swelling or Edema Girth Measurement

To assess for the extent of any swelling or edema present:

- Use a tape measure to record the **swelling or edema girth**, or the circumference of the limb where the swelling or edema is located.

- To ensure that the girth is measured at the same location each time, record the distance from a bony landmark to the point of girth measurement. This same distance is used in each subsequent girth assessment. For example, with a thigh injury, the head of the fibula or the anterior superior iliac spine may be used as a landmark.

Swelling and edema should be differentiated from each other:

- ✦ A painful **swelling** that occurs between a few minutes and an hour after an acute injury often indicates a **hematoma** (Hertling, Kessler, 1990; Brukner, Khan, 1993).

- ✦ **Swelling** that takes eight to 24 hours to develop following an acute injury to a joint may indicate **synovial effusion** (Magee, 1992). Both these conditions indicate referral for **immediate medical attention.**

- ✦ **Edema** is an accumulation of fluid in the interstitial spaces of the tissue and may present with acute or chronic conditions.

Pitted Edema Test

To assess for the presence of chronic pitted edema:

- Apply firm finger pressure to the edematous area for 10 to 20 seconds, then release

the pressure.
+ If an indentation remains where the pressure was applied, the test is **positive** for pitted edema.

Trigger Point Compression Test

To assess for pain caused by latent trigger points which are activated by movement, not by rest:

- Compress the painful, affected muscle, or the skin above the affected muscle, in a pincer grasp, while the muscle is actively contracting.
  + If the pain diminishes or disappears on compression, the test is **positive** for a latent trigger point *(Travell, Simons, 1983)*.

Tendinitis Differentiation

To assess for tendinitis anywhere in the body using active resisted isometric contraction:

- Test the affected musculotendinous unit thoroughly; instruct the client to resist isometrically at discrete intervals throughout the entire range of the affected muscle.
  + A **positive** test for tendinitis is indicated by pain at the lesion site on the tendon, which **increases** with the force of the isometric contraction. There may also be muscle weakness.

Bursitis Differentiation

To assess for bursitis using active resisted isometric contraction:

- Instruct the client to isometrically contract the muscles and tendons surrounding the affected bursa.
  + A **positive** test is indicated by pain at the site of the bursa that is **constant**, even if the force of the isometric contraction is increased. The pain is caused by the surrounding muscles and tendons compressing the inflamed bursa as they contract. Since the bursa is noncontractile, the pain begins as it is compressed and remains constant. This is unlike the pain of a tendinitis, which increases as the tendon contracts.

Stress Fracture Test

Although a definitive diagnosis for stress fracture is made medically by X-ray, to assess for the possibility of this fracture:

- Apply direct compression to the site of the suspected stress fracture with the thumb.
  + The area of the stress fracture is extremely point tender to compression, whereas solid bone a few centimetres away from the fracture site lacks this extreme tenderness. Severe local pain on direct compression from the thumbs is **positive** for a stress fracture.

A variation:

- Take a tuning fork and strike it on a solid surface to initiate its vibration.

- Gently touch the end of the tuning fork to the point-tender area of the suspected stress fracture.
  - ✦ Severe local pain is a **positive** sign for stress fracture *(Buschbacher, 1994)*; refer the client for **medical assessment**.

Tinel's Sign

To assess nerve compression or the amount of regeneration of a peripheral nerve or the presence of a neuroma at the severed end of a complete nerve lesion:

- Locate the specific nerve to be assessed and gently tap or percuss the nerve.
  - ✦ In the case of nerve compression, a **positive** test is paresthesia or tingling along the distribution of the nerve, distal to where the nerve is percussed. This is a common test for carpal tunnel syndrome, where the percussion is applied over the median nerve at the carpal tunnel.

Other specific locations for Tinel's test:

- Tap the **brachial plexus** superior to the clavicle.
- Tap the **ulnar nerve** at the elbow between the olecranon and the medial epicondyle.
- Tap the infrapatellar branch of the **saphenous nerve** medial to the tibial tubercle.
- Tap the **common peroneal nerve** posterior to the head of the fibula.
- Tap the anterior branch of the **deep peroneal nerve** at the anterior ankle.
- Tap the **posterior tibial nerve** just posterior to the medial malleolus *(Magee, 1992)*.

To determine how far a peripheral nerve has regenerated after a trauma (axonotmesis or neurotmesis):

- Apply Tinel's test along the path of the affected nerve, going from proximal to distal.
  - ✦ A **positive** test is indicated by paresthesia or a tingling sensation, which the client will feel up to the most distal point that the nerve has regenerated. Beyond that point the test will not yield a response. With the presence of a neuroma that is the result of a trauma or severance of a peripheral nerve, a **positive** Tinel's test is indicated by pain at the site of the neuroma *(Stewart, 1993; Hoppenfeld, 1976; Chusid, 1985)*.

Muscle Strength Grading

Assessment of the client's muscle strength is useful in determining a baseline of strength and in designing a remedial exercise program. The strength can then be regularly reassessed to chart the client's progress during the recovery process. Conditions that result in primary symptoms of muscle weakness include peripheral nerve lesions, degenerative disc disease, spinal cord injury and multiple sclerosis. Muscle weakness may also be present following muscle strain, tendinitis, inflammatory joint diseases such as rheumatoid arthritis and disuse or immobilization of a body part, such as with frozen shoulder, osteoarthritis, fracture, burns and amputation.

Manual muscle strength testing will not yield clear results with clients who have spasticity due to upper motor neuron lesions, such as cerebral palsy or hemiplegia. Here, the muscles are hypertonic; movement frequently occurs in larger synergistic patterns. This makes isolating the individual joint motions difficult or impossible, so a specific muscle cannot be tested. In addition, the effects of reflexes and the position of the client's head, body and proximal joints influence the client's muscle tone and, therefore, the ability to perform specific movements. For example, a client with hemiplegia will have reinforced flexor spasticity patterns in the affected upper limb if the head is rotated away from the affected side *(Bobath, 1990)*.

With muscle weakness resulting from disuse or peripheral nerve injuries:

- Begin with gravity-decreased testing, grading the client's ability to move affected structures through the full range of motion. These motions are performed on a horizontal plane to reduce the effects of gravity on the muscle.

- For example, ask a supine client to abduct the affected humerus to assess the strength of the deltoid and supraspinatus.

- If possible, progress towards testing with gravity, where the movement occurs on the vertical plane and gravity provides resistance.

- In the above example, instruct the seated client to abduct the humerus against gravity.

- Finally, if possible, apply some additional resistance to the muscle using the hand or fingers.

To assess the strength of a normally innervated muscle:

- Place the client in a position that allows for fixation of the trunk. Depending on the muscle to be assessed, this position may be prone, supine, sidelying or seated.

- Generally, stabilize proximal to the muscle to be tested with one hand, while applying the testing force with the other hand. This force is applied gradually and smoothly, without jerking the muscle.

- For more accurate testing, instruct the client to avoid shifting the body while performing the movement. This applies to all forms of strength testing.

- Specifically palpate the muscle as the client attempts to contract it. This helps to identify that the correct muscle is being used and if contraction is possible at all.

The results can be graded as follows:

GRADE	MEANING OF GRADE
Zero	No response palpated
One	Trace of a response only; the muscle palpably contracts but there is no joint movement
Two	Complete range of motion only if gravity is decreased
Three	Complete range of motion against gravity
Four	Complete range of motion against gravity and moderate resistance
Five	Complete range of motion against gravity and full resistance

(Kendall et al., 1993; Pedretti, Zoltan, 1990; Magee, 1992)

- If you have experience with muscle strength testing, you can also use positive or negative grades to be more precise. For example, describe a client with more than a trace of response (Grade one), but less than complete range of motion with gravity decreased (Grade two), as having Grade two-minus or incomplete range of motion with gravity reduced.

- It may be difficult to accurately determine strength using this scale with a client who has musculoskeletal injuries or joint pathologies. Such a client can move against gravity (Grade three) but have some weakness, falling somewhere in Grade four. Strength can be measured more accurately using a blood pressure cuff. The cuff is rolled loosely into a cylinder and secured by elastic bands. The rolled cuff is inflated to 100 mm Hg, then deflated to 20 mm Hg. The cuff is then placed between the therapist's palm and the distal portion of the limb to be tested. For example, when asking a seated client to abduct the affected humerus to assess the strength of the deltoid and supraspinatus, the cuff is held at the lateral elbow. Resistance is held for three seconds and the highest pressure is recorded. A rise in pressure of 20 mm Hg is equivalent to 2 kg (5 lbs) of force (*Walker, Helewa, 1996*).

- Be alert for the client substituting other muscles for the muscle being tested. This is called "muscle recruitment". For example, with shoulder abduction, the client may substitute lateral trunk flexion instead of pure glenohumeral abduction if the supraspinatus or deltoid is weak.

- There can be spontaneous muscle fibre movements associated with lower motor neuron degeneration or irritation. Do not confuse these with conscious muscular contraction. In the case of muscle fasciculations, the innervation to the muscle is intact but is hyperexcitable due to infection or irritation of the nerve cell body or axon. This results in spontaneous twitching on the muscle's surface. These contractions of muscle fibre groups can be seen and palpated (*Porth, 1990; Chusid, 1985*). Fasciculations are most prominent in disorders such as polio, amyotrophic lateral sclerosis and spinal cord injuries.

Deep Tendon Reflex Test

Deep tendon reflexes are tested to assess the functioning of the nerve or nerve roots supplying the reflex. Deep tendon reflexes are caused by stretching of the muscle spindle, which synapses through the sensory neurons to the spinal cord and then back through the motor neurons, contracting the muscle.

To assess the reflex:

- Tap the tendon with a reflex hammer and watch for a sudden muscular contraction or reflex jerk.

- To eliminate the possibility of a fading response due to a developing nerve root lesion, tap the tendon five or six times or repeat the test several times to ensure that the response is consistent.

  + With central nervous system damage, the reflex response is hyperreflexive or exaggerated, and generally bilateral.

  + With a peripheral nerve lesion, the abnormal or lost peripheral nerve conductivity results in a hyporeflexive (weakened) or areflexive (lost) deep tendon reflex and the specific limb is affected.

1122

- Reflexes are graded as:

  - ✦ zero (absent)
  - ✦ one (diminished)
  - ✦ two (average)
  - ✦ three (exaggerated)
  - ✦ four (clonus).

- The neurological levels tested and the tendons commonly used are as follows:

LEVEL, TENDON AND NORMAL RESPONSE

C5, Distal biceps tendon, biceps contracts

C6, Brachioradialis tendon, elbow flexes

C7-C8, Distal triceps tendon, elbow extends

L3-L4, Patellar tendon, knee extends

L4 L5, Tibialis posterior tendon, ankle plantarflexes, foot inverts

L5-S1, Semimembranosis tendon, knee flexes

S1-S2, Achilles tendon, ankle plantarflexes

(Hoppenfeld, 1976; Magee, 1992)

Muscle Spasticity Grading, AF

To assess the degree of spasticity present with central nervous system lesions:

- Place the client in a comfortable seated or supine position.
- Instruct the client to move the limb through the cardinal planes of motion of each affected joint. The degree of spasticity present will affect the voluntary movements of the client. The more extreme the spasticity, the less controlled the active movement will be.
- Note that the client's effort to make particular movements of the affected side often in itself will increase spasticity. For other factors that increase spasticity, see the chapter Strategies: Central Nervous System Conditions.
- Spasticity in active free movement is generally graded as mild, moderate or severe:

  - ✦ **Mild spasticity** allows for the client to complete movements in a regular manner but more slowly and with somewhat more effort.
  - ✦ **Moderate spasticity** enables the client to manage parts of the movement or sometimes all of the movement, but with excessive effort and the movement is not smooth.
  - ✦ **Severe spasticity** results in the client's inability to perform active free movements in the affected limbs.

Muscle Spasticity Grading, PR

To passively test for spasticity present with central nervous system lesions:

- Place the client in a comfortable seated or supine position.

- **Slowly**, passively move the affected joint **away** from the pattern of spasticity and assess the resistance to the movement.

- Note that the client will have excessive involuntary **assisted** movement when the limb is moved **into** the patterns of spasticity. In both cases, the client is unable to control the movement.

- Note that several factors can increase spasticity. Passive movements performed quickly can increase spasticity, whereas slow passive movements allow for full movement after some initial resistance. For more factors that increase spasticity, see the chapter Strategies: Central Nervous System Conditions.

There is no agreed-upon objective scale for measuring spasticity readily available to therapists. Instead, a general assessment is performed based on the amount of passive movement available at a joint. This information will be supplemented by the results of active free range of motion testing (*Johnstone, 1991*).

- Spasticity in passive movement is generally graded as mild, moderate or severe:

> ✦ **Mild spasticity** reflects only slight resistance to fairly "normal" movement, though usually the movement must be performed more slowly.
>
> ✦ **Moderate spasticity** will require increased effort to move the limb through some stages of the movement. Motion will be less smooth and likely in a less "normal" pattern.
>
> ✦ **Severe spasticity** interferes with the therapist's ability to move the limb because of strong resistance.

Bradykinesia Test

To assess for bradykinesia (increasingly difficult movement or lack of coordination):

- Place the client in a seated position.

- Instruct the client to alternate pronation and supination of the forearm. Specifically, instruct the client to touch the thigh repeatedly, first with the palm and then with the back of the hand.

  - ✦ A **positive** test will result in the movement becoming slower and increasingly difficult.

Sensory Testing

There is no consensus as to the location on the body and the direction in which sensory testing should be performed. Some sources suggest that the therapist should begin in the area where there is likely no sensory disturbance, or move from proximal, unaffected areas to distal, more likely affected areas on the involved limb. This will allow the client to experience "normal sensation" first *(Mumenthaler, 1992).*

Other sources believe this will encourage the client to imagine sensation that is not present. These sources state that therapists are to move from distal to proximal, or areas of likely sensory impairment to areas of less sensory impairment in the testing protocol *(Wale, 1980).*

In general:

- Place the client in a comfortable seated position during the assessment.

- To eliminate the possibility of visual clues, instruct a sighted client to keep the eyes closed during these assessments.

- Apply the tests so the client cannot detect a pattern.

- If sensory loss or reduction is a consideration, perform a general scan of the potentially affected area and its bilateral counterpart. The area of lost or altered sensation is then clearly mapped out in order to determine if the loss follows a peripheral nerve distribution or a dermatomal distribution. This allows you to determine if the lesion is of a peripheral nerve or of the nerve root.

   ✦ A **positive** test is indicated if the client says the stimulus to the affected area feels different from stimulus to the unaffected area.

- To record test results, use a plus sign to indicate the response is accurate, a minus sign to indicate an inaccurate or delayed response and a zero to indicate a complete lack of response.

- Peripheral nerve patterns are distinct and consistent, whereas dermatomal patterns are variable. Note that, except in cases of very severe lesions, the sensory impairment is often confined to the most distal region. For example, instead of sensory impairment along the entire median nerve distal to the lesion, carpal tunnel symptoms are usually experienced in the fingertips alone *(Stewart, 1993).* It is possible that the tests will cause the client to experience paresthesia, which is often perceived as pain.

Touch Perception Test

Touch perception testing is divided into light touch and deep pressure assessment. For light touch assessment:

- Lightly touch the client's skin with a cotton ball or Q-Tip.

   ✦ If the client does not report perceiving this sensation, the test is **positive** for light touch perception loss.

For deep pressure assessment:

- Apply pressure with the pad of the thumb. Pressure is sufficient to dent the skin.

   ✦ The test is **positive** for deep touch perception loss if the client cannot feel this stimulus.

Temperature Perception Test

To assess the client's temperature perception:

- Fill one test tube or metal container with water that is comfortably hot and another with water that is comfortably cold.

- Apply the test tubes to the affected area on the client's skin.
- Ask the client to report which is hot and which is cold.
    - ✦ If the client cannot differentiate between the two, the test is **positive** for temperature perception loss.

Pain Perception Test

To assess the client's pain perception:

- Use a pinwheel to gently prick the affected area on the client's skin.
- Do **not** break the skin with this procedure.
- Use both blunt and sharp objects to further differentiate between dull and sharp pain perception.
    - ✦ If the client cannot distinguish the sensation as pain, the test is **positive.**
- Since pain and temperature perception follow the same sensory tracts, it is possible to use either the test for temperature perception or the test for pain perception.

Two-Point Discrimination Test

To assess for sensation impairment:

- Use a paper clip bent into a U-shape or the dulled points of a protractor. Set the two points of either instrument two to three millimetres apart.
- Touch the points to the affected area on the client's skin.
- Ask the client if one point or two points are felt.
- If necessary, set the points farther apart and repeat the test. Normal two-point discrimination in the fingertip pads is two to three millimetres.
    - ✦ If the client is unable to determine two points at a distance greater than two to three millimetres, this is a **positive** test for sensation impairment.
    - ✦ With the finger pads, an inability to discriminate two points set 15 millimetres or more apart indicates severe sensation impairment (*Pedretti, Zoltan, 1990*).

Proprioception Test

To assess for proprioception loss:

- Grasp the client's affected finger or toe and passively move it into flexion or extension.
- Ask the client what position the digit is in, bent or straight. The client should answer without hesitation.
    - ✦ An incorrect answer or hesitation before answering indicates a **positive** test for proprioception loss.
- If the test is positive, repeat the test using the next proximal joint, such as the wrist or ankle.

Piloerector Response Test

To assess for loss of the piloerector response:

- Stroke the client's back or upper chest with something cold, such as an ice cube, to elicit a general piloerector response or goosebumps.

- Note any areas where there is no response.

  - ✦ The absence of the piloerector response in a particular area is a **positive** sign for a complete peripheral nerve lesion, while an increase in the response can indicate a partial peripheral nerve lesion.

Appendix D:

VISCERAL AND OTHER SYSTEMIC PATHOLOGY PAIN REFERRAL PATTERNS

Fiona Rattray

Although massage therapists cannot diagnose a condition, an educated assessment of the client's condition can be made. This information is gathered from the client's written health history form, answers to health history questions, observations and the outcome of palpation and orthopedic testing. Therefore, the therapist should be able to recognize when the client is presenting with a pain that does not suggest a neuromusculoskeletal origin but rather points to a possible underlying systemic pathology as the cause.

If results from the assessment and testing are inconclusive or negative for a neuromusculoskeletal source of the pain, the therapist must recognize that massage therapy is inappropriate or contraindicated at this point and that referral to a physician is the next step. If the client is not in pain, it may be possible to perform a relaxation massage following the inconclusive assessment as long as the client is referred to a physician after the treatment. However, continuing with massage therapy for an unknown condition without referring the client to a physician for diagnosis is not being responsible to the client.

The answers to health history questions may give clues to the condition. For example, back pain due to an underlying systemic disorder such as a tumour usually is not relieved by lying down or resting; it may get worse at night. The client with systemic back pain will be restless or will adopt a curled-up posture when sitting. The pain does not vary on activity and frequently is felt in both the back and abdomen at the same level. There may be fever, fatigue, nausea, vomiting or diarrhea. The pain may increase after eating. Sweating and dyspnea may occur after little effort on the client's part. The onset and progression of the pain may be insidious *(Goodman, Snyder, 1995)*.

The client may also present with a combination of a neuromusculoskeletal condition and the symptoms of an undiagnosed pathology. The therapist again needs to recognize that a medical referral is appropriate.

In addition, if the client has a systemic disorder that is referring pain to the abdomen, shoulders or back, and massage is not contraindicated, the therapist must understand that the hypertonicity, muscle guarding and pain are symptomatic to the underlying pathology. Therefore, the therapist should not overwork the area of referred pain. For example, trigger points can be activated by referred visceral pain and it may not be possible to completely inactivate them in the viscerally triggered referral zone. The client may benefit more from having the overall sympathetic nervous system firing reduced through a relaxation treatment.

In summary, a client complaining of pain who has no history of neuromusculoskeletal trauma or overuse may be experiencing systemic pain. The presence of other systemic complaints and the quality of the pain, especially in someone over 45 years of age, indicate the need for medical referral.

Some pathologies, their common pain referrals and a few signs and symptoms are listed below *(Goodman, Snyder, 1995; Porth, 1990)*. This is not meant as a comprehensive listing but as a **guideline** of some warning signs. See also the section on contraindications to massage for more information.

Angina

Perceived as a mild to moderate vice-like pressure, lasting usually less than 10 minutes, the pain is located mostly along the sternum and left shoulder and down the left medial arm to the fingers. Rest or nitroglycerine relieves the pain.

Pericarditis

The pain is continuous, moderate to severe, and sharp. Leaning forward or sitting upright relieves the pain, which is concentrated over the sternum.

Myocardial Infarction

Pain may be along the sternum and left shoulder and down the left medial arm, and also localized to the sternum, anterior neck and upper abdomen. The pain is burning, vice-like and severe, lasting for approximately 30 minutes to one hour. There are no relieving factors.

Anxiety Attack

This is localized, non-radiating stabbing pain, pressure or burning that is commonly located over the substernal area. The pain is relieved by relaxation, rest and medication.

Pleural

This sharp pain is located close to the chest wall and is made worse by coughing, inspiration and movement. Palpation will not localize the pain. Possible causes include infectious disease, rib fractures, pneumothorax and pulmonary embolism.

Breast

This is a sharp, intermittent to constant aching pain, with possible signs of inflammation and edema of the breast tissue. The pain is located in the breast itself and down the medial side to the affected arm. Relief is gained temporarily through ice and rest. Possible causes include mastitis and benign or malignant tumours.

Esophagus

The client feels a sharp, burning pain often associated with eating. The pain is projected around the anterior thorax at the level of the lesion. An esophageal stricture due to reflux or spasm may be the cause.

Stomach and Duodenum

This is experienced as mild to severe waves of aching, cramp-like pain, inferior to the xiphoid process, which are occasionally referred to the T6 through T10 vertebral level. The pain is associated with eating. Possible causes are peptic ulcers and carcinoma, including Kaposi's sarcoma.

Small Intestine

Cramping and intermittent, this pain is located anteriorly around the umbilicus and posteriorly in the lumbar area. The pain may not be relieved by defecation. Symptoms may be due to Crohn's disease, an increase in intestinal motility or neoplasm.

Large Intestine

This is a poorly localized, lower abdominal pain of a cramping, dull nature. There may be constipation or diarrhea, with relief often occurring after defecation. Crohn's disease, ulcerative colitis, irritable bowel syndrome, long-term antibiotic use or carcinoma may be causes.

Appendix

The client has a well-localized, moderate to severe aching pain over the right lower quadrant of the abdomen. Pain is first referred around the umbilicus, then to the right groin and upper thigh. The pain worsens over time and is associated with nausea, vomiting and fever.

Liver

Liver pain is dull and constant, increasing over time or after exertion. It is local to the right upper quadrant of the abdomen with a possible referral to the right shoulder and associated pain between the scapulae. Possible causes include hepatitis A or B, cystic tumours, abscesses and cirrhosis. There may be fever, jaundice, fatigue and myalgias with hepatitis. Pallor and bleeding disorders are associated with cirrhosis and carcinomas.

Gall Bladder

The pain is located below the xiphoid process and into the right upper quadrant of the abdomen. There is a possible referral pattern to the right shoulder and between the scapulae. The pain is dull and aching, and increases over two to three hours to become severe. Movement and respiratory inspiration increase the pain. With gall stones, the pain and nausea occur several hours after eating, while with gall bladder inflammation, the pain strikes immediately upon eating. There is an intolerance of fatty food. With a prolonged obstruction, the skin may be jaundiced or appear greenish.

Common Bile Duct

The location and referral pattern are similar to gall bladder pain. Dull and aching at first, the pain steadily and constantly increases over a three- to four-hour period. Other symptoms include nausea after eating, fatty food intolerance and jaundice. Choledocholithiasis (gall stones), common bile duct stricture and pancreatic carcinoma are possible causes.

Pancreas

The pain is located inferior to the xiphoid process and typically is also referred to the left shoulder or low back. Constant burning, gnawing, severe pain of sudden onset can be accompanied by vomiting. If the symptoms are related to digestion, pancreatitis may be a cause. If the symptoms are not related to digestion, the cause may be carcinoma.

Kidney

Chronic problems exhibit poorly localized, constant, dull and aching pain, usually located in the posterior costovertebral and subcostal region, on the side of the affected kidney. There may be a referral to the ipsilateral abdomen. With acute problems, the pain is intense and severe, sometimes accompanied by nausea. Changing position does not relieve the pain, and hyperesthesia of the T9 and T10 dermatomes occurs. The pain may arise from a pre-renal impairment of blood flow, such as hypertension or heart failure, renal tissue damage from infection, diabetes mellitus or lupus and post-renal blockage due to calculi or tumours of the ureters or urethra.

Ureter

Excruciating waves of colicky pain at the costovertebral angle and referring into the ipsilateral lower abdomen and upper thigh are associated with passing calculi (kidney stones). Hyperesthesia of T10 and L1 dermatomes is present. The pain is unrelieved by changing position.

Bladder

A localized sharp pain is felt in the lower abdomen and the suprapubic area. The pain is intermittent and may be relieved by urination, which may be urgent and accompanied by a burning sensation. Some possible causes are infection, tumour and an enlarged prostate gland.

Primary and Metastatic Cancer

The pain is continuous, progressive and unrelieved by any activity or by lying down. The location of the pain may be the back or neck. The onset may occur over one or two months. With metastatic cancer, the client is often over 45 years old and may have a history of cancer. The pain of a lumbar metastasis starts centrally and then worsens and spreads in a bilateral sciatica pattern. Marked weakness with no pain may also indicate cancer. Back pain may exist with a secondary metastases from the breast, lung, thyroid, kidney or prostate. Primary or secondary cervical bone cancer creates a neck pain that is constant, unrelieved by rest and present through the night. In contrast, an osteoid osteoma may not exhibit the characteristic night pain but may bring on hamstring spasm and reduced hip flexion during a straight leg raise test.

Vasculogenic Pain

Cramping, aching vasculogenic pain is felt at the level of the vascular pathology. For example, an obstruction at the aortic bifurcation will give rise to bilateral gluteal and leg pain, with an absence of the femoral pulse. The extremities are cold and there is a change of skin colour. The leg muscles are weak and may atrophy. Iliac artery symptoms include numbness and pain in the low back, gluteals and leg. Pathologies of the femoral artery exhibit thigh and lower leg pain, with an absence of the pulse below the femoral artery.

Appendix E:

SKIN PATHOLOGIES AND CONDITIONS

Fiona Rattray, Linda Ludwig

The skin is the largest organ of the body, functioning to protect the body from infection, to regulate the body's internal temperature and to register sensory input such as touch and pressure.

Although skin lesions are frequently the result of primary skin diseases, the health and appearance of the skin may be an indicator of possible underlying systemic diseases, such as thyroid conditions, systemic lupus erythematosus and cancer. There is increasing medical awareness of the connection between the mind and the body, and of how emotional states can influence, or be reflected in, the health of the skin (Porth, 1990). For example, an increase in stress can exacerbate psoriasis.

In terms of massage and skin lesions, the therapist should be alert for any skin conditions that contraindicate *local* treatment. In such a case, massage is appropriate for the rest of the body; in other words, it is not *generally contraindicated.*

When large areas of the skin are affected, massage may be *absolutely contraindicated.* It is appropriate to refer the client to her physician if the lesion is recent and the client is unable to identify it.

Some of the more common lesions are described in this appendix. These include conditions that are contagious and that contraindicate either local or general massage because they may be spread to other parts of the client's skin, to the therapist's hands and, possibly, to a subsequent client if proper precautions are not taken. If general massage is appropriate, the lesion itself should be avoided altogether to prevent spread. The therapist should wear vinyl or latex gloves when working near the affected area. Vinyl gloves are used if the client has a latex allergy; health history questions are asked to determine this. An example of an infectious condition where local massage is contraindicated but general massage is appropriate is a plantar wart.

Non-contagious skin conditions that can be irritated by some lubricant oils and by techniques that stretch or rub over the skin are also included in this appendix. With these lesions, such as psoriasis, massage may be contraindicated locally or involve only gentle strokes to apply an emollient. To help with differential assessment, non-infectious conditions of varying skin pigmentation are listed as well.

✦ The therapist should maintain a record of any change in size or colour of skin lesions. The ABCDEF criteria is used to assess any pigmented lesion: **A**symmetric shape, irregular **B**order, multiple **C**olours, **D**iameter more than 7 millimetres, changes in **E**levation and **F**eeling of itching or tingling *(Johnson et al., 1998; Goldstein, Goldstein, 1997)*. Two or more of these changes may indicate the presence of a melanoma. The client should be referred to a physician for a diagnosis if such changes are noted. Because the therapist is assessing a change, not diagnosing a condition, the referral should be made in a way that informs, rather than alarms, the client. An example is, "I think this mole looks a little different from the last time you were here. The next time you see your doctor, ask her to take a look at this."

Skin Lesion Terms

✦ A *crust* is a scab or dried exudate.

✦ A *cyst* is an enclosed cavity that contains a semisolid or liquid.

✦ *Fissures* are linear breaks in the skin that are sharply defined.

✦ *Lichenification* is a diffuse area of thickening and scaling skin with an increase in skin lines and markings.

✦ A *macule* is a small flat spot that is a different colour from the surrounding skin.

✦ A *papule* is a small (less than 5 millimetres in diameter), solid, elevated area of the skin that is well defined. A nodule is a large papule (5 to 20 millimetres in diameter).

✦ A *plaque* is a large (greater than 5 millimetres in diameter), superficial, circumscribed, elevated, flat lesion.

✦ *Pruritis* is severe itching.

✦ A *pustule* is a small skin elevation containing pus; pustules vary in size.

✦ A *scale* is a superficial area of dead epidermal cells that are cast off the skin.

✦ A *telangiectasia* is an area of dilated superficial blood vessels.

✦ A *tumour* is a large nodule. It may be neoplastic, or new, abnormal tissue formation which grows at the expense of other tissues and serves no useful function.

✦ A *vesicle* is a small blister up to 1 centimetre in diameter containing serum. A bulla is a blister containing serous fluid that is larger than 1 centimetre in diameter.

Viral Infections

Herpes Simplex

Herpes simplex, or a cold sore, is a highly contagious viral infection. It is very common. Vesicles, pustules, redness, edema, crusts, erosions and ulcers may be present. There are two main types, herpes simplex virus 1 (non-genital) and herpes simplex 2 (genital). The virus is able to survive up to three days on moist gauze and toilet seats. However, it cannot survive in extremely chlorinated water. Herpes simplex is transmitted by direct skin contact during the vesicular stage; it enters the body through mucous membranes or cuts and scrapes. Genital herpes simplex is sometimes passed from mother to infant during birth.

The virus incubates for four to 10 days, at which point groupings of painful vesicles on an edematous red base appear. These lesions may be anywhere on the body; most commonly they affect the mouth, lips and face. In half of those affected, headache, fever and sore throat occur. Lesions heal within two weeks, then the virus lies dormant in the basal ganglia.

Reactivation of the virus occurs with emotional stress, fatigue, sunlight exposure, trauma and fever. The latent virus is conducted through peripheral nerves to the skin. Recurrence of herpes is signalled by itching, burning and pain before the vesicles appear; subsequent episodes are not as severe as the initial one. People who have recurrent herpes simplex may shed the virus from their skin even when no symptoms or lesions are present.

Medically, topical anesthetics and acyclovir medication, as well as sun screen, are used. Prevention remains the best approach.

✦ Massage is locally contraindicated due to the possibility of infection and the local pain. Intraoral massage is contraindicated while a lesion on the mouth is present; although the therapist is wearing vinyl gloves for intraoral massage, pressure around the lesion is painful.

Varicella

Varicella, or chicken pox, is a contagious infection that produces vesicles and papules over the trunk, face and limbs.

The virus is spread by airborne droplets. A fever and malaise occur 10 to 20 days after infection. The red vesicles eventually crust over; commonly, lesions in all stages of progression occur at the same time. Chicken pox is caused by herpesvirus varicella. Most cases occur in children during the winter time. In children the disease is self-limiting; however, in adults the condition is more systemic and severe. Pregnant women and those persons who are immunosuppressed require immediate medical referral.

Vaccines are available.

✦ Massage is completely contraindicated until the symptoms disappear.

Herpes Zoster

Herpes zoster, or shingles, is the reactivation of the varicella virus. The virus lies dormant in a nerve root ganglion. It is reactivated when the person is fatigued, under stress, immunosuppressed, elderly, or experiencing trauma or surgery. The onset of an attack is signalled by itching, aching or neuralgia in the affected dermatome. Vesicles, pustules, crusts, edema and redness occur in the dermatomal distribution. The pain becomes increasingly sharp, hot and localized in the affected area; the person may have fever and muscle pain. The lesions heal within three weeks. The person may experience postherpetic neuralgia, or pain, four weeks or more after the lesions resolve. Immunity usually occurs after one outbreak. Shingles mostly strikes those over 50 years of age, although persons with HIV disease may be affected.

Medically, herpes is treated with analgesics and topical lotions to soothe the skin. Involvement of the optic nerve and the tip of the nose indicates immediate medical referral.

✦ Although herpes zoster has a low contagion rate, massage is locally contraindicated due to the possibility of infection and the local neuralgia.

Verruca

Verrucas, or warts, are contagious papules or nodules of the epidermis. Warts begin as smooth, skin-coloured areas. Over time, thickening of the skin, or hyperkeratosis, occurs and the normal skin lines are absent. Within the wart, small capillaries thrombose; this gives the characteristic black dot appearance of many plantar warts. A wart may become tender or may enlarge with repeated irritation. They may be single or multiple in occurrence.

Warts are caused by the human papillomavirus. There are more than 50 types of this virus. *Common warts* are found on the hands and trauma sites. *Plantar* and *palmar warts* are found on the soles of the feet and the palms of the hands. *Flat warts* are found on the face and hands, while *filiform warts* are finger-like projections often occurring on the face.

Warts are passed on by skin-to-skin contact or through cuts or scrapes on the skin. They are most common in persons 12 to 16 years of age. They are believed to be on the increase over the past 20 years; a person with warts may have a decreased immune response.

Sixty per cent of warts in children disappear on their own within two years *(Hooper, Goldman, 1999)*.

Medically they are treated by liquid nitrogen, salicylic acid or excision; treatment may take months and the wart may recur if any of the virus is left in the skin.

✦ Massage therapy is locally contraindicated.

Acute Bacterial Infections

Impetigo

Impetigo is a superficial skin condition, usually caused by a staphylococcal infection. It is highly contagious and commonly transmitted by direct contact.

It appears as a red sore on affected areas such as around the mouth, legs, hands, genitalia and scalp. There may be blistering which causes a golden-coloured crust over the lesion. The condition can easily spread from a localized lesion to other skin surfaces of the body in a few days. Impetigo tends to affect prepubescent children. It can occur in teens and adults, often over areas of other skin disorders, especially eczema *(Marks, 1993)*.

Medical treatment involves antibacterial washes along with topical compounds such as betadine or polysporin. Unless the area affected is small, systemic antibiotics are taken internally to further combat the infection *(Hooper, Goldman, 1999)*.

✦ Massage over the affected area is contraindicated. Gloves should be worn by the therapist if massage is to be performed on the area not affected. This is only possible if the client has a localized outbreak. The sheets are bagged and laundered separately; the table is cleaned with an antiseptic solution as usual. In the case of an outbreak that has spread over various parts of the body, the therapist may wish to have the client reschedule when the condition is resolved; impetigo generally responds well to medical treatment within a few days *(Marks, 1993)*.

Cellulitis

Cellulitis is a deep inflammatory condition affecting the superficial to subcutaneous skin layers. It can be caused by staphylococcal or streptococcal infection. Cellulitis usually affects the face or the limbs, especially the legs, where there is lymphedema or a break in the skin integrity such as an ulcer or wound. The condition is painful, with diffuse swelling and redness observed over the infected part. Fever, chills, headache, malaise and vomiting may occur. Once a person has had cellulitis, the client is predisposed to future episodes. Most at risk are young children, older adults or those in poor health; malnutrition, alcoholism, recent infections or edema can increase one's risk for cellulitis.

Medical treatment involves hospitalization. The limb is elevated. Hot or cool compresses may be applied to the affected area and analgesics taken to decrease pain *(Hooper, Goldman, 1999)*. Antibiotics are essential and may be given intravenously. If left untreated, cellulitis may have serious consequences with the development of lymphadenopathy and septicemia *(Hooper, Goldman, 1999)*.

✦ If this condition is suspected, medical attention is required as soon as possible. Massage is safe to perform once the condition has resolved and provided there are no other contraindications, such as an open ulcer or wound. If edema were a predisposing factor, reducing the edema should be included in the aims of treatment. The therapist should also remain vigilant to any recurrence of the condition by noticing any local increase in temperature and redness.

Fungal Infections

Ringworm and Athlete's Foot

Fungal infections referred to as *ringworm* affect the superficial layers of the skin. A warm moist environment is suitable for the fungus to invade the skin and flourish. They release enzymes that digest the keratin in the tissue and an inflammatory response follows. This process is increased at the edges of the inflammation resulting in raised, defined areas. The infected ring-like patches of skin are itchy and flaky. Fungal infections affect various areas of the body.

- *Tinea pedis* (athlete's foot) is the most common superficial fungal infection. This condition affects up to 70 per cent of the population at some time and the possibility increases with age *(Hooper, Goldman, 1999)*. Tight and non-breathing footwear, poor hygiene or sweating, a hot and humid environment, and use of communal baths, showers and pools can contribute to the chance of developing athlete's foot. Recurrence is common. Prevention of athlete's foot includes wearing cotton socks and changing them frequently, keeping the feet dry, wearing well ventilated shoes and avoiding walking barefoot in public places. There is minimal inflammation, with scaling and hyperkeratosis observed on the soles and lateral aspect of the foot. Variations of tinea pedis include more serious infections which cause pustules or vesicles on the instep of the foot.

Medical treatment is with antifungal powders, creams and washes. Oral antifungals may also be prescribed.

- *Tinea corporis* (ringworm of the body) affects the chest, back, shoulders, neck, arms or legs. It is frequently found in children who contract it from pets; less commonly, adults may get tinea corporis from direct human contact or from infected objects. Multiple lesions are observed that are fairly similar in size. They vary from pustules to scaly patches. For some the condition is asymptomatic but for others, such as those who are immunosuppressed, the condition may be more severe.

Medical treatment includes both topical antifungal agents and systemic medication.

- *Tinea capitis* (ringworm of the scalp) affects primarily children, with boys five times more affected that girls. It causes pink, scaly patches on the scalp and some local hair loss.

Medically, topical antifungal medication is used.

✦ Massage is not generally contraindicated for fungal infections, but because these types of infections are contagious through direct contact, the area local to and surrounding the lesion is avoided during massage because fungus spreads outward *(Hooper, Goldman, 1999)*. The therapist is advised to wear gloves during the massage. Tea tree essential oil has antifungal properties and may be used at a 2.5 per cent dilution; 25 drops of pure essential oil are added to 50 ml. of carrier oil *(Balch, Balch, 1997)*. The sheets should be bagged and laundered separately, with the table disinfected as usual.

Candidiasis

This common fungal infection is caused by a yeast, candida albicans. It normally resides in the gastrointestinal tract, genital tract, mouth, esophagus and throat. Candida is held in check when the body is healthy, but with certain conditions it multiplies, weakens the immune system and causes the infection, candidiasis. Candidiasis may be observed in infants who were infected by yeast in the birth canal. In children and adults this condition is associated with immune deficiencies (such as HIV and AIDS), endocrine disorders (such as diabetes and hypothyroidism), nutritional deficiencies and pregnancy. The use of broad spectrum antibiotics, corticosteroids and immunosuppressive agents can also lead to this condition.

Candidiasis can lead to lesions in the mouth, the vaginal area, the skin, the nails, the lungs and the gastrointestinal tract. Depending on the area affected and the severity of the infection, the lesions are accompanied by a wide range of symptoms including pain and itching.

- *Cutaneous candidiasis* affects the skin.

- With *candidal paronychia,* there is painful, red swollen skin around the nail bed. If the condition is chronic the nails thicken and harden. It is observed in people who frequently immerse their hands in water.

- *Candidal intertrigo* presents as red eroded patches; scaly pustular lesions with an undefined border of satellite papules are observed. Often areas of large skin folds are affected such as the area beneath breasts, overhanging abdominal folds, the axilla, genital and anal areas as well as the webs of the toes and fingers. This type of infection develops during hot humid weather, when tight underclothing is worn and among those with diabetes or who use systemic antibiotics. The fingers are affected in those whose occupation involves frequent immersion of the hands in water.

- Mucous membrane candidiasis, also called *oral candidiasis* (thrush) affects the oropharyngeal cavity. White flakes, described as looking like cottage cheese, appear over the red and inflamed buccal membrane, tongue, gingiva, palate and pharynx. Over time and with severe cases, erosions or ulcers may develop. This type of candidiasis is especially common in people with AIDS. It also manifests more frequently and severely in this population because of their increased susceptibility to opportunistic infections *(Marks, 1993).*

Medical treatment of candidiasis includes elimination of predisposing factors, if possible. Topically, antifungal and anti-inflammatory creams are used *(Helm, Marks, 1998).* For thrush, the antifungal and antibiotic medication, nystatin, may be prescribed as well as stronger antifungal medications such as ketoconazole (Nizoral) or fluconazole (Diflucan).

✦ Massage is locally contraindicated.

Infestations

Scabies

Scabies is the result of a mite infestation. This is a contagious condition which can be transmitted through prolonged direct contact with an infected person but may also be transmitted through contact with clothing, linens or towels (the female *sarcoptes scabei humani* mite can survive for two to three days off its human host). Once on the host, the female mite will burrow into the outer layer of the epidermis to deposit eggs. The eggs will hatch and mature over a period of a month; most people develop a sensitivity to the organism and its waste over the course of a month or two. Intense itching is a classic symptom of a scabies infestation. The condition will continue unless treatment is received. The crusted papules are itchy; itching is worse at night. Secondary infection can result from excessive scratching. The lesions are found on the wrists, finger webs, buttocks, axilla, breasts, genitals and around the umbilicus. While the face is not affected in adults, it may be involved with younger infants. The mites' burrows are 0.5 to 2 millimetres long and resemble s-shaped ridges; these are most commonly observed on the wrist. Red-brown nodular lesions may also develop around the axilla and genitalia *(Arndt et al., 1997).* Papules, pustules and vesicles develop. Crusting, scaling and redness occur secondary to scratching the lesions.

Medical treatment is with Kwell, or some other scabicide, which is applied repeatedly to the entire body below the neck, even under the nails. Antipruritic creams and antihistamines are prescribed for the itching, which can continue for days or weeks after treatment *(Hooper, Goldman, 1999)*. Treatment of the entire household is recommended to completely eradicate the mite and prevent cross-infestation.

✦ Massage is completely contraindicated to avoid contacting the scabies mites. If contact occurs before medical diagnosis, the therapist should seek treatment. Linens and towels should be washed in hot water and dried on a hot cycle to effectively kill any mites *(Goldstein, Goldstein, 1997)*.

Premalignant and Malignant Neoplasms

A malignant neoplasm is a new, abnormal formation of tissue that grows at the expense of the healthy organism; it is potentially life-threatening. A premalignant neoplasm has not yet become malignant; however, it has the potential for malignancy.

Actinic Keratosis

Actinic keratosis is a premalignant plaque, scale or papule occurring as a result of chronic sun exposure. These lesions are found on the face, scalp and backs of the hands. Actinic keratoses are common in fair skinned people; occasionally they may progress to squamous cell carcinomas.

Medically the lesions are removed by cryosurgery.

✦ Massage is not generally contraindicated. However, techniques which rub or torque the skin, such as frictions or fascial spreading, are avoided directly over the lesion. The appearance of any suspicious lesion indicates referral to a physician for assessment.

Basal Cell Carcinoma

Basal cell carcinoma is a malignancy of the epidermal basal cells. It is often found in sun-exposed areas such as the face. It occurs most commonly in men between ages 40 and 80 years; darker skinned people are less likely to develop this cancer than fair skinned persons. Basal cell carcinoma rarely metastasizes *(Dollinger et al., 1995)*.

Basal cell carcinomas are classified according to appearance. The most common type is *nodular basal cell carcinoma*; this waxy, translucent papule has a central ulceration and a raised border. Other forms of basal cell carcinomas are in plaque or ulcerous forms; hyperpigmentation or erythema may be present.

Medically, basal cell carcinoma is excised or treated with radiation therapy. Due to the high rate of recurrence, reassessment is recommended yearly.

✦ Massage is locally contraindicated. The appearance of any suspicious lesion indicates referral to a physician for assessment.

Malignant Melanoma

A malignant melanoma is a proliferation of melanocytes. Three per cent of all cancers are melanomas; this lesion is on the increase at a faster rate than any other cancer *(Dollinger et al., 1995).* Melanomas can spread to almost any tissue in the body and are potentially fatal; yet if detected early, they have an excellent prognosis.

Malignant melanomas affect fair skinned persons more frequently than darker skinned persons. The causes are not completely understood. Melanomas in fair skinned persons may be related to intermittent, intense exposure to sunlight causing sunburns. However, the majority of melanomas found in Blacks, Asians and Native Americans occurs in non-sun-exposed areas such as the palmar and plantar surfaces *(Johnson et al., 1998).*

Melanomas are classified according to clinical and microscopic changes.

- A *superficial spreading melanoma* is a macule with variable pigmentation, irregular borders and increasing size. It is the most common of these types of lesions, occurring in people between 40 to 60 years of age. It may develop from a new or existing nevus, usually on the back, face, arms or legs. There is an initial horizontal spreading phase that may last for years, followed by a nodular phase where the melanoma grows vertically and becomes invasive.

- *Lentigo maligna melanoma* is a macule with irregular pigmentation and, over several years, slowly expanding borders. It is commonly found in sun-exposed areas such as the face and in elderly, fair skinned people. Raised areas, often several centimetres in diameter, indicate the invasive stage.

- *Nodular melanoma* is a blue-black elevated plaque or nodule. It develops anywhere on the body, usually in people between 50 to 70 years of age. This melanoma is rapidly invasive.

Medically, any malignant melanoma is excised; the person is tested for several years to determine if the melanoma has metastasized. In terms of massage therapy, any suspicious lesion indicates referral to a physician for assessment.

- ✦ If a melanoma is medically diagnosed, massage is locally contraindicated and may be generally contraindicated. The client's physician should approve the massage before treatment.

Squamous Cell Carcinoma

Squamous cell carcinoma is a tumour of malignant keratinocytes (cells that produce keratin). Papules, plaques and nodules may have crusty, eroded ulcerous portions. It is more common in persons over 55 years of age. This form of cancer is the most common skin cancer in Black persons; it is often found in non-sun-exposed areas of the body. In white persons, squamous cell carcinoma is often found in sun-exposed areas, or may develop from actinic keratosis. Other causes of this cancer are immunosuppression, smoking and exposure to arsenic and coal tars. Three per cent of squamous cell carcinomas metastasize; these are usually lesions on the lower lip or on old burn scars, and lesions that are large and invasive *(Dollinger et al., 1995).*

Medically, excision of the tumour and yearly observation for the development of new lesions are performed. Any suspicious lesion indicates referral to a physician for assessment.

- ✦ If a carcinoma is medically diagnosed, massage is locally contraindicated and may be generally contraindicated. The client's physician should approve the massage before treatment.

Benign Neoplasms

Benign neoplasms are new proliferations of cells that are not life-threatening.

Cherry Angioma and Venous Lake

A cherry angioma is a superficial capillary proliferation, usually affecting middle-aged to elderly people. It forms a dome-shaped papule up to 4 millimetres in diameter, most commonly on the trunk. When compressed, a cherry angioma blanches; it bleeds profusely if ruptured. A venous lake is a dark blue, soft, compressible area of dilated capillaries on the lips, face and ears of elderly people; it also bleeds if traumatized.

Medically, either of these condition may be removed by laser or cauterization.

✦ Massage is not generally contraindicated; however, techniques which stretch the skin, such as fascial spreading, are avoided over the lesion site.

Dermatofibroma

A dermatofibroma is a benign proliferation of fibroblasts. These firm, discrete papules or nodules are not tender. In darker skinned people, dermatofibromas are hyperpigmented; in lighter skinned people they are reddish. Dermatofibromas are usually found on the legs but may appear elsewhere. Often idiopathic, they may also result from trauma or insect bites. Dermatofibromas dimple if the surrounding skin is pinched together.

Unless the lesion has recently changed colour or is bleeding, medical removal is not indicated as surgery often results in a scar that is worse than the original lesion.

✦ Massage is not locally contraindicated.

Epidermal Inclusion Cyst

Epidermal inclusion cysts are raised nodules filled with odiferous white material; often a central pore is visible. They may become inflamed. Epidermal inclusion cysts are frequently idiopathic, sometimes due to trauma.

Medically, if the cyst is in an irritating area, it is excised.

✦ Massage is not generally contraindicated; however, cysts should not be irritated by massage techniques that drag on the skin, such as fascial spreading, or invasive techniques such as frictions.

Hemangioma

A hemangioma is a superficial proliferation of blood vessels, or telangiectasis. There are several types of hemangiomas.

• A *nevus flammus* (port wine stain) is a red to purple macule or papule on the face or head; it is present at birth and usually resolves by five years of age.

• *Salmon patches* (stork bites) are red macules, usually on the back of the neck; they occur in up to 10 per cent of fair skinned infants; they usually disappear by puberty.

- *Capillary hemangiomas* (strawberry marks) are telangiectatic macules that may develop into soft nodules or tumours; they develop in the first few days or months of life and usually resolve by puberty.

✦ Massage is not contraindicated with nevus flammus or salmon patches. Local massage is avoided with capillary hemangiomas.

Medically, none of these conditions require treatment. While capillary hemangiomas are usually benign, if they occur on the face or the eyes, or are obstructing an airway, a medical treatment is indicated.

Lipoma

A lipoma is a benign proliferation of fatty tissue below the dermis and epidermis. These mobile, soft, slightly compressible tumours are from one to several centimetres in size. They often occur in people 40 years of age or more. The cause of these slow-growing tumours is unknown *(Hooper, Goldman, 1999)*. Lipomas are commonly located on the back, shoulders, legs and arms. They may be single or multiple.

Medically, lipomas are not treated unless for cosmetic appearance or because they cause an irritation to the person.

✦ Massage is not generally contraindicated; however, lipomas should not be irritated by massage techniques that drag on the skin, such as fascial spreading, or invasive techniques such as frictions.

Nevus

A nevus, or mole, is a benign proliferation of normal skin components. They are found everywhere on the body, with the size varying from small (6 millimetres in diameter) to extensive. Everyone has at least one nevus, although they are more common in fair skinned than darker skinned individuals. The number of nevi a person has peaks in early adulthood and decreases afterwards.

- Nevi are described according to the layer of the skin affected. A *melanocytic nevus* is a macule of melanocytes, or dark pigmentation cells, that occurs in childhood. A *congenital nevus* is present at birth; it may extend down into the subcutaneous fat. A *nevus of Ota* affects the dermal layer of the face in the distribution of the trigeminal nerve; primarily affecting Asian and Black persons, this macule is present at birth or soon after. A *junctional nevus* is a macule of melanocytes at the junction of the epidermis and the deeper dermis. A *compound nevus* is a papule of melanocytes that extends deeper than the junction, into the dermis itself. A *dermal nevus* is a papule that occurs only in the dermis and it lacks melanocytes *(Johnson et al., 1998; Goldstein, Goldstein, 1997)*.

Medically, a benign nevus may be removed for cosmetic reasons.

✦ There are no massage contraindications to flat nevi; a raised nevus should not be irritated by techniques that drag on the skin, such as fascial spreading applied directly over it.

- *Dysplastic nevi* are irregularly shaped, pigmented macules with raised areas. They are larger (1 centimetre in diameter) than most nevi. Pigmentation may be brown, tan, red-pink or sometimes black. Atypical, isolated lesions have a low risk of developing melanoma, whereas higher numbers of dysplastic nevi run a higher risk *(Goldstein, Goldstein, 1997)*. A *halo nevus* is a pigmented nevus with a surrounding lighter coloured halo. While halo nevi are common and benign in adolescents, in adults they may indicate melanoma or skin cancer.

Medically, dysplastic nevi and halo nevi in adults are excised and assessed for the possibility of cancer.

✦ In terms of massage therapy, there are no local contraindications, but both of these nevi types indicate referral to a physician for assessment.

Seborrheic Keratosis

Seborrheic keratosis is a benign proliferation of keratinocytes, cells that produce the tough protein keratin. The keratosis forms a pigmented, scaly plaque with well-defined borders; the raised lesion appears stuck on the skin. The lesions range up to 2 centimetres in size, occasionally larger. They are commonly found on the trunk, arms and face. Seborrheic keratoses are most common in those over 50 years of age; they may be inherited.

Medically, seborrheic keratoses may be removed for cosmetic reasons; usually they are left alone unless they become irritated.

✦ Massage is not locally contraindicated. However, techniques which rub or torque the skin, such as frictions or fascial spreading, are avoided directly over the lesion.

Skin Tags

A skin tag is an outgrowth of normal skin; it may have darker pigmentation than the surrounding skin. A skin tag forms a papule or nodule on a narrow stalk, often in areas of friction such as the axilla. There may be numerous skin tags in one area.

Medically, they are treated by excision if the lesions are irritated by clothing or if the person wants them removed for cosmetic reasons.

✦ Massage is not generally contraindicated. However, techniques which rub or torque the skin, such as frictions or fascial spreading, are avoided directly over the lesion.

Solar Lentigo

Solar lentigo, commonly called liver or age spots, are benign proliferations of normal melanocytes as a result of chronic sun exposure and damage. The macules have darker pigmentation that is even throughout. They are found in areas of chronic sun exposure, such as the hands, face and shoulders. No medical treatment is necessary unless the person wishes removal for cosmetic reasons.

✦ Massage is not contraindicated.

Non-Infectious Inflammatory Disorders

Acne

Acne is a disorder of the sebaceous gland. An overproduction of oil from the gland may block the hair follicle, allowing bacteria to multiply and produce a local inflammation. Blackheads, whiteheads, papules, pustules and cysts may be present; scarring may occur. While the occasional blemish or pimple may happen anywhere on the body, a number of such lesions which recur over months or years are termed acne.

There are several forms of acne, which may appear on the face, neck, back, anterior trunk and buttocks. *Acne vulgaris* occurs during puberty, while *acne conglobata* is chronic and occurs later in life. *Acne rosacea* exhibits erythema, usually on the face, and occurs in middle-aged adults. Exposure to irritating chemicals, hair oils, cosmetics and, occasionally, to sunlight can also cause acne.

Medically, treatment includes the use of skin cleansers and topical lotions, and the removal of any irritants.

+ Although acne is not a contagious condition per se, the bacterial infection present in the inflamed hair follicle can be spread if a pimple is ruptured in the course of a massage; therefore, massage is locally contraindicated. Some massage oils can irritate an acne condition; lotion or gel may be less irritating.

Dermatitis and Eczema

Dermatitis is a general term used to describe a wide variety of non-contagious, inflammatory skin disorders. It is frequently used interchangeably with eczema, although some sources suggest eczema is a type of dermatitis *(Arndt et al., 1997)*. The term *eczematous dermatitis* is often used to describe red, scaly and inflamed skin *(Goldstein, Goldstein, 1997)*. Therefore, the terminology can lead to some confusion.

With these types of disorders, the key commonality is inflammation of the skin accompanied by itchiness. The condition can be acute and severe, with edema, vesicles and bullae; subacute, with scaling plaques; or chronic, with lichenification, scales and changes in pigmentation of the affected skin.

+ Massage is not completely contraindicated for dermatitis and eczema. If the lesions are open and oozing, they are avoided. If open lesions are not observed, and with agreement from the client, gentle massage using essential oils over the lesions may be helpful. Essential oils such as mélissa or chamomile may be used at a one per cent dilution; that is 10 drops of pure essential oil to 50 ml. of carrier lotion. Lavender essential oil may be used at a dilution of 25 drops of essential oil to 50 ml. of carrier lotion *(Davis, 1998)*. Care is taken to ensure that the client does not react to the carrier lotion or oil. Synthetic fragrances are avoided as they may cause or worsen dermatitis *(Watt, 1992)*.

Contact and Allergic Contact Dermatitis

Both contact dermatitis conditions result from direct contact with an irritating substance. A toxic agent may cause injury through contact with the skin, referred to as *primary irritant contact dermatitis*. There may be a delayed hypersensitivity reaction because of an allergy to the substance or agent, called *allergic contact dermatitis*. Dermatitis is among the most common causes of occupational disability *(Goldstein, Goldstein, 1997)*.

In both conditions, the reaction goes through acute, subacute and chronic stages. Initially, the area of contact is itchy with red vesicles, epidermal edema leading to vesicles and bullae; when these rupture, oozing and crusting result. In the chronic stages, lichenifications, scaling and fissures develop *(Helm, Marks, 1998)*. In some cases, the fissures are painful and can make movement difficult *(Marks, 1993)*.

- *Contact dermatitis* develops after contact with an irritating agent. The hands are a common site. After a repeated minor destruction of the epidermis from exposure to this agent, the tissue experiences *epidermal failure* and a reaction occurs. If the substance is very toxic the reaction is more severe, resulting in exudate and increased inflammation local to the dermatitis.

  Those who work with alkalis, organic solvents, detergents, cement and particulate waste are frequently affected; mechanics, builders, hairdressers, cooks, laundry workers and massage therapists are occupational examples.

- *Allergic contact dermititis* reactions occur with varying speed, due to the allergic nature of the condition. For example, after first contact with a particular substance, sensitivity occurs within 10 to 14 days. During this time the T-lymphocytes develop a memory for the substance. In the future, each time the skin is in contact with this specific substance again, the lymphocytes respond much faster, often within 12 to 72 hours *(Helm, Marks, 1998)*. The reaction can occur on any part of the body in contact with the allergen.

  Many substances can be allergens. Nickel, present in stainless steel, is a common example. A person with an allergy to nickel cannot wear stainless steel jewellery; there is irritation when the skin is in contact with steel studs, buckles and clips common in clothing such as jeans. Other common allergens are plant oils such urushiol, found in poison oak, ivy and sumac; rubber chemicals; cosmetic and shampoo ingredients such as fragrances and preservatives; and dyes such as those in fabric and hair colour. A thorough health history is taken to determine what substance exposure caused the reaction; a referral is appropriate for allergy testing.

Medical treatment includes avoidance of the irritating substance or prevention of contact with it. Wearing gloves or protective clothing is recommended. Sometimes a less irritating substance can be substituted, such as a milder soap. When it is impossible to avoid the irritating substance, the person should thoroughly remove it from the skin surface and apply emollients over the tissue. Topical or oral corticosteroids may be prescribed. Antihistamines are also suggested to control itching.

Within 30 minutes of contact with an irritating substance, the substance should be removed using soap and water or alcohol to reduce the severity of the reaction. This is especially important with poison ivy, oak or sumac. During the first few days after contact, in the blistering stage, cool wet compresses can be applied frequently and short, cool baths using colloidal oatmeal (Aveeno) are recommended.

✦ Massage is contraindicated over areas affected by contact and allergic dermatitis, specifically, open lesions, blisters or if it is uncomfortable for the client. Substances irritating for that client are avoided.

Atopic Dermatitis

Atopic dermatitis is a chronic form of dermatitis in those people with a familial predisposition to dermatitis, allergic rhinitis (hay fever) and asthma. These people are usually referred to as having sensitive skin. Atopic dermatitis is likely due to a combination of immunological response, epidermal dysfunction and genetic susceptibility (*Goldstein, Goldstein, 1997*). There is an association between atopic dermatitis and increased susceptibility to herpes simplex and wart viruses and sensitivity to wool and lanolin.

The lesions are very itchy. Cutaneous hypersensitivity, chronic redness, scaling, skin eruptions, plaques and papules are present. Atopic dermatitis can start as early as six weeks of age and may occur in childhood or in adolescence. Areas affected vary with the age of the person affected. The face and extensor surfaces of the arm are susceptible in infants. The hands and the flexor surfaces of the arms, namely the antecubital area and popliteal fossa, are affected in children and adults.

The course of this condition is variable, though symptoms tend to lessen with age. There may be a period of disappearance and reappearance; occasionally, there is a complete resolution.

Medical treatment is with topical corticosteroids and topical antibiotics, oral antibiotics and antihistamines, and cool compresses.

✦ Massage is locally contraindicated with open lesions or if it is uncomfortable for the client.

Hand and Foot Eczema

Eczema is a chronic, often pruritic, inflammatory skin disorder ranging from an acute to chronic presentation. Redness, vesicles, papules and plaques are present. People affected are those with their hands frequently immersed in water such as cooks or nurses. The presence of atopic dermatitis or contact dermatitis may predispose the person to this type of eczema (*Goldstein, Goldstein, 1997*). Usually, the palms of the hands including the sides of the fingers or the soles of the feet are symmetrically affected. If the eczema involves the nail, dystrophy may occur.

Medical treatment includes the use of milder cleansers and soaps as well as frequent applications of lanolin-free and fragrance-free emollients. The person is also advised to avoid constant contact with water by wearing cotton-lined protective gloves. Topical corticosteroids may be prescribed.

✦ Massage is locally contraindicated if open lesions are present or if it is uncomfortable for the client.

Venous Eczema

Venous eczema, or stasis dermatitis, affects the lower limbs of people with chronic venous stasis. Women are more often affected than men, as are persons over 50 years of age

(Goldstein, Goldstein, 1997).

Predisposing factors include varicose veins, thrombophlebitis, cardiac failure, hypoalbuminemia, surgery or trauma to the limb, pregnancy and long periods of immobility.

In the early stage, hyperpigmentation occurs on the medial aspect of the ankles and on the lower limb from the ankle to the calf. There may be an acute-chronic cycle. In the acute portion of the cycle, sensations of itchiness, aching or burning in the affected area are common. Red, scaly and itchy patches become vesicular and crusty due to scratching. Secondary infections often occur. This is followed by a decrease in venous circulation which then leads to an increase in calf edema. During this portion of the cycle, any small break in the skin could result in a stasis ulceration. This is serious since chronic ulcerations are associated with an increase in morbidity due to uncontrolled secondary infection *(Arndt et al., 1997).*

With chronic stasis dermatitis, there are thickened brownish-red plaques over dystrophic skin; they are generally asymptomatic during this time. An acute flare-up can occur secondary to a local infection, trauma, thrombophlebitis or deep vein thrombosis.

Medical treatment involves the reduction of edema and improvement of venous return. This is achieved through elevation of the affected limb, wearing of support hose and encouraging lower limb use by walking or isometric contractions. Topical corticosteroids are used and oral antibiotics are prescribed for secondary infections.

✦ Massage and lymphatic drainage can be used proximal to the affected area, to decrease edema and facilitate venous return, if no other contraindications are present, such as an ulcer or local infections.

Xerotic Eczema

Xerotic eczema is an inflammatory disorder of severely dry skin, with plaques, scales, redness and fissures into the skin. The legs, hands and arms are often affected. This common disorder of dry skin may be caused by a decrease in surface skin lipids; why this happens is unknown. *Nummular eczema* describes coin-shaped, extremely itchy xerotic lesions. Xerotic eczema affects older adults, often those with a history of atopic dermatitis; low humidity is a predisposing factor.

Medical treatment includes avoiding irritating substances and the use of emollient creams.

✦ Massage is not locally contraindicated unless open lesions are present or if it is uncomfortable for the client.

Psoriasis Vulgaris

Psoriasis is a chronic, hyperproliferating, scaling, inflammatory condition affecting the skin and, occasionally, the mucous membranes. This condition appears to be inherited; the inheritability rate is about 65 per cent *(Hooper, Goldman, 1999).* Psoriasis is not contagious. Most commonly, the lesions are well demarcated red papules and plaques with silver-white scales. The condition may involve only a few coin-sized lesions or extensive, thick lesions covering much of the body.

Psoriasis usually occurs on the limbs with an affinity for the extensor surfaces such as the knees and elbows, as well as the scalp, back, genitalia, intergluteal fold and nails. Areas of previous trauma are also affected *(Goldstein, Goldstein, 1997)*.

While some lesion are asymptomatic, pruritic lesions may occur in up to 20 per cent of people *(Marks, 1993)*. If these lesions dry and split, they become painful and susceptible to secondary infection; if the scaling plaque is removed bleeding can occur. The nails are pitted, with yellow discolouration, separation of the nail plate from the nail bed and general dystrophy. An associated arthritis of the finger and toe joints occurs in up to 30 per cent of those with psoriasis.

There is an exacerbation and remission cycle with psoriasis. Flare-ups seem to occur more in the winter (probably due to low humidity and lack of sunlight) and may be precipitated by emotional stress, trauma to the skin and medications, such as lithium and beta blockers, and steroid withdrawal. Improvement in the condition often occurs in the summer; occasionally, there may be a spontaneous remission.

Medical treatments of topical corticosteroids and vitamin D preparations may be used to control the lesions. If the condition is widespread or pustular, drugs such as cyclosporin, an immunosuppressant, may be used or ultraviolet radiation treatments may be given.

✦ Massage is not locally contraindicated unless open lesions are present or if it is uncomfortable for the client. Full body massage, with the aim of relaxation, is appropriate. Bergamot essential oil may be used at a 2.5 per cent dilution; that is 25 drops of essential oil to 50 ml. of carrier lotion *(Davis, 1998)*.

Differentiating Between Scaly Skin Conditions

✦ **Acute contact** or **allergic contact dermatitis** has vesicles present; medical patch tests to the allergen are positive *(Helm, Marks, 1998)*.

✦ **Atopic dermatitis** is associated with dermatitis, hay fever and asthma, and a chronic history since childhood; the lesions are itchy and often appear on the flexor surface of the arm in children and adults.

✦ **Psoriasis** lesions have distinct margins surrounding them; they often appear at trauma sites; with nail involvement, pitting is present. There is an affinity to the extensor surface such as knees and elbows.

✦ **Ringworm** is usually not symmetrical; there is diffuse redness and silvery scaling; medical tests for fungus are positive.

✦ **Venous dermatitis** has a history of predisposing conditions; areas affected are the lower limbs; hyperpigmentation is present.

Pigmentation Disorders

Vitiligo

Vitiligo is an acquired skin depigmentation condition. Well-defined depigmented macules of varying sizes appear. These are usually on the face and on the skin surrounding joints, such as the hands and knees. The condition is usually slow and progressive. Vitiligo is thought to be the result of an autoimmune disorder where anti-melanocyte antibodies are present. Genetic factors and exposure to certain chemicals may also play a part. Conditions associated with vitiligo include thyroid diseases and diabetes mellitus.

Vitiligo affects about one per cent of the world's population, both women and men. It is particularly striking in darker skinned persons. Vitiligo can occur at any age, although it is more common between the ages of 10 and 30. Repigmentation may occur spontaneously in 10 per cent of those affected (*Goldstein, Goldstein, 1997*).

Medically, repigmentation is achieved through the use of corticosteroids and photochemotherapy. Left untreated, the affected areas tend to burn easily if they are exposed to sunlight or ultraviolet rays. The client is recommended to use a sunblock or to cover the affected areas in the sun.

✦ Massage, whether local or general, is not contraindicated with vitiligo.

Post-inflammatory Hyperpigmentation

Post-inflammatory hyperpigmentation is an overproduction of melanin granules as a result of the inflammatory process. While all races can acquire this condition, it is more common and severe in darker skinned people. Causes of this condition include trauma (cuts, burns), acne, eczema and a response to certain medications. Phytophotodermatitis, or exposure to sunlight after exposure of the skin to certain plant juices or essential oils, such as lime juice or essential oil of lemon, may also cause the condition (*Johnson et al., 1998; Watt 1992*).

These dark macules occur either in the epidermis (a brownish colour) or the dermis (a bluish or greyish colour). The hyperpigmented area occurs at the exact location of the previous inflammation. Resolution of this condition may take months or years; or it may never resolve.

Medically, prevention of further trauma is recommended over treatment of existing lesions.

✦ Massage is not contraindicated.

REFERENCES AND SELECTED BIBLIOGRAPHY

Achauer, Bruce, M. 1987. *Management of the Burned Patient.* Norwalk: Appleton and Lange.

Ada, Louise, and Colleen Canning. 1990. *Key Issues in Neurological Physiotherapy.* London: Butterworth and Heinemann.

AIDS Committee of Toronto. 1999. *HIV/AIDS Complimentary Therapists.*

AIDS Committee of Toronto. 1998. *Frequently Asked Questions (FAQs) about HIV and AIDS.*

AIDS Council of New South Wales. N.d. *Fact Sheet 4: Women and HIV.*

AIDS: Let's Talk Women and AIDS. 1989. Queen's Printer for Ontario.

Alexander, Douglas. 1996/7. "Guidelines for Massage Therapy Referral in Whiplash Cases." *Journal of Soft Tissue Manipulation* Vol. 4, no. 2:3-8.

Alexander, Douglas. 1996. "The Importance of the Quebec Task Force on Whiplash-Associated Disorders (WAD) for Massage Therapy." *Journal of Soft Tissue Manipulation* Vol. 3, no. 4:4-12.

Alexander, Douglas. 1995a. "Case Presentation: Deep Vein Thrombosis." *Journal of Soft Tissue Manipulation* Vol. 3, no. 1:2-16.

Alexander, Douglas. 1995b. "Soft Touch Palpation." *Journal of Soft Tissue Manipulation* Vol. 2, no. 6:2-4.

Alexander, Douglas. 1994. "When Headache Is Ominous." *Ontario Massage Therapist Association Newsletter* October/November:4-8.

Alexander, Douglas. 1992. "Deep Vein Thrombosis and Massage Therapy." *Ontario Massage Therapist Association Newsletter* August/September:1.

Alviso, D. J., J. T. Dong, and G. L. Lentell. 1988. "Intertester Reliability for Measuring Pelvic Tilt in Standing." *Physical Therapy* Vol. 68:1347-51.

American College of Obstetricians and Gynecologists. 1996. *Planning for Pregnancy, Birth, and Beyond, 2nd Ed.* New York: Dutton.

American Heart Association. 1994. *How Stroke Affects Behaviour.*

American Massage Therapy Association (AMTA). 1999. *State Boards Administering Massage Practice Laws.* June 10.

American Massage Therapy Association. 1998. *Massage Therapy Journal* Vol. 37, no. 2:99.

Aminoff, Michael. 1995. *Neurology and General Medicine.* New York: Churchill Livingstone.

Anderson, Bob. 1980. *Stretching.* Bolinas: Shelter Publications.

Anderson, Dale L. 1992. *90 Seconds to Muscle Pain Relief: The Fold and Hold Method.* Minneapolis: Comp Care.

Andrews, James R., and Kevin E. Wilk. 1994. *The Athlete's Shoulder.* New York: Churchill Livingstone.

Apley, A. Graham, and Louis Solomon. 1993. *Apley's System of Orthopaedics and Fractures, 7th Ed.* Oxford: Butterworth and Heinemann.

Arat, Arsavir. 1973. *Neck Sprains as Muscle Injury, Tension Headache and Related Concerns, 2nd Ed.* El Paso: Guynes.

Arndt, Kenneth A., Bruce U. Wintroub, June K. Robinson, and Philip E. Leboit. 1997. *Primary Care Dermatology.* Philadelphia: W. B. Saunders Company.

Arthritis Foundation. 1997. *Scleroderma.*

Arthritis Foundation. 1993. *Lyme Disease.*

REFERENCES AND SELECTED BIBLIOGRAPHY

Arthritis Foundation. 1992. *Reiter's Syndrome.*

Arthritis News. N.d. *As Seen on TV... Glucosamine: "The Next Big Thing" for OA of the Knee?* Vol. 14, no. 4:8-9.

Arthritis Society. 1998a. "Arthritis." *Living Well with Arthritis* June.

Arthritis Society. 1998b. "Fibromyalgia." *Living Well with Arthritis* June.

Arthritis Society. 1998c. "Healthy Eating and Arthritis." *Living Well with Arthritis* June.

Arthritis Society. 1998d. "Lupus." *Living Well with Arthritis* June.

Arthritis Society. 1996a. *Ankylosing Spondylitis.*

Arthritis Society. 1996b. *Gout and Pseudogout.*

Arthritis Society. 1988. *Infectious Arthritis.*

Atwood, Glenna Wotton. 1991. *Living Well with Parkinson's.* New York: John Wiley and Sons.

Bach, John R. 1996. *Pulmonary Rehabilitation: The Obstructive and Paralytic Conditions.* Philadelphia: Hanley and Belfus Inc.

Bader, Dan. 1990. *Pressure Sores: Clinical Practice and Scientific Approach.* London: Macmillan Press.

Balch, James F., and Phyllis A. Balch. 1997. *Prescriptions for Nutritional Healing, 2nd Ed.* New York: Avery Publications.

Barnes, Thomas A. 1988. *Respiratory Care Practice.* Chicago: Year Book Medical Publishers.

Barral, Jean Pierre. 1991. *The Thorax.* Seattle: Eastland Press.

Barral, Jean Pierre. 1989. *Visceral Manipulation 2.* Seattle: Eastland Press.

Barral, Jean Pierre, and Pierre Mercier. 1988. *Visceral Manipulation.* Seattle: Eastland Press.

Basmajian, John. 1985. *Manipulation, Traction and Massage, 3rd Ed.* Baltimore: Williams and Wilkins.

Basmajian, John. 1984. *Therapeutic Exercise, 4th Ed.* Baltimore: Williams and Wilkins.

Basmajian, John, and Carlo J. DeLuca. 1985. *Muscles Alive: Their Functions Revealed by Electromyography, 5th Ed.* Baltimore: Williams and Wilkins.

Basmajian, John, and Rich Nyberg. 1993. *Rational Manual Therapies.* Baltimore: Williams and Wilkins.

Basmajian, John, and Steven J. Wolf. 1990. *Therapeutic Exercise, 5th Ed.* Baltimore: Williams and Wilkins.

Bateman, J. R. M., K. M. Daunt, S. P. Newman, D. Pavia, and S. W. Clarke. 1979. "Regional Lung Clearance of Excessive Bronchial Secretions During Chest Physiotherapy of Patients with Stable Chronic Airway Obstruction." *Lancet* Vol. 1:294-7.

Bates, Barbara. 1987. *A Guide to Physical Examination and History Taking, 4th Ed.* Philadelphia: J. B. Lippincott.

Bennett, R. M. 1990. "Myofascial Pain Syndrome and Fibromyalgia Syndrome: A Comparative Analysis." In J. R. Fricton and E. Awad, eds. *Advances in Pain Research and Therapy, Vol 17.* New York: Raven Press.

Bennett, V. Ruth, and Linda K. Brown. 1993. *Myles Textbook for Midwives, 12th Ed.* Edinburgh: Churchill Livingstone.

Benson, Herbert, and Miriam Z. Klipper. 1975. *The Relaxation Response.* New York: William Morrow.

Bergan, John J., and Mitchell P. Goldman. 1993. *Varicose Veins and Telangiectasias: Diagnosis and Treatment.* St. Louis: Quality Medical Publishing.

Bernhardt, Roslyn Turner. 1994. "Massage Therapist as Doula." *Massage Therapy Journal* Vol. 33, no. 3:46- 8.

Bergqvist, David. 1994. *Prevention of Venous Thromboembolism.* London: Med-Orion.

Bleck, Eugene. 1979. *Orthopedic Management of Cerebral Palsy.* London: W. B. Saunders Company.

Bleton, J. P. 1994. *Spasmodic Torticollis.* Paris: Frisons Roche.

Bloom, R. A., D. Gheorghiu, A. Verstandig, H. Pogrund, and E. Libson. 1990. "The Psoas Sign in Normal Subjects Without Bowel Preparation: The Influence of Scoliosis on Visualization." *Clinical Radiology* 41:204- 5.

Bobath, Berta. 1990. *Adult Hemiplegia: Evaluation and Treatment, 3rd Ed.* Oxford: Butterworth and Heinemann.

Bollinger, A., H. Partsch, and J. H. N. Wolfe. 1985. *The Initial Lymphatics.* New York: Thieme-Stratton.

Booher, James, and Gary Thibodeau. 1989. *Athletic Injury Assessment.* St. Louis: Times Mirror/Mosby.

Bourne, Gordon. 1995. *Pregnancy, 4th Ed.* London: Cassell.

Bowers, Mark. 1997. *Peripheral Neuropathy.* San Francisco AIDS Foundation: *BETA* 3:1-9.

Boyle, Wade, and Andre Saine. 1988. *Lectures in Naturopathic Hydrotherapy.* East Palestine: Buckeye Press.

Boyling, Jeffery, and Nigel Palastanga. 1994. *Grieve's Modern Manual Therapy, 2nd Ed. The Vertebral Column.* Singapore: Churchill Livingstone.

Braddon, Randall. 1996. *Physical Medicine and Rehabilitation.* Philadelphia: W. B. Saunders Company.

Brannon, Frances J., Margaret Foley, Julie Ann Starr, and Mary Geyer Black. 1993. *Cardiopulmonary Rehabilitation: Basic Theory and Application, 2nd Ed.* St. Louis: Mosby.

Brandt, Kenneth D., Michael Doherty, and L. Stefan Lohmander. 1998. *Osteoarthritis.* Oxford: Oxford University Press.

Brayshaw, Eileen, and Pauline Wright. 1994. *Teaching Physical Skills for the Childbearing Years.* Cheshire: Books for Midwives Press.

Brennan, M. J., and J. Weitz. 1992. "Lymphedema 30 Years After Radical Mastectomy." *American Journal of Physical Medicine Rehabilitation* 71:12-4.

Beighton, Peter, Rodney Grahame, and Howard Bird. 1989. *Hypermobility of Joints, 2nd Ed.* London: Springer Verlag.

Brillhart, Allen. T. 1994. *Arthroscopic Laser Surgery: Clinical Applications.* New York: Springer Verlag.

Brodin, Harald. 1984. "Cervical Pain and Mobilization." *International Journal of Rehabilitation Research* 7:190-1.

Brooks, Debra, Denise Borreli, Robert King, Ralph Stephens, and Mitchell Coven. 1996. "Boston Panel on Fibromyalgia and CFS." *Massage Therapy Journal* Summer:71-104.

Brown, Catherine Caldwell. 1984. *Pediatric Round Table 10: The Many Facets of Touch.* Johnson and Johnson Baby Products Co.

Bruggemann, W. 1982. *Kneipp Vademecum Pro Medico.* Wurtzburg: Sebastian Kneipp.

Brukner, Peter, and Karim Khan. 1993. *Clinical Sports Medicine.* New York: McGraw-Hill.

Bullard-Dillard, R., J. Chen, S. Peluse, V. Dao, and P. F. Agris. 1993. "Dietary Factors May Aggravate Lupus." *Lupus News* Vol. 13, no. 1:148.

Bunch, Wilton, and Avinash Patwardhan. 1989. *Scoliosis: Making Clinical Decisions.* St. Louis: C. V. Mosby.

Bunker, Timothy, and W. Angus Wallace. 1991. *Shoulder Arthroscopy.* London: Martin Dunitz.

Burns, Ethel, and Caroline Blamey. 1994. "Soothing Scents in Childbirth." *The International Journal of Aromatherapy* Vol. 6, no. 1:24-8.

Buschbacher, Ralph. 1994. *Musculoskeletal Disorders: A Practical Guide for Diagnosis and Rehabilitation.* Stoneham: Butterworth and Heinemann.

Cady, Roger K., and Anthony W. Fox. 1995. *Treating the Headache Patient.* New York: Marcel Dekker.

Cailliet, Rene. 1995. *Low Back Pain Syndrome, 5th Ed.* Philadelphia: F.A. Davis.

Cailliet, Rene. 1993. *Pain: Mechanisms and Management.* Philadelphia: F.A. Davis.

Cailliet, Rene. 1988. *Soft Tissue Pain and Disability, 2nd Ed.* Philadelphia: F.A. Davis.

Cailliet, Rene. 1981. *Shoulder Pain, 2nd Ed.* Philadelphia: F.A. Davis.

Cailliet, Rene. 1980. *The Shoulder in Hemiplegia.* Philadelphia: F.A. Davis.

Cailliet, Rene. 1975. *Scoliosis: Diagnosis and Management.* Philadelphia: F.A. Davis.

Caird, Francis. 1991. *Rehabilitation of Parkinson's Disease.* London: Chapman, Hall.

Calais-Germain, Blandine. 1993. *Anatomy of Movement.* Seattle: Eastland Press.

Calne, Susan, Trevor Hurwitz, Beverly McConnell, Carole Shaw, Karen Poulin, Barbara Purves, and Wayne Wright. 1995. *Taking Charge: A Guide to Living with Parkinsonism.* Toronto: Parkinson Foundation of Canada.

Calvert, Robert. 1992. "Paul St. John and His Neuromuscular Therapy, Part 2." *Massage* 35:56-65.

Campbell, A. H., J. M. O'Connell, and F. Wilson. 1975. "The Effect of Chest Physiotherapy upon the FEV1 in Chronic Bronchitis." *Medical Journal of Australia* 1:33-5.

Canadian Cancer Society. 1998a. *Facts on Prostate Cancer.*

Canadian Cancer Society. 1998b. *Radiation Therapy and You: A Guide to Self-Help During Treatment*

Canadian Cancer Society. 1998c. *Surgical Options for Breast Cancer.*

Canadian Cancer Society. 1997a. *After Lumpectomy: A Woman's Guide.*

Canadian Cancer Society. 1997b. *After Mastectomy: A Woman's Guide.*

Canadian Cancer Society. 1997c. *Exercise Guide after Breast Surgery.*

Canadian Cancer Society. 1997d. *Facts on Skin Cancer.*

Canadian Cancer Society. 1996a. *Chemotherapy and You: A Guide to Self Help During Treatment.*

Canadian Cancer Society. 1996b. *Colorectal Cancer: What You Need to Know.*

Canadian Cancer Society. 1996c. *Detecting Changes in the Prostate.*

Canadian Cancer Society. 1996d. *Finding Cancer in the Prostate.*

Canadian Cancer Society. 1996e. *Facts on Breast Cancer.*

Canadian Cancer Society. 1996f. *Facts on Colorectal Cancer.*

Canadian Cancer Society. 1996g. *Facts on Lung Cancer.*

Canadian Cancer Society. N.d. *Breast Cancer: What You Need to Know as a Woman, Friend, Daughter.*

Canadian Diabetes Association. 1997a. *Diabetes Risks and Symptoms.*

Canadian Diabetes Association. 1997b. *Prevalence of Diabetes.*

Canadian Diabetes Association. 1997c. *Seriousness of Diabetes.*

Canadian Medical Association Journal. 1998a. "Clinical Practice Guidelines for the Diagnosis and Management of Osteoporosis" Vol. 155, no. 8:1113-33.

Canadian Medical Association Journal. 1998b. "A Patient's Guide to Choosing Unconventional Therapies" Vol. 158, no. 9:1161-5.

Canadian Medical Association Journal. 1998c. "Prevention and Management of Osteoporosis: Consensus Statements from the Scientific Advisory Board of the Osteoporosis Society of Canada" Vol. 155, no. 7:921-65.

Canadian Pharmaceutical Association. 1996. *Compendium of Pharmaceuticals And Specialties, 30th Ed.* Toronto: Southam Mirror.

Cantu, Robert I., and Alan J. Grodin. 1992. *Myofascial Manipulation: Theory and Clinical Application.* Gaithersburg: Aspen Publications.

Cafarelli, E., and F. Flint. 1992. "The Role of Massage in Preparation for and Recovery from Exercise." *Sports Medicine* Vol. 14, no. 1:1-9.

Cariol, Francis. 1991. *Rehabilitation of Parkinson's Disease.* London: Chapman, Hall.

Carpi, John. 1996. "Stress: It's Worse than You Think." *Psychology Today* Vol. 29, no. 1:33-41.

Carroll, Roz. 1995. "Supporting the Immune System: Psychoneuroimmunology and the Role of Massage." *Continuum* Vol. 3, no. 3:6-9.

Casley-Smith, J. R., and M. O. Bjorlin. 1985. "Some Parameters Affecting the Removal of Oedema by Massage: Mechanical or Manual." *Progress in Lymphology* X:82-4.

Casley-Smith, J. R., and Judith R. Casley-Smith. 1986. *High-Protein Oedemas and the Benzo-Pyrones.* Sydney: J. B. Lippincott.

Cawson, Roderick, A. Alexander, W. McCracken, Peter B. Marcus, and Ghazi Zaatari. 1998 *Pathology: The Mechanism of Disease.* St. Louis: C.V. Mosby.

Cawson, Roderick A., Alexander W. McCracken, and Peter B. Marcus. 1982. *Pathologic Mechanisms and Human Disease.* St. Louis: C.V. Mosby.

Chaitow, Leon. 1988. *Soft Tissue Manipulation.* Hong Kong: Healing Arts Press.

Chaitow, Leon. 1980. *NeuroMuscular Technique: A Practitioner's Guide to Soft Tissue Manipulation.* Willingborough: Thorsons.

Chalmers, Andrew, Geoffrey Owen Littlejohn, Irving Salit, and Frederick Wolfe. 1995. *Fibromyalgia, Chronic Fatigue Syndrome and Repetitive Strain Injury: Current Concepts in Diagnosis, Management, Disability and Health Economics.* New York: Haworth.

Chapman, John. 1995. *Asthma: Alternative Ways to Treat the Causes of Asthma.* London: Thorson Press.

Chapman-Smith, L. 1996. "Measuring Results with Pain Questionnaires." *Journal of Soft Tissue Manipulation* Vol. 3, no. 4:13-26.

Chapman-Smith, L. 1994. "The New Importance Of Pain Questionnaires." *Journal of Soft Tissue Manipulation* Vol. 1, no. 5:8-11.

Chard, Tim, and Richard Lilford. 1998. *Basic Sciences for Obstetrics and Gynaecology, 5th Ed.* New York: Springer Verlag.

Chatelaine. 1995. "The Icing on the Pain" Vol. 10:192.

Chusid, Joseph G. 1985. *Correlative Neuroanatomy and Functional Neurology, 19th Ed.* Los Altos: Lange Medical Publications.

Ciullo, Jerome V. 1996. *Shoulder Injuries in Sport.* Champaign: Human Kinetics.

Clark, Tim, and John Rees. 1996. *Practical Management of Asthma, 2nd Ed.* London: Martin Dunitz.

Clarkson, Hazel, and Gail Gilewich. 1989. *Musculoskeletal Assessment: Joint Range of Motion and Manual Muscle Strength.* Baltimore: Williams and Wilkins.

Clement, Sarah. 1998. *Psychological Perspectives on Pregnancy and Childbirth.* Edinburgh: Churchill Livingstone.

Clodius, M., and M. Foldi. 1984. "Therapy for Lymphedema Today." *Int. Angiology* 3:207-13.

Cochrane, G. Mac, William F. Jackson, and P. John Rees. 1996. *Asthma: Current Perspectives.* London: Mosby Wolfe.

Coffman, Jay. 1989. *Raynaud's Phenomenon.* New York: Oxford University Press.

Cohen, Andrea, and William Weiner. 1994. *The Comprehensive Management of Parkinson's Disease.* New York: Demos Publications.

Colman, Libby L., and Arthur D. Colman. 1991. *Pregnancy: The Psychological Experience.* New York: Noonday Press.

College of Family Physicians of Canada. 1995a. *Migraine Headaches: Ways to Deal With the Pain.*

College of Family Physicians of Canada. 1995b. *Stress: How to Cope Better with Life's Challenges.*

College of Massage Therapists of Ontario. 1996. *Code of Ethics; Standards of Practice.*

College of Massage Therapists of Ontario. 1991. *Contraindications for Massage Therapy Treatment.*

Conwell, H. Earle. 1982. *Injuries to the Wrist.* Summit: CIBA Pharmaceutical Clinical Symposia Vol. 22, no. 1.

Cooke, Ernest D., Andrew N. Nicholaides, and John M. Parker. 1991. *Raynaud's Syndrome.* London: Med-Orion.

Copeland, Stephen A. 1997. *Shoulder Surgery.* London: W.B. Saunders.

Coulter, Jackie. 1994. "Charting Progress Is Essential." *Journal of Soft Tissue Manipulation* Vol. 1, no. 5:4-7.

Curties, Debra. 1994. "Could Massage Therapy Promote Cancer Metastasis?" *Journal of Soft Tissue Manipulation* Vol. 1, no. 6:3-7.

Curties, Debra. 1993. "Breast Massage: Discussion Paper and Suggested Guidelines." *Journal of Soft Tissue Manipulation* Vol. 1, no. 1:4-6.

Cyriax, James, and Margaret Coldham. 1984. *Textbook of Orthopaedic Medicine, Volume 2, Treatment by Manipulation, Massage And Injection, 11th Ed.* London: Baillière Tindall.

Cyriax, James. 1991. *Textbook Of Orthopaedic Medicine, Volume 1, Diagnosis Of Soft Tissue Lesions, 8th Ed.* London: Baillière Tindall.

D'Amico, Ron. 1998. "Latest Opportunistic Infection Guidelines." *Positively Aware* January/February: 43-4.

Danneskiold-Samsoe, B., E. Christiansen, and R. B. Andersen. 1986. "Myofascial Pain and the Role of Myoglobin." *Scandinavian Journal of Rheumatology* Vol. 15:174-178.

Davidoff, Robert A. 1995. *Migraine: Manifestations, Pathogenesis and Management.* Philadelphia: F. A. Davis.

Davis, Pat. 1998. *Aromatherapy: An A-Z, New Revised Edition*. Cambridge: C.W. Daniel.

Davis, Patricia. 1988. *Aromatherapy: An A-Z*. Cambridge: C.W. Daniel.

Dawson, David, Mark Hallett, and Lewis H. Millender. 1990. *Entrapment Neuropathies, 2nd Ed*. Boston: Little, Brown and Company.

Dealey, Carol. 1994. *The Care of Wounds: A Guide for Nurses*. Oxford: Blackwell Scientific Publications.

deGroot, Jack. 1991. *Correlative Neuroanatomy, 21st Ed*. Norwalk: Appleton and Lange.

Dellon, Lee, and Michael Jabaky. 1982. "Reeducation of Sensation in the Hand Following Nerve Suture." *Clinical Orthopaedics and Related Research*. Vol. 163:75-9.

DeFranca, George G. and Linda J. Levine. 1996. *Pelvic Locomotor Dysfunction: A Clinical Approach*. Gaithersburg: Aspen Publications.

DeLisa, Joel A., and Bruce M. Gans. 1993. *Rehabilitation Medicine: Principles and Practice, 2nd Ed*. Philadelphia: J. B. Lippincott.

DeSmet, Arthur. 1985. *Radiology of Spinal Curves*. St. Louis: C.V. Mosby.

Desouza, Lorraine. 1990 *Multiple Sclerosis: Approaches to Management*. London: Chapman, Hall.

Dettenmeier, Patricia A. 1992. *Pulmonary Nursing Care*. St. Louis: Mosby Year Book.

DiGregorio, Vincent R. 1984. *Rehabilitation of the Burn Patient*. New York: Churchill Livingstone.

Dollinger, Martin, Ernest H. Rosenbaum, and Greg Cable. 1995. *Everyone's Guide to Cancer Therapy: How Cancer Is Diagnosed, Treated and Managed Day to Day*. Toronto: Somerville House.

Donatelli, Robert. 1991. *Physical Therapy of the Shoulder, 2nd Ed*. New York: Churchill Livingstone.

Doran, James P. 1993. "The Vertebral Artery Test." *Journal of Soft Tissue Manipulation* Vol. 1, no. 1:8-9.

Douglas, D. M. 1963. *Wound Healing and Management*. Edinburgh: Churchill Livingstone.

Duncan, Pamela W., and Mary Beth Badke. 1987. *Stroke Rehabilitation: The Recovery of Motor Control*. Chicago: Year Book Medical Publishers.

Dunne, Lavon J. 1990. *Nutrition Almanac, 3rd Ed*. New York: McGraw-Hill.

Duvoisin, Roger. 1991. *Parkinson's Disease: A Guide for Patient and Family*. New York: Raven Press.

Dvorak, Jiri, and Vaclav Dvorak. 1990. *Manual Medicine: Diagnostics*. Stuttgart: Georg Thieme.

Ebner, Maria. 1980. *Connective Tissue Massage*. Huntington: Robert Krieger.

Edeling, Joy. 1994. *Manual Therapy for Chronic Headache. 2nd Ed*. London: Butterworth and Heinemann.

Edmond, Susan. 1993. *Manipulation and Mobilization*. St. Louis: Mosby Yearbook.

Edwards, Peter, and Mark S. Myerson. 1996. "Exertional Compartment Syndrome of the Leg." *The Physician and Sportsmedicine* Vol. 24, no. 4:31-46.

Edwardson, Barbara M. 1995. *Musculoskeletal Disorders: Common Problems*. San Diego: Singular Publishing Group.

Elble, Rodger, and William Koller. 1990. *Tremor*. Baltimore: The Johns Hopkins University Press.

Eliska, O., and M. Eliskova. 1995. "Are Peripheral Lymphatics Damaged by High-Pressure Manual Massage?" *Lymphology* Vol. 28:21-3.

Evjenth, Olaf, and Jern Hamberg. 1985a. *Muscle Stretching in Manual Therapy: A Clinical Manual: The Extremities, Vol. 1*. Milan: New Interlitho.

Evjenth, Olaf, and Jern Hamberg. 1985b. *Muscle Stretching in Manual Therapy: A Clinical Manual: The Spinal Column and the TM Joint, Vol. 2*. Milan: New Interlitho.

Farfan, H. F. 1996. *The Sciatic Syndrome*. New Jersey: SLACK Inc.

Fehr, K., and H. Krueger. 1992. *Occupational Musculoskeletal Disorders: Occurrence, Prevention and Therapy*. Basel: EULAR Publishers.

Feldman, Robert G., Robert Young, and Werner P. Koella 1980. *Spasticity Disordered Motor Control*. Chicago: Year Book Medical Publishers.

Fernandez, Sylvia. 1987. "Physiotherapy Prevention and Treatment of Pressure Sores." *Physiotherapy*. Vol. 73, no. 9:450-4.

Field, Tiffany. 1995. "Massage Therapy for Children." *Touchpoints* Vol. 2, no. 1:1-2.

Field, Tiffany, T. Henteleff, M. Hernandez-Reif, C. Kuhn, E. Martinez, K. Mavunda, and S. Schanberg. 1997a. "Asthmatic Children Have Improved Pulmonary Functions After Massage Therapy." *Touchpoints* Vol. 4, no. 1:2.

Field, Tiffany, C. Kuhn, A. LaGreca, K. Shaw, and S. Schanberg. 1997b. "Adherence and Glucose Levels Improved after Giving Massage Therapy to Children with Diabetes." *Touchpoints* Vol. 4, no. 1:2.

Field, Tiffany, T. Henteleff, M. Hernandez-Reif, E. Martinez, K. Mavunda, C. Kuhn and S. Schanberg. 1996. "Asthmatic Children Benefit From Massage." *Touchpoints* Vol. 3, no. 4:2.

Field, Tiffany, T. Henteleff, K. Mavunda, C. Kuhn, and S. Schanberg. 1995a. "Asthmatic Children Have Less Anxiety and Respiratory Problems After Touch Therapy." *Touchpoints* Vol 2, no. 1:3.

Field, Tiffany, G. Ironson, J. Pickens, N. Fox, F. Scafidi, T. Nawrocki, A. Goncalves, S. Schanberg, and C. Kuhn. 1995b. "Massage Therapy Reduces Job Stress and Enhances EEG Pattern of Alertness and Math Computations." *Touchpoints* Vol. 2, no. 2:3.

Field, T., Delamater, Shaw, and LaGreca. 1995c. "Diabetes." *Touchpoints* Vol. 2, no. 4:2.

Field, Tiffany, M. Seligman, F. Scafidi, and S. Schanberg. 1995d. "Posttraumatic Stress Disorder." *Touchpoints* Vol. 2, no. 4:2.

Field, Tiffany, N. Grizzle, F. Scafidi, and S. Schanberg. 1995e. "Massage and Relaxation Therapies Effects on Depressed Adolescent Mothers." *Touchpoints* Vol. 2, no. 4:2.

Field, Tiffany, S. M. Schanberg, F. Scafidi, C. R. Bauer, N. Vega-Lahr, R. Garcia, J. Nystrom, and C. M. Khun. 1986. "Tactile /Kinesthetic Stimulation Effects on Preterm Neonates." *Pediatrics* Vol. 77, no. 5:654-8.

Flanagan, Madeleine. 1997. *Wound Management.* New York: Churchill Livingstone.

Fleetcroft, J. P. 1982. *The Musculoskeletal System: Orthopaedics, Rheumatology and Fractures.* Edinburgh: Churchill Livingstone.

Foldi, E., 1995a. "Massage and Damage to the Lymphatics." *Lymphology* Vol. 28:1-3.

Foldi, Michael. 1995b. "Book Review: Modern Treatment for Lymphodema." *Lymphology* Vol. 28:147-9.

Foldi, Ethel, M. Foldi, and H. Weissleder. 1985. "Conservative Treatment of Lymphoedema of the Limbs." *Angiology: Journal of Vascular Diseases*:171-9.

Foldi, M. 1985. "Complex Decongestive Physiotherapy." *Progress in Lymphology* X:165-7.

Foreman, Stephen M., and Arthur Croft. 1995. *Whiplash Injuries: The Cervical Acceleration/Deceleration Syndrome, 2nd Ed.* Baltimore: Williams and Wilkins.

Fox, James, and Wilson Del Pizzo. 1993. *The Patellofemoral Joint.* New York: McGraw-Hill.

Freeman, Michael D., Arthur C. Croft, and Annette M. Rossignol. 1998. "'Whiplash Associated Disorders: Redefining Whiplash and Its Management' by the Quebec Task Force: A Critical Evaluation." *Spine* Vol. 23, no. 9:1043-9.

Fried, Robert. 1990. *The Breath Connection.* New York: Plenum Press.

Frisch, Herbert. 1994. *Systemic Musculoskeletal Examination: Including Manual Medicine Diagnostic Techniques.* Berlin: Springer Verlag.

Fritz, Sandy Cochrane, and Jennifer Noltie. 1992. "Massage Therapy and Intimacy." *Massage Magazine* no. 37:58-61.

Frownfelter, Donna L. 1987. *Chest Physical Therapy and Pulmonary Rehabilitation: An Interdisciplinary Approach, 2nd Ed.* Chicago: Year Book.

Gabbe, Steven G., Jennifer R. Niebyl, and Joe Leigh Simpson. 1996. *Obstetrics: Normal and Problem Pregancies, 3rd Ed.* New York: Churchill Livingstone.

Gelb, Harold. 1985. *Clinical Management of Head, Neck and TMJ Pain and Dysfunction, 2nd Ed.* Philadelphia: W. B. Saunders Company.

Gerard, Janet A., and Steven Kleinfield. 1993. *Orthopaedic Testing: A Rational Approach to Diagnosis.* New York: Churchill Livingstone.

Gerhardt, John, and Jules Rippstein. 1990. *Measuring and Recording of Joint Motion: Instrumentation and Techniques.* Toronto: Hogrefe and Huber.

Gianni, Sandro, Fabio Catani, Maria Grazia Benedetti, and Alberto Leardini. 1994. *Gait Analysis: Methodologies and Clinical Applications.* Amsterdam: IOS Press.

Glinz, Werner. 1987. *Diagnostics and Operative Arthoscopy of the Knee Joint, 2nd Ed.* Toronto: Hogrefe and Huber.

Globe and Mail. 1995. "Stethoscopes Risky, Study Finds." October 21.

Goldberg, Burton. 1998. *Chronic Fatigue, Fibromyalgia and Environmental Illness: Alternative Medicine Guide.* Tiburon: Future Press.

Goldberg, F. K., and Dudley F. Rochester. 1980. "Techniques of Respiratory Physical Therapy." *American Review of Respiratory Disorders* Vol. 122, no. 5: 133-46.

Goldstein, Beth G., and Adam O. Goldstein. 1997. *Practical Dermatology, 2nd Ed.* St. Louis: Mosby.

Goodman, Catherine, and Teresa Snyder. 1995. *Differential Diagnosis in Physical Therapy, 2nd Ed.* Philadelphia: W. B. Saunders Company.

Gracovetsky, Serge. 1988. *The Spinal Engine.* Vienna: Springer Verlag.

Graham, Judy. 1989. *Multiple Sclerosis: A Self-Help Guide to Its Management.* Rochester: Healing Arts Press.

Grant, Ruth. 1988. *Physical Therapy of the Cervical and Thoracic Spine.* New York: Churchill Livingstone.

Greenberg, Jerrold S. 1996. *Comprehensive Stress Management, 5th Ed.* Madison: Brown and Benchmark.

Greenman, Philip E. 1989. *Principles of Manual Medicine.* Baltimore: Williams and Wilkins.

Gregory, Brenda. 1994. *Orthopaedic Surgery.* St. Louis: Mosby.

Grimes, David, J., Peggy A. Gray, and Kelly Grimes Ohman. 1994. *Parkinson's: One Step at a Time, 2nd Ed.* Ottawa: Creative Bound Inc.

Grodin, Allan. 1989. *Soft Tissue Mobilization Vol. 2, No. 2.* Baltimore: Williams and Wilkins.

Guyton, Arthur. 1984. *Textbook of Medical Physiology, 7th Ed.* Philadelphia: W. B. Saunders Company.

Haldane, Sean. 1984. *Emotional First Aid.* Barrytown: Station Hill Press.

Hammell, Karen W. 1995. *Spinal Cord Injury Rehabilitation.* London: Chapman, Hall.

Hammer, W. I. 1991. *Functional Soft Tissue Examination and Treatment by Manual Methods: The Extremities.* Aspen: Rockville.

Hanak, Marcia, and Anne Scott. 1993 *Spinal Cord Injury: An Illustrated Guide for Health Care Professionals.* New York: Springer Verlag.

Hartley, Anne. 1995a. *Practical Joint Assessment Upper Quadrant. 2nd Ed.* St. Louis: Mosby.

Hartley, Anne. 1995b. *Practical Joint Assessment Lower Quadrant. 2nd Ed.* St. Louis: Mosby.

Harries, Richard. 1987. "Personal Experience of Pressure Sores." *Physiotherapy* Vol. 73, no. 9:448-450.

Harris, Robert. 1996. Personal Correspondence.

Harris, Robert. 1994. "Edema and Its Treatment in Massage Therapy."*Journal of Soft Tissue Manipulation* Vol. 1, no. 4:4-6.

Hawkins, Richard, and Gary Misamore. 1966. *Shoulder Injuries in the Athlete: Surgical Repair and Rehabilitation.* New York: Churchill Livingstone.

Heart and Stroke Foundation of Canada. 1993. *Strokes: A Guide for the Family.*

Heart and Stroke Foundation of Canada. N.d.a. *Congestive Heart Failure: Information on Congestive Heart Failure for Patients and Their Families.* Cat. 26059522.

Heart and Stroke Foundation of Canada. N.d.b. *Know Your Blood Pressure by Heart: How to Keep Your Blood Pressure Healthy.*

Heart and Stroke Foundation of Ontario. N.d.a. *Heart and Stroke: Women Should Know Their Blood Pressure...by Heart.*

Heart and Stroke Foundation of Ontario. N.d.b. *Strokefacts: Caution: Brain Attack.*

Heart and Stroke Foundation of Ontario. N.d.c. *Strokefacts: Communicating with a Stroke Survivor.*

Heart and Stroke Foundation of Ontario. N.d.d. *Strokefacts: Preventing a Stroke.*

Heart and Stroke Foundation of Ontario. N.d.e. *Strokefacts: The Role of the Stroke Caregiver.*

Hecox, Bernadette, Tsega Mehreteab, and Joseph Weisberg. 1994. *Physical Agents: A Comprehensive Text for Physical Therapists.* Norwalk: Appleton Lange.

Hellman, D. B. 1995. "Arthritis and Musculoskeletal Disorders." In L.M. Tierny, S. J. McPhee, and M. A. Papadakis, eds. *Current Medical Diagnosis and Treatment, 34th Ed.* Norwalk: Appleton Lange.

Helliwell, P. S., P. F. Evans, and V. Wright. 1994. "The Straight Cervical Spine: Does It Indicate Muscle Spasm?" *The Journal of Bone and Joint Surgery* 76B:103-6.

Helm, Klaus F., and James G. Marks, Jr. 1998. *Atlas of Differential Diagnosis in Dermatology.* New York: Churchill Livingstone.

Henche, Hans Rudolf, and Jorg Holder. 1988. *Arthroscopy of the Knee Joint, 2nd Ed.* London: Springer Verlag.

Hertling, Darlene, and Randolph M. Kessler. 1996. *Management of Common Musculoskeletal Disorders, 3rd Ed.* Philadelphia: J.B. Lippincott.

Hertling, Darlene, and Randolph M. Kessler. 1990. *Management of Common Musculoskeletal Disorders, 2nd Ed.* Philadelphia: J.B. Lippincott.

Hickey, Noel, and Ian M. Graham. 1988. *Hypertension.* London: Croom Helm.

Hill, Judy P. 1986. *Spinal Cord Injury: A Guide to Functional Outcomes in Occupational Therapy.* Rockville: Aspen Publications.

Hogenhuis, L. A. H., and T. J. Steiner. 1994. *Headache and Migraine 3.* Utrecht: Wetenschappelijke Uitgeverij Bunge.

Holmes, Gary. 1988. "Chronic Fatigue Syndrome: A Working Case Definition." *Annals of Internal Medicine* Vol. 108, no. 3:387-9.

Hooper, Bonnie J., and Mitchel P. Goldman. 1999. *Primary Dermatology Care.* St. Louis: Mosby.

Hooper, G. 1992. *Colour Guide Orthopaedics.* Edinburgh: Churchill Livingstone.

Hooper, Paul D. 1996. *Physical Modalities: A Primer for Chiropractic.* Baltimore: Williams and Wilkins.

Hooshmand, Hooshang. 1993. *Chronic Pain: Reflex Sympathetic Dystrophy Prevention and Management.* Boca Raton: CRC Press.

Hopkins, Anthony. 1994. *Clinical Neurology: A Modern Approach.* Oxford: Oxford University Press.

Hoppenfeld, Stanley. 1976. *Physical Examination of the Spine and Extremities.* New York: Appleton-Century-Crofts.

Hoppenfeld, Stanley. 1967. *Scoliosis: a Manual of Concept and Treatment.* Philadelphia: J. B. Lippincott.

Hosenpud, Jeffrey D., and Barry H. Greenberg. 1994. *Congestive Heart Failure.* New York: Springer Verlag.

Hough, Alexandra. 1996. *Physiotherapy in Respiratory Care: A Problem-Solving Approach to Respiratory and Cardiac Care, 2nd Ed.* London: Chapman, Hall.

Howard, Nigel. 1995. *Irritable Bowel Syndrome: A Comprehensive Guide to Effective Treatment.* Shaftsbury: Element.

Hueston, John T., and Raoul Tubiana. 1985. *Dupuytren's Disease, 4th Ed.* New York: Churchill Livingstone.

Hunt, Gary C., and Thomas G. McPoil. 1995. *Physical Therapy of the Foot and Ankle, 2nd Ed.* New York: Churchill Livingstone.

Immen, Wallace. 1996. "Drug Offers Hope to Women Suffering from Osteoporosis." *Globe and Mail* September 12.

Immen, Wallace. 1995. "A Swell System of Tiny Hearts." *Globe and Mail* June 28.

Ingram, Jay. 1995. *The Burning House: Unlocking the Mysteries of the Brain.* Toronto: Penguin.

Interagency Coalition on AIDS and Development. 1998. *AIDS in the World: Regional Distribution of the Pandemic.*

Ironson, G., T. Field, and M. Fletcher. 1995. "Massage Therapy and Immunity". *Touchpoints* Vol. 2, no. 1:2.

Irwin, Scott, and Jan Stephen Tecklin. 1995. *Cardiopulmonary Physical Therapy, 2nd Ed.* St. Louis: Mosby.

Jacobs, Rae, ed. 1984. *Pathogenesis of Idiopathic Scoliosis.* Chicago: Scoliosis Research Society.

Jacobson, Alan L., and William C. Donlon. 1990. *Headache and Facial Pain: Diagnosis and Management.* New York: Raven Press.

Jamer, Roderick. N.d. "Suffer the Little Children: Kids Get Fibromyalgia Too." *Arthritis News* Vol. 11, no. 1:8-11.

Janda, Vladimir. 1991. "Muscle Spasm: A Proposed Procedure for Differential Diagnosis." *Journal of Manual Medicine* 6:136-139.

Janda, Vladimir. 1984. *Muscle Function and Testing.* London: Butterworth.

Johnson, Bernett L., Ronald L. Moy, and Gary M. White. 1998. *Ethnic Skin: Medical and Surgical.* St. Louis: Mosby.

Johnstone, Margaret. 1991. *Therapy for Stroke.* Edinburgh; Churchill Livingstone.

Johnstone, Margaret. 1987. *Restoration of Motor Function in the Stroke Patient, 3rd Ed.* Edinburgh; Churchill Livingstone.

Jones, Francis. 1972. *Management of Constipation.* Oxford: Blackwell Scientific Publications.

Jones, Lawrence H. 1993. *Strain and Counter Strain.* Indianapolis: The American Academy of Osteopathy.

Jones, Peter. 1968. *Torticollis in Infancy and Childhood.* Springfield: Charles Thomas.

Juhan, Deane. 1987. *Job's Body: A Handbook for Bodywork.* Barrytown: Station Hill Press.

Kaiser, Jon. 1997. "Medical Matters: How to Prevent and Treat Peripheral Neuropathy." *PWAC New York Newsline* July/August:36-7.

Kaliner, Michael, Peter Barnes, and Carl Pesson. 1990. *Asthma: Its Pathology and Treatment.* New York: Marcel Dekker.

Kamm, Michael A., and John E. Lennard-Jones. 1994. *Constipation.* Petersfield: Wrightson Biomedical Publications.

Kapandji, A. 1974. *The Physiology of the Joints, Vol. 3: The Trunk and Vertebral Column.* Edinburgh: Churchill Livingstone.

Kapit, Wynn, and Lawrence M. Elson. 1977. *The Anatomy Coloring Book.* New York: Harper and Row.

Kaplan, Norman M., and C. Venkata S. Ram. 1995. *Individualized Therapy of Hypertension.* New York: Marcel Dekker.

Kaplan, Paul, and Leonard Cerullo. 1986. *Stroke Rehabilitation.* Boston: Butterworth.

Kart, Cary, Eileen Metress, and Seamus Metress. 1992. *Human Aging and Chronic Disease.* Boston: Jones and Bartlett.

Kendall, Florence, Elizabeth McCreary, and Patricia Provance. 1993. *Muscles: Testing and Function, 4th Ed.* Baltimore: Williams and Wilkins.

Kendall, Florence, and Elizabeth McCreary. 1983. *Muscles: Testing and Function, 3rd Ed.* Baltimore: Williams and Wilkins.

Kettenbach, Ginge. 1990. *Writing SOAP Notes.* Philadelphia: F.A. Davis.

Kirschmann, John D. 1979. *Nutrition Almanac: Revised Edition.* New York: McGraw-Hill.

Kisner, Carolyn, and Lynn Allen Colby. 1996. *Therapeutic Exercise: Foundations and Techniques, 3rd Ed.* Philadelphia: F.A. Davis.

Kisner, Carolyn, and Lynn Allen Colby. 1990. *Therapeutic Exercise: Foundations and Techniques, 2nd Ed.* Philadelphia: F.A. Davis.

Klimas, Nancy, and Roberto Patarca. 1995. *Clinical Management of Chronic Fatigue Syndrome.* New York: Haworth.

Kline, David G., and Alin R. Hudson. 1995. *Nerve Injuries: Operative Results for Major Nerve Injuries, Entrapments and Tumors.* Philadelphia: W. B. Saunders Company.

Kloth, Luther C., Joseph M. McCulloch, and Jeffery A. Feeder. 1990. *Wound Healing: Alternatives in Management.* Philadelphia: F.A. Davis.

Knaster, Mirka. 1994. "Researching Massage as Real Therapy." *Massage Therapy Journal* Vol. 33, no. 3:56-112.

Knuppel, Robert A., and Joan E. Drukker. 1993. *High-Risk Pregnancy: A Team Approach, 2nd Ed.* Philadelphia: W. B. Saunders Company.

Kottke, Frederic J., G. Keith Stillwell, and Justus F. Lehmann. 1982. *Kreusen's Handbook of Physical Medicine and Rehabilitation, 3rd Ed.* Philadelphia: W. B. Saunders Company.

Krakoff, Lawrence R. 1995. *Management of the Hypertensive Patient.* New York: Churchill Livingstone.

Krasner, Diane. 1990. *Chronic Wound Healing: A Clinical Source Book for Healthcare Professionals.* Pennsylvania: Health Management Publications.

Kraus, Hans. 1988. *Diagnosis and Treatment of Muscle Pain.* Chicago: Quintessence.

Kuchera, William, and Michael Kuchera. 1993. *Osteopathic Principles in Practice, Revised, 2nd Ed.* Columbus: Greyden Press.

Kunz, Jeffery, and Asher Finkel. 1987. *The American Medical Association Family Medical Guide.* New York: Random House.

Kuprian, Werner. 1995. *Physical Therapy for Sports, 2nd Ed.* Philadelphia: W. B. Saunders Company.

Kurz, Ingrid. 1990. *Textbook of Dr. Vodder's Manual Lymph Drainage Volume 3: Treatment Manual, 2nd Revised Ed.* Heidelburg: Karl F. Haug Verlag.

Kurz, Ingrid. 1989. *Textbook of Dr. Vodder's Manual Lymph Drainage Volume 2: Therapy, 2nd Ed.* Heidelburg: Karl F. Haug Verlag.

Kuettner, Klaus E., and Victor M. Goldberg. 1995. *Osteoathritic Disorders.* Rosemont: American Academy of Orthopedic Surgeons.

Lanasky, Kathleen. 1993. *Prevention of Secondary Conditions Conference: Cerebral Palsy: The Adult Experience.* Ontario Federation for Cerebral Palsy.

Lane, Joseph, M. 1987. *Fracture Healing.* New York: Churchill Livingstone.

Langer, Ellen J. 1989. *Mindfulness.* Reading: Addison-Wesley Publishing.

Larson, Robert L., and William A. Grana. 1993. *The Knee: Form, Function, Pathology and Treatment.* Philadelphia: W. B. Saunders Company.

Latimer, Paul R. 1983. *Functional Gastrointestinal Disorders: A Behavioural Approach.* New York: Springer.

Lawless, Julia. 1995. *The Illustrated Encyclopedia of Essential Oils.* Shaftesbury: Element Books.

Lawless, Julia. 1992. *The Encyclopedia of Essential Oils.* Longmead: Element Books.

Leung, Kwok-sui, Hung Leung-Kim, and Leung Ping-chung. 1994. *Biodegradable Implants in Fracture Fixation.* Singapore: World Scientific Publishing Company.

Lewit, Karel. 1993. *Manipulative Therapy in Rehabilitation of the Locomotor System, 2nd Ed.* Linacre House: Butterworth.

Lewit, Karel, and David G. Simons. 1984. "Myofascial Pain: Relief by Post-isometric Relaxation." *Archives of Physical Medicine and Rehabilitation* Vol. 65.

Lieberman, A., and Frank Williams. 1993. *Parkinson's Disease: The Complete Guide for Patients and Caregivers.* New York: Fireside Press.

Licht, Sidney M. 1963. *Medical Hydrology.* New Haven: Licht.

Lipovenko, Dorothy. 1995. "Study Links Paints, Glues to Onset of Parkinson's." *Globe and Mail* September 21:A8.

Lohnert, Johannes, and Jurgen Raunest. 1988. *Arthroscopic Surgery of the Knee.* New York: Thieme Medical Publications.

Lorig, Kate, and James F. Fries. 1995. *The Arthritis Helpbook: A Tested Self-Management Program for Coping with Arthritis and Fibromyalgia, 4th Ed.* Reading: Addison-Wesley Publishing.

Lowe, Whitney W. 1995. "Looking in Depth: Orthopedic Assessment Skills." *Orthopedic and Sports Massage Reviews* Vol. 7:4-5.

Lundborg, Goran. 1988. *Nerve Injury and Repair.* Edinburgh: Churchill Livingstone.

Lynch, Mary, and Vivian Grisogono. 1991. *Strokes and Head Injuries.* London: John Murray Publishers.

MacDonald, Kathy, and Christine Sutherland. N.d. *Sutherland Chan Massage Treatments Workbook.* Toronto: Sutherland Chan.

Macnab, Ian, and John McCulloch. 1994. *Neck Ache and Shoulder Pain.* Baltimore: Williams and Wilkins.

Magee, David J. 1997. *Orthopedic Physical Assessment. 3rd Ed.* Philadelphia: W.B. Saunders Company.

Magee, David J. 1992. *Orthopedic Physical Assessment, 2nd Ed.* Philadelphia: W.B. Saunders Company.

Maigne, Robert. 1996. *Diagnosis and Treatment of Pain of Vertebral Origin: A Manual Medicine Approach.* Baltimore: Williams and Wilkins.

Marks, R. 1993. *Roxburgh's Common Skin Diseases, 16th Ed.* London: Chapman, Hall Medical.

Masellis, M., and S. W. A. Gunn. 1995. *The Management of Burns and Fire Disasters: Perspectives 2000.* Dordrecht: Klumer Academic Publications.

Mastalgia, Frank, and John Walton. 1982. *Skeletal Muscle Pathology.* Edinburgh: Churchill Livingstone.

Matsen, Frederick. 1992. *The Shoulder: A Balance of Mobility and Stability.* Rosemont: AAOS.

Matsen, Frederick, Steven Lippett, John Sidles, and Douglas Harryman. 1994. *Practical Evaluation and Management of the Shoulder.* Philadelphia: W. B. Saunders Company.

Mattingly, Gary E., and Paul J Mackarey. 1998. "Optimal Methods of Shoulder Tendon Palpation: A Cadaver Study." *Orthopaedic Division Review* March/April: 36-41.

May, D. B., and P. W. Munt. 1979. "Physiological Effects of Chest Percussion and Postural Drainage in Patients with Chronic Stable Bronchitis." *Chest* Vol. 75:29-32.

McAtee, Robert. 1993. *Facilitated Stretching: PNF Stretching Made Easy.* Champaign: Human Kinetics.

McCain, Glenn. 1990. "Fibromyalgia: A Real (and Common) Cause of Muscular Aches and Pains." *Ontario Medicine* Vol. 9, no. 4, article 5.

McKenzie, Robin. 1989. *The Lumbar Spine: Mechanical Diagnosis and Therapy.* Upper Hutt: Wright and Carman.

McKinney, L. A. 1989. "Early Mobilization Outcome in Acute Sprains of the Neck." *British Journal of Medicine* Vol. 229:1006-8.

McKinney, L. A., J. O. Dornan, and M. Ryan. 1989. "The Role of Physiotherapy in the Management of Acute Neck Sprains Following Road-Traffic Accidents." *Archives of Emergency Medicine* Vol. 6:27-33.

McRae, Ronald. 1990. *Clinical Orthopaedic Examination, 3rd Ed.* Edinburgh: Churchill Livingstone.

Mealy, K., H. Brennan, and G. C. C. Fenelon. 1986. "Early Mobilization of Acute Whiplash Injuries." *British Medical Journal* Vol. 292: 656-7.

Menard, Martha Brown. 1994. "An Introduction to Research Methods for Massage Therapists." *Massage Therapy Journal* Vol. 33, no. 3:113-8.

Mennell, John. 1964. *Joint Pain: Diagnosis and Treatment Using Manipulative Techniques.* Boston: Little, Brown and Company.

Migraine Foundation of Canada. 1992. *Living with Migraine: You and Your Medication.*

Miller, James A. A. 1984. "Mechanical Factors in Idiopathic Scoliosis." In Rae Jacobs, ed. *Pathogenesis of Idiopathic Scoliosis.* Chicago: Scoliosis Research Society:61-9.

Milne, Robert D., Blake More, and Burton Goldberg. 1997. *An Alternative Medicine Definitive Guide to Headaches.* Tiburon: Future Medicine Publishing.

Mohr, J. P., and J. C. Gautier. 1995. *Guide to Clinical Neurology.* New York: Churchill Livingstone.

Moon, S. D., and S. L. Sauter. 1996. *Beyond Biomechanics: Psychosocial Aspects of Musculoskeletal Disorders in Office Work.* London: Taylor and Francis.

Mooney, Maureen, and Lorrie Maffey-Ward. 1995. "All Heel Pain Is Not Plantar Fasciitis." *Physiotherapy Canada* Vol. 47, no. 3:185-99.

Moor, Fred B., Stella C. Peterson, Ethel M. Manwell, Mary C. Noble, and Getrude Muench. 1964. *Manual of Hydrotherapy and Massage.* Mountain View: Pacific Press.

Moore, Keith. 1985. *Clinically Oriented Anatomy, 2nd Ed.* Baltimore: Williams and Wilkins.

Morgan, Susan. 1989. *Plaster Casting: Patient Problems and Nursing Care.* Oxford: Heinemann.

Muggeridge, Peter. 1997. "For the Health of It." *Diabetes Dialogue* Vol. 44, no. 4:58.

Mumenthaler, Mark. 1992. *Neurological Differential Diagnosis.* New York: Thieme Medical Publications.

Mumenthaler, Mark, and Hans Schliack. 1991. *Peripheral Nerve Lesions: Diagnosis and Therapy.* New York: Thieme Medical Publications.

Murphy, Joseph G. 1997. *The Mayo Clinic Cardiology Review.* Armonk: Futura Publishing Co.

Murray, Michael T. 1995. *Stress, Anxiety and Insomnia: How You Can Benefit from Diet, Vitamins, Minerals, Herbs , Exercise and Other Natural Methods.* Rocklin: Prima Publishers.

Nachemson, Alf. "Future Research in Scoliosis: Possible Neuromuscular Causes." In Rae Jacobs, ed. *Pathogenesis of Idiopathic Scoliosis.* Chicago: Scoliosis Research Society:143-52.

National AIDS Awareness Campaign Resource Guide. 1998/9a. *General Facts on AIDS.* Module 2:18-9.

National AIDS Awareness Campaign Resource Guide. 1998/9b. *General Facts on AIDS: The Faces of HIV/AIDS in Canada.* Module 2:1-2.

National Cancer Institute of Canada. 1998. *Canadian Cancer Statistics 1998.* Toronto: Statistics Canada.

Netter, Frank H. 1989. *Atlas of Human Anatomy.* West Caldwell: CIBA GEIGY Corporation.

Neumann, Heinz-Dieter. 1989. *Introduction to Manual Medicine.* New York: Springer Verlag.

Nightingale Research Foundation. 1992. *A Physicians Guide to Myalgic Encephalomyelitis Chronic Fatigue Syndrome (M.E./CFS), Revised.* Vol. 1, no. 7.

Oldenburg, F. A., G. A. Traver, and L. M. Taussig. 1979. "Maximal Expiratory Flows after Postural Drainage." *American Review of Respiratory Dysfunctions* Vol. 119:239-45.

Olesen, Jes, and Robert F. Schmidt. 1993. *Pathophysiological Mechanisms of Migraine.* Wenheim: VCH.

Oloff, Lawrence M. 1994. *Musculoskeletal Disorders of the Lower Extremities.* Philadelphia: W. B. Saunders Company.

Omer, George E., and Morton Spinner. 1980. *Management of Peripheral Nerve Problems.* Philadelphia: W. B. Saunders Company.

Ontario. *Health Care Consent Act.* 1996. Queen's Printer for Ontario.

Ontario. *Massage Therapy Act.* 1991a. Queen's Printer for Ontario.

Ontario. *Regulated Health Professions Act.* 1991b. Queen's Printer for Ontario.

Ontario Federation for Cerebral Palsy. 1993. *Health, Aging and Cerebral Palsy.*

Ontario Federation for Cerebral Palsy. N.d.a. *A Guide to Cerebral Palsy.*

Ontario Federation for Cerebral Palsy. N.d.b. *Cerebral Palsy Overview.*

Ontario Federation for Cerebral Palsy. N.d.c. *Perspective on Aging and Cerebral Palsy.*

Osteoporosis Society of Canada. 1997. *Osteoporosis: Let's Talk About It! A Preventive Guide for Women.*

Osteoporosis Society of Canada. N.d.a. *Building Better Bones: A Guide to Active Living.*

Osteoporosis Society of Canada. N.d.b. *Fact Sheet Series, No. 1: Pain Management, Ways to Cope with Chronic Pain.*

Osteoporosis Society of Canada. N.d.c. *Fact Sheet Series, No. 2: Physical Activity, the Role of Exercise in the Prevention and Treatment of Osteoporosis.*

Osteoporosis Society of Canada. N.d.d. *Fact Sheet Series, No. 3: Calcium, an Essential Element of Bone Health.*

Osteoporosis Society of Canada. N.d.e. *Fact Sheet Series, No. 4: How Strong Are Your Bones? Assessing Your Risk and Testing for Bone Loss.*

Osteoporosis Society of Canada. N.d.f. *Fact Sheet Series, No. 5: Calcium Supplementation, When You Can't Get Enough From Food.*

Osteoporosis Society of Canada. N.d.g. *Fact Sheet Series, No. 6: Men and Osteoporosis, Not Just Women's Disease.*

Osteoporosis Society of Canada. N.d.h. *Fact Sheet Series, No. 7: Secondary Osteoporosis, Medications that Cause Secondary Bone Loss.*

Osteoporosis Society of Canada. N.d.i. *Fact Sheet Series, No. 8: Hormone Therapy, the Role of Hormone Therapy in the Prevention and Treatment of Osteoporosis.*

Osteoporosis Society of Canada. N.d.j. *Fact Sheet Series, No. 9: Bisphosphonates, an Alternative Therapy for Established Osteoporosis.*

Osteoporosis Society of Canada. N.d.k. *Osteoporosis to the Third Millennium: Priorities for Prevention and Treatment.*

Ozer, Mark N. 1988. *Management of Persons with Spinal Cord Injuries.* New York: Demos.

Pansky, Ben. 1979. *Review of Gross Anatomy, 4th Ed.* New York: Macmillan Press.

Pappas, Arthur M. 1995. *Upper Extremity Injuries in the Athlete.* New York: Churchill Livingstone.

Pascarelli, Emil, and Deborah Quilter. 1994. *Repetitive Strain Injury: A Computer User's Guide.* New York: John Wiley and Sons.

Patient Care. 1989. "Recognizing Fibromyalgia" 07/15.

Patterson, David, and Tom Treasure. 1993. *Disorders of the Cardiovascular System.* London: Edward Arnold.

Pauls, Julie A., and Kathlyn L. Reed. 1996. *Quick Reference to Physical Therapy.* Gaithersburg: Aspen Publications.

Pavia, Cedelia. 1995. "Navigating the Choppy Seas of Dual Relationships." *The Journal of Soft Tissue Manipulation* Vol. 3, no. 1:9-14.

Pecina, Marko, Jelena Krmpotic-Nemanic, and Andrew D. Markiewitz. 1991. *Tunnel Syndromes.* Boca Raton: CRC Press

Pedersen, Ejner. 1969. *Spasticity: Mechanism, Movement, Management.* Springfield: Charles C. Thomas.

Pedretti, Lorraine, and Barbara Zoltan. 1990. *Occupational Therapy Practical Skills for Physical Dysfunction, 3rd Ed.* St. Louis: C. V. Mosby.

Persad, Randall. 1995a. "Pharmacological Considerations in Massage Therapy: Aspirin and the NSAIDS." *Journal of Soft Tissue Manipulation* Vol. 2, no. 6:8-12.

Persad, Randall. 1995b. "The Skeletal Muscle Relaxants." *Journal of Soft Tissue Manipulation* Vol. 3, no. 1:6-8.

Persad, Randall. 1995c. "The Corticosteroids." *Journal of Soft Tissue Manipulation* Vol. 3, no. 2:6-10.

Persing, Gary. 1994. *Advanced Practitioner Respiratory Care Review: Written Registry and Clinical Simulation Exam.* Philadelphia: W. B. Saunders Company.

Pick, Marc. 1995. "The Short Term Effect of a Cranial Manipulation." *Journal of Soft Tissue Manipulation* Vol. 2, no. 6:13.

Pillemer, Stanley. 1994. *The Fibromyalgia Syndrome: Current Research and Future Directions in Epidemiology, Pathogenesis and Treatment.* New York: Haworth.

Pinder, Ruth. 1990. *The Management of Chronic Illness: Patient and Doctor Perspectives on Parkinson's Disease.* London: Macmillan Press.

PI Perspective. 1997a. "HIV Neuropathy" July:12-13.

PI Perspective. 1997b. "Update on Opportunistic Infections" November:16.

Pirsig, Robert M. 1974. *Zen and the Art of Motorcycle Maintenance.* New York: William Morrow and Company.

Pollack, Erich. 1986. *Thoracic Outlet Syndrome.* New York: Futura.

Porro, G. Bianchi, and N. W. Read. 1990. *Irritable Bowel Syndrome: One Disease, Several or None?* New York: Raven Press.

Porth, Carol Mattson. 1990. *Pathophysiology 3rd Ed.* Philadelphia: J. B. Lippincott.

Positively Aware. 1998. "Latest Opportunistic Infection Prevention Guidelines" January/February:43-4.

Prudden, Bonnie. 1980. *Pain Erasure: The Bonnie Prudden Way.* New York: M. Evans and Company.

Pryor, Jennifer A. 1991. *Respiratory Care.* Edinburgh: Churchill Livingstone.

Rachlin, Edward. 1994. *Myofascial Pain and Fibromyalgia: Trigger Point Management.* St. Louis: Mosby.

Read, Nicholas W. 1991. *Irritable Bowel Syndrome.* Oxford: Blackwell Scientific Publications.

Read, Nicholas W. 1985. *Irritable Bowel Syndrome.* London: Grune and Stratton.

Richard, Reginald L., and Marlys J. Staley. 1994. *Burn Care Rehabilitation: Principles and Practice.* Philadelphia: F.A. Davis.

Richmond, John C., and Edward J. Shahady. 1996. *Sports Medicine for Primary Care.* Ann Arbour: Blackwell Scientific Publications.

Ritson, Fenella, and Shona Scott. 1996. "Physiotherapy for Osteoporosis; A Pilot Study Comparing Practice and Knowledge in Scotland and Sweden." *Physiotherapy* Vol. 82, no. 7:309-4.

Robbins, Stanley L., Ramzi S. Cotran, and Vinay Kumar. 1984. *Pathologic Basis of Disease, 3rd Ed.* Philadelphia: W. B. Saunders Company.

Robin, Gordon C. 1990. *The Aetiology of Idiopathic Scoliosis: A Review of Current Research.* Boca Raton: CRC Press.

Rochester, Dudley F., and S. K. Goldberg. 1980. "Techniques of Respiratory Physical Therapy." *American Review of Respiratory Diseases* Vol. 122, no. 5:133-46.

Rockwood, Charles A., David P. Green, and Robert W. Bucholz. 1991. *Fractures in Adults, Vol. 2.* Philadelphia: J. B. Lippincott.

Rockwood, Charles A., David P. Green, and Robert W. Bucholz. 1984. *Fractures in Adults. Vol. 1.* Philadelphia: J. B. Lippincott.

Rodrigues, Jimmy. N.d. "1.2 Billion People Can't Be Wrong, Can They?" *Arthritis News* Vol. 15, no. 4.

Roscovitch, Dale. 1987. "Acceleration/Deceleration Injuries and Massage Therapy." *The Verdict* Vol. 1:15-16.

Rosenbaum, Richard, B., and Jose L. Ochoa. 1993. *Carpal Tunnel Syndrome and Other Disorders of the Median Nerve.* Boston: Butterworth and Heinemann.

Rowland, Lewis. 1995. *Merritt's Textbook of Neurology, 9th Ed.* Baltimore: Williams and Wilkins.

Rudolph, Ross, and Joel M. Noe. 1983. *Chronic Problem Wounds.* Boston: Little, Brown and Company.

Rupp, Ned T. 1996. "Diagnosis and Management of Exercise-Induced Asthma." *Physician and Sports Medicine* Vol. 1:77-87.

Samii, M. 1990. *Peripheral Nerve Lesions.* Berlin: Springer Verlag.

Sammarco, James. 1995. *Rehabilitation of the Foot and Ankle.* St. Louis: Mosby.

Sandler, Merton, Michael Ferrari, and Sara Harnett. 1996. *Migraine: Pharmacology and Genetics.* London: Altman.

Sauer, Gordon C., and John C. Hall. 1996. *Manual of Skin Diseases, 7th Ed.* Philadelphia: Lippincott-Raven.

Savage, Peter A. 1983. *Problems in Peripheral Vascular Disease.* Lancaster: MTP.

Scafidi, F., and T. Field. 1995. "Massage Effects on the Development of HIV-Exposed Infants." *Touchpoints* Vol. 2, no. 1:2.

Schapiro, Randall T. 1994. *Symptom Management of Multiple Sclerosis.* New York: Demos Publications.

Schaumburg, Herbert, Allen R. Berger, and P. K. Thomas. 1992. *Disorders of Peripheral Nerves, 2nd Ed.* Philadelphia: F. A. Davis.

Schneider, Werner, Jiri Dvorak, Vaclav Dvorak, and Thomas Tritschler. 1988. *Manual Medicine: Therapy.* New York: Thieme Medical Publications.

Schumacher, H. Ralph. 1993. *Primer on the Rheumatic Diseases, 10th Ed.* Atlanta: Arthritis Foundation.

Scully, Rosemary M., and Marylou Barnes. 1989. *Physical Therapy.* Philadelphia: J. B. Lippincott.

Seddon, Herbert. 1972. *Surgical Disorders of the Peripheral Nerves, 2nd Ed.* Edinburgh: Churchill Livingstone.

Sellar, Wanda. 1992. *The Directory of Essential Oils.* Essex: C. W. Daniel and Company.

Selye, Hans. 1974. *Stress Without Distress.* New York: J. B. Lippincott.

Settle, John A. D. 1996. *Principles and Practice of Burn Management.* New York: Churchill Livingstone.

Silberstein, Stephen, Richard B. Lipton, and Peter J. Goadsby. 1998. *Headache in Clinical Practice.* Oxford: Isis Medical Media.

Siliski, John. 1994. *Traumatic Disorders of the Knee.* New York: McGraw-Hill.

Simpson, Alison, Kate Bowers, and Dickon Weir-Hughes. 1996. *Pressure Sore Prevention.* London: Whurr Publishers Ltd.

Smith, Ruth. 1994. "Lavender Helps Burned Boy." *The International Journal of Aromatherapy* Vol. 5, no. 4:6-9.

Snow, Christine. 1996/7. "Massage Therapist as Doula." *The Journal of Soft Tissue Manipulation* Vol. 4, no. 2:14-5.

Snyder, Stephen J. 1994. *Shoulder Arthroscopy.* New York: McGraw-Hill.

Sobel, Barry J., and George L. Bakris. 1995. *Hypertension: A Clinician's Guide to Diagnosis and Treatment.* Philadelphia: Hanley and Belfus.

Somers, Martha F. 1992. *Spinal Cord Injury: Functional Rehabilitation.* Norwalk: Appleton and Lange.

Souza, Thomas. 1997. *Differential Diagnosis for the Chiropractor.* Gaithersburg: Aspen Publications.

Souza, Thomas. 1994. *Sports Injuries of the Shoulder: Conservative Management.* New York: Churchill Livingstone.

Spake, A. 1995. "Osteoporosis Awareness." *Journal of Soft Tissue Manipulation* Vol. 2, no. 5:10.

Speer, Frederick. 1983. *Food Allergies, 2nd Ed.* Boston: John Wright.

Spitzer, W. O. 1995. *Whiplash-Associated Disorders (WAD): Redefining "Whiplash" and Its Management.* Quebéc: Société d'assurance automobile du Quebéc.

St. John, Paul. 1994. *Neuromuscular Components of Scoliosis and Cranial Decompression: Study Guide.* St. Petersburg: St. John NMT Seminars.

St. John, Paul. 1991. *Cervical Injuries, Postural Analysis and Pelvic Stabilization: Study Guide.* St. Petersburg: St. John NMT Seminars.

Steinberg, Charles L. 1990. "Integrating Traditional Medicine with Other Therapies in the Treatment of HIV-Infected Individuals." *Modern Medicine Journal* Vol. 39, no. 2:183-8.

Stern, Gerald. 1990. *Parkinson's Disease: The Facts.* Oxford: Oxford University Press.

Stewart, John. 1993. *Focal Peripheral Neuropathies, 2nd Ed.* New York: Raven Press.

Stewart, Mel. 1996. "Researches into the Effectiveness of Physiotherapy in Rheumatoid Arthritis of the Hand." *Physiotherapy* Vol. 82, no. 12:666-71.

Stillerman, 1994. "Mothermassage: Massage During Pregnancy." *Massage Therapy Journal* Vol. 33, no. 3:42-48.

Stillwell, G. K. 1969. "Treatment of Postmastectomy Lymphedema." *Modern Treatments* :396-412.

Streetnen, David. 1987. *Orthostatic Disorders of the Circulation: Mechanisms, Manifestations and Treatment.* New York: Plenum.

Sullivan, S. John. 1991. "Effects of Massage on Alpha Motoneuron Excitability." *Physical Therapy* Vol. 71, no. 8:555-60.

Sunderland, Sydney. 1991. *Nerve Injuries and Their Repair: A Critical Approach.*

Edinburgh: Churchill Livingstone.

Sunderland, Sydney. 1978. *Nerves and Nerve Injuries, 2nd Ed.* Edinburgh: Churchill Livingstone.

Sunshine, W., T. M. Field, S. Schanberg, C. Kuhn, O. Quintino, K. Fierro, T. Kilmer, and I. Burman. 1995a. "Chronic Fatigue Syndrome: Massage Therapy Effects on Depression and Somatic Symptoms." *Touchpoints* Vol. 2, no. 2:3.

Sunshine, W., T. M. Field, S. Schanberg, C. Kuhn, O. Quintino, K. Fierro, T. Kilmer, and I. Burman. 1995b. "Massage Therapy and Transcutaneous Electrical Stimulation Effects on Fibromyalgia." *Touchpoints* Vol. 2, no. 2:4.

Swedborg, I. 1985. "Reduction of Arm Edema in Postmastectomy Patients by Different Methods of Physiotherapy." *Progress in Lymphology* X:176-7.

Szabo, Robert M. 1989. *Nerve Compression Syndromes: Diagnosing and Treatment.* New Jersey: SLACK Inc.

Taber's Cyclopedic Medical Dictionary, 14th Ed. 1981. Philadelphia: F.A. Davis.

Tanser, Paul H. 1994. *Heart Failure: Management Issues and Primary Care.* Montreal: Grosvenor House Publishers.

Tappan, Francis. 1961. *Massage Techniques: A Case Method Approach.* New York: Macmillan Press.

Terzis, Julia, and Kevin Smith. 1990. *The Peripheral Nerve: Structure, Function and Reconstruction.* New York: Raven Press.

Theisler, Charles W. 1990. *Migraine Headache Disease: Diagnostic and Management Strategies.* Gaithersburg: Aspen.

Thompson, Diana. 1993. *Hands Heal: Documentation for Massage Therapy.* Washington: Thompson.

Thompson, W. Grant. 1979. *The Irritable Gut: Functional Disorders of the Alimentary Canal.* Baltimore: University Press.

Thomson, Ann, Alison Skinner, and Joan Piercy. 1991. *Tidy's Physiotherapy, 12th Ed.* Oxford: Butterworth Heinemann.

Tiran, Denise. 1996. *Aromatherapy in Midwife Practice.* London: Ballière Tindall.

Tiran, Denise, and Sue Mack. 1995. *Complementary Therapist for Pregnancy and Childbirth.* London: Baillière Tindall.

Today's Health. 1991. "Headaches: A Special Report." Vol. 4:4.

Tortora, Gerard J., and Nicholas P. Anagnostakos. 1981. *Principles of Anatomy and Physiology.* New York: Harper and Row.

Travell, Janet G., and David Simons. 1992. *Myofascial Pain and Dysfunction: The Trigger Point Manual, Vol. 2: The Lower Extremities.* Baltimore: Williams and Wilkins.

Travell, Janet G., and David Simons. 1983. *Myofascial Pain and Dysfunction: The Trigger Point Manual.* Baltimore: Williams and Wilkins.

Tucker, Evelyne, Sylvia Krueger, and Eunice Mooney. 1998. "A Study on the Effects of Manual Lymph Drainage on Fibromyalgia." *Journal of Soft Tissue Manipulation* Vol. 5, no. 3: 8-13.

Turk, Margaret, and Richard Machemer. 1993. *Aging and Developmental Disabilities of Cerebral Palsy.* New York: University of Rochester Press.

Turnbull, George. 1992. *Physical Therapy Management of Parkinson's Disease.* New York: Churchill Livingstone.

Turnbull, Wendy. 1994/5. "Massage and Medicine Merging." *Ontario Massage Therapist Association Newsletter* no. 8.

Turner, Janice. 1995. "Controversial Surgery Provides Hope for Relief from Parkinsons." *Toronto Star* March 13:D7.

Turner, Oscar, Norman Taslitz, and Steven Ward. 1990. *Handbook of Peripheral Nerve Entrapment.* New Jersey: Humana Press.

Twomey, L., and J. R. Taylor. 1987. *Physical Therapy and the Low Back.* New York: Churchill Livingstone.

Umphred, Darcy Ann. 1985. *Neurological Rehabilitation Volume 3.* St. Louis: C. V. Mosby.

Upledger, John E. 1991. *Cranio Sacral 1 Study Guide.* UI Publishing.

Upledger, John E. 1987. *Cranio Sacral Therapy 2: Beyond the Dura.* Seattle: Eastland Press.

Upledger, John E., and Jon D. Vredevoogd. 1983. *Craniosacral Therapy.* Seattle: Eastland Press.

Valnet, Jean. 1990. *The Practice of Aromatherapy.* Rochester: Healing Arts Press.

Vander, Arthur, James Sherman, and Dorothy Luciana. 1994. *Human Physiology: The Mechanisms of Body Function, 6th Ed.* New York: McGraw-Hill.

Vermeire, P., M. Demedts, and J. C. Yernault. 1989. *Progress in Asthma and COPD.* Oxford: Exerpta Medica.

Wale, J.O. 1980. *Tidy's Massage and Remedial Exercises, 11th Ed.* Bristol: John Wright and Sons.

Walker, Joan M., and Antonine Helewa. 1996. *Physical Therapy in Arthritis.* Philadelphia: W. B. Saunders Company.

Warner, Jon J. P., Joseph P. Iannotti, and Christian Gerber. 1997. *Complex and Revision Problems in Shoulder Surgery.* Philadelphia: Lippincott-Raven.

REFERENCES AND SELECTED BIBLIOGRAPHY

Watt, Martin. 1992. *Plant Aromatics: A Data and Reference Manual on Essential Oils and Aromatic Plant Extracts.* Witham: Beeleigh Litho Ltd.

Waylett-Rendall, J. 1981. "Sensibility Evaluation and Rehabilitation." *Orthopaedic Clinics of North America* Vol. 19, no. 1:53-5.

Webster, J. G. 1991. *Prevention of Pressure Sores; Engineering and Clinical Aspects.* Bristol: Adam Hilger.

Weed, Lawrence. 1991. *Knowledge Coupling: New Premises and New Tools for Medical Care and Education.* New York: Springer Verlag.

Weed, Lawrence. 1976. *Implementing the Problem-Oriented Medical Record, 2nd Ed.* Seattle: MCSA.

Weiner, William, and Christopher Goetz. 1989. *Neurology for the Non-Neurologist, 2nd Ed.* Philadelphia: J. B. Lippincott.

Weinstein, James. 1995. "Redefining Whiplash and Its Management: Scientific Monograph of the Quebec Task Force on Whiplash-Associated Disorders." *Spine* Vol. 20, no. 85:1S-73S.

Wexner, Steven D., and David C. C. Bartolo. 1995. *Constipation: Etiology, Evaluation and Management.* Oxford: Butterworth.

Whalley-Hammell, Karen. 1995. *Spinal Cord Injury Rehabilitation.* London: Chapman, Hall.

Wheeden M. S., F. Scafidi, T. Field, G. Ironson, C. Valedon, and E. Brandstra. 1995. "Massage Effects on Cocaine-Exposed Preterm Neonates." *Touchpoints* Vol. 2, no. 2:2-4.

Wilkinson, J. D., S. Shaw, and D. A. Fendon. 1987. *Dermatology.* New York: Churchill Livingstone.

Wilson, Robert L. 1981. "Management of Pain Following Peripheral Nerve Lesions." *Orthopaedic Clinics of North America* Vol. 12, no. 2:343-55.

Winter, P. Anne. 1993/4. "Effects of Massage on Blood Flow and Survival of Ischaemic Musculocutaneous Flaps in Rats." *Canadian Massage Therapy Association Newsletter* no. 6:4.

Wittlinger, Gunther, and Hildegard Wittlinger. 1990. *Introduction to Dr. Vodder's Manual Lymph Drainage, Vol. 1, Revised Edition.* Heidelberg: Karl F. Haug Verlag.

Wittlinger, Gunther, and Hildegard Wittlinger. 1985. *Introduction to Dr. Vodder's Manual Lymph Drainage, Vol. 1.* Heidelberg: Karl F. Haug Verlag.

Wood, Elizabeth, and Paul Becker. 1981. *Beard's Massage, 3rd Ed.* Philadelphia: W.B. Saunders Company.

Woolf, Neville. 1988. *Cell, Tissue and Disease: The Basis of Pathology, 2nd Ed.* London: Baillière Tindall.

Wu, Kent K. 1987. *Techniques in Surgical Casting and Splinting.* Philadelphia: Lea and Fabian.

Yarkony, Gary M. 1994. *Spinal Cord Injury: Medical Management and Rehabilitation.* Gaithersburg: Aspen Publications.

Yarom, R., E. Wolf, A. Muhlrad, and G.C. Robin. 1984. "Neuromuscular Causes of Idiopathic Scoliosis." In Rae Jacobs, ed. *Pathogenesis of Idiopathic Scoliosis.* Chicago: Scoliosis Research Society:153-62.

Yates, John. 1990. *A Physician's Guide to Therapeutic Massage: Its Physiological Effects and Their Application to Treatment.* Vancouver: Massage Therapist's Association of British Columbia.

Young, Jess, Robert Graor, Jeffrey Olin, and John Bartholomew. 1991 *Peripheral Vascular Diseases.* St. Louis: Mosby Yearbook.

Yehuda, Shlomo, and David I. Mostofsky. 1997. *Chronic Fatigue Syndrome.* New York: Plenum Press.

Yeung, Ella. 1996. "Whiplash Injuries of the Cervical Spine: The Relationship Between the Mechanism of Injury and Neural Tissue Involvement." *Physiotherapy* Vol. 82, no. 5:286-90.

Zadai, Cynthia Coffin. 1992. *Pulmonary Management in Physical Therapy.* New York: Churchill Livingstone.

Zohn, David, and John Mennell. 1976. *Musculoskeletal Pain: Diagnosis and Physical Treatment.* Boston: Little, Brown.

Index

INDEX